Clinical Practice
of the
Dental Hygienist

Clinical Practice
of the
Dental Hygienist

ESTHER M. WILKINS, B.S., R.D.H., D.M.D.

*Department of Periodontology, Tufts University, School of
Dental Medicine, Boston, Massachusetts*

FIFTH EDITION

Lea & Febiger   Philadelphia

Lea & Febiger
600 Washington Square
Philadelphia PA 19106
U.S.A.

Library of Congress Cataloging in Publication Data

Wilkins, Esther M.
  Clinical practice of the dental hygienist.

  Bibliography: p.
  Includes index.
  1. Dental hygiene.   I. Title.   [DNLM: 1. Dental
hygienists.   2. Preventive dentistry.   WU 90 W684c]
RK60.5.W5   1982   617.6'01   82-8966
ISBN 0-8121-0844-2   AACR2

Translations:
  Fourth Edition—
    Japanese Edition by Ishiyaku Publishers, Inc., Tokyo, Japan, 1982(?)

PRINTED IN THE UNITED STATES OF AMERICA

Print No.   4

Preface

Thoughtful retrospection over the nearly 25 years since the first edition of *Clinical Practice of the Dental Hygienist* reveals notable changes in the scope of dental hygiene education and practice. A significant factor in the changes is the effect of the application of new research in the prevention and control of oral diseases on the professional health care requirements of individual patients. Health care has become an important national issue, and people are expecting more and better health services. The health care providers, including dental auxiliaries, have acquired broader functions and need greater insight and knowledge to identify and deliver necessary services.

Dental hygienists have demonstrated their willingness to accept the challenge of increased responsibilities as members of the dental team. Dentists rely more and more on the competence of auxiliary co-workers, whose specialized knowledge is of vital importance in the recognition and treatment of oral conditions.

Dental hygiene care, interrelated as it is with a patient's self-care and all phases of treatment by general and specialized dentists, is able to provide necessary links to unify an individual's total oral care and maintenance. For comprehensive preventive, educational, and therapeutic services, the dental hygienist must be prepared to assess and evaluate the oral health needs of each patient and to plan immediate and long-range dental hygiene care within the total treatment supervised and conducted by the dentist.

Within the above framework, the first objective of this book is to make available comprehensive information and major reference sources fundamental to clinical dental hygiene practice. The second objective is to present practical material about patients with oral, systemic, physical, or other problems that require special additional knowledge and adaptations of basic techniques.

As a result of many helpful comments by students, faculty members, practicing dental hygienists, and dentists, this fifth edition incorporates a number of specific changes as well as a considerable body of new information. Each chapter has been carefully updated and expanded as needed, and several chapters were completely rewritten. New concepts and terminology have been introduced, references and suggested readings have been made current, new chapters and new subsections for other chapters added, and many new illustrations prepared.

The overall format has not been changed. The book is still sequenced in a general way to follow steps in patient care, starting with preparation for appointments, followed by patient assessment and evaluation, patient instruction for self-care, professional treatment procedures, and evaluation and recall for maintenance of health. The final part is devoted to patients with special needs.

The revision represents an effort to aid individual dental hygienists, whether student, practicing, or returning to practice after a period of interruption, to gain and maintain integrity and competency in patient care. It is hoped the approach to dental hygiene used in this book will increase understanding and sensitivity as the dental hygienist engages in the most challenging and rewarding of tasks, namely, helping patients to cope with their own oral health problems, and providing safe and effective individualized professional care.

Boston, Massachusetts   Esther M. Wilkins

Acknowledgments

The contributions of knowledge, encouragement, and generously-given time by many individuals are gratefully and humbly acknowledged. Expertise in certain areas has been obtained by seeking consultation as needed, and by having parts of the drafts read by individuals with specialized knowledge and experience.

The author is particularly indebted to those who reviewed whole chapters and identified essential content. In the general order of chapters as they appear in the book, special notes of gratitude go to Prof. Martha Shouldis, West Virginia Institute of Technology (Chapters 3 and 4, prevention of disease transmission); Prof. Barbara Wilson, University of Rhode Island (Chapter 7, vital signs, and sections of numerous other chapters); Dr. Nicholas Darzenta, Tufts University School of Dental Medicine, and Dr. Anthony Michelich, Mayo Clinic (Chapter 9, radiography); Prof. Linda Saline, University of Minnesota at Duluth (Chapter 15, occlusion); Profs. Patricia Connolly-Atkins, Forsyth School for Dental Hygienists, and Sharon Gravois, University of California at San Francisco (Chapter 19, indices); Dr. Dan Nathanson, Tufts University School of Dental Medicine (Chapter 30, sealants); Dr. Gordon Pattison, University of California at Los Angeles and Prof. Anna Pattison, University of Southern California (Chapter 35, acute lesions, and many other areas); and Prof. Corine Barone, Forsyth School for Dental Hygienists (Chapter 41, amalgam finishing and polishing).

In the areas of special patient needs, the following deserve particular recognition: Prof. Sandra Saunders, University of Rhode Island; Dr. Joseph Yacovone and Bonnie Houle, Division of Dental Health, State of Rhode Island (Chapter 45, gerodontics); Dr. James Gallagher, Tufts University School of Dental Medicine (Chapters 24, 25, and 40, sections on care of removable prostheses, and Chapter 46, edentulous patient); Prof. Suzanne Box, Cape Cod Community College (Chapter 48, oral surgery, and sections of other chapters); Dr. Thomas Quinn, Tufts University School of Dental Medicine (Chapter 48, section on fractured jaw, and Chapter 58, emergencies); Dr. Arthur Miller, Temple University, Department of Pathology (Chapter 8, intraoral and extraoral examination, and Chapter 49, oral cancer); and Ardath Rynning, Veterans Administration Hospital, Atlanta (Chapter 49, oral cancer).

The large new chapter on care of patients with disabilities was initiated by members of the staff of the Tufts Dental Facility at the Belchertown State School, Belchertown, Massachusetts. They are An Nicolaci, Evelyn Matysczyk, and Nancy Stover, dental hygienists, and Dr. David Tessini. Their motivation, advice, and practical critique of the initial drafts were invaluable. The chapter was also thoroughly reviewed by Dr. Arthur Nowak, University of Iowa, School of Dentistry; Prof. Susan Trusselle, Forsyth School for Dental Hygienists; and Prof. Suzanne Boundy, Northampton County Area Community College. Material and expert advice for the chapter on epilepsy was provided by Patricia Gibson, Comprehensive Epilepsy Program Director, Bowman-Gray School of Medicine, Winston-Salem. Additional thanks go to the following for certain reviews: Profs. Susan Trusselle and Suzanne Boundy (Chapter 54, physical and sensory handicaps); Prof. Janet Towle, Forsyth School for Dental Hygienists (Chapter 55, cardiovascular); Patricia Griffiths, Columbus, Ohio (Chapter 55, section on the cardiac pacemaker);

and Prof. Debra Heysek, Forsyth School for Dental Hygienists (Chapter 58, emergencies).

A particular expression of appreciation goes to Dr. Jerome Smulow, Chairman, Department of Periodontology, Tufts University School of Dental Medicine, for his thoughtful regard for the problems and time-consuming efforts of manuscript preparation.

The new art work for this edition has been prepared by two talented artists, Susan Smyth, R.D.H. and John Giunta, D.M.D., M.S. Such a combination of professional dental knowledge and artistic skill as possessed by each is rare.

And finally, thanks to my husband, Dr. James Gallagher, whose patience is amazing and measureless.

Contents

I

Orientation to Clinical Dental Hygiene Practice

1

The Professional Dental Hygienist

The registered dental hygienist is a licensed, professional, oral health educator and clinical operator who, as an auxiliary to the dentist, uses preventive, educational, and therapeutic methods for the control of oral diseases to aid individuals and groups in attaining and maintaining optimum oral health. The services of the dental hygienist are utilized in general and specialty dental practices, in the armed services, and in programs for research, professional education, public health, school health, industrial health, hospital, and institutional care.

The term *dental hygiene care* is used to denote all integrated preventive and treatment services administered to a patient by a dental hygienist. This term is parallel to the commonly used term *dental care* which refers to the services performed by the dentist.

Clinical services, both dental and dental hygiene, have limited long range probability of success if the patient does not understand the need for cooperation in daily procedures of personal care and diet, and for regular appointments for professional care. Educational and clinical services are, therefore, mutually dependent and inseparable in the total dental hygiene care of the patient.

Dr. Alfred C. Fones, who initiated the active use of the dental hygienist and founded the first formal course of professional study in 1913, emphasized the important role of education. In the first textbook for dental hygienists he wrote:

It is primarily to this important work of public education that the dental hygienist is called. She must regard herself as the channel through which dentistry's knowledge of mouth hygiene is to be disseminated. The greatest service she can perform is the persistent education of the public in mouth hygiene and the allied branches of general hygiene.[1]

Dental hygiene has been studied and the scope of practice has developed from Dr. Fones' original concept. Scientific information about the prevention of oral diseases has been advancing steadily. The public has become increasingly aware of the need for dental hygiene care and the importance of oral health instruction. The clinical practice of the dental hygienist integrates specific care with instructional services required by the individual patient.

I. Role in Patient Care

The dental hygienist may be responsible for gathering and assembling information for use by the dentist in diagnosis and treatment planning. The personal, medical, and dental histories, the radiographic survey, study casts, photographs, and charts of oral conditions observed during the oral inspection, and dental and periodontal examinations may be prepared. These data become part of the patient's permanent record and are used by the dentist and the dental hygienist throughout the treatment procedures and for comparison during continuing recall evaluations.

3

The role of the dental hygienist is to implement and coordinate the treatment and preventive program prescribed for each patient. Specific clinical services are required and the dental hygienist teaches, motivates, and guides the patient in the performance of measures for disease control. The success of each phase of treatment, whether periodontic, orthodontic, restorative, or prosthodontic, depends on the patient's cooperative daily performance of the recommended measures. Dental hygiene care as provided by the dental hygienist becomes an integral part of the total care of the patient.

II. Special Practice Areas

A wide range of settings is available for the practice of a dental hygienist. Likewise a wide range of patient needs emphasizes the necessity for specialized knowledge and skills.

There are eight areas of dentistry in which a dentist may conduct an ethical limited practice. They are the following: dental public health, endodontics, oral pathology, oral and maxillofacial surgery, orthodontics, pedodontics (dentistry for children), periodontics, and prosthodontics.[2] Education and training for certification in the dental specialties require a minimum of two years of graduate or postgraduate study and the successful completion of written and practical examinations. Masters and doctoral degrees require three or more years beyond basic dental education.

Although dental hygienists have not been required to complete examinations for practice within a specialty, there are educational curricula for certain areas. For example, advanced degree programs to prepare for dental hygiene education or public health have been available for many years.

In other special areas, short-term courses have been developed, such as for instruction in the care of patients with disabilities. In-service training may be available in long-term care institutions, hospitals, and skilled nursing facilities. Some dental hygienists have learned how to practice in a specialty through private study, special conferences, and personal experience.

Dental hygienists are needed to practice with dentists in specialty areas, particularly orthodontics, pedodontics, and periodontics. Others are involved in special clinics with a variety of health specialists, where patients with dental deformities, such as cleft lip and/or palate, or patients with oral cancer are under care. In other facilities, dental hygienists serve with a combined medical and dental team in the treatment of patients with severe systemic diseases, patients with physical, mental, or emotional handicapping conditions, or combinations of any of the problems mentioned.

III. Factors Influencing Clinical Practice

A. Legal

The law of a state must be studied and respected by each dental hygienist practicing within that state. Although the various practice acts have certain basic similarities, differences in scope and definition exist. Terminology varies, but each practice act regulates the patient services which may be delegated by the dentist to auxiliary personnel. Changes may be made from time to time.

All states are consistent in the provision that a dental hygienist may practice only under the direction and supervision of a licensed dentist. Definitions for "direction," "supervision," "direct supervision," and "indirect supervision," should be checked for each practice location.

B. Ethical

Professional people in the health services are set apart from others by virtue of the dignity and responsibility of their work. Service is the primary objective of the dental hygienist and is the reason for the existence of the profession. Others look to the professional person for leadership and expect more than ordinary demonstration of good human relations. Being professional requires interpersonal, professional, interprofessional, and community relationships of a high standard.

The American Dental Hygienists' Association has defined the principles of ethics for the professional dental hygienist. Understanding of and loyalty to these principles is essential to successful practice.

PRINCIPLES OF ETHICS OF THE
AMERICAN DENTAL HYGIENISTS'
ASSOCIATION[3]

Each member of the American Dental Hygienists' Association has the ethical obligation to subscribe to the following principles:

To provide oral health care utilizing highest professional knowledge, judgment, and ability.

To serve all patients without discrimination.

To hold professional patient relationships in confidence.

To utilize every opportunity to increase public understanding of oral health practices.

To generate public confidence in members of the dental health profession.

To cooperate with all health professions in meeting the health needs of the public.

To recognize and uphold the laws and regulations governing this profession.

To participate responsibly in this professional Association and uphold its purposes.

To maintain professional competence through continuing education.

To exchange professional knowledge with other health professions.

To represent dental hygiene with high standards of personal conduct.

C. Personal

Each dental hygienist may represent the entire profession to the patient being served. The dental hygienist's expressed or demonstrated attitudes toward dentistry, dental hygiene, and other health professions, as well as toward health services and preventive measures, are very apt to be reflected in the subsequent attitude of the patient toward other dental hygienists, and dental hygiene care in general.

Members of health professions need to exemplify the traits they hold as objectives for others if response and cooperation are to be expected. There are many personal factors of general physical health, oral health, cleanliness, appearance, and mental health to be considered. A few of these are mentioned below.

1. *General Physical Health.* Optimum physical health depends primarily upon a well-planned diet, a sufficient amount of sleep, and an adequate amount of exercise. A routine plan for complete physical examination is important, since the maintenance of personal health is a necessity for continued service. Because of the occupational hazards of dental personnel, routine examinations at least annually should include tests for hearing, sight, tuberculosis, urinary mercury, and hepatitis B surface antigen for persons not immune to hepatitis B.[4,5] Immunizations are described on page 49.

2. *Oral Health.* The maintenance of a clean, healthy mouth demonstrates by example that the dental hygienist follows the teachings of the dental and dental hygiene professions relative to prevention and control of disease. Freedom from offensive odors is important because the hygienist works in close proximity to patients.

3. *Cleanliness and Appearance.* A professional appearance includes a fresh uniform, and clean hose and shoes. Hair must be worn in a neat arrangement to prevent it from falling toward the patient or the instruments while working.

Jewelry other than a professional pin should be avoided since the crevices of pieces such as rings and watchbands harbor microorganisms and make thorough hand washing and scrubbing impossible. A trim dental hygiene cap and moderation in make-up contribute to increased respect for the female dental hygienist.

From the point of view of avoiding infection for both the operator and the patient, daily care of the hands and the fingernails is required. The nails are trimmed short and the hands protected by lotions to keep them soft and smooth.

The skin should be clear and impressively clean. Frequent baths and hair shampoos prevent bodily odors and aid in maintaining cleanliness.

4. *Mental Health.* The mental health of the dental hygienist is reflected in interpersonal relationships and the ability to inspire confidence through a display of professional and emotional maturity. Adequate physical health, recreation, and participation in professional and community activities contribute to optimum mental health.

IV. Objectives for Practice

The hygienist's self-assessment is essential in attaining goals of perfection in service to the patient and assistance to the dentist in the total dental and dental hygiene care program. Personal objectives need to be outlined and reviewed frequently in a plan for continued self-improvement. The goal with respect to patients was included in the definition of the dental hygienist at the beginning of this chapter: *to aid individuals and groups in attaining and maintaining optimum oral health*. Other objectives are related to this primary one.

The professional dental hygienist will:

A. Strive toward the highest degree of professional ethics and conduct.

B. Plan and carry out effectively the dental hygiene services essential to the total care program for an individual patient.

C. Apply knowledge and understanding of the basic and clinical sciences in the intelligent recognition of oral conditions and prevention of oral diseases during clinical practice.

D. Apply scientific knowledge and skill to all clinical techniques and instructional procedures.

E. Recognize each patient as an individual and adapt techniques and procedures accordingly.

F. Identify and care for the needs of patients who have unusual general health problems which affect dental hygiene procedures.

G. Demonstrate interpersonal relationships which permit attending the patient with assurance and presenting dental health information effectively.

H. Provide a complete and personalized instructional service to help each patient to become motivated toward changes in oral health behavioral practices.

I. Practice safe and efficient procedures pertaining to the care and sterilization of instruments and to general clinical routines.

J. Apply a continuing process of self-development and self-evaluation in clinical practice throughout professional life.

  1. Be objective and critical of procedures used in order to perform the best possible service.

  2. Appreciate the need for acquiring new knowledge and skills as current advancements require them.

V. Factors to Teach the Patient

A. The role of the dental hygienist as an auxiliary in the dental profession.

B. The scope of service of the dental hygienist as defined by state practice acts.

C. The interrelationship of instructional and clinical services in dental hygiene care.

D. The individual's potential state of oral health and how it can be developed and maintained.

References

1. Fones, A.C., ed.: *Mouth Hygiene*, 4th ed. Philadelphia, Lea & Febiger, 1934, p. 248.
2. American Dental Association: *ADA Principles of Ethics and Code of Professional Conduct*, Chicago, American Dental Association, 1980.
3. American Dental Hygienists' Association, House of Delegates: *Professional Code of Ethics for the Dental Hygienist*, Revised November, 1974.
4. Gravois, S.L. and Stringer, R.B.: Survey of Occupational Health Hazards in Dental Hygiene, *Dent. Hyg., 54*, 518, November, 1980.
5. Goldman, H.S.: Hazards in the Dental Workplace. Prevention for the Dentist, *Clin. Prev. Dent., 2*, 18, September-October, 1980.

Suggested Readings

Blau, M.A.: Expanded Use of Auxiliary Personnel in Orthodontic Practice, *Am. J. Orthod., 64*, 137, August, 1973.

Brine, P., Rossman, P.P., and Mescher, K.D.: A New Career Emphasis for Baccalaureate Dental Hygiene Education, *Dent. Hyg., 53*, 269, June, 1979.

Butler, N.P. and Carroll, B.M.: An Analysis of the Titles and Job Specifications of Operating Dental Auxiliaries, *Quintessence Int., 8*, 63, August, 1977.

Calisti, L.J.P., Silversin, J.B., and Wechsler, H.: *Handbook of Dental Specialties*. Wellesley, Arandel Pub., 1979.

Deuben, C.J., Sumner, W.L., and Johns, R.M.: Expanded Functions: Future Roles for Dental Hygienists, *Dent. Hyg., 54*, 29, January, 1980.

Feldman, S.M. and Scheetz, J.P.: Motivating Dental Auxiliaries: Theories and Applications, *J. Am. Coll. Dent., 46*, 162, July, 1979.

Gladstone, R.N.: International Dental Nurse Programs, *Dent. Hyg., 49*, 169, April, 1975.

Granger, B.: Legal Aspects of Dental Hygiene Practice, *Dent. Hyg., 54*, 337, July, 1980.

Hunter, E.L. and Rossman, P.P.: Baccalaureate Dental Hygiene Graduates' Perceptions of Community Dental Health Employment, *J. Public Health Dent., 40*, 134, Spring, 1980.

Jones, P.F.: The Changing Role of the Dental Hygienist, in Boundy, S.S. and Reynolds, N.J., eds.: *Current Concepts in Dental Hygiene*. St. Louis, The C.V. Mosby Co., 1977, pp. 1–20.

Lobene, R.R. and Kerr, A.: *The Forsyth Experiment; An*

Alternative System for Dental Care. Cambridge, Harvard University Press, 1979, 149 pp.

Logan, H., Hayden, H., and Jakobsen, J.: Role Expectations of Dental Hygienists, *Dent. Hyg.*, *54*, 321, July, 1980.

Rowat, J.A.: Utilization of the Dental Hygienist in Preventive Private Practice, *Dent. Surv.*, *56*, 42, June, 1980.

Sisty, N.L., Henderson, W.G., and Paule, C.L.: Review of Training and Evaluation Studies in Expanded Functions for Dental Auxiliaries, *J. Am. Dent. Assoc.*, *98*, 233, February, 1979.

World Health Organization: *World Directory of Schools for Dental Auxiliaries*. Geneva, WHO Health & Biomedical Information Programs, 1977.

Professionalism and Ethics

Fleming, W.C.: The Attributes of a Profession and Its Members, *J. Am. Dent. Assoc.*, *69*, 390, September, 1964.

Hine, M.K.: The Professional Concept—Its History and Meaning to Health Service, *J. Am. Coll. Dent.*, *37*, 19, January, 1970.

MacQuarrie, E.E.: Factors in the Development of Professional Attitude, *J. Am. Dent. Hyg. Assoc.*, *45*, 86, March-April, 1971.

Motley, W.E.: *Ethics, Jurisprudence and History for the Dental Hygienist*, 2nd ed. Philadelphia, Lea & Febiger, 1976, 185 pp.

2

Planning Dental Hygiene Care

The dental hygienist participates with the other members of the dental team to promote, maintain or restore the oral health of the patient. Together they must help the patient learn about his or her oral health needs, how these needs can be dealt with to bring the health of the oral cavity to an optimum level, and then how to maintain the optimum level to prevent future disease. As an operating auxiliary with formal training and licensure for performing intraoral procedures, the dental hygienist has a key position in the total care of the patient.

I. Types of Services

The services the dental hygienist performs can be divided into three basic categories, namely, preventive, educational, and therapeutic. The three are inseparable and overlapping as patient care is planned and accomplished.

A. Preventive

Preventive services fall into two groups, primary and secondary. *Primary prevention* refers to measures carried out so that disease does not occur and is truly prevented. *Secondary prevention* involves the treatment of early disease to prevent further progress of potentially irreversible conditions which, if not arrested, may lead eventually to extensive rehabilitative treatment or loss of teeth. An example of a primary preventive measure is the application of a topical agent for dental caries prevention. Removal of subgingival calculus and smoothing the root surface in a relatively shallow pocket is an example of a secondary prevention procedure in that the treatment of a small pocket contributes to the prevention of a deep pocket with marked bone loss.

B. Educational

Educational aspects of dental hygiene service permeate the entire patient care system. The preparation for specific treatment, the success of treatment, and the long-term success of both preventive and therapeutic services are dependent on the patient's understanding of each procedure and daily care of the oral cavity.

C. Therapeutic

Dental hygiene treatment services are an integral part of the total treatment procedures. All scaling, root planing, and curettage procedures, along with the steps in postoperative care, are parts of the therapeutic phases in the treatment of periodontal diseases. Restorative procedures are involved in the treatment of dental caries.

II. Purposes in Planning Care

Planning dental hygiene care for a patient means preparing a schedule to guide the preventive, educational, and therapeutic activities prescribed by the dentist and delegated to the dental hygienist. Initially, the dental hygienist plays a major role in the collection of data to be used by the dentist in formulating the diagnosis on which the total treatment plan is based.

The dental hygienist must have a clear understanding of the patient's needs, the nature of the oral illness, and the principles relating to the treatment of the illness. The dental hygienist should be aware of the patient's emotional needs and psychological reactions to the oral conditions. It is important to create an atmosphere in which the patient can respond to instruction, carry out the necessary procedures to supplement professional treatment, and cooperate during dental and dental hygiene appointments for the specific services.

STEPS IN PATIENT CARE

A purpose of this chapter is to bring into focus aspects to be considered in the planning and execution of competent dental hygiene care. Because much of the text is concerned with details of how to perform services for the patient, it is important to keep services and techniques in their proper perspective. Much more is involved in dental hygiene care than the performance of technical procedures.

In general, the sections of the book are arranged in an order to correspond with a sequence in which dental hygiene services may logically be performed. A brief descriptive outline of the sequence is presented here.

I. Preliminary Preparation for Appointments

Supervision of the operatory, equipment, instruments, and all measures for the prevention of disease transmission constitutes a basic essential phase in patient care. A neat, clean operatory contributes to the development of confidence and appreciation on the part of the patient.

Clean, sanitized equipment and sterile instruments are prerequisite to the patient's safety. Dental personnel must make every effort to prevent disease transmission.

II. Diagnostic Work-up

The diagnostic work-up is a name applied to the collection of data about the patient, which is to be used by the dentist for the diagnosis and treatment plan and by the dentist and dental hygienist as a guide to treatment and its follow-up. The diagnostic work-up is discussed in more detail on pages 79–80.

The initial step is to determine the present state of the patient's general and oral health. The medical and dental histories, oral examination, radiographic examination, and other sources of information are used. The findings of dental and periodontal examinations are charted, study casts are made, vital signs recorded, and other tests made as indicated.

III. Treatment Plan

The dentist uses the data collected to formulate a diagnosis and outline a treatment plan. The many factors taken into consideration in treatment planning are described in Chapter 21, pages 325–329. The objective is to plan a sequence of treatment that will lead to the restoration to health.

Within the overall treatment plan, the dental hygiene plan is organized with preventive, educational, and therapeutic phases, all designed to supplement parts of the treatment carried out by the dentist. The plan, then, is an outline of the essential procedures to be followed by the dentist, dental hygienist, and the patient.

IV. Preventive Services

Essential preventive measures are revealed during the collection of data for the diagnostic work-up. The history, examinations, dietary analysis, and radiographs can bring out the specific preventive measures related to dental caries, periodontal diseases, oral habits, or other area where change is important. The preventive plan is outlined for those measures to be carried out in the dental office and those for the patient to conduct on a daily basis. Suggestions for the preventive plan may be found on page 333.

V. Educational Services

In conjunction with the preventive and therapeutic programs, the patient needs to become well informed concerning the disease process and how it can be arrested. Each step in the treatment plan must be explained. Specific measures for the prevention of recurrence have to be demonstrated and practiced, redemonstrated, and reviewed as much as needed until appropriate habits of self-care have been established. Education may extend beyond the single patient, to the family, as well as into the community.

VI. Treatment

Treatment begins with patient involvement in *therapeutic plaque control*. Elimination and control of inflammatory disease of the periodontal tissues and of dental caries depend on the patient's efforts to minimize the plaque microorganisms that cling to the tooth and gingival surfaces.

The therapeutic phase encompasses all of the dental hygiene techniques, and, depending on the state or country in which the hygienist practices, may include restorative and periodontal procedures. The procedures may involve *initial* treatment, in which the teeth and gingiva are prepared for the additional treatment performed by the dentist, or *definitive* treatment. With definitive treatment, the hygienist's procedures may be the total treatment required, as is often the case in a young patient with gingivitis, when a combination of preventive, educational, and therapeutic treatment is conducted by the dental hygienist. Follow-up treatment procedures are essential, and recall at appropriate intervals is directed at the preservation of the healthy state acquired during initial phases.

VII. Recall

Upon completion of the inital treatment phase, each patient's recall program is determined. Future appointments are reserved.

The recall appointment is for the purpose of evaluation of the current state of oral health, and the steps follow the same pattern as the original diagnostic work-up. Each finding is charted, recorded, and reported to the dentist for re-evaluation. A new treatment plan is outlined. Preventive and educational phases are evaluated and renewed.

VIII. The Challenge of Planning Patient Care

Advancement in dental science has made it imperative for the professional dental hygienist to be able to adapt dental hygiene care to changing concepts with understanding and flexibility. Dental hygiene care needs to be modified intelligently according to the patient, the oral condition and disease, and the personal problems.

Each patient is an individual with specific problems of oral care which need consideration. Good dental hygiene care is patient-centered.

The professional dental hygienist must be a self-directed person who can apply scientific knowledge to problem solving. The questions are: What is the status of this patient's oral health? Why and how did it happen? What can I do to supplement that which the dentist does for the patient? What can the patient learn to do as a result of my teaching and guidance? What will be the outcome?

In the effort to deliver more effective and comprehensive health service, a set pattern of dental hygiene care, one which was memorized or learned by rote, cannot always be used. Knowledge must be applied to meet the individual needs of each patient.

II

Preparation for Dental Hygiene Appointments

3

Prevention of Disease Transmission: Methods of Sterilization and Disinfection

The transmission of disease is an insidious process. Infection and communicable diseases can lead to illness, disability, and loss of work time. In addition, other patients, family members, and community contacts become exposed and may become ill and lose productive time or suffer permanent after-effects.

In dental and dental hygiene practice, the objective is to protect patients and dental personnel from acquiring infection in the environment of the office or clinic. Health services facilities, including dental facilities, must be places for the cure and prevention, not the dissemination of disease due to inadequate precautionary measures and habits of the professional personnel.

A group responsibility of a dental team is first to organize and maintain a system for the sterilization, disinfection, and care of instruments and equipment. The second step is to conduct all appointments in a manner that will prevent direct or indirect cross-infections between dental personnel and patients, and from one patient to another.

Pathogenic (disease producing), potentially pathogenic, or nonpathogenic microorganisms may be present in the oral cavity of each patient. Pathogenic organisms may be transient. Patients may be carriers of certain diseases. Inadvertent transmission to subsequent susceptible patients or to dental personnel may occur as a result of careless handwashing and unhygienic personal habits or by inadequate sterilization or handling of sterile instruments.

I. Microorganisms of the Oral Cavity

At birth the oral cavity is sterile, but within a few hours to one day a simple oral flora develops. In a mature mouth, bacterial counts of the saliva are close to six billion per milliliter and are composed of at least 30 species. Most of the salivary bacteria come from the dorsum of the tongue, while some are from other mucous membranes. Much larger counts, up to 200 billion microorganisms per gram, are found in dental plaque and in the gingival sulcus.[1,2]

The intact mucous membrane of the oral cavity protects against infection to a degree. However, when the gingival tissues are manipulated during instrumentation, microorganisms can be introduced into the underlying tissues by way of the gingival sulcus or periodontal pocket.

II. Mechanisms for Transfer of Infectious Material

Recognition of the many possibilities for the transfer of infection in a dental office or clinic provides a basis for planning the system of sterilization, disinfection, and handling of instruments and equipment. The patient becomes the center of the many potential sources of infection as shown in figure 3–1. Several terms that apply to the transfer of infectious material are defined here.

A. Cross-contamination

Cross-contamination refers to the spread of microorganisms from one source to another: person to person, or person to an inanimate object and then to another person.

B. Direct Contact Transmission

When infection is spread from one person to another without an intermediate object, it is called direct contact.

C. Indirect Contact Transmission

Infection spread from one person to another person by way of an environmental surface, droplets, or other vehicle, is known as indirect contact.

D. Droplet Infection

Infection may be acquired by inhalation of droplets or aerosols that contain microorganisms or viruses from another person.

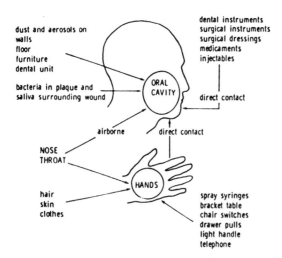

Figure 3–1. Sources of infection. The dental and dental hygiene patient is the center for environmental, autogenous, and interpersonal infection carried by the hands of a dental team member or airborne from the nose and throat. (From Crawford, J.J., *In* Block, S.S.: Disinfection, Sterilization, and Preservation, 2nd ed. Philadelphia, Lea & Febiger, 1977.)

E. Vehicle

The term vehicle is used when referring to a substance or object that carries infectious material from one person to another, directly or indirectly. Saliva on the hands of a dentist or dental auxiliary or in the splatter from a patient's mouth is an example of the most common vehicle for cross-contamination in a dental setting.

AIRBORNE INFECTION

I. Microorganisms of the Air

Transmission of microorganisms occurs by direct droplets from patient to operator or operator to patient, by way of hands and instruments that have made contact with the patient's oral cavity, or indirectly from the hands to other objects, such as the equipment or records, from which organisms may be picked up and brought to an oral cavity or skin break.

In addition, organisms enter the air of the operatory and thus provide another means for indirect transmission to a susceptible person, a subsequent patient, or a member of the dental team.

A. Dust-borne Organisms

Clostridium tetani (tetanus bacillus), *Staphylococcus aureus*, and enteric bacteria are among the organisms that may travel in the dust brought in from outside and that moves in and about dental operatories. When doors are opened and closed and people pass in and out, dust is set into motion which can settle on instruments, other objects, or people.

Infectious microorganisms also reach dust from the oral cavities of patients by way of large airborne particles which are described as splatter further on. Dust-borne organisms can be sources of contamination for dental instruments and the hands of dental personnel.

Surface disinfection of all equipment contacts during a dental appointment contributes to control of dust-borne pathogens. Procedures for surface disinfection are described on pages 58–61.

B. Aerosol Production[3]

Airborne particles are usually classified by

size as either aerosols or splatter. They are constantly being produced.

1. *Aerosols.* An aerosol is an artificially generated collection of particles suspended in air and capable of causing an airborne infection. A particle of a true aerosol is less than 50 microns in diameter. Aerosols are biologic contaminants that occur in solid or liquid form, are invisible, and remain suspended in air for long periods.

   Aerosol particles that are five microns or smaller may be breathed deep into the lungs. Larger particles get trapped higher in the respiratory tree. In the tiny particles, there may be respiratory disease-producing organisms or traces of mercury or amalgam, which collect in the lung since they are not biodegradable.

2. *Splatter.* Heavier, larger particles may remain airborne a relatively short time because of their own size and weight and drop or splatter on objects, people, and the floor. The splatter is composed of particles greater than 50 microns in diameter.

   In contrast to aerosols, splatter may be visible, particularly after it has landed on skin, hair, clothing, or environmental surfaces where gross contamination can result.

3. *Origin.* Aerosols and splatter are created during breathing, speaking, coughing, or sneezing. They are produced during all intraoral procedures, including examination and manual scaling. When produced by air-spray, air-water-spray, handpiece activity, or ultrasonic scaling, the number of aerosols increases to tremendous proportions.[3,4,5,6]

4. *Contents*
   a. Microorganisms. An aerosol may contain a single organism or a clump of microorganisms adhered to a dust or debris particle. The organisms may be contained within a liquid droplet.
   b. Particles from cavity preparation. Tooth fragments, microorganisms from saliva, plaque, and/or oropharynx/nasopharynx, oil from a handpiece, and water from the cooling equipment, may be in aerosols, following cavity preparation.
   c. Ultrasonic scaling. Great numbers of microorganisms have been found in the aerosols from ultrasonic scalers including *Staphylococcus aureus, albus,* and *pyogenes, Streptococcus viridans,* lactobacilli, Actinomyces, pneumococci, and diphtheroids.[5,6] Viruses also may be spread by ultrasonic instruments.

5. *Concentration.* Bacteria-laden aerosols and splatter are in greater concentration close to the scene of operation; the quantity decreases with distance. The aerosols travel with air currents and, therefore, move from room to room.

II. Prevention of Transmission[3]

The control of airborne infection depends on elimination or limitation of the organisms at their source, interruption of transmission, and protection of the potentially susceptible recipient.

Carefully monitored procedures are necessary for the patient who is known to have hepatitis B antigen, active tuberculosis, or other severe communicable disease. A list of procedures appears on pages 63–65.

A. Limitation of Organisms

Organisms can be limited by postponement of elective treatment for a patient known to have specific communicable organisms in the oral cavity. Patients can be asked to change their appointments when they are suffering from respiratory or other communicable disease.

B. Preoperative Oral Hygiene Measures

Toothbrushing with water or a mouthrinse or rinsing with water or a mouthrinse have been shown to reduce the numbers of bacteria contained in aerosols. Preparation of the patient is described on pages 62–63.

C. Interruption of Transmission

1. Use rubber dam, high volume evacuation, and manual instrumentation as much as possible.
2. Install air-control methods to supply adequate ventilation, filtration, and relative humidity.

3. Employ vacuum cleaning to remove dirt and microorganisms rather than dust-arousing housekeeping methods. The cleaner must have a filter to prevent the escape of organisms after they are suctioned.[7]

D. Clean Water

Run water through all tubings to handpieces, ultrasonic, and air/water spray for at least two minutes at the start of the day and at least 30 seconds after each appointment during the day. Contamination of splatter and aerosols will be reduced by this method.[8]

E. Protection of the Recipient

The use of masks and protective eyeglasses can prevent direct contact of splatter and aerosols with the faces of the dental team. These and other measures are described in Chapter 4.

AUTOGENOUS INFECTION[9,10]

An autogenous infection is one that originates within a person when the normal defense mechanisms are modified. The microflora of the oral cavity may become pathogenic when, for example, the organisms are forced into the tissues during instrumentation.

I. Normal Defenses

The body responds to or resists bacterial and viral invasion in different ways, such as those listed below.

A. Nutritional Status

In health, disease is resisted; whereas in a deprived state, the body can be susceptible to infection.

B. Antibody Response

After certain types of infection, antibodies are produced that provide resistance against a second attack of the same organism.

C. Physical Barrier

The intact skin and mucous membranes serve as barriers to prevent microorganisms from invading susceptible tissues.

D. Defense Cell Reaction

Phagocytes and white blood cells, particularly polymorphonuclear leukocytes respond to inflammation and collect at the site of infection to defend the body against disease.

II. Sources of Autogenous Infection

A. Bacteremia

Bacteremia is a condition in which bacteria or other microorganisms are in the blood stream. In the oral cavity, bacteria can enter the blood stream by way of a break in the mucosa, or through a gingival or periodontal pocket. When scaling or other instrumentation is performed, the microbial flora is disturbed and may be forced into the underlying tissues.

B. Injection Site

An abscess can occur at the site of injection when microorganisms are picked up by the needle as it is carried to the injection site. Organisms from bacterial plaque or those residing on the mucosal surface can be carried into the underlying tissues as the needle is inserted.

III. Factors That Alter Normal Defenses

The patient's complete medical and dental history must be reviewed in order that specific problems be identified and necessary precautions taken. Examples of situations that alter the normal defenses are included under the topics below.

A. Abnormal Physical Conditions

A heart valve may be defective due to a congenital or acquired condition. Such a valve may be susceptible to infective endocarditis resulting from a bacteremia created during dental or dental hygiene instrumentation. Prevention of infective endocarditis is described on pages 99 and 780.

B. Systemic Diseases

Examples of systemic conditions in which there is an increased susceptibility to infection are diabetes mellitus, alcoholism, leukemia, and glomerulonephritis.

C. Drug Therapy

Certain drugs used in the treatment of

systemic disease alter the body's defenses. Examples are steroids and chemotherapeutic agents that are immunosuppressive. Special precautions such as prophylactic antibiotics are needed to prevent infection.

D. Prostheses and Implants

A patient with, for example, a joint replacement, cardiac prosthesis, ventriculoatrial shunt for hydrocephalus, or an organ transplant, can be particularly susceptible to infection.

IV. Prevention of Autogenous Infection

A. Give Antibiotic Premedication

For the patient who is at risk for infection that may result from bacteremia, antibiotic premedication may be indicated. A list of patients who are medically compromised and potentially endangered during treatment appears on pages 99–100. For the American Heart Association recommendations for antibiotic premedication see page 100.

B. Lower the Surface Microbial Count

Suggested procedures for lowering the numbers of microorganisms at the treatment site just prior to treatment, are described on page 62. They include plaque removal procedures, particularly toothbrushing and flossing, rinsing with an antibacterial rinse, and the application of a topical antiseptic. By lowering the numbers of surface microorganisms, the potential for autogenous infection is decreased.

C. Prepare the Injection Site[9,11]

After drying the tissue surface with a sterile sponge, a topical antiseptic is swabbed over the surface. A povidone-iodine preparation (0.5 to 1%) is recommended. Maintain retraction to prevent contact of other tissues or saliva.

Disposable needles are required for disease control. Particular care must be taken to avoid contacting the needle with anything prior to injection. Contact with a tooth or tissue can contaminate the needle with microorganisms which can then be injected as the needle is inserted.

PATHOGENS TRANSMISSIBLE BY THE ORAL CAVITY

The organisms of many communicable diseases enter the body by way of the oral cavity. A few infectious diseases have specific oral manifestations such as the chancre and mucous patches of syphilis and the Koplik's spots of measles. Pathogens can be present within the oral cavity without an oral manifestation, a fact that is of particular importance to the total consideration of disease transmission.

Selected pathogens that may be transmitted by way of the oral cavity with their disease manifestations, mode of transfer, incubation and communicability periods are listed in table 3–1. Several of the so-called "children's diseases" are included.

When studying the diseases that may be acquired by members of the dental staff from patients, consideration should be given to the tremendous amount of time, energy, and potential long-range effect on, or permanent loss to, general health, which can result from illness. Knowledge and application of principles of sanitation and aseptic technique are necessary for the prevention and control of diseases.

Tuberculosis and viral hepatitis will be described in detail because of the special problems they create in personal and patient care. The general preventive measures described for these diseases can be applied during all appointments.

TUBERCULOSIS

Mycobacterium tuberculosis, the etiologic factor in tuberculosis, is a resistant organism that requires special consideration when sterilization and disinfection methods are selected and administered. Tuberculosis is a serious disease which can involve many months and years of lost time during the active stages of illness and the convalescence following. Clinical procedures must be planned to prevent exposure and infection from this debilitating disease.

Tuberculosis is a common communicable disease throughout the world. In the United States, it is no longer a leading cause of death as it was before preventive public health and medical measures were developed. Among reportable bacterial infections, however, it is still high, with a rate of approximately 2 deaths per 100,000. High incidence areas relate to urban slums and economically depressed areas.[12]

Table 3–1. Infectious Diseases of Oral Transmission

Infectious Agent	Disease Produced	Route or Mode of Transmission	Incubation Period	Communicability
Hepatitis A virus (HAV)	"Infectious" hepatitis Chronic liver disease	Fecal-oral Blood during acute stage Food, water, shellfish	2 to 6 weeks	2 to 3 weeks before onset of jaundice through 8 days after
Hepatitis B virus (HBV)	"Serum" hepatitis Chronic liver disease	Blood Saliva and all body fluids Semen	2 to 6 months	Before, during, and after clinical signs Carrier state: indefinite
Herpes Simplex virus Type I	Herpes labialis (fever blister, cold sores) Acute herpetic gingivostomatitis Keratoconjunctivitis Finger lesion (whitlow)	Saliva Direct contact Indirect contact (on objects, brief survival)	14 to 16 days up to 21 days	Carrier state in persons with latent virus One day before onset to 6 days after the macules appear; until all lesions are crusted
Mycobacterium tuberculosis	Tuberculosis	Droplet nuclei Sputum Saliva	Up to 6 months	Long, repeated exposure usually needed
Influenza viruses	Influenza	Droplet nuclei Nasal discharge	24 to 72 hours	3 days from clinical onset
Beta-hemolytic Streptococci (Streptococcus pyogenes)	Tonsillitis Strep throat Scarlet fever Impetigo Rheumatic fever	Droplet nuclei Direct contact	1 to 3 days	24 hours when treated 10 to 21 days when untreated Carrier state
Staphyloccus aureus	Abscesses Postoperative infections Boils (furuncle) Impetigo Bacterial pneumonia	Saliva Exudates Skin contact Angular cheilitis	4 to 10 days Variable	As long as lesions drain and carrier state persists

Organism	Disease	Mode of transmission	Incubation period	Period of communicability
Treponema pallidum	Syphilis	Direct contact Transplacental	Primary: 10 to 90 days Secondary: 2 weeks to 6 months Tertiary Years, decades	Variable and indefinite Highly infectious during the chancre stage Mucous patches of oral mucosa are highly infectious
Neisseria gonorrhoeae	Gonorrhea	Direct contact Indirect (short survival of organisms) Skin Saliva	2 to 5 days usually; may be 9 days or longer	During incubation and continued for months, years
Rubeola RNA paramyxovirus	Rubeola (measles)	Droplet nuclei Direct contact (saliva) Dust	9 to 14 days (10 days to fever, 14 days to rash)	4 days before to 5 days after the rash appears
Rubella Togavirus	Rubella (German measles)	Droplet nuclei Direct contact (saliva) Dust	14 to 21 days	From early signs of illness to 7 days after rash Highly communicable
Mumps virus Myxovirus	Infectious or epidemic parotitis (Mumps)	Droplet nuclei Direct contact (saliva)	14 to 28 days	From 1 to 7 days before symptoms until 9 days after swelling has gone
Varicella virus	Chickenpox	Direct contact Indirect contact Droplet nuclei	14 to 16 days	5 days prior to appearance of rash until crusting of the vesicles
Poliovirus	Poliomyelitis	Direct contact Saliva Droplet nuclei	7 to 14 days	Most infectious 7 to 10 days before and after the onset of symptoms

I. Transmission

Tuberculosis is contracted by the inhalation of fresh droplets containing tubercle bacilli. The organisms are disseminated from sputum and saliva by coughing, breathing heavily, or sneezing (figure 3–2). During the use of ultrasonic, other handpieces, and water and air spray, aerosols are created that can carry the bacilli. Aerosol production was described on pages 16–17.

When the organisms are in tiny aerosols they can pass readily into the lungs and the respiratory bronchioles. There, they can invade the tissue and establish an infection.

Transmission of tuberculosis is dependent on the following: (1) the degree to which the diseased person produces infectious droplets, (2) the amount and duration of exposure, and (3) the susceptibility of the recipient. Some patients are more contagious than others. Maximum communicability is usually just before the disease is diagnosed when there may be a severe cough and other respiratory symptoms.

The tubercle bacillus may enter the body by ingestion or direct inoculation as well as by inhalation. A person may have or may have had an infection, and therefore have a positive tuberculin test. Many adults have positive tuberculin tests without ever having had disease symptoms.

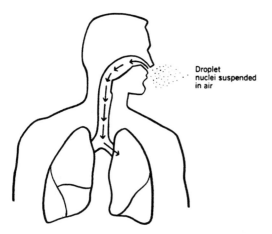

Figure 3–2.   Droplet nuclei. Many potentially pathogenic microorganisms are disseminated by aerosols and splatter. The primary mode of transmission of tubercle bacilli is by droplet nuclei breathed directly into the lung. (From McInnes, M.E.: Essentials of Communicable Disease, 2nd ed. St. Louis, The C.V. Mosby Co., 1975.)

II. Disease Process

A. Predisposing Factors

Any debilitating or immunosuppressive condition can predispose to invasion by the tubercle bacillus. Systemic conditions that lower the resistance to infection include diabetes, congenital heart disease, chronic lung disease, and alcoholism.

B. Incubation Period

As shown in table 3–1, the incubation period may be as long as six months. After such an extended period, it is difficult or impossible to trace the origin.

C. Early Symptoms

In the early stages before marked symptoms appear, the patient may have a low grade fever, loss of appetite, weight loss, and may tire easily. There may be a slight cough, and eventually sputum, indicating the possible presence of tubercle bacilli in the throat and saliva.

D. Later Symptoms

Definite temperature elevation, particularly in the afternoons, night sweats, weakness, and a persistent cough become apparent. Diagnosis is by chest radiograph and tuberculin testing.

III. Clinical Management

A. Patient History

1. *Questions About Symptoms.* In early disease, there may not be a suspicion of tuberculosis to alert the dental hygienist to assume precautions to prevent personal exposure. Careful history-taking and review of previous histories for comparison, may provide essential information.

2. *High Incidence Groups.* Information may be available for specific residence groups. For example, in comparison to the prevalence of tuberculosis in the United States of approximately 25 cases per 100,000 population, the prevalence rate among Indochinese refugees entering the United States in 1979 and 1980 was approximately 1500 per 100,000.[13] Pre-

ventive therapy has been administered to thousands of the refugees who have been exposed, as well as treatment therapy for those with known active disease.

B. **Extraoral and Intraoral Examination**

Tuberculosis is primarily a lesion of the lungs, but any organ or tissue may be involved.
1. *Oral Lesion.*[14] An oral lesion is a nodule at first, which then develops into an ulcer. It is usually located on or under the tongue. As with examination for all oral lesions, the hands should be protected by gloves (pages 57–58).
2. *Lymphadenopathy.* Regional lymph node enlargement may be found associated with an oral tuberculous ulcer.

C. **Patient Under Treatment**

Chemotherapy can control the patient's contagious condition. Isoniazid is used for long periods, sometimes supplemented by streptomycin. After a few weeks from the beginning of therapy, bacilli in the sputum and the cough are decreased. Disease transmission is rare after satisfactory treatment is started, and the patient can be safely managed with basic precautions.[15]

D. **Aseptic Technique**

Strict aseptic procedures must be followed for the active case, as described on page 64. Dental hygienists employed in hospital situations where patients with communicable diseases are treated, learn and practice full operating room aseptic procedures.[16]

VIRAL HEPATITIS

Hepatitis means inflammation of the liver. Viruses cause a variety of types of hepatitis. Some of the viruses have been specifically identified, and hepatitis A, hepatitis B, and hepatitis non A/non B are described in this section.

The incidence of hepatitis B has increased significantly over the past 20 years. It has been a serious occupational hazard for health workers. Among professional personnel, both medical and dental, the incidence has reached startling proportions, to the point where the use of strict sterilization of equipment and materials, aseptic

techniques, and self-protection measures are mandatory. With the advent of the newly developed hepatitis B vaccine, immunization for health workers and other frequently exposed individuals is available.[17]

TERMINOLOGY AND SYMBOLS[18]

Hepatitis A

HAV	Hepatitis A virus
anti-HAV	Antibody to hepatitis A virus

Hepatitis B

HBV	Hepatitis B virus. The hepatitis B virus has three antigens.
HBsAg	Hepatitis B surface antigen (formerly known as Australia antigen). It is the diagnostic indicator or serum marker of infection and is found in the blood during (a) acute hepatitis B (b) chronic hepatitis B (c) carrier state (currently asymptomatic)
HBcAg	Hepatitis B core antigen, found within the inner core of the virus.
HBeAg	Hepatitis B "*e*" antigen, associated with an infective contagious state; may be a marker of chronic liver disease. When present in a carrier it indicates very high ability to transmit the disease.
anti-HBs*	Antibody to hepatitis B surface antigen. Its presence indicates previous infection with immunity to hepatitis B.
anti-HBc	Antibody to hepatitis B core antigen. With anti-HBs, it indicates immunity.
anti-HBe	Antibody to hepatitis B "*e*" antigen.

Hepatitis Non A/non B

NANB	Non A/non B hepatitis

Immune Globulins

IG	Immune globulin. Former names include ISG, immune serum globulin, and gamma globulin.
HBIG	Hepatitis B immune globulin

HEPATITIS A[18,19,20]

Hepatitis A occurs much more frequently in children and young adults than in older adults. It is more severe in adults.

I. **Transmission**

A. **Fecal–Oral Route**

The most common transmission is through

---

*HBsAb has also been used to abbreviate the antibody to hepatitis B surface antigen; HBcAb for the antibody to the core antigen; and HBeAb for the antibody to the "e" antigen.

close contact when there are unsanitary conditions. Unwashed hands of an infected person can contaminate anything touched.

B. Water-borne and Food-borne

Epidemics may occur when sanitation is inadequate. Contaminated water may carry hepatitis A virus directly to those using the water, or may contaminate shellfish grown in the water.

Infected food handlers can contaminate uncooked food or food handled after cooking.

C. Blood

In the earliest days of active disease, the blood contains transient hepatitis A viruses; however, transmission by blood transfusion is rare.

II. Disease Process

A. Incubation and Communicability

The incubation period is from 2 to 6 weeks, with an average of 25 days. During the 2- to 3-week period before the onset of jaundice, the infection is communicable. Shortly after jaundice appears, the communicability begins to diminish. There is no carrier state.

B. Signs and Symptoms

The stages are defined by the incidence of jaundice, as preicteric (before jaundice appears) and icteric (while jaundice is present). Hepatitis A without jaundice (anicteric) is two to three times more prevalent than icteric. A diagnosis of hepatitis has not always been made, since without jaundice, symptoms may resemble influenza or other diseases.

1. *Preicteric* (before jaundice). Typically, there is an abrupt onset of an influenza-like illness, with fever, headache, fatigue, nausea, vomiting, and abdominal pain. The liver may be enlarged and tender to palpation.
2. *Icteric Phase.* Jaundice may appear in adults, but rarely in children. Other symptoms become prolonged, and the patient may be ill for a few days to a month. Occasionally chronic hepatitis

follows, but 85 to 90 percent recover completely.

III. Immunity

Anti-HAV is usually detectable in the serum within 2 weeks of the onset. Immunity to reinfection follows with recovery.

In addition to those that are known to have had the disease, many more people acquire immunity from undetected disease. In the United States, an estimated 25 to 30 percent of healthy adults are immune. In other countries where hepatitis A is endemic, as many as 90 percent of the population may have anti-HAV antibodies at an early age.[20]

IV. Prevention[18,21]

A. Sanitation and Personal Hygiene

Because the principal means of transmission is by way of the feces, prevention on that level is indicated.
1. Public health control of food handlers and water contamination.
2. Personal hygiene control through scrupulous handwashing by a patient and all contacts, as well as by all health workers involved in patient care.

B. Application in Dental Setting

Instrument sterilization, use of disposable materials, and all related precautions for persons and objects contacted by the patient. Such procedures must be the same for all patients, since the presence of hepatitis A viruses is not usually known. Clinic procedures are described in Chapter 4.

V. Passive Immunization

A. IG

Standard immune globulin (IG) is used for the prevention or modification of hepatitis A in a person known to be susceptible, who is accidentally exposed. Since the incubation period may be as short as 2 weeks, IG must be given within the first few days following exposure.

B. Indications[21]

1. *Individual Exposure.* Exposure sufficient for need of IG requires close per-

sonal, physical contact, such as by the members of the patient's household and other intimate contacts.

2. *Institution for Custodial Care* (Examples: prisons, facilities for developmentally disabled). Hepatitis A may be endemic in certain institutions. IG may be used during outbreaks, for new admissions, and for all employees who have direct contact.

3. *Day-Care Centers.* When there is evidence of HAV transmission in a day-care center, particularly where children are in diapers, IG should be administered to staff, children, and family members with whom the children reside. Thorough handwashing after diaper changing is emphasized.

4. *Traveler to Endemic Area.* If a stay is to be longer than 3 months, and especially outside ordinary tourist routes, in a tropical area, or an area known to have endemic hepatitis A, IG may be indicated. A second dose may be recommended for a stay longer than 5 months. A subclinical infection may be acquired that would confer immunity.

HEPATITIS B[18,19,20,22]

Hepatitis B differs in many respects from hepatitis A, particularly in mode of transmission, the length of the incubation period, the onset, and the existence of a chronic carrier state. Hepatitis B occurs at any age.

I. Transmission

The major sources of hepatitis B virus are patients with acute hepatitis B infection and symptomless chronic carriers.

A. Blood

Parenteral inoculation is a usual mode of transfer. Blood transfusion from infected donors, use of contaminated instruments by medical and dental professionals, contaminated needles used by drug abusers, and accidental self-inoculation by health workers, are examples.

B. Other Body Fluids

Hepatitis B viruses have been found in nearly all body fluids including saliva, se-

men, menstrual blood, tears, urine, sweat, and nasopharyngeal secretions. The transfer of disease may occur by oral and sexual routes or other close physical contact. Salivary transmission by way of hands and aerosols is of particular importance to dental personnel.

C. Perinatal Transmission

An infected mother can transmit hepatitis B to her baby. The exact mechanism of spread is not certain, but infection in utero appears to be rare. The baby can become a persistent carrier. The use of hepatitis B immune globulin (HBIG) immediately after birth may provide some protection.[18,21]

II. Disease Process

A. Incubation and Communicability

The incubation period is longer than that for hepatitis A, and ranges from 2 months to 6 months, with an average at about 70 days. The period of communicability varies, but HBsAg may be detected by laboratory examination of the blood as early as 30 days after exposure to the disease.

The presence of serum HBsAg indicates communicability. HBsAg may no longer be detected in the blood from a few days to 3 months after the icteric or jaundice stage of illness. After 6 months, a persistent detection of HBsAg indicates a chronic carrier state.

B. Signs and Symptoms

Hepatitis B cannot be distinguished from other viral hepatitis infections on the basis of the clinical signs and symptoms. The onset, which is typically acute for hepatitis A, is slower and more insidious for hepatitis B, and there also may be skin rash, itching, and joint pains.

A majority of patients do not have an icteric stage, but have subclinical disease. Many may remain undiagnosed for hepatitis.

The period of illness extends from 4 to 6 weeks for hepatitis A and may be even longer for hepatitis B.

C. Carrier State

Between 5 and 10 percent of recovering

patients develop a chronic carrier state. It is more likely to follow hepatitis infection in children than in adults. A carrier state may also result following a subclinical undiagnosed exposure and, therefore, be unknown to the individual.

It is to be hoped that the HBsAg status can be determined so that dental and dental hygiene procedures can be carried out safely. However, as summarized on page 48, information from the most carefully prepared medical histories reveals only a portion of the risk patients. For those patients who do not know their status, but who may be included in one of the high-risk groups listed below, a diagnostic serologic test for HBsAg should be requested.

D. High-Risk Individuals

High carrier incidence has been found associated with certain factors, including place of residence, occupation, life style, confinement to an institution, geographic location, presence of certain other diseases, and treatment associated with other diseases. The individuals listed below are examples of those most likely to have been exposed to hepatitis B and associated with high carrier frequency.[9,22,23,24]

1. Patients with past history of jaundice or hepatitis
2. Patients treated by
   renal dialysis
   chemotherapy and other immunosuppressive therapy
   radiation therapy
   frequent blood transfusions or blood products (hemophilia, hematologic disorders)
3. Drug addicts who inject themselves
4. Institutional clients (current or previous), particularly individuals with Down's Syndrome (those with mental retardation who have always lived at home are not special risks)
5. Military populations, particularly those stationed in countries with high incidences of hepatitis B
6. Residents from areas of high incidence of hepatitis and hepatitis carriers, particularly refugees[25]

7. Returned travelers who stayed in area of high incidence of hepatitis 3 months or longer or were treated medically by transfusion while there
8. Personnel employed in medical and dental environments such as clinical laboratories, dialysis units, drug abuse treatment centers, dental clinics
9. Male homosexuals; prostitutes
10. Families and close associates of hepatitis patients.

III. Immunity

The presence of anti-HBs in the serum shows that the person had a previous hepatitis B infection and is immune to reinfection. An estimated 15 percent of adults in the United States have HBsAg antibodies, although many of them are unknown because their immunity was acquired following a subclinical, anicteric, or otherwise unrecognized case of hepatitis B.

IV. Prevention[18,21,25]

A. Public Health

1. *Blood Transfusion Safety.* Testing of each unit of blood for the presence of HBsAg has been required for several years. As a result, a large number of post-transfusion cases have been avoided (page 28).
2. *Education.* Information about the modes of transmission of HBV and how to control the disease must be provided to all carriers, their families, and other close contacts. Health care professionals and all persons working in settings where there may be continual danger of repeated exposure need to learn and practice strict methods for self-protection and prevention of transmission.
3. *Disease Reporting.* Physicians are responsible for having all cases of hepatitis tested for classification and then reporting viral hepatitis to the state or local health department. Community-wide education can be initiated when indicated. A patient who is found to be HBsAg positive from testing requested by the dentist or dental hygienist, should also be reported.

B. **Dental Office or Clinic**

1. *Testing for HBsAg and anti-HBs*
   a. Dental personnel: should be tested periodically. A person with HBsAg positive blood must defer from working until released by the physician.

      A person with anti-HBs, who is therefore immune, can concentrate efforts to prevent transfer of hepatitis from patient to other patients or susceptible dental personnel.
   b. Patients: serum testing should be requested for all high-risk patients. When patients are HBsAg positive, special handling with maximum precautions (page 64) or referral to a clinic equipped for operating room sterilization and decontamination is mandatory.[22] Referral of HBsAg positive patients to a physician is indicated for those not currently under medical care.
2. *Personal Protection.* Until patient serum testing is refined and more widely used, attention to wearing gloves (rubber or plastic), mask, and protective eyeglasses is important during all appointments.
3. *Sterilization and Disinfection.* Methods for sterilization are described on page 33 and chemicals acceptable for disinfection on page 39. All instruments that are reusable must be routinely sterilized, not only when a communicable disease is known to be present.

   Decontamination of environmental surfaces immediately following each appointment is necessary to prevent splatter, discharges, and aerosols from drying on the surfaces. Procedures for disinfection are outlined on pages 58–61.
4. *Reduction of Aerosols.* Avoidance of use of aerosol-producing instruments, including high-speed handpieces and ultrasonic scalers as well as a water and air spray syringe can prevent the dispersal of pathogenic microorganisms to environmental surfaces, dental personnel, and hence to subsequent patients. The use of high power evacuation aids in preventing the spread of microorganisms.

5. *Care of Waste and Disposable Materials.* After treating a high risk patient, the disposable items must be sterilized before discarding them into the general waste.

V. **Passive Immunization**[21]

A. **Hepatitis B Immune Globulin (HBIG)**

High titer anti-HBs immunoglobulin HBIG, has been available, following research over recent years. Its primary use is for postexposure prophylaxis.

IG, described for passive immunization for hepatitis A (page 24), contains low titer anti-HBs of varying amounts. It is effective against HBV for preexposure prophylaxis to a lesser degree than HBIG, but should be used when HBIG is not available.

B. **Postexposure Prophylaxis Using HBIG**

Examples of single exposures to HBV that may occur are the accidental inoculation by needle or other instrument (scaler, explorer), or by oral ingestion of splatter of the patient's saliva, blood, or nasopharyngeal secretions.

1. *Source Known; HBsAg Status Positive.* HBIG should be given to a susceptible recipient within 24 hours of exposure. The second dose is given in one month.
2. *Source Known; HBsAg Status Not Known*
   a. When the source is a high-risk individual (page 26),
      (1) Request serum analysis for HBsAg of the patient.
      (2) When test results can be available within 7 days, IG is given within 24 hours, preferably immediately. With a return of positive test results, HBIG is given immediately, and again in one month.
      (3) When test results cannot be ready before 7 days of exposure, HBIG may be used immediately.
   b. When the source is not believed to be a high risk individual, postexposure prophylaxis is optional. When given, IG is used within 24 hours.

VI. Active Immunization

An HBV vaccine composed of highly purified inactivated HBsAg particles derived from the plasma of chronic carriers of the antigen has been produced after extensive research. The use of the vaccine promotes anti-HBs development in the serum of the vaccinated individual, which in turn, means protection against the infectious hepatitis B surface antigen.[17,26]

NON A/NON B VIRUSES[18,27]

A major complication of blood transfusion has been post-transfusion hepatitis. Screening of blood donors and exclusion of those with HBsAg, after HBsAg was identified as the serum disease marker for hepatitis B, contributed to a reduction of incidence of post-transfusion hepatitis. Rarely is post-transfusion hepatitis caused by hepatitis A.

Continuing research showed that hepatitis can occur as a result of transfusion of HBsAg-negative blood. That and other findings led to the realization that other viruses were involved in post-transfusion hepatitis. Until the causative agents are characterized, they have been referred to as Non A/non B viruses.

I. Transmission

The Non A/non B viruses are believed to account for up to 95 percent of post-transfusion hepatitis. There is a high incidence among immunosuppressed patients and those who are dependent on support blood products.

II. Disease Process

A. Incubation Period

The incubation period is 7 to 8 weeks, between that of hepatitis A and hepatitis B. The range is from 2 to 35 weeks.

B. Signs and Symptoms

The onset and symptoms are similar to hepatitis B. Laboratory diagnosis is made by ruling out the other types of hepatitis.

C. Carrier State

The development of a carrier state may be more frequent than after hepatitis B. Chronic liver disease can result.

III. Postexposure Prophylaxis[21]

In the absence of specific tests for Non A/non B hepatitis, recommendations for passive immunization or postexposure prophylaxis have not been defined. The recommendations for hepatitis A should be applied when indications for protection are apparent.

TERMINOLOGY FOR ASEPTIC TECHNIQUE

Clarification of terms is important to understanding the objectives to be attained in the use of various methods applied for the control of disease transmission. In addition to the procedures described here, other terms are defined in the glossary.

I. Sterilization

The process by which all forms of life, including bacterial spores and viruses, are destroyed by physical or chemical agents.

II. Disinfection

Any process, chemical or physical, by means of which pathogenic agents or disease-producing microorganisms can be destroyed. *Disinfectants* are applied to inanimate objects in contrast to *antiseptics* which are applied to living tissues. As ordinarily employed, most disinfectants do not destroy spores, tubercle bacilli, or viruses, particularly hepatitis viruses.

III. Sanitization

The process by which the number of organisms on inanimate objects is reduced to a safe level. It does not imply freedom from microorganisms, and generally refers to a cleaning process.

IV. Surface Disinfection

The process by which microorganisms that contaminate environmental surfaces of implements and equipment are removed by vigorous scrubbing with a germicidal disinfectant.

V. Contamination

The presence of microorganisms on a body surface or on inanimate articles or substances.

VI. Aseptic Technique

The use of aseptic technique refers to procedures carried out in the absence of pathogenic microorganisms, techniques that avoid contamination of patients, and the careful use of sterilized instruments and materials to avoid contamination.

A. Sepsis

A condition in which disease-producing (pathogenic) microorganisms are present.

B. Asepsis

A condition in which living pathogenic microorganisms are absent.

C. Chain of Asepsis

A chain of asepsis means a procedure that avoids transfer of infection. "Chain" implies that each step, related to the previous one, continues to be carried out without the presence of pathogenic microorganisms.

D. Strict Aseptic Technique[28]

Procedures used during strict aseptic technique are similar to those used in a hospital operating room, conducted with the highest level of asepsis for the treatment area, the personal cleanliness of the operators and their auxiliaries, instrument sterilization, and surface decontamination.

E. Sterile-Clean Technique

In dental and dental hygiene practice, strict aseptic techniques are needed for periodontal and general oral surgery, as well as for other patients with an active or carrier state of communicable disease, such as tuberculosis or hepatitis.

For a routine *sterile-clean* procedure, patient and operator protection is essential, and absolute sterility is necessary for instruments and other items that have the greatest potential for disease transmission. Other materials and equipment with a lower potential for transmitting infection must be thoroughly decontaminated.

PREPARATION FOR INSTRUMENT STERILIZATION

A consistent system for the removal of used instruments and equipment from the treatment area at the completion of a patient appointment should be worked out to assure safety measures against self-contamination. Cycling to keep used instruments in one area and sterile trays or packages in another can be planned. A good rule is to learn the most effective method to prevent cross-contamination, and then to always follow that method without exception.

I. Handling

Heavy-duty household gloves should be worn. A transfer or handling forceps may be kept especially for use during the handling of nonsterile instruments.

During processing for cleaning and sterilization, careless handling of instruments with delicate working ends such as scalers and explorers can lead to fracture of the tips. Rubbing or rough contact of blades or tips with other instruments contributes to their dullness. Pressure or bending will distort various instruments.

Attention to glassware such as dappen dishes is necessary to prevent chipping or breakage. In addition, during careful handling, prevention of injury to the hands is of particular importance to prevent cuts or abrasions which permit entry of microorganisms from contaminated instruments.

To prevent rusting or discoloration, instruments should be cleaned as soon as possible after use. Even stainless steel can acquire a tarnish that is difficult to remove. If there is an unavoidable delay, or when instruments are accumulated to be cared for after a series of appointments, they should be rinsed with cold water to remove blood and debris and then immersed in warm water containing a blood solvent or detergent.

Instruments used for a patient with active disease must be isolated and sterilized before cleaning (page 65).

II. Manual Cleaning[9]

A. Rinse

Rinse or soak in cold water to remove blood and debris. Avoid splashing because splatter can contain blood, saliva, or other contaminated material.

B. Decontaminate

Immerse in trisodium phosphate solution (one tablespoon per quart of water) or glutaraldehyde 2%. Rinse thoroughly under running water.

C. Dismantle Instruments

Dismantle instruments with detachable parts, such as the porte polisher or a mouth mirror with handle, and open instruments with joints, such as scissors.

D. Clean by Scrub Technique

1. Apply a solvent to remove greases or oils.
2. Scrub with a stiff brush with detergent and running water to remove all particles of dried blood or debris.
3. Use a detergent, not ordinary soap.
   a. Soap can form insoluble alkalies in hard water that can enmesh and protect the bacteria from the sterilizing effect later.
   b. Cake soap can harbor microorganisms and become a potential source of transfer.
   c. Avoid use of abrasives or sharp cleaners as they may roughen the instrument surface and affect the stainless properties of the metal.
4. Apply individual measures for problem areas.
   a. Grooves and joints where debris can collect and harden; for example, the mouth mirror with grooves at the attachment of the shank as well as around the mirror rim.
   b. Saliva ejector. Slide a pipe cleaner dipped in detergent through a wide opening, or use a fine twisted wire through a narrow opening; use an instrument tip such as a broken explorer to clean around the small openings in the receiving end.

E. Rinse

Rinse in hot water to remove all detergent.

F. Dry

1. Purposes
   a. To prevent instrument discoloration if there is an interval before sterilization.
   b. Water will dilute the pre-autoclaving emulsion or cold disinfection solution.
2. Air dry. Prevents need for extra handling.
3. Dry carefully with paper towels when time does not permit air drying.

G. Care of Scrub Brushes

1. Wash contaminated brushes in detergent, rinse thoroughly, and sterilize.
2. Label brushes or identify by using a specific size or shape only for instrument care to prevent inadvertent mixing with hand-scrubbing brushes.

III. Ultrasonic Cleaning

Ultrasonic cleaning prior to sterilization is safer than manual cleaning. Risk of injury to hands and of infection is not as great.

Manual cleaning of instruments is a difficult and time-consuming procedure with numerous disadvantages. When ultrasonic equipment is adjusted for optimum performance and those using it are properly informed and adhere to the manufacturer's instructions, the quality of cleaning is much better than by the hand-scrub technique. *Ultrasonic processing is not a substitute for sterilization: it is only a cleaning process.*

A. Advantages

Benefits from the use of ultrasonic cleaning include the following:
1. Increased efficiency in obtaining a high degree of cleanliness.
2. Reduced potential danger to operator from direct contact with hepatitis viruses and other pathogens.
3. Improved effectiveness for disinfection.
4. Elimination of possible dissemination of microorganisms through release of aerosols and droplets which can occur during the scrubbing process.
5. Penetration into areas of the instruments where the bristles of a brush are too coarse to contact.
6. Removal of tarnish.

B. Principles of Action

Ultrasonic vibrations initiate cavitation in the cleansing solution. Cavitation means that minute bubbles are generated, which expand until they are unstable, then collapse by bursting inward. This creates minute vacuum areas which are responsible for the cleaning process by dislodging, dispersing, or dissolving the material that has adhered to the surface of the instrument.

Cleaning is accomplished by both the physical agitation and chemical dissolution. Soluble material goes into solution and heavier material sinks to the bottom of the cleaning tank.

C. Procedure

1. Select the proper agent from the various concentrates available from the manufacturers. Selection is based on the specific use; for example, one solution is prepared for general instrument cleaning and another for removal of denture stains.
2. Wear heavy-duty rubber gloves to protect against infection and chemicals.
3. Place instruments in the carrier tray or basket and submerge in the solution.
   a. Guard against overloading and crowding, which can prevent the solution from reaching all surfaces.
   b. Open jointed instruments; dismantle detachable parts.
   c. Space instruments to avoid contacts between easily damaged surfaces, which may lead to bending or dulling.
   d. Do not mix various metals in the same bath; for example, separate stainless steel, aluminum, copper, and brass.
4. Time from 1 to 10 minutes, depending on the unit, the solution, and the material being treated. Consult manufacturer's chart.
5. Remove, drain, then rinse thoroughly with warm water.
6. Dry in air thoroughly.

D. Care of Unit

Change solution and clean the unit daily to maintain its efficiency.
1. The solution does not contain a disinfectant and becomes heavily contaminated.
2. The unit should be kept covered to prevent contamination from air and splatter.

3. The container is emptied at the end of each day.
   a. Clean the container with 1% hypochlorite.
   b. Let dry overnight.
   c. Refill each morning.

IV. Packaging

A. Methods for Instrument Arrangement

The three general ways for arrangement of instruments and equipment for sterilization after manual or ultrasonic cleansing and drying are as follows:
1. They may be placed on an open tray which fits into the sterilizer, and may be transferred directly to the treatment area after sterilization, to be used immediately. No provision for storage is included.
2. They may be arranged in metal trays with fitted covers. Each tray is planned to contain a complete set-up for a given procedure. The covers are left ajar during sterilization to permit access by steam or gas, and then the covers are slipped on immediately after opening the sterilizer. Preprepared trays are to be described in the next section.
3. They may be packaged in various materials, depending on which of the sterilizing methods will be used. The packaging material must permit steam or gas penetration. Acceptable and unacceptable wrappers will be listed as each of the sterilizing methods is described. A package is sealed to preserve the sterile state and not opened until ready to be used.

B. Suggestions for Packaging[28]

1. Insert sharp tips into a small piece of a cotton roll
   a. to protect the sharp tip from damage by other instruments.
   b. to prevent it from puncturing a bag or wrapper during sterilization. A punctured package can no longer be considered sterile.
2. Place a strip of sterilizer indicator tape inside each package on the instruments to show that the package contents have

been raised to the proper temperature for sterilization and that the wrapper did not hinder penetration.

3. Label and date each package. To prevent puncturing the bag while writing, the label should be placed before loading the bag.

4. Seal each package securely by folding the material twice and sealing with an indicator tape.

5. Gauze sponges, cotton rolls, and other accessories can be packaged in small lots for individual appointments.

PREPREPARED TRAYS

Preprepared or preset covered trays are preplanned trays, arranged to contain all of the items usually needed for a particular appointment. They are sterilized and assembled and ready for delivery at the dental chair at the time of the appointment.

The trays are prepared in advance, so that either a half day's or an entire day's appointments may be conducted without the confusion frequently related to the preparation for individual appointments. With analysis and experimentation, a tray system can be adapted to the specific needs of an individual practice.

I. Characteristics

A. Trays should be as large as possible but small enough to fit into the sterilizer and provide ample surrounding space.

B. Instruments should be arranged in an orderly manner on the tray, in sequence for use, with accessory materials conveniently placed. Instruments and materials to be used throughout the appointment are grouped in contrasting position to those such as floss or cotton roll holders, which may be used once or twice during the appointment.

C. An excess of instruments should be avoided. Double-ended instruments conserve space and limit the need for repeated changing. The basic tray should meet the basic needs.

D. Extra instruments to replace a dulled or dropped instrument, or to supplement when a particular problem requires a special instrument, are sterilized separately in labeled wrappers, and kept sealed in a convenient place within reach of the operating position.

E. Trays should be marked for identification of contents; for example, *Adult Scaling and Curettage, Small Child Examination*.

F. Specially designed cabinets with slots for sterile covered trays are available or may be constructed for temporary storage purposes.

II. Advantages

A. Increases efficiency and conserves time.
  1. Between-appointment preparation is minimized; delays for the patient are lessened.
  2. Instruments and materials are readily available and arranged for effective utilization.

B. Preserves sharpness of instruments since they can be arranged and kept apart from other instruments, in an orderly manner. When placed in a bag or canister, contact with other instruments can dull them.

C. Trays may be positioned at the convenience of the dental hygienist working alone, or the assistant in a team plan (page 76).

D. Sterilizing procedures can be systematized.

III. Preprepared Tray Arrangements

Examples of contents for trays are listed here. Specific names and numbers for explorers, probes, scalers, curets, or other instruments are not included because of individual variation. However, specific lists should be made and posted where instruments are prepared for sterilization, so that all concerned with tray preparations can have immediate reference.

The specific tray contents vary with the type of practice. In a specialty practice as, for example, periodontics, trays for dressing and suture removal would be needed more frequently than in a general practice; therefore, more trays would be prepared in advance.

A. **Initial Appointment: Examination Tray**

  Mouth mirror
  Explorers
  Probe
  Cotton pliers
  Saliva ejector tip
  Air syringe tip
  Gauze sponges
  Cotton-tip applicator
  Impression trays for study casts
  Radiographic film holder, if made of a

nondisposable material that can
be sterilized

B. Adult Scaling and Root Planing

Mouth mirror
Explorers
Probe
Cotton pliers
Scalers
Curets
Dappen dishes
Aspirator or evacuator tip
Air syringe tip
Saliva ejector tip
Gauze sponges
Dental floss lengths
Cotton rolls
Cotton-tip applicator

C. Topical Fluoride Application

Cotton roll holders
Cotton rolls cut to appropriate lengths
Cotton pellets and cotton pliers or
    applicators
Dappen dish
Saliva ejector tip
Air syringe tip

METHODS OF STERILIZATION

The method for sterilization that is selected
must provide complete destruction of all microorganisms, viruses, and spores, and yet must not
damage the instruments and other materials
treated. In addition, the procedures must not
be complex, with many chances for errors in the
processing.

The four methods of sterilization that are acceptable and that can be controlled and monitored are *steam under pressure, dry heat, chemical vapor pressure,* and *ethylene oxide gas.* The
four will be described in detail in this section.

Careful, specific use of sterilizing equipment
in accord with the manufacturer's specifications
is necessary. Incomplete sterilization is most frequently due to inadequate preparation of the
materials to be sterilized or to misuse of the
equipment.

I. Moist Heat: Steam Under Pressure[9,28,29]

Destruction of microorganisms by heat takes
place as a result of inactivation of essential cel-

lular proteins or enzymes. Moist heat causes coagulation of protein.

A. Use

Moist heat may be used for all materials
except oils, waxes, and powders that are impervious to steam, or materials that cannot
be subjected to high temperatures, such as
plastics.

B. Principles of Action

1. Sterilization is achieved by action of heat
   and moisture; pressure serves only to
   attain high temperature.
2. Sterilization depends on the penetrating
   ability of steam.
   a. Air must be excluded, otherwise
      steam penetration and heat transfer
      are prevented.
   b. Space between objects is essential to
      assure access for the steam.
   c. Materials must be thoroughly
      cleaned since adherent material can
      provide a barrier to the steam.
   d. Air discharge occurs in a downward
      direction; load must be arranged for
      free passage of steam toward bottom
      of autoclave.

C. Preparation of Materials

Linens are laundered; instruments are
scrubbed or cleaned in ultrasonic cleaner
and dried (pages 30–31).

1. *Protection of Metal Instruments from
   Corrosion.* Use a corrosion inhibitor such
   as 2% sodium nitrite.[30] Immerse, drain,
   and wrap or place in tray. This procedure is needed primarily for carbon steel
   instruments.
2. *Wrapping.* Bundles may be made with
   paper, muslin, see-through plastic and
   paper bags, or metal trays (with covers
   ajar), or dialysis tubing. Steam will not
   penetrate closed metal containers, canvas, cellophane, plastic cloth, or aluminum foil.[28]

   Tie or seal with autoclave tape; do not
   use pins for fastening paper because the
   pinholes leave openings for contamination. Label with date and list of contents.
3. *Autoclave Tape.* Bundle is sealed with
   tape which develops colored stripes at

121° C (250° F). The tape serves as a chemical monitor to identify packages that have been put through the sterilizer.[31]

4. *Autoclave Bags.* These are commercially available; they should not be overloaded.

5. *Packing Autoclave.* Pack loosely to permit steam to reach all instruments in all packages; place jars or tall vessels on their sides to permit air to leave as steam enters.

D. Operation

Follow manufacturer's specifications for use of autoclave.

The two ranges generally used when unwrapped instruments are treated are:

1. 121° C (250° F) at 15 pounds pressure for 15 minutes.
2. 134° C (270° F) at 30 pounds pressure for 3 to 7 minutes.
3. Wrapped instruments: add 5 to 10 minutes, depending on the thickness of the wrapper.

E. Cooling

1. *Dry Materials.* Release steam pressure, turn operating valve, and open the door; required time for drying, about 15 minutes.
2. *Liquids.* Reduce chamber pressure slowly at an even rate over 10 to 12 minutes to prevent boiling or escape of fluids into the chamber; preferable to turn off the autoclave and let the pressure fall before opening the door. Check heat sensitivity of each solution and avoid prolonged exposure, as indicated.

F. Care of Autoclave

1. *Daily.* Maintain proper level of distilled water; wash trays and interior surfaces of chamber with water and a mild detergent; clean removable plug, screen, or strainer.
2. *Weekly.* Flush chamber discharge system with an appropriate cleaning solution such as hot trisodium phosphate.

G. Biologic Indicator or Spore Test[31]

The chemical indicator color change or monitor is related to temperature, not time. For a real test of sterilization, a daily or weekly spore test is recommended for clinics and hospitals, while a weekly or monthly test may be sufficient for a smaller practice situation, depending on the amount of use. A spore test should also be made on a new machine, following repairs, and when there is a change of personnel who operate the equipment.

Ampules containing living resistant spore plus a color indicator are available. Sources are listed in the Technical Hints at the end of this chapter.

An ampule is placed in the center of a package between instruments and that package placed in the middle of a load of packages to be autoclaved. After sterilization has been completed by the usual time-temperature, the ampule and one that was not autoclaved are incubated according to the manufacturer's instructions. Unautoclaved spores will change the color indicator, whereas the autoclaved spores will not germinate. Certain companies provide spore strips which are returned to the company for culturing.

H. Evaluation of Steam Under Pressure

1. *Advantages*
   a. All microorganisms, spores, and viruses destroyed quickly and efficiently.
   b. Wide variety of materials may be treated; most generally economical.
2. *Disadvantages*
   a. May corrode carbon steel instruments if precautions are not taken; tends to reduce cutting edges slightly.
   b. Unsuitable for oils or powders that are impervious to heat.
   c. Rubber products may deteriorate after repeated exposures.

II. Dry Heat[9,28,29]

The action of dry heat is oxidation.

A. Use

1. Primarily for materials that cannot safely be sterilized with steam under pressure.
2. Oils and powders when they are thermostabile at the required temperatures.
3. For small metal instruments enclosed in special containers or that might be corroded or rusted by moisture, such as endodontic instruments.

B. Principles of Action

1. Sterilization is achieved by heat which is conducted from the exterior surface to the interior of the object; the time required to penetrate varies between materials.
2. Sterilization can result when the whole material is treated for a sufficient length of time at the specified temperature: timing for sterilization must therefore start when the entire contents of the sterilizer have reached the peak temperature needed for that load.
3. Oil, grease, or organic debris on instruments insulates and protects microorganisms from the sterilizing effect.

C. Preparation of Materials

1. *Instruments*, glassware, or other materials must be thoroughly cleaned and dried to prevent corrosion.
2. *Packaging.* Small packages permit greater access to the heat. Materials that may be used for packaging are paper bags, muslin towels, aluminum trays, pans, or aluminum foil.[28]
3. *Packing the Sterilizer.* Allow space for access to heat around each item; never load to the limit.

D. Operation

1. *Temperature.* 160° to 170° C (320° to 340° F) held for 1 or 2 hours. Timing must start after the desired temperature has been reached.
2. *Penetration Time.* Heat penetration varies with different materials, and the nature and properties of various materials must be considered.
3. *Care* must be taken not to overheat as certain materials can be affected: temperatures over 160° C (320° F) may destroy the sharp edges of cutting instruments; over 170° C, paper and cotton materials will begin to scorch.
4. *Spore Tests.* Procedures for testing sterilization are similar to those for a steam autoclave, but spores of different microorganisms are used.[31]

E. Evaluation of Dry Heat

1. *Advantages*
   a. Useful for materials that cannot be subjected to steam under pressure.
   b. When maintained at correct temperature, it is well suited for sharp instruments.
   c. No corrosion as found with steam under pressure.
2. *Disadvantages*
   a. Long exposure required; penetration slow and uneven.
   b. High temperatures critical to certain materials.

III. Chemical Vapor Sterilizer[28,29,32]

A combination of alcohols, formaldehyde, ketone, water, and acetone heated under pressure produces a gas that is effective as a sterilizing agent.

A. Use

Chemical vapor sterilization cannot be used for materials or objects that can be altered by the chemicals that make the vapor, or that cannot withstand the high temperature. Examples are low-melting plastics, liquids, or heat-sensitive handpieces.

B. Principles of Action

Microbial and viral destruction results from the permeation of the heated formaldehyde and alcohol. Heavy, tightly wrapped or sealed packages would not permit the penetration of the vapors.

C. Preparation of Materials

1. *Protection from Corrosion.* Rusting is not to be expected if instruments are dried before they are placed in the sterilizer.
2. *Wrapping*
   a. Penetration into and around the in-

struments is necessary. Sealed tubes
or jars or multiple thick cloth wrap-
pings would hinder the circulation of
the vapor.
  b. Acceptable for packaging are paper,
     perforated metal trays, and metal
     trays with covers, if the covers are
     left ajar. Plastic bags compatible with
     the gases as advised by the manufac-
     turer may also be used.
  c. Instruments may be placed on a ster-
     ilizer tray without wrapping when the
     sterilized materials will be used di-
     rectly and therefore do not need the
     protection of a wrapper.

D. Operation

  1. *Temperature.* 127° to 132° C (260° to
     270°F) with 20 to 40 pounds pressure in
     accord with the manufacturer's direc-
     tions.
  2. *Time.* Minimum of 20 minutes after the
     correct temperature has been attained.
     Time should be extended for a large load
     or a heavy wrap.

E. Cooling at the Completion of the Cycle

  Instruments are dry. Larger instruments
  may need a short period for cooling.

F. Care of Sterilizer

  Depending on the amount of use, refilling
  will be needed by at least every 30 cycles.
  In accord with manufacturers' instructions,
  the condensate tray is removed, the ex-
  hausted solution emptied, and the tray
  cleaned.

G. Spore Test for Sterilization

  A spore test strip is placed inside a typical
  package on a regular basis, weekly in a busy
  clinical situation. Procedures are similar to
  those described previously for a steam autoclave. Each type of sterilizer requires selected types of organisms in the spore test
  strip.[31]

H. Evaluation of Chemical Vapor Sterilizer

  1. *Advantages*
    a. Corrosion- and rust-free operation for
       carbon steel instruments.
    b. Ability to sterilize in a relatively short
       total cycle.
    c. Easy to operate and care for the
       equipment.
  2. *Disadvantages*
    a. Adequate ventilation is needed; can-
       not use in a small room.
    b. Slight odor, which is rarely objec-
       tionable.

IV. Ethylene Oxide[28,29,33]

  Gaseous sterilization using ethylene oxide is
  not commonly found in a private dental office
  or clinic, but rather in hospitals and larger clinics. As compact units are developed, ethylene
  oxide will be more widely used in dentistry.

A. Use

  Nearly all materials, whether metal, plastic, rubber, or cloth, can be sterilized in
  ethylene oxide with little or no damage to
  the material.

B. Principles of Action

  Ethylene oxide vapor is effective against
  all types and forms of microorganisms provided sufficient time is allowed.

C. Preparation of Materials

  1. *Instruments* must be completely cleaned
     and dried.
  2. *Wrapping*
    a. Penetration around and on all sur-
       faces is necessary for sterilizing ac-
       tion. Sealed metal containers are not
       acceptable for packaging.
    b. Acceptable for packaging are paper,
       perforated trays, metal trays with
       covers, if the covers are left ajar.

D. Operation

  Specific operation is related to the type
  of equipment. Operation in a well-ventilated room is necessary. Overnight processing is usually the most practical.
  1. *Time and Temperature.* The time may
     vary from 2 to 12 hours depending on
     both the temperature and the concen-
     tration of ethylene oxide used.
  2. *Aeration After Completion of the Cycle.*
     Plastic and rubber products need to be

aerated at least 24 hours. Metal instruments can be used immediately.

E. Spore Test

Effectiveness of sterilization must be tested regularly. A system similar to that described for steam autoclave is used, but does not contain the same type of spores.

F. Evaluation of Ethylene Oxide

1. *Advantages*
   a. Many types of materials can be sterilized with minimum or no damage to the material itself. There is no damage to the finest instruments.
   b. Low temperature for operation.
2. *Disadvantages*
   a. High cost of the equipment.
   b. Problems of dispersement of gaseous exhaust. Need for planned and tested ventilation.
   c. Increased time of operation.
   d. Gas absorption requires airing of plastic, rubber, and cloth goods for several hours.

METHODS OF DISINFECTION

Disinfection does not accomplish complete destruction of all forms of microorganisms; therefore it is not a substitute for sterilization. Physical or chemical means are used for disinfection.

The effect of disinfection is coagulation, precipitation, or denaturation of the protein, particularly the enzymes, of microorganisms.

I. Boiling Water[29]

A. Use

Boiling water may be used for the disinfection of metal instruments, glassware, or other materials which can be subjected to water.

B. Principles of Action

1. Disinfection is accomplished by heat.
2. Objects must be completely submerged for a sufficient length of time.
3. Bactericidal effect is increased by the addition of an alkali such as 2% sodium carbonate.

4. Distilled water should be used to supply the boiler.

C. Preparation of Materials

1. Scrub thoroughly, or use ultrasonic cleaner (pages 30–31).
2. Disassemble or open jointed instruments.
3. Arrange items carefully in metal basket of boiler to protect delicate and sharp edges and provide access of the boiling water; instruments must be completely submerged.

D. Operation

1. Minimum of 30 minutes at boiling (100° C or 212° F at sea level).
2. When instruments are added to those already boiling, the time cycle must be repeated.
3. An increase of heat does not increase the temperature of boiling water. Action is more vigorous and evaporation is increased.
4. Instruments should be removed with sterile transfer forceps while hot and dried promptly to prevent rusting.

E. Care of Unit

To decrease corrosive action on instruments and the formation of scaly deposit on the sides of the unit, use distilled water and add an antirust agent such as trisodium phosphate, sodium carbonate, or borax. Daily cleaning is necessary for units in constant use. Add a small amount of acetic acid (vinegar) and boil for 10 minutes to loosen the scale, then apply scrub brush and water, and rinse before filling.

F. Evaluation

1. *Advantages.* Relatively short time required for disinfection, and the preparation of materials is simple.
2. *Disadvantages.* Limited usefulness in a dental office or clinic because of the resistance of certain organisms, reduction in sharpness of instruments, and the tendency for instruments to corrode.

II. Hot Oil[29]

A hot oil unit that utilizes a hydrocarbon or

silicone oil has been used for jointed instruments, oilstones for sharpening, and for certain handpieces and prophylaxis angles that can not be sterilized.

A. Principles of Action

1. Disinfection is achieved by heat.
2. Item must be completely submerged for a sufficient length of time.

B. Preparation of Materials

Items must be cleaned of debris and oral contaminating substances in order to keep the oil in the unit clean and provide access to the surfaces being disinfected.

C. Operation

The manufacturer's directions should be followed carefully, as timing varies with the temperature.
1. Disinfection can be attained at 150° C (300° F) for 15 minutes or at 125° C (260° F) for 30 minutes. When at least 160° C (320° F) is used, spores and hepatitis viruses will be destroyed if held for a minimum of 1 hour.
2. Timing must start after the desired temperature has been reached.
3. When instruments are added to others already in a unit, the time cycle must be repeated for all.

D. Evaluation

1. *Advantages*
   a. Sharp edges are not dulled.
   b. Hot oil does not rust or corrode metals.
   c. Oilstones for sharpening do not dry out, become brittle, and chip, as they may when steam sterilized.
2. *Disadvantages*
   a. Oil may produce unpleasant odors.
   b. Cleaning the unit may be inconvenient and unpleasant.

III. Chemical Disinfectants[29,34]

The term "cold sterilization," which has been rather commonly used, is a misnomer which can be misleading. There is no cold chemical agent at the present time that can be considered a substitute for sterilization accomplished by steam under pressure, dry heat, chemical vapor, or ethylene oxide.

Chemical agents that have been tried in the past or are in current use have not been shown completely effective in killing resistant tubercle bacilli, hepatitis viruses, or bacterial spores. Many of the chemical solutions are only bacteriostatic, which, for certain preparations, may depend on concentration. Some agents are bactericidal at one concentration and bacteriostatic at another. Since chemical solutions do not destroy certain pathogens, viruses, and spores, it is important to recognize that the solution itself can become contaminated and thus contaminate instruments placed in it.

The American Dental Association has outlined provisions for acceptance of chemicals proposed for the disinfection of instruments, and lists those approved in the *Accepted Dental Therapeutics*. For acceptance, a disinfectant must be effective in killing vegetative forms of pathogenic organisms, influenza and enteroviruses, and the tubercle bacillus within 30 minutes. The label must include statements to clarify the inability of the agent to kill spores and hepatitis viruses, the unsuitability for disinfection of hypodermic needles, and other specific regulatory information.[35]

A. Uses

1. For stop-gap measure, to use only until sterilizable instruments can be obtained: disinfection of instruments or other items that cannot be sterilized because of their incompatibility with the sterilizing agent (heat or chemical). This does not imply disinfection for items intended to be disposable.
2. For disinfection of environmental surfaces contacted during an appointment.
3. For disinfection of dental appliances prior to insertion into a patient's mouth. Selection of a disinfectant depends on compatibility with oral tissues, although thorough rinsing with water after use of disinfection is indicated. Solution is used for one patient only.
4. For use in surgical handwashing preparations.

B. Principles of Action

1. Disinfection is achieved by coagulation,

precipitation, or oxidation of protein of microbial cells or denaturation of the enzymes of the cells.

2. Disinfection depends on the contact of the solution at the known effective concentration for the optimum period of time.

3. Items must be thoroughly cleaned and dried, since action of the agent is altered by foreign matter and dilution.

4. A solution has a specific shelf life. Some may be altered by changes in pH, or the active ingredient may decrease. Length of time may depend on amount of use; check manufacturer's directions.

5. Indicators are not available for chemical or biologic monitoring of disinfectants.

C. Preparation of Materials

1. *Scrub* thoroughly or use ultrasonic cleaner (pages 30–31) to eliminate organic matter (blood, debris, oil, grease) which interferes with the action of the chemical. Use wire brush for grooved metal instruments such as files or burs.

2. *Rinse* thoroughly to eliminate soap or detergent that is incompatible with the chemical.

3. *Dry* thoroughly. Dilution of the chemical solution will lessen or eliminate its effect. Place on paper towels to blot dry.

D. Operation

1. Place instruments in solution and immerse completely; solution must contact all parts. Care must be taken to prevent overloading.

2. Temperature: usually room temperature.

3. Time: follow manufacturer's instructions. Time varies from 30 minutes to 10 hours.

4. Do not add other instruments without starting timing over again.

5. When time is complete, drain the instruments, remove with sterile transfer forceps, and dry with a sterile towel. When a solution is known to be irritating to tissue or distasteful, instruments should be rinsed with sterile water to remove the chemical.

E. Care of Equipment

1. Keep the container covered to prevent contamination of the solution from dust- or airborne microorganisms.

2. Clean the container and change the solution on a regular schedule to maintain its cleanliness, proper dilution and potency in accord with the shelf life of the chemical.

F. Recommended Chemical Disinfectants[23,29,36]

The agents that have been shown adequate for use in dentistry are glutaraldehyde, iodophores, certain chlorine compounds, and formaldehyde. These will be described below.

Alcohols, phenolic compounds, and quaternary ammonium compounds are not approved for instrument or environmental surface disinfection. They are not effective against hepatitis B viruses or bacterial spores, and some have undesirable chemical or physical properties. The alcohols, ethanol and isopropanol, have been widely accepted and used for the preparation of the skin prior to injections or blood-taking procedures.[37]

1. *Glutaraldehyde*
   a. Action. Buffered 2% glutaraldehyde has a two-week shelf life. It is effective against fungi, some viruses (not hepatitis), and bacteria, including the tubercle bacillus, in 10, preferably 15, minutes, and against spores when the time is extended to 10 hours.
   b. Precautions. Buffered 2% glutaraldehyde can cause irritation of the eyes and skin. It should be handled carefully to prevent skin contact and used in a well-ventilated area. Rinsing with water immediately following contact is necessary. Carbon steel instruments may corrode if left in the solution over 24 hours.
   c. Clinical care. Rinse instruments with sterile water or 70% isopropyl alcohol after removing from the disinfecting solution to prevent contact of the solution with the patient's oral cavity.
   d. Example: Cidex (buffered 2% glutaraldehyde).

2. *Iodine Complex: Iodophors*[38]
   a. Action. Iodine is slowly liberated to provide effective antibacterial, antiviral action. Povidone-iodine preparations are widely used for disinfecting purposes in the forms of surgical scrub, surgical liquid soap, mouthrinse, and surface antiseptics prior to hypodermic injection.
   b. Environmental surface disinfectant. As a surface disinfectant and for treating instruments when sterilization is not possible, an iodophore solution prepared in a 1:20 dilution of iodine surgical scrub (one part) with isopropyl alcohol (20 parts) for a 30-minute exposure can be considered effective.[9] Most infectious agents including hepatitis viruses will be destroyed. The disinfection of environmental surfaces is described on page 60. Stronger solutions at 1:1 ratio are used when dealing with a patient for whom maximum precautions are taken (page 65).
   c. Precautions. An occasional person is sensitive to iodine. Residual iodine on environmental surfaces can be removed with alcohol to prevent possible contact of the sensitive individual.

      Instruments left in the solution can become corroded. The recommended 30-minute exposure time should be the limit.
   d. Examples: Betadine Surgical Scrub; Vestal Iodine Scrub. Addresses are included with the Technical Hints at the end of this chapter.
3. *Sodium Hypochlorite*
   a. Action. Chlorine compounds have been used in a variety of ways for disinfection. Water purification action is well known. Solutions of sodium hypochlorite are used in cleaning dentures (pages 387–388).

      When sterilization of instruments is not possible, a solution of sodium hypochlorite can be used for 30 minutes.[29] The proportions call for a 1:10 dilution of 5% household bleach in water.[28]
   b. Precautions. Hypochlorite solutions can harm the eyes, skin, and clothing, deteriorate on standing, and corrode metal instruments. The strong odor may be offensive. Careful handling to prevent splashing is needed. Thorough rinsing of instruments is indicated.

      Organic matter can inactivate chlorine rapidly; therefore, thorough cleaning and drying of instruments before placing them in the hypochlorite solution is important.
4. *Formaldehyde*
   a. Action. Used in 2 to 3% aqueous solution, formaldehyde is germicidal after 20 to 30 minutes exposure. The use as a surface disinfectant is therefore generally limited except at the end of a day. An 8% solution has a high antibacterial action, whereas the 3% solution has a moderate action.

      When formaldehyde is mixed with isopropyl alcohol, there is a more rapid action than when in aqueous solution. A 3 to 4 percent solution of formaldehyde in isopropyl alcohol is an effective disinfectant.[29]
   b. Precautions. Skin and mucosal irritation, fumes with a pungent odor that may lead to coughing, and a severe, serious contact dermatitis in sensitive individuals, indicate the need for careful handling of the solutions. A residue is left after surface application, and materials should be aired or cleaned with sterile water or alcohol before use.

HANDPIECE CARE

With the manufacture of handpieces and prophylaxis angles that can be sterilized, a major hurdle in the attempt to control cross-infection in dental clinics and offices has been overcome. Handpieces and angles have always been difficult to manage because of the materials and intricate parts that could not be subjected to sterilization processes, particularly high temperatures.

Problems have centered around handpieces, prophylaxis angles, and ultrasonic handpieces, not only because it was not possible to sterilize them, but also because of the contaminated water that passes through them, and the splatter and aerosols they create. Difficulties related to unit water lines are described on page 42, and aerosols on page 17.

Other equipment, such as nondetachable air/water three-way syringes, also presents complications for sterilization. Methods such as those described for handpieces can be applied to the air/water syringe.

I. Handpiece Preparation for Sterilization

A. General Procedures

1. Clean the instrument soon after use. When saliva, blood, and other organic debris is allowed to dry on the surfaces of an instrument, sterilization is incomplete because the film of saliva and debris can form a protective covering for viable microorganisms. Scrubbing tenacious, hardened material in the attempt to completely clean the surfaces is time consuming.

2. Rotate several handpieces and prophylaxis angles. Time is an important factor in the outcome of each sterilization method. The specified length of time for sterilization should not be compromised because of a close schedule of patient appointments. The initial investment for obtaining several handpieces may be greater, but the life of an individual instrument is not altered.

B. Cleaning

1. Follow the manufacturer's instructions relative to disassembling and cleaning prior to sterilizing.

2. Scrub with a brush, using iodophore surgical scrub.[39] Pay particular attention to cleaning out the grooves and markings (knurling) that retain microorganisms because of inaccessibility to wiping with a sponge.

3. Extend the handpiece hose and tubings for air, water, and suction to a sink, when possible, to facilitate scrubbing with a brush and iodophore surgical scrub.

4. Lather with the surgical scrub and leave it in place for 3 minutes. Scrub under

running water. By leaving the handpiece running while brushing under running water, the water will be prevented from entering the inner parts of the handpiece.

5. Dry the instruments prior to gaseous forms of sterilization.

6. Dip in antirust solution prior to steam pressure autoclave.

II. Sterilization

A. Heat-Sterilizable

The steam pressure autoclave or dry heat may be used for those instruments that can withstand the heat and steam, as specified by the manufacturer. Nearly all manufacturers now have handpieces of materials that can be sterilized.[40] The manufacturer's instructions are followed relative to lubrication before or after sterilizing.

B. Non-Heat-Sterilizable

Ethylene oxide sterilization is recommended for certain other handpieces and prophylaxis angles that can not withstand heat.

III. Disinfection

Until such time as only sterilizable handpieces, prophylaxis angles, ultrasonic handpieces, and detachable air and water syringes are available, stop-gap measures for careful disinfection are needed. A quick, however vigorous, wiping of the outer sleeve of a handpiece is not adequate to satisfy requirements for disinfection, since contact is limited both in surface and in time.

A. Separate the Parts that Can Be Sterilized

Examples of removable parts are the outer sheath from certain handpieces and the tips from air and water syringes. Clean these parts as previously described and prepare them for sterilization.

B. Scrub with a Brush[11]

All parts that cannot be sterilized must be disinfected. A few handpieces and other pieces of equipment may withstand submerging and soaking for a period of time.

1. Use an iodine-alcohol disinfecting scrub mixture. Prepare the disinfectant by combining 1:20, one part iodophore surgical scrub and 20 parts isopropyl alcohol. Scrub thoroughly and vigorously, using a brush.
2. Leave a coating of iodine on the instruments for 3 to 30 minutes. Rinse thoroughly and wipe clean with alcohol on a sponge. When there is no objection, the iodine does not have to be wiped off.
3. Dry and lubricate.

C. Wrap in a Sponge

1. After mechanical cleansing, wrap a 4 × 4 inch sterile sponge, which has been saturated in the disinfectant, around the handpiece and/or prophylaxis angle, and cover with a clean finger cot. The cot prevents volatilization of the disinfectant and maintains the sponge in place.
2. Protection from airborne contamination becomes especially important when the aerosols remain in the room from a previous patient. The cot and sponge should remain in place until time for the next use.

IV. Belt-Driven Handpiece

A. Cleaning

1. Remove outer sheath (figure 3–3B).
2. Wipe spindle (covering of inner part) with a clean dry cloth.
3. Ultrasonic cleaning may be used.

B. Sterilization

1. Use method in keeping with manufacturer's instructions.
2. Use corrosion-preventive agent to coat the handpiece prior to autoclaving.[30]
3. Scrub with iodophore surgical scrub and alcohol (1:20) as described previously.

C. Lubrication

Ordinarily, the handpiece should be lubricated each morning because the oil will drip out while it hangs overnight. When the handpiece is laid flat, it may be lubricated at the end of the day. Caution should be used when applying oil, as an excessive amount causes increased heat production and unnecessary wear.

1. Lubricate handpiece after sterilization.
2. Apply sterile oil with sterile swab or pipe cleaner.
3. Oil chuck opening (at working end of spindle) with pipe cleaner dipped in oil. Insert pipe cleaner into the opening as far as it will go.
4. Hold handpiece with chuck opening up, and apply two drops of oil to tip of spindle. Draw the oil-moistened pipe cleaner across the back of the spindle once.
5. Apply a small amount of oil to wrist joint of handpiece attachment with cotton pliers; press ball of joint as oil is applied.
6. Replace sheath slowly to avoid splashing oil.

V. Dental Motor and Arm

A. Daily Care

Wipe arm, including pulleys.

B. Weekly Care

Oil pulley with end of pipe cleaner dipped in oil.

C. Monthly Care

Place *one* drop of oil in each oil hole of motor in accord with the manufacturer's specifications.

D. Belt

1. Adjust tension of belt for smooth running.
2. Replace belt when it begins to fray to avoid its breaking during an appointment.
3. Wash handpiece belt occasionally with mild soap and water to remove grease and oil. Grease and oil cause loss of traction and attract dust. Replace belt while it is still partially dry.

VI. Unit Water Lines

High counts of microorganisms have been found in the waterline tubings after overnight standing. Tests have been made on tubings to handpieces, water syringes, and ultrasonic scalers.[8,41,42,43] When the lines were flushed for 2 minutes, the microbial counts were reduced.[8]

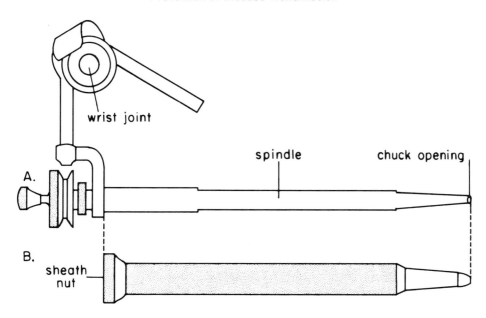

Figure 3–3. Parts of a belt-driven handpiece. A. Handpiece with sheath removed. B. Sheath.

A. Procedures for Clinical Use

1. Flush all waterlines at least 5 to 6 minutes at the beginning of each day.
2. Operate handpieces and waterspray over a sink or cuspidor for 30 seconds before and 30 seconds after each patient appointment.

B. Testing Water Lines

Cultures can be made to test the microbial counts in water samples from each tubing.[44]

C. Corrective Measures

Research has been conducted to find new types of filters to reduce the bacterial counts.[44,45]

Sterile water reservoirs can be installed.[11] Contaminated water should not be used for surgical purposes or during the irrigation of pocket areas, since infective microorganisms can be introduced. If contaminated water were directed forcefully into a pocket, microorganisms could enter the tissue and bacteremia result.

D. Water Retraction System

To correct saliva and debris suck-back in the water line of a handpiece, the water retraction valve should be removed and a check valve or antiretractor valve installed.[46,47] Originally, handpieces were made with a retraction valve to prevent dripping when the instrument was turned off. Material sucked into the line, possibly filled with microorganisms including hepatitis viruses, tubercle bacilli, and other pathogens, will then be discharged when the handpiece is used for the succeeding patient.

TECHNICAL HINTS

I. Handpiece Maintenance

Keep records of handpiece purchase, maintenance, and other information pertinent to the longevity and effectiveness. Maintain a sufficient number of handpieces to permit rotation and thorough sterilization.

II. Sterilization Monitoring

Keep a written record of dates when processing tests and biologic monitor tests were performed for each sterilizer. Indicate advance dates for the next testing clearly on a calendar or other reference point. Tests made weekly should be performed on the same day to simplify remembering.

III. Sources of Test Materials

A. Biologic Monitor and Chemical Indicator

Amsco Medical Products Division (*Spordi*)
American Sterilizer Company
2820 West 23rd St.
Erie, Pennsylvania 16512

Medical Products Division/3M (*Attest*)
3 M Center
St. Paul, Minnesota 55101

Sybron Corporation (*Unispore*)
Medical Products Division
P.O. Box 23077
Rochester, New York 14692

B. Iodophore Scrubs

Amsco Medical Products Division
(*Prepodyne*)
American Sterilizer Company
2820 West 23rd St.
Erie, Pennsylvania 16512

Parke-Davis & Company (*Deseret Iodophore E–Z Scrub*)
P.O. Box 1506
Greenwood, S.C. 29646

Purdue Frederick Company (*Betadine* products)
50 Washington St.
Norwalk, Connecticut 06856

Vestal Laboratories (*Vestal Surgical Scrub*)
Division of Chemed Corporation
St. Louis, Missouri 63110

References

1. Burnett, G.W. and Schuster, G.S.: *Oral Microbiology and Infectious Disease*, Student edition. Baltimore, The Williams & Wilkins Co., 1978, p. 141.
2. Socransky, S.S. and Manganiello, S.D.: The Oral Microbiota of Man from Birth to Senility, *J. Periodontol.*, 42, 485, August, 1971.
3. Miller, R.L. and Micik, R.E.: Air Pollution and Its Control in the Dental Office, *Dent. Clin. North Am.*, 22, 453, July, 1978.
4. Miller, R.L.: Generation of Airborne Infection—by High Speed Dental Equipment, *J. Am. Soc. Prev. Dent.*, 6, 14, May/June, 1976.
5. Larato, D.C., Ruskin, P.F., and Martin, A.: Effect of an Ultrasonic Scaler on Bacterial Counts in Air, *J. Periodontol.*, 38, 550, November-December, 1967.
6. Holbrook, W.P., Muir, K.F., MacPhee, I.T., and Ross, P.W.: Bacteriological Investigation of the Aerosol from Ultrasonic Scalers, *Br. Dent. J.*, 144, 245, April 18, 1978.
7. Pokowitz, W. and Hoffman, H.: Dental Aerobiology, *N.Y. State Dent. J.*, 37, 337, June-July, 1971.

8. Gross, A., Devine, M.J., and Cutright, D.E.: Microbial Contamination of Dental Units and Ultrasonic Scalers, *J. Periodontol.*, 47, 670, November, 1976.
9. Crawford, J.J.: *Clinical Asepsis in Dentistry*, 2nd ed. Mesquite, Texas, R.A. Kolstad, Publisher, 1978, 40 pp.
10. Whitacre, R.J., Robins, S.K., Williams, B.L., and Crawford, J.J.: *Dental Asepsis*. Seattle, Stoma Press, 1979, pp. 46–51.
11. Crawford, J.J.: Sterilization, Disinfection and Asepsis in Dentistry, in Block, S.S., ed.: *Disinfection, Sterilization, and Preservation*, 2nd ed. Philadelphia, Lea & Febiger, 1977, pp. 685–704.
12. Robbins, S.L. and Cotran, R.S.: *Pathologic Basis of Disease*, 2nd ed. Philadelphia, W.B. Saunders Co., 1979, pp. 396–404.
13. United States Department of Health and Human Services, Public Health Service, Tuberculosis Control Division, Bureau of State Services, Center for Disease Control: Follow-up on Tuberculosis Among Indochinese Refugees, *MMWR*, 29, 573, November 28, 1980.
14. Shklar, G. and McCarthy, P.L.: *The Oral Manifestations of Systemic Disease*. Boston, Butterworths, 1976, pp. 56–59.
15. Rowe, N.H. and Brooks, S.L.: Contagion in the Dental Office, *Dent. Clin. North Am.*, 22, 491, July, 1978.
16. Hooley, J.R. and Phillips, R.E.: The Operating Room, in Hooley, J.R. and Daun, L.G.: *Hospital Dental Practice*. St. Louis, The C.V. Mosby Co., 1980, pp. 192–214.
17. Szmuness, W., Stevens, C.E., Harley, E.J., Zang, E.A., Oleszko, W.R., William, D.C., Sadovsky, R., Morrison, J.M., and Kellner, A.: Hepatitis B Vaccine. Demonstration of Efficacy in a Controlled Clinical Trial in a High-Risk Population in the United States, *New Engl. J. Med.*, 303, 833, October 9, 1980.
18. World Health Organization: *Advances in Viral Hepatitis*, WHO Technical Report Series, Number 602. Geneva, World Health Organization, 1977, 62 pp.
19. Krugman, S. and Gocke, D.J.: *Viral Hepatitis*. Philadelphia, W.B. Saunders Co., 1978, pp. 20–29, 37–45.
20. Robbins and Cotran: op. cit., pp. 1035–1038.
21. United States Department of Health and Human Services, Immunization Practices Advisory Committee: Immune Globulins for Protection Against Viral Hepatitis, *MMWR*, 30, 423, Number 34, September 4, 1981.
22. Whitacre, Robins, Williams, and Crawford: op. cit., pp. 30–43.
23. Expert Group on Hepatitis in Dentistry: Hepatitis in Dentistry, *Br. Dent. J.*, 146, 123, February 20, 1979.
24. Krugman and Gocke: op cit., p. 78.
25. American Dental Association, Council on Dental Therapeutics, and United States Hepatitis Laboratories Division, Bureau of Epidemiology, and Tuberculosis Control Division, Bureau of State Services, Center for Disease Control: Viral Hepatitis Type B, Tuberculosis, and Dental Care of Indochinese Refugees, *MMWR*, 29, 1, Number 1, January 11, 1980.
26. Dienstag, J.L.: Toward the Control of Hepatitis B, *New Engl. J. Med.*, 303, 874, October 9, 1980.
27. Krugman and Gocke: op. cit., pp. 82–90.
28. Whitacre, Robins, Williams, and Crawford: op. cit., pp. 57–104.
29. American Dental Association, Council on Dental Therapeutics: *Accepted Dental Therapeutics*, 39th ed. Chicago, American Dental Association, 1982, pp. 100–116.
30. Bertolotti, R.L. and Hurst, V.: Inhibition of Corrosion during Autoclave Sterilization of Carbon Steel Dental Instruments, *J. Am. Dent. Assoc.*, 97, 628, October, 1978.
31. Runnells, R.R. and Schmoegner, J.C.: The Need to

Monitor Use and Function of Sterilizers, *Dent. Surv.*, 56, 20, October, 1980.

32. Harvey, Chemiclave, MDT Corporation, 1 Continental Plaza, El Segundo, California, 90245.

33. Phillips, C.R.: Gaseous Sterilization, in Block, S.S., ed.: *Disinfection, Sterilization, and Preservation*, 2nd ed. Philadelphia, Lea & Febiger, 1977, pp. 594–602.

34. Spaulding, E.H., Cundy, K.R., and Turner, F.J.: Chemical Disinfection of Medical and Surgical Materials, in Block, S.S., ed.: *Disinfection, Sterilization, and Preservation*, 2nd ed. Philadelphia, Lea & Febiger, 1977, pp. 654–684.

35. American Dental Association, Council on Dental Therapeutics: op. cit., p. xxi.

36. Cianco, S.G. and Bourgault, P.C.: *Clinical Pharmacology for Dental Professionals*. New York, McGraw-Hill, 1980, pp. 131–138.

37. American Dental Association, Council on Dental Therapeutics: op. cit., pp. 267–268.

38. Gershenfeld, L.: Iodine, in Block, S.S., ed.: *Disinfection, Sterilization, and Preservation*, 2nd ed. Philadelphia, Lea & Febiger, 1977, pp. 196–208.

39. Crawford, J.J.: Office Sterilization and Asepsis Procedures in Endodontics, *Dent. Clin. North Am.*, 23, 717, October, 1979.

40. Sanger, R.G., Bradford, B.A., and Delaney, J.M.: An Inquiry into the Sterilization of Dental Handpieces Relative to Transmission of Hepatitis B Virus, *J. Am. Dent. Assoc.*, 96, 621, April, 1978.

41. Abel, L.C., Miller, R.L., Micik, R.E., and Ryge, G.: Studies on Dental Aerobiology: IV. Bacterial Contamination of Water Delivered by Dental Units, *J. Dent. Res.*, 50, 1567, November-December, 1971.

42. Clark, A.: Bacterial Colonization of Dental Units and the Nasal Flora of Dental Personnel, *Proc. R. Soc. Med.*, 67, 1269, December (Part 1), 1974.

43. McEntegart, M.G. and Clark, A.: Colonisation of Dental Units by Water Bacteria, *Br. Dent. J.*, 134, 140, February 20, 1973.

44. Sawyer, D.R., Page, D.G., Sweeney, W.T., and Dalton, H.P.: Bacterial Contamination and Disinfection of the High-speed Dental Handpiece and the Water It Delivers, *Va. Dent. J.*, 53, 14, December, 1976.

45. Dayoub, M.B., Rusilko, D.J., and Gross, A.: A Method of Decontamination of Ultrasonic Scalers and High Speed Handpieces, *J. Periodontol.*, 49, 261, May, 1978.

46. Crawford, J.J. and Fine, J.: Infection Control in Hospital Dentistry, in Hooley, J.R. and Daun, L.G., eds.: *Hospital Dental Practice*, St. Louis, The C.V. Mosby Co., 1980, pp. 119–154.

47. American Dental Association, Council on Dental Materials and Devices and Council on Dental Therapeutics: Infection Control in the Dental Office, *J. Am. Dent. Assoc.*, 97, 673, October, 1978.

Suggested Readings

Adrian, J.C. and Gross, A.: A New Method of Sterilization: the Carbon Dioxide Laser, *J. Oral Pathol.*, 8, 60, February, 1979.

American Dental Association, Council on Dental Materials, Instruments, and Equipment: Current Status of Sterilization Instruments, Devices, and Methods for the Dental Office, *J. Am. Dent. Assoc.*, 102, 683, May, 1981.

American Dental Association, Council on Dental Materials, Instruments and Equipment: *Dentist's Desk Reference: Materials, Instruments and Equipment*, 1st ed. Chicago, American Dental Association, 1981, pp. 314–324.

Christensen, R.P.: Effectiveness of Glutaraldehyde as a Chemosterilizer Used in a Wrapping Technique on Simulated Metal Instruments, *J. Dent. Res.*, 56, 822, July, 1977.

Custer, F. and Coyle, T.: Instrument Changes During Sterilization, *J. Dent. Res.*, 49, 487, May-June, 1970.

Ernst, R.R.: Sterilization by Heat, in Block, S.S., ed.: *Disinfection, Sterilization, and Preservation*, 2nd ed. Philadelphia, Lea & Febiger, 1977, pp. 481–521.

Ernst, R.C.: Biohazards in Dentistry. Part II. Infections, *Dent. Assist.*, 48, 23, March/April, 1979.

Ernst, R.C.: Biohazards in Dentistry. Part IV. Sterilization, *Dent. Assist.*, 48, 39, July/August, 1979.

Gillespie, J. and Eisenbud, L.: Disinfection and Sterilization of Dental Instruments in a Hospital Dental Clinic, *J. Hosp. Dent. Pract.*, 13, 96, 3rd Quarter, 1979.

Goldman, H.S. and Hartman, K.S.: Their Disease, Our Unease: Infectious Diseases and Dental Practice, *Ann. Dent.*, 38, 62, Fall, 1979.

Green, E.J.: An Efficient Approach to Patient Care, in Clark, J.W., ed.: *Clinical Dentistry, Volume 5*, Chapter 28. Hagerstown, Maryland, Harper & Row, 1980, pp. 1–9.

MacFarlane, T.W.: Cross Infection and Sterilisation in Dental Practice, *Br. Dent. J.*, 141, 213, October 5, 1976.

Matis, B.A., Christen, A.G., Young, J.M., and Sellers, W.R.: *Infection Control in Air Force Dental Clinics*, Aeromedical Review 3-80. Brooks Air Force Base, USAF School of Aerospace Medicine, Texas 78235, December, 1980, 24 pp.

McLundie, A.C.: The Effects of Various Methods of Sterilization and Disinfection on Tungsten-carbide Burs, *Br. Dent. J.*, 137, 49, July 16, 1974.

Mostafa, S.M.: Adverse Effects of Buffered Glutaraldehyde on the Heidbrink Expiratory Valve, *Br. J. Anaesth.*, 52, 223, February, 1980.

Pelleu, G.B.: Antiseptics and Disinfectants, in Holroyd, S.V., ed.: *Clinical Pharmacology in Dental Practice*, 2nd ed. St. Louis, The C.V. Mosby Co., 1978, pp. 221–227.

Project Acorde: *Sanitization, Disinfection, Sterilization of Dental Instruments and Equipment*. Castro Valley, California, Quercus Corporation, 1979, 112 pp.

Rothstein, S.S. and Goldman, H.S.: Sterilizing and Disinfecting for Hepatitis B Virus in the Dental Operatory, *Clin. Prev. Dent.*, 2, 9, November-December, 1980.

Simpson, J.P. and Whittaker, D.K.: Serum Contamination of Instruments in Dental Practice, *Br. Dent. J.*, 146, 76, February 6, 1979.

Stapff, K.-H.: Is Ultrasonic Cleaning of Instruments Rational? (I), *Quintessence Int.*, 5, 73, November, 1974.

Walsh, M.M.: The Effect of Various Sterilizing Wraps on the Corrosion of Instruments During Autoclaving, *Dent. Hyg.*, 53, 504, November, 1979.

Aerosols

Ernst, R.C.: Biohazards in Dentistry. Part I. Splatter and Aerosols, *Dent. Assist.*, 48, 28, January/February, 1979.

Grayson, B.H., Li, W.K.P., and Benjaminson, M.A.: Viability of Bacteria in High-Speed Dental Drill Aerosols with Antimicrobial Agents in the Water Coolant System, *J. Dent. Res.*, 52, 7, January-February, 1973.

Lu, D.P. and Zambito, R.F.: Aerosols and Cross Infection in Dental Practice—A Historic View, *Gen. Dent.*, 29, 136, March-April, 1981.

Miller, R.L., Micik, R.E., Abel, C., and Ryge, G.: Studies on Dental Aerobiology: II. Microbial Splatter Discharged from the Oral Cavity of Dental Patients, *J. Dent. Res.*, 50, 621, May-June, 1971.

Muir, K.F., Ross, P.W., MacPhee, I.T., Holbrook, W.P., and Kowolik, M.J.: Reduction of Microbial Contamination from Ultrasonic Scalers, *Br. Dent. J.*, *145*, 76, August 1, 1978.

Pollok, N.L., Williams, G.H., Shay, D.E., and Barr, C.E.: Laminar Air Purge of Microorganisms in Dental Aerosols, *J. Am. Dent. Assoc.*, *81*, 1131, November, 1970.

Shreve, W.B., Wachtel, L.W., and Pelleu, G.B.: Air Cleaning Devices for Reduction in Number of Airborne Bacteria, *J. Dent. Res.*, *49*, 1078, September-October, 1970.

Wenner, J.H., Greene, V.W., and King, K.J.: Monitoring Microbial Aerosols in an Operating Room During Restorative Dentistry, *J. Dent. Child.*, *44*, 25, January-February, 1977.

Williams, G.H., Pollok, N.L., Shay, D.E., and Barr, C.E.: Laminar Air Purge of Microorganisms in Dental Aerosols: Prophylactic Procedures with the Ultrasonic Scaler, *J. Dent. Res.*, *49*, Suppl., 1498, November-December, 1970.

Handpieces

Besford, J.: Handpiece Sterilization in General Practice, *Proc. R. Soc. Med.*, *67*, 1265, December, 1974.

Gross, A., Devine, M.J., and Cutright, D.E.: Microbial Contamination of Dental Units and Ultrasonic Scalers, *J. Periodontol.*, *47*, 670, November, 1976.

Hegna, I.K., Kardel, K., and Kardel, M.: Autoclaving of Lubricated Dental Instruments, *Scand. J. Dent. Res.*, *86*, 130, March, 1978.

Mooney, P.E.: Care and Feeding of Handpieces, *Dent. Assist.*, *47*, 35, January/February, 1978.

Pelzner, R.B., Kempler, D., Stark, M.M., Barkin, P.R., and Graham, D.A.: Laser Evaluation of Handpiece Contamination, *J. Dent. Res.*, *56*, 1629, December, 1977.

Peyton, F.A., American Dental Association, Council on Dental Materials and Devices: Status Report on Dental Operating Handpieces, *J. Am. Dent. Assoc.*, *89*, 1162, November, 1974.

Wirthlin, M.R., Shklair, I.L., Northerner, R.A., Shelton, S.W., and Bailey, G.L.: The Performance of Autoclaved High-speed Dental Handpieces, *J. Am. Dent. Assoc.*, *103*, 584, October, 1981.

Hepatitis

Alexander, R.E.: Hepatitis Risk: A Clinical Perspective, *J. Am. Dent. Assoc.*, *102*, 182, February, 1981.

American Dental Association, Council on Dental Therapeutics: Type B (serum) Hepatitis and Dental Practice, *J. Am. Dent. Assoc.*, *92*, 153, January, 1976.

Behr, M.T.: Dental Considerations of Most Common Medical Therapy, in Boundy, S.S. and Reynolds, N.J., eds.: *Current Concepts in Dental Hygiene, Volume 2*, St. Louis, The C.V. Mosby Co., 1979, pp. 138–154.

Bond, W.W., Petersen, N.J., and Favero, M.S.: Viral Hepatitis B: Aspects of Environmental Control, *Health Lab. Sci.*, 14, 235, October, 1977.

Brown, B.S.: Non-A, Non-B Hepatitis: Implications for Health Care Professionals, *Horizons*, *2*, 10, April, 1981.

Crawford, J.J.: New Light on the Transmissibility of Viral Hepatitis in Dental Practice and its Control, *J. Am. Dent. Assoc.*, *91*:829, October, 1975.

Ernst, R.: Serum Hepatitis: The Hidden Menace to the Dental Team, *Dent. Assist.*, *47*, 22, May/June, 1978.

Follett, E.A.C. and MacFarlane, T.W.: Infectivity in Hepatitis B Surface Antigen (Australia Antigen) Positive Patients, *Br. Dent. J.*, *150*, 92, February 17, 1981.

Goebel, W.M. and Gitnick, G.L.: Hepatitis B Virus Infection in Dental Students. A Two-year Evaluation, *J. Oral Med.*, *34*, 33, April-June, 1979.

Hollinger, F.B., Grander, J.W., Nickel, F.R., and Suarez, M.: Hepatitis B Prevalence Within a Dental Student Population, *J. Am. Dent. Assoc.*, *94*, 521, March, 1977.

Hribar, D.L.A.: Viral Hepatitis: A Review of Clinical Laboratory and Research Aspects, *Aust. Dent. J.*, *22*, 471, December, 1977.

Hurlen, B., Jonsen, J., Netland, A., and Osnes, S.: Salivary HBsAg in Hepatitis B Infection, *Acta Odontol. Scand.*, *38*:51, Number 1, 1980.

James, S.P. and Sampliner, R.E.: Hepatitis B in the Dental Setting: Dental Hygienists, *J. Maryland State Dent. Assoc.*, *21*, 26, April, 1978.

Koga, Y.T. and Penland, L.R.: Guidelines: Hepatitis Patients and Dental Hygiene Practice, *Educ. Dir. Dent. Aux.*, *2*, 21, February, 1977.

Norkrans, G., Frösner, G., Hermodsson, S., and Iwarson, S.: Multiple Hepatitis Attacks in Drug Addicts, *J. Am. Med. Assoc.*, *243*, 1056, March 14, 1980.

Petersen, N.J., Bond, W.W., and Favero, M.S.: Air Sampling for Hepatitis B Surface Antigen in a Dental Operatory, *J. Am. Dent. Assoc.*, *99*, 465, September, 1979.

Pollack, A. and Wright, A.D.: Viral Hepatitis, *Br. Dent. J.*, *144*, 146, March 7, 1978.

Ratcliff, R.: Hepatitis and the Dental Hygienist, *Dent. Hyg.*, *51*, 493, November, 1977.

Ross, J.W. and Clarke, S.K.R.: Hepatitis B in Dentistry: the Current Position, *Br. Dent. J.*, *150*, 89, February 17, 1981.

Rothstein, S.S., Goldman, H.S., and Arcomano, A.S.: Hepatitis B Virus: An Overview for Dentists, *J. Am. Dent. Assoc.*, *102*, 173, February, 1981.

Sachs, H.L.: Dentistry and Hepatitis B: the Legal Risks, *J. Am. Dent. Assoc.*, *102*, 177, February, 1981.

Shields, W.B.: Dentistry and the Issue of Hepatitis B, *J. Am. Dent. Assoc.*, *102*, 180, February, 1981.

Sims, W.: The Problem of Cross-infection in Dental Surgery with Particular Reference to Serum Hepatitis, *J. Dent.*, 8, 20, March, 1980.

Tullman, M.J., Barrett, R.A., Boozer, C.H., Hamrick, J.T., and Rayson, J.H.: Prevalence of Hepatitis B Surface Antigen in a Dental School Patient Population, *J. Public Health Dent.*, *38*, 4, Winter, 1978.

Vogel, C.: Hepatitis: New Dangers for the Dental Team, *Quintessence J.*, *2*, 35, March, 1980.

Withers, J.A.: Hepatitis. A Review of the Disease and Its Significance to Dentistry, *J. Periodontol.*, *51*, 162, March, 1980.

4

Prevention of Disease Transmission: Clinical Applications

The success of a planned system for control of disease transmission depends on the cooperative effort of each member of the dental health team. The objective should be to provide the highest level of sterile procedures possible and practical in order to protect all patients and members of the dental health team from cross-infection.

When a patient is known to have a condition that involves communicable pathogenic microorganisms, special precautions can be taken before instruments and other nondisposable items are used for another patient. The presence of disease-producing organisms is not always known; therefore, there is a need for application of protective, preventive procedures prior to, during, and following *all* patient appointments.

Basic factors involved in the conduct of safe practice include the material in Chapter 3, and the following, which will be described in this chapter:

1. Application of information from the medical history of each patient.
2. Individual safety of dental health team members
   a. Immunizations
   b. Personal hygiene; clothing coverage for protection from splatter and aerosols
   c. Use of eyeglasses and mask

d. Hand hygiene; use of correct hand-washing procedures and gloves
3. Environmental control
   a. Housekeeping and maintenance of equipment
   b. Disinfection of environmental surfaces
4. Sterilization and effective handling of instruments and equipment
   a. Efficient sterilizing equipment, which is monitored regularly
   b. Use of disposable presterilized items
   c. Safe storage of sterilized items
5. Patient preparation and care
   a. Protection for clothing, hair, and eyes
   b. Oral hygiene and mouthrinse to lessen contamination in aerosols and field of operation in the oral cavity
   c. Surface disinfectant to prevent autogenous infection following anesthetic administration
6. Definitive postoperative decontamination
   a. Instrument cleaning
   b. Safe disposal of waste

MEDICAL HISTORY

Chapter 6 is devoted to content and types of patient histories. Items from the histories that call for immediate application are described on page 99. One of the items for immediate attention relates to the patient's status relative to infectious disease.

Before an oral examination or any clinical procedure is performed, screening for possible contagious disease is needed. Prevention of cross-contamination begins at the very start of the appointment, even prior to seating the patient.

I. Key Questions to Include in a History

Questions concerning a basic history of past disease and current disease that is under treatment are typically included in a medical history. For a patient who gives no history of certain communicable diseases, or is uncertain, additional leading questions are needed to determine possible exposure.

In the case of hepatitis B, for example, questions can be included that may reveal those individuals who have a high risk potential as listed on page 26. When infection is suspected, the antigen test for HBsAg and other serologic tests can be requested.

Examples of questions not found on some history forms that may aid in the detection of hepatitis carriers, potential carriers, or other diseases, such as tuberculosis, are listed here.[1]

1. Do you presently have a cough, chest or head cold, or sore throat?
2. Do you presently have any lip or mouth sores?
3. Have you had or do you have liver disease, hepatitis, chronic diarrhea, or jaundice?
4. Have you had close contact at home or socially with anyone with hepatitis, especially during the past 6 months?
5. When have you received blood products, a transfusion, kidney dialysis, or hemodialysis?
6. Have you ever had a positive test for hepatitis, or had your blood refused for donation to a blood bank?
7. Have you ever had to stay in a hospital or other institution for a long period of time?
8. Are you a health care professional exposed to hepatitis patients?
9. Have you traveled or lived in any other countries for 3 months or longer? Were you ill while there, and did you require

hospitalization and/or blood transfusions?
10. Have you recently had any unexpected weight loss and tiredness?
11. Have you recently had night sweats or a slight fever?

II. Limitations of a Medical History

For the safety of the patient and the dental health team, correct and current information about communicable diseases which a patient may be able to transmit is vital. Problems arise because a patient does not always have or give complete information about past disease and present status of communicability. Frequently, the word of the patient is all that is available, and consultation with the patient's physician is needed for confirmation and supplementation.

Studies have been conducted to determine the reliability of the medical history as a means of identifying patients likely to transmit hepatitis.[2,3,4] In the research, by comparing serologic test findings with data from medical histories provided by patients, it was found that comprehensive questioning for a dental and medical history is insufficient to identify all patients who carry HBsAg. Many patients did not know that they had had hepatitis at all, and others who knew they had had hepatitis had no knowledge of whether they had type A, type B, or Non A/non B.[2,3,4] As described on pages 25–26, individuals can become carriers of hepatitis B surface antigen (HBsAg) following a subclinical case that was not diagnosed as hepatitis.

Dental personnel are placed in a hazardous position. When a patient's history does not provide the necessary information, serologic testing is advisable, at least for individuals in one of the risk groups (page 26).

III. Use of the Medical History[5]

A. Screen All Patients

All patients should be screened for potential communicable disease before any clinical instrumentation for examination or treatment. Avoid exposure to an unknown infectious disease by wearing mask, glasses, and gloves. Other basic precautions are listed on page 63.

B. New Patient

1. Obtain a complete medical history; sup-

plement it with information from the patient's physician as indicated.

2. Request serologic or other laboratory tests; plan future appointment after information is returned.

C. Current Patient on Recall or Continuing Care

1. Update the patient history regularly.
2. Avoid exposure to current infectious disease by rescheduling after the communicability period. Common cold, influenza, and other respiratory diseases may be more serious than is initially realized.
3. Request periodic laboratory tests as changes in the disease history occur.

D. Emergency Patient

1. Complete the medical history.
2. Follow precautions with strict sterile procedures when the patient status is not known and when immediate pain-relieving treatment is required.

PERSONAL PROTECTION OF THE DENTAL TEAM

The continuing health and productivity of dental health personnel depend to a large degree on the control of cross-contamination. Loss of work time, personal suffering, long-term systemic effects, and even exclusion from continued practice are possible results from communicable diseases. The only safe procedure is to practice defensively at all times, with specific precautions for personal protection.

In this section, topics include immunizations and periodic tests, clothing, barriers to infectious microorganisms such as face mask, eyeglasses, and gloves, and personal hygiene, handwashing, and habits.

IMMUNIZATIONS AND PERIODIC TESTS

Dental personnel in a hospital setting are subject to the rules and regulations for all hospital employees. Policies usually require certain immunizations for new employees if written proof of vaccinations is not available and tests for antibodies prove to be negative.

In private dental practices, individual initiative is required to maintain standards of safety

for all dentists and auxiliaries. All staff members should be well aware of the signs and symptoms of diseases that are occupational hazards. All must be encouraged to seek early diagnosis and treatment of a seemingly minor condition that could be the initial symptom of a more serious communicable disease.

At the time of employment, it is reasonable for a dentist-employer to request of auxiliaries a record of current immunizations and their most recent updating, as well as specific tests, such as for tuberculosis (Mantoux test) and hepatitis B (serum HBsAg and anti-HBs). Immunization for rubella is particularly important for female employees of child-bearing age.

Following are listed the infectious diseases for which immunization is usually provided during infancy and childhood. Booster or reimmunization requirements are specific for each disease.

I. Immunizations

A. Basic Schedule

The immunization schedule for infants and children may include protection against poliomyelitis, diphtheria, tetanus, pertussis (whooping cough), measles, mumps, and rubella (German measles).[6,7]

B. Booster and Reimmunization

Each agent requires booster or reimmunization on a specific plan, which may range from 1 to 10 years, or reimmunization only upon intimate contact or exposure. The needs differ in different climates, countries, and locations. Persons moving or traveling need to become aware of specific precautions.

C. Other Immunizations

Annual influenza immunization can provide needed protection for health personnel. Pneumococcal vaccine is recommended for susceptible groups at certain intervals. Hepatitis vaccine is available for health professionals.

II. Management Program

A. Recommended Tests

1. Six months' tests for hepatitis B surface antigen (HBsAg) and antibody (anti-Hbs).

2. Annual tuberculin test (Mantoux); chest radiograph as indicated.
3. Periodic throat culture for possible hemolytic streptococcus carrier.
4. Serologic test for herpes simplex virus-I (HSV-1) antibodies to determine susceptibility to primary HSV.[8]

B. Obtaining Tests

Obtain tests promptly when exposed to certain infectious diseases and seek prophylactic immunization as indicated and available.

C. Written Records

Keep written records of immunizations, boosters, and reimmunizations; plan for regular follow-up. When the status of current immunizations is known, time is saved by not needing a susceptibility test prior to initiating passive immunizations when accidental exposure occurs.

CLINICAL ATTIRE

The wearing apparel of clinical operators and their assistants is vulnerable to contamination from splash, splatter, aerosols, and patient contact. The gown or uniform should be designed and cared for in a manner that will minimize cross-contamination.

I. Strict Aseptic Procedures

In a *strict aseptic* technique, with the highest level of asepsis (pages 29, 64), one-use gowns and other attire may come from sterile packages. Also in strict aseptic technique, the use of coverings for hair, beards, and shoes becomes part of customary routines.

Procedures for use when treating a patient with a suspected or known contagious disease, such as one who has active tuberculosis or one who is a hepatitis B carrier, are outlined on pages 64–65.

II. Sterile-Clean Procedure

When a *sterile-clean* technique is followed in routine practice, personal hygiene and cleanliness do not differ from that in the strict aseptic technique. Gowns or uniforms are not packaged sterile, but are expected to be clean, and maintained as free as possible from contamination. Certain characteristics and habits contribute to

the sterile-clean situation and are described below.

A. Design of Clinical Attire[9]

1. *Solid, Closed Front.* Gowns or jacket-style uniforms that may be left open in front do not provide adequate protection for clothes worn underneath. Dentists and male hygienists who wear short clinic coats, or any dental person who wears an open coat-style uniform over street clothes, should be aware of the exposure of the street clothes to infectious material.
2. *No Pockets.* Pockets are too readily available for placing contaminated objects such as writing implements or keys. Washed hands, prepared for clinical treatment, must be kept from touching objects or being placed in pockets.
3. *Short Sleeves.* Complete hand and wrist washing cannot be accomplished with long sleeves. Long sleeves become soiled and readily contaminated, and can serve to carry infectious material from patient to patient.

B. Protection of Uniform

A plastic washable or a disposable apron may be used when clinical services are performed that usually involve blood, splatter, or aerosols.

C. Outside Wear

Clinic uniforms and shoes should not be worn outside the clinic practice setting.[10] When clinic clothing is worn outside, it carries contamination from, and brings contamination into, the treatment area.

Another problem is that contamination is taken into the home when uniforms are worn to and from the work area. When laundered at home, the items from a dental office or clinic should be kept separate and treated with household bleach for disinfection.

USE OF FACE MASK

In the attempt to control airborne infections, it has been common practice to wear a mask when either the patient or the operator has been known to have an acute respiratory infection. Such a practice has its own value, but does not take into account the fact that many diseases are transmittable during the incubation period when no clinical signs are apparent.

Dispersion of particles of debris, polishing agents, calculus, and water, all of which are contaminated by the patient's oral flora, occurs regularly during all instrumentation. The greatest aerosols are created following the use of a handpiece, prophylaxis angle, or ultrasonic scaler. Evidence of the spread of particles appears on the splashed face, glasses, and uniform, and on the coverall placed over the patient for protection from the spray. Aerosol production was described on pages 16–17.

I. Mask Efficiency

A. Essential Characteristics

Undesirable characteristics that minimize the comfort with which a mask will be worn are the ability to create irritation to the nose, heat leading to perspiration, and pressure or a tight feeling about the ears and face, which may leave marks on the face. Unfortunately, discomfort is a common reason for neglect in wearing a mask that can make an important contribution to the total disease control plan.

The shape, material, and degree of absorption will influence the efficiency. A scientifically effective mask will
1. Prevent inward and outward passage of microorganisms.
2. Filter particles produced during dental and dental hygiene procedures.
3. Have minimal marginal leakage.

B. Materials

A variety of materials have been used for masks, including gauze and other cloth, plastic foam, fiberglass, synthetic fiber mat, and paper. In one research study, foam, paper, and cloth were found to be the least adequate filters of aerosols, whereas glass fiber and synthetic fiber mat were shown to be the most effective.[11,12]

II. Indications for Use[13]

Wearing a mask and protective glasses is recommended for all appointments (figure 4–1). Many office and clinic groups have a policy of wearing protective glasses during all appointments, but limit the required use of masks to the situations indicated below.

As more members of dental teams become aware of the effects of thoughtless exposure to potential disease, there will be increased use of all safety measures for self-protection and patient protection. A minimum use of a mask is suggested by the following indications:
A. Patient history shows potential or existing communicable disease; for examples, tuberculosis, hepatitis, or a sore throat. The procedures for a known hepatitis carrier are on page 64.
B. Current infection; for example, when either a dental team member or a patient have a respiratory infection.
C. Aerosol production. Whenever aerosols or splatter will be generated during the examination or treatment procedures, particularly from an ultrasonic scaler, handpiece, prophylaxis angle, and air/water spray.
D. During all surgical procedures, including subgingival scaling, root planing, and gingival curettage.
E. Protection of facial hair from splatter. Beards and other facial hair are not as readily washed as skin, and, if left unprotected, may collect a wide assortment of splatter, saliva, microorganisms, and other infectious material.[9]

III. Use of a Mask

A. Tie on the mask before a scrub or handwash.

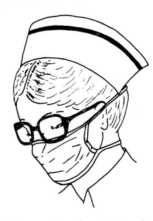

Figure 4–1. Face mask with protective glasses. The mask fits over nose and chin and is tied securely to prevent slipping. A mask should be changed for each patient appointment. Glasses are worn over the edge of the mask to help prevent fogging of the glass. When a dental team member does not require prescription lens, clear plastic eyeglasses are essential for protection from aerosols and general debris from the mouths of patients.

B. Use a fresh mask for each patient. When a mask becomes wet it should be changed, because a wet mask is no longer effective.
C. Keep the mask on after completing a procedure, while staying in the operatory in the presence of aerosols. Particles under 5 micrometers remain suspended longer (up to 24 hours) than larger particles and can be inhaled directly into terminal lung alveoli. Removal of a mask in the operatory immediately following the use of aerosol-producing procedures permits direct exposure to airborne organisms.

USE OF PROTECTIVE EYEGLASSES

Eye protection during dental and dental hygiene appointments for the dentist, auxiliaries, and patients is necessary to prevent physical injuries and infections of the eyes. A list of measures for eye accident prevention is included on page 832 in conjunction with emergency treatment.

Severe and disabling eye accidents and infections have been reported.[14,15,16] Eye involvement may lead to pain, discomfort, loss of work time, and, in certain instances, permanent injury. Accidents can occur at any time, and as with most accidents, they occur when least prepared for or expected.

Eye infections can follow the accidental dropping of an instrument on the face or the splashing of various materials from a patient's oral cavity into the eye. Contamination can be introduced from saliva, plaque, carious material and pieces of old restorative materials during cavity preparation, bacteria-laden calculus during scaling, and any other microorganisms contained in aerosols or splatter as described on page 17. An aerosol created by an ultrasonic scaler is heavily contaminated with oral microorganisms.

Careful, deliberate techniques and instrument management, with evacuation and other procedures for the control of oral fluids, contribute to the prevention of accidents and infections of the eyes. All measures described for prevention of airborne disease transmission by aerosols and splatter apply to eye protection (page 17). The most effective defense is the use of protective eyeglasses by all concerned, dental team and patients.

I. Indications for Use of Eyeglasses

A. Dental Team Members

Glasses should be worn at all times (figure 4-2). For dental personnel who do not require corrective lens for vision, protective glasses with clear lens should become a routine part of clinical dress.

If glasses are intended to be worn only when a handpiece, ultrasonic instrument, or other aerosol-producing instrument is used, they can easily be forgotten or misplaced. Even without power-driven instruments, pieces of calculus and splatter from air and water spray can reach the eyes.

B. Patients

Protective eye coverage is recommended for each patient at each appointment. Patients with their own prescription lens may

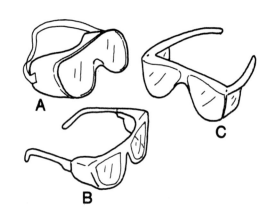

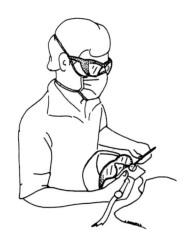

Figure 4-2. Protective eyeglasses for patient and operator. **A.** Goggles-style. **B.** and **C.** Glasses with side shields.

prefer to wear them, but for the safety of the patient's glasses, the use of the protective glasses provided in the office or clinic is advisable.

II. Protective Glasses

A. General Features of Acceptable Glasses

1. Wide coverage to protect around the eye.
2. Shatterproof; made of strong, sturdy plastic.
3. Light weight.
4. Flexible and with rounded smooth edges to prevent discomfort if pressed against the nose or ears.
5. Easily disinfected
   a. Surface areas should be smooth to prevent accumulation of infectious material.
   b. Frames and lens should not be damage or distorted by the disinfectant used.
6. Lens color. A clear or lightly tinted lens will permit the dental team members to watch the patient's reactions and maintain contact and response.
7. Protection against glare. Certain patients may request tinted lens or prefer to wear their own sunglasses when their eyes are especially sensitive to the dental light.

B. Types of Glasses

Many styles, including regular glasses shapes and those described below have been used. A list of sources is provided in the Technical Hints at the end of the Chapter.

1. *Goggles (figure 4–2A)*. Shielding on all sides of the glasses may give the best protection, provided they fit closely around the edges. Goggle-style coverage is especially necessary for protection during laboratory work.
2. *Glasses with Side Shields (figure 4–2B and C)*. A side shield can provide added protection. For the member of the dental team, it may be possible to wear this type over regular prescription glasses.
3. *Spectacles with Curved Frames*. When the sides of the glasses are curved back at the sides, they may provide a protec-

tion somewhat similar to those with the side shield.
4. *Postmydriatic Spectacles Used by Ophthalmologist*. Disposable glasses are available that are made of flexible plastic. They may be especially useful for patients with a known communicable disease or carrier state.
5. *Child-Size*. Child-sized sunglasses and children's play spectacles have been used.

C. Availability

Several pairs of goggles or glasses are maintained to facilitate cleaning and disinfecting after each use.

III. Suggestions for Clinical Application

A. Patient Instruction

A patient who has not been asked to wear protective glasses before needs a simple explanation of the reasons for the glasses.

B. Contact Lens

1. Dental team members who wear contact lens should always wear protective glasses over them.
2. Patients with contact lens should be asked to remove them, and then use the protective glasses that are provided.

C. Care of Protective Glasses

1. Disinfect by rubbing vigorously with, or soaking in, an acceptable disinfectant solution; place on a clean towel during the drying stage.
2. Check periodically for scratches, and replace appropriately. When polishing agents or other abrasives have splattered the lens, clean thoroughly under running water first before rubbing, as rubbing the abrasive agent over the plastic glass will create scratches.

HAND CARE

Hands, through direct contact with a patient's saliva, become contaminated, and therefore are sources for cross-infection. Cross-infection can be prevented by making a conscious effort to keep the hands from touching objects other than the instruments and disinfected parts of equipment prepared for the immediate patient.

Emphasis has always been placed on the need for thorough washing or scrubbing prior to starting; now increased emphasis must also be placed on immediate postappointment washing and after any interruptions during an appointment. Through contact with the patient's record, the dental chair, operating stool, telephone, or a multitude of other items, many opportunities occur for the spread of microorganisms.

I. Bacteriology of the Skin[17,18]

A. Resident Bacteria

Large numbers of relatively stable bacteria inhabit the surface epithelium or deeper areas in the ducts of skin glands or depths of hair follicles; they are ultimately shed with the exfoliated surface cells, or with excretions of the skin glands. They may be altered by newly introduced pathogens, or reduced by washing and disinfection procedures.

B. Transient Bacteria

These reflect the continuous contamination by routine contacts: some are pathogens and may act temporarily as residents, may be washed away, or in the event that a skin break exists, may cause an autogenous infection. Most transients can be readily removed with soap and water.

C. Handwashing

1. *Rationale.* Effective and frequent handwashing can reduce the overall bacterial flora of the skin and prevent the organisms acquired from a patient from becoming skin residents. It is impossible to sterilize the skin, but every attempt must be made to reduce the bacterial flora to a minimum.
2. *Purposes.* The objective of all scrub procedures is to reduce the bacterial flora of the hands to an absolute minimum. An effective scrub procedure can be expected to accomplish the following:
   a. Removal of surface dirt and bacteria.
   b. Dissolution of the normal greasy film on the skin.
   c. Destruction of surface bacteria when an antiseptic accompanies or follows the scrub.
   d. Rinse and remove all loosened debris and microorganisms.

II. Principles for Handwashing

A. Hand Care

1. Maintain clean, smoothly trimmed, short fingernails with well-cared-for cuticles to prevent breaks where microorganisms can enter.
2. Remove hand and wrist jewelry at the beginning of the day. Microorganisms can become lodged in crevices of rings, watchbands, and watches, where scrubbing is impossible.
3. After hand washing, keep hands away from face, hair, clothing (pockets), dental chair, operating stool (manipulate by foot motions), telephone, patient records, and other objects that cannot be sterilized or disinfected.
4. Never expose open skin lesions or abrasions to a patient's oral tissues and fluids. The use of gloves is described on pages 57–58.

B. Facilities

1. *Sink*
   a. Use a sink with a foot pedal for water flow control to avoid contamination from faucet handles.
   b. Adaptation for regular sink: turn on water at the beginning and leave on throughout the entire procedure. Turn faucets off with the towel after drying hands.
   c. Use a sink of sufficient size so that contact with the inside of the wash basin can be avoided easily. A sink cannot be sterilized and is highly contaminated.
   d. Prevent contamination of uniform by not leaning against the sink.
   e. Use a separate area and sink reserved for instrument washing. Contaminated instruments should be removed from the operatory prior to preparation for the next patient.
2. *Soap*

a. Use a liquid detergent surgical scrub. A povidone-iodine (iodophore) preparation is recommended.[19]

b. Apply from a foot- or knee-activated dispenser to avoid contamination to and from a hand-operated dispenser or cake soap.

c. Do not substitute the use of foam hand preparations, alcohol wipes, or other substitutes for handwashing, since many pathogenic microorganisms cannot be destroyed by disinfecting preparations. Rinsing is a very important part of the handwashing procedure.[9]

3. *Scrub Brushes*

a. Clean brushes with a detergent, and sterilize after each use.

b. Avoid over-vigorous use of a brush to minimize skin abrasion. Skin irritation and abrasion can leave openings for additional cross-contamination.

c. Disposable sponges and sponges containing iodophore detergent are available commercially and may be preferred when a scrub brush is traumatic to the skin.

d. Identify brushes by label or color-code for handwashing to prevent mixing with instrument scrub brushes; however, both types will be sterilized. Handwashing and instrument cleaning should be accomplished at separate sinks.

4. *Towels*

a. Obtain towel from a dispenser that requires no contact except with the towel itself which hangs down from the container (figure 4–3).

b. When a cloth towel is used, it must be used for only one patient.

III. Methods of Handwashing

The three methods that will be described here are called the *short scrub, handwashing,* and the *surgical scrub.* Handwashing techniques are usually defined by numbers of latherings and rinsings, whereas scrub techniques are completed in time periods or by specific numbers of scrub brush strokes.[20]

The two commonly used systems for scrub

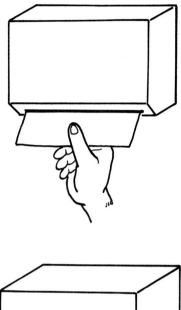

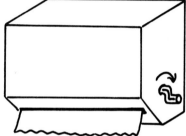

Figure 4–3. Towel dispenser. **Above,** correct type dispenser which requires no contact except with the towel itself which hangs down from the container. **Below,** incorrect type which requires contact with handle to advance towel.

techniques are the "stroke-count" method and the "time" method. In the *stroke-count* method, a specific number of brush strokes is applied to each surface, and each finger and part of the hand is considered to have four surfaces. In the *time* method each surface is scrubbed for a certain number of seconds.

When learning to perform a scrub, it is helpful to combine the stroke-count and the time methods, to assure complete coverage and to develop a sequence of performance that can be completed in a minimum of time.

A. Short Scrub

The short scrub is recommended for the beginning of the day just prior to the first patient appointment, and just prior to the first appointment of the second half of the day. It is also used following an appointment for a patient with a known communicable disease, and following any major interruption that may have caused unusual contamination of the hands and forearms.

When the time method is used, a short scrub may vary from a minimum of 3 minutes to 5 minutes. Approximately one half of the time is used for scrubbing each hand. For a 3-minute scrub, the time may be divided as follows:[20]

Nails and fingertips
    1/2 minute (15 seconds each hand)
Fingers and hands
    1 1/2 minutes (45 seconds each hand)
Wrists and forearms
    1 minute (30 seconds each hand)

The procedure outlined below may be expected to take 3 minutes when five stroke-counts are applied to each surface.

1. Don eyeglasses and mask, and fix hair securely back. Remove watch and all jewelry.
2. Wash hands and arms briefly, using surgical scrub soap. Leave water running at a moderate speed that will not allow splashing from base and sides of sink.
3. Clean under finger nails with orangewood stick from sterile package. Orangewood stick and scrub brush may be packaged together for sterilization.
4. Rinse from finger tips to hands, wrists to elbows. Keep hands higher than elbows throughout the entire procedure.
5. Lather hands and arms again. Leave the soap lather on the hands and arms during the scrub to increase exposure time to the antimicrobial ingredient of the scrub soap.
6. Remove scrub brush from the previously opened sterile package, apply several measures of soap. Note the time, and start scrubbing in an orderly sequence without returning to areas already scrubbed.
7. First hand
   a. Brush back and forth across nails and finger tips five times.
   b. Begin with the thumb, use small circular strokes (five strokes each area) on each side of thumb and each finger, then palm, and back of hand. Extend fingers to gain access to each crevice and line.
   c. Scrub wrist on all sides and move to forearm.
   d. When completed, rinse well, from finger tips on up the arm; let water run off at the elbow.
8. Rinse the brush and transfer to other hand; repeat entire procedure.
9. Rinse brush and drop it into the sink.
10. Rinse the hand and arm generously and thoroughly to wash away all transient microorganisms.
11. Dry hands
    a. Take care not to recontaminate hands while drying them.
    b. Use a separate paper towel for each hand.
    c. Cloth towel: use one end of a large towel for one hand and the other end for the other hand, taking care not to drag the towel over unwashed parts or clothing. Two small towels may be used, one for each hand.
12. Maintain cleanliness by touching only sterile or disinfected instruments and surfaces.

B. Handwashing

Handwashing is used after the first appointment of the day and before and after each succeeding appointment. It is also used before and after handling records, radiographs, telephone, and other items. It is the general procedure for all times except those indicated under the short scrub technique.

Handwashing is considered the most important single procedure for the prevention of cross-contamination and is a basic requirement before and after hospital patient care.[18]

1. Don eyeglasses and mask and fix hair securely back. Remove watch and all jewelry.
2. Use comfortably warm water and surgical scrub soap (iodophore preparation).
3. Lather hands, wrists, and forearms quickly, rubbing all surfaces vigorously. Interlace fingers and rub back and forth with pressure.
4. Rinse thoroughly, running the water from fingertips down the hands. Keep water running.

5. Repeat three times. One lathering for 3 minutes is less effective than three short latherings and rinsing three times in 30 seconds.[9] The lathering serves to loosen the debris and microorganisms and the rinsings wash them away.
6. Use paper towels for drying, taking care not to recontaminate.

C. Surgical Hand Scrub

Each hospital or oral surgery clinic will have rules and regulations for scrub procedures. These should be posted over the scrub sinks.

A surgical scrub performed as the initial scrub of a day would be 10 minutes and subsequent scrubs may be 3 to 5 minutes. Following a contagious or isolated patient, the scrub would be at least 5 minutes.[20]

The outline for a long scrub presented below is similar to the short scrub described previously. The major differences are in the number of strokes when the stroke-count method is used, and the longer time spent.

1. Don eyeglasses, mask, hair and beard coverings. Make sure hair is completely covered. Watch and jewelry are removed.
2. Wash hands and arms over the elbows using surgical soap to remove gross surface dirt before using the scrub brush. Lather vigorously with strong rubbing motions, 10 on each side of hands, wrists, arms. Interlace the fingers and thumbs to clean the proximal surfaces.
3. Rinse thoroughly from finger tips across hands and wrists. Hold hands higher than elbows throughout the procedure. Leave water running.
4. Use orangewood stick or file from the sterile package to clean nails. Rinse.
5. Lather the hands and arms and leave the lather on during the scrub to increase the exposure time to the antimicrobial ingredient.
6. Remove sterile scrub brush from previously opened sterile package, apply surgical soap, and begin the brush procedure. Note the time and scrub in an orderly sequence without returning to areas previously scrubbed.
7. First hand

a. Brush back and forth across nails and finger tips, passing the brush under the nails (30 seconds).
b. Fingers and hand. Use small circular strokes on all sides of the thumb and each finger, overlapping strokes for complete coverage ($2^{1}/_{2}$ minutes).
c. Continue to wrist. Rinse brush and arms at each level. Apply more soap to maintain a good lather (2 minutes for wrist and forearm).
d. When arm is completed over the elbow, rinse thoroughly, starting at the finger tips and letting water pass down over the arm.
8. Rinse the brush thoroughly. Some systems require the use of a second sterile brush for the second hand. When this is so, discard the first brush into the proper container, and obtain second brush.
9. Repeat entire procedure for the second hand and arm.
10. Rinse the hand and arm thoroughly; wash and discard brush.
11. Rinse both arms for a final rinse; turn off the water.
12. Hold hands up and clasped together. Proceed to dressing area for gowning and gloving.

IV. Gloves

The wearing of gloves is part of the total plan for control of cross-contamination. Skin lesions should never be left exposed to contamination.

Although indications for wearing gloves are outlined below, certain factors dictate the need for protection at all times. The need for hand protection becomes evident when the unknown potentials for acquiring infection are realized. Examples are the patient who has been exposed to a communicable disease and may be in the incubation period without clinical disease symptoms, but who is infectious; and the hepatitis carrier who did not have a recognized case of hepatitis B and has never been tested for hepatitis B surface antigen.

A. Indications for Wearing Surgical Gloves[13]

When gloves are not worn as part of the regular daily uniform, they are indicated for use at least during the following situations:

1. While making an initial extraoral/intraoral examination, or for reexamination after a period of time.
2. When a facial lesion is apparent such as a herpes lesion (cold sore) of the lip. Never touch herpes lesions or other open lesions with bare fingers. In most cases, the appointment would best be postponed.
3. When breaks or cuts in the hands of the dental person provide portals of entry for microorganisms from a patient's oral flora, particularly transient pathogenic or potentially pathogenic microorganisms.
4. During all procedures that bring the operator's and assistant's hands into contact with a patient's blood, saliva, plaque, and other contaminated material. Examples are during oral surgery and periodontal therapy, including subgingival scaling, root planing, and gingival curettage.
5. When a patient presents with signs and symptoms of a communicable disease. Gloves and a mask are worn by the dental team in attendance.
6. When the dentist or dental auxiliary is positive for hepatitis B surface antigen (HBsAg).
7. When the patient is suspected of being, or has been shown to be, positive for HBsAg. Complete procedures are outlined on page 64.

B. **Types of Gloves**
   1. Disposable latex or plastic.
   2. Sterilizable rubber gloves. Rubber gloves are packaged before sterilizing and kept sealed until ready to use. After a surgical hand scrub, the gown and glove procedure follows.[20] Sterile gloves may also be used at other times without complete hospital routine.

C. **Suggestions for Use of Gloves**
   1. *Cover for Hand Abrasions.* Whole gloves are preferred over finger cots. Unless a finger cot is very tight, there will be leakage of fluids while washing, and saliva and blood from a patient's mouth.
   2. *Need for Hand Scrub Before Donning Gloves.* Because gloves are susceptible

to tears and pin holes from instrument sticks, infection can be introduced inadvertently. In addition, bacteria may multiply profusely under gloves where a warm damp medium is provided. Long fingernails under gloves are a potential cause of breaks in the gloves.[20]

3. *Repeated Washing.* Gloves can be washed cleaner with fewer latherings than bare hands because gloves have no crevices and grooves for microbial accumulation.[19] When gloves are worn for consecutive appointments, lather and rinse two or three times thoroughly after and before each appointment. If this procedure is used, gloves must be checked for pinpoint holes. Using disposable gloves and changing between patients is preferred.
4. *Hand Wash Before Glove Removal.* Before removing gloves, lather and rinse thoroughly to
   a. reduce possible contamination to hands during removal and disposal.
   b. reduce contamination in the waste, particularly following a patient known to have a communicable disease.
   c. clean reusable gloves prior to resterilizing.

ENVIRONMENTAL SURFACES

The cleanliness and neatness of the treatment room reflect the character and conscientiousness of the dental personnel. The patient, with limited knowledge of dental science, may judge the ability of the dental personnel by the appearance of the office or clinic.

The patient's attitude is important, but more important is the relationship of cleanliness to the presence of microorganisms and the need for performing techniques in a situation that minimizes cross-contamination.

The orderliness and immaculate cleanliness of the operatory result from continuing care. An excellent test for the effects of care and any minor oversights is for the dentist or dental auxiliary to sit in the dental chair occasionally and look around at what the patient sees from that vantage point.

I. Objectives

Effective care of instruments and equipment contributes to the following:

A. Control of disease transmission by way of environmental surfaces.
B. An increase in the operating efficiency of the office personnel.
C. An atmosphere of cleanliness and orderliness that will contribute to the patient's well-being.
D. An increase in the patient's confidence in the ability of the dental personnel.
E. The maintenance of the working efficiency of office equipment and instruments
   1. To prolong their span of usefulness.
   2. To contribute to patient safety (see Pacemaker, pages 789–790).
F. A decrease in the occurrence of unpleasant odors in the office.

II. Preparation for an Appointment

The preparation of environmental surfaces for an appointment is, in reality, the disinfection after the previous appointment. Indeed, at the end of the final appointment of a day, the steps for disinfection should be carried out so that splatter and microorganisms are not left to dry on the contaminated surfaces overnight.

During appointments, the dental furniture, equipment, and the room fixtures may become contaminated by the contact of the hands of members of the dental team carrying saliva, blood, plaque, organisms, and other potentially infectious material from the patient's oral cavity (figure 3–1, page 16). In addition, aerosols and splatter created during the treatment procedures are spread throughout the area.

Pathogenic as well as other organisms can survive on environmental surfaces. Transfer of microorganisms is, therefore, possible from one patient to a subsequent patient by contact with a chair arm, headrest, or other surface. A patient may use a telephone that was previously contaminated by the hands of the dentist or auxiliary. Hepatitis B viruses can remain active for transmission for weeks and months on environmental surfaces.

III. Planning for Decontamination

To decontaminate the treatment room when time between appointments is limited requires an efficient procedural system and an effective disinfecting agent. When a dentist uses several operatories, preparation time can be a designated part of the rotating system. Dental hygienists frequently are confined to one room, so that a continuing orderly arrangement for decontamination is necessary.

Planning for a system of disinfection can be accomplished by first making a list of all the surfaces contacted during a usual appointment.[9,21] Each contact can then be placed in one of the categories listed below. The list can be studied for possible changes to increase efficiency, save time, and decrease cross-contamination.

A. Unnecessary Hand Contacts

Only contacts essential to the service to be performed should be made. Planning ahead to have materials ready so that cabinet knobs or drawer handles do not have to be contacted is an example.

B. Sterilizable Items

Removable tips for air and water that can be cleaned and sterilized by one of the available methods (pages 33–37) are examples. Changing the tips is faster than scrubbing with a disinfectant. Handpieces and prophylaxis angles that can be sterilized are important additions to the list. Several handpieces are needed for rotation. Much time is saved, and a safer instrument is used.

C. Disposable Items

An object used that is not currently disposable may be replaced by one that is. Time and effort are saved.

D. Items That May Be Covered

Coverings, particularly plastic-backed patient napkins, aluminum foil, and clear plastic wrap or bags can prevent contamination from reaching surfaces. Covers for light handles, counter tops, x-ray cone (using see-through plastic), and water faucet (using aluminum foil) are examples. Care must be taken when removing the covers not to contaminate the object beneath.

E. Items That Require Chemical Disinfection

Objects and surfaces that cannot be included in one of the above categories must be treated with a chemical disinfectant. If the material is not compatible with the chemical action of the disinfectant, a substitute item which is either disposable or coverable will be needed.

IV. Disinfection of Environmental Surfaces

A. Agent

1. *Preparation.* The approved effective agents were described on pages 39–40. The preparation of choice for surface disinfection is iodine surgical scrub with isopropyl alcohol in a concentration of 1:20 (page 40). A stronger solution of 1:1 would be indicated after a patient with a known communicable disease or carrier state.[21]
2. *Action.* The effectiveness of the disinfection procedure is the result of two actions, which are the physical rubbing and removal of contaminated material and the chemical inactivation of the living microorganisms.
3. *Care of Solution.* Do not store gauze sponges in the solution. A reaction can deactivate the agent.

B. Procedure[9,13,21]

1. Wash hands before starting the disinfecting process. At the beginning of the day, handwashing will lessen the microorganisms brought into the clinical area. Between patients, handwashing will help control cross-contamination.
2. Use several large gauze sponges. Small sponges are time wasting. A disinfectant-soaked sponge in each hand can decrease time while doing certain objects, and contaminated objects such as tubings can be held with one sponge while scrubbing with the other sponge.

   Spraying a disinfectant must be followed by vigorous scrubbing. When applied only by spray without scrubbing, the agent does not penetrate or remove the film of microorganisms.
3. Scrub the disinfectant over the entire surface with attention to irregularities where contaminated material can aggregate. Leave the surfaces wet. The alcohol evaporates and a film of the iodine detergent remains, which should be left in place whenever possible.
4. Use an alcohol sponge to remove the iodine film when it is unattractive or unacceptable, but a minimum of 3 minutes contact of the solution should be allowed. For heavily contaminated surfaces, allow 30 minutes contact.
5. Surfaces to be covered should be wiped after the disinfectant before positioning the cover. Examples are the headrest (disposable cover to be placed) and the tray where the instruments will be placed.

C. Surfaces to Disinfect[19,22]

The list of surfaces will vary from one clinic or office to another because of different equipment and availability of sterilizable and disposable items. The list must include all surfaces that are contacted if they are not sterilized, covered, or disposable. A typical list of surfaces would include the following:

1. All hose ends (e.g., saliva ejector, evacuator, handpiece, ultrasonic).
2. Non-sterilizable air/water syringe (removable tip is sterilized).
3. Forked holder for hanging suction device, handpiece, or air/water syringe.
4. Bracket tray, Mayo stand, or other instrument tray holder (will be covered).
5. Control knobs and switches (including dental chair, light, ultrasonic unit).
6. Cuspidor. A cuspidor will require special handling. Use paper towels to first wash with soap and water, and rinse off the soap. Disinfect first the outside, then the inside. Discard sponges and towels used, and wash hands before going on to other items.[19]
7. Headrest (after disinfection, place the headrest disposable cover).
8. Dental chair arms. When of a color that may become stained by an iodine preparation, alcohol may be used, followed by placing a plastic or paper cover.
9. Sink
   a. Manually operated faucets. Scrub with disinfectant and then cover handles with aluminum foil.
   b. Manually operated soap dispenser. Scrub with disinfectant and then

cover release knob with plastic or aluminum foil.

  c. Rim of sink. The outer rim where clothes may contact should be scrubbed with disinfectant.

10. X-ray. All contact areas should be scrubbed, including control knobs, machine head and cone, and film dispenser. Plastic covers may be placed over the head and cone. Nondisposable film holder must be sterilized.

11. Inhalant anesthetic masks and tubing. These must be sterilized by autoclave, ethylene oxide, or at least thoroughly washed, rinsed, and dried before soaking at least 30 minutes in 0.1% iodine or chlorine (diluted iodophore or hypochlorite).

12. Miscellaneous items. Other materials and equipment that will be contacted should be included on the list of items to be treated during disinfection of environmental surfaces. The stethoscope endpiece is an example.

CARE OF STERILE INSTRUMENTS

After the effort has been made to sterilize and disinfect, procedures are then conducted to prevent contamination and to control the transfer of pathogenic microorganisms. Although a strict procedure for sterile technique such as is practiced in a hospital operating room would be difficult or even impossible in a dental office, it is possible to preserve the chain of sterility through effective handling and storage procedures.

I. Tray Preparation[23]

The instrument tray is reserved for sterile instruments. Other equipment that has been disinfected needs its own special area. Educational devices and materials that are neither sterile nor disinfected are kept apart.

The tray is disinfected (if not a sterilizable tray) and covered over the rims. Currently available plastic-back towels, which are also used for a patient's clip-on bib-napkin, are useful for the tray cover. The plastic back aids to keep liquid contaminants from leaking through and contaminating the tray underneath. A paper tray liner is placed on the open towel to receive the sterilized instruments.

II. Handling Instruments and Materials

A. Opening a Sterile Package

1. Do not open a sterile package until ready to use.
2. Touch only the outer surfaces of the wrapper.
3. Cloth wrapper can be laid back to become the sterile instrument tray cover, with contents exposed on the top.
4. Paper container is opened by tearing off an end and sliding the sterile instruments on to the prepared tray cover.

B. Transfer Forceps

When a transfer forceps is to be used, it must be sterilized for each patient. A transfer forceps container must also be sterilized after each use.

C. Transfer of Sterile Items from a Closed Container

1. Hold cover of container in nondominant hand in a downward direction while using a sterile forceps to remove the item from the inside (figure 4–4). Return cover promptly.
2. When it is necessary to place the cover down, turn it up with the sterile inside surface away from the tabletop to prevent contamination to the inner surface.

III. Storage

Instruments stored without sealed wrappers are only momentarily sterile because of airborne contamination.[22]

A. Prepared Trays

Trays may have fitted covers which are sterilized with them and slid into position as the tray is removed from the sterilizer. Trays without fitted covers, which are covered with a sterile towel immediately, are sterile for only a short period of time. When that system is used, the tray should be sterilized on the same day as the appointment in which it will be utilized. Until used, trays should be stored in a closed cabinet to exclude dust, aerosols, or other contaminants.

B. Individual Instrument Packages

Individual instrument packages are la-

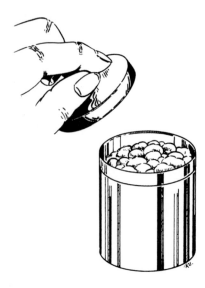

Figure 4–4. Removing the cover from a container of sterile supplies. When the cover is held while contents are removed with a sterile forceps, the cover should be held with inner surface downward as shown. When the cover must be placed on the table, the cover is turned over and the outer surface is placed downward to prevent contamination to the inner surface.

beled prior to sterilization and kept in a closed cabinet or other container unless used immediately. Paper wrappers must be handled carefully to prevent puncture.

C. Dating

All stored packages should be dated and used in rotation.

D. Factors Affecting Contamination of Sterile Wrapped Supplies

1. Porosity of the wrapping material.
2. Method of wrapping and sealing.
3. Changes in the atmospheric conditions surrounding the package.

PATIENT PREPARATION

The use of preoperative rinsing and toothbrushing has been shown to lower the numbers of oral bacteria, and hence to lower the numbers of infected aerosols created during instrumentation.

Oral procedures that require penetration of tissues, such as giving anesthesia by injection or scaling and curetting subgingival pocket surfaces, can introduce bacteria into the tissues and hence into the blood stream. Enough organisms

injected into the tissue could multiply and create an abscess. Because of natural resistance, the body can handle and destroy invading microorganisms, provided the numbers can be kept to a minimum. Autogenous infection was described on page 18.

Practical procedures for the preparation of a patient include preoperative oral hygiene measures and the application of a surface disinfectant. These contribute to the prevention of disease transmission.

I. Preoperative Oral Hygiene Measures

A. Toothbrushing

Toothbrushing disturbs and removes microorganisms. When a patient is being trained in plaque control measures and needs supervision at each appointment, a double purpose can be accomplished. Demonstration of plaque removal from the teeth, tongue, and gingiva contributes to surface degerming prior to treatment procedures.

B. Rinsing

The numbers of bacteria on the gingival or mucosal surfaces can be reduced by the use of an antiseptic mouthrinse. In studies using povidone-iodine mouthrinse, the bacterial counts on mucosal surfaces were reduced before and during scaling and gingivectomy.[24,25] Aerosol contamination was also reduced.[26,27] Reduction of surface and total bacteria in the oral cavity during oral procedures can contribute to surgical cleanliness and more favorable healing after treatment.

II. Application of a Surface Disinfectant[19]

A. Prior to Injection of Anesthetic

As a needle is introduced into the mucosa for penetration to deeper tissues, microorganisms on the surface can be carried into the tissue (page 19). During positioning of the instrument for injection, the needle might accidentally contact a tooth surface and pick up some plaque which could be carried to and into the injection site. Reduction of surface microorganisms by rinsing with a germicidal mouthrinse can reduce the hazards related to the injection of bacteria with a needle.

B. Prior to Scaling and Other Dental Hygiene Instrumentation

1. Instrumentation in the sulcus or pocket and around the gingival margin can create breaks in the tissue where bacteria can enter. Subgingival instrumentation in a pocket with broken down sulcular epithelium can contribute to the entrance of bacteria into the underlying tissues. Local infection or bacteremia can be created.
2. Procedure. Dry the surface and swab the area prior to instrumentation. Use the antiseptic solution to irrigate the sulci and pockets carefully to prevent forcing the solution into the tissues. Research has shown povidone-iodine to be an effective prophylactic germicide for this purpose.[24]

SUMMARY OF PROCEDURES FOR THE PREVENTION OF DISEASE TRANSMISSION

Basic procedures for clinical management are listed here. For many items, a detailed description has been provided in either Chapter 3 or 4.

I. Patient Factors

A. Prepare a comprehensive patient history. Refer suspected patients for laboratory tests available for symptomless carriers. When a patient has a history of jaundice, treat the patient as a hepatitis carrier.
B. Request diagnostic tests for patients who may be carriers of hepatitis B, syphilis, or tuberculosis.
C. Avoid elective procedures for a patient suffering from a communicable disease such as a respiratory infection. When emergency care must be provided, precautions and strict adherence to environmental, personal, and sterilization factors are needed.
D. Have the patient rinse with germicidal mouthrinse to reduce the numbers of oral microorganisms.
E. Provide protective eyeglasses.

II. Clinic Preparation

A. Run water through all water lines including the air/water syringe, handpieces, and ultrasonic unit for 5 to 6 minutes at the start of the day and at least 30 seconds before and after each use during the day (pages 42–43).
B. Cover or disinfect all environmental surfaces that may be touched during the appointment (pages 59–60). Make an orderly sequence for surface disinfection.
C. Sterilize instruments and all other equipment that can be sterilized by one of the four methods for complete sterilization (pages 33–37). Use specific sterilization procedures for all patients, not only those suspected or known to have an existing communicable disease or to be in a carrier state.

III. Factors for the Dental Team

A. Have medical examinations; keep immunizations up to date; have tests for hepatitis B antigen and antibody, syphilis, tuberculosis, and any other appropriate testing on a periodic basis.
B. Always use mask, protective eyeglasses, gloves, and a clean, closed-front uniform.
C. Wash hands using a short scrub at the start of the day and handwashes with three latherings and thorough rinsings before and after appointments and all interruptions.
D. Develop habits that minimize contacts with switches and other parts of the dental unit, dental chair, light, and operating stool, and avoid all possible environmental contacts unrelated to the procedure at hand.

IV. Treatment Factors

A. Hypodermic Needles

1. Use disposable injection needles and other disposables when treatment involves penetration of tissue.
2. Keep needles capped on the instrument tray at all times to avoid accidental penetration or self-inoculation.
3. Destroy needles when disposing of them to prevent unauthorized access and infection of custodial workers.
4. Dispose of all partially emptied carpules of anesthetics.

B. Manual Instruments

Use manual instruments to minimize use

of instruments and procedures that create aerosols (handpiece, prophylaxis angle, ultrasonic scaler, air/water spray) to control the spread of microorganisms over the room, people, equipment, and other objects. Use rubber dam for applicable procedures.

C. Removable Oral Appliances

Routinely, gloves should be worn to receive a septic appliance from a patient. Rinse the appliance under running water, brush, and disinfect in an effective germicide for 30 minutes (pages 38–40). Use a fresh solution of 1:4 iodine scrub and water or a fresh solution of 5% sodium hypochlorite diluted 1:4 parts water.[19]

When a lathe is used for cleaning the denture, wear a mask and use a sterile ragwheel and fresh pumice. Pumice is used only once and caught on a disposable paper liner in the dustbin.

V. Post-Treatment

A. Fold tray cover over instruments to transport them to the sterilization area. Use heavy household gloves to handle used instruments.
B. Follow routines on pages 29–32 to disinfect, clean in ultrasonic cleaner, and prepare for sterilization.
C. Contaminated waste is secured in plastic disposal bags.
D. Disinfect safety glasses for patient and dental team members.

MAXIMUM PRECAUTIONS AND PROCEDURES FOR HEPATITIS B CARRIER[1,10,21]

When maximum precautions are necessary because a patient has a communicable disease, particularly for a patient who has been shown to be HBsAg positive, and when the office or clinic is not prepared to manage this level of precaution, it is advisable to refer the patient to a facility that is equipped to handle the problem.[1,28,29,30] Many of the required procedures for maximum prevention that are listed below are similar to the procedures of the daily routine but are applied with increased intensity.

Members of the dental team who have immunity to hepatitis B (or the communicable disease of the particular patient) should be trained to take over the appointments for the special carrier patients. Without the threat of personal exposure, attention can be concentrated on control of transmission to other members of the team and to subsequent patients.

Whether or not any team member has immunity, rehearsals of the proper procedures are needed. A list of the items to receive covers, those to be avoided, and others to maintain in sterile packages, can be placed in the procedures manual along with other office or clinic policies. Drawings, flow charts, and other descriptive material can be prepared as specific guides. As new research findings and new materials become available, the procedures manual can be revised.

I. Clinical Features Essential to Maximum Precautions

A. Enclosed, confined treatment area.
B. Adequate sterilization equipment and approved disinfectant solution.
C. Unit with smooth plastic hoses.
D. Handpiece waterlines with check valves installed (pages 42–43).
E. Handpieces and air/water syringe that can be steam autoclaved or sterilized in gas (ethylene oxide).
F. All possible disposable items available.

II. Preparation of Treatment Area

A. Schedule the patient for the last appointment of the day to allow time for room decontamination and preparation for the next appointment in that room.
B. Use a self-contained room that can be closed off so that confinement is possible. Materials and all necessities should be readied and in the treatment room to prevent the need for any traffic. Only those attending the patient should be allowed in the room.
C. Disinfect and drape all environmental surfaces
   1. Cover the entire dental chair. A drape of disposable plastic such as is used by painters for drop cloths is suggested.
   2. Bracket, light handles, and other smaller items may be covered with clear plastic wrap or bags.
   3. Hand controls can be covered with clear plastic taped on; they can be operated through the plastic. Hand controls of

unit, light, dental chair, x-ray machine, viewbox, all are included.

4. Cover x-ray machine, head, cone.

D. Use disposable materials wherever possible.

E. Sterilized instruments, handpieces, air/water syringe, and all tips are readied. Extra packages of sterile scalers and curets are available to open when instruments are dulled, to prevent need for sharpening equipment.

F. Place available radiographs on viewbox and cover radiographs and viewbox with transparent plastic.

III. Preparation of the Dental Team

Even the dental hygienist who routinely does not have the help of a dental assistant should not attempt treatment for a maximum precautions patient alone. Appointment management can be greatly improved when two people work together, and strict asepsis can be maintained with increased efficiency.

A. Wear a cloth gown that can be sterilized or a disposable paper gown. Operating-room-style overshoes and hair cover can also be obtained.

B. Wear protective glasses with side shields (figure 4–2 B or C). For those who require prescription eyeglasses, protective glasses should be placed over them.

C. Wear two pairs of surgical gloves, donned after a scrub procedure. Care must be taken during instrumentation to avoid procedures that can injure the hands or cut the gloves.

D. Wear double tie-on masks. Facial hair must be covered.

IV. Patient Preparation

A. Cover the patient's hair with a disposable cap.

B. Use a long disposable drape to cover the patient's clothes.

C. Provide protective disposable eyeglasses.

D. Have the patient rinse for 30 to 60 seconds with a germicidal mouthrinse.

V. Treatment Factors

A. In all procedures, touch only areas draped or otherwise covered.

B. Use a disposable radiographic film holder (pages 144, 146).

C. Submerge exposed x-ray plastic film packets in iodine surgical scrub with isopropyl alcohol 1:1 for 30 minutes. Rinse and dry before processing.[1,21]

D. Use disposable trays for making impressions. Place impression in iodine surgical scrub with isopropyl alcohol 1:1 for 30 minutes. Rinse before taking to the laboratory. Stone models can be sterilized with ethylene oxide.[21]

VI. Post-Treatment

A. Place instruments directly in the sterilizer without cleaning them. They may be wrapped in the draping material, or submerged in a basin of water and placed in the sterilizer.[31] After sterilization, they will be ready to clean, package, and sterilize again.

B. Place all disposable contaminated covers, sponges, needles, gloves, and other materials into a bag for direct incineration, or sterilize them.

C. Disinfect all surfaces not draped but touched, using iodine surgical scrub with isopropyl alcohol 1:1 and keep the surfaces wet with the disinfectant for 30 minutes.

D. Disinfect all eyeglasses in undiluted iodine scrub.

E. Wash face, hands, and exposed arms with undiluted surgical scrub by lathering and rinsing three times.[1,21]

TECHNICAL HINTS

I. Check and clean the exposed parts of the face not covered by mask or eyeglasses, where splatter collects, as an aid to disease control as well as for general sanitation. The face should be cleaned several times each day, and washed before eating. When washing the face, an effort should be made not to spread splatter material into the eyes or the mouth.

II. Smoking or eating should not be permitted in treatment areas.

III. Select toys and other reception area items that can be cleaned and disinfected.

IV. Small abrasions or cracks of the hands can be covered with a clear liquid bandage for safety under gloves in case the glove is damaged.

V. Include in the clinic or office policy manual outlines of procedures to follow for special precautions, such as for a patient who is a hepatitis carrier. Addresses for sources of various materials can be kept in a special reference section of the manual. Emergency procedures to follow when accidentally exposed should also be defined clearly (Passive Immunization, page 27).

VI. Investigate the regulations of each town or city sanitation division for rules concerning disposal of contaminated waste. The safety of the workers has been protected in many areas by the refusal to pick up bags of waste from hospitals and dental clinics unless the contents of the bags have been pre-sterilized.

VII. Sources for Protective Eyeglasses

C.L. Crump Company
Box 161, Winnetka, Illinois 60093

Dri-Clave Corporation
54 Kinkel Street
Westbury, Long Island, New York 11590

Lactona
Academy and Red Lion Roads
Philadelphia, Pennsylvania 19114

Pickering & Edwards
P.O. Box 13066
Oakland, California 94661

Silverman's Catalog
5 Apollo Road
Plymouth Meeting, Pennsylvania 19462

G. Taylor
P.O. Box 15352
Milwaukee, Wisconsin 53215

VIII. Sources for Face Masks

Deseret Operating Room Products
P.O. Box 1506
Greenwood, South Carolina 29646

Medical Products Division / 3M
555-2S 3M Center
St. Paul, Minnesota 55101

FACTORS TO TEACH THE PATIENT

I. Importance of the patient's complete history to the protection of both the patient and the operator.

II. Facts about the normal oral flora and the factors that influence an increased number of bacteria on the tongue, mucosa, and in the plaque.

III. Methods for personal daily control of the oral bacteria through plaque control and tongue brushing.

IV. Reasons for preoperative brushing, rinsing, and irrigating.

V. Method for thorough rinsing (page 369).

VI. Reasons for use of protective eyeglasses.

References

1. Crawford, J.J., Graham, J.B., Hines, R.N., Jessup, P.W., and Mohorn, H.W.: Suggested Guidelines for Asepsis in the Dental Office Environment, *North Carolina Dent. J.*, *63*, 16, Winter-Spring, 1980.
2. Goebel, W.M.: Reliability of the Medical History in Identifying Patients Likely to Place Dentists at an Increased Hepatitis Risk, *J. Am. Dent. Assoc.*, *98*, 907, June, 1979.
3. Tullman, M.J. and Boozer, C.H.: Past Infection with Hepatitis B Virus in Patients at a Dental School, *J. Am. Dent. Assoc.*, *97*, 477, September, 1978.
4. Tullman, M.J., Boozer, C.H., Villarejos, V.M., and Feary, T.W.: The Threat of Hepatitis B from Dental School Patients, A One-year Study, *Oral Surg.*, *49*, 214, March, 1980.
5. Whitacre, R.J., Robins, S.K., Williams, B.L., and Crawford, J.J.: *Dental Asepsis.* Seattle, Stoma Press, 1979, p. 17.
6. Berkow, R., ed.: *Merck Manual of Diagnosis and Therapy*, 13th ed. Rahway, N.J., Merck, Sharp & Dohme Research Laboratories, 1977, pp. 1823–1827.
7. Department of Health, Education, and Welfare, Public Health Service, Center for Disease Control: General Recommendations on Immunization, *MMWR*, *29*, 76, February 22, 1980.
8. Brooks, S.L., Rowe, N.H., Drach, J.C., Shipman, C., and Young, S.K.: Prevalence of Herpes Simplex Virus Disease in a Professional Population, *J. Am. Dent. Assoc.*, *102*, 31, January, 1981.
9. Whitacre, Robins, Williams, and Crawford: op. cit., pp. 57–80.
10. Federation Dentaire Internationale, Commission on Dental Practice: Technical Report: Recommendations for Hygiene in Dental Practice, *Int. Dent. J.*, *29*, 72, March, 1979.
11. Micik, R.E., Miller, R.L., and Leong, A.C.: Studies on Dental Aerobiology: III. Efficacy of Surgical Masks in Protecting Dental Personnel from Airborne Bacterial Particles, *J. Dent. Res.*, *50*, 626, May–June, 1971.
12. Miller, R.L. and Micik, R.E.: Air Pollution and Its Control in the Dental Office, *Dent. Clin. North Am.*, *22*, 453, July, 1978.
13. Groll, L.S.: *Dental Asepsis. Sanitization, Disinfection, and Sterilization.* San Antonio, Texas, University of Texas Health Center at San Antonio, Dental Hygiene Program, 28 pp.
14. Colvin, J.: Eye Injuries and the Dentist, *Aust. Dent. J.*, *23*, 453, December, 1978.

15. Cooley, R.L., Cottingham, A.J., Abrams, H., and Barkmeier, W.W.: Ocular Injuries Sustained in the Dental Office: Methods of Detection, Treatment, and Prevention, *J. Am. Dent. Assoc.*, 97, 985, December, 1978.
16. Hartley, J.L.: Eye and Facial Injuries Resulting from Dental Procedures, *Dent. Clin. North Am.*, 22, 505, July, 1978.
17. Altemeier, W.A.: Surgical Antiseptics, in Block, S.S., ed.: *Disinfection, Sterilization, and Preservation*, 2nd ed. Philadelphia, Lea & Febiger, 1977, pp. 641–653.
18. Steere, A.C. and Mallison, G.F.: Handwashing Practices for the Prevention of Nosocomial Infections, *Annals Int. Med.*, 83, 683, November, 1975.
19. Crawford, J.J.: Sterilization, Disinfection and Asepsis in Dentistry, in Block, S.S.: *Disinfection, Sterilization, and Preservation*, 2nd ed. Philadelphia, Lea & Febiger, 1977, pp. 685–704.
20. Hooley, J.R. and Phillips, R.E.: The Operating Room, in Hooley, J.R. and Daun, L.G.: *Hospital Dental Practice*. St. Louis, The C.V. Mosby Co., 1980, pp. 192–214.
21. Crawford, J.J.: *Clinical Asepsis in Dentistry*, 2nd ed. Mesquite, Texas, R.A. Kolstad, Publisher, 1978, 40 pp.
22. Crawford, J.J.: Office Sterilization and Asepsis Procedures in Endodontics, *Dent. Clin. North Am.*, 23, 717, October, 1979.
23. Whitacre, Robins, Williams, and Crawford: op. cit., pp. 102–107.
24. Randall, E. and Brenman, H.S.: Local Degerming with Povidone-iodine. I. Prior to Dental Prophylaxis, *J. Periodontol.*, 45, 866, December, 1974.
25. Brenman, H.S. and Randall, E.: Local Degerming with Povidone-iodine. II. Prior to Gingivectomy. *J. Periodontol.*, 45, 870, December, 1974.
26. Litsky, B.Y., Mascis, J.D., and Litsky, W.: Use of Antimicrobial Mouthwash to Minimize the Bacterial Aerosol Contamination Generated by the High-speed Drill, *Oral Surg.*, 29, 25, January, 1970.
27. Wyler, D., Miller, R.L., and Micik, R.E.: Efficacy of Self-administered Preoperative Oral Hygiene Procedures in Reducing the Concentration of Bacteria in Aerosols Generated During Dental Procedures, *J. Dent. Res.*, 50, 509, March–April, 1971.
28. Whitacre, Robins, Williams, and Crawford: op. cit., pp. 28–43.
29. Adams, D. and Zwink, R.: Treating Australia Antigen Positive Patients. Practical Experience, *Br. Dent. J.*, 141, 341, December, 7, 1976.
30. Expert Group on Hepatitis in Dentistry: Hepatitis in Dentistry, *Br. Dent. J.*, 146, 123, February 20, 1979.
31. Ernst, R.: Biohazards in Dentistry. Part III. Procedures for Clean vs. Contaminated Cases, *Dent. Assist.*, 48, 31, May/June, 1979.

Suggested Readings

American Dental Association, Council on Dental Materials, Instruments and Equipment: *Dentist's Desk Reference: Materials, Instruments and Equipment*. 1st ed. Chicago, American Dental Association, 1981, pp. 15–17.
American Dental Association, Council on Dental Materials and Devices, Council on Dental Therapeutics: Infection Control in the Dental Office, *J. Am. Dent. Assoc.*, 97, 673, October, 1978.
Autio, K.L., Rosen, S., Reynolds, N.J., and Bright, J.S.: Studies on Cross-contamination in the Dental Clinic, *J. Am. Dent. Assoc.*, 100, 358, March, 1980.
Codino, R.J. and Marshall, W.E.: Control of Infection in the Dental Operatory, *Dent. Surv.*, 52, 42, May, 1976.
Furuhashi, M.: A Study on the Microbial Filtration Efficiency of Surgical Face Masks–With Special Reference to the Non-woven Fabric Mask, *Bull. Tokyo Med. Dent. Univ.*, 25, 7, March, 1978.
Hesselgren, S-G.: The Spread of Infection by Dental Suction Devices, *Quintessence Int.*, 10, 79, June, 1979.
Hunt, M and Yagiela, J.A.: Bacterial Contamination and Transmission by Nitrous Oxide Sedation Apparatus, *Oral Surg.*, 44, 367, September, 1977.
Jokinen, M.A.: Prevention of Postextraction Bacteremia by Local Prophylaxis, *Int. J. Oral Surg.*, 7, 450, October, 1978.
Lilley, J.D. and Russell, C.: Contamination and Sterilisation of Local Anaesthetic Cartridges, *Br. Dent. J.*, 139, 391, November 18, 1975.
Norris, C.: If Saliva Were Red, *Dent. Surv.*, 55, 24, June, 1979.
Parker, R.B.: Sterilization, Disinfection, and Control of Infection in the Dental Office, in Clark, J.W., ed.: *Clinical Dentistry, Volume I*, Chapter 23, Hagerstown, Maryland, Harper & Row, 1981, pp. 1–7.
Rylander, R., Myrback, K.-E., Verner-Carlson, B., and Ohrstrom, M.: Bacteriological Investigation of Wall-to-wall Carpeting, *Am. J. Public Health*, 64, 163, February, 1974.
Schön, F.: Dealing with Refuse, *Quintessence Journal*, 3, 85, February, 1981.
Schön, F. and Gierl, B.: Improving Hygiene in the Dental Office, *Quintessence Journal*, 2, 21, March, 1980.
Tolman, D.E.: Modification of Operating Light: Addition of Removable Handle for Use During Surgical Procedures, *J. Oral Surg.*, 31, 353, May, 1973.
White, S.C. and Glaze, S.: Interpatient Microbiological Cross-contamination after Dental Radiographic Examination, *J. Am. Dent. Assoc.*, 96, 801, May, 1978.
Yagiela, J.A., Hunt, L.M., and Hunt, D.E.: Disinfection of Nitrous Oxide Inhalation Equipment, *J. Am. Dent. Assoc.*, 98, 191, February, 1979.

Hands

Eigener, U.: Hand Hygiene in Dental Practice, *Quintessence Journal*, 1, 25, January, 1979.
Furuhashi, M. and Miyamae, T.: Effect of Pre-operative Hand Scrubbing and Influence of Pinholes Appearing in Surgical Rubber Gloves during Operation, *Bull. Tokyo Med. Dent. Univ.*, 26, 73, June, 1979.
Skaug, N.: Micropunctures of Rubber Gloves Used in Oral Surgery, *Int. J. Oral Surg.*, 5, 220, October, 1976.
Tucci, V.J., Stone, A.M., Thompson, C., Isenberg, H.D., and Wise, L.: Studies of the Surgical Scrub, *Surg. Gynec. Obstr.*, 145, 415, September, 1977.

Protective Eyeglasses

Casey, D.M. and Casey, E.P.: Patient Eye Protection in the Dental Office, *N.Y. State Dent. J.*, 45, 460, November, 1979.
Casey, D.M.: Eye Injuries in Dental Office (Letter to Editor), *J. Am. Dent. Assoc.*, 91, 502, September, 1975.
Colvin, J.: Eye Protection (Letter to Editor), *Aust. Dent. J.*, 24, 371, October, 1979.
Cunningham, P.J.: Eye Protection (Letter to Editor), *Aust. Dent. J.*, 23, 502, December, 1978.
Folk, J.C. and Lobes, L.A.: Intraocular Complications (Letter to Editor), *J. Am. Dent. Assoc.*, 102, 161, February, 1981.
Needleman, M.S., McLaughlin, D.K., Orner, G., and Mumma, R.D.: Eye Hazards Among a Dental School Population, *J. Dent. Educ.*, 41, 573, September, 1977.

Dental Laboratory Hygiene

Engelhardt, J.P.: Hygiene in the Dental Laboratory, *Quin-*

tessence Dent. Technol., *1*, 95, September–October, 1976.

Firtell, D.N., Moore, D.J., and Pelleu, G.B.: Sterilization of Impression Materials for Use in the Surgical Operating Room, *J. Prosthet. Dent.*, *27*, 419, April, 1972.

Katberg, J.W.: Cross-contamination via the Prosthodontic Laboratory, *J. Prosthet. Dent.*, *32*, 412, October, 1974.

Larato, D.C.: Disinfection of Pumice, *J. Prosthet. Dent.*, *18*, 534, December, 1967.

Rowe, A.H.R. and Forrest, J.O.: Dental Impressions. The Probability of Contamination and a Method of Disinfection, *Br. Dent. J.*, *145*, 184, September 19, 1978.

Trevelyan, M.R.: The Prosthetic Treatment of Hepatitis B Antigen Positive Patients, *Br. Dent. J.*, *137*, 63, July 16, 1974.

Wakefield, C.W.: Laboratory Contamination of Dental Prostheses, *J. Prosthet. Dent.*, *44*, 143, August, 1980.

Orthodontics

Matlack, R.E.: Instrument Sterilization in Orthodontic Offices, *Angle Orthod.*, *49*, 205, July, 1979.

Starnbach, H. and Biddle, P.: A Pragmatic Approach to Asepsis in the Orthodontic Office, *Angle Orthod.*, *50*, 63, January, 1980.

Thompson, R.P. and Bogues, W.H.J.P.: An Investigation into Methods Used to Clean and Sterilize Orthodontic Instruments and Bands, *Br. J. Orthod.*, *4*, 201, October, 1977.

5

Patient Reception and Positioning in the Dental Chair

The patient's well-being is the all-important consideration throughout the appointment. At the same time, the operator must function effectively and efficiently by applying work simplification principles to reduce stress and fatigue.

The physical arrangement and interpersonal relationships provide the setting for specific services to be performed. The patient's presence in the office is an expression of confidence in the dentist and the auxiliary personnel. This confidence is inspired by the reputation for professional knowledge and skill, the appearance of the office, and the action of the workers in it.

I. Preparation for the Patient

A. Treatment Area

The procedures for the prevention of disease transmission were summarized on page 63. Additional requirements for maximum precautions in the presence of a patient with a known communicable disease are listed on page 64.

1. *Environmental Surfaces.* All contact areas must be thoroughly disinfected to control cross-contamination. Appointment preparation was described on pages 58–61.

2. *Instruments.* When a preprepared tray is used, it is uncovered in front of the patient. Packaged instruments remain sealed until the start of the appointment.

3. *Equipment.* Prepare and make ready other materials that will be used, such as for the determination of blood pressure and patient instruction. Anticipate specific needs for assessment procedures for a new patient.

B. Records

By leaving the record open for possible reference, the need for handling the record after hand scrubbing for instrumentation may be avoided. Radiographs can be placed on the viewbox and the light left on.

1. Review the patient's medical and dental history for pertinent appointment information and need for updating.

2. Read previous appointment case records to focus the current treatment needs.

3. Anticipate examination procedures and new record making for a new patient.

C. Position Chair

1. Upright, in low position.
2. Chair arm adjusted for access.
3. Pre-adjustment of traditional chair when

size of patient is known will contribute to ease while making final adjustments.

D. Clear Path

Clear pathway to chair of obstacles: rheostat, operating stool.

II. Patient Reception

A. Introductions

1. The dental assistant or the dentist may introduce the new patient to the dental hygienist, but more frequently, a self-introduction is in order. The patient is greeted by name and the hygienist's name is clearly stated, for example, "Good morning, Mr. Smith; I am Miss Jones, the dental hygienist." Wearing a name-tag for the patient's convenient observation is helpful.
2. Procedure for introducing the patient to others:
   a. A lady's name always precedes a gentleman's.
   b. An older person's name precedes the younger person's (when of the same sex and when the difference in age is obvious).
   c. In general, the patient's name precedes that of a member of the dental personnel.
3. An older patient is not called by the first name unless requested by the patient.

B. Procedures

1. Invite patient to be seated.
   a. For the average patient, stand ready to adjust the chair.
   b. Assist the elderly, infirm, or very small children; guide into the chair with support to the patient's arm.
2. Assist with wheelchair. Bring wheelchair adjacent to the dental chair and provide assistance when indicated. Wheelchair transfers and assistance for a patient with a walker or crutches are described on pages 691–694.
3. Place handbag within the patient's view.
4. Apply drape and napkin. A female patient's legs may be draped and an elderly patient may need a blanket. Stabilization

aids for patients with handicaps are described on pages 694 and 710.

5. Receive removable prosthetic appliances and place in water in a protective container.
6. Provide protective eyeglasses. For details of the types and care of protective eyeglasses, see page 52. When a patient removes personal corrective eyeglasses to substitute those provided by the office or clinic, make sure the personal glasses are safely placed in their case in the patient's handbag.

POSITION OF THE DENTAL HYGIENIST

The adjustment for the position of the patient is contingent upon the position of the dental hygienist. Attention to the patient's comfort must always be foremost, but when the working arrangement is considered, it is realistic to remember that the patient's position will be assumed for a relatively short time compared with that of the dental hygienist, who may conduct a major portion of a full day's professional activity in close proximity to the chairside. The patient, therefore, is positioned to permit the dental hygienist to accomplish a thorough, biologically oriented dental hygiene service conveniently and efficiently within a reasonable length of time.

I. Objectives

Objectives concern the health of the dental hygienist, the service to be performed, and the effect on the patient. The *preferred* working position is one which will attempt to accomplish the following:

A. Contribute to rather than detract from the health of the dental hygienist.
B. Provide physical comfort and mental tranquility.
C. Apply principles of body mechanics which will reduce fatigue and maintain stamina for prolonged periods of peak efficiency.
D. Contribute to ease and efficiency of performance, which will produce complete, thorough results for effective treatment; this, in turn, will have long-range benefits for the patient.
E. Transmit to the patient a sense of well-being, security, and confidence, as well as a need for cooperation with dental personnel.

F. Develop better patient–dental hygienist relationships because of greater comfort, lessened physical stress, and reduced appointment time.
G. Be flexible in relation to individual needs of patients with special health problems, where limitations of physiologic or pathologic conditions require variations in chair positions.
H. Be flexible in relation to studying and utilizing, where applicable, new concepts of patient care and new developments in dental equipment which will contribute to all objectives of service.

II. The Seated Dental Hygienist

In keeping with current concepts, it is expected that the dental hygienist will utilize an operating stool. Benefits to the dental hygienist can result which relate to general health, productivity, and the manner in which work is accomplished. Greater comfort and opportunity to relax is afforded the patient when the dental hygienist is seated and the patient must necessarily be lowered back to a reclining or supine position.

A. Characteristics of an Acceptable Operating Stool[1]

1. *Base.* Broad and heavy for stability, with no fewer than four casters. A stool with five casters has greater stability.
2. *Mobility.* Completely mobile; not connected to other dental equipment; built with free-rolling casters; without tipping hazards.
3. *Seat.* Relatively large to provide complete body support; padded firmly, yet not too hard; without a welt on the leaning edge which could dig into the upper part of the thigh.
4. *Rotating Support.* May be applied to the operator's back, side, or abdomen for support.
5. *Height.* Adjustable to provide exactly the correct level for the individual so that feet can be flat on the floor and thighs parallel with the floor.
6. *Assistant's Stool.* Needs additional support at the base with at least five casters recommended for maximum stability; should be freely adjustable for height. A footrest is needed at the base of the chair

since the assistant is positioned 4 to 6 inches higher than the operator, and generally the feet could not reach the floor.

B. Use of the Operating Stool

Once the operating stool is adjusted for the individual, it does not need changing, unless other personnel also use it. Once adjusted, the height remains constant, and other dental equipment is arranged to accommodate for optimum usage at the convenience of the seated dental hygienist. Positioning that incorporates principles of good body mechanics will benefit both dental hygienist and patient. Basic positioning includes the following features related to posture and the field of operation.

1. Feet are flat on the floor; thighs parallel with the floor (figure 5–1A).
2. Back is straight; head is relatively erect; shoulders are relaxed and parallel with floor.
3. Body weight is completely supported by the chair; balancing on the edge of the stool should be avoided (figure 5–1B).
4. Eyes are directed downward in a manner that prevents neck strain and eye strain; it is not necessary to bend the head.
5. Operating distance from the patient's mouth to the eyes of operator should be 14 to 16 inches.

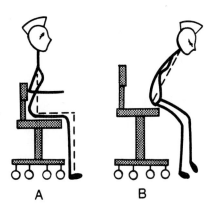

Figure 5–1. Use of operating stool. **A.** Correct position with feet flat on the floor, thighs parallel with floor, and body weight supported by chair. **B.** Incorrect position with seat high, body balanced on the edge of the stool, and back bent forward.

6. With elbows close to the sides, the field of operation (patient's mouth) is adjusted to elbow height.

III. The Standing Dental Hygienist

As in the seated position, the standing posture also requires application of principles of good body mechanics.

A. Distribution of Balance

1. Both feet are flat on the floor with toes forward.
2. Back is straight; head relatively erect; shoulders relaxed and parallel with floor.
3. Weight is centered over the balls of the feet and distributed evenly to both feet; knees are slightly flexed.

B. Relation to Field of Operation

1. With elbows close to sides, the field of operation (patient's mouth) is adjusted to elbow height.
2. Eyes are directed downward in a manner that prevents neck strain and eye strain; it is not necessary to bend the head.
3. Operating distance from the patient's mouth to the eyes of operator should be 14 to 16 inches.

POSITION OF THE DENTAL CHAIR

Once the height of operation is established by the height of the dental hygienist's elbow, dental chair positioning relates directly to the type of dental chair. The sequence of procedures for effective, efficient adjustment of the traditional or conventional dental chair and of the contour chair is outlined here.

I. Traditional Dental Chair

The back of the chair is adjusted first, then the headrest; the chair is inclined, to adjust the seat; and finally, the whole chair is lowered or raised to bring the field of operation to the correct level and angulation. For most patients, the footrest remains in a constant position, but it should be adjusted to meet individual needs.

A. Prepositioning for Patient Reception

1. Seat parallel with floor.

2. Back slightly inclined back and away from the upright position.
3. Headrest tilted back to prevent its bumping the patient during seating.
4. Location of base of chair on the floor should permit access to the dental unit when chair is inclined (figure 5–2).

B. Backrest

1. Raise or lower until the curvature of the chair back corresponds with the curvature in the middle of the patient's back.
2. When correctly positioned, the top border of many traditional chairs will be at a level approximating the lower third of the patient's scapulae. Other chairs have taller backs which may reach nearer the upper third of the scapulae.

C. Headrest

1. Request the patient to hold the head erect with chin slightly up.
2. Bring the headrest to a position almost touching the back of the head under the occipital protuberances before securing it.

D. Chair Seat

1. Incline the whole chair back as a unit. For the correct position, usually the chair will be tilted as far as it will go.
2. The "V" formed between the seat and the back prevents the patient from sliding forward (figure 5–3A).

E. Final Adjustment

1. *The Seated Dental Hygienist*
   a. Lower the chair to its lowest level and incline the chair back as far as it will go.
   b. To lower the field of operation further, it may be necessary to lower the back of the chair.
2. *The Standing Dental Hygienist.* With the chair inclined as far back as possible, raise or lower the whole chair until the patient's mouth is at elbow height of the operator.
3. *Basic Position of the Patient.* When correctly positioned, the spinal cord of the patient should be straight from the brain to the hips. An imaginary straight line

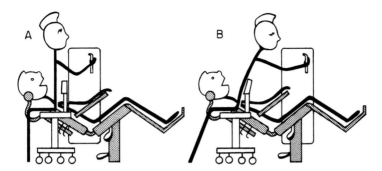

Figure 5–2. Relation of patient in dental chair to traditional dental unit and seated dental hygienist. **A.** Correct position with patient's mouth at elbow height, convenient to unit without stretching, **B.** Incorrect position with dental chair too far removed. Dental hygienist must stretch across patient to reach unit.

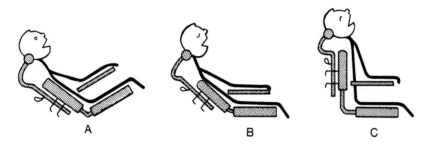

Figure 5–3. Traditional dental chair adjustment, **A.** Correct position with backrest and headrest adjusted so that the body is straight from hip to top of head and the whole chair is tilted back. **B.** Incorrect position with headrest too far forward and chair seat flat which encourages the patient to slide forward. **C.** Incorrect with headrest too far back.

can be drawn from the top of the ear to the hips to test this.

F. Effects of Chair Maladjustment

1. *Backrest Too Low or Too High.* Curvature of the spine will cause muscle tension and restlessness, and the patient will attempt to slide into a more comfortable posture out of appropriate operating position.

2. *Headrest Too High or Too Far Forward.* Chin moves toward chest, there is difficulty in maintaining accessibility and vision; dental hygienist must lean forward and bend neck sidewards (figure 5–3B).

3. *Headrest Too Low or Too Far Back.* Patient's neck muscles can be stretched and become fatigued; swallowing may be difficult; patient will slide down (figure 5–3C).

4. *Chair Seat Parallel with Floor.* Patient will slide forward and down (figure 5–3B).

II. Contour Dental Chair

A contour chair differs from a traditional chair in many ways. It has advantages in that it provides complete body support for the patient, which increases patient relaxation. The operator can be in a better working position with better access, light, and visibility, which in turn, contribute to a more efficient performance in less time.

The adjustment of a contour chair is easier than for the traditional chair with its many separate parts. Once the basic goal is learned, contour chair adjustment does not vary for different sized patients as much as does the traditional chair adjustment.

In a supine position, a patient is ideally situated for support of the circulation; rarely could a patient faint while lying with the feet slightly higher than the head. Research has shown that astronauts, for example, withstand the most stress in a supine, contoured, body-supported position.[2]

A. Characteristics of a Contour Chair for Efficient Utilization

1. Provides complete body support.
2. Seat and leg support work as a unit; back and headrest work as a unit; both are power controlled.
3. Has a thin back without protruding adjustment devices so that the chair may be lowered close to the dental hygienist's lap for proper positioning of the field of operation.
4. Has supports that hold the patient's arms as the chair is lowered into the supine position; otherwise the hands hang down or the patient must hold them up forcibly.
5. Chair base should be as shallow as possible to permit the chair to be lowered as close to the floor as needed for correct operating position.
6. Chair base should be power driven with pedal access from the working position on the dental operating stool. Likewise, the switches for the back and seat should be readily available to both the assistant and operator.

B. Prepositioning for Patient Reception

1. Chair at low level; back upright.
2. Chair arm raised on side of approach.

C. Adjustment Steps

1. Patient is first seated with back upright.
2. Female patient's legs are draped.
3. Chair seat and foot portion is raised first to help the patient settle back.
4. Backrest is lowered until the patient reaches the supine position with the knees on a level with the nose.
5. Patient is requested to slide up until the head is at the upper edge of the backrest and on the side next to the dental hygienist. Note patient's head position in figure 5–5 shown for a right-handed operator.

D. Final Adjustment

1. Lower or raise the total chair until the field of operation (patient's mouth) is at hygienist's elbow level, as previously described.

2. Basic position of patient: back level and parallel with floor; for maxillary instrumentation, complete supine position with feet slightly higher than the head (figure 5–4).
3. When working on the mandibular arch from the 9:00 or 7:30 position (left-handed operator at 3:00 or 4:30) (figure 5–5), it is sometimes helpful to raise the back of the patient slightly. The whole chair must then be lowered to bring the field of operation back to elbow height. An alternate method for adjustment is to place a small plastic cushion under the head. Certain dental chair models have separate head cushions for this purpose.

E. Conclusion of Appointment

1. Raise backrest slowly.
2. Tilt chair forward.
3. Have patient sit in upright position briefly to avoid possible effects of postural hypotension. Symptoms of dizziness and faintness may occur.

III. Chair Position for Small Child

A. Traditional Chair

1. Use a portable seat or a large firm cushion to raise seat level.
2. Cover the seat with a cloth to protect the finish from the child's shoes.
3. Lower back and headrest to lowest levels with back at right angles to chair seat.
4. Incline chair back.
5. Final adjustment: child's head will rest as near the headrest as possible; legs may be crossed to give support.

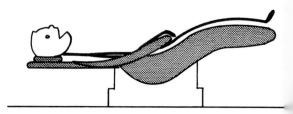

Figure 5–4. Contour chair. For maxillary instrumentation, patient is in supine position with back of chair parallel with floor and feet slightly higher than the head. For mandibular instrumentation, adjust chair back to a 20-degree angle with the floor.

B. Contour Chair

Adjustment the same as for an adult. Child will slide up so that the head is near the top of the backrest and on the side toward the dental hygienist (figure 5–5).

FUNCTIONAL FACTORS

I. Lighting

During treatment, visibility of specific areas of the oral cavity is prerequisite to thoroughness without undue trauma to the tissues. With inadequate light, inefficiency increases and leads to prolonged operating time, which reduces patient cooperation.

The position of the dental light or lights and the intensity of the beam affect the illumination. A study of the operating room can be made that includes measurement of the total light at the patient's face in working position. Selection of an operating light that meets certain standards can assure intensity sufficient for good visibility and yet safe for the eyes.

A. Dental Light: Suggested Features

1. The light should be readily adjustable

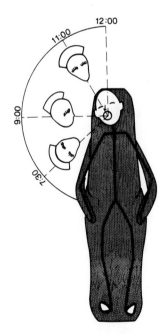

Figure 5–5. Operating positions. Patient's head is placed at the upper edge of the backrest and on the side next to the dental hygienist. The right-handed dental hygienist is positioned between 7:30 and 11:00 for access to the patient's oral cavity from the side-front, side, or side-back. The left-handed hygienist is positioned between 1:00 and 4:30.

both vertically and horizontally and the beam capable of being focused.

2. The size must be small enough so that it may be brought close to the operating area without being in the way, blocking the room light, or being a hazard for movement of people in its vicinity.

3. Intensity of room light should be sufficient to prevent a marked contrast between it and the illuminating beam of the dental light. An all-luminous ceiling contributes to evenly distributed room lighting.

B. Dental Light: Location

1. *Attachment.* The most versatile arrangement is a ceiling-mounted light on a track, which permits the light to move over a range from behind the patient's head in supine to a position anterior to the patient's chin.

2. *Dual Lighting.* With the use of a supine patient position in a contour chair, advantages to the use of two operating lights have been demonstrated. One light directed from the front of the patient may be attached to the dental chair or unit; the other light mounted on a ceiling track as described above.

C. Dental Light: Adjustment

Direct the light first on the napkin under the patient's chin, then rotate the light up to the mouth to avoid flashing light in the patient's eyes.

II. Working Positions

A. Objectives

1. The operator must see the field of operation clearly without having to assume body positions that are harmful if held over long periods.

2. When an assistant participates, the field of operation must be accessible and visible to both dental hygienist and dental assistant.

3. Instruments and equipment must be within reach without stretching.

B. Basic Zone for Operation

The dental hygienist may perform patient

services from a position that permits access to the patient's oral cavity from the side-front, the side, or the side-back. The hours of a clock have been used to designate positions at the dental chair and zones of operation. With 12:00 directly over the top of the patient's head and 6:00 toward the feet, the side-front position is 7:30 to 8:00, the side is at 9:00, and the side-back at 11:00 for the right-handed operator (figure 5–5). Certain procedures require positions between these numbers. The left-handed dental hygienist operates between 1:00 and 4:00 to 4:30.

C. Dental Hygienist without Assistant

1. Arrange necessary items for immediate access without leaving operating stool.
2. Cervical tray may be used and positioned conveniently around the patient.
3. Height of tray for instruments should be at or slightly below the elbow of the dental hygienist, so that no effort need be expended when instruments are changed.

D. Dental Hygienist with Assistant

1. Position of assistant: seated with eye level 4 to 6 inches above the dental hygienist's eye level and facing toward the head of dental chair (figure 5–6).
2. Assistant applies principles of good body mechanics: body weight supported by

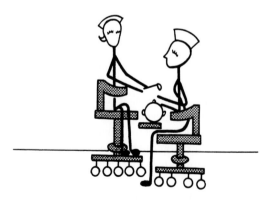

Figure 5–6. Dental hygienist with dental assistant. The dental assistant is seated with eye level 4 to 6 inches above the dental hygienist's eye level. The sterile preprepared tray is placed on a portable cabinet in front of the assistant within easy reach for passing instruments.

operating stool; feet are rested on the base of the operating stool.

3. Instruments and other essential materials are kept within arm's length and the portable cabinet with sterilized preprepared tray is in front of the dental assistant.[3]
4. Four-handed dentistry procedures are practiced with instrument transfers and evacuation during operations.

TECHNICAL HINTS

I. The face of the dental hygienist should not be in close proximity to that of the patient. If it is difficult to keep working distance at 14 to 16 inches, an eye examination may be indicated.

II. Keep body contact at a minimum. A good operator does not lean on the patient or rest the forearms on the patient's shoulders, or rest the hands on the patient's face or forehead. Unnecessary contact can be very unpleasant to certain patients, and, more importantly, it contributes to disease transmission.

III. Conditions that contraindicate use of the supine position include congestive heart, cerebral vascular insufficiency, and any condition associated with breathing difficulty such as emphysema, severe asthma, or sinusitis.

FACTORS TO TEACH THE PATIENT

I. Orientation of patients, particularly previous patients, is important when changes in equipment and operating procedures are introduced.

II. Give specific instruction on the parts of a dental chair or other equipment which will be of concern to the patient to prevent embarrassment or adverse reactions.

References

1. Sinnett, G.M. and Wuehrmann, A.H.: The Dental Operatory of the Future, in Peterson, S., ed.: *The Dentist and His Assistant*, 3rd ed. St. Louis, The C.V. Mosby Co., 1972, pp. 392–401.
2. Tarsitano, J.J.: Contour Configuration, *J. Am. Dent. Assoc.*, 70, 1194, May, 1965.
3. Sinnett, G.M., McDevitt, E.J., Robinson, G.E., and Wuehrmann, A.H.: Four-handed Dentistry: a New Mobile Dental Cabinet Design, *J. Am. Dent. Assoc.*, 78, 305, February, 1969.

Suggested Readings

American Dental Association, Council on Dental Materials, Instruments, and Equipment: *Dentist's Desk Reference: Materials, Instruments and Equipment,* 1st ed. Chicago, American Dental Association, 1981, pp. 304–313.

Davis, M.H. and Eccles, J.D.: Attitudes of Patients to Conservation Treatment in Different Chair Positions, *J. Dent.,* 6, 294, December, 1978.

Forsyth, W.D., Allen, G.D., and Everett, G.B.: An Evaluation of Cardiorespiratory Effects of Posture in the Dental Outpatient, *Oral Surg.,* 34, 562, October, 1972.

Glenner, R.A.: The Dental Chair—A Brief Pictorial History, *J. Am. Dent. Assoc.,* 86, 38, January, 1973.

Glenner, R.A.: Components of the Dental Unit, *J. Am. Dent. Assoc.,* 89, 1012, November, 1974.

Hilborn, L.B., Campbell, E.M., and Hall, W.R.: Facility Design and Equipment Considerations for the Team Practice of Dentistry, *Dent. Clin. North Am.,* 18, 873, October, 1974.

Jeffrey, I.W.M. and Butchart, D.G.M.: The Use of Television in Studying Postural Operative Positions, *Br. Dent. J.,* 139, 193, September 2, 1975.

Kilpatrick, H.C.: Dental Equipment Selection, in Clark, J.W., ed.: *Clinical Dentistry, Volume 5,* Chapter 25. Hagerstown, Maryland, Harper & Row, 1981, pp. 1–21.

Rasmus, B.J. and Wulf, B.R.: Work Simplification for the Dental Hygienist, *Educ. Dir. Dent. Aux.,* 5, 11, August, 1980.

Ruby, J.D.: A Dental Chair Design for Pediatric Dentistry, *J. Pedod.,* 3, 52, Fall, 1978.

Scanlan, D.: A Dental Chair Modification for Children, *Can. Dent. Assoc. J.,* 45, 165, April, 1979.

Schön, F.: The Incorrectly Programmed Patient Treatment Chair, *Quintessence Int.,* 10, 57, December, 1979.

Stombaugh, E.F.: The Reduction of Stress and Fatigue in the Dental Operatory, *Quintessence Journal,* 1, 13, November/December, 1979.

Weinert, A.M.: An Evaluation of the Modern Dental Lounge Chair, *Dent. Clin. North Am.,* 15, 129, January, 1971.

Four-handed Procedures

Castano, F.A. and Alden, B.A., eds.: *Handbook of Expanded Dental Auxiliary Practice,* 2nd ed. Philadelphia, J.B. Lippincott Co., 1980, pp. 27–42.

Cooper, T.M.: Four-handed Dentistry in the Team Practice of Dentistry, *Dent. Clin. North Am.,* 18, 739, October, 1974.

Handelman, S.L., Kwasman, R., MacIntyre, B.A., and Barrett, G.V.: Factors Affecting Dental Team Performance, *J. Am. Dent. Assoc.,* 89, 880, October, 1974.

Hirsch, S.M. and Anson, R.A.: A Seated, Four-handed Team Approach, in Ward, H.L. and Simring, M., eds.: *Manual of Clinical Periodontics,* 2nd ed. St. Louis, The C.V. Mosby Co., 1978, pp. 205–224.

Kryger, L.K. and Zender, B.H.: Chairside Assisting Techniques, in Peterson, S., ed.: *The Dentist and the Assistant,* 4th ed. St. Louis, The C.V. Mosby Co., 1977, pp. 157–186.

Paul, E.: A Practical Guide to Assisted Operating. 1. Principles of Assisted Operating, *Br. Dent. J.,* 133, 258, September 19, 1972; 2. Aspiration, *Br. Dent. J.,* 133, 305, October 3, 1972; 3. Instrument Handling (1), *Br. Dent. J.,* 133, 348, October 17, 1972; 4. Instrument Handling (2), *Br. Dent. J.,* 133, 384, November 7, 1972; 5. Instrument Handling (3), *Br. Dent. J.,* 133, 437, November 21, 1972.

Pipe, P., Kryger, L.K., Underwood, B., and MacIntyre, M.: *Introduction to Four-handed Dentistry, A Multimedia Self-instructional Program for Dental Assistants.* Philadelphia, J.B. Lippincott Co., 1974.

Robinson, G.E.: Utilization of Dental Auxiliaries, in Clark, J.W., ed.: *Clinical Dentistry, Volume 5,* Chapter 31. Hagerstown, Maryland, Harper & Row, 1981, pp. 1–40.

Robinson, G.E., McDevitt, E.J., Sinnett, G.M., and Wuehrmann, A.H.: *Four-Handed Dentistry Manual,* 2nd ed. Birmingham, University of Alabama School of Dentistry, 1971.

Schmid, W. and Stevenson, S.B.: Dynamic Instrument Placement, and Operator's and Assistant's Stool Placement, *Dent. Clin. North Am.,* 15, 145, January, 1971.

Schulgen, G.: Four-handed Dental Hygiene, in Boundy, S.S. and Reynolds, N.J., eds.: *Current Concepts in Dental Hygiene.* St. Louis, The C.V. Mosby Co., 1977, pp. 21–30.

Spencer, P.R.: Chairside Procedures for the Dental Assistant, in Park, V.R., Ashman, J.R., and Shelly, G.J.: *A Textbook for Dental Assistants,* 2nd ed. Philadelphia, W.B. Saunders Co., 1975, pp. 394–422.

Strickland, W.D.: Operative Dentistry, in Richardson, R.E., Barton, R.E., and Brauer, J.C., eds.: *The Dental Assistant,* 5th ed. New York, McGraw-Hill, 1978, pp. 564–574.

Lighting

Cutler, M. and Cutler, J.: Office Space and Facilities, in Clark, J.W., ed.: *Clinical Dentistry, Volume 5,* Chapter 24. Hagerstown, Maryland, Harper & Row, 1981, pp. 1–30.

Preston, J.D., Ward, L.C., and Bobrick, M.: Light and Lighting in the Dental Office, *Dent. Clin. North Am.,* 22, 431, July, 1978.

Price, D.L. and Shaw, W.A.: Illumination of the Dental Operatory, *J. Am. Dent. Assoc.,* 98, 925, June, 1979.

Viohl, J.: Dental Operating Lights and Illumination of the Dental Surgery, *Int. Dent. J.,* 29, 148, June, 1979.

III

Patient Evaluation

INTRODUCTION

Before treatment begins, information must be obtained about the patient's general and oral health from which a diagnosis and treatment plan can be formulated. The gathering, organizing, and assembling of all data from observations, patient questioning, and clinical and radiographic examination may be called a *diagnostic work-up*. Basically, it is a collection of all pertinent facts and materials for the dentist to use during diagnosis and treatment planning and for use during all treatment as a guide.

The chapters in this section, *Patient Evaluation*, include descriptions for the preparation of materials that make up a diagnostic work-up. While a dental hygienist prepares specific parts of the work-up, comments on or reactions to any findings must be withheld until after the diagnosis and treatment plan are finalized by the dentist. Even a simple, well-intentioned remark can be misleading to the patient and create misunderstandings which can be difficult to clarify later.

I. Parts of a Diagnostic Work-up

A. Basic Procedures

The essential information for assessment of a patient prior to formulation of the diagnosis and treatment plan by a dentist is derived from the following:
1. Patient histories (personal, medical, and dental).
2. Determination of vital signs.
3. Extraoral and intraoral examination.
4. Radiographic survey.
5. Study casts.

6. Examination of the gingival and periodontal tissues, including clinical signs of disease involvement, pocket measurement and charting, and mobility evaluation.
7. Examination of the teeth to determine and record deposits, restorations, carious lesions, structural defects, pulp vitality, and occlusion factors.

B. Diagnostic Work-up for Preventive Treatment Plan

A preventive program is planned to meet individual needs. Therefore, information to be obtained depends on the particular oral problems and could include:
1. Dental or periodontal indices.
2. Dietary analysis.
3. Caries activity test.

C. Additional Procedures

In addition to the basic procedures, other parts of a diagnostic work-up will be selected depending on the individual needs of a patient, as well as the specialty area and special emphasis of the dentist. Selection of procedures to be used may be influenced by the age group to which the patient belongs.

Certain procedures may be of an emergency examination category. For example, if during the intraoral examination of the oral mucosa a suspicious lesion was found for which a biopsy was indicated, such a diagnostic procedure would take precedence over any other.

In accord with the policy or special re-

quest of the dentist, a diagnostic work-up may include some or all of the following:
1. Photographs.
2. Biopsy or cytologic smear.
3. Tests for suspected systemic conditions such as bleeding tendencies, sickle cell anemia, or diabetes.
4. Special consultations or referrals to a physician.

II. Purposes

The diagnostic work-up can benefit the patient, aid the dentist, and provide an overall perspective from which the dental hygienist can conduct a patient-oriented dental hygiene care program. Basic objectives of a diagnostic work-up are to

A. Organize information and materials for the dentist to use while making the diagnosis and outlining the treatment plan for the patient.
B. Aid the dental hygienist in
  1. Planning dental hygiene preventive care and instruction for the patient.
  2. Guiding techniques during dental hygiene appointments.
  3. Correlating dental hygiene care with dental care.
C. Provide a permanent, documented, continuing record of the patient's oral and general health for
  1. Evaluating the response to treatment which may be compared with future observations at follow-up and recall appointments.
  2. Protecting the dental practice in case of misunderstandings or evidence in legal matters should questions arise.
D. Increase the scope of contribution of the dental hygienist to comprehensive patient care by the dental health team.

EXAMINATION PROCEDURES

A specific objective of patient examination as a part of the total diagnostic work-up is the recognition of deviations from normal which may be signs and symptoms of disease. The importance of careful, thorough examination cannot be overstressed. Concentration and attention to detail are necessary in order that each slight deviation from normal may be entered on the record for review by the dentist. Signs and symptoms of disease are the deviations from normal that must be recorded.

I. Signs and Symptoms

A. Sign

A *sign* is any abnormality that may be indicative of a deviation from normal or of disease that is discovered by a professional person while examining a patient. A sign is an objective symptom.

Examples of signs are changes in color, shape, or consistency of a tissue not observable by the patient. Other signs are findings revealed by the use of a probe, explorer, radiograph, or vitality tester of the dental pulp.

B. Symptom

A *symptom* is also any departure from the normal that may be indicative of disease. Symptoms may be subjective or objective.
1. *Subjective symptom:* when observed by the patient. Examples are pain, tenderness, or itching.
2. *Objective symptom:* when observed by the professional person during an examination. As described above, objective symptoms are frequently called *signs.*

C. Pathognomonic Signs and Symptoms

Some signs and symptoms are general and may occur during various disease states. An increase in body temperature, for example, accompanies many infections.

Other signs and symptoms are *pathognomonic*, which means that the sign or symptom is unique to a particular disease and can be used to distinguish that disease or condition from other diseases or conditions.

II. Types of Examination

A. Complete

A complete examination means that a thorough comprehensive diagnostic work-up is prepared.

B. Screening

Screening implies a brief examination

using only parts of the complete diagnostic work-up. Screening is used for initial evaluation and classification. In a community health program, when a survey of a population is made to single out people with a particular condition, it is called screening.

C. Limited

A limited examination is usually made for an emergency. It may be used in the management of acute conditions.

D. Follow-up

A follow-up examination is a type of limited examination. It is used to observe the effects of treatment after a period of time during which the tissue or lesion could recover and heal. Indications for the need for additional or alternate treatment are apparent at a follow-up examination.

E. Recall

A recall examination is made after a specified period of time following the completion of treatment and the restoration to health. A recall examination is a complete examination with a comprehensive diagnostic work-up. The purpose of the recall examination is to evaluate the maintenance of health.

III. Examination Methods

A patient is examined by various visual, tactile, manual, and instrumental methods. General types are defined briefly here, and other specific methods are found throughout the book as they apply to a certain area under consideration.

A. Visual Examination

1. *Direct Observation.* Visual examination is made in a systematic order to note surface appearance (color, contour, size, etc.) and to observe movement and other evidence of function.
2. *Radiographic Examination.* The use of radiographs can reveal deviations from the normal not notable by direct observation.
3. *Transillumination.* A strong light directed through a soft tissue or a tooth to enhance examination is especially useful

for detecting irregularities of the teeth and locating calculus.

B. Palpation

Palpation is examination using the sense of touch through tissue manipulation or pressure on an area with the fingers or hand. The method used depends on the area to be investigated. Types of palpation are described on page 114.

C. Instrumentation

Examination instruments such as the explorer and probe are used for specific examination of the teeth and periodontal tissues. They are described in detail on pages 211–225.

D. Percussion

Percussion is the act of tapping or striking a surface or tooth with the fingers or an instrument. Information about the status of health of the part is determined either by the response of the patient or by the sound. Example: A metal mirror handle is used to tap each tooth successively. When a tooth is known to be painful to movement, percussion should be avoided.

E. Electrical Test

An electrical pulp vitality tester is used to detect the presence or absence of vital pulp tissue. The technique for use is described on page 244.

F. Auscultation

Auscultation is the use of sound. An example is the sound of clicking or snapping of the temporomandibular joint when the jaw is moved.

TOOTH NUMBERING SYSTEMS

There are three tooth designation systems in general use. They are the *Continuous Numbers 1 through 32* as adopted by the American Dental Association;[1] the *F.D.I. Two-digit*, adopted by the Federation Dentaire Internationale;[2] and the use of *Quadrant Numbers 1 through 8*. Since dentists have learned different systems, it behooves each auxiliary person to be familiar with all.

I. Continuous Numbers 1 Through 32

This tooth numbering method is referred to as the *universal* or *ADA* system.

A. Permanent Teeth

Start with the right maxillary third molar (Number 1) and follow around the arch to the left maxillary third molar (16); descend to the left mandibular third molar (17), and follow around to the right mandibular third molar (32). Figure III–I shows the crowns of the teeth with the corresponding numbers.

B. Primary or Deciduous Teeth

Use continuous upper case letters A through T in the same order as described for the permanent teeth: right maxillary second molar (A) around to left maxillary second molar (J); descend to left mandibular second molar (K), and around to the right mandibular second molar (T).

II. F.D.I. Two-Digit

The *FDI* system is also called the *International*.

A. Permanent Teeth

The first digit indicates the quadrant; starting with the maxillary right (quadrant 1) to maxillary left (quadrant 2), mandibular left (quadrant 3) and mandibular right (quadrant 4). The second digit indicates the number of the tooth within the quadrant, starting with number one at the midline and counting to number eight, the third molar (figure III–2).

It is recommended that the digits be pronounced separately. For example, "two-five" means the maxillary left second premolar, and "four-two" is the mandibular right lateral incisor.

B. Primary or Deciduous Teeth

The quadrants for the primary teeth are numbered to continue with the permanent teeth. The maxillary right quadrant is Number 5, maxillary left is 6, mandibular left is 7, and mandibular right is 8. Second numbers are 1 through 5 to correspond with the primary teeth from the midline (Figure III–2). For example, "eight-three" is the mandibular right primary canine, and "six-five" is the maxillary left second primary molar.

III. Quadrant Numbers 1 Through 8

Names to identify this method are the *symbolic* or *Palmer system*.

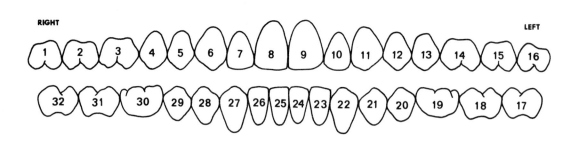

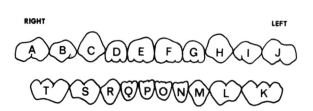

Figure III–1. **Upper.** Tooth Numbering System: Continuous Numbers 1 through 32. Each tooth is designated by a specific number starting with the right maxillary third molar (Number 1), and following around to the left maxillary third molar (Number 16), to the left mandibular third molar (17), back around to the right mandibular third molar (32). **Lower.** Primary teeth are designated by letters.

PERMANENT TEETH

Maxillary right

Maxillary left

1–8	1–7	1–6	1–5	1–4	1–3	1–2	1–1	2–1	2–2	2–3	2–4	2–5	2–6	2–7	2–8
4–8	4–7	4–6	4–5	4–4	4–3	4–2	4–1	3–1	3–2	3–3	3–4	3–5	3–6	3–7	3–8

Mandibular right

Mandibular left

PRIMARY TEETH

Maxillary right

Maxillary left

5–5	5–4	5–3	5–2	5–1	6–1	6–2	6–3	6–4	6–5
8–5	8–4	8–3	8–2	8–1	7–1	7–2	7–3	7–4	7–5

Mandibular right

Mandibular left

Figure III–2. Tooth Numbering System: F.D.I. Two-digit. Each quadrant is numbered 1 through 4, Number 1 the maxillary right, Number 2 the maxillary left, 3 the mandibular left, and 4 the mandibular right. Each tooth is numbered by the quadrant number and by the number of the tooth within the quadrant, starting with number 1 at the midline, to 8 the third molar. The quadrants of the primary teeth continue with the permanent teeth, from 5 (maxillary right) through 8 (mandibular right).

PERMANENT TEETH

Maxillary right

Maxillary left

8	7	6	5	4	3	2	1	1	2	3	4	5	6	7	8
8	7	6	5	4	3	2	1	1	2	3	4	5	6	7	8

Mandibular right

Mandibular left

PRIMARY TEETH

Maxillary right

Maxillary left

E	D	C	B	A	A	B	C	D	E
E	D	C	B	A	A	B	C	D	E

Mandibular right

Mandibular left

Figure III–3. Tooth Numbering System: Quadrant Numbers 1 through 8. With Number 1 for each central incisor, the teeth in each quadrant are numbered to 8 the third molar. See text for quadrant designation method. Primary teeth are identified by upper case letters A through E.

A. Permanent Teeth

With Number 1 for each central incisor, the teeth in each quadrant are numbered to 8, the third molar (figure III–3). To identify individual teeth, horizontal and vertical lines are used, drawn to indicate the quadrant. For example, the left maxillary first premolar is ⌊4, the right mandibular first and second molars are 76⌉. An entire quadrant may be represented by the use of the letter Q, for example the maxillary right quadrant is Q⌋.

B. Primary or Deciduous Teeth

Upper case letters A through E are used instead of the numbers. Examples are the mandibular left canine ‾C, and the maxillary right first primary molar D⌋.

References

1. American Dental Association: System of Tooth Numbering and Radiograph Mounting, Approved by the American Dental Association House of Delegates, October, 1968.
2. New F.D.I. Two-Digit Tooth-Recording System, *F.D.I. Newsletter* (London), No. 74, 1971.

Suggested Readings

Allen, D.L., McFall, W.T., and Hunter, G.C.: *Periodontics for the Dental Hygienist,* 3rd ed. Philadelphia, Lea & Febiger, 1980, pp. 97–138.

American Dental Association, Council on Dental Care Programs: Code on Dental Procedures and Nomenclature, *J. Am. Dent. Assoc., 104,* 351, March, 1982.

Brightman, V.J.: Rational Procedures for Diagnosis, in Lynch, M.A., ed.: *Burket's Oral Medicine, Diagnosis and Treatment,* 7th ed. Philadelphia, J.B. Lippincott Co., 1977, pp. 2–26.

Goldman, H.M. and Cohen, D.W.: *Periodontal Therapy,* 6th ed. St. Louis, The C.V. Mosby Co., 1980, pp. 303–377.

Ibsen, O.A.: Application of Diagnostic Methods in Oral Disease, *N.Y. J. Dent., 48,* 209, August-September, 1978.

Kerr, D.A., Ash, M.M., and Millard, H.D.: *Oral Diagnosis,* 5th ed. St. Louis, The C.V. Mosby Co., 1978, pp. 3–15, 85–89.

Komensky, A.M.: Ownership and Maintenance of Dental Records, *J. Am. Dent. Assoc., 97,* 44, July, 1978.

McCarthy, F.M. and Malamed, S.F.: Physical Evaluation System to Determine Medical Risk and Indicated Dental Therapy Modifications, *J. Am. Dent. Assoc., 99,* 181, August, 1979.

Mitchell, D.F., Standish, S.M., and Fast, T.B.: *Oral Diagnosis/Oral Medicine,* 3rd ed. Philadelphia, Lea & Febiger, 1978, pp. 1–2, 111–124.

Ramfjord, S.P. and Ash, M.M.: *Periodontology and Perio-* *dontics.* Philadelphia, W.B. Saunders Co., 1979, pp. 247–309.

Dental Photography

DeVore, D.T.: Radiology and Photography in Forensic Dentistry, *Dent. Clin. North Am., 21,* 69, January, 1977.

Freehe, C.L.: Clinical Dental Photography: Equipment and Techniques, in Clark, J.W., ed.: *Clinical Dentistry, Volume 1,* Chapter 1. Hagerstown, Maryland, Harper & Row, 1981, pp. 1–50.

Hurtgen, T.: Kodak Instant Close-up Camera. The Newest Close-up Camera, *Dent. Radiogr. Photogr., 52,* 20, Number 1, 1979.

Kaiser, D.A. and Walters, G.R.: Intraoral Photographic Survey, *J. Prosthet. Dent., 40,* 457, October, 1978.

Llewelyn, J. and Addy, M.: A Photographic Method for the Assessment of Examiner Accuracy and Variability for the Scoring Criteria of the Debris Index, *J. Periodontol., 50,* 84, February, 1979.

Lorson, E.L.: Simplified Approach to Clinical Photography, *J. Oral Surg., 34,* 1035, November, 1976.

Nuckles, D.B., McCall, W.J., and Jones, C.R.: Close-up Photography in the Dental Office, *J. Am. Dent. Assoc., 90,* 152, January, 1975.

Smith, G.E. and Hodson, J.T.: Serial Photography for Operative Dentistry, *J. Am. Dent. Assoc., 88,* 1004, May, 1974.

Stutts, W.F.: Clinical Photography in Orthodontic Practice, *Am. J. Orthod., 74,* 1, July, 1978.

Woodall, I.R., Dafoe, B.R., Young, N.S., Weed-Fonner, L., and Yankell, S.L.: *Comprehensive Dental Hygiene Care.* St. Louis, The C.V. Mosby Co., 1980, pp. 175–192.

6

Personal, Medical, and Dental History

For safe, scientific dental and dental hygiene care, a meaningful, complete patient history is necessary. The history directs and guides steps to be taken in preparation for, during, and following appointments.

At least a part of the history is needed before oral examination procedures with periodontal probe and explorer are carried out. The use of instruments that would manipulate the soft tissue around the teeth may be contraindicated in certain instances until after a medical consultation to determine whether protective, precautionary measures are needed.

When there is a question about the medical history as described by the patient or when an unusual or abnormal condition is observed, consultation with the patient's physician, or referral for examination of the patient who does not have a physician, is mandatory. Even emergency treatment such as for the relief of pain should be postponed tentatively or kept to a minimum until the patient's status is determined.

The significance of the history cannot be overestimated. Oral conditions reflect the general health of the patient. Dental procedures may complicate or be complicated by existing pathologic or physiologic conditions elsewhere in the body. General health factors influence response to treatment, such as tissue healing, and thereby affect the outcomes that may be expected from oral care.

The state of the patient's health is constantly changing. Therefore, the history represents the period in the patient's life in which the history was made. With successive recall appointments the history must be reviewed and considered along with other new findings.

I. Purposes of the History

Carefully prepared personal, medical, and dental histories are used in comprehensive patient care to

A. Provide information pertinent to the etiology and diagnosis of oral conditions and the total treatment plan.

B. Reveal conditions that necessitate precautions, modifications, or adaptations during appointments to assure that dental and dental hygiene procedures will not harm the patient and that emergency situations will be prevented.

C. Aid in the identification of possible unrecognized conditions for which the patient should be referred for further diagnosis and treatment.

D. Permit appraisal of the general health and nutritional status, which in turn, contributes to the prognosis of success in patient care and instruction.

E. Give insight into emotional and psychologic factors, attitudes, and prejudices, which may affect present appointments as well as continuing care.

85

F. Document records for reference and comparison over a series of appointments for periodic follow-up.

G. Furnish evidence in legal matters should questions arise.

II. History Preparation

The general methods in current use are the *interview*, the *questionnaire*, or a combination of the two. There are several systems for obtaining the history.

A. Alternative Appointment Procedures

1. *Complete history* made at the initial visit: may be a combination of interview and questionnaire.

2. *Brief history* of vital items obtained at the initial visit; complete history obtained at a succeeding appointment.

   a. Purposes of brief history: to prepare for emergency care and to learn of any condition that may contraindicate instrumentation in and around the gingival sulcus during dental and periodontal examinations.

   b. Brief history may be in the form of a questionnaire, while an interview for follow-up provides opportunity for individual evaluation.

3. *Self-history* prepared at home: the history form may be mailed to the patient in advance or given at the first appointment to complete and bring in at the second appointment. Such a form might include some checking, as in a questionnaire, and some space to allow free expression by the patient.

B. Record Forms

1. *Types.* Many varying forms are in current use. Forms are available commercially or from the American Dental Association,[1] but many dentists and dental hygienists prefer to prepare their own design and have the form printed to their specifications.

2. *Characteristics of an Adequate Form.* The number of items or questions included is not necessarily indicative of the value of the form. The extensive and involved form may be as practical or impractical as the brief checklist that permits no detailed description. Success in use depends on function and a clear common understanding of the meaning of the recorded information to all who will refer to it.

Some characteristics of an adequate form are that it should

a. Provide for convenient notation of important details in a logical sequence.

b. Permit quick identification of special needs of a patient when the history is reviewed prior to each appointment.

c. Allow ample space to record the patient's own words whenever possible in the interview method, or for self-expression by the patient on a questionnaire.

d. Have space for notes concerning attitudes and knowledge as stated or displayed by the patient during the history-taking or other later appointments.

e. Be of a size consistent with the complete patient record forms for filing and ready availability.

C. Introduction to the Patient

The patient needs to realize why the information requested in the histories is essential before treatment can be undertaken. Dental personnel must convey the idea that oral health and general health are interrelated, without creating undue alarm concerning potential ill effects or harmful sequelae from required treatment.

For building rapport, children may participate in their history preparation, but most of the information will need to be supplied by a parent. The signature of the responsible adult on the record is advisable.

D. Limitations of a History[2,3,4]

Many patients cannot or will not provide complete or, in certain cases, correct information when answering medical or dental history questions. There may be problems related to the method of obtaining the histories, how the questions are worded, or an inadvertent lack of neutrality in attitude of the person preparing the history. Some patients may have difficulty in comprehending a self-administered test, or there may be a language barrier.

Another reason for inaccuracy or incompleteness is that patients may not understand a relationship between certain diseases or conditions and having dental treatment. Information may seem irrelevant, so it is withheld. Occasionally, a patient will not want to tell about a condition that may be embarrassing to discuss. The patient may fear refusal of treatment, particularly if there had been previous experiences in other dental practices.

Studies conducted to determine the reliability of a medical history in identifying patients who are positive for hepatitis B antigen were described on page 48.

III. The Questionnaire

Positive findings on a completed questionnaire need supplementation in a personal interview. A questionnaire by itself cannot be expected to satisfy the overall purposes of the history, but can be adapted best to phases of the personal history, some aspects of the dental history, and factual information in the medical history.

A. Types of Questions

The Health Questionnaire available from the American Dental Assocation (figure 6–1) provides useful examples of questions essential to patient evaluation.[1] In addition, there is a short form available in which questions are directed to provide information on drug use, allergies, and current medical treatment for preliminary or emergency use.*

1. *System-oriented.* Direct questions or topics to check whether or not the patient has had a disease of, for example, the digestive system, respiratory system, or urinary system may be used. The questions may contain specific body parts, for example the stomach, lungs, kidneys. Specific questions can then be

directed to the specific disease state and the dates of duration.

2. *Disease-oriented.* A typical set of questions for the patient to check may start with "Do you have, or have you had, any of the following diseases or problems?" A listing under that question contains items such as diabetes, asthma, rheumatic fever, arranged alphabetically or grouped by systems or body organs.

Follow-up questions can determine dates of illness, severity, and outcome. Suggested questions for determining information related to communicable diseases were listed on page 48.

3. *Symptom-oriented.* In the absence of previous or current disease states, questions may lead to a suspicion of a condition, which, in turn, can provide an opportunity to recommend and encourage the patient to schedule an examination by a physician. Samples of the symptom-oriented question appear in figure 6–1; for example, "Are you thirsty much of the time?" "Does your mouth frequently become dry?" or "Do you have to urinate (pass water) more than six times a day?" the positive answers for which could lead to tests for diabetes detection.

B. Advantages of a Questionnaire

1. Broad in scope: useful during the interview to identify positive areas that need additional clarification.
2. Time saving.
3. Consistent: all selected questions are included, and none omitted because of time or other factors.
4. Patient has time to think over the answers: not under pressure, nor under the eyes of the interviewer.
5. Patient may write information that might not be expressed directly in an interview.
6. Legal aspect of a written record with patient's signature.

C. Disadvantages of a Questionnaire (if used alone without a follow-up interview)

1. Impersonal: no opportunity to develop rapport.

---

*Copies of the questionnaires are obtainable in quantity. Request the A.D.A. Catalog and order form from the Order Department, American Dental Association, 211 E. Chicago Ave., Chicago, Ill. 60611. The catalog numbers are: Health Questionnaire P1-HQ (Long Form) and P1-HQ 1 (Short Form).

MEDICAL HISTORY

Date _____

Name _____ Address _____
 Last   First   Middle   Number & Street

City   State   Zip Code   Home & Business Phone

Date of Birth_____ Sex _____ Height _____ Weight _____ Occupation_____

Married   Spouse _____ Single _____

Closest Relative _____ Phone _____

If you are completing this form for another person, what is your relationship to that person?_____

In the following questions, circle yes or no, whichever applies. Your answers are for our records only and will be considered confidential.

1. Are you in good health . . . . YES   NO
2. Has there been any change in your general health within the past year . . . . YES   NO
3. My last physical examination was on _____
4. Are you now under the care of a physician . . . . YES   NO
     a. If so, what is the condition being treated _____
5. The name and address of my physician is   _____
                                                 _____
                                                 _____
                                                 _____
6. Have you had any serious illness or operation . . . . YES   NO
     a. If so, what was the illness or operation _____
7. Have you been hospitalized or had a serious illness within the past five (5) years . . . . YES   NO
     a. If so, what was the problem _____
8. Do you have or have you had any of the following diseases or problems.
     a. Rheumatic fever or rheumatic heart disease . . . . YES   NO
     b. Congenital heart lesions . . . . YES   NO
     c. Cardiovascular disease (heart trouble, heart attack, coronary insufficiency, coronary occlusion,
        high blood pressure, arteriosclerosis, stroke) . . . . YES   NO
        1) Do you have pain in chest upon exertion . . . . YES   NO
        2) Are you ever short of breath after mild exercise . . . . YES   NO
        3) Do your ankles swell . . . . YES   NO
        4) Do you get short of breath when you lie down, or do you require extra pillows when you sleep . . . . YES   NO
        5) Do you have a cardiac pacemaker . . . . YES   NO
     d. Allergy . . . . YES   NO
     e. Sinus trouble . . . . YES   NO
     f. Asthma or hay fever . . . . YES   NO
     g. Hives or a skin rash . . . . YES   NO
     h. Fainting spells or seizures . . . . YES   NO
     i. Diabetes . . . . YES   NO
        1) Do you have to urinate (pass water) more than six times a day . . . . YES   NO
        2) Are you thirsty much of the time . . . . YES   NO
        3) Does your mouth frequently become dry . . . . YES   NO
     j. Hepatitis, jaundice or liver disease . . . . YES   NO
     k. Arthritis . . . . YES   NO
     l. Inflammatory rheumatism (painful swollen joints) . . . . YES   NO
     m. Stomach ulcers . . . . YES   NO
     n. Kidney trouble . . . . YES   NO
     o. Tuberculosis . . . . YES   NO
     p. Do you have a persistent cough or cough up blood . . . . YES   NO
     q. Low blood pressure . . . . YES   NO
     r. Venereal disease . . . . YES   NO
     s. Other _____

(over)

Figure 6–1. Health Questionnaire. From *Accepted Dental Therapeutics*. Copyright by the American Dental Association. Reprinted by permission.

9. Have you had abnormal bleeding associated with previous extractions, surgery, or trauma .... YES   NO

    a. Do you bruise easily .... YES   NO

    b. Have you ever required a blood transfusion .... YES   NO

       If so, explain the circumstances _____

10. Do you have any blood disorder such as anemia .... YES   NO

11. Have you had surgery or x-ray treatment for a tumor, growth, or other condition of your head or neck .... YES   NO

12. Are you taking any drug or medicine... YES   NO

    If so, what _____

13. Are you taking any of the following:

    a. Antibiotics or sulfa drugs .... YES   NO

    b. Anticoagulants (blood thinners) .... YES   NO

    c. Medicine for high blood pressure... YES   NO

    d. Cortisone (steroids) .... YES   NO

    e. Tranquilizers .... YES   NO

    f. Antihistamines .... YES   NO

    g. Aspirin .... YES   NO

    h. Insulin, tolbutamide (Orinase) or similar drug .... YES   NO

    i. Digitalis or drugs for heart trouble .... YES   NO

    j. Nitroglycerin .... YES   NO

    k. Oral contraceptive or other hormonal therapy .... YES   NO

    l. Other _____

14. Are you allergic or have you reacted adversely to:

    a. Local anesthetics .... YES   NO

    b. Penicillin or other antibiotics .... YES   NO

    c. Sulfa drugs .... YES   NO

    d. Barbiturates, sedatives, or sleeping pills .... YES   NO

    e. Aspirin .... YES   NO

    f. Iodine.. YES   NO

    g. Codeine or other narcotics .... YES   NO

    h. Other _____

15. Have you had any serious trouble associated with any previous dental treatment .... YES   NO

    If so, explain _____

16. Do you have any disease, condition, or problem not listed above that you think I should know about .... YES   NO

    If so, explain _____

17. Are you employed in any situation which exposes you regularly to x-rays or other ionizing radiation .... YES   NO

18. Are you wearing contact lenses .... YES   NO

WOMEN

19. Are you pregnant .... YES   NO

20. Do you have any problems associated with your menstrual period .... YES   NO

CHIEF DENTAL COMPLAINT:

_____
SIGNATURE OF PATIENT

_____
SIGNATURE OF DENTIST

P1 HQ

Figure 6–1. (Continued)

2. Inflexible: no provision for additional questioning in areas of specific importance to an individual patient.

IV. The Interview

In long-range planning for the patient's health, much more is involved than asking questions and receiving answers. The rapport established at the time of the interview contributes to the continued cooperation of the patient.

A. Participants

The dental hygienist is alone with the patient or parent of the child patient. The history should never be taken in a reception room when other patients are present.

B. Setting

1. A consultation room or office is preferred; the patient should be away from the atmosphere of the operatory where thoughts may be on the techniques to be performed.
2. Operatory: may be the only available place where privacy is afforded.
   a. Seat patient comfortably in upright position.
   b. Turn off running water and dental light, and close the door.
   c. Sit on operating stool to be at eye level with the patient.

C. Pointers for the Interview

Interviewing involves communication between individuals. Communication implies the transmission or interchange of facts, attitudes, opinions, or thoughts, through words, gestures, or other means. Through tactful but direct questioning, communication can be successful and the patient will give such information as is known. Frequently the patient is unaware of a health problem.

The attitude of the dental personnel should be one of friendly understanding, reassurance, and acceptance. Genuine interest and willingness to listen when a patient wishes to describe symptoms or complaints not only aids in establishing the rapport needed, but frequently provides insight into the patient's real attitudes and prejudices. By asking simple questions at first, and more

personal questions later after rapport has developed, the patient will be more relaxed and frank in answering.

Self-confidence and gentle efficiency on the part of the dental hygienist help to give the patient a feeling of confidence. Skill is required, since tact, ingenuity, and judgment are taxed to the fullest in the attempt to obtain both accurate and complete information from the patient.

D. Interview Form

The interviewer may use a structured form with places to check and fill in, or record on blank sheets from questions created from a guide list of essential topics. Either may involve reference to the positive or negative answers on a previously completed questionnaire. Familiarity with the items on the history will permit the interviewer to be direct and informal without reading from a fixed list of topics, a method that may lack the personal touch necessary to gain the patient's confidence. When appropriate, the patient's own words are recorded.

E. Advantages of the Interview

1. Personal contact contributes to development of rapport for future appointments.
2. Flexibility for individual needs: details obtained can be adapted for supplementary questioning.

F. Disadvantages of Interview

1. Time-consuming when not prefaced with questionnaire.
2. Unless a list is consulted, items of importance may be omitted.
3. Patient may be embarrassed to talk about personal conditions and may hold back significant information.

V. Items Included in the History

Information obtained by means of the history is directly related to how the goals of dental and dental hygiene care can and will be accomplished. In tables 6–1, 6–2, and 6–3, items are listed with suggested influences on appointment procedures. Objectives for the items to include in the various parts of the history are listed below.

In specialized practices, objectives may require increased emphasis on certain aspects. The age group most frequently served would influence the material needed. Parental history and pre- and postnatal information may take on particular significance for the treatment of a small child; in a pedodontist's practice, a special form could be devised to include all essential items.

Insight and awareness shown while preparing the patient history depends on background knowledge of the oral manifestations of systemic diseases, medications for various conditions, and drug–drug interactions.[5,6,7] Interpretation of findings and alertness to immediate needs for application are described on page 99.

A. **Personal History** (table 6–1)

The basic objectives in gathering the personal information about the patient are:
1. Data essential for appointment planning and business aspects.
2. Approval of care of a minor, and other legal aspects.
3. Patient's physician: for consultation relative to interrelations between general and oral health.

B. **Medical History** (table 6–2)

Objectives of the medical history are to determine whether the patient has any conditions in the following categories.
1. Diseases that may contraindicate certain kinds of dental and dental hygiene treatment.
   Examples. Leukemia, because of lowered resistance to infection; uncontrolled hypertensive patient with blood pressure reading 180/105 or greater; congestive heart failure requires treatment before stressful procedures, particularly surgery, can be performed.
2. Diseases that require special precautions or premedication prior to treatment.
   Examples. Antibiotic coverage for patient with a history of rheumatic fever or congenital heart defect to prevent infective endocarditis; patient subject to convulsions who may need increased sedation to prevent a seizure if treatment is to be stressful.
3. Diseases under treatment by a physician which require medicating drugs which may influence or contraindicate procedures of the dental or dental hygiene appointments.
   Examples. Tranquilizers in daily use could contraindicate premedication with sedatives; anticoagulant therapy requires consultation with physician; antihypertensive drug may alter the general or local anesthetic used.
4. Allergic or untoward reactions to drugs.
   Examples. All drugs that may possibly be used or recommended to the patient for postoperative care should be checked with the patient as to previous use and reaction.
5. Diseases and drugs with manifestations in the mouth.
   Examples. Hematologic disorders; phenytoin-induced gingival overgrowth.
6. Diseases that endanger the dental personnel.
   Examples. Active tuberculosis; hepatitis, herpes, syphilis.
7. Physiologic state of the patient.
   Examples. Pregnancy, puberty, menopause.

C. **Dental History** (table 6–3, page 97)

The dental history should contribute to knowledge of
1. The immediate problem, chief complaint, cause of present pain, or discomfort of any kind in the oral cavity.
2. The previous dental care as described by the patient, including extent of restorative and prosthetic replacement, as well as any adverse effects.
3. The attitude of the patient toward oral health and care of the mouth as may be indicated by previous periodic dental and dental hygiene treatment.
4. The personal daily care exercised by the patient as evidence of knowledge of the purposes of continuing care and of the value placed on the teeth and their supporting structures.

Table 6–1.   Items for the Personal History

Items to Record in Patient History	Considerations	Influences on Appointment Procedures

1. **Name**
   Addresses: Residence and Business
   Telephone Numbers
   Sex
   Marital Status
   For Child: Name of Parent or Guardian
   For Parent: Ages and Sex of Children
	Accurate recording necessary for business aspects of dental practice	Aids in establishing rapport
		
		Instruction applicable to entire family
		Advice concerning fluorides for children

2. **Birthdate**	Whether of age or a minor Oral conditions related to age changes; diseases, healing, and other possible characteristics	Approval of parent or guardian necessary for care of minor or person with a mental handicap; signature must be obtained Approach to patient instruction
3. **Birthplace and Residence in Early Years**	Presence of fluoride in drinking water. Food and eating patterns Conditions endemic to certain areas	Effects of fluoride on teeth Instruction in dietary needs adapted to cultural practices

4. **Occupation: Present and Former**
 	
   Spouse's Occupation
 	
   For Children: Parent's Occupation
	May be a factor in etiology of certain diseases, dental stains, occlusal wear
	
	May affect diet, oral habits, general health
		Instruction applied to specific needs
		
		Dexterity in use of self-care devices related to dexterity gained from occupation
		
		Influence on oral care of entire family
		For child: which parent will supervise and assist child in oral care

5. **Physician**	Name, address, and telephone number For consultation	Consultation indicated: (1) for condition which may require premedication (2) when disease symptoms are suspected but patient does not state (3) in an emergency
6. **Referred by and Address**	To whom to send referral acknowledgment and appreciation	Contribution to rapport with patient Patient referred by another patient may have concept of the office procedures

Table 6–2. Items for the Medical History

Item to Record in the History	Considerations	Influences on Appointment Procedures
1. **General Health and Appearance**	Disabilities Overall impression of well-being Patient's appraisal of own health	Response, cooperation and attitude to expect during appointments
2. **Medical Examination**	Date most recent examination Reason for the examination Tests performed; results Anticipated surgery	May need verification with the physician if questions exist Need for superior state of oral health in advance of surgery (1) when long recovery is expected and patient may miss recall (2) prior to transplant, heart surgery or prosthesis
3. **Major Illnesses and Hospitalizations**	Causes of illness Type and duration of treatment Anesthetics used Convalescence Course of healing: normal, not normal	Influence of illnesses on health and care of the oral cavity Anesthetic choice Healing to anticipate following gingival treatments
4. **Height and Weight**	Weight changes over past years or months Obesity Undernourishment Child growth pattern	Marked weight change may be a symptom of undiagnosed disease; suggest referral for medical examination Influence on dietary instructions for oral health
5. **Current Treatment by Physician**	Nature and duration of illness	Effects on dental and dental hygiene procedures and personal care
6. **Radiation Therapy**	Reason, location, duration Head and neck radiation: susceptibility to osteoradionecrosis	Effect on oral radiographic survey: prevention of over-exposure Caries: preventive measures Xerostomia: substitute saliva
7. **Medication: prescribed by physician**	Drugs, medicine, injections, tonics, vitamins, pills: past and present, purpose Drug-drug interactions with possible dental prescriptions Effects on oral tissues	Consultation with physician concerning adjustments in dosage for dental or dental hygiene appointments Indications for premedication Problem of xerostomia associated with many drugs (diuretics, tranquilizers, estrogens, antihistamines are examples) Inhibition of inflammatory response (steroid therapy, for example)

Table 6–2. *continued*

Item to Record in the History	Considerations	Influences on Appointment Procedures
8. Self-medication	Type and frequency Drug abuse	Information not revealed by patient could complicate treatment Lack of interest in oral health, only pain relief
9. Familial Medical History	Predisposition to certain diseases (example: diabetes) History of diseases which occur in the family	May help patient seek medical examination when symptom suggests possible disease
10. Daily Diet	Recommendations of patient's physician, past and present Vitamin supplements Appetite Regularity of meals Food likes and dislikes	Instructions to be given relative to oral health Prognosis for healing after treatment Need for dietary review and analysis (page 423)
11. Use of Alcohol	Frequency Quantity	Excessive use: effect on anesthesia; increased healing time Poor nutritional state is common; lack of oral care May result in poor patient cooperation
12. Communicable Disease	Stage of disease; current therapy Degree of communicability; susceptibility of dental personnel Residences or extended vacations in countries with high endemic incidences of certain diseases	Request laboratory tests for unknown disease or suspected carrier state Wear face mask, gloves, or other precautionary measure Consultation with physician
A. Hepatitis	If patient had jaundice whether diagnosed as hepatitis or not, treat as a carrier Date of termination of disease Likelihood of carrier state	Observe maximum precautions (page 64) Postpone elective treatment when possible
B. Venereal Disease	Oral lesion may be present May not obtain history	Wear gloves for oral examination (pages 57–58)
C. Tuberculosis	Active or passive Current treatment	Passive: use supplementary aseptic technique; wear face mask Active: techniques performed under hospital sterile procedures
13. Allergies	Determine substances to which the patient is allergic Anesthetics Penicillin Medicaments Foods Iodine	Avoid use of substances to which the patient is allergic Consider allergies when planning dietary recommendations

Table 6–2. *continued*

Item to Record in the History	Considerations	Influences on Appointment Procedures
14. Respiratory Problems Asthma Bronchitis Bronchiectasis Emphysema	Agents which may bring on attack Prevention measures Breathing problems Coughing spells	Chair position for appointments Anesthesia choice
15. Diabetes	Uncontrolled requires antibiotic premedication Ask patient when insulin was taken Diet and medication requirements Family incidence: identification of susceptible but undiagnosed	Appointment time related to insulin therapy and mealtime Avoid tissue trauma Need frequent recall Preparation for emergencies (pages 826, 848–849)
16. Cardiovascular Diseases	Category and history of disease (page 775) Type of treatment; medication Consultation with physician Pacemaker Prosthetic heart valves Low salt diet	Short appointment to prevent fatigue Selection of anesthesia; premedication Preparation for emergencies Emphasis on preventive oral care measures Avoid hot salt rinses for patient on low salt diet
A. High Blood Pressure	May be a symptom of other disease state Current therapy Choice of anesthetic	Length of appointment Allay fears to prevent apprehension
B. Congenital Heart Disease and Rheumatic Heart Disease	History of rheumatic fever Current therapy Consultation with physician	Prophylactic antibiotic to prevent infective endocarditis (pages 99–100)
17. Blood Diseases	Type and duration Current therapy Consultation with physician Need for high level of oral health	Serious condition: palliative treatment may be all that is possible Frequent recall to prevent long, tiring appointments and to administer preventive service
18. Bleeding	Previous experiences: causes, treatment History of disorder with coagulation problem History of transfusions or other blood products Check use of aspirin (relation to bleeding tendency) Laboratory tests for bleeding time, coagulation, may be needed	Emergency prevention through pre-appointment precautions Avoid tissue trauma Test for HBsAg Carrier May need to apply dressing after scaling to provide pressure Special measures for hemophilia (pages 813–815)

Table 6–2. **continued**

Item to Record in the History	Considerations	Influences on Appointment Procedures
19. Eyes	Purpose for correction with eyeglasses, contact lenses Manifestations of systemic disease	Protection of eyes during instrumentation, especially handpiece and ultrasonic scaler Adaptations for blind or partially sighted (pages 765–766) Use of glasses during patient instruction
20. Ears	Deafness or degree of hearing impairment Infections, operations	Adaptations for instruction (pages 770–771)
21. Nasal Sinuses, Tonsils, Adenoids	Mouthbreathing as a possible factor in gingival disease Breathing problems during appointment	Chair positioning for gagging or breathing problem Personal care emphasis for effects of mouthbreathing
22. Gastrointestinal Disease	Nature and treatment of the disease Diet restrictions prescribed by physician	Patient instruction in accord with prescribed diet and medication
23. Epilepsy	Frequency of seizures Medications prescribed Consultation may be indicated Minimize stress during appointment	Gingival overgrowth from phenytoin therapy (page 725) Preparation for emergency (pages 727, 850)
24. Endocrine Influences	Nature of possible problem related to age group Possible oral manifestations Current therapy Effect of birth control pills, estrogens	Emphasis on high level of plaque control Adaptations of procedures during appointments (pages 617–618, 621)
25. Pregnancy	Month, parturition date Possible oral manifestations History of previous pregnancies	Adjust physical arrangements for patient comfort Adapt techniques (pages 610–611) Need for frequent recall

26. Physical Disabilities	Extent of disability
	Nature, cause, treatment
	  Cerebral palsy
	  Multiple sclerosis
	  Arthritis
	  Poliomyelitis
	  Other (Chapter 54)
	Consult physician for special precautions; possible effects related to current medications
	Prosthetic joint replacement
		Adjustment of physical arrangements
		Wheelchair accessibility and transfer
		Adaptations of techniques and instruction needs
		
		Need for prophylactic antibiotic premedication

27. Mental, psychiatric, psychological	Emotional problems expressed by patient Medications	Mental retardation: special adaptations (pages 735, 738–739) Attitudes toward personal care

Table 6–3. Items for the Dental History

Items to Record in the History	Considerations	Influences on Appointment Procedures
1. **Reason for Present Appointment**	Chief complaint in patient's own words Pain or discomfort Onset, symptoms, duration of an acute condition	Need for immediate treatment Attitude toward dentistry and preventive care
2. **Previous Dental Appointments**	Date last treatment Services performed Regularity	Patient knowledge concerning regular dental care Cooperation anticipated
3. **Anesthetics Used**	Local, general Adverse or allergic reactions	Choice of anesthetic
4. **Radiographs**	Date most recent survey Availability from previous dentist Amount of exposure considered with exposure for medical purposes	Amount of exposure: limitations Patient's appreciation for need and use of radiographs
5. **Family Dental History**	Parental tooth loss or maintenance	Attitude toward saving teeth and preventive dentistry
6. **Previous Treatment**	Type of treatment; frequency of recall Whether referred to specialist	Attitude toward specialized care Previous familiarity with role of dental hygienist
A. Periodontal	History of acute infection (necrotizing ulcerative gingivitis, page 535) Surgery; postoperative healing	Attitude toward self-care and disease control
B. Orthodontic	Age during treatment; completion Previous problem Habit correction	For current treatment, consultation with orthodontist needed to determine instructions
C. Endodontic	Dates, etiology	Periodic recheck
D. Prosthodontic	Types of prostheses	Care of prostheses and abutment teeth
E. Other	Extent of restorations	Understanding toward prevention
7. **Injuries to Face or Teeth**	Causes and extent Fractured teeth or jaws	Limitation of opening Special care during healing (pages 667–670)
8. **Temporomandibular Joint**	History of discomfort, disease, dislocation Previous treatment	Effect on opening; accessibility during instrumentation

Table 6–3. *continued*

Items to Record in the History	Considerations	Influences on Appointment Procedures
9. Habits	Clenching, bruxism, doodling Mouth breathing Biting objects: fingernails, pipe stem, thread, other Cheek or lip biting Patient awareness of habits	Tension of patient Instruction relative to effects of habits
10. Smoking	Form of tobacco, amount used Frequency Knowledge of effects on oral tissues	Instruction concerning oral effects Need for frequent observation to detect tissue changes if patient continues at same rate Tooth stains; dentifrice selection
11. Fluorides	Systemic, topical, dates Residences during tooth development years Amount of fluoride in drinking water	Current preventive procedures and need for reevaluation
12. Plaque Control Procedures	Toothbrushing: current procedures Type of brush (manual or powered) Texture of bristles Frequency of use Age of brush; frequency of having a new brush Dentrifrice Name How selected; reason Additional cleansing devices and frequency of use Dental floss Water irrigation Perio-aid, rubber tip, or other Mouthrinse or other agents: frequency, purpose Source of instruction in care of oral cavity	Present practices and previous instruction New instruction needed; reception by patient Relation of techniques to prevention of dental caries and periodontal diseases Supervision of child by parent: current practices Problems of habit change

VI. Review of History

Updating the history at each recall evaluation appointment is essential. Changes in health status revealed by interim medical examinations or evidenced by reported illness or hospitalizations must be recorded and considered during continuing treatment.

Following a review of the previously recorded history, the questions can be directed to the patient to compare the present condition with the previous one and to determine at least the following:
A. Interim illnesses: changes in health.
B. Visits to physician: reasons and results.
C. Laboratory tests performed and the results: blood, urine, or other analyses.
D. Current medications.
E. Changes in the oral soft tissues and the teeth, observed by the patient.

IMMEDIATE APPLICATION OF PATIENT HISTORIES

Together with information from all other parts of the diagnostic work-up, the patient histories are essential to the treatment plan. Treatment planning for an individual patient is described on pages 326–331.

Prior to that, immediate evaluation of the histories is necessary before proceeding to succeeding steps in the preparation of materials for the complete diagnostic work-up. Any one of the objectives for the medical history (V., B., page 91) could alter the procedures to be accomplished.

The list that follows is not intended to be exhaustive, but rather suggestive. From these items, it is expected that the dental personnel will be alerted to precautions that may be needed.

I. Identification of Conditions That Require Medical Consultation

A. Dentist and physician need to consult relative to current therapy, medications, or health status of the patient. Immediate consultation may be needed, for example, for a patient who is taking antihypertensive medication and presents with a blood pressure reading of 180/105 or greater.
B. Patient referred for physical examination when signs of possible disease condition are apparent.
C. Patient referred for laboratory tests.

II. Communicable Disease

A history of communicable disease, either current, in the past, or recent past, requires attention to the prevention of disease transmission through direct contact, instruments, and other materials used during examination. Methods for precautions related to hepatitis and other diseases were described on page 64. Self-protection restrictions by all dental personnel are mandatory.

III. Radiation

When a patient is receiving radiation therapy, or has had recent radiation for other purposes, a complete oral radiographic survey may be contraindicated. Conference with the physician or oncologist involved may be necessary to determine the quantity of radiation received.

IV. Prophylactic Premedication

Patients susceptible to infective endocarditis must have antibiotic premedication prior to any tissue manipulation that could create a bacteremia. Tissue manipulation, particularly the use of a probe and an explorer subgingivally, must be withheld until the condition has been discussed with the patient's physician. Bacteremia created by instrumentation is described on page 508 and infective endocarditis on page 778.

Other patients who may need prophylactic premedication are those with marked reduced capacity to resist infection. There is no indication for generalized use of antibiotics in healthy persons for the purpose of preventing infection.[7]

A. **Indications for Prophylactic Premedication to Prevent Infective Endocarditis**

1. Rheumatic and congenital heart disease.[8,9]
2. Rheumatic fever and other febrile disease that predispose to valvular damage. When a patient has a heart murmur, it may be necessary to determine from the patient's physician whether the murmur is considered functional or organic. As advised by the physician, a functional murmur may not require premedica-

tion, whereas an organic murmur that is based on a defect in the structure of the heart does require antibiotic coverage.[10]

3. Prior cardiac surgery and valvular prosthesis. The patient with intracardiac prosthesis requires extensive antibiotic coverage and should be managed only under orders of the attending physician. Coverage also may be indicated for a patient with a pacemaker which has implanted wires (page 790).

4. History of previous case of infective endocarditis.

B. Other Indications for Prophylactic Premedication

1. Uncontrolled, unstable diabetes. Controlled diabetics are treated as healthy patients (pages 826–827).
2. Grossly contaminated traumatic facial injuries and compound fractures.
3. Reduced capacity to resist infection
   a. Anticancer chemotherapy.
   b. Blood disease, particularly acute leukemia and agranulocytosis.
   c. Irradiation.
   d. Corticosteroid or immunosuppressive therapy.
4. Renal transplant and hemodialysis; glomerulonephritis or other active renal disorder.[11,12]
5. Prosthetic joint replacements.[13,14]

V. Prophylactic Antibiotic Regimens

Regimens A and B are the recommendations of the American Heart Association and accepted by the American Dental Association.[8] They are reviewed periodically and updated in accord with current research findings.

Regimen A or B may be selected by the dentist or physician for any of the conditions just listed under IV except prosthetic heart valves. Regimen B is definitely indicated for patients with prosthetic heart valves.

Regimen A—Penicillin

1. *Parenteral-oral combined:*
   Adults: Aqueous crystalline penicillin G (1,000,000 units intramuscularly) **mixed with** *Procaine Penicillin G*

(600,000 units intramuscularly). Give 30 minutes to 1 hour prior to procedure and then give penicillin V (formerly called phenoxymethyl penicillin) 500 mg orally every 6 hours for 8 doses.†

Children: * *Aqueous crystalline penicillin G* (30,000 units/kg intramuscularly **mixed with** *Procaine Penicillin G* (600,000 units intramuscularly). Timing of doses for children is the same as for adults. For children less than 60 lbs. the dose of penicillin V is 250 mg orally every 6 hours for 8 doses.†

2. *Oral:‡*
   Adults: Penicillin V (2.0 gm orally 30 minutes to 1 hour prior to the procedure and then 500 mg orally every 6 hours for 8 doses.)†

   Children: * *Penicillin V* (2.0 gm orally 30 minutes to 1 hour prior to procedure and then 500 mg orally every 6 hours for 8 doses.† For children less than 60 lbs use 1.0 gm orally 30 minutes to one hour prior to the procedure and then 250 mg orally every 6 hours for 8 doses.)†

For Patients Allergic to Penicillin:

Use *either* Vancomycin (see Regimen B)

or use

Adults: Erythromycin (1.0 gm orally 1½ to 2 hours prior to the procedure and then 500 mg orally every 6 hours for 8 doses.)†

Children: Erythromycin (20 mg/kg orally 1½ to 2 hours prior to the procedure and then 10 mg/kg every 6 hours for 8 doses.)†

Regimen B—Penicillin plus Streptomycin

Adults: Aqueous crystalline penicillin G (1,000,000 units intramuscularly) **mixed with** *Procaine penicillin G* (600,000 units intramuscularly)
PLUS
Streptomycin (1 gm intramuscularly).

Give 30 minutes to 1 hour prior to the procedure; then penicillin V 500 mg orally every 6 hours for 8 doses.†

*Children:** *Aqueous crystalline penicillin G (30,000 units/kg intramuscularly)*

mixed with

Procaine penicillin G (600,000 units intramuscularly)

PLUS

Streptomycin (20 mg/kg intramuscularly).

Timing of doses for children is the same as for adults. For children less than 60 lbs. the recommended oral dose of penicillin V is 250 mg every 6 hours for 8 doses.†

For Patients Allergic to Penicillin:

Adults: Vancomycin (1 gm intravenously over 30 minutes to 1 hour). Start initial vancomycin infusion $^1/_2$ to 1 hour prior to procedure; then *erythromycin* 500 mg orally every 6 hours for 8 doses.†

*Children:** Vancomycin* (20 mg/kg intravenously over 30 minutes to 1 hour).** Timing of doses for children is the same as for adults. *Erythromycin* dose is 10 mg/kg every 6 hours for 8 doses.†

TECHNICAL HINTS

I. Date all records.

II. Keep permanent records in ink.

III. Provide a specific line on a health history form for the signature of the patient.[15] The completed history for a minor should be signed by a parent or guardian.

IV. All information obtained for a patient history must be maintained in strictest confidence.

Footnotes to Regimens:

†*In unusual circumstances or in the case of delayed healing, it may be prudent to provide additional doses of antibiotics even though available data suggest that bacteremia rarely persists longer than 15 minutes after the procedure. The physician or dentist may also choose to use the parenteral route of administration for all of the doses in selected situations.*

**Doses for children should not exceed recommendations for adults for a single dose or for a 24-hour period.*

***For vancomycin the total dose for children should not exceed 44 mg/kg/24 hours.*

‡*For those **patients receiving continuous oral penicillin for secondary prevention of rheumatic fever**, alpha hemolytic streptococci which are relatively resistant to penicillin are occasionally found in the oral cavity. While it is likely that the doses of penicillin recommended in Regimen A are sufficient to control these organisms, the physician or dentist may choose one of the suggestions in Regimen B or may choose oral erythromycin.*

V. For patients with special health problems that require premedication or other adaptation of procedure, print in red ink with a fine pen in $^1/_2$ to $^3/_4$ inch letters diagonally across all permanent record pages the identifying word such as DIABETIC, HEPATITIS, CARDIAC, or RHEUMATIC.

VI. Analyze the usefulness of items on the patient history form periodically and plan for revision as scientific research reveals new information that must be applied.

VII. A medical history update plaque is available for posting in an appropriate place in a dental office or clinic. It reads: *Please Advise Us of Any Change in Your Medical History Since Your Last Visit.* It is ADA Catalog Number P35L and is available from the American Dental Association, Order Department, 211 East Chicago Avenue, Chicago, Illinois 60611

FACTORS TO TEACH THE PATIENT

I. The need for having the personal, medical, and dental history prior to performance of dental and dental hygiene procedures.

II. The relationship between oral health and general physical health.

III. The interrelationship of medical and dental care.

IV. Advantages of cooperation in furnishing information that will help dental personnel to interpret observations accurately and to assure the dentist that the correct diagnosis and treatment plan have been made.

V. All patients who require antibiotic premedication need special emphasis on the importance of preventive dentistry, the imperative need for regular dental care, and the necessity for precautions to be taken whenever dental or dental hygiene treatment is to be given.

References

1. American Dental Association, Council on Dental Therapeutics: *Accepted Dental Therapeutics*, 39th ed. Chicago, American Dental Association, 1982, pp. 8–10.

2. Brady, W.F. and Martinoff, J.T.: Validity of Health History Data Collected from Dental Patients and Patient Perception of Health Status, *J. Am. Dent. Assoc.*, 101, 642, October, 1980.

3. Goebel, W.M.: Reliability of the Medical History in Identifying Patients Likely to Place Dentists at an In-

creased Hepatitis Risk, *J. Am. Dent. Assoc.*, 98, 907, June, 1979.
4. Pecoraro, R.E., Inui, T.S., Chen, M.S., Plorde, D.K., and Heller, J.L.: Validity and Reliability of a Self-administered Health History Questionnaire, *Pub. Health Rep.*, 94, 231, May–June, 1979.
5. American Dental Association, Council on Dental Therapeutics: op. cit., pp. 80–90.
6. Cowan, F.F.: *Pharmacology for the Dental Hygienist*. Philadelphia, Lea & Febiger, 1978, pp. 285–305.
7. Matukas, V.J. and McCallum, C.A.: The use of Antibiotics, in Clark, J.W., ed.: *Clinical Dentistry, Volume 1*, Chapter 28. Hagerstown, Maryland, Harper & Row, 1981, pp. 1–7.
8. American Heart Association: Prevention of Bacterial Endocarditis, *Circulation*, 65, 139A, July, 1977; *J. Am. Dent. Assoc.*, 95, 600, September, 1977.
9. American Dental Association, Council on Dental Therapeutics: op. cit., p. 11.
10. Kerr, D.A., Ash, M.M., and Millard, H.D.: *Oral Diagnosis*, 5th ed. St. Louis, The C.V. Mosby Co., 1978, p. 364.
11. Westbrook, S.D.: Dental Management of Patients Receiving Hemodialysis and Kidney Transplants, *J. Am. Dent. Assoc.*, 96, 464, March, 1978.
12. Heard, E., Staples, A.F., and Czerwinski, A.W.: The Dental Patient with Renal Disease: Precautions and Guidelines, *J. Am. Dent. Assoc.*, 96, 792, May, 1978.
13. Mulligan, R.: Late Infections in Patients with Prostheses for Total Replacement of Joints: Implications for the Dental Practitioner, *J. Am. Dent. Assoc.*, 101, 44, July, 1980.
14. Jacobsen, P.L. and Murray, W.: Prophylactic Coverage of Dental Patients with Artificial Joints: A Retrospective Analysis of Thirty-three Infections in Hip Prostheses, *Oral Surg.*, 50, 130, August, 1980.
15. Sheppard, G.A.: Medical-legal Considerations, in Malamed, S.F.: *Handbook of Medical Emergencies in the Dental Office*. St. Louis, The C.V. Mosby Co., 1978, p. 54.

Suggested Readings

Baumgartner, J.C. and Plack, W.F.: Dental Treatment and Management of a Patient With a Prosthetic Heart Valve, *J. Am. Dent. Assoc.*, 104, 181, February, 1982.
Brooks, S.L.: Survey of Compliance with American Heart Association Guidelines for Prevention of Bacterial Endocarditis, *J. Am. Dent Assoc.*, 101, 41, July, 1980.
Chow, M.H. and Peterson, D.S.: Dental Management for Children with Chronic Renal Failure Undergoing Hemodialysis Therapy, *Oral Surg.*, 48, 34, July, 1979.
Cottone, J.A. and Kafrawy, A.H.: Medications and Health Histories: A Survey of 4,365 Dental Patients, *J. Am. Dent. Assoc.*, 98, 713, May, 1979.
Grant, D.A., Stern, I.B., and Everett, F.G.: *Periodontics*, 5th ed. St. Louis, The C.V. Mosby Co., 1979, pp. 438–451.

Halpern, I.L.: Patient's Medical Status—A Factor in Dental Treatment, *Oral Surg.*, 39, 216, February, 1975.
Kerr, D.A., Ash, M.M., and Millard, H.D.: *Oral Diagnosis*, 5th ed. St. Louis, The C.V. Mosby Co., 1978, pp. 36–77.
Lewis, D.P., Casterline, C.L., and Stein, M.: Aspirin Idiosyncrasy, *J. Am. Dent. Assoc.*, 98, 737, May, 1979.
Macedo-Sobrinho, B.: Infective Endocarditis: Is it Being Neglected Within the Dental Profession? *Clin. Prev. Dent.*, 1, 14, November-December, 1979.
Mitchell, D.F., Standish, S.M., and Fast, T.B.: *Oral Diagnosis/Oral Medicine*, 3rd ed. Philadelphia, Lea & Febiger, 1978, pp. 89–110.
Pepin, J.I.: Medicodental History, in Boundy, S.S. and Reynolds, N.J., eds.: *Current Concepts in Dental Hygiene*. St. Louis, The C.V. Mosby Co., 1977, pp. 195–204.
Rosenbaum, C.H. and Barton, D.H.: Use of a Continuing Health History in Dental Practice: A Survey, *J. Dent. Child.*, 45, 371, September-October, 1978.
Rubin, R., Salvati, E.A., and Lewis, R.: Infected Total Hip Replacement after Dental Procedures, *Oral Surg.*, 41, 18, January, 1976.
Santinga, J.T., Fekety, R.F., Bottomley, W.K., Else, B., and Willis, P.W.: Antibiotic Prophylaxis for Endocarditis in Patients with a Prosthetic Heart Valve, *J. Am. Dent. Assoc.*, 93, 1001, November, 1976.
Schuckit, M.A.: Overview of Alcoholism, *J. Am. Dent. Assoc.*, 99, 489, September, 1979.
Tocker, J. and Weibert, E.: The Dental Significance of Corticosteroids, Antihypertensive Drugs and Anticoagulants, *Dent. Hyg.*, 49, 11, January, 1975.
Wallace, J., Barrett, R.A., and Boozer, C.H.: Personal Health Information, in Clark, J.W., ed.: *Clinical Dentistry, Volume 1*, Chapter 3. Hagerstown, Maryland, Harper & Row, 1981, pp. 1–19.

Medical Consultation

Abbey, L.M.: Dealing with the Hypertensive Patient–Dentist–Physician Interaction, *Dent. Surv.*, 54, 26, May, 1978.
Brasher, W.J. and Rees, T.D.: The Medical Consultation: Its Role in Dentistry, *J. Am. Dent. Assoc.*, 95, 961, November, 1977.
Halpern, I.L.: Medical Consultation: Essential in Today's Dental Practice, *Dent. Surv.*, 55, 26, February, 1979.
Odenheimer, K.J., Jacobs, S., and Odenheimer, B.J.: The Importance of Developing Teamwork Between Dentists and Physicians, *J. Am. Dent. Assoc.*, 95, 322, August, 1977.

Interview

Croft, J.J.: Interviewing in Physical Therapy, *Physical Therapy*, 60, 1033, August, 1980.
Froelich, R.E. and Bishop, F.M.: *Clinical Interviewing Skills*, 3rd ed. St. Louis, The C.V. Mosby Co., 1977, 203 pp.
Mansky, M.: The Dental Interview Can Be Constructive, *J. Am. Soc. Prev. Dent.*, 5, 13, November-December, 1975.
Trieger, N. and Goldblatt, L.: The Art of History Taking, *J. Oral Surg.*, 36, 118, February, 1978.

7

Vital Signs

The vital signs are the body temperature, pulse and respiratory rates, and blood pressure. Table 7–1 summarizes the normal values for adults.

Recording vital signs contributes to the proper systemic evaluation of a patient in conjunction with the complete medical history. Treatment planning and appointment sequencing are directly influenced by the findings. Proficiency in determination of the vital signs is essential for monitoring during emergency treatment (pages 832 and 835).

Abnormal vital signs must be regarded with suspicion since they may indicate undetected systemic problems. For example, a patient's life may be saved because of medical treatment initiated as a result of a high blood pressure determination during a dental hygiene appointment.

When vital signs are not within normal range, they are called to the dentist's attention. The patient should be informed and the findings discussed with a physician. When the patient does not have a personal physician, a recommendation for referral for additional diagnostic procedures is indicated.

BODY TEMPERATURE

While preparing the patient history and making the extraoral and intraoral examinations, the need for taking the temperature may become apparent, or the dentist may have requested the procedure in conjunction with current oral dis-

Table 7–1. Vital Signs

VITAL SIGN	VALUES OF SIGNIFICANCE in dental and dental hygiene appointments		
BODY TEMPERATURE (oral)	Normal 37.0°C (98.6°F) Normal Range 35.5° to 37.5°C (96.0° to 99.5° F)		
PULSE RATE	Normal Range 60 to 90 per minute		
RESPIRATION	Normal Range 14 to 20 per minute		
BLOOD PRESSURE		*Systolic/ Diastolic*	*Diastolic Range*
	Low	90/60	60–79
	Average	120/80	80–89
	Mild Hypertension	140/90	90–104*
	Moderate Hypertension	180/105	105–114*
	Severe Hypertension	200/115	115 and higher†
	* Refer for additional medical evaluation † Refer for immediate medical evaluation; reappoint for dental or dental hygiene therapy.		

ease. When the temperature is to be taken along with the other vital signs, the pulse and respiratory rates are determined concurrently while the thermometer is in the patient's mouth.

A temperature above the normal range indicates the presence of infection. Patients can have an elevated body temperature due to oral causes such as an apical or periodontal abscess or acute pericoronitis. Determination of the temperature

103

of a patient with an oral infection may be necessary for diagnosis and treatment planning.

For the protection of the health of the personnel in the dental office or clinic, to prevent loss of working time due to illness, as well as for the protection of subsequent patients who may be indirectly exposed, it is important to detect the presence of a systemic, contagious condition. Screening for elevated temperature among patients may have particular significance during certain seasons or epidemics. When a definite increase in temperature is found, the patient can be dismissed by the dentist to prevent further contamination of the office or clinic. The patient can be advised to seek medical care.

I. Maintenance of Body Temperature

A. Normal Adult

The normal average temperature is 37.0° C (98.6° F) with a range from 35.5° to 37.5° C (96.0° to 99.5° F).

B. Temperature Variations

1. Fever (pyrexia): values over 37.5° C (99.5° F)
2. Hyperthermia: values over 41.0° C (105.8° F)
3. Hypothermia: values below 35.5° C (96.0° F)

C. Factors That Alter Body Temperature

1. Time of day: highest in late afternoon and early evening; lowest during sleep and early morning.
2. Temporary increase: exercise, hot drinks, smoking, or application of external heat.
3. Pathologic states: infection, dehydration, hyperthyroidism, myocardial infarction, tissue injury from trauma.
4. Decrease: starvation, hemorrhage, or physiologic shock.

II. Methods of Determining Temperature

A. Oral: Most commonly used.
1. Indications for use: An oral thermometer is used for the patient who
   a. Can follow instructions.
   b. Can keep the mouth closed to hold the thermometer.
   c. Will not bite or otherwise break the thermometer (which could happen with small children or confused patients of any age).
   d. Has no mouth injuries or problem breathing through the nose.
2. Contraindications: The oral thermometer cannot be used for a patient who is unconscious, confused, irrational or restless, infants or small children, or a patient with a very dry mouth.

B. Rectal: Generally applicable when the oral thermometer is contraindicated.

C. External: Axillary and groin positions are the least accurate but occasionally the oral or rectal methods are impossible to use.

D. Types of Thermometers

1. Mercury-column clinical thermometer: consists of a bulb containing mercury which, when heated by the body temperature, expands and rises in the hollow center of the glass stem. The bulb of the oral thermometer is usually tapered, whereas the rectal thermometer has a blunt, round mercury bulb.
2. Electronic: some hospitals use electronic thermometers which require less time for taking the temperature, are more easily cared for because of their disposable tips, and which decrease the possibility of cross-contamination.

E. Comparison of Readings

Rectal readings are about one degree above oral readings, and oral readings are about one degree above axillary or groin readings.

III. Procedure

A. Equipment: clinical thermometer, tissues, clock or watch with second hand, sheath.

B. Prepare Patient

1. Tell patient what is to be done.
2. Wait 15 minutes for the patient who has just had a hot or cold beverage or has smoked within 10 minutes, as the surface temperature of the oral mucosa can

alter the accuracy of the thermometer reading.

C. Prepare the Thermometer

1. Hold the thermometer only by the stem, never by the bulb.
2. Wipe with a tissue.
3. Check the reading: it must be below 35.6° C (96° F).
4. Shake down the mercury level if not already below 35.6° C (96° F). The thermometer maintains the highest temperature previously registered, and remains there until the force of shaking lowers the mercury level.
   a. Move away from furniture or other hard objects to prevent accidental forceful contact of the thermometer.
   b. Grasp stem firmly and shake with a firm, even, downward motion one or two times.
   c. Recheck the reading and reshake when indicated.
5. Place the thermometer into a thermometer sheath (a disposable cover available from a medical supply) to prevent contact with the patient's oral microflora.

D. Take the Temperature

1. Insert the bulb under the patient's tongue, with stem outside of the mouth.
2. Instruct patient to hold the thermometer gently with the lips, to avoid biting, and to breathe through the nose.
3. Observe watch or other timer, and remove thermometer after 3 clocked minutes.

E. Read and Record

1. Stand with back to light source and hold the thermometer by the stem at eye level to read.
2. Roll the thermometer slowly between the fingers to find the solid column of mercury.
3. Read at the point where the mercury ends. Each long line represents a degree of temperature, and short lines between are at two-tenths (0.2) of a degree.
4. Retake the temperature when the reading is unusually high or low.
   a. Reshake the mercury column down.

b. Watch the patient to make certain that the thermometer is in position during the 3 minutes.
5. Record date, time of day, and temperature on the patient's record.
6. Inform the dentist of a temperature over 37.5° C (99.5° F).

F. Care of the Thermometer

1. Disposable thermometer sheath: remove and dispose in waste.
2. Conventional
   a. Wash with soap and slightly warm water; rinse with clear cool water; dry. Hot water can raise the temperature and force the mercury to break the thermometer.
   b. Soak in disinfectant solution, completely covered (pages 38–40).
   c. Rinse with water and dry before placing in container or using again. Container should be sterilizable.

IV. Care of Patient With Temperature Elevation[1,2]

A. Temperature Over 41.0° C (105.8° F)

1. Treat as a medical emergency.
2. Transport to a hospital for medical care.

B. Temperature 37.6° to 41.0° C (99.6° to 105.8° F)

1. Check possible temporary or factitious cause such as hot beverage or smoking, and observe patient while repeating the determination.
2. Review the dental and medical history.
3. Call to the attention of the dentist.
4. Provide no elective care when there are signs of respiratory infection or other possible communicable disease.

PULSE

The pulse is the intermittent throbbing sensation felt when the fingers are pressed against an artery. It is the result of the alternate expansion and contraction of an artery as a wave of blood is forced through by the heartbeat. The pulse rate is the count of the heartbeats. Irregularities of strength, rhythm, and quality of the pulse should be noted while counting the pulse rate.

I. Maintenance of Normal Pulse

A. Normal Pulse Rates

1. Children: At birth the pulse rate is between 130 and 160 beats per minute, and in the young child it is usually over 100, until about the third year. Older children range from 80 to 100.
2. Adults: There is no absolute normal. The adult range is 60 to 90 beats per minute, slightly higher for women than for men.

B. Factors That Influence Pulse Rate

An unusually fast heartbeat (over 150 beats per minute in an adult) is called tachycardia; an unusually slow beat (below 50) is bradycardia.

1. Increased pulse: caused by exercise, stimulants, eating, strong emotions, extremes of heat and cold, and some forms of heart disease.
2. Decreased pulse: caused by sleep, depressants, fasting, quieting emotions, and low vitality from prolonged illness.
3. Emergency situations: listed in table 58-1, pages 845-852.

II. Procedure for Determining Pulse Rate

A. Sequence

The pulse rate is conveniently obtained at the same time that the thermometer is in the patient's mouth to determine body temperature. Respirations are counted immediately following the pulse rate.

B. Sites

The pulse may be felt at several points over the body. The one most commonly used is on the radial artery at the wrist and is called the *radial pulse* (figure 7–1). Other sites convenient for use in a dental office or clinic are the *temporal* artery on the side of the head in front of the ear, or the *facial* artery at the border of the mandible.

C. Prepare the Patient

1. Tell the patient what is to be done.
2. Have the patient in a comfortable position with arm and hand supported, palm down.

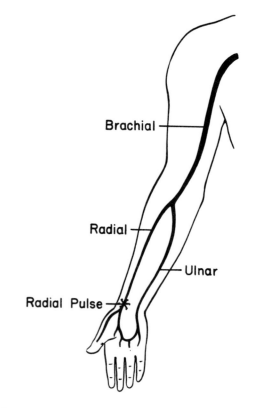

Figure 7–1. Arteries of the arm. Note location of radial pulse. The brachial pulse may be felt just before the brachial artery branches into the radial and ulnar arteries.

3. Locate the radial pulse on the thumb side of the wrist with the tips of the first three fingers (figure 7–2). Do not use the thumb as it contains a pulse that may be confused with the patient's pulse.

D. Count and Record

1. When the pulse is felt, exert light pressure and count for one clocked minute. Use the second hand of a watch or clock. Check with a repeat count.
2. While taking the pulse, observe the following:
   a. Rhythm: regular, regularly irregular, irregularly irregular.
   b. Volume and strength: full, strong, poor, weak, thready.
3. Record on patient's record: date, pulse rate, other characteristics.
4. Call unusual findings to the dentist's attention. A pulse rate over 90 should be considered abnormal for an adult and over 120 abnormal for a child.

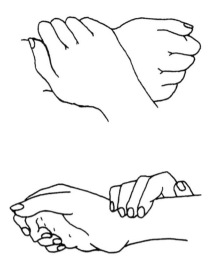

Figure 7–2. Determination of pulse rate. **Upper,** correct position of hand. **Lower,** the tips of the first three fingers are placed over the radial pulse located on the thumb side of the ventral surface of the wrist.

RESPIRATION

The function of respiration is to supply oxygen to the tissues and to eliminate carbon dioxide. Variations in normal respirations may be shown by characteristics such as the rate, rhythm, depth, and quality and may be symptomatic of disease or emergency states.

I. Maintenance of Normal Respirations

A respiration is one breath taken in and let out.

A. Normal Respiratory Rate

1. Children: The number of respirations per minute may be as high as 80 at birth. During the first year the normal range is considered from 20 to 40.
2. Adults: The adult range is from 14 to 20 per minute, slightly higher for women.

B. Factors That Influence Respirations

Many of the same factors that influence pulse rate also influence the number of respirations. A rate of 12 per minute or fewer is considered subnormal for an adult; over 28 is accelerated; and rates over 60 are extremely rapid and dangerous.

1. Increased by work and exercise, excitement, nervousness, strong emotions, pain, hemorrhage, shock.
2. Decreased by sleep, certain drugs, pulmonary insufficiency.

3. Emergency situations are listed in table 58–1, pages 845–846.

II. Procedures for Observing Respirations

A. Determine Rate

1. Make the count of respirations immediately after counting the pulse.
2. Maintain the fingers over the radial pulse.
3. Respirations must be counted so that the patient is not aware, as the rate may be voluntarily altered.
4. Count the number of times the chest rises in one clocked minute. It is not necessary to count both inspirations and expirations.

B. Factors to Observe

1. *Depth.* Describe as shallow, normal, or deep.
2. *Rhythm.* Describe as regular (evenly spaced) or irregular (with pauses of irregular lengths between).
3. *Quality.* Describe as strong, easy, weak, or labored (noisy). Poor quality may have an effect on body color; for example, a bluish tinge of the face or nailbeds may mean an insufficiency of oxygen.
4. *Sounds.* Describe deviate sounds made during inspiration, expiration, or both.
5. *Position of Patient.* When the patient assumes an unusual position to secure comfort during breathing or prefers to remain seated upright, mark records accordingly.

C. Record

Record all findings on the patient's record.

D. Notify

Call to the attention of the dentist any unusual findings.

BLOOD PRESSURE

Information about the patient's blood pressure is essential during dental and dental hygiene appointments, since special adaptations may be needed. Screening for blood pressure in dental offices has been shown to be an effective health service for all ages. Many people may make regular visits to their dentists, but see their physicians infrequently.[3]

I. Components of Blood Pressure

Blood pressure is the force exerted by the blood on the blood vessel walls. When the left ventricle of the heart contracts, blood is forced out into the aorta and travels through the large arteries to the smaller arteries, arterioles, and capillaries. The pulsations extend from the heart through the arteries and disappear in the arterioles. During the course of the cardiac cycle the blood pressure is changing constantly.

A. Systolic Pressure

Systolic pressure is the peak or the highest pressure. It is caused by ventricular contraction. The normal systolic pressure ranges from 100 to 140 mm. Hg.

B. Diastolic Pressure

Diastolic pressure is the lowest pressure. It is the effect of ventricular relaxation. The normal diastolic pressure ranges from 60 to 90 mm. Hg.

C. Boundaries

More than one reading is needed within a few minutes to determine an average and assure a correct reading. That should be followed by serial readings at least every six months and always before surgery or other stressful treatment.

D. Pulse Pressure

The pulse pressure is the difference between the systolic and the diastolic pressures. The normal or safe range is between 30 and 60 mm. Hg.

II. Factors That Influence Blood Pressure

Cardiovascular diseases are described in Chapter 55, and the causes, predisposing factors, and treatment of hypertension on pages 781–783. That information can be a helpful introduction and is recommended for reading in conjunction with this section on the techniques for obtaining blood pressure.

A. Maintenance of Blood Pressure

Blood pressure depends on

1. Force of the heart beat (energy of the heart).
2. Peripheral resistance; condition of the arteries; changes in elasticity of vessels, which may occur with age.
3. Volume of blood in the circulatory system.

B. Factors That Increase Blood Pressure

1. Exercise, eating, stimulants, and emotional disturbance.
2. Menopause: In general, women have recorded blood pressure 4 to 5 mm. Hg less than men until menopause, when there is usually an abrupt rise to slightly more than the average male.

C. Factors That Decrease Blood Pressure: fasting, rest, depressants, and quiet emotions.

D. Pathology

1. *Hypertension:* sustained abnormal elevation
   a. Age and history need consideration when classifying normal and abnormal for an individual.
   b. Systolic pressure over 140 mm. Hg and diastolic over 90 mm. Hg bear watching and rechecking. Pressures over 150 mm. Hg systolic and 100 mm. Hg diastolic are reportable, and the patient with such readings must be referred to a physician for examination.
   c. Increased diastolic is more significant than increased systolic.
2. *Hypotension:* abnormally low blood pressure. In shock, the systolic pressure may drop to 70 or 80 mm. Hg (page 847).

III. Equipment for Determining Blood Pressure

The mercury manometer is usually considered the most reliable recorder of blood pressure. Electronic devices are available, but additional research is needed before their reliability can be fully assured. Another type is the aneroid which has a round gauge. It requires frequent calibration.

A. **Sphygmomanometer** (blood pressure machine): consists of an *inflatable cuff* and *two tubes*, one connected to the *pressure hand control bulb*, and the other to the *pressure gauge*.
   1. *Cuff*
      a. Material. The cuff is made of a non-elastic material and is fastened by a velcro overlap. The inflatable bladder is located within the material of the cuff.
      b. Size. The diameter of the arm, not the age of the patient, determines the size of the cuff selected. There are four cuff sizes available: child size, regular adult, large adult, and thigh. The thigh size is needed for grossly obese persons.
      c. Dimension. The cuff width that is used should be 20 percent greater than the diameter of the arm to which it is applied (figure 7–3). It should cover approximately two thirds of the upper arm.

      When a cuff is too narrow, the blood pressure reading will be too high; when the cuff is too wide, the reading will be too low.[4]
   2. *The Mercury Manometer*
      a. Gauges are marked with long lines at each 10 mm. Hg, with shorter lines at 2 mm. intervals between each long line.
      b. The level of the column of mercury of the manometer should be at eye level for accurate reading and must not be tilted.

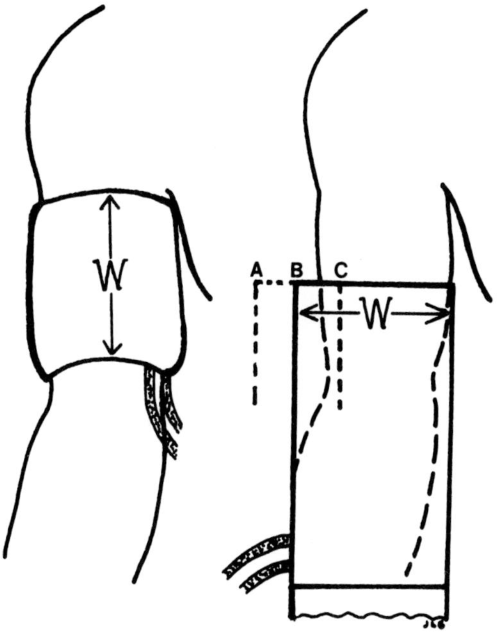

B. **Stethoscope** (a listening aid that magnifies sound): consists of an *endpiece* which is connected by tubes to carry the sound to the *earpieces*.
   1. Types of endpieces: bell-shaped or flat (diaphragm). The bell shape is used for medical examinations, particularly for chest examination.
   2. Care of earpieces: clean by rubbing with gauze sponge moistened in disinfectant.

IV. Procedure for Determining Blood Pressure

A. **Prepare Patient**
   1. Tell patient briefly what is to be done. Detailed explanations are to be avoided since they may excite the patient and change the blood pressure.
   2. Seat patient comfortably with the arm slightly flexed, with palm up and the whole forearm supported on a level surface at the level of the heart.
   3. Use either arm unless otherwise indicated, for example, by a handicap. Repeat blood pressure determinations should be made on the same arm since there may be as much as 10 mm. Hg difference between arms.
   4. Take pressure on bare arm, not over clothing. A tight sleeve should be loosened or the garment removed.

B. **Apply Cuff**
   1. With the patient's arm resting on the arm of the dental chair with the elbow at or below the level of the heart, apply the completely deflated cuff. The portion of the cuff that contains the inflatable bladder is placed directly over the

Figure 7–3. Selection of arm cuff for blood pressure determination. The correct width (W) is 20% greater than the diameter of the arm to which it is applied. **A.** too wide, **B.** correct width, **C.** too narrow.

brachial artery. The cuff may have an arrow to show the point that should be placed over the artery. The lower edge of the cuff is placed one inch above the antecubital fossa (figure 7–4). Fasten the cuff evenly and snugly.

2. Adjust the position of the gauge for convenient reading but so that the patient cannot see the mercury.

3. Palpate one inch below the antecubital fossa to locate the brachial artery pulse (figure 7–1). The stethoscope endpiece

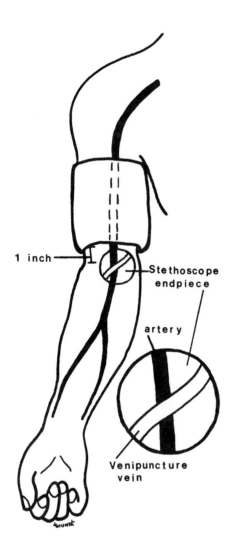

Figure 7–4. Blood pressure cuff in position. The lower edge of the cuff is placed approximately one inch above the antecubital fossa. The stethoscope endpiece is placed over the palpated brachial artery pulse point approximately one inch below the antecubital fossa and slightly toward the inner side of the arm.

will be placed over the spot where the brachial pulse is felt.

4. Position the stethoscope earpieces in the ears, with the tips directed forward.

C. **Locate the Radial Pulse** (figures 7–1 and 7–2)

Hold the fingers on the pulse.

D. **Inflate the Cuff**

1. Close the needle valve (air lock) attached to the hand control bulb firmly but so it may be readily released.

2. Pump to inflate the cuff until the radial pulse stops. Note the mercury level at which the pulse disappears.

3. Look at the dial, and pump to 20 or 30 mm. Hg beyond where the radial pulse was no longer felt. This is the maximum inflation level (MIL). It means that the brachial artery is collapsed by the pressure of the cuff and no blood is flowing through.

Unless the MIL is determined, the level to which the cuff is inflated will be arbitrary. Excess pressure can be very uncomfortable for the patient.

E. **Position the Stethoscope Endpiece**

Place the endpiece over the palpated brachial artery, one inch below the antecubital fossa, and slightly toward the inner side of the arm (figure 7–4). Hold lightly in place.

F. **Deflate the Cuff Gradually**

1. Release the air lock slowly (2 to 3 mm. per second) so that the dial drops very gradually and steadily.

2. Listen for the first sound: *systole* ("tap tap"). Note the number on the dial which is the *systolic pressure*. This is the beginning of the flow of blood past the cuff.

3. Continue to release the pressure slowly. The sound will continue, first becoming louder, then diminishing and becoming muffled until finally disappearing. Note the number on the dial where the last distinct tap was heard. That number is the *diastolic pressure.*

4. Release further (about 10 mm.) until there is a cessation of all sounds. That is the second diastolic point. In some clin-

ics and hospitals the last sound is taken as the diastolic pressure.

5. Let the rest of the air out rapidly.

G. **Repeat for Confirmation**

Wait 30 seconds before inflating the cuff again.

H. **Record**

1. Write date and arm used.
2. Record blood pressure as a fraction, for example 120/80. When both diastolic points are recorded, it can be written 120/80/72.

I. **Notify**

Call to the prompt attention of the dentist any unusual variation from normal or from previous readings noted in the patient's permanent record.

A blood pressure reading of 140/90 or over is considered mild hypertension, 180/105 is moderate hypertension, and 200/115 or over, severe hypertension (table 7–1, page 103).

TECHNICAL HINTS

I. When a patient's sleeve is drawn back for blood pressure determination, observe the sleeve and the arm for small blood stains or evidence of an injection which may reveal a mainliner drug addict. The patient may request, even insist, that a particular arm be used. When suspicion of drug abuse has been previously aroused because of physical observation or items in a medical history, determine the blood pressure on both arms to permit observation. Tell the patient that the pressure should always be measured on both sides.

II. Sources of Materials
National High Blood Pressure Education Program
High Blood Pressure Information Center
120/80 National Institutes of Health
Bethesda, Maryland 20205

American Heart Association
7320 Greenville Avenue
Dallas, Texas 75231

FACTORS TO TEACH THE PATIENT

I. How vital signs can influence dental and dental hygiene appointments.
II. The importance of having a blood pressure determination at regular intervals.

References

1. Soltero, D.J. and Whitacre, R.J.: *Vital Signs.* Seattle, Instructional Services, 1978, 48 pp.
2. McCarthy, F.M.: Vital Signs—the Six-minute Warnings, *J. Am. Dent. Assoc.,* *100,* 682, May, 1980.
3. Abbey, L.M.: Screening for Hypertension in the Dental Office, *J. Am. Dent. Assoc.,* *88,* 563, March, 1974.
4. Geddes, L.A. and Whistler, S.J.: The Error in Indirect Blood Pressure Measurement with the Incorrect Size of Cuff, *Am. Heart J.,* *96,* 4, July, 1978.

Suggested Readings

Abbey, L.M.: Dealing with the Hypertensive Patient—Dentist-Physician Interaction, *Dent. Surv.,* *54,* 26, May, 1978.

Abbey, L.M., Keener, L.H., and Raper, A.J.: Hypertension Screening Among Dental Patients, *J. Am. Dent. Assoc.,* *93,* 996, November, 1976.

Berman, C.L., Guarino, M.A., and Giovannoli, S.M.: High Blood Pressure Detection by Dentists, *J. Am. Dent. Assoc.,* *87,* 359, August, 1973.

Berman, C.L., Stewart, A.V., Ramazzotto, L.J., and Davis, F.D.: High Blood Pressure Detection: A New Public Health Measure for the Dental Profession, *J. Am. Dent. Assoc.,* *92,* 116, January, 1976.

Blozis, G.G.: Blood Pressure, in Boundy, S.S. and Reynolds, N.J., eds.: *Current Concepts in Dental Hygiene,* Volume 2. St. Louis, The C.V. Mosby Co., 1979, pp. 37–46.

Cutright, D.E., Carpenter, W.A., Tsaknis, P.G., and Lyon, T.C.: Survey of Blood Pressure of 856 Dentists, *J. Am. Dent. Assoc.,* *94,* 918, May, 1977.

Malamed, S.F.: Blood Pressure Evaluation and the Prevention of Medical Emergencies in Dental Practice, *J. Prev. Dent.,* *6,* 183, June, 1980.

Maloney, K.L.: The Role of the Auxiliary in Hypertension Screening, *Quintessence Journal,* *3,* 245, May, 1981.

Merchant, H.W. and Carr, A.A.: Blood Pressure Measurement: Problems and Solutions, *J. Am. Dent. Assoc.,* *95,* 98, July, 1977.

Newkirk, C.: The Hypertensive Dental Patient: Detection and Treatment, *Dent. Hyg.,* *51,* 205, May, 1977.

Silverberg, D.S.: The Dentist's Role in Hypertension Detection, *Can. Dent. Assoc. J.,* *42,* 549, November, 1976.

Stout, F.W.: The Sphygmomanometer: Its Development, Use, and Abuse, *J. Prev. Dent.,* *6,* 169, June, 1980.

United States Department of Health and Human Services, National High Blood Pressure Coordinating Committee: *The 1980 Report of the Joint National Committee on Detection, Evaluation, and Treatment of High Blood Pressure.* NIH Publication Number 81–1088, December, 1980, National Heart, Lung, and Blood Institute, National High Blood Pressure Education Program, 120/80 National Institutes of Health, Bethesda, Maryland 20205.

Wessberg, G.: Role of Screening for Hypertension in Patient Management, *J. Am. Dent. Assoc.,* *96,* 1040, June, 1978.

8

Extraoral and Intraoral Examination

A careful overall observation of each patient and a thorough examination of the oral cavity and adjacent structures is essential to total evaluation prior to treatment. A variety of lesions may be observed for which the patient may or may not report subjective symptoms. Recognition, treatment, and follow-up of specific lesions may be of definite significance to the present and future general and oral health of the patient.

Despite the occurrence of many seemingly minor lesions, the danger of oral malignancies remains a definite possibility. Approximately six percent of all male cancers and two percent of female cancers occur in the area of the oral cavity.[1] Every effort must be made to detect potentially cancerous lesions early.

Each area of the mucous membrane must be examined, and minor deviations from normal must be given prompt attention. A life may depend on a dental hygienist's oral examination. Routine inspection for each new patient and at each recall appointment provides a realistic approach to the control of oral disease.

The oral tissues are sensitive indicators of the general health of the individual. Changes in these structures may be the first indication of subclinical disease processes in other parts of the body.

Although not legally permitted to diagnose, the dental hygienist has the responsibility to observe, record, and call to the attention of the dentist deviations from the normal appearance of the oral cavity. Prerequisite to accomplishing this are knowledge and understanding of the normal morphology and function (anatomy and physiology) of the oral cavity and the surrounding area which can be applied in the intelligent recognition of oral conditions.

OBJECTIVES

A thorough examination is essential to the total care of the patient as suggested by the following objectives:

I. To observe the patient overall as well as all areas in and about the oral cavity and to record and call to the attention of the dentist those areas that appear to deviate from normal and that may be evidence of disease.

II. To screen each patient at least annually to detect lesions suspicious of cancer.

III. To recognize a need for postponement of the current appointment because of evidence of communicable disease or in deference to the need for urgent medical consultation and/or treatment.

IV. To prevent the development of advanced, irreversible, or untreatable oral disease by early recognition of initial lesions.

V. To identify suspected conditions which require additional testing or other diagnostic aids which the dentist may use or may direct the dental hygienist to use under supervision.

VI. To identify extraoral and intraoral deviations from normal which are related to and for which dental hygiene care and instruction may need special adaptations.

VII. To provide a means of comparison of individual oral examinations over a series of recall appointments, and thus to determine the effects of dental and dental hygiene care and the success of patient instruction.

VIII. To provide information for continuing records of the patient's diagnosis and treatment plan for legal purposes.

COMPONENTS OF EXAMINATION

The current concept of patient care is that the total patient is being treated, not only the oral cavity, and particularly not only the teeth and their immediately surrounding tissues. The examination must be, therefore, an all-inclusive one to include any detectable physical, mental, or psychologic influences of the whole patient on the oral health.

Certain parts of the examination may be carried out by the dentist. Other parts will be delegated to the dental hygienist. Thorough examination must become a routine part of each patient recall appointment if treatment for the control and prevention of oral diseases is to be effective.

I. Methods of Examination

The various examination methods were de-

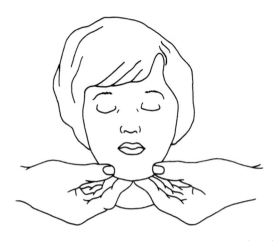

Figure 8–2. Palpation of the submandibular area. Bilateral palpation is used to examine corresponding structures on opposite sides of the body.

scribed on page 81. The extraoral and intraoral examination is accomplished primarily by direct observation and palpation, but other methods are also used.

A. Direct Observation

Patient position, optimum lighting, and effective retraction for accessibility contribute to the accuracy and completeness of the examination. Visual examination is made in conjunction with other methods.

B. Palpation

Fingers or hands are used to move or press tissue to detect changes in consistency and size. Types of palpation include the following:

1. *Digital.* Use of a single finger. Example: index finger applied to inner border of the mandible beneath the canine-premolar area to determine the presence of a torus mandibularis.

2. *Bidigital.* Use of finger and thumb of the same hand. Example: palpation of the lips (figure 8–1).

3. *Bimanual.* Use of finger or fingers and thumb from each hand applied simultaneously in coordination. Example: index finger of one hand palpates on the floor of the mouth inside, while a finger or fingers from the other hand press on

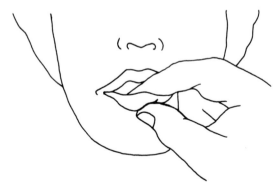

Figure 8–1. Palpation of the lip. Bidigital palpation is applied to detect deviations from normal particularly induration.

the same area from under the chin externally.

4. *Bilateral.* The two hands are used at the same time to examine corresponding structures on opposite sides of the body. Comparisons may be made. Example: fingers placed beneath the chin to palpate the submandibular lymph nodes (figure 8–2).

II. Order of Examination

A recommended order for examination is outlined in table 8–1, in which factors to consider during appointments are related to the actual observations made and recorded. The sequence presented in table 8–1 is adapted from the *Oral Cancer Examination Procedure* available from the American Cancer Society.[2]

A. Systematic Sequence for Examination

The advantages of following a routine order for examination include:

1. Minimal possibility of overlooking an area and missing details of importance.
2. Increased efficiency and conservation of time.
3. Maintenance of a professional atmosphere which will inspire the patient's confidence.

B. Steps for Thorough Examination (table 8–1)

1. Observe patient during reception and seating to note physical characteristics and abnormalities, and make an overall appraisal.
2. Observe head, face, eyes, and neck, and evaluate the skin of the face and neck.
3. Palpate the salivary glands and lymph nodes.
4. Examine mandibular movement and palpate the temporomandibular joint.
5. Make a preliminary examination of the lips and intraoral mucosa, using a mouth mirror or a tongue depressor. Do not retract directly with ungloved fingers in the event of an open lesion which may be communicable.
6. View and palpate lips, labial and buccal mucosa, and mucobuccal folds.
7. Examine and palpate the tongue, including the dorsal and ventral surfaces, lateral borders, and base. Retract to observe posterior third (figure 8–3).
8. Observe mucosa of the floor of the mouth. Palpate the floor of the mouth.
9. Examine hard and soft palates, tonsillar areas, and pharynx. Use mirror to observe oropharynx, nasopharynx, and larynx.
10. Note amount and consistency of the saliva and evidences of dry mouth.

C. Compare with Expected Normal Appearance.

Note deviations from normal.

D. Corroborate Findings

Corroborate findings with information from the patient's history.

E. Consult Dentist

Call questionable areas to the dentist's attention promptly.

III. Description of Observations

A. Record Form

1. Contain adequate space for complete descriptions of lesions observed; not merely a check sheet.
2. Contain spaces for successive examinations at periodic recall intervals.

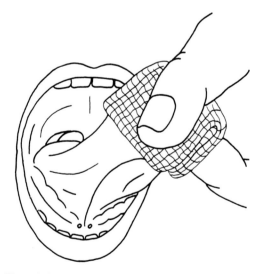

Figure 8–3. Tongue examination. To observe the posterior third of the tongue and the attachment to the floor of the mouth, hold the tongue with gauze, retract the cheek and move the tongue first out to the right, then the left, as each section of mucosa is carefully inspected.

B. Information to Include

1. Location. Describe the location in words or use a printed diagram on the record form to mark specific location of deviations from normal (figure 8–4).
2. History
   a. Whether the lesion is known to the patient or not known.
   b. Duration; changes in size and appearance.
   c. Symptoms.
3. Physical Characteristics
   a. Size: indicate width and depth in millimeters.
   b. Shape or contour: define whether the lesion is elevated (papillary) or depressed (ulcer-like); pedunculated, cracked, fissured.
   c. Color: compared with other areas of the patient's mouth.
   d. Resiliency, consistency: firm, indurated, soft, spongy.
   e. Surface texture: smooth, irregular.

C. Definitions

1. Descriptive Terminology
   a. *Discrete:* separate, not running together or blending.
   b. *Confluent:* running together, blended. Originally separate but subsequently formed into one.
   c. *Pedunculated:* elevated, papillary-type lesions having a narrow part (stem) which acts as a support and connector.
   d. *Verrucose:* covered with or full of wart-like growths.
   e. *Papillary:* small nipple-like elevation or projection.
   f. *Erythema:* red area of variable size and shape.
   g. *Petechia(e):* minute round red spot.
   h. *Induration:* hardened area of tissue.
2. Types of Lesions
   a. *Macule (macula):* circumscribed spot, not elevated above the surrounding level and distinguished by a different color.
   b. *Papule:* small (pinhead to 5 mm.), circumscribed, solid elevated area which may be pointed, rounded, or flattened.
   c. *Vesicle:* small (2 to 5 mm.), circumscribed, elevated lesion having a thin surface covering and containing fluid (small blister).
   d. *Bulla:* large (5 mm. to several cm.) vesicular-type lesion filled with fluid (large blister or bleb). A bullous lesion may develop individually or result from the union of several vesicles.
   e. *Pustule:* vesicular-type lesion containing purulent material rather than clear fluid.
   f. *Ulcer:* defect or break in continuity of the epithelium to produce a de-

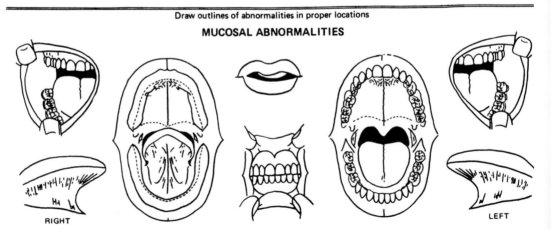

Draw outlines of abnormalities in proper locations

MUCOSAL ABNORMALITIES

RIGHT

LEFT

Figure 8–4. Record form for clinical findings. In this section of a clinical examination record form, outline of a deviation from normal may be drawn to show the location and relative size. (Courtesy, University of Southern California School of Dentistry.)

pressed area. It may result from the rupture of a vesicle or a bulla, and usually has some degree of erythema at the margin.

g. *Erosion:* shallow defect that does not extend through the epithelium into underlying tissue.

h. *Nodule:* solid elevated lesion (5 mm. to 2 cm. wide).

i. *Tumor:* solid growth of varying size which arises from the mucosa and projects out; swelling or overgrowth of cells independent of normal growth.

j. *Torus:* bony elevation or prominence usually found on the midline of the hard palate (torus palatinus) and the lingual surface of the mandible (torus mandibularis) in the premolar area.

k. *Leukoplakia:* white keratotic patch-like lesion on the mucosa which cannot be rubbed off.

l. *Crust:* an outer layer, covering, or scab, which may have formed from coagulation or drying of blood, serum, or pus, or a combination. A crust may form after a vesicle breaks; for example, the skin lesion of chicken pox is first a macule, then a papule, then a vesicle, and then a crust.

Table 8–1. Extraoral and Intraoral Examination

Order of Examination	*To Observe*	*Influences on Diagnosis and Appointments*
1. Overall Appraisal of Patient	Posture, gait General health status; size Hair Breathing, state of fatigue Voice, cough, hoarseness	Response, cooperation, attitude toward treatment Length of appointment possible
2. Face	Expression: evidence of fear or apprehension Shape, twitching, paralysis Profile for occlusion classification Jaw movements during speech Injuries, signs of abuse	Need for alleviation of fears Use of face mask when evidence of upper respiratory infection Enlarged masseter muscle may relate to bruxism or clenching habit
3. Skin	Color, texture, blemishes Traumatic lesions Eruptions, swellings Growths, moles	Skin color may relate to systemic factors; need for additional medical history and referral Skin lesions may require biopsy Open lesions need treatment before oral treatment Influence on instruction in diet and health
4. Eyes	Size of pupil (figure 8–5) Color of sclera Eyeglasses (corrective; sunglasses) Protruding eyeballs	Pupils dilated or pinpoint as a result of certain emergency situations (shock, heart failure, Table 58–1, pages 845–848) Eyeglasses essential during instruction to patient Hyperthyroidism
5. Nodes (figure 8–6) Palpate: a. Auricular (anterior, posterior, inferior) b. Submental c. Submaxillary d. Cervical	Adenopathy; lymphadenopathy Induration Coordinate with intraoral examination	Need for referral for biopsy

Table 8–1.   continued

Order of Examination	To Observe	Influences on Diagnosis and Appointments
6. Temporomandibular joint	Limitations or deviations during movement Tenderness, sensitivity Crepitation	Disorder of the joint Opening for plaque control
7. Lips a. Observe closed, then open b. Palpate using thumb and index finger (figure 8–1)	Color, texture, size Cracks, angular cheilosis Blisters, ulcers Traumatic lesions Irritation from biting habit Limitation of opening; muscle tone, elasticity Evidences of mouthbreathing or tongue thrusting Induration	Wear gloves Need for biopsy; referral Immediate need for postponement of appointment when lesions may be contagious or could interfere with procedures Care during retraction Difficulty of accessibility or visibility during intraoral procedures Patient instructions: dietary, special plaque control procedures for mouthbreather
8. Breath Odor	Severity Relation to oral hygiene and overall gingival state	Possible relation to systemic condition Emphasis on oral care and plaque control
9. Labial and Buccal Mucosa (left and right examined systematically) a. Observe vestibule, mucobuccal fold, frena, opening to Stensen's duct b. Palpate the entire cheek areas	Color, size, texture, contour Abrasions, traumatic lesions cheekbite, lip bite Effects of tobacco Ulcers, growths Moistness of membranes Relation of frena to free and attached gingiva Flexibility of cheeks Induration	Need for biopsy, referral, or cytologic smear Frena and other anatomical parts that need adaptation of impression tray Avoidance of sensitive areas during retraction, radiographic film placement, or plaque control instruction
10. Tongue and Floor of Mouth a. Dorsum (1) at rest with mouth slightly open (2) protruded b. Base of tongue Hold tip of tongue with gauze sponge Place mirror gently against uvula to view downward c. Lateral borders Hold tongue with sponge: extend to left then right (figure 8–3)	Color, size, texture, consistency Papillae, fissures Coating Lesions: ulcers, traumatic Deviation or straight Asymmetry Mobility; limitation of movement Attachments to floor of mouth and back to the anterior pillar Swelling, ulceration, color changes	Need for biopsy, referral, or cytologic smear Large muscular tongue affects retraction, gag reflex, and accessibility for instrumentation and film placement Instruction: tongue brushing, dietary factors

Table 8–1. *continued*

Order of Examination	To Observe	Influences on Diagnosis and Appointments
d. Ventral Surface Ask patient to touch the palate with the tip of the tongue	Undersurface of tongue Varicosities Lesions on floor of the mouth Duct openings from submandibular and sublingual glands Lingual frenum attachments Freedom of movement of tongue	Biopsy, referral, cytologic smear Care of sensitive areas during instrumentation Depth of floor of mouth and elasticity influence placement of radiographic films, and cotton roll holders Tonguetie
e. Ask patient to swallow. f. Palpate the entire tongue including the base.	Observe with lips slightly apart for evidence of tongue thrust. Induration, enlargements	
g. Palpate floor of mouth. (Place index finger of one hand in the mouth, other hand outside under the chin.)	Induration, enlargements	
11. **Saliva**	Quantity Evidence of dry mouth shown by lip wetting, tongue protrusion, excess plaque Quality of saliva: watery, ropy, mucoid	Reduced in certain diseases and by certain drugs Corroborate with items from the history Excess can influence instrumentation techniques
12. **Hard Palate** Observe and palpate	Height, contour, color Appearance of rugae Tori, growths, ulcers	May need biopsy, referral, or cytologic smear Signs of tongue thrust and deviate swallow Influence radiographic placement
13. **Soft Palate and Uvula** Observe: depress tongue with mirror or tongue depressor	Color, size, shape Petechiae Ulcers, growths	Biopsy, referral, smear Large uvula can affect gag reflex
14. **Tonsillar Region** a. Depress tongue with mirror or tongue depressor b. Ask patient to say "Ah" to open the oropharynx c. Place mirror behind uvula, glass up, to observe nasopharynx. (Request patient to breathe through the nose and mouth.)	Anterior and posterior pillars Tonsils, size, shape Color, surface characteristics Lesions, trauma	Biopsy, referral, smear may be indicated Adjustment of procedures for effect of enlarged tonsils on gag reflex Need for face mask when patient has a throat infection (or possible postponement of the appointment) Instruction: adapt plaque control procedures in posterior region when patient has sensitivity to gagging

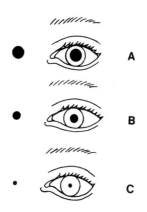

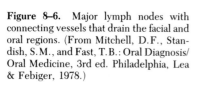

Figure 8–5. Examination of the pupils. **A.** *Dilated,* occurs in shock, heart failure, and other emergencies, and drug overdose of hallucinogens and amphetamines; **B.** *Normal* **C.** *Pinpoint,* occurs in drug overdose of morphine and related drugs, and barbiturates. (Adapted from American National Red Cross, *Standard First Aid and Personal Safety.*)

Figure 8–6. Major lymph nodes with connecting vessels that drain the facial and oral regions. (From Mitchell, D.F., Standish, S.M., and Fast, T.B.: Oral Diagnosis/Oral Medicine, 3rd ed. Philadelphia, Lea & Febiger, 1978.)

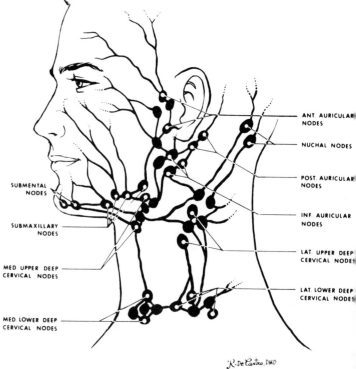

ORAL CANCER

The objective is to detect cancer of the mouth the earliest possible stage. Discovered early, is likely to have a high cure rate, whereas when cancer extends into adjacent structures and to the lymph nodes of the neck, the prognosis is poor.

Since the early lesions are generally symptomless, they may go unnoticed and unreported by the patient. Observation by the dentist or dental hygienist, therefore, is the principal method for the control of oral cancer. The first step in accomplishing this is to examine the entire oral mucous membrane for each patient at the initial examination and at each recall appointment.

The dental hygienist needs to know how to make the oral examination, where oral cancer occurs most frequently, what an early cancerous lesion may look like, and what to do when such lesion is found.

Location

Tumors may arise at any site in the oral cavity. The most common sites are the floor of the mouth, tongue, lower lip, and the anterior and posterior fauces (pillars). Figure 8–7 diagrams the oral cavity to show the areas where most cancers occur.

Although patients may be instructed in self-examination to watch for changes in oral tissues, it is difficult for a person to see his or her own tissues, particularly the entire floor of the mouth and base of the tongue, by the usual mirror and lighting systems available in a private home. Self-examination needs routine supplementation with professional examination.

I. Appearance of Early Cancer

Early oral cancer takes many forms and may resemble a variety of common oral lesions. All types should be looked at with suspicion. Five basic forms are listed here.

A. White Areas (Leukoplakia)

These may vary from filmy, barely visible changes in the mucosa to heavy, thick, heaped up areas of dry white keratinized tissue. Fissures, ulcers, or areas of induration in a white area are most indicative of malignancy.

B. Red Areas (Erythroplakia)

Lesions of red, velvety consistency, sometimes with small ulcers, should be identified.

C. Ulcers

These may be with flat or raised margins which may appear similar to aphthous ulcers. Palpation may reveal induration.

D. Masses

Papillary masses, sometimes with ulcerated areas, occur as elevations above the surrounding tissues. Other masses may occur below the normal mucosa and may be found only by palpation.

E. Pigmentation

This occurs as brown or black pigmented areas located on mucosa where pigmentation does not normally occur.

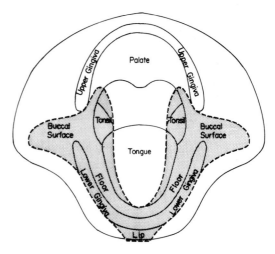

Figure 8–7. Sites of oral cancer. The shaded area represents the most frequent sites of squamous cell carcinoma of the oral cavity. Most of this area is not visible by self-examination and requires regular professional supervision. (From Burket, L.W.: Oral Medicine, 6th ed. Philadelphia, J.B. Lippincott Co., 1971.)

III. Procedure for Follow-up of a Suspicious Lesion

As designated by the dentist, a lesion may be biopsied immediately, a cytologic smear may be made, or the patient may be referred for additional diagnosis and biopsy.

A. Biopsy

1. *Definition.* Biopsy is the removal and examination, usually by microscope, of a section of tissue or other material from the living body for the purposes of diagnosis.
2. *Indications for Biopsy*[3]
   a. Any unusual oral lesion that cannot be identified with clinical certainty must be biopsied.
   b. Any lesion that has not shown evidence of healing in two weeks should be considered malignant until proven otherwise.
   c. A persistent, thick, white, hyperkeratotic lesion, and any mass (elevated or not) that does not break through the surface epithelium should be biopsied.

B. Cytologic Smear

1. *Definition.* The cytologic smear technique is a diagnostic aid in which surface cells of a suspicious lesion are removed for microscopic evaluation.
2. *Indications for Smear Technique*
   a. In general, a lesion for which a biopsy is not planned may be examined by smear. An exception is a white keratotic lesion (leukoplakia) that is not suitable for exfoliative cytology.
   b. A lesion that looks like potential cancer should be examined by smear if the patient refuses to have a biopsy specimen taken. A positive report from a smear should convince the patient of the need for treatment or biopsy.
   c. The smear technique is used for follow-up examination of patients with oral cancer treated by radiation.
   d. In mass screening programs for cancer detection, smears may be taken.

   However, all lesions of high suspicion should be referred for biopsy.
   e. Research studies to show changes in surface cells, for example the effect of topical agents, may use a smear technique.

3. *Limitations of Smear Technique*
   a. When a clear-cut lesion, recognized as pathologic, is present, treatment must not be delayed by waiting for cytologic smear analysis.
   b. The smear detects only surface lesions.
   c. It is difficult or impossible to scrape deep enough to obtain representative cells from a heavily keratinized lesion.
   d. Treatment cannot be determined by smear technique results only. After a positive smear, a biopsy is needed for definitive diagnosis.
   e. Because research has shown that the smear technique is not diagnostically reliable (there can be "false negatives" which turn out to be positive biopsies), a negative report should not be considered conclusive.

EXFOLIATIVE CYTOLOGY

Stratified squamous cells are constantly growing toward the epithelial surface of the mucous membrane where they are exfoliated. Exfoliated cells and cells beneath them are scraped off, and when prepared on a slide, changes in the cells can be detected by staining and studying them microscopically. The cells of a malignancy stain differently than normal cells and take on unusual, abnormal forms.

I. Procedure

A. Materials

Gauze sponges
Glass microscopic slides with frosted end
Plain lead pencil
Paper clips
Blade to scrape lesion (flexible metal spatula)
Fixative (70% alcohol)
Protective mailing container
History form or data sheet

B. Steps

1. *Prepare Materials.* Write the patient's name on the frosted ends of two glass slides (two for each lesion), and place a paper clip on the end of one slide to prevent contact between the slides when packaged for mailing to the laboratory.
2. *Prepare the Lesion.* Irrigate the surface to remove debris. Wipe the surface gently with a wet gauze sponge as needed to remove debris or blood. Do not dry.
3. *Scrape the Lesion.* Use a flexible metal spatula. Scrape the entire surface of the lesion firmly several times (all strokes in the same direction) (figure 8–8A).
4. *Smear the Glass Slide.* Spread the collected material on the glass slide. Start at the center of the clear end of the slide and smear evenly across the surface. Cover an area approximately 20 mm. wide. Handle all glass slides by their edges to prevent finger prints or other contamination (figure 8–8B).
5. *Fix the Cells.* Immediately, to prevent drying of the cells, place the slide on a flat surface and flood with generous drops of 70% alcohol.
6. *Obtain Second Smear.* Duplicate previous smear technique. Apply fixing agent immediately.
7. *Complete the Fixation.* Leave slides for 30 minutes. After 20 minutes, tip the slide to let remaining alcohol run off. Air dry where dust or other foreign material cannot contaminate the smear.
8. *Prepare History or Data Sheet.* Basic information includes the following:
   Dentist: name and address
   Patient: name and address
   Lesion: description (size, color, location, shape, consistency, and duration).
   Other related clinical findings or pertinent history.
9. *Prepare for Mailing.* Wrap slides in facial tissue to prevent breakage. Pack with the history or data sheet.

II. Laboratory Report

The pathologist makes the microscopic examination and classifies the specimen in one of the following categories:

Unsatisfactory	Slide is inadequate for diagnosis. The specimen may have been too thick or thin, or the cells may have dried before fixation. Another smear should be made promptly.
Class I	Normal
Class II	Atypical, but not suggestive of malignant cells
Class III	Uncertain (possible for cancer)
Class IV	Probable for cancer
Class V	Positive for cancer

III. Follow-up

A. Report of Class IV or V

Refer for biopsy.

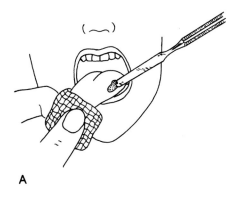

A

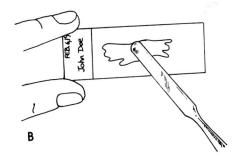

B

Figure 8–8.   Oral cytology technique. **A.** Tongue is held out with gauze sponge while a metal spatula is used to scrape a lesion. **B.** Collected material is spread evenly on a glass slide. See text for details.

B. **Report of Class III**

Re-evaluate clinical findings; biopsy usually indicated.

C. **Report of Class I or II**

1. The patient must not be dismissed until the lesion has healed.
2. When lesion persists, the dentist will either re-evaluate the clinical findings and request a repeat cytologic smear, or perform a biopsy.

D. **Negative Report**

Either biopsy or smear requires careful follow-up when a negative report is obtained for an oral lesion that appears suspicious by clinical examination. It is possible to have a false negative report; that is, a malignancy may be present but the sample examined in the smear or biopsy may not have included cancerous cells.

SPECIAL APPLICATIONS FOR THE EXTRAORAL AND INTRAORAL EXAMINATION

In Section VI of this book, many types of patients with special needs for adapted techniques are described. Some of them have general physical and oral characteristics that can be identified during an extraoral and intraoral examination. Facial and oral tissue examinations for pathology apply to all patients.

With certain patients, the recognition of particular characteristics has another dimension which may have social and legal implications. One example is the group of intraoral and extraoral signs that may reveal a child who is a victim of abuse or neglect. Another patient who may not be identified by questions from a medical and dental history is a drug addict. A variety of treatment problems are related to the care of a patient who misuses drugs. Identification of the patient's addiction can be essential to successful treatment. Characteristics for recognition of these two special patients are described here.

CHILD ABUSE

Recognition of a child who has been abused or neglected should be important to the entire dental team. They need to be aware of the problem of child abuse, be able to identify and report suspected cases, and document the injuries observed for future reference and comparison.

During the extraoral and intraoral examination various findings may lead to a suspicion of child abuse. Head, facial, or oral trauma occur in 50 to 65 percent of child abuse cases.[4] Some of the patients may be seen in dental offices or clinics, while others are taken to a hospital emergency clinic because other serious bodily injuries have been inflicted.

I. Definition

Child abuse and neglect can be defined as repeated mistreatment or neglect of a child by the parent(s) or other guardian which results in injury or harm to the child. The harm may be physical (including nutritional), emotional, verbal, sexual, or a combination of two or more.

Children ranging from infants through teenage are involved. Several thousands a year die as a result of the severe physical damage inflicted, while others suffer permanent brain damage or physical deformities.

II. Recognition[5,6,7,8]

Recognition of signs of suspected neglect or abuse is the first step toward protection of the child. As the child enters the reception area and then goes into the treatment room, there may be identifiable characteristics suggestive of abuse.

A. **General Signs**

1. Behavioral. An abused child may be one of two extremes: very fearful with excessive crying, or no fear at all and extremely withdrawn. The child may act differently when the parent is present than when alone, which may provide clues to the type of relationship that exists.
2. Overall appearance
   a. Failure to thrive; malnutrition.
   b. Uncleanliness and other signs of lack of care.
   c. Clothing with long sleeves and long pants even in warm weather, which may suggest that bruises and lacerations are being covered.

3. Abrasions and lacerations of varying degrees of healing; inconsistent with explanations given by the parent.
4. Burns, bite marks, trauma to the eyes, external ears, or the neck.

B. Oral Signs

1. Bruised and swollen lips; scars on lips may show previous trauma.
2. Abrasions at the corners of the mouth, such as from a gag tied around the head.
3. Lacerations of lingual and labial frena, possibly from forced feeding, or related to external traumatic blows.
4. Teeth
   a. Avulsed, fractured, darkened.
   b. Radiograph: signs of fractures in different degrees of healing.
5. Jaw fracture.
6. Tongue injuries: evidence of scarring and recent healing.
7. Signs of dental neglect.
   a. Untreated disease, including rampant caries, pain, inflammation, bleeding gingiva.
   b. Lack or irregularity of professional care; may have been primarily for tooth removal.

C. Parental Attitude

Parents who abuse their children are frequently immature and not prepared to accept the responsibilities of parenting. On the other hand, they may have been abused by their own parents. Drug abuse and alcoholism are sometimes involved.

Child abuse is very complex. A few of the possible parental attitudes and behavior patterns are mentioned here.

1. Disinterest or denial in relationship to the child; may be critical, scolding, or belittling in front of others, including dental personnel.
2. Lack of interest in proposed dental and dental hygiene treatment plan, with a tendency to want only pain relief for the child. Such an attitude may not be shown toward other children in the family.
3. Unavailable for consultation. Does not usually accompany the child for dental appointments, but sends the child with another sibling.

4. Provides inconsistent information about the sources and causes of damaged teeth, bruises, or other signs of trauma.

III. Reporting

Professional people have a particular responsibility to report suspected child abuse to the proper authorities. Each state in the United States has laws defining and governing child abuse and neglect. In certain states the failure to report can lead to legal involvement. The failure to recognize and act in behalf of the child may be dangerous, even fatal, for the child involved.

DRUG ABUSE

It is usually impossible to determine from a patient's medical and dental history whether the patient is a drug addict. A few of the common characteristics of drug abusers, which may aid in general identification, are listed here. Several significant relationships and precautions need application during patient care.

I. Definition

A *drug* is a chemical substance that can alter the structure or function of living cells. In drug use and misuse, mood, perception, consciousness, and stress-response mechanisms are altered.

The term *habituation* is applied when there is psychologic dependence on the drug to provide a continued sense of well being. On the other hand, when there is physical *dependence* or *addiction*, the individual cannot function normally without repeated use of the drug. Withdrawal leaves the person with severe physical and psychic disturbances.

II. Recognition

There are many addictive drugs, each with characteristic effects on the user. Specific identification is difficult or impossible without information from the patient. Physical and behavioral factors are listed below, which are common signs of drug abuse.

A. General Signs

1. Personal appearance
   a. Careless in appearance, with apparent lack of interest in dress and per-

sonal hygiene; particularly a person who previously was neatly dressed.
  b. Wears long sleeves to cover needle marks.
  c. May have small blood stains on clothes or skin left from previous injections.
2. Eyes
  a. Wears sunglasses to conceal dilated or constricted pupils, eye redness, or to avoid bright light because of eye sensitivity.
  b. Pupils dilated (amphetamine, LSD, cocaine, marijuana) (figure 8–5).
  c. Pupils constricted (heroin, morphine, methadone).
  d. Red, inflamed, bloodshot (marijuana).
3. Needlemarks on arms. These may be noted when sleeve is raised to determine the blood pressure.
4. Unusual behavior[9]
  a. Sneezing; itching.
  b. Tendency to gaze into space; moodiness.
  c. Drowsiness; yawning.
  d. Appearance of intoxication without odor of alcohol; slurred speech.
  e. Changes in habits, attitudes, and efficiency or irregular attendance at appointments by a previously conscientious, regular patient.
5. Possession of pills, capsules.
6. Hallucinations or convulsions: indicate need for immediate medical emergency care.

B. Oral Characteristics

1. Poor oral hygiene; lack of personal care or interest in care.
2. Higher incidence of periodontal diseases than peers.[10,11,12]
3. High dental caries incidence with open rampant carious lesions and tooth loss; few if any restorations. The abuse of analgesic drugs which reduce pain helps the addict to become indifferent to pain.[13,14]

III. Appointment Factors

A. Drug Interactions

Possible drug interactions should be checked. For example, epinephrine-containing products should not be used when treating habitual marijuana users.[15] Methadone masks the effects of narcotics, so other drugs must be used for pain relief.[12]

B. Postponement of Appointment

When a patient is under the influence of a drug, only limited procedures should be performed. Not advised are procedures requiring anesthesia or those that involve soft tissue healing.

C. Prophylactic Antibiotic Premedication[9]

For addicts who inject their drugs, antibiotic premedication has been advised. See page 100 for the regimen.

D. Hepatitis

There is a high incidence of hepatitis B carriers among addicts who inject their drugs (page 26). Maximum precaution procedures are described on page 64.

E. Attempt of Addicts to Obtain Prescriptions

Addicts frequently use dentists to obtain prescriptions of various pain-relieving drugs. By having a toothache, refusing to have the tooth removed but needing pain relief, a prescription can be obtained. Prescription pads should be kept out of sight, as addicts have been known to steal a pad and forge the dentist's signature.

Drugs kept in the dental office or clinic should be locked in a place inaccessible and unknown to patients to prevent theft. Drugs kept for emergency purposes are described on pages 833–835.

TECHNICAL HINTS

I. Wear protective gloves when making an intraoral examination to avoid contact with contagious lesions.
II. Learn the state and community regulations for reporting suspected child abuse and the specific agency that should receive the report.
III. Source of materials for information on cancer is the American Cancer Society, 219 East 42nd Street, New York, New York,

10017. Local or state societies are usually preferable as a direct source.

FACTORS TO TEACH THE PATIENT

I. Reasons for a careful extraoral and intraoral examination at each recall.
II. Method for self-examination.[16,17] Examination should include the face, neck, lips, gingiva, cheeks, tongue, palate, and throat. Any changes should be reported to the dentist and the dental hygienist.
III. The Warning Signs of Oral Cancer
   A. A swelling, lump, or growth anywhere; with or without pain.
   B. White scaly patches, or red velvety areas.
   C. Any sore that does not heal promptly (within two weeks).
   D. Numbness or tingling.
   E. Excessive dryness or wetness.
   F. Prolonged hoarseness, sore throats, persistent coughing, or the feeling of a "lump in your throat."
   G. Difficulty with swallowing.
   H. Difficulty in opening your mouth.
IV. General dietary and nutritional influences on the health of the oral tissues.
V. How the oral cavity tends to reflect the general health.
VI. Relationship of Smoking, Oral Health, and Oral Cancer
   A. Oral Effects of Smoking
     1. Increased risk of oral cancer.
     2. Increased severity and incidence of periodontal diseases.
     3. More stain and calculus on the teeth.
     4. Halitosis.
     5. Dulls senses of taste and smell.
   B. Educational Booklets
     1. American Dental Association: *Smoking and Your Oral Health* (G8), *Smoking and Teeth?* (G37), and *Smoking and Oral Cancer* (G27). Send for ADA Catalog, Order Department, 211 East Chicago Avenue, Chicago, Illinois 60611.
     2. United States Department of Health, Education, and Welfare: *Let's Help Smokers Quit,* a kit containing a variety of materials for professional use. Write to the Office of Cancer Communications, National Cancer Institute, Building 31, Room 10A18, Bethesda, Maryland 20205

References

1. Cancer Statistics, 1981, *CA—A Cancer Journal For Clinicians, 32,* 15, January-February, 1982.
2. Engelman, M.A. and Schackner, S.J.: *Oral Cancer Examination Procedure.* Published by Oral Cancer Prevention and Detection Center, St. Francis Hospital, Poughkeepsie, N.Y. Distributed by American Cancer Society, 219 E. 42nd Street, New York, N.Y. 10017.
3. Kerr, D.A., Ash, M.M., and Millard, H.D.: *Oral Diagnosis,* 5th ed. St. Louis, The C.V. Mosby Co., 1978, pp. 332–333.
4. Becker, D.B., Needleman, H.L., and Kotelchuck, M.: Child Abuse and Dentistry: Orofacial Trauma and Its Recognition by Dentists, *J. Am. Dent. Assoc., 97,* 24, July, 1978.
5. Davis, G.R., Domoto, P.K., and Levy, R.L.: The Dentist's Role in Child Abuse and Neglect, *J. Dent. Child., 46,* 185, May-June, 1979.
6. Herschaft, E.E.: Dental Implications of Child Abuse, in Clark, J.W., ed.: *Clinical Dentistry, Volume 1,* Chapter 19, Addendum. Hagerstown, Maryland, Harper & Row, 1981, pp. 19–21.
7. Laskin, D.M.: The Recognition of Child Abuse (Editorial), *J. Oral Surg., 36,* 349, May, 1978.
8. ten Bensel, R.W. and King, K.J.: Neglect and Abuse of Children: Historical Aspects, Identification and Management, *J. Dent. Child., 42,* 348, September-October, 1975.
9. Rosenbaum, C.H.: Dental Precautions in Treating Drug Addicts: A Hidden Problem Among Teens and Preteens, *Pediatric Dentistry, 2,* 94, June, 1980.
10. Shapiro, S., Pollack, B.R., and Gallant, D.: The Oral Health of Narcotic Addicts, *J. Public Health Dent., 30,* 244, Fall Issue, 1970.
11. Shapiro, S., Pollack, B.R., and Gallant, D.: Periodontal Disease in Narcotic Addicts, *J. Dent. Res., 49,* 1556, November-December, 1970.
12. Rosenstein, D.I. and Stewart, A.V.: Dental Care for Patients Receiving Methadone, *J. Am. Dent. Assoc., 89,* 356, August, 1974.
13. Picozzi, A., Dworkin, S.F., Leeds, J.G., and Nash, J.: Dental and Associated Attitudinal Aspects of Heroin Addiction: A Pilot Study, *J. Dent. Res., 51,* 869, May-June, 1972.
14. Rosenstein, D.I.: Effect of Long-term Addiction to Heroin on Oral Tissues, *J. Public Health Dent., 35,* 118, Spring, 1975.
15. Horowitz, L.G. and Nersasian, R.R.: A Review of Marijuana in Relation to Stress-response Mechanisms in the Dental Patient, *J. Am. Dent. Assoc., 96,* 983, June, 1978.
16. Bednarsh, H.S.: Oral Cancer Self-examination, *J. Texas D.H. Assoc., 17,* 11, November-December, 1979.
17. Glass, R.T., Abla, M., and Wheatley, J.: Teaching Self-examination of the Head and Neck: Another Aspect of Preventive Dentistry, *J. Am. Dent. Assoc., 90,* 1265, June, 1975.

Suggested Readings

Adams, R.J., Pullon, P.A., and Lee, F.: Expanding the Role

of the Dentist in the Detection of Oral and Laryngeal Cancer, *J. Am. Dent. Assoc.*, 89, 607, September, 1974.

Antoon, J.W. and Miller, R.L.: Aphthous Ulcers—A Review of the Literature on Etiology, Pathogenesis, Diagnosis, and Treatment, *J. Am. Dent. Assoc.*, 101, 803, November, 1980.

Bernstein, M.L. and Miller, R.L.: Oral Exfoliative Cytology, *J. Am. Dent. Assoc.*, 96, 625, April, 1978.

Bhaskar, S.N.: *Synopsis of Oral Pathology*, 6th ed. St. Louis, The C.V. Mosby Co., 1981, pp. 8–47, 373–460, 473–538.

Chue, P.W.Y.: Gonorrhea—Its Natural History, Oral Manifestations, Diagnosis, Treatment, and Prevention, *J. Am. Dent. Assoc.*, 90, 1297, June, 1975.

Colby, R.A., Kerr, D.A., and Robinson, H.B.G.: *Color Atlas of Oral Pathology*, 3rd ed. Philadelphia, J.B. Lippincott Co., 1971, pp. 91–168.

Eversole, L.R., Silverman, S., Tolley, P., and Polly, M.: The Dental Hygienist as a Comprehensive Head and Neck Cancer Screener, *Educ. Dir. Dent. Aux.*, 5, 25, December, 1980.

Geiger, B.: The Importance of an Examination of the Lymph Nodes of the Head and Neck, *Dent. Hyg.*, 53, 213, May, 1979.

Grabau, J.C. and Scott, S.J.: Early Detection of Head and Neck Cancer Using Oral/Facial Self-examination, *J. Prev. Dent.*, 4, 47, September-October, 1977.

Grabau, J.C. and Kaufman, S.: Oral Soft-Tissue Examination by Dental Hygienists, *N.Y. State Dent. J.*, 46, 23, January, 1980.

Hart, D.: Dental Hygienist's Responsibility in Preliminary Diagnosis, *Dent. Hyg.*, 53, 29, January, 1979.

Kerr, D.A., Ash, M.M., and Millard, H.D.: *Oral Diagnosis*, 5th ed. St. Louis, The C.V. Mosby Co., 1978, pp. 90–167.

Krolls, S.O. and Hoffman, S.: Squamous Cell Carcinoma of the Oral Soft Tissues: A Statistical Analysis of 14,253 Cases by Age, Sex, and Race of Patients, *J. Am. Dent. Assoc.*, 92, 571, March, 1976.

Mashberg, A. and Garfinkel, L.: Early Diagnosis of Oral Cancer: The Erythroplastic Lesion in High Risk Sites, *CA-A Cancer Journal for Clinicians*, 28, 297, September/October, 1978.

McCarthy, P.L. and Shklar, G.: *Diseases of the Oral Mucosa*, 2nd ed. Philadelphia, Lea & Febiger, 1980, pp. 18–34, 470–506.

Mitchell, D.F., Standish, S.M., and Fast, T.B.: *Oral Diagnosis/Oral Medicine*, 3rd ed. Philadelphia, Lea & Febiger, 1978, pp. 22–46, 111–124, 199–205.

Olszewski, V.: The Role of the Dental Hygienist in Oral Cancer Detection, *Dent. Hyg.*, 50, 169, April, 1976.

Sapp, J.P.: Diagnostic Laboratory Tests for Dentists, *Can. Dent. Assoc. J.*, 45, 533, October, 1979.

Seffrin, J.R. and Stauffer, D.J.: Patient Education on Cigarette Smoking: The Dentist's Role, *J. Am. Dent. Assoc.*, 92, 751, April, 1976.

Shafer, W.G.: Initial Mismanagement and Delay in Diagnosis of Oral Cancer, *J. Am. Dent. Assoc.*, 90, 1262, June, 1975.

Shklar, G. and McCarthy, P.L.: *The Oral Manifestations of Systemic Disease*. Boston, Butterworth Publishers, 1976, pp. 283–310.

Stalker, T.: Clinical Conduct Related to Oral Pathology Findings, *Dent. Hyg.*, 51, 399, September, 1977.

Zegarelli, E.V., Kutscher, A.H., and Hyman, G.A., eds.: *Diagnosis of Diseases of the Mouth and Jaws*, 2nd ed. Philadelphia, Lea & Febiger, 1978, pp. 1–19, 296–298 (with color plates).

Alcoholism

Becker, C.E.: Review of Pharmacologic and Toxicologic Effects of Alcohol, *J. Am. Dent. Assoc.*, 99, 494, September, 1979.

Grondin, D.M.: The Female Alcoholic, *Dent. Assist.*, 48, 19, March/April, 1979.

Hillman, R.W. and Kissin, B.: Oral Cytologic Patterns and Nutritional Status: Some Relationships in Alcoholic Subjects, *Oral Surg.*, 49, 34, January, 1980.

Molina, M.P.: Treating the Alcoholic Dental Patient, *Dent. Hyg.*, 55, 29, March, 1981.

Schuckit, M.A.: Overview of Alcoholism, *J. Am. Dent. Assoc.*, 99, 489, September, 1979.

Szymaitis, D.W.: Dental Considerations for Treatment of the Alcohol-consuming Patient, *J. Am. Dent. Assoc.*, 95, 592, September, 1977.

Weber, F.L., Sherman, P.M., and Stoopack, J.C.: Consider the Alcoholic Patient, *N.Y. J. Dent.*, 49, 3, January, 1979.

Child Abuse

American Dental Association, Bureau of Economic and Behavioral Research and Council on Dental Practice: *The Dentist's Responsibility in Recognizing and Reporting Child Abuse*. Chicago, American Dental Association, 1980, 40 pp.

Axelband, A.A. and Travin, M.S.: Child Abuse and What You Should Do About It, *N.Y. State Dent. J.*, 46, 76, February, 1980.

Beckstead, J.W., Rawson, R.D., and Giles, W.S.: Review of Bite Mark Evidence, *J. Am. Dent. Assoc.*, 99, 69, July, 1979.

Bowen, P.L.: Child Neglect Identification: The Hygienist and Child Advocacy, *Dent. Hyg.*, 54, 71, February, 1980.

Giovannoni, J.M. and Becerra, R.M.: *Defining Child Abuse*. New York, MacMillan, 1979, 302 pp.

Kempe, C.H., Silverman, F.N., Steele, B.F., Droegemueller, W., and Silver, H.K.: The Battered Child Syndrome, *J. Am. Med. Assoc.*, 181, 17, July 7, 1962.

Kenney, J.P.: Recognizing Child Abuse and Neglect—A Professional Responsibility, *Quintessence Journal*, 3, 269, May, 1981.

Kittle, P.E., Richardson, D.S., and Parker, J.W.: Two Child Abuse/Child Neglect Examinations for the Dentist, *J. Dent. Child.*, 48, 175, May-June, 1981.

McNeese, M.C. and Hebeler, J.R.: The Abused Child. A Clinical Approach to Identification and Management, *CIBA Clinical Symposia*, 29, Number 5, 1977, 36 pp.

Primosch, R.E. and Young, S.K.: Pseudobattering of Vietnamese Children (cao gio), *J. Am. Dent. Assoc.*, 101, 47, July, 1980.

Schwartz, S., Woolridge, E., and Stege, D.: Oral Manifestations and Legal Aspects of Child Abuse, *J. Am. Dent. Assoc.*, 95, 586, September, 1977.

Sopher, I.M.: The Dentist and the Battered Child Syndrome, *Dent. Clin. North Am.*, 21, 113, January, 1977.

Tomasetti, B.J., Walker, L., Gormley, M.B., Berger, J., and Gold, B.D.: Human Bites of the Face, *J. Oral Surg.*, 37, 565, August, 1979.

Drug Abuse

American National Red Cross: *Advanced First Aid and Emergency Care*, 2nd ed. New York, Doubleday, 1979, Chapter 8.

Ayer, W.A. and Cutright, D.E.: Dental Treatment and Heart Valve Complications in Narcotic Addicts, *Oral Surg.*, 37, 359, March, 1974.

Colon, P.G.: Dental Disease in the Narcotic Addict, *Oral Surg.*, 33, 905, June, 1972.

Gambera, S.E. and Clarke, J-A.K.: Comments on Dietary

Intake of Drug-dependent Persons, *J. Am. Dietet. Assoc.*, *68*, 155, February, 1976.

Roth-Schechter, B.F.: Drug Abuse, in Holroyd, S.V., ed.: *Clinical Pharmacology in Dental Practice*, 2nd ed. St. Louis, The C.V. Mosby Co., 1978, pp. 328–335.

United States Drug Enforcement Administration: What You Should Know About Drug Abuse and Misuse, (I) *Quintessence Journal*, *1*, 27, October, 1979; (II) *1*, 19, November/December, 1979; (III) *2*, 21, January, 1980.

9

Dental Radiographs

Radiographs are an essential adjunct to other means of oral diagnosis for treatment planning in the complete care program for a patient. The dentist is responsible for determining the need for radiographs and the number and type to be prepared. Excessive exposure of a patient to low levels of ionizing radiation from dental radiation cannot be justified. Designation of the number and types of dental exposures must be made selectively.

Preparation of radiographs may be one of the first procedures to be accomplished for a patient following a partial or complete history and a preliminary extraoral and intraoral examination. The radiographs are then available for use during the subsequent complete oral examination and charting. Later, during dental hygiene treatment appointments, the radiographs serve to guide instrumentation and to aid in patient instruction.

*The objective in radiography is to use techniques that require the least amount of radiation exposure possible to produce radiographs of the greatest interpretive value.*This can be accomplished first through the limitation of number of exposures to those that are determined to be necessary for the specific requirements of the patient. Once the *need* has been determined, then the above objective can be accomplished

by application of known safety measures for the patient and operator, through analysis of techniques to prevent making repeated inadequate radiographs, and through continuing study to keep informed of research developments.

Patients ask questions about safety factors, and occasionally a patient may refuse to have any radiographs made. The patient must be reassured with confidence, be instructed as to why radiographs are necessary at this time, and be informed about how modern equipment and techniques are in accord with minimum radiation standards.

The American Dental Association has stated that dental and general health treatment requirements must be assessed first. After that, the role of diagnostic radiographs and the minimum exposure of the patient can be determined. Selection of the number of film exposures involved in a radiographic examination should be justifiable in terms of the expected yield of diagnostic information.[1]

This chapter is designed to serve as a summary of terminology, fundamentals of x-ray production, techniques of exposure and processing, safety factors, analysis of the completed radiograph, and suggestions for patient instruction. A comprehensive bibliography is provided to allow for additional study.

131

TERMS USED IN RADIOGRAPHY*

I. Radiology

That branch of medicine dealing with the diagnostic and therapeutic applications of ionizing radiation.

II. Radiation

The emission and propagation of energy through space or a material medium in the form of waves; for example, electromagnetic waves. **Ionizing radiation** is any electromagnetic or particulate radiation capable of producing ions, directly or indirectly, in its passage through matter.

III. Radiography

The art or science of making radiographs.

IV. Radiograph

An image or picture produced on a radiation-sensitive film emulsion by exposure to ionizing radiation directed through an area or region or substance of interest, followed by chemical processing of the film (noun). To make a radiograph (verb).

V. Xeroradiography

Xeroradiography is the technique in which electrostatically charged plates (selenium plates) sensitive to x-rays are used in diagnostic radiology in place of conventional film. A bibliography is included in the Suggested Readings at the end of this chapter.

VI. Types of Radiation

A. Primary

Radiation coming directly from the target of the anode of an x-ray tube. Except for the useful beam, most of this radiation is absorbed in the tube housing.

B. Useful Beam

That part of the primary radiation that is permitted to emerge from the tube housing

---

*All definitions in this chapter are taken from or adapted from and in accord with the *Glossary of Dental Radiology,* 2nd ed. prepared by the Committee on Nomenclature, American Academy of Dental Radiology, 1978. Additional definitions to those included in this chapter may be found in the Glossary.

as limited by the aperture, cone, or other collimating devices.

C. Leakage

Radiation other than the useful beam; it escapes through the protective shielding of the x-ray tube housing.

D. Secondary

Radiation emitted by any matter being irradiated with x-rays. It originates mainly in the irradiated soft tissues of the patient's face, the pointed plastic cone, and the filter.

E. Scattered

Radiation that, during the passage through a substance, has been deviated in direction and may have been modified with an increase in wavelength. It is one form of secondary radiation.

F. Stray

A term used in a broad sense to include all radiation emitted in directions other than that of the useful beam; for example, leakage radiation, secondary radiation, scattered radiation.

VII. Irradiation

The exposure of material to x-ray or other radiation. One speaks of radiation therapy, but of irradiation of the patient.

ORIGIN AND CHARACTERISTICS OF X-RAY

X-rays were first discovered by Wilhelm C. Roentgen in 1895, who called them x rays after the mathematical symbol "x" for an unknown. "Roentgen rays" is a term often applied to mechanically generated x-rays.

Professor Roentgen used a Crookes tube, and it was not until 1913 that William D. Coolidge designed a tube in which electricity was used instead of gas. Modern x-ray tubes have the same principles of construction as the Coolidge tube. The historical development of the science of radiology and radiography provides a realistic monument to the early researchers and their efforts.[2]

I. Definition and Properties of X-Ray

A. X-ray

Electromagnetic, ionizing radiation of

very short wavelength resulting from the bombardment of a material (usually tungsten) by highly accelerated electrons in a high vacuum.

B. Properties

1. Short wave length
   a. Hard x-rays: shorter wavelengths, high penetrating power.
   b. Soft x-rays: relatively longer wavelengths, relatively less penetrating; more likely to be absorbed into the tissue through which the x-rays pass.
2. Speed of travel same as visible light.
3. Power to penetrate opaque substances.
4. Invisible.
5. Ability to affect the emulsion of a photographic film.
6. Ability to produce fluorescence on contact with certain crystals.
7. Ability to stimulate or destroy living cells.

II. How X-Rays are Produced[3,4,5,6]

With reference to the definition of x-ray above, essential to x-ray production are (1) a source of electrons, (2) a high voltage to accelerate the electrons, and (3) a target to stop the electrons. The parts of the tube and the circuits within the machine are designed to provide these.

A. The X-ray Tube (figure 9–1)

1. *Protective Tube Housing.* X-ray tube enclosure that reduces the primary radiation to permissible exposure levels; highly vacuated glass tube surrounded by a specially refined oil with high insulating powers.
2. *Cathode*
   a. Tungsten filament, which is heated to give off a cloud of electrons.
   b. Molybdenum cup around the filament to focus the electrons toward the anode.
3. *Anode*
   a. Copper arm containing a tungsten button, the target, positioned opposite the cathode.
   b. Focal spot: that part of the target on the anode bombarded by the focused electron stream when the tube is energized.
4. *Aperture.* Where the useful beam emerges from the tube; covered with a permanent seal of glass or aluminum.

B. Circuits

1. *Autotransformer.* Voltage compensator that adjusts variations in line voltage.
2. *Filament Circuit:* step-down.
   a. Voltage of line current is decreased to approximately three volts.
   b. Purpose: to heat the tungsten filament to produce electrons.
3. *High Voltage Transformer:* step-up.
   a. Voltage of line current (110 volts) is increased to 65,000–90,000 volts (65–90 kVp).
   b. Purpose: to give the electrons high speed.
4. *Tube Circuit.* The flow of electrons from the cathode to the anode, activated when the timer button is depressed.

C. Machine Control Devices

Machines vary, but in general, in operating an x-ray machine there are four factors to control: the line switch (to electrical outlet), the kilovoltage, the milliamperage, and the time. Certain machines operate at a

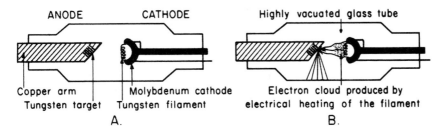

Figure 9–1. X-ray tube. **A.** Inactive, and **B.** In function. Highly accelerated electrons are propelled from the cathode to the anode. X-rays are produced as the electrons strike the tungsten target.

standard kilovoltage (for example, 65 kVp) and milliamperage (10 mA), whereas others permit a range of selection.

1. *Voltage Control* (may be 1 or 2 meters, depending on the machine).
   a. Circuit voltmeter; registers line voltage before voltage is stepped up by the transformer (with alternating current this is 110 volts); or may register the kilovoltage that will result after step-up.
   b. KVp selector (kilovoltage peak): to change the line voltage to a selected kilovoltage (65 to 90 kVp).
2. *Milliamperage Control.* Milliammeter: to select the actual current through the tube circuit used during the time of exposure (10 to 20 mA).
3. *Time Control*
   a. X-ray timer: a time switch mechanism used to complete the electrical circuit so that x-rays will be produced for a predetermined time.
   b. Mechanical timer: spring-activated device; range from $\frac{1}{4}$ to 10 or 15 seconds; does not reset itself; will not accommodate new high-speed film and techniques.
   c. Electronic timer: vacuum tube device; will reset itself automatically to the last-used exposure time. The timer is calibrated in seconds with 60 *impulses* in each second (in a 60 cycle AC current).

D. Steps in the Production of X-Rays[4,6]

1. Tungsten filament is heated and a cloud of electrons produced.
2. Difference in electrical potential is developed between the anode and the cathode.
3. Electrons attracted to anode from cathode at high speed during the intervals of the alternating current when the anode is charged positive and the cathode negative. (During the alternating half of the cycle the electrons are attracted back into the filament in a self-rectifying tube.)
4. Curvature of the molybdenum cup controls the direction of the electrons and causes them to be projected on the focal spot.

5. Reaction of the electrons as they strike the tungsten target; loss of energy.
   a. Approximately one percent of the energy of electrons is converted to electromagnetic energy of an x-ray. (Greater percent at higher kilovoltages.)
   b. Approximately 99 percent of the energy is converted to heat which is dissipated through the copper anode and oil of the protective tube housing.
6. X-rays leave the tube through the aperture to form the useful beam.

FACTORS THAT INFLUENCE THE FINISHED RADIOGRAPH

As the beam leaves the x-ray tube it is collimated, filtered, and allowed to travel a designated source-film (or focal spot-film) distance before reaching the film of a selected speed. The quality or diagnostic usefulness of the finished radiograph as well as the total exposure of the patient and operator are influenced by the collimation, filtration, source-film distance, film speed, kilovoltage, and milliampere seconds.

Film processing (pages 155–159) also influences directly the quality of the radiograph, and indirectly the total exposure, since re-exposure would be necessary should the film be rendered inadequate during processing.

I. Characteristics of an Acceptable Radiograph

A. All Parts of the Image: shown as close to their natural size and shape as possible with a minimum of distortion and superimposition.

B. Area to be Examined: shown completely with sufficient surrounding tissue included to provide for comparative interpretation.

C. Highest Film Quality

1. *Density.* The degree of darkening of exposed and processed x-ray film.
2. *Contrast.* The visual differences in density between adjacent areas on the radiograph.
3. *Definition.* The property of the projected images relating to their sharpness, distinctness, or clarity of outline.

II. Collimation[7,8]

Collimation is the technique or mechanism for reducing the size and shape of the beam of radiation emitted through the aperture of the tube. A *collimator* is a diaphragm or system of diaphragms made of an absorbing material designed to define the dimensions and direction of a beam of radiation.[9]

A. Purposes

1. Eliminate peripheral or more divergent radiation.
2. Minimize exposure to patient's face.
3. Minimize secondary radiation which can fog the film and expose the bodies of patient and operator.

B. Method

A diaphragm usually of lead and pierced with a central aperture of the smallest practical diameter for making radiographic exposure is used; located between x-ray tube and cone.
1. Recommended thickness of lead: $1/8$ inch.
2. Recommended size of aperture: to permit a diameter of the beam of radiation equal to $2^3/_4$ inches at the end of the plastic cone next to the patient's face.
3. Use of rectangular collimation: when a rectangular diaphragm is used, it should be approximately $1^1/_2 \times 2$ inches at the skin. A rectangular diaphragm must be rotated to accommodate for films positioned horizontally or vertically.

    Rectangular collimation has been shown to reduce the exposure and absorbed dose in the bone marrow of the head and neck areas by as much as 60 percent.[10]

C. Relation to Techniques

The dimensions of the largest periapical film are $1^1/_4$ by $1^5/_8$ inches. Precise angulation techniques are required to eliminate cone-cut of film, particularly when rectangular collimation is used.

III. Filtration[1,7]

Filtration is the insertion of layers of aluminum for selective removal of x-rays of longer wavelengths from the primary beam.

A. Purpose

To minimize exposure of the patient's skin to unnecessary radiation that will not reach and expose the film.

B. Methods

1. *Inherent Filtration.* Accomplished by internal barriers built into the x-ray tube, including the glass wall of the tube and the insulating oil surrounding the tube.
2. *Added Filtration.* Thin, commercially pure aluminum disks inserted between the lead diaphragm and the x-ray tube.
3. *Total Filtration.* The sum of inherent and added filtration.
    a. Recommended total: equivalent of 0.5 mm. (below 50 kVp); 1.5 mm. (50–70 kVp); and 2.5 mm. (over 70 kVp) of aluminum.[1]
    b. Check the inherent filtration of the individual x-ray machine; then add a sufficient amount of commercially pure aluminum to bring the total to the recommended level.

C. Disadvantage of Added Filtration

Some secondary radiation is produced which scatters in all directions.

IV. Kilovoltage

A. Amount of Kilovoltage

Determines the quality of the x-radiation.
1. Kilovoltage creates a difference in potential between the anode and the cathode for the production of x-rays.
2. The higher the kilovoltage, the greater the acceleration of the electrons, the greater the force with which they bombard the target; therefore, the shorter the wavelength.
3. The shorter the wavelength, the greater the penetrating power at the skin surface.

B. Use of High Kilovoltage (90 kVp)[7]

1. Density of the finished radiograph increases with increased kilovoltage (other factors remaining constant).
2. To maintain the proper film density, the milliampere seconds must be decreased as the kVp is increased.

3. Variation in contrast
   a. Low kilovoltage: high contrast, with sharp black-white differences in densities between adjacent areas, but small range of distinction between subject thicknesses recorded.
   b. High kilovoltage: low contrast, with wide range of subject thicknesses recorded; greater range of densities from black to white (more gray tones), which, when examined under proper viewing conditions, provide more interpretive details.
4. Advantages
   a. Permits shorter exposure time.
   b. Reduces exposure to tissues lying in front of the film packet.
5. Disadvantages
   a. Increased radiation to tissues outside the edges of the film.
   b. More scattered radiation at 90 kVp than at 65 kVp.

V. Milliampere Seconds

A. Milliamperage

The measure of the electron current passing through the x-ray tube; it regulates the heat of the filament, which determines the number of electrons available to bombard the target.

B. Quantity of Radiation

Quantity of radiation is expressed in milliampere seconds (mAs).
1. MAs is the milliamperes multiplied by the time seconds of exposure.
2. Example: at 10 milliamperes for one half second the exposure of the film would be 5 mAs.

C. Radiographic Density

Radiographic density increases with increased milliamperage and/or time of exposure (other factors remaining constant).

VI. Distance

Several distances are involved in x-ray film exposure. The source-surface, the source-film, and the object-film distances must be considered for film placement. In addition, there is the distance the operator stands from the patient's head during film exposure, which is outlined on page 140 in connection with safety factors.

A. Object-Film Distance

In a technique where x-ray films are placed against the teeth being radiographed, the object-film distance is negligible. Close adaptation of the film to the tooth is essential to obtain a sharp image when an 8-inch source-film distance is utilized.

With the paralleling or right-angle technique and use of a longer source-film distance (16 to 20 inches), there is an increased object-film distance for most radiographs. A collimated beam and increased source-film distance compensate to preserve definition and film quality.

B. Source-Film Distance

The directing cone on the x-ray machine is designed to indicate the direction of the central axis of the x-ray beam and to serve as a guide in establishing a desired source-surface and source-film distance. Techniques using 8- and 16-inch source-film distances are commonly used.

The source-film distance is the sum total of the distance from the source to the cone within the tube housing, the length of the directing cone, and the distance from the end of the cone (at the face) to the film. Directions in technique call for lightly touching the skin with the end of the cone to standardize the source-film distance.

Principles related to source-film distance are:
1. The intensity of the x-ray beam varies inversely as the square of the source-film distance. Example: if a film of the same speed were used at a 16-inch source-film distance as at 8 inches, with all other factors such as kVp and mAs remaining constant, the film at 16 inches would require four times the exposure (time) to maintain the same density in the finished radiograph.
2. The exposure decreases as the distance increases: when the distance is made twice as great, the radiation exposure to the patient is reduced to one-fourth.

3. To maintain film density, an increase in mAs, kVp, or film speed is required when distance is increased.

C. Advantages in the Use of an Extended Source-Film Distance

1. Definition or distinctness and clarity of detail improve (because the image is produced by the more central rays).
2. Enlargement or magnification of image decreases (because at shorter distances the outer, more divergent rays tend to enlarge or magnify the image).
3. Skin exposure of the patient is reduced.
4. There is less tissue within the primary beam of radiation, since there is less spreading of the x-ray beam.

VII. Films[11]

With optimum filtration, collimation, and fast film, the skin dose to the face can be reduced significantly. Within recent years, the manufacture of very slow-speed films has been discontinued, the speed of many films has been doubled, and the use of higher speed films has gained increasing acceptance by the dental profession.

A. Film Composition

A thin, transparent sheet of cellulose acetate or similar material coated on one or both sides with an emulsion sensitive to radiation and light.

1. *Emulsion.* Gelatin containing a suspension of countless tiny crystals of silver halide salts.
2. *Film Packet.* Small, light-proof, moisture-resistant, sealed paper envelope containing an x-ray film (or two), and a thin sheet of lead foil.
   a. Two-film packet: useful for processing one film differently than the other to make diagnostic comparisons; for sending to specialist to whom patient may be referred; for legal evidence.
   b. Purpose of lead foil backing: prevent exposure of the film by scattered radiation that could enter from back of packet; protection of patient's tissues lying in the path of the x-ray.

B. Film Speed

Film speed or film emulsion speed refers to the sensitivity of the film to radiation exposure. The speed is the amount of exposure required to produce a certain image density.

1. *Factors Determining*
   a. Grain size: the smaller the grain size, the slower the film speed.
   b. Use of double or single emulsion: slower have single, on one side only. Nearly all present-day films have two emulsions.
2. *Classification.* Films have been classified by the American National Standard Institute (ANSI) in cooperation with the American Dental Association (ADA). The ANSI/ADA Specification Number 22 designates six groups, A through F. Speed groups A, B, and C, the slowest, are associated with excess radiation exposure and are not used. Only film speeds D or faster are used for dental purposes. E film requires only one-half the exposure time used for D film.

EXPOSURE TO RADIATION

A number of factors influence the biologic effects of radiation, including the quality of the radiation, the chemical composition of the absorbing medium, the tissues irradiated, the dose (total and rate per unit of time), the blood supply to the tissues, and the size of the area exposed. Generally, radiation of a specific area is less harmful than whole body radiation. Biologic effects of radiation are either somatic (of the general body cells) or genetic (heritable changes, chiefly mutations, produced by the absorption of ionizing radiation by reproductive cells).[8]

I. Ionization

The phenomenon of separation of electrons from molecules which changes their chemical activity is called ionization. The organic and inorganic compounds that make up the human body may be altered by exposure to ionizing radiation. The biologic effects following irradiation are secondary effects in that they result from physical, chemical, and biologic action set in motion by the absorption of energy from radiation.

II. Permissible Exposure

A. Exposure

A measure of the x-radiation to which a

person or object, or a part of either, is exposed at a certain place; this measure being based on its ability to produce ionization.

1. *Threshold Exposure.* The minimum exposure that will produce a detectable degree of any given effect.
2. *Entrance or Surface Exposure.* Exposure measured at the surface of an irradiated body, part, or object. It includes primary radiation and backscatter from the irradiated underlying tissue material. The term skin exposure is used with reference to the exposure measured at the center of an irradiated skin surface area.
3. *Erythema Exposure.* The radiation necessary to produce a temporary redness of the skin. The exposure required will vary with the quality of the radiation to which the skin is exposed.

B. Exposure Units

1. *Roentgen (R):* unit of quantity of radiation derived from the ionizing effect of x-rays on air.
2. *Other Units: rad* (unit of absorbed dose); *rem* (unit of the RBE or Relative Biological Effectiveness).

C. Dose

The amount of energy absorbed per unit mass of tissue at a site of interest. The gonadal dose is the dose of radiation absorbed by the gonads.

D. Permissible Dose

The amount of radiation that may be received by an individual within a specified period without expectation of any significantly harmful result.

1. Assumptions on which permissible doses are calculated.
   a. That no irradiation is beneficial.
   b. There is a dose below which no somatic change will be produced.
   c. Children are more susceptible than older people.
   d. There is a dose below which, even though it is delivered before the end of the reproductive period, the probability of genetic effects will be slight.

E. Radiation Hazard

A condition under which persons might receive radiation in excess of the maximum permissible dose or radiation damage might be caused to materials.

F. National Council on Radiation Protection and Measurements[12]

1. Limits for dentists and dental personnel (table 9–1).
2. Limits for patients: exposure to x-ray radiation shall be kept to the minimum level consistent with clinical requirements. This limitation is determined by the professional judgment of the dentist.

III. Sensitivity of Cells[8,13]

A. Factors Affecting

1. *Maturity of Cell.* Immature cells are most sensitive.
2. *Reproductive Capacity.* Rapidly reproducing are more sensitive; most sensitive when undergoing mitosis.
3. *Metabolism.* More sensitive in periods of increased metabolism.

B. Radiosensitive Tissues

Blood-forming tissues, reproductive cells, lymphatic tissues, young bone tissue, and skin.

C. Radioresistant Tissues

Most glandular tissues, muscle tissue, nerve tissue, and mature bone tissue.

D. Tissue Reaction

1. *Latent Period.* Lapse between the time of exposure and the time when effects are observed. (May be as long as 25 years or relatively short, as in the case of the production of a skin erythema.)
2. *Cumulative Effect*
   a. Amount of reaction depends on dose: less reaction when radiation is received in fractional doses than with one large dose.
   b. There will be partial or total repair as long as there is not complete destruction.
   c. There may be some irreparable damage which is cumulative as, little by

Table 9–1. **Maximum Permissible Dose Equivalent Values (MPD)* to Whole Body, Gonads, Blood-Forming Organs, Lens of Eye**[12]

Average Weekly Exposure†	*Maximum 13-week Exposure*	*Maximum Yearly Exposure*	*Maximum Accumulated Exposure‡*
0.1 R	3 R	5 R	5(N-18)R§

Exposure of persons for dental or medical purposes is not counted against their maximum permissible exposure limits.

Used only for the purpose of designating radiation barriers.

When the previous occupational history of an individual is not definitely known, it shall be assumed that the full dose permitted by the formula 5(N-18) has already been received.

N = Age in years and is greater than 18. The unit for exposure is the roentgen (R).

little, more is added (examples: hair loss, skin lesions, falling blood count).

RULES FOR RADIATION PROTECTION[1]

Dental X-ray Protection prepared by the National Council on Radiation Protection and Measurements[12] provides specific information about radiation barriers, film speed group rating, film badge service sources, x-ray equipment data, and operating procedure regulations.

In the application of procedures for protecting the operator and the patient from excessive radiation, particular attention should be paid to unnecessary radiation which may result from the need for an unusual number of retakes due to inadequate technical procedures. Perfecting techniques contributes to the accomplishment of minimum exposure for maximum safety.

I. Protection of Operator

A. Protection from Primary Radiation

1. Avoid the useful beam of radiation. When this is not possible, stand behind a protective barrier.
2. Never hand-hold the film during exposure.
3. Fluorescent mirrors shall not be used in dental examination.

B. Protection from Leakage Radiation

1. Do not hand-hold the tube housing or the directing cone of the machine during exposures.
2. Test machine for leakage radiation. Surpak is a film device for surveying dental x-ray machines which can be obtained at no cost from a State Health Department. The survey determines the size of the beam, the output of the machine, the total filtration, the beam symmetry, and the presence of leakage radiation occurring in a forward direction.

C. Protection from Secondary Radiation

The major sources of secondary radiation are the filter, the pointed plastic cone, and the irradiated soft tissues of the patient's face. The face produces the greatest amount. Methods of protection are related to these three sources.

1. *Minimization of Total X-Radiation*
   a. Use high-speed films. When attempting to use high-speed films with older x-ray machines, the original mechanical timers may prove inadequate. Replacement timers are available.
   b. Replace older x-ray machines with modern shockproof equipment.
2. *Collimation of Useful Beam.* Use diaphragms or cones to collimate the useful beam to an area no larger than three inches in diameter when measured at the end of the directing cone. Rectangular collimation has been shown to be more effective than round.
3. *Type of Cone.* Use an open-ended, shielded (lead-lined) cone in place of the pointed plastic cone. The scattered secondary radiation from the filter and the plastic cone are controlled and eliminated respectively.

4. *Position of Operator While Making Exposures.* The operator shall stand behind the patient's head behind the three major sources of secondary radiation, to prevent direct exposure.

    a. Exposure of the region of the central incisors: stand at a 45-degree angle to the path of the central ray. This position is approximately behind either the left or the right ear of the patient (figure 9–2).

    b. Exposure of other regions: stand behind the patient's head and at an angle of 45 degrees to the path of the central ray of the x-ray beam.

5. *Distance*

    a. Safety increases with distance. A long cord on the timer will permit greater freedom of movement.

    b. The operator shall stand as far as practical from the patient, at least 6 feet, and outside the path of the useful beam, or behind a suitable barrier.

    c. When space limitations within the dental office prevent occupying the safer positions listed above, the operator should step out of the room and stand behind a thick wall.

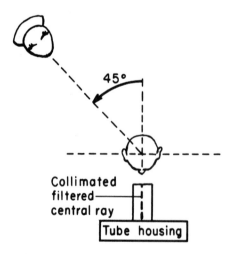

Figure 9–2. Safer position of operator during film exposure. The operator stands behind the patient's head at a 45° angle to the path of the central ray. The irradiated tissues of the patient's face are the greatest source of secondary radiation.

D. Monitoring

Monitoring refers to the periodic or continuous determination of the amount of ionizing radiation or radioactivity present at a given location, usually for considerations of health protection.

The amount of x-ray radiation that reaches the body of the dentist or dental personnel can be measured economically with a film badge. Badges can be obtained from one of several laboratories. The film badge is worn on the clothing for one, two, or four weeks and is then returned by mail to the laboratory where it was purchased. At the laboratory, the film in the badge is carefully processed and its exposure evaluated. The amount of radiation recorded by the film badge is a measure of the exposure of the wearer who is notified by mail of the amount of exposure.

II. Protection of Patient

A. Films

Use high-speed films.

B. Collimation

Use diaphragms or cones to collimate the useful beam.

C. Filtration

Use filtration of the useful beam to recommended levels (page 135).

D. Processing

Process films according to the manufacturer's directions. When a choice of two periods of development is offered, the exposure of the patient can be reduced if the longer development time is employed.

E. Film Size

Use the largest intraoral film that can be skillfully placed in the mouth. Maximum coverage is provided in this manner with one exposure, whereas two exposures may be required if smaller films are used to examine the same area of the mouth. This factor is especially important when examining the mouths of children.

F. **Total Exposure**

Do not expose the patient unnecessarily. There must be a good and valid reason for each exposure.

G. **Leaded Apron**

A leaded apron for general body coverage, including the gonads, and a thyroid shield or collar provide significant protection from exposure.

The use of a leaded apron on each patient is required by law in several states and countries.

H. **High Voltage**

The use of high voltages has been over-emphasized. High voltages permit shorter exposure times and reduce the exposure of tissues lying in front of the film packet, but the exposure of the gonads and the tissues lying behind the film packet can increase with increased voltage.

TECHNIQUES FOR FILM PLACEMENT AND ANGULATION OF RAY

The characteristics of the acceptable finished radiograph have been listed, (page 134) and certain technical factors, including collimation, filtration, kilovoltage, milliampere seconds, distance, and films have been described. For consideration next in the procedure for preparation of radiographs is the placement of the film and the angulation of the useful beam.

Intraoral techniques for periapical, bite-wing, and occlusal radiographs are included in this chapter. The principles and uses of panoramic radiographs are also described.

Two fundamental periapical techniques are used in practice: the *paralleling* or right-angle and the *angle bisection*. The paralleling technique is sometimes referred to as the "long" or "extension cone" and the angle bisection as the "short cone" technique. However, the long cone may be employed with angle bisection procedures.

Operators vary in their application of the principles of the two techniques. Basically, the primary ray should pass through the region to be examined and the film should be placed in relation to the ray so that all parts of the image

are shown as close to their natural size and shape as possible with a minimum of distortion in the finished radiograph.

As with other techniques, the development of a systematic procedure is essential. A comfortable, smooth operation saves time and energy for both patient and operator, increases the confidence of the patient in the operator, and allows for consistency in technique which produces consistent results. A basic objective during radiographic technique is to minimize the length of time the film packet remains in the patient's mouth.

I. **Film Selection for Intraoral Surveys**

A. **Periapical**

1. *Purpose:* to obtain a view of the entire tooth and its periodontal supporting structures.
2. *Films*
   a. Child size: Number 0 (1.0) ($7/8 \times 13/8$ inches) for primary teeth and small mouths.
   b. Anterior: Number 1 (1.1) ($15/16 \times 19/16$ inches) for anterior regions where width of arch makes positioning of standard film difficult or impossible.
   c. Standard: Number 2 (1.2) ($11/4 \times 15/8$ inches) may be used for all positions.
3. *Number of Films Used in a Complete Survey:* for the adult mouth it will vary from 14 to 30 depending on the operator's preferences, objectives for showing specific areas, anatomy of the patient's mouth, and the size of the films used. For children see page 154.

B. **Bite-wing (Interproximal)**

1. *Purpose:* to show the crowns of the teeth, the alveolar crest, and the interproximal area.
2. *Films with Tab Attached*
   a. Anterior teeth ($15/16 \times 19/16$ inches): three films are generally used.
   b. Adult posterior teeth, standard film size: four films, one for molar region and one for premolar, each side.
   c. Child posterior teeth, with first permanent molar erupted, standard size film; one on each side.

d. Adult posterior teeth using longer, narrower film: Number 3 ($1^1/_{16}$ × $2^1/_8$ inches) designed to include molars and premolars; one on each side.

3. *Commercial Tabs:* to be attached to standard or child-size films; two types, one a loop to slide over the film packet and the other with an adhesive to attach directly to the film packet.

C. **Occlusal**

1. *Purpose:* to show large areas of the maxilla, mandible, or floor of the mouth.
2. *Film:* Number 4 ($2^1/_4$ × 3 inches) for use in self packet or in intraoral cassette.
3. *Standard Film:* ($1^1/_4$ × $1^5/_8$ inches) for child or individual areas of adult.

II. Preliminary Preparation

A. **Equipment**

1. *Surface Disinfection* of patient surroundings includes wiping the parts of the x-ray machine that are handled in conjunction with oral contact (directing cone, handle of tube housing, timer). Cross-contamination by way of the hands of the operator and the radiographic equipment has been demonstrated.[14]
2. *Advanced Readiness:* the patient should not be kept waiting for procedures such as setting the x-ray machine or placing bite-wing tabs on film packets.
3. *Timer:* check automatic reset or adjust mechanical timer for exposure prior to film placement. Manufacturer's chart is consulted for exposure time at given source-film distance, kilovoltage, and milliamperes.

B. **Patient Preparation**

1. Remove eyeglasses and removable dental appliances.
2. For panoramic radiography, earrings must be removed.

C. **Oral Examination**

1. *Purpose:* to determine necessary adaptations during film placement.
2. *Factors of particular interest*
   a. Position of teeth and edentulous areas.

b. Apparent size of teeth as compared to average size of teeth.
c. Accessibility: height and shape of palate, flexibility of muscles of orifice, floor of the mouth, possible gag reflex, size of tongue.
d. Unusual features: tori, sensitive areas of the mucous membranes.

III. Patient Cooperation: Prevention of Gagging[15]

Gagging may be the result of psychologic or physiologic factors. It presents some problem in the placement of all films for molar radiographs and may be initiated in the patient who ordinarily does not gag if techniques are not carried out efficiently. Many of the factors related to the prevention of gagging may be applied for the comfort and cooperation of all patients.

A. **Causes of Gagging**

1. *Hypersensitive oral tissues,* particularly of posterior region of oral cavity.
2. *Anxiety and apprehension*
   a. Fear of unknown, of the film touching a sensitive area.
   b. Previous unpleasant experiences with radiographic techniques.
   c. Failure to comprehend the operator's instructions.
   d. Lack of confidence in the operator.
3. *Techniques:* film moved over the oral tissues or retained in the mouth longer than necessary.

B. **Preventive Procedures**

1. Inspire confidence in ability to perform the service.
2. Alleviate anxiety: explain procedures carefully.
3. Film placement: firmly and positively without sliding the film over the tissue.
4. Film retention: use a film holder on which the patient can bite to distract from the procedure.
5. Instruct patient to breathe through the nose with quick, short breaths during film placement and to hold the breath during exposure.
6. Use of premedicating agent prescribed by the dentist.
7. Use of topical anesthetic.

a. Cold water or ice cube held in the mouth for a short time before film placement dulls the sensory nerve endings.

b. Salt: one-half teaspoonful placed on the tongue has an anesthetic effect. It may be swallowed or rinsed after radiographs are made.

c. Prepared topical anesthetics, in the form of an ointment (applied with cotton swab), troche, or rinse give up to 20 minutes of surface anesthesia (pages 521–523).

IV. Definitions and Principles Related to Techniques

A. Planes

1. *Sagittal or Median.* The plane that divides the body in the midline into right and left sides.

2. *Occlusal.* The mean occlusal plane represents the mean curvature from the incisal edges of the central incisors to the tips of the occluding surfaces of the third molars. The occlusal plane of the premolars and first molar may be considered as the mean occlusal plane.

   When it is specified in techniques that the occlusal plane of the teeth being radiographed shall be parallel to the floor, at least three head positions are involved for the maxillary: for anterior teeth, the head must be tipped forward; for premolars, held at the mean occlusal plane; and for molars, tipped back.

B. Angulation

1. *Horizontal.* The angle at which the central ray of the useful beam is directed within a horizontal plane. Inadequate horizontal angulation results in overlapping or superimposition of parts of adjacent teeth in the radiograph.

2. *Vertical.* The plane at which the central ray of the useful beam is directed within a vertical plane. Inadequate vertical angulation results in elongation or foreshortening in the image.

C. Long Axis of a Tooth

An imaginary line passing longitudinally through the center of the tooth.

Because of marked variations in tooth position and root curvature, estimation of the long axis of a tooth is difficult. Clinically, it can be considered that the long axis of a posterior tooth is at right angles to the occlusal surface plane. For single-rooted teeth the long axis would ordinarily pass from the center of the incisal edge to the tip of the apex, but it is not possible to observe this during clinical examination. It must be remembered that the line from the incisal to the cervical on the labial surface should not be confused with the long axis.

PERIAPICAL SURVEY: PARALLELING TECHNIQUE

The paralleling or right-angle technique is based on the principles that *the film is placed as nearly parallel to the long axis of the tooth as the anatomy of the oral cavity will permit and the central ray is directed at right angles to the film.* In figure 9–3 A the parallel relationship of the film with the long axis of the tooth and the right-angle direction of the central ray are shown.

The distance between the crown of the tooth and the film is increased to attain parallelism. In the majority of positions for individual films, the edge of the film against the soft tissues is approximately in the same position on the palate or the floor of the mouth as when the film is placed against and close to the tooth, for example, in the angle bisection technique. In other words, the distance between the root apex and the film is not materially different in the paralleling technique than in the angle bisection technique. Figure 9–3 A and B shows the comparative projection of the parts of the tooth on the film to produce the image in the radiograph.

I. Patient Position

As long as the film is parallel to the long axis of the tooth and the central ray is directed at right angles to the film, the head may be in any position convenient to the operator and comfortable for the patient. Slight modification of positioning may be needed for making radiographs in a supine position.[16,17]

New x-ray units have been developed in which an extra-long arm permits equal ease of angulation whether the patient is in an upright or a supine position. With the use of the supine pa-

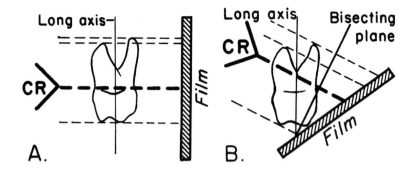

Figure 9–3. Comparison of paralleling and angle bisection techniques. **A.** Paralleling technique. The film is parallel with the long axis of the tooth and the central ray (CR) is directed perpendicular to both the film and the long axis of the tooth. **B.** Angle bisection. The central ray (CR) is directed perpendicular to an imaginary line which bisects the angle formed by the film and the long axis of the tooth.

tient position, less radiation to body areas below the neck has been demonstrated.[18]

The use of a film holder facilitates obtaining the correct angulation of the ray, since the directing cone for the central ray can be lined up with the part of the film holder that extends from between the teeth and that is designed to be at right angles to the film.

For the inexperienced operator, horizontal angulation may be visualized more readily when the occlusal plane of the teeth being radiographed is parallel with the floor and the sagittal plane is perpendicular to the floor.

II. Film Placement

A. Film Position and Angulation of the Central Ray

Instructions for film placement and angulation are included in this section. In addition to the references associated with specific parts of this section, other references will be helpful in studying and perfecting techniques.[19,20,21]

1. *Basic principles* for film placement and angulation of the central ray are shown in figures 9–5 and 9–6. The image objective in the completed radiograph is also illustrated.
2. *Horizontal Angulation.* The ray is directed approximately at the center of the film and through the interproximal area.
3. *Vertical Angulation.* The ray is directed at right angles to the film.

B. Film Positioning Devices

1. *Purposes.* The use of a beam-guiding, field-size-limiting film-holding instrument provides important advantages. There will be dose reduction, film quality, and consistently adequate diagnostic radiographs without frequent retakes. Sanitation is improved, and lack of need for patient involvement in holding film is helpful.

2. *Characteristics.* An effective film positioning device will have characteristics such as the following:
   a. Adaptable to all necessary positions for obtaining diagnostic radiographs of the entire dental arches.
   b. Weight and other properties that do not hinder placement or holding without requiring the patient to hand-hold the device.
   c. Comfortable for the patient during the necessary time interval.
   d. Simplicity of placement; minimal complexity for learning.
   e. Aid in alignment of x-ray beam for correct exposure of film.
   f. Disposable or conveniently sterilized. To this end, more than one device should be maintained to permit sterilization between patients.

3. *Types*[22]
   a. *Hemostat* is inserted through a rubber bite block and film is positioned and held in claws of the hemostat. The film is positioned in the mouth and held by the patient biting on the bite block.

b. *Bite blocks:* plastic or wooden (short and long for different areas of the mouth).

c. *Styrofoam disposable film holder* (Stabe).[23] Simple, comfortable, light weight device; assists in beam alignment by the end that protrudes after the teeth are closed down to hold the device in place (figure 9–4). The film holder may be taped to a tongue depressor to aid in the proper alignment of the central ray.[24]

d. *Precision X-ray device.* Has a facial shield attached to the bar which holds the film in position parallel to the shield. A rectangular hole in the shield permits the passage of only the x-rays that will reach the film. (Distributed by the Precision X-ray Company.)

e. *Snap-A-Ray.* Plastic film holder with two ends for positioning anterior and posterior films. It is held between the teeth. (Rinn Corporation.)

f. *X-C-P (X-tension C-one P-aralleling).* Has an adjustable circular ring that permits film alignment with the primary beam by bringing the open end of the cone in contact with the ring.[25] (Rinn Corporation.)

g. *V.I.P. (Versatile Intraoral Positioner).* Film-holding, beam-directing, with a target attachment for alignment of the open-end tube. It is called versatile because it has holders to accommodate three film sizes and it can be used for periapical and bite-wing surveys.[26] (UP-RAD Corporation.)

4. *Supplements*

a. Removable denture may be needed in place in opposite jaw to stabilize a film holder.

b. A cotton roll between the film holder or bite block and the biting surface can aid in paralleling when teeth are short and/or the palatal vault is low.

III. Paralleling Technique: Advantages

A. Accuracy

The paralleling technique gives truer size

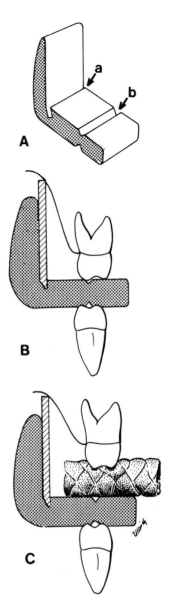

Figure 9–4. Styrofoam disposable film holder. **A.** Empty holder to show **a,** slot for insertion of film, and **b,** break off point to shorten the bite surface for use in mandibular posterior positions; **B.** Film placement for maxillary molar radiograph for patient with high palatal vault; **C.** Film placement for low palatal vault using a cotton roll to lower the film holder.

and shape of dental structures with less distortion than when angle bisection is used.

1. Buccal and lingual aspects can be shown in proper relation to each other.

2. Zygomatic bone can be shown in its normal position above the root apices of the molars and premolars.

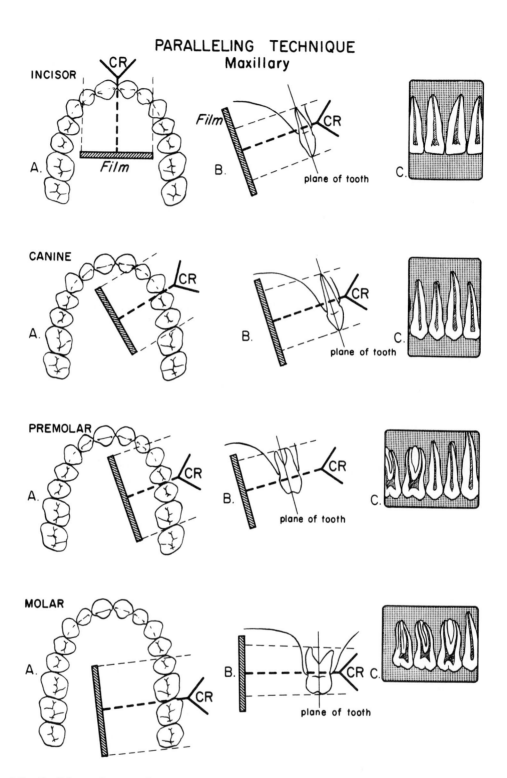

Figure 9–5. Paralleling technique. Film positioning for the four major maxillary positions. Two additional radiographs are frequently made centered at the right and left lateral incisors. **A.** Horizontal angulation with film placed parallel to the long axes of the teeth; central ray (CR) directed parallel with a line through the interproximal. **B.** Vertical angulation with central ray (CR) directed at right angles to the film. **C.** Image objective for the completed radiograph.

PARALLELING TECHNIQUE
Mandibular

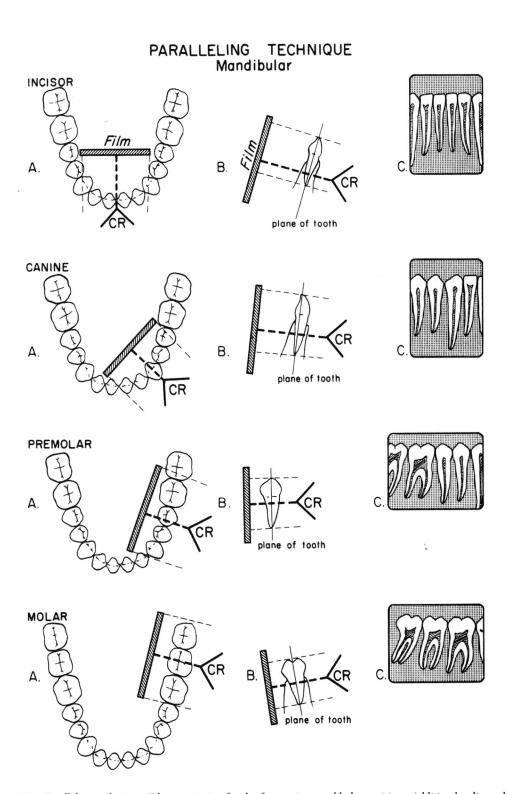

Figure 9–6. Paralleling technique. Film positioning for the four major mandibular positions. Additional radiographs are frequently made centered at the right and left lateral incisors. **A.** Horizontal angulation with film placed parallel to the long axes of the teeth; central ray (CR) directed through the interproximal. **B.** Vertical angulation with central ray (CR) directed at right angles to the film. **C.** Image objective for the completed radiograph.

B. Bite-wing Radiographs May Not Be Required

In a complete survey, the right angle view of proximal surfaces in paralleling technique radiographs is the same as in the bite-wing. Time and effort as well as radiation to patient are saved.

C. Simpler to Perform

Bisection of the angle between the long axis and the film in the bisection technique can be difficult to visualize.

D. Standardized Results Obtained That Can Be Duplicated

E. Horizontal Ray Direction

No rays are directed toward the thyroid, whereas with angle bisection several radiographs require a relatively steep vertical angulation.

BITE-WING SURVEY

The bite-wing or interproximal survey is used as an adjunct to the periapical survey. It has been used at the time of patient recall to detect proximal surface caries.

Standard bite-wing radiographs do not provide adequate information about periodontal conditions. Periapical radiographs prepared by the paralleling technique are more useful. A vertical periapical bite-wing made with a standard Number 2 (1.2) film has been suggested.[27,28] The crestal bone of a patient with advanced bone loss can be viewed to better advantage than when a standard bite-wing radiograph is used.

As with all other radiographic surveys, a bite-wing survey should be made only when a need is demonstrated for specific diagnostic purposes.

When the angle bisection technique is used for the periapical radiographs, the bite-wing survey is essential, since an accurate view of all proximal surfaces cannot otherwise be obtained. The angulation for the bite-wing radiographs is based on the same principle as that for periapical surveys made with the paralleling or right-angle technique.

I. Preparation for Film Placement

A. Patient Position

1. *Traditional*. Sagittal plane perpendicu-
lar to the floor and occlusal plane parallel with the floor.
2. *Patient in Supine Position*. The plane are reversed in their relation to the floor

B. Vertical Angulation

Set at +10 degrees.

C. Patient Instruction

Request patient to practice closing o posterior teeth prior to positioning film fo posterior bite-wings, and edge-to-edge (figure 15–3 page 251) for anterior.

II. Film Placement and Central Ray Angulation

Figure 9–7 shows in diagram form the position of the molar bite-wing film in relation to the teeth, the horizontal and vertical angulation, and the image objective for both the premolar and molar completed radiographs when standard film is used.

A. Position of Film

1. *Molar* (standard film): mesial border o film at mesial of maxillary second premolar or more distal as needed to include the distal surface of the third molar when it is erupted and in position.
2. *Premolar* (standard film): mesial border of film at center or mesial of maxillary canine.
3. *Anterior*: center of film at mesial surface of maxillary canine for the two lateral bite-wings; center of film at midline for central bite-wing.

B. Position of Directing Cone

With the vertical angulation at +10 degrees, the horizontal angulation is adjusted to direct the central ray to the center of the film. The ray must pass through the interproximals or parallel to a line through the interproximals.

C. Maintain Film Flat During Exposure

Although slight curving of the film may be needed for certain patients depending on the oral anatomy and tissue sensitivity, the basic rule is to keep the film as flat as possible to prevent distortion.

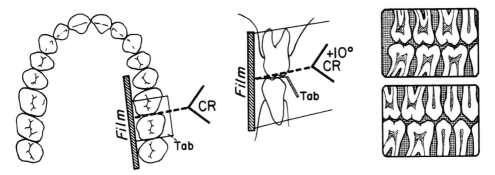

Figure 9–7. Bite-wing radiograph. **Left,** film position showing horizontal angulation for molar bite-wing with the central ray (CR) directed through the interproximals to the center of the film. **Middle,** vertical angulation set at + 10 degrees. **Right,** image objective for molar (above) and premolar (below) regions.

PERIAPICAL SURVEY: ANGLE BISECTION TECHNIQUE

The angle bisection technique is based on the geometric principle that *the central ray is directed perpendicular to an imaginary line which is the bisector of the angle formed by the long axis of the tooth and the plane of the film.* Figure 9–3 B illustrates in diagram form the relationship of the long axis of the tooth, the film, and the bisector of the angle formed by these two.

I. Patient Position

A. Traditional

1. *Sagittal Plane:* perpendicular to the floor.
2. *Occlusal Plane:* parallel with the floor.

B. Patient in Supine Position

The planes are reversed in their relation to the floor.

II. Film Placement and Position

Instructions for film placement and angulation are included in this section. Additional references will be helpful in studying and perfecting techniques.[19,20,21]

A. Basic Considerations

1. Center of film: at center of teeth being radiographed. The exception to this rule is the maxillary canine film which is placed slightly distal to accommodate film positioning.
2. Border of film: $1/8$ to $1/4$ inches beyond occlusal or incisal.
3. Film must be kept as flat as possible. A cotton roll may be used with the anterior

and maxillary molar films to aid in accomplishing this.

B. Film Position in Relation to Angulation of the Central Ray

Figures 9–8 and 9–9 show the position of the individual films, the horizontal and vertical angulations, and the image objective in the completed radiograph.

III. Direction of the Central Ray

A. Direct the Ray Through the Apical Third of the Teeth Being Radiographed

1. *Maxillary.* To determine location of the apices of the teeth, draw an imaginary line from the ala of the nose to the tragus of the ear, and the apices will be approximately at that level.
2. *Mandibular.* Apices are located approximately $1/2$ inch above the lower border of the mandible.

B. Horizontal Angulation

The ray should pass through the interproximal or parallel to a line through the interproximal, at approximately the center of the area being radiographed.

C. Vertical Angulation

Bisect the angle formed by the film and the long axes of the teeth, and direct the ray perpendicular to this line.

D. Average Angles for Vertical Angulation

1. *Uses*
   a. For the anatomically ideal mouth: it

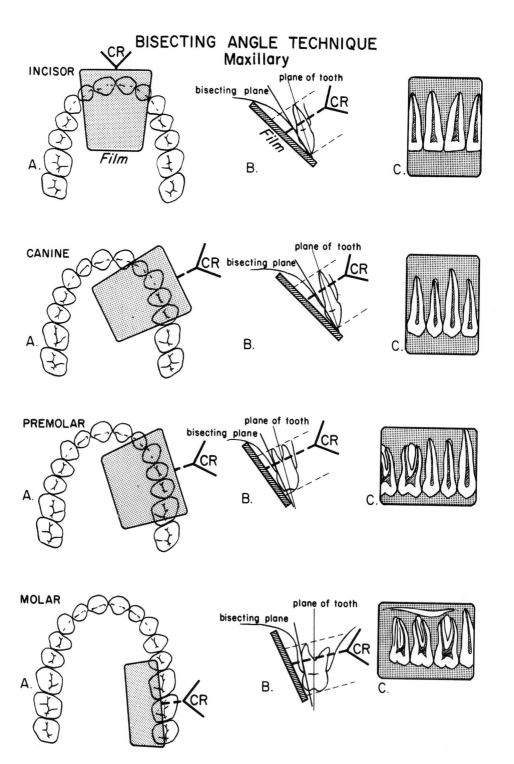

Figure 9–8. Angle bisection technique. Film positioning for the four major maxillary radiographs. Additional radiographs may be made centered at the right and left lateral incisors. **A.** Horizontal angulation with central ray (CR) directed through the interproximal. **B.** Vertical angulation with central ray (CR) directed perpendicular to the bisector of the angle formed by the film and the long axes of the teeth. **C.** Image objective for the completed radiograph.

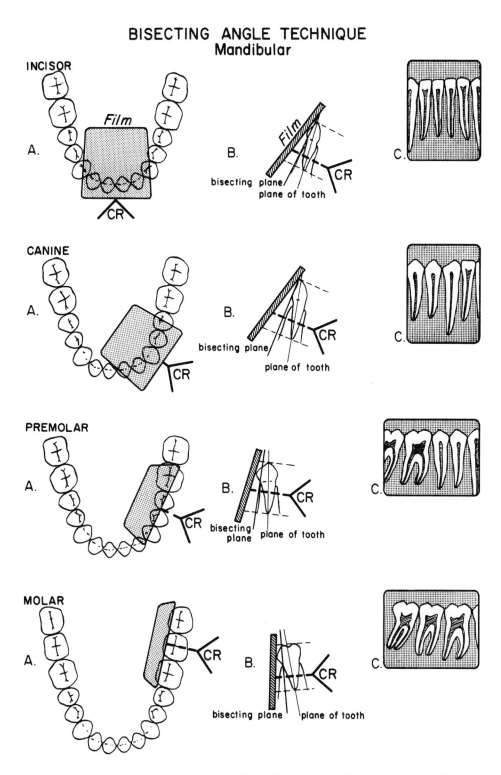

BISECTING ANGLE TECHNIQUE
Mandibular

Figure 9-9. Angle bisection technique. Film positioning for the four major mandibular radiographs. Additional radiographs may be made centered at the right and left incisors. **A.** Horizontal angulation with central ray (CR) directed through interproximal. **B.** Vertical angulation with central ray (CR) directed perpendicular to the bisector of the angle formed by the film and the long axes of the teeth. **C.** Image objective for the completed radiograph.

would be expected that the average angle and the angle determined by the bisection principle would be the same.

b. As a point from which to begin when bisecting the angle: usually the angle of the bisection would be within 5 to 10 degrees of the average angle.

c. As a time saver in angle bisection technique: prior to placing the film in the patient's mouth, the cone is positioned at the average angle to facilitate angulation and prevent undue discomfort on the part of the patient.

d. For the beginner, as a first technique, while developing concepts of angle bisection.

2. *The Average Angles*

Maxillary		Mandibular	
Central	+40–45	Central	−15–20
Canine	+45–50	Canine	−20–25
Premolar	+30–35	Premolar	−10–15
Molar	+20–25	Molar	− 5– 0

OCCLUSAL SURVEY

The use of occlusal films is particularly important for observing areas that cannot be completely or conveniently shown on other film, in cases where positioning periapical films is difficult or impossible, to supplement the angulation provided by other films for such conditions as fractures, impacted teeth, or salivary duct calculi, and as a specific part of a complete survey for edentulous or very young patients.

The central midline films for maxillary and mandibular are described in this section. A variety of positions for the occlusal films is possible, depending on the area to be examined. Additional references will be helpful as a guide.[19,29]

I. Maxillary Midline

A. Position of Patient's Head

The line from tragus of the ear to ala of the nose is parallel with floor.

B. Position of Film

The emulsion side is toward the palate; posterior border of film is brought back close to third molar region; film is held between the teeth with edge-to-edge closure.

C. Angulation

The cone is directed toward the bridge of the nose at a 65-degree angle.

D. Exposure

Consult chart of film manufacturer's specifications for exposure related to source-film distance, kilovoltage, and milliamperage. When a cassette is used, exposure time is reduced, an advantage in prevention of movement of the film.

II. Mandibular Midline

A. Position of Patient's Head

The head is tilted directly back.

B. Position of Film

Emulsion side is toward floor of mouth, posterior border of film is in contact with soft tissues of retromolar area, and the film is held between teeth in an edge-to-edge bite.

C. Angulation

For incisal region, the cone is pointed at the tip of the chin at an angle of approximately 55 degrees. For the floor of the mouth, the cone is directed from under the chin, perpendicular to the film.

D. Exposure

Consult chart of film manufacturer's specifications.

PANORAMIC RADIOGRAPHS

Panoramic radiography refers to techniques that produce films showing large areas of the maxillary and mandibular arches with adjacent structures on one or more extraoral films. This type of radiograph is a supplement to a periapical survey but not a substitute because of less sharpness and detail in the panoramic radiograph. The derived benefit must be weighed against the additional exposure to a wide area of tissues outside the oral tissues.

I. Types of Panoramic Techniques[29,30]

A. Tomography or Curved-surface Laminography

Lamina means layer, and in this technique a single layer of the teeth and surrounding structures appears in the radiograph. Other structures do not appear superimposed as they do in traditional extraoral techniques. The head is stabilized with a chin support or one of several types of head holders characteristic of each machine. Two methods are used in laminography.

1. Film and x-ray source rotate around the patient's head. Examples are the Panorex (S.S. White), Panelipse II (General Electric), and the Orthopantograph (Siemens).
2. Patient is rotated between the x-ray source and the film. An example is the Rotagraph (Watson, England).

B. Still-picture Technique

An intraoral fine-focus x-ray tube is placed within the patient's mouth.

1. Film in cassette is molded to the face, using separate films for the mandible and the maxilla. An example is the Status-X (Siemens).
2. Head and film positioners are used to make a series of lateral jaw radiographs. An example is the Orthoramix (Dental Corporation of America) which attaches to a conventional x-ray machine. With the Orthoramix, four overlapping exposures are made to cover the entire maxillary and mandibular arches.

II. Uses

Because definition and detail are inferior to periapical radiographs and because there is distortion, panoramic radiographs provide an overall view, not a detailed one. They do not show proximal carious lesions except for large cavities, which can be seen by direct examination. They are also inadequate for examination of periodontal supporting structures.

Routine use of panoramic radiographs for patients seeking general oral care cannot be recommended.[31,32] Possible uses are listed here.

A. Oral Pathology

The area surveyed in oral examination increases with the use of a panoramic radiograph, but the number of pathologic lesions found has been shown to be small.[31] Rarely

is it possible to base a diagnosis on a panoramic radiograph alone.[33]

B. Edentulous Patient

A panoramic survey prior to making complete dentures can usually provide sufficient information for most patients.[34]

C. Orthodontics

The overall view of growth, development at the beginning of orthodontic observation, diagnosis, and treatment, and during the treatment to assess periodic progress, can be helpful to the orthodontist.

D. Patients For Whom Conventional Radiographs Cannot be Used

For patients with handicaps or systemic conditions which hinder cooperation, such as patients with trismus, temporomandibular joint disability, Parkinson's disease, facial paralysis, intermaxillary fixation, or with facial trauma, when examination may not be possible by intraoral techniques.

E. Oral Surgery

Use of a panoramic radiograph has been shown to be sufficient for many treatment procedures.

III. Limitations

A. Inferiority of Definition and Detail

Causes of poor definition are
1. Use of intensifying screens.
2. Increased object-film distance.
3. Movement of x-ray tube and film.

B. Distortion

1. Magnified images are produced because of increased film-object distance.
2. Overlapping. In periapical techniques, each film is angulated with the central ray so that when a tooth is out of line, adjustment is made to prevent overlapping. With panoramic technique, the head and teeth remain fixed, and the ray and film are positioned for the average only.

IV. Technique[29]

Learning to use panoramic equipment is not

difficult. Each machine has its own characteristics which can be readily learned from the manufacturer's instructions.

A. Patient Preparation

The use of a leaded apron with a collar or a separate thyroid shield is important.[35,36,37]

B. Film

Film sizes are usually either 5 × 12 or 6 × 12 inches. Speed film should be used to minimize radiation. The new master control panoramic radiography can be performed at 4 mA for increased patient safety, compared with 8 mA of previous machines.

C. Processing

Regular processing solutions are used for panoramic film. Special film holders may be obtained.

CHILD PATIENT SURVEY

For all ages, the frequency for making a radiographic survey as well as the selection of type, size, and number of films to be used is based on individual patient evaluation. The objective is to minimize exposure of children to radiation. Low levels of x-radiation are associated with the induction of cancer, and children are more sensitive than adults.[33]

The need for radiographs in a healthy child is limited when the oral cavity appears free from disease as shown by direct clinical examination.[38] A specific rule of frequency for making complete surveys is not in keeping with current knowledge of radiation hygiene and safety.

With consideration for risk and benefit, five categories have been suggested for which radiographs may be indicated. These are the detection of congenital dental anomalies in the mixed dentition of children undergoing complete dental care or needing orthodontic treatment, detection of proximal surface dental caries when close contacts do not permit direct examination, third molar evaluation, infection, and trauma to the teeth or jaws.[33] In addition, periodontal radiographic evaluation may be needed after probing reveals the presence of bone loss and periodontal pockets.

The aim for a young child is to make as thorough a clinical evaluation of the teeth and the surrounding structures as possible. The real need for radiographs can then be determined.

I. Primary Dentition

When radiographs are indicated, various combinations of periapical, bite-wing, occlusal, panoramic, and extraoral films have been recommended by the specialists.[39,40,41] Film size is suggested that will be consistent with the size of the mouth, the cooperation of the patient, and the ability of the operator. Examples of number and size of films for three effective surveys are listed here.
A. Occlusal views of anterior maxillary and mandibular (standard film) and posterior bite-wings (child or adult anterior film); total of four films.
B. Occlusal views of anterior maxillary and mandibular and maxillary posterior (standard film), posterior bite-wings (child or standard film) and extraoral lateral jaw films (5 × 7 inches).
C. Periapical views for each posterior quadrant and one each for anterior (child size film); total six films.

II. Mixed Dentition (6 to 9 Years)

When a complete survey is determined necessary, 12 to 14 exposures using standard film are suggested. These include two posterior bite-wings, four molar (to include first permanent and primary molars), four canine, and two or four incisor periapical views.

III. Technique with Children

A. Use of Leaded Apron and Thyroid Collar

Children are more susceptible than adults to low-level radiation.

B. Orientation to Lessen Apprehension

1. For a young child's first visit to the dental office, making the radiographic survey may be a necessary first procedure. When the child is not able to cooperate, the survey may be delayed until the second or even the third visit except in an emergency.
2. Explain procedures carefully; rehearse to show what is to be done; repeat instructions with each film placement.

C. **Sequence**

Make the easiest, most comfortable exposures first (extraoral, panoramic, occlusal).

D. **Periapical Films**

Use film holder.

EDENTULOUS SURVEY

I. Types of Surveys

Periapical, occlusal, and panoramic surveys have been used alone and together for edentulous patients. The periapical series, usually of 14 films, has been shown to be the most complete and accurate for diagnosis. Radiographic examination of an edentulous mouth is frequently used to detect residual pathology, foreign bodies, and retained teeth or root tips prior to denture construction.

In research to compare three techniques, panoramic, two occlusal films, one maxillary and one mandibular, and a 14-film periapical survey, total residual and potential pathology was found in 37 percent of the periapical surveys, 17 percent of the occlusal radiographs, and 31 percent of the panoramic.[42] A detailed review of the retained root tips in the same study proved that the occlusal films were of little value, whereas the periapical survey revealed 115 tips to only 71 in the panoramic.[43] The research makes it clear that panoramic and occlusal films by themselves cannot be relied upon to provide complete information.

II. Techniques for Periapical Survey

A. **Film Placement**

1. *Paralleling Technique.* A film holder adjusted to provide a wider biting area is needed.
   a. Rubber bite block on a hemostat: turn bite block around so that the broader dimension is in the vertical plane.
   b. XCP holder can be padded with cotton rolls.[25]
2. *Angle Bisection Technique.* Use cotton rolls to aid in positioning the films and increase the angulation to accommodate flattened film.

B. **Exposure Time**

The time is reduced by approximately 25 percent.[25]

PARACLINICAL PROCEDURES

Supplemental to the chairside clinical procedures are the processing of the films and the mounting of radiographs for diagnostic and clinical use. Standard procedures are outlined in the following sections.

Film processing is the chemical transformation of the latent image, produced in a film emulsion by exposure to radiation, into a stable image visible by transmitted light. The usual procedure is basically a selective reduction of affected silver halide salts to metallic silver grains (development), followed by the selective removal of unaffected silver halide (fixation), washing to remove the processing chemicals, and drying.

CONVENTIONAL PROCESSING

Standardization of processing procedure goes hand in hand with standardized exposure techniques if consistently acceptable radiographs are to be prepared. Processing should be treated as an exacting chemical operation in which each step has specific objectives for the finished product. Fast and extra-fast film are even more sensitive to variations in temperature, light, and processing chemicals than medium and slow film formerly in general use; hence, the need for fastidious attention to detail.

I. Essentials of an Adequate Darkroom

Cleanliness and orderliness are mandatory. Since the films are handled in near darkness, materials must be available at the fingertips and each piece of equipment kept in its own place.

The work area must be free from chemicals, water, dust, and other substances that can contaminate the film either by splashing or direct contact should a film touch the bench. The processing room should not be used as a storage room or for other dental procedures in which dust or fumes might be produced.

Convenience and ease in carrying out precision techniques can be provided through good planning for the location and arrangement of equipment.

A. **Lighting**

1. Darkroom completely void of white light
   a. All possible light leaks found and eliminated.
   b. Do not use fluorescent overhead light because of afterglow.
2. Safelight[44]

   By following a manufacturer's instructions on a film package, the correct and safe lighting can be used. Different films require different light filters. A 7.5 watt bulb is used in a light fixture 4 feet above the working surface, and a filter selected for the light in accord with the type of film, whether screen film or intraoral.
   a. Filter Type GBX: primarily for automatic processor
   b. Filter Type ML-2: for intraoral film. It should not be used for extraoral film.
3. Safe lighting test[19,45]
   a. Expose a periapical film under usual clinical circumstances.
   b. Unwrap film in totally dark darkroom.
   c. Place film on work tabletop and place a coin on the film.
   d. Turn on safelight and leave for maximum amount of time (such as 20 to 25 minutes) typical of that required when preparing several surveys to be processed together.
   e. Turn off safelight, remove coin, process film.
   f. Observe radiograph: if any evidence of light circle where coin was placed, the darkroom safelight is excessive.
4. Lock on door of darkroom; signal light on outside to show room in use.

B. **Basic Equipment and Facilities**

1. Tanks for developer and fixer with water bath between
   a. Removable tanks made of stainless steel with joints welded and polished to prevent reactions with the processing chemicals.
   b. Close-fitting, light-proof cover for tank.
   c. Stirring paddles identified specifically for developer and fixer.
   d. Water bath with connecting water flow and temperature control indicator.
   e. Floating tank thermometer (kept in developer tank).
2. Workbench: covered with linoleum or Formica for easy cleaning.
3. Drying facilities: rod to hold hangers over drip pan; electric fan to facilitate drying.
4. Utility sink.
5. Interval timing clock.
6. Storage area beneath workbench for materials to change solutions.
7. Waste receiver: conveniently located for ready disposal of film wrappers to prevent losing films in midst of paper wrappers.

C. **Care of Solution**

1. Factors affecting life of solution
   a. Original quality (care in preparation).
   b. Age.
   c. Care received (temperature, whether kept covered, contamination).
   d. Number of films processed.
2. Changing solutions: at least every three weeks.
3. Preparation of new solution
   a. Tanks must be thoroughly scrubbed with water and a soft brush and then thoroughly rinsed.
   b. Label tanks as well as stirrers and mixing jars to prevent possibility of interchange.
   c. Follow manufacturer's specifications and directions precisely.

D. **Protection of Solution**

1. Use same position for tank cover so that same cover routinely is used for the same solution.
2. Purposes for covering tanks
   a. Prevent evaporation: which can change the concentration of the solutions and lower the level so the top film on rack is not covered during processing.
   b. Prevent oxidation: reduces useful life of solution.
   c. Prevent contamination: dust, drippings.

3. Temperature: keep cool when not in use: heated solutions can oxidize rapidly.
4. Replenisher: between changing of solutions, freshness may be maintained by replenishment according to manufacturer's specifications.

II. Processing

A. Preparation

1. Stir solutions and check temperature of solutions and water bath: all should be 20° C (68° F) (within 2°)
   a. Lower temperatures: chemical reactions too slow.
   b. Higher temperatures: cause fogging and may soften the emulsion.
2. Check cleanliness of workbench and film racks; wash hands to prevent film contamination.
3. Plan number of films to be processed so that facilities will not be overcrowded: films must hang individually out of possible contact with other films, sides of tanks, or wall in drying area.
4. Prepare labels for identification of radiographs.
5. Extinguish white lights; turn on safelight; lock door.
6. Load film hangers
   a. Hold film by edges to avoid finger marks, scratches, or bending.
   b. Clip firmly: test by pulling gently on film.

B. Developing

1. Set timer. (Refer to time-temperature chart provided by the film manufacturer.*)
2. Completely immerse rack with films in developer; turn on timer.
3. Agitate racks (without splashing) to eliminate air bubbles and assure contact of solution with all film surfaces.
4. When timer rings, remove racks to water or to a stop bath.

---

*The time-temperature method of processing is the only way to be assured of dependable results. Processing by the "visual inspection" method is not recommended because of the lack of standardization.

C. Rinsing

1. Immerse in freely running water for at least 30 seconds: agitate to provide contact of water with film.
2. Stop bath: a 10% acetic acid may be preferred in place of running water: immerse for 30 to 45 seconds.
3. Remove and drain for several seconds to prevent carrying an excess of water or acetic acid to the fixing bath.

D. Fixing

1. Immerse completely; set and start timer.
2. Agitate racks to remove air bubbles and assure contact of the solution with all parts of the film surfaces.
3. Clearing time: time needed for complete disappearance of white or milky opaqueness.
4. Total fixing time: minimum of twice clearing time
   a. Check manufacturer's specifications.
   b. Minimum of ten minutes and maximum of one hour are safe; excess time will produce a light radiograph.
5. Negatives may be viewed for limited time after clearing when needed for immediate use; return to fixer promptly for completion of fixing process.

E. Washing

1. Place in running water bath for minimum of 20 minutes.
2. Temperature: 20° C (68° F)
   a. Too warm: gelatin will swell, thus hindering diffusion.
   b. Drastic temperature changes cause reticulation (network of wrinkles or corrugations in the emulsion); retake necessary.

F. Drying

1. Drain off water and place in dryer.
2. Radiographs become brittle when left in a heated drying cabinet too long.

III. How the Image is Produced

A. The Chemistry of Processing

1. Film emulsion contains crystals of silver halides (bromide and iodide).
2. X-ray exposure changes the silver halides to silver and halide ions.

3. Developer reacts with the halide ions, leaving only the metallic silver in a specific arrangement corresponding with the radiolucency and radiopacity of the tissue being radiographed.
4. Fixer removes only those crystals of silver halide that were not affected by the action of the x-rays. Fixer has no effect on the black metallic silver produced by the developer.
5. End result: a negative, showing various degrees of lightness and darkness (microscopic grains of black metallic silver).

B. **Developer Action**
1. Purpose: to remove the halides from the metallic silver.
2. Constituents
   a. Developing agents (reducers): *elon* brings out detail and *hydroquinone* reacts slowly and brings out contrast.
   b. Preservative: sodium sulfite: to protect the developing agents from oxidizing rapidly in air.
   c. Restrainer: potassium bromide: inhibits the fogging tendency of the solution and slows the reaction of the reducers.
   d. Activator (alkali): sodium carbonate: initiates the action of the reducers with the halides.
3. Transfer to water bath at completion of developing time: if racks are shaken or allowed to drip over the developer, the solution falling back into the tank will be highly oxidized, which will shorten the life of the solution.

C. **Rinsing Purposes**
1. To stop the developing process.
2. To remove the developing solution from the emulsion to reduce carry-over of alkaline developer to the acid fixing bath.
3. To preserve the acidity of the fixer, and hence, make a more efficient, longer lasting fixing bath.

D. **Fixer Action**
1. Purpose; to remove the undeveloped halide salts.
2. Constituents
   a. Fixing agent: sodium thiosulfate

("hypo"): to dissolve the silver halides.
   b. Acidifer: acetic acid: to neutralize the alkali from the developer.
   c. Hardener: potassium alum: to shrink and harden the emulsion.
   d. Preservative: sodium sulfite: to counteract surface oxidation and stabilize the solution.

E. **Washing Purpose**

To remove residual chemicals from the negative.

AUTOMATIC AND ACCELERATED PROCESSING

Equipment that can provide accelerated or automatic processing (or both) is available.[46,47] Manufacturer's instructions must be followed and routine care and cleaning attended to for maintenance.[48,49]

I. **Objectives and Advantages**

Although cost and maintenance factors may be greater than with a traditional darkroom procedure, an automatic and/or rapid processing machine has advantages, including those listed below.
A. Time conservation by dental personnel.
B. Finished radiographs in from $1^1/_2$ to 8 minutes depending on the machine used. Some have automatic dryers.
C. Consistency of results through automatic control of temperature and time.
D. Available radiographs for immediate use during diagnosis, which is particularly important in emergencies, during endodontic therapy, and certain surgical procedures.

II. **Principles of Operation**

Automatic or accelerated processing (or both) is accomplished by one or a combination of the following:

A. **Automatic Film Transport**

Rollers or tracks are used to carry the film through developing and washing and fixing, washing, and forced drying. Certain machines produce wet films and do not have hot-air drying chambers. The various machines available are built to carry different sizes of film. Some machines may process only standard intraoral films, while others may also accommodate extraoral sizes.

B. High Temperature

Increased temperature decreases processing time. Special solutions are needed for the rapid processors, because with conventional solutions the excess temperature causes deterioration and fogging of the film. Solution temperatures in the automatic and rapid processors may be from 17° to 38° C (62° to 100° F), and with drying temperatures up to 65° C (150° F), the total processing and drying may be cut to 1½ minutes.

C. Use of Special Films and Processing Solutions

1. *Concentrated Processing Solution.* Solutions with increased chemical reactivity decrease developing time. In one type of machine, a combined developer-fixer is used which elminates the need for film to pass through two solutions. The film diagnostic quality is generally less with the special solutions.[50]
2. *Films.* Films with special emulsions have been developed which process best at higher temperatures and with the special processing solutions.

D. Agitation

Mechanically controlled movement of the film and/or movement of the solution is built into some units to provide fresh solution continuously at the film surface. This decreases the processing time.

ANALYSIS OF COMPLETED RADIOGRAPHS

The completed radiographs are mounted and examined at a viewbox or other adequate light source. The characteristics of the acceptable finished radiograph (page 134) serve as a basis for analysis. Nothing less than the ideal should satisfy, and errors must be studied in order to improve techniques for future surveys. Interpretation of radiographs is difficult for the dentist and the determination of pathology requires keen evaluation, but to attempt to base interpretation on inadequate, insufficient radiographs is guesswork rather than true, timely diagnosis.

I. Mounting

A. Legibly mark the mount with the name of patient, date, name of dentist; printing preferred.
B. Handle radiographs only by the edges with clean, dry hands, or wear clean cotton gloves.
C. Keep films clean, free from dust, liquids, or other contaminants.
D. Place a clean, dry towel or paper in front of the illuminator where mounting is to be done; arrange radiographs on this or mount one by one directly as they are removed from the rack.
E. The embossed dot near the edge of the negative is the guide to mounting: the depressed side of the dot is on the lingual.
F. Identify individual negatives by the teeth and other anatomic landmarks.
G. Approved mounting system:[51] looking at the teeth from outside the mouth, the teeth are viewed and mounted in the same manner as the approved numbering system (figure III–I, page 82).

II. Anatomic Landmarks

A. Definition

An anatomic landmark is an anatomic structure, the image of which may serve as an aid in the localization and identification of the regions portrayed by a radiograph. The teeth are the primary landmarks.

B. Landmarks That May Be Seen in Individual Radiographs

1. *Maxillary Molar:* maxillary sinus, zygomatic process, zygomatic (malar) bone, hamular process, coronoid process of the mandible, maxillary tuberosity.
2. *Maxillary Premolar:* maxillary sinus.
3. *Maxillary Canine:* maxillary sinus, junction of the maxillary sinus and nasal fossa (Y-shaped, radiopaque).
4. *Maxillary Incisors:* incisive foramen, nasal septum and fossae, anterior nasal spine (V-shaped), median palatine suture, symphysis of the maxillae.
5. *Mandibular Molar:* mandibular canal, internal oblique line, external oblique ridge, mylohyoid ridge.

6. *Mandibular Premolar:* mental foramen.
7. *Mandibular Incisors:* lingual foramen, mental ridge, genial tubercles, symphysis of the mandible. Nutrient canals are seen most frequently in this radiograph.

III. Identification of Inadequacies in Radiographs

Inadequacies are related to film placement, angulation, exposure, processing, care and handling of the film, and, indeed, any step in the entire procedure. Errors appear as problems of inadequate density, contrast, incomplete or distorted images, fogging, artifacts, or stains. Table 9–2 outlines the more common inadequacies and their causes, the keys to correction.

IV. Interpretation

Radiographs are used in conjunction with clin-

Table 9–2. Analysis of Radiographs: Causes of Inadequacies

Inadequacy	*Cause: Factors in Correction*
Image	
Elongation	Insufficient vertical angulation
Foreshortening	Excessive vertical angulation
Superimposition (overlapping)	Incorrect horizontal angulation (central ray not directed through interproximal)
Partial Image	Cone-cut (incorrect direction of central ray or incorrect film placement)
	Incompletely immersed in processing tank
	Film touched other film or side of tank during processing
Blurred or Double Image	Patient, tube, or packet movement during exposure
	Film exposed twice
Stretched Appearance of Trabeculae or Apices	Bent film
No Image	Machine misfunction from time switch to wall plug
	Failure to turn on the machine
	Film placed in fixer before developer
Density	
Too Dark	Excessive exposure
	Excessive developing
	Developer too warm
	Unsafe safelight
	Accidental exposure to white light (may be completely black)
Too Light	Insufficient exposure
	Insufficient development or excessive fixation
	Too cool solutions
	Use of old, contaminated, or poorly mixed solutions
	Film placement: leaded side toward teeth
	Film used beyond expiration date
Fog	
Chemical Fog	Imbalance or deterioration of processing solutions
Light Fog	Unintentional exposure to light to which the emulsion is sensitive, either before or during processing.
	(1) Unsafe safelight
	(2) Darkroom leak

Table 9–2. *continued*

Inadequacy	*Cause: Factors in Correction*
Radiation Fog	Improper storage of unused film Film exposed prior to processing
eticulation (puckered or pebbly surface)	Sudden temperature changes during processing, particularly from warm solutions to very cold water

rtifacts
  Dark Lines
	Bent or creased film
	Static electricity
	  (1) Film removed from wrapper with excessive force
	  (2) Wrapper sticking to film when opened with wet fingers or if there was excessive moisture from patient's mouth
	Fingernail used to grasp film during opening

Herringbone Pattern (light film)	Packet placed in mouth backwards with foil next to teeth
Stains and Spots	Unclean film hanger Splatterings of developer, fixer, dust Finger marks Insufficient rinsing after developing before fixing Splashing dry negatives with water or solutions Air bubbles adhering to surface during processing (insufficient agitation) Overlap of film on film in tanks or while drying Paper wrapper stuck to film (film not dried when removed from patient's mouth)
Discoloration at later date after storage of completed radiographs	Incomplete processing or rinsing Storage in too warm a place Storage near chemicals

cal examination for a complete program of treatment. Periodic radiographs permit continuing evaluation. As part of the permanent record, radiographs help to document the oral condition for comparative purposes as well as legal.

The quality of the radiographs determines their usability for diagnostic interpretation. Techniques for the preparation of radiographs must be perfected in order that radiographs have maximum interpretability with minimum radiation exposure of the patient.

A. Prerequisites for Interpretation

1. *Mounting.* Mount radiographs in an opaque mount to prevent light between each radiograph from creating glare and producing a blinding effect.

2. *Viewbox.* Use an adequately lighted viewbox. Dimmed room light improves visibility for contrasting radiolucent and radiopaque areas.

   Holding the radiographs up to view by window, room, or unit light is inadequate and only gross interpretation can be accomplished. When a viewbox is larger than the mount used, cover the edges to block out peripheral light.

3. *Hand Magnifying Glass.* Examine radiographs on a viewbox through a magnifying glass. A viewbox is available with a built-on magnifying glass.

B. Systematic Examination

1. Observe one radiographic feature at a time. Examine all of the radiographs for

that feature, rather than taking each radiograph separately to find everything. It is important to note comparisons for each change over the entire survey.

2. When examining a particular tooth, compare the appearance of that tooth in each radiograph in which it appears, including bite-wings. At different angulations, different findings may become apparent.

C. Coordination with Clinical Examination

A description of radiographic examination of the teeth may be found on page 242 and of the periodontal tissues, on page 226. Correlation of radiographic findings with the clinical examination, using probe and explorer, is basic to an understanding of the true oral condition of the patient.

TECHNICAL HINTS

I. Holding Film

Never hold a film in a patient's mouth during exposure.

II. Question Radiation Exposure

Inquire whether the patient is receiving radiation treatment. It may be necessary to minimize the number of exposures. The patient's physician should be consulted.

III. Film Placement

Dot on film packet is placed toward the occlusal or incisal to prevent the embossed dot on the film from superimposing over the image on the negative.

IV. Check State Radiation Protection Laws

Many states have regulations concerning x-ray unit registration, inspection, safety requirements, and limitations for use of x-rays.

V. Record in Patient's Permanent Record

When a patient refuses to have radiographs made, record this in the patient's permanent record. Obtain patient's signature to a statement indicating such refusal in the event a legal iss should arise related to an operation performe

VI. Who Owns Dental Radiographs?

They are part of the dentist's record and main as professional property the same as oth parts of the case record.[52,53] The first rule is nev to give radiographs to a patient. If they are be loaned to another dentist, they should be se or delivered directly, preferably with a lett indicating, if known, when they will next needed and should be returned. Conservatis should be exercised in loaning radiographs other dentists. As a part of valuable permane records, it is never known when they will needed as evidence of the careful diagnosis ar treatment provided.

VII. Film Storage

Film should always be stored in a clean, d place. Keep in lead-lined container. Watch e piration dates. Store oldest film in front for ne use. Purchase as needed, not in excess quantit

VIII. Study Informational Sheets

It is important to study the information sheets provided in the film package. This appli particularly when a new brand of film is bein used.

IX. Stain Removal from Clothes
A. Do not launder before spot removal.
B. Commercially Prepared Spot Remover (Available from dental supply companies.
C. Removal of Spots in Nylon Materials
  1. Prepare solution containing
     Sodium hypochlorite $^{1}/_{2}$ oz. (15 m
       (5% solution)
       (household bleach)
     Acetic acid $^{1}/_{2}$ oz. (15 m
       (5% solution)
       (household vinegar)
     Water at about 38° C (100° F) 1 gal (3.8 I
  2. Soak the stained portion in the solutio for 5 to 10 minutes, then soak in *fres* fixer.
  3. Rinse thoroughly in plain water. Dry.

X. X-ray Film Contamination by Stannous Fluoride

Stannous fluoride can cause artifacts on a fin ished radiograph. When radiographs are to b made following a topical application of stannou fluoride solution, it is recommended that citric acid be used for washing the hands. Stannous fluoride contamination of the hands is impossible to remove by ordinary handwashing procedures.[54]

FACTORS TO TEACH THE PATIENT

I. When the Patient Asks About the Safety of Radiation

A. Adapt the answer to the patient. Certain patients will have more fear; others will have more knowledge about x-rays. If the hygienist expresses confidence, this will aid in allaying fears. Hesitation will increase the patient's doubt.

B. Radiographs are essential to diagnosis and treatment. Without the information provided, the dentist can only guess at conditions not visible clinically.

C. The benefits resulting from the intelligent use of x-rays outweigh any possible negative effects.

D. Modern x-ray machines are equipped for safety. For the patient who will understand, details about filtration, collimation, film speed, and short exposure times can be explained.

II. Educational Features in Dental Radiographs

(Avoid diagnosis. For teaching, it may be advisable to use radiographs of someone other than the patient.)

A. Position of unerupted permanent teeth in relation to primary teeth.

B. Detection of early carious lesions not visible by clinical examination.

C. Effects of loss of teeth and the importance of having replacements.

D. Periodontal changes and other pathology appropriate to an individual patient.

References

1. American Dental Association, Council on Dental Materials, Instruments and Equipment: *Dentist's Desk Reference: Materials, Instruments and Equipment,* 1st ed. Chicago, American Dental Association, 1981, pp. 10–12.
2. Glenner, R.A.: 80 Years of Dental Radiography, *J. Am. Dent. Assoc.,* 90, 549, March, 1975.
3. Manson-Hing, L.R.: *Fundamentals of Dental Radiography.* Philadelphia, Lea & Febiger, 1979, pp. 1–13.
4. Wuehrmann, A.H. and Manson-Hing, L.R.: *Dental Radiology,* 5th ed. St. Louis, The C.V. Mosby Co., 1981, pp. 4–21.
5. American Dental Association, Council on Dental Materials, Instruments and Equipment: op. cit., pp. 295–299.
6. Barr, J.H. and Stephens, R.G.: *Dental Radiology: Pertinent Basic Concepts and Their Applications in Clinical Practice.* Philadelphia, W.B. Saunders Co., 1980, pp. 27–42.
7. Wuehrmann and Manson-Hing: op. cit., pp. 35–53, 76–85.
8. Manson-Hing: op. cit., pp. 89–103.
9. Barr and Stephens: op. cit., pp. 35, 89, 407.
10. White, S.C. and Rose, T.C.: Absorbed Bone Marrow Dose in Certain Dental Radiographic Techniques, *J. Am. Dent. Assoc.,* 98, 553, April, 1979.
11. American Dental Association, Council on Dental Materials, Instruments and Equipment: op. cit., pp. 215–218.
12. National Council on Radiation Protection and Measurements: *Dental X-ray Protection.* NCRP Report Number 35, March 9, 1970, 50 pp.
13. De Lyre, W.R.: *Essentials of Dental Radiography for Dental Assistants and Hygienists,* 2nd ed. Englewood Cliffs, New Jersey, Prentice-Hall, 1980, pp. 57–60.
14. White, S.C. and Glaze, S.: Interpatient Microbiological Cross-contamination after Dental Radiographic Examination, *J. Am. Dent. Assoc.,* 96, 801, May, 1978.
15. Langland, O.E.: Radiologic Examination, in Clark, J.W., ed.: *Clinical Dentistry, Volume 1,* Chapter 4. Hagerstown, Maryland, Harper & Row, 1981, pp. 14–15.
16. Park, J.K.: Radiographic Technique in the Contour Dental Chair, *J. Am. Dent. Hyg. Assoc.,* 46, 351, September-October, 1972.
17. Venokur, P.C., Einbender, S., and Myers, B.S.: Modified X-ray Technique for Dentistry with Patients in the Supine Position, *Oral Surg.,* 38, 148, July, 1974.
18. Baum, A.T. and Morgan, E.: Reduction of X-ray Dose by Variable Rectangular Collimation and Reflex Optical Direction of Dental X-ray Beams and by Supine Position of the Patient, *J. Am. Dent. Assoc.,* 85, 1091, November, 1972.
19. Eastman Kodak Company: *X-rays in Dentistry.* Rochester, Eastman Kodak, 1977, 84 pp.
20. De Lyre: op. cit., pp. 208–235.
21. Manson-Hing: op. cit., pp. 39–64.
22. Manson-Hing: op. cit., pp. 65–69.
23. STABE Disposable Dental Film Holder, Greene Dental Products, Inc., 12801 Arroyo Street, San Fernando, California, 91342.
24. Silha, R.E.: Paralleling Technic With a Disposable Film Holder, *Dent. Radiogr. Photogr.,* 48, 27, Number 2, 1975.
25. *Utilization of the Extension Cone Paralleling, Bisecting Angle and Interproximal Techniques with Rinn Instruments.* Elgin, Illinois, Rinn Corporation, 1975, 51 pp.
26. Updegrave, W.J.: Dental Radiography With the Versatile Intraoral Positioner System, *J. Prev. Dent.,* 4, 14, May-June, 1977.
27. Updegrave, W.J.: Vertical Interproximal Radiography, *Dent. Radiogr. Photogr.,* 51, 56, Number 3, 1978.
28. Green, M.L. and Green, B.L.: The Vertical Periapical Bite-wing: A Better Radiograph for Periodontal Diagnosis, *Dent. Hyg.,* 52, 477, October, 1978.
29. Manson-Hing: op. cit., pp. 113–145.
30. De Lyre: op. cit., pp. 304–319.
31. White, S.C. and Weissman, D.D.: Relative Discernment of Lesions by Intraoral and Panoramic Radiography, *J. Am. Dent. Assoc.,* 95, 1117, December, 1977.

32. Stephens, R.G., Kogon, S.L., Reid, J.A., and Ruprecht, A.: A Comparison of Panorex and Intraoral Surveys for Routine Dental Radiography, *Can. Dent. Assoc. J.*, *43*, 281, June, 1977.
33. Valachovic, R.W. and Lurie, A.G.: Risk-benefit considerations in Pedodontic Radiology, *Pediatr. Dent.*, *2*, 128, June, 1980.
34. Perrelet, L.A., Bernhard, M., and Spirgi, M.: Panoramic Radiography in the Examination of Edentulous Patients, *J. Prosthet. Dent.*, 37, 494, May, 1977.
35. Block, A.J., Goepp, R.A., and Mason, E.W.: Thyroid Radiation Dose During Panoramic and Cephalometric Dental X-ray Examinations, *Angle Orthod.*, *47*, 17, January, 1977.
36. Myers, D.R., Shoaf, H.K., Wege, W.R., Carlton, W.H., and Gilbert, M.A.: Radiation Exposure during Panoramic Radiography in Children, *Oral Surg.*, *46*, 588, October, 1978.
37. Whitcher, B.L., Gratt, B.M., and Sickles, E.A.: A Leaded Apron for Use in Panoramic Dental Radiography, *Oral Surg.*, *49*, 467, May, 1980.
38. White, G.E. and Tsamtsouris, A.: The Use and Abuse of Radiographs of the Primary Dentition, *Quintessence Int.*, *8*, 59, August, 1977.
39. De Lyre: op. cit., pp. 262–276.
40. O'Brien, R.C.: *Dental Radiography: An Introduction for Dental Hygienists and Assistants*, 4th ed. Philadelphia, W.B. Saunders Co., 1982, pp. 177–194.
41. Manson-Hing: op. cit., pp. 152–158.
42. Scandrett, F.R., Tebo, H.G., Miller, J.T., and Quigley, M.B.: Radiographic Examination of the Edentulous Patient. Part I. Review of the Literature and Preliminary Report Comparing Three Methods, *Oral Surg.*, *35*, 266, February, 1973.
43. Scandrett, F.R., Tebo, H.G., Quigley, M.B., and Miller, J.T.: Radiographic Examination of the Edentulous Patient, *Oral Surg.*, *35*, 872, June, 1973.
44. Hurtgen, T.P.: Safelighting in the Dental Darkroom, *Dent. Radiogr. Photogr.*, *52*, 78, Number 4, 1979.
45. Manson-Hing: op. cit., pp. 184–185.
46. American Dental Association, Council on Dental Materials, Instruments and Equipment: op. cit., pp. 301–302.
47. Manson-Hing: op. cit., pp. 27–30.
48. Fortier, A.P.: Preventive Care and Maintenance of the Automatic Dental Film Processor, *J. Prev. Dent.*, *4*, 20, November-December, 1977.
49. Thunthy, K.H., Fortier, A.P., and Knapp, W.B.: Automatic Film Processing for Optimal Results: Proper Procedure and Maintenance, *Quintessence Journal*, *1*, 17, April, 1979.
50. Pestritto, S.T., Anderson, S.J., and Braselton, J.A.: Comparison of Diagnostic Quality of Dental Radiographs Produced by Five Rapid Processing Techniques, *J. Am. Dent. Assoc.*, *89*, 353, August, 1974.
51. American Dental Association: System of Tooth Numbering and Radiograph Mounting, Approved by the American Dental Association House of Delegates, October, 1968.
52. Terezhalmy, G.T. and Bottomley, W.K.: General Legal Aspects of Diagnostic Dental Radiography, *Oral Surg.*, *48*, 486, November, 1979.
53. Department of National Health and Welfare, Working Group on Oral Radiological Services: *Oral Radiological Services*. Minister of National Health and Welfare, Ottawa, Canada, December, 1979, 108 pp.
54. Yamane, G.M., Meskin, L.H., and Mehaffey, P.: Stannous Ion Contamination of Radiographic Films. Etiology

and Prevention, *J. Am. Dent. Hyg. Assoc.*, *42*, 147, 3 Quarter, 1968.

Suggested Readings

Alcox, R.W.: Biological Effects and Radiation Protection the Dental Office, *Dent. Clin. North Am.*, *22*, 517, July 1978.
Anderson, V.K.: Radiological Hygiene, in Boundy, S.S. an Reynolds, N.J., eds.: *Current Concepts in Dental H giene, Volume 2*. St. Louis, The C.V. Mosby Co., 197 pp. 82–92.
Antoku, S., Kihara, T., Russell, W.J., and Beach, D.F Doses to Critical Organs from Dental Radiography, *Or Surg.*, *41*, 251, February, 1976.
Beeching, B.W., Ismail, A., and Smith, N.J.D.: Exposu to Scattered Radiation in the Vicinity of Dental X-ra Sets, *Br. Dent. J.*, *143*, 367, December 6, 1977.
Bengtsson, G.: Maxillo-facial Aspects of Radiation Prote tion, Focused on Recent Research Regarding Critic Organs, *Dentomaxillofac. Radiol.*, *7*, 5, Number 1, 1978
Brown, G.E.: ADHA Continuing Education Self-stud Course, *Dental Radiology*, *Dent. Hyg.*, *52*, 15, Januar 1978; 52, 65, February, 1978; 52, 113, March, 1978; 5. 161, April, 1978; 52, 225, May, 1978; 52, 273, Jun 1978.
Ciola, B.: Clinical Manifestations of Human Skin Expose to X-radiation, *Dent. Radiogr. Photogr.*, *50*, 29, Num ber 2, 1977.
Crabtree, C.L.: Factors That Influence Quality of the Dent Radiograph, *J. Prev. Dent.*, *4*, 8, November-Decembe 1977.
Eliasson, S.T. and Haasken, B.: Radiopacity of Impressio Materials, *Oral Surg.*, *47*, 485, May, 1979.
Holyoak, B.: Radiological Protection in the Dental Profe sion, *Br. Dent. J.*, *146*, 189, March 20, 1979.
Johnson, O.N. and Barone, G.J.: What the Federal X-ra Regulations Mean to the Dentist, *J. Am. Dent. Assoc* 95, 810, October, 1977.
Matteson, S.R.: Dental Radiology, in Richardson, R.E. an Barton, R.E.: *The Dental Assistant*, 5th ed. New York McGraw-Hill, 1978, pp. 341–374.
Oishi, T.T. and Parfitt, G.J.: Effects of Varying Peak Kilc voltage and Filtration on Diagnostic Dental Radic graphs, *Can. Dent. Assoc. J.*, *42*, 449, September, 197€
Overend, J.K.: Dose Reduction in Dental Radiography Control of Exposure Time and Film Processing, *B Dent. J.*, *141*, 87, August 3, 1976.
Smith, N.J.D.: Radiation Protection. The Administrativ and Legal Framework in the United Kingdom, *Br. Den J.*, *144*, 47, January, 17, 1978.
Triolo, K., Konicki, D.L., and Struba, R.J.: Radiation Hy giene: An Overview, *Dent. Hyg.*, *53*, 359, August, 1979
Updegrave, W.J.: Simplified and Standardized Intraoral Ra diography with Reduced Tissue Irradiation, *J. Am. Dent Assoc.*, *85*, 861, October, 1972.
White, S.C. and Frey, N.W.: An Estimation of Somati Hazards to the United States Population from Denta Radiography, *Oral Surg.*, *43*, 152, January, 1977.
Wuehrmann, A.H.: Preventive Dental Radiology, in Cald well, R.C. and Stallard, R.E.: *A Textbook of Preventiv Dentistry*. Philadelphia, W.B. Saunders Co., 1977, pp 250–264.

Techniques

Alcox, R.W. and Jameson, W.R.: Patient Exposures from Intraoral Radiographic Examinations, *J. Am. Dent. As soc.*, *88*, 568, March, 1974.
Fortier, A.P.: Common Errors in Dental Radiography, *J Dent. Educ.*, *43*, 683, December, 1979.

nglais, R.P., Langland, O.E., and Morris, C.R.: Radiographic Localization Technics, *Dent. Radiogr. Photogr.*, *52*, 69, Number 4, 1979.

anson-Hing, L.R.: What's the Angle: A Study of the Angle Bisected in Intraoral Radiography, *Oral Surg.*, *49*, 86, January, 1980.

tel, J.R.: A Step by Step Description of the Mounting of a Complete Mouth Radiographic Survey, *Dent. Hyg.*, *53*, 114, March, 1979.

tel, J.R.: Intraoral Radiographic Errors, *Oral Surg.*, *48*, 479, November, 1979.

eid, J.A. and Ruprecht, A.: Simple Methods of Accommodating to Fast Dental X-ray Films, *Can. Dent. Assoc. J.*, *42*, 447, September, 1976.

eid, J.A. and Ruprecht, A.: Duplication of Radiographs: Simple Methods to be Used in the Dental Office, *Can. Dent. Assoc. J.*, *43*, 278, June, 1977.

eid, J.A. and Stephens, R.G.: Paralleling Radiographic Technique Without the Long Cone, *Can. Dent. Assoc. J.*, *43*, 289, June, 1977.

ichards, A.G.: The Buccal Object Rule, *Dent. Radiogr. Photogr.*, *53*, 37, Number 3, 1980.

nawkat, A.H., Nolting, F.W., Phillips, J.D., and Banks, T.E.: Evaluation of the Utilization of the Supine Position in Intraoral Radiology, *Oral Surg.*, *43*, 963, June, 1977.

hort, T.: Back to the Basics in Bitewing Radiology, *R.D.H.*, *1*, 22, March, 1981.

ilha, R.E. and Simon, W.J.: The Processing of Radiographic Films, *Dent. Assist.*, *45*, 17, April, 1976.

hunthy, K.H.: Automatic Film Processing, *J. Prev. Dent.*, *4*, 18, November-December, 1977.

hunthy, K.H.: Radiographic Illusions Due to Faulty Angulations, *Dent. Radiogr. Photogr.*, *51*, 1, Number 1, 1978.

hunthy, K.H. and Weinberg, R.: Comparison of Films Processed in Automatic and Manual Processors, *Oral Surg.*, *50*, 479, November, 1980.

alachovic, R.W., Reiskin, A.B., and Kirchhof, S.T.: A Quality Assurance Program in Dental Radiology, *Pediatr. Dent.*, *3*, 26, March, 1981.

an Aken, J. and Verhoeven, J.W.: Factors Influencing the Design of Aiming Devices for Intraoral Radiography and Their Practical Application, *Oral Surg.*, *47*, 378, April, 1979.

Vagner, M.: Pitfalls in Processing Radiographs, *Quintessence Journal*, *1*, 19, January, 1979.

Vhaley, C.: The Paralleling Technique of Intraoral Radiography, An American Dental Assistants Association Continuing Education Course, *Dent. Assist.*, *48*, 27, March/April, 1979.

Vhitcher, B.L., Gratt, B.M., and Sickles, E.A.: Leaded Shields for Thyroid Dose Reduction in Intraoral Dental Radiography, *Oral Surg.*, *48*, 567, December, 1979.

Vierich, A.: Radiographic Techniques and the Dental Assistant, *Quintessence Journal*, *2*, 11, May, 1980.

Villiamson, G.F.: Alternatives to Full Mouth Radiographs, *Dent. Hyg.*, *53*, 118, March, 1979.

Children

Bachman, L.H.: Pedodontic Radiography, *Dent. Radiogr. Photogr.*, *44*, 51, Number 3, 1971.

Bean, L.R. and Isaac, H.K.: X-ray and the Child Patient, *Dent. Clin. North Am.*, *17*, 13, January, 1973.

Benusis, K.P.: The Buccal Bitewing Radiograph for the Child Patient, *Northwest Dent.*, *56*, 186, July-August, 1977.

Darzenta, N.C. and Tsamtsouris, A.: Radiography in Pedodontics, *J. Pedodont.*, *2*, 228, Spring, 1978.

Howard, H.E.: Rethinking Pedodontic Radiology, *J. Dent. Child*, *48*, 192, May-June, 1981.

Khanna, S.L. and Harrop, T.J.: A Five-film Oral Radiographic Survey for Children, *J. Dent. Child.*, *40*, 42, January-February, 1973.

Kogon, S.L., Stephens, R.G., and Reid, J.A.: The Selection of the Most Efficient Radiographic Survey for Young Adult Patients, *Can. Dent. Assoc. J.*, *44*, 317, July-August, 1978.

Matlock, J.F.: Radiographic Techniques, in McDonald, R.E. and Avery, D.R.: *Dentistry for the Child and Adolescent*, 3rd ed. St. Louis, The C.V. Mosby Co., 1978, pp. 94–114.

Silha, R.E.: Special Radiographic Surveys, *Dent. Radiogr. Photogr.*, *45*, 23, Number 2, 1972.

Panoramic Radiography

American Dental Association, Council on Dental Materials and Devices: Advantages and Disadvantages of the Use of Dental Tomographic Radiography, *J. Am. Dent. Assoc.*, *94*, 147, January, 1977.

Frome, K., Dickert, P., Silko, K., and Miller, A.S.: Panographic Survey, *Dent. Hyg.*, *51*, 208, May, 1977.

Hurlburt, C.E. and Wuehrmann, A.H.: Comparison of Interproximal Carious Lesion Detection in Panoramic and Standard Intraoral Radiography, *J. Am. Dent. Assoc.*, *93*, 1154, December, 1976.

Jerman, A.C., Kinsley, E.L., and Morris, C.R.: Absorbed Radiation from Panoramic plus Bitewing Exposures vs. Full-Mouth Periapical plus Bitewing Exposures, *J. Am. Dent. Assoc.*, *86*, 420, February, 1973.

Manson-Hing, L.R. and Greer, D.F.: Radiation Exposure and Distribution Measurements for Three Panoramic X-ray Machines, *Oral Surg.*, *44*, 313, August, 1977.

Matteson, S.R. and Sanders, S.S.: Localization of Objects in the Anterior Areas with a Single Panorex Radiograph, *Oral Surg.*, *42*, 847, December, 1976.

Smith, C.J. and Fleming, R.D.: A Comprehensive Review of Normal Anatomic Landmarks and Artifacts as Visualized on Panorex Radiographs, *Oral Surg.*, *37*, 291, February, 1974.

Stallard, J.A. and Stallard, R.E.: Panoramic Radiography, *Dent. Assist.*, *43*, 12, October, 1974.

Weissman, D.D. and Longhurst, G.E.: Comparative Absorbed Doses in Periapical Radiography. II Panorex, *Oral Surg.*, *33*, 661, April, 1972.

Xeroradiography

Binnie, W.H., Cawson, R.A., Davis, R., and Stacey, A.J.: Applications of Xeroradiography in Dentistry—a Review, *Int. Dent. J.*, *29*, 34, March, 1979.

Binnie, W.H., Stacey, A.J., Davis, R., and Cawson, R.A.: Applications of Xeroradiography in Dentistry, *J. Dent.*, *3*, 99, May, 1975.

Gratt, B.M., Sickles, E.A., and Armitage, G.C.: Use of Dental Xeroradiographs in Periodontics, *J. Periodontol.*, *51*, 1, January, 1980.

Gratt, B.M., Sickles, E.A., and Nguyen, N.T.: Dental Xeroradiography for Endodontics: A Rapid X-ray System that Produces High-quality Images, *J. Endodont.*, *5*, 266, September, 1979.

Gratt, B.M., Sickles, E.A., and Parks, C.P.: Xeroradiography of Dental Structures. I. Preliminary Investigations, *Oral Surg.*, *44*, 148, July, 1977.

Gratt, B.M., White, S.C., Sickles, E.A., and Jeromin, L.S.: Imaging Properties of Intraoral Dental Xeroradiography, *J. Am. Dent. Assoc.*, *99*, 805, November, 1979.

Jeromin, L.S., Geddes, G.F., White, S.C., and Gratt, B.M.: Xeroradiography for Intraoral Dental Radiology, A Process Description, *Oral Surg.*, *49*, 178, February, 1980.

Lopez, J.: Xeroradiography in Dentistry, *J. Am. Dent. Assoc.*, *92*, 106, January, 1976.

Nakasima, A., Nakata, S., Shimizu, K., and Takahama, Y.:

Radiologic Exposure Conditions and Resultant Skin Doses in Application of Xeroradiography to the Orthodontic Diagnosis, *Am. J. Orthod.*, 78, 646, December, 1980.

Snyder, M.B., Stacey, A.J., Davis, R., Cawson, R.A., and Binnie, W.H.: The Advantages of Xeroradiography for Panoramic Examination of the Jaws and Teeth. *J. Periodontol.*, 48, 467, August, 1977.

Thunthy, K.H.: Comparison of Xeroradiographs with Occlusal and Screen Films, *Oral Surg.*, 45, 959, June, 1978.

White, S.C. and Gratt, B.M.: Clinical Trials of Intraoral Dental Xeroradiography, *J. Am. Dent. Assoc.*, 99, 810, November, 1979.

10

Study Casts

As accurate reproductions of the teeth, gingiva, and adjacent structures, study casts can be useful and frequently indispensable adjuncts in the care of the patient. The study casts, radiographs, and clinical examination with recordings and chartings, together with the medical and dental histories, are utilized in the diagnosis, total treatment planning, treatment, and subsequent maintenance through recall by the dentist and the dental hygienist.

I. Purposes and Uses of Study Casts

A. To serve as a permanent record of the patient's present condition.

B. To give sharper delineation and corroboration of the observations made during the oral examination.

C. To observe normal conditions, the variations of and departures from the normal at the outset of treatment, and, by comparison with subsequent periodic casts, to compare and evaluate certain aspects of treatment.

D. During charting of the teeth to note missing teeth, anomalies of size, shape, or number, partial eruption, tooth positions such as drifting, tilting, and open or closed spacing, and other factors.

E. During examination of the occlusion to observe the static relations (Angle's classification, malrelations of groups of teeth, and malpositions of individual teeth; pages 250–255) and other features such as wear

patterns and the effects of premature loss of teeth.

F. During periodontal charting to record anatomic features such as the position, size, and shape of the gingiva and interdental papillae, and the position of freni.

G. To be an effective visual aid to use when the oral conditions are explained and the dental and dental hygiene treatment plan is presented; to enable the patient to visualize and understand the need for the specific care outlined.

H. To serve as a guide to clinical treatment procedures.

I. To supplement clinical observations in the selection of an oral disease and plaque control program for the patient's own treatment, and to serve as a visual aid in teaching aims and procedures of the recommended measures to the patient.

II. Terms Used*

A. **Cast** (also called a model)

Positive likeness of some desired form.

B. **Study Cast or Diagnostic Cast**

Positive likeness of part or parts of the

---

*Definitions are taken or adapted from and in accord with the *Glossary of Prosthodontic Terms*, fourth edition, Journal of Prosthetic Dentistry, *38*, 70, July, 1977. Additional definitions to those included in this chapter may be found in the Glossary.

oral cavity for the purpose of study and treatment planning.

C. **Impression**

An imprint or negative likeness of the teeth and/or edentulous areas where the teeth have been removed, made in a plastic material which becomes relatively hard or set while in contact with the tissues. Impressions are named or classified by the type of material used to make the impression, such as reversible or irreversible hydrocolloid, plaster, or wax.

D. **Interocclusal Record**

A record of the positional relation of the opposing teeth or jaws to each other made in a plastic material such as wax.

III. **Steps in the Preparation of Study Casts**

The steps noted here are detailed in the sections following.

A. **Clinical Procedures**
1. Assemble materials and equipment.
2. Prepare the patient.
3. Select and prepare the impression trays.
4. Make the mandibular impression.
5. Make the maxillary impression.
6. Make the interocclusal record for occluding the casts.

B. **Paraclinical Procedures**
1. Assemble materials and equipment.
2. Prepare the impressions for pouring.
3. Pour the casts.
4. Trim and finish the casts.
5. Polish the casts.

CLINICAL PREPARATION

The need for and uses of study casts are explained to the patient when the steps in diagnosis and treatment planning are outlined. As with any procedure not familiar to a patient, an explanation is in order. The reactions of patients who have had an impression made previously may range from indifference to dread, and the conversation and approach can be directed accordingly.

When the radiographic survey has been made for the new patient prior to the study casts, it will have been determined as to whether precautions to prevent gagging require special application. With all patients, a calm approach, an exhibition of confidence, a direct and efficient procedure, and a gentle handling of the patient's oral tissues will increase rapport and contribute to a satisfactory result.

I. **Assemble Materials and Equipment**

A. Coverall (plastic drape), towel, and mouthwash.
B. Impression Trays
   1. Perforated type generally used: small, medium, and large sizes are available.
   2. Care of trays: for use in the patient's mouth; trays must be clean, shiny, and sterilized.
C. Mixing bowl: clean, dry, flexible rubber or plastic with smooth, unscratched surface.
D. Spatula: clean, dry, stiff, with a smooth, rounded end that will reach every part of the bowl without scraping or cutting its surface.
E. Saliva ejector.
F. Dental materials
   1. Wax for preparation of tray rim: soft utility wax.
   2. Alginate: irreversible hydrocolloid.
G. Water thermometer.

II. **Prepare the Patient**

A. **Antibiotic Premedication**

Research has not demonstrated the production of bacteremia following an impression using irreversible hydrocolloid.[1] However, when a high-risk patient has moderate to severe periodontitis with mobile teeth, clinical judgment must be used by the dentist when deciding on the need for antibiotic premedication.

Impressions can be planned for an appointment when the patient is protected and has received antibiotic coverage for other procedures. The medical and dental histories must be reviewed for all possible precautionary needs.

B. **Explain the Procedure to be Performed**

C. **Position the Patient**

Position the patient for maximum visibility and accessibility and to minimize gagging.

D. Receive Removable Appliances

Provide a container with water in which the patient can place removable oral appliances.

E. Drape the Patient

Drape patient with a protective coverall and towel.

F. Examine the Oral Cavity

Note labially and buccally displaced teeth, height of palate, undercut areas, mandibular tori, and other factors that may influence the size or preparation of the impression tray and the procedures to be carried out during impression making.

G. Free the Mouth of Debris

1. Spray proximal areas; use dental floss.
2. When there is excess, tenacious debris, plaque control instruction should be started so that debris and plaque can be removed during brushing by the patient.

H. Request Patient to Use Mouthrinse

1. To aid in the removal of saliva and debris and lessen the numbers of surface microorganisms.
2. To lower the surface tension; aids in preventing bubbles in the impression.
3. To provide a pleasant taste and feeling for the patient.
4. To distract an anxious patient while the trays are being prepared.

I. Dry the Teeth

Use a cotton roll or compressed air stream to remove saliva from the teeth to prevent irregularities in the surface of the study cast.

J. Prevent Gagging

1. Approach with confidence to reassure the patient.
2. Work as quickly and efficiently as possible.
3. Use a topical anesthetic (pages 521–523)
   a. Cold water or an ice cube held in the mouth has some anesthetic effect.
   b. Salt: a small amount ($\frac{1}{4}$ teaspoon) on the tongue to swallow just before the tray is to be inserted may relieve tissue reactions.
   c. Apply topical anesthetic to posterior palatal area, or patient may rinse with a commercial topical agent. A spray topical preparation is contraindicated because of proximity to throat where coughing may be initiated.
4. Technique considerations
   a. Avoid excessive impression material in the tray.
   b. Seat the maxillary tray from posterior to anterior as described in section II, A, 3 (page 174).
   c. Instruct patient to breathe deeply through the nose before the tray is inserted and to continue after insertion; bring head forward.

PREPARATION OF IMPRESSION TRAYS

I. Selection of Proper Size and Shape

A. Width

1. Objectives: to allow an adequate thickness of impression material on the facial and lingual of each tooth to provide strength and rigidity to the impression.
2. Tray flanges may be spread to accommodate for extra width in the molar regions, particularly lingual to the mandibular molars in the mylohyoid region.
3. When a tooth is in prominent labio-, bucco-, or linguoversion, a minimum thickness of $\frac{1}{8}$ to $\frac{1}{4}$ inch is suggested, but even then the fragility of the impression material in that area is increased.
4. The tray that is too wide may appear in correct relation to the facial surfaces but may impinge on the lingual cusps of molars.

B. Length

1. Objective: to allow coverage of the retromolar area of the mandible and the tuberosity of the maxilla.
2. Anteriorly there should be at least $\frac{1}{4}$ inch clearance labial to the most protruded incisor without impingement on lingual gingiva.

II. Maxillary Tray Try-in

A. Operator position: side back of patient

B. Retraction

1. With index finger of nondominant hand retract the patient's lip and cheek.
2. At the same time, use the side of the tray to distend the other side of the patient's mouth to gain entry (figure 10–1).

C. Insertion

1. With a rotary motion, insert the tray.
2. Orient the tray beneath the arch and center it using the tray handle and the midline (usually between the central incisors and in line with the middle of the nose) as guides for positioning.
3. Bring the front of the tray to a position $1/4$ inch labial to the most labially inclined incisor.
4. Seat the tray by bringing the posterior up before the anterior; retract the lip as the anterior is brought into place.

D. Evaluation

Evaluate the size of the tray: gently lower the front of the tray while holding the posterior border in place (figure 10–2) and examine the relationship of the posterior border to the most posterior molars and the tuberosity areas to determine whether there will be ample coverage. By moving the tray up and down it is possible to observe the relation to the facial surfaces of all teeth, malaligned teeth, protuberances, and other features to assay the space allowed for the impression material.

III. Mandibular Tray Try-in

A. Operator Position: at side front of patient

B. Retraction

1. With index and middle fingers of nondominant hand retract the patient's lip and cheek.
2. At the same time, use the side of the tray to distend the side of the mouth to gain entry, similar to the procedure illustrated in figure 10–1 for the maxillary tray.

C. Insertion

1. With a rotary motion insert the tray.
2. Orient the tray over the dental arch and center it using the tray handle and the midline (usually between the central incisors and in line with the center of the chin) as guides for positioning.
3. Bring the tray rim to about $1/4$ inch anterior to the most labially positioned incisor; instruct the patient to raise the

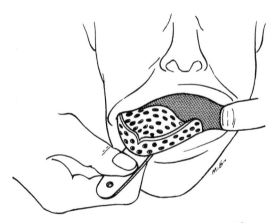

Figure 10–1. Maxillary impression tray insertion. The patient's lip and cheek are retracted with the fingers of the nondominant hand, while the side of the tray is used to distend the other lip and cheek to gain entry. The tray is inserted with a rotary motion. The procedure for the mandibular tray insertion is similar.

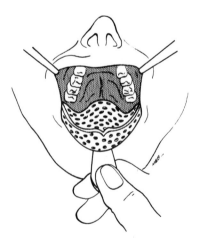

Figure 10–2. Selection of impression tray. To determine adequate coverage, the posterior border of the tray is held in position while the front of the tray is lowered to observe the relationship of the posterior border to the maxillary tuberosity areas which are to be covered by the impression. The mandibular tray position is examined similarly by lifting the tray to observe coverage of the retromolar areas.

tongue to permit the lingual flange of the tray to pass by the lateral borders of the tongue without interference.

4. As the tray is lowered, retract the cheeks in the posterior regions to make certain the buccal mucosa is not caught beneath the edge of the tray; hold the lip out to ascertain that there is clearance to the base of the vestibule.

D. Evaluation

1. Evaluate the size of the tray. Lift the tray handle while keeping the posterior in position, similar to the procedure illustrated in figure 10–2 for the maxilla, to determine whether there will be ample coverage posteriorly to include the retromolar areas, and laterally to allow for $1/4$ inch thickness of impression material on the facial and lingual aspects of the teeth.

2. Reselect larger or smaller trays as indicated and repeat try-in. When in doubt, the larger tray is used rather than the smaller.

V. Application of Wax Rim Around Borders of Trays (Beading)

A. Purposes

1. To position the loaded trays without the metal rims causing discomfort to the soft tissues.

2. To seat the vestibular periphery firmly into position with reduced pressure on the displaced tissues.

3. To prevent penetration of the incisal or occlusal surfaces through the impression material and thus prevent a defective cast.

4. To provide a slight undercut at the rim as an aid in the retention of the alginate in the tray during placement and removal.

5. To create a posterior palatal seal to aid in preventing excess material from passing into the throat.

B. Procedure

1. Attach a strip of soft utility wax firmly around the entire periphery of each tray (figure 10–3).

2. Mandibular tray: add extra layers from canine to canine labially and notch the wax, to fit about the labial frenum.

3. Maxillary tray

   a. Add extra layers as needed to extend the tray into the vestibule above the anterior teeth and notch the wax to fit about the labial frenum (figure 10–4).

   b. Apply extra thickness across the posterior palatal seal area.

   c. When a patient has a high palatal vault, apply extra wax to support the impression material in that area.

4. Try the rimmed trays in the mouth and examine by retraction of the lips and cheeks and by use of a mouth mirror for lingual areas; hold the tray in position.

5. Characteristics of the completed molding: when the tray is held firmly, the wax will contact all borders of the mucous membrane, will displace the soft tissue outward and upward, and the teeth will not touch the tray.

THE IMPRESSION MATERIAL

I. Factors Related to the Impression Material That Contribute to a Satisfactory Impression

Texts on dental materials should be reviewed for complete information about the irreversible hydrocolloids.[2,3,4,5] ANSI/ADA (American National Standards Institute/American Dental Association) Specification No. 18 applies to the requirements expected for an approved product.[6,7] Properties related to the clinical procedures essential to making an accurate impression are listed here.

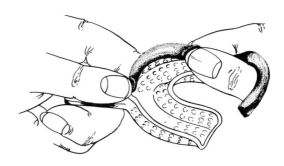

Figure 10–3. Beading the tray. A strip of soft utility wax is applied around the periphery of each tray.

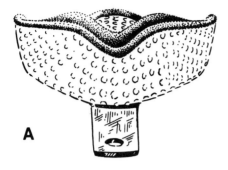

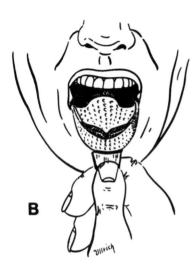

Figure 10–4. **A.** Tray with double layer of beading wax about the labial frenum. The extra wax extends the tray, protects the soft tissue from the metal rim, and provides a more complete impression of the area. **B.** Try-in after beading. The wax should contact all borders of the mucous membrane, displace the soft tissue outward, and prevent the teeth from contacting the tray.

A. Powder

The alginate material deteriorates on standing, particularly at higher temperatures and humidity.

1. Keep metal container tightly closed; store in a cool place.
2. Use individually sealed packages except when large numbers of impressions are made regularly; powder is preweighed for the packages, since measuring is less accurate than weighing; heat and moisture are eliminated.
3. Individual package may be refrigerated in hot weather, provided the powder is

used immediately on opening. If left exposed, water condenses on the powder. The bulk container cannot be refrigerated for that reason.

B. Water

Temperature controls gelation time.

1. At room temperature 20–21° C (68–70° F) an ideal gelation time between 3 to 4 minutes provides adequate working time.
2. Temperature of the water should be measured with a thermometer at the time of mixing.
3. Control in hot, humid weather: use cooler water and refrigerate the bowl and spatula.

C. Strength and Quality

The strength and quality of the finished impression depend on the following factors:

1. Powder-water ratio accurately weighed and measured.
2. Spatulation (one minute) to allow chemical reactions to proceed uniformly.
3. Holding the impression material in position for an optimum period (two clocked minutes after the mix on the spatula has lost its stickiness). The elasticity of most alginates improves with time; therefore, a superior reproduction can be obtained by waiting. Distortion can result when the impression is left in the mouth too long.

D. Surface Accuracy

The cast must be poured immediately to prevent loss of water from the impression. Permanent distortion can result.

II. Mixing the Impression Material

Follow manufacturer's specifications precisely: total time lapse for mixing and insertion is approximately 2 minutes.

A. Place measured water 20–21° C (68–70° F, measured with a thermometer) in a clean, dry mixing bowl.
B. Sprinkle measured powder (from individually sealed package or premeasured from large container) into the water.
C. Quickly incorporate the powder and water using a clean, dry, stiff spatula.

). Mix for 1 minute (clocked) vigorously, incorporating powder into the water, until a smooth, creamy mix is obtained.

II. Tray Preparation

The mandibular impression is made first to introduce the patient to the procedure in an area where discomfort or gagging may be the least likely.

ᴀ. Working Time

The working time is 30 seconds.

ʙ. Filling the Tray

1. Fill the tray from one end to the other, being careful not to trap air bubbles.
2. Adapt the material to the tray thoroughly; press slightly through the perforations in the tray.
3. Do not overload; fill to a level just below the edge of the wax rim.
4. Wet index finger with cold water and pass lightly over the surface of the impression material; smooth the surface and make a slight indent where the dental arch will insert.

ᴄ. Excess Material

Quickly gather the excess material from the bowl and bring the material on the spatula near to patient.

THE MANDIBULAR IMPRESSION

. Precoat Potential Areas of Air Entrapment

This prevents air bubbles in the finished impression.

ᴀ. Take a small amount of impression material from the spatula on the index finger.

ʙ. Apply quickly with a positive pressure to:
1. Undercut areas, such as distal surfaces of teeth adjacent to edentulous areas, cervical areas of erosion or abrasion, or gingival surfaces of fixed partial dentures.
2. Vestibular areas, particularly anterior areas about the freni.
3. Occlusal surfaces.

II. Insertion of Tray

A. Steps

1. Follow the procedure for try-in of mandibular tray described on page 170, III. Briefly, from the front of the patient, retract patient's lip and cheek with fingers of nondominant hand; use side of tray to distend the other lip and cheek; rotate the tray into position, center it over the teeth, introduce the tray $1/4$ inch anterior to the labial surface of the most anterior incisor. Instruct patient to raise tongue while tray is lowered; retract cheeks and lip to clear the way for impression material to reach the base of the vestibule.
2. Seat the tray directly downward with a slight vibratory motion to aid in filling all crevices between the teeth.
3. Instruct the patient to extrude the tongue briefly to mold the lingual borders of the impression.
4. Apply equal bilateral pressure firmly, holding the middle fingers over the premolar regions and using the thumbs to support the mandible; or, if equal pressure can be maintained with one hand, place an index finger over the patient's premolar area on one side and the middle finger over the opposite side with the thumb under the edge of the mandible for stabilization. Mold cheeks around buccal.
5. Saliva ejector: when the impression tray is held with one hand or when assistance is available, a saliva ejector may be slipped in over the tray and then removed before the tray is removed.

B. Setting Time

When the leftover material on the spatula has lost its surface stickiness (tackiness), the impression is held in position two more clocked minutes.

III. The Completed Impression

A. Removal of Impression

1. Hold tray with thumb and fingers.
2. Retract cheek and lip with fingers and release the edge of the impression by depressing the buccal mucosa.

3. Do not rock the impression back and forth to release it as these movements may cause permanent distortion.
4. Remove the impression with a sudden jerk or snap.

B. Rinse

Rinse under cool running water to remove saliva.

C. Examine and Evaluate the Impression

Observe surface detail, proper extension over retromolar area, and the peripheral roll (rounded border of the impression) generally.

D. Repeat the Procedure

Correct mistakes, rather than be satisfied with a substandard impression.

E. Wrap Mandibular Impression in a Wet Towel while making the maxillary impression.

THE MAXILLARY IMPRESSION

I. Preparation

A. Request Patient to Rinse

To clear particles left from the mandibular impression, and to relax the oral muscles.

B. Examine the Maxillary Teeth

Teeth should be examined for particles of mandibular impression material: remove. Request patient to use mouthrinse.

C. Prepare the Alginate

Fill the tray as described previously for the mandibular impression.

D. Precoat Undercut Areas

Precoat undercut areas, vestibular areas, and occlusal surfaces (see procedure for mandibular impression).

II. Insertion of Tray

A. Steps

1. Follow the procedure for insertion of maxillary tray described on page 170. Briefly, from the side back position, retract the patient's lip with the fingers of the nondominant hand; use side of tray to distend the lip and cheek; insert the tray with a rotary motion; center it over the teeth using the small gap in the red wax border to relate to the labial frenum.
2. Introduce the material to the teeth so that the wax rim is about $1/4$ inch labial to the most labially inclined incisor.
3. Seat the tray
   a. Seat the tray from posterior to anterior to direct the impression material forward and thus prevent irritation to the soft palate area.
   b. Retract the lip and bring the tray to place with a slight vibratory motion to allow the material to flow into crevices and proximal areas.
   c. The middle finger of each hand is placed over the premolar region to support and guide the tray; the index fingers and thumbs hold the lip out.
   d. Request the patient to form a tight "O" with the lips to mold the impression material.
   e. Maintain equal pressure on each side of the tray throughout the setting of the alginate. If assistance is available or if the pressure to hold the tray can be maintained with one hand, a saliva ejector can be inserted.

B. Setting Time

When the material on the spatula has lost its surface stickiness, the impression is held in place for two more clocked minutes.

III. The Completed Impression

A. Remove Impression

Hold the tray handle with the thumb and fingers of the dominant hand and retract the opposite lip and cheek with the fingers of the other hand. Elevate the cheek over the edge of the impression to break the seal, and remove the impression with a sudden jerk.

B. Rinse

Rinse under cool running water to remove saliva.

C. Examine

Examine surface detail and proper extension to include tuberosity areas and a complete reproduction of the height of the vestibule.

D. Repeat Procedure

Repeat procedure rather than be satisfied with a substandard impression.

E. Wrap Impression in a Damp Towel

This is to prevent dehydration and distortion; however, impressions should be poured promptly.

F. Check Manufacturer's Specifications

Check for use of a fixative.

THE INTEROCCLUSAL RECORD (WAX BITE)

I. Purposes

A. To relate the maxillary and mandibular casts correctly.

B. To place between the casts during trimming and storage to prevent breakage of teeth.

C. Indication for Special Need. Many, if not most, casts will orient to each other readily in only one position, but when there are problems such as openbite, crossbite, edentulous areas, end-to-end, or edge-to-edge relations which may interfere with direct occlusion of the casts, a wax bite is generally needed.

II. Procedure

A. Have patient practice opening and closing on the posterior teeth to assure that the correct position can be obtained easily.

B. Ask patient to rinse with cold water.

C. Shape a double layer of soft baseplate wax in the form of the arch, warm slightly over a gas burner, and place over the maxillary occlusal surfaces.

D. Request patient to close; press the wax against the facial surfaces of the teeth to shape it accurately to the arch.

E. Remove carefully to prevent distortion; chill in cold water.

PARACLINICAL PROCEDURES

Supplemental to the chairside clinical procedures is the laboratory work involved in the production of the study casts from the impressions.

These duties may be the responsibility of the dental laboratory technician or other dental auxiliary, as directed by the dentist.

The most frequent error in the use of the alginates for impressions is in delay in pouring the cast. Undue dehydration or water loss from the alginate will cause permanent distortion, an uneven surface, and hence an inaccurate cast. Regard for the sensitive properties of the dental materials, precision and practice in laboratory procedures, and pride in the production of neat, smooth, well-proportioned study casts determine the finished product's appearance, usefulness, and accuracy.

I. Equipment and Materials

A. Mixing bowl: clean, dry, flexible rubber or plastic, with smooth, unscratched surface.

B. Spatula: clean, dry, stiff, with a smooth, rounded end that will reach every part of the bowl without scraping or cutting its surface.

C. Plaster knife: sharp.

D. Vibrator.

E. Mechanical mixer.

F. Model-base formers, glass or ceramic slab, wax paper or other nonabsorbent-surfaced material.

G. Dental materials
1. Baseplate wax (and wax spatula).
2. White dental stone.

H. Model trimmer.

I. Compass or dividers.

J. Plastic ruler.

K. Waterproof sandpaper.

L. Soap solution.

II. Preparation of the Impressions

A. Rinse impressions under cool running water; shake out excess water gently and apply gentle blast of compressed air.

B. Mandibular: create an artificial floor of the mouth in the impression to facilitate pouring and trimming of the cast.
1. Trim the lingual impression material all around so that there is a consistent height from the occlusal and incisal surfaces to the base of the impression.
2. Using alginate
   a. Mix a small portion of alginate.
   b. Hold the mandibular impression upright in the left hand with the middle

and ring fingers extended from under the tray into the tongue area.

   c. Apply alginate over the fingers to form a flat bridge slightly above the lingual flanges of the impression.

   d. Smooth the surface with a finger moistened with cool water; hold until the alginate sets.

   e. When assisted at the chair, the floor for the mandibular impression can be made while the maxillary impression is being held for setting. There is usually sufficient alginate mixed with that for the maxillary impression to use for this purpose.

3. Using baseplate wax

   a. Cut a piece of baseplate wax to the shape of the lingual periphery of the impression.

   b. Seal into place with a warm spatula, taking care that no heat is applied to the anatomic portions of the impression.

   c. Cool under running water.

III. Pouring the Casts: Mixing the Stone

A. Factors Related to Dental Stone That Contribute to a Successful Cast

Texts on dental materials should be reviewed for complete information about gypsum products.[8,9,10,11] Some pertinent properties are listed here as reference points.

1. *Dental Stone.* Sensitive to changes in the relative humidity of the atmosphere.

   a. Store in airtight container; close soon after use; do not let water enter the container.

   b. Keep the spoon or scoop used to remove the powder clean and dry.

2. *Water.* Controls the strength, rigidity, and hardness of the cast.

   a. Temperature: generally, cooler water decreases the setting time and warmer water increases it.

   b. Quantity: follow manufacturer's proportions exactly. Increasing the water over the specifications prolongs the setting time and reduces the strength.

3. *Spatulation.* Prolonged or very rapid mixing can hasten the chemical reaction and shorten the setting time.

B. The Mix

1. Measure the water and powder by the manufacturer's specifications.

   a. White stone is generally preferred for study casts. Plaster produces a cast more susceptible to breakage.

   b. Ratio of 30 to 40 ml. water to 100 g stone.

2. Place measured water (room temperature) in a clean, dry, mixing bowl.

3. Sift in the powder gradually to prevent air trapping and to allow each particle to become wet.

4. Wait briefly until all powder is wet, then vibrate to release large bubbles.

5. Spatulation: with clean, stiff spatula.

   a. Hand spatulate for not less than 30 and not more than 60 seconds.

   b. Contact the entire inner surface of the bowl so no powder is left unincorporated.

   c. Do not whip or beat as this encourages bubble formation.

   d. Vibrate during and after spatulation to remove bubbles.

   e. Mechanical mixer or vacuum mixer may be used when available.

6. Result: smooth, homogeneous, creamy mix.

C. Pouring the Cast

1. Shake water out of the impression.

2. Hold the impression tray by the handle and press handle against the vibrator.

3. With a small amount of stone mix on the end of the spatula, start at one posterior corner and allow the mix to flow through the impression. Use small amounts and vibrate continually.

   a. Tip the impression so that the material will pass into the tooth indentations and flow slowly down the side, across the occlusal or incisal, and up the other side of the impression of each tooth.

   b. Air will be trapped if the process is hurried or if too large a quantity of mix is poured in at one time without attentive control of the flow.

4. When all tooth indentations are covered, larger amounts of mix are added to fill the impression slightly over the periphery. Vibrate.

One-Step Method for Forming the Base of the Cast

1. Fill rubber model-base former with the remainder of the mix, or form a mass of stone on a glass or ceramic slab or other nonabsorbable surface (wax paper on a smooth surface). Add excess stone at the heel areas.
2. Invert the poured impression onto the base
   a. Use a slight back-and-forth motion to secure the two parts together.
   b. Common error: inverting the impression before the stone is firm enough to prevent the mix from flowing out of the impression.
3. Adjust tray to proper position
   a. Occlusal plane (at premolars) should be parallel with the base of the model-base former or tabletop.
   b. Midline (anterior as judged by handle of impression tray) centered at the midline of the model-base former.
   c. Accommodate position so that a tooth in labio- or buccoversion will not protrude over the trimming line of the art portion (figure 10–6).
4. Add stone on peripheral and heel areas to provide a smooth surface; remove excess so that wax periphery of the tray is visible. When excess stone above the edge of the tray rim is permitted to set, it is difficult to separate the tray, and the use of a knife to carve the excess from the tray may damage the cast.
5. Final set occurs within one hour. Separate one hour after pouring to prevent damage to the surface of the cast.

Other Methods for Forming the Base of the Cast

1. *Two-step or Double-pour.* Both maxillary and mandibular impressions are poured and left upright (Steps III, C, 1 through 4, above). Stone is then prepared separately for the bases, and the model-base formers are filled or the mass is placed on the smooth nonabsorbent surface.

   The impression is inverted and held on the surface of the new stone while the sides and periphery are shaped and smoothed. An advantage in this method is that there is no danger of inverting the poured impression too soon; in which case, the unset stone can fall away from the occlusal and incisal portions and leave bubbles in strategic places.
2. *Boxing Technique.* The object is to form a wall around the impression before pouring to provide a shape for the base as well as to prevent the need for inverting the poured impression. A cylinder of utility wax is attached slightly below the periphery of the impressions and completely around the entire impression. Boxing wax or baseplate is applied around the rope of utility wax and attached to it by means of a warm spatula at a height that allows for proper thickness of the final cast, about $1/_2$ inch. Care must be taken not to displace the impression dimensionally, or to touch the anatomic portions with the warm spatula. Pouring is carried out as described previously.

   Work-model formers with side walls to provide the boxing effect are available. Such a mold has a slot through the rubber where the handle of the impression tray can be inserted.

F. Separation of the Impression and the Cast

1. Objective: to remove tray and impression material without breaking the teeth.
2. When model-base former is used, remove it first.
3. Cut away stone from the periphery to free the margin of the tray.
4. Remove the tray by itself.
5. Cut the impression material along the line of the occlusal surfaces and peel off the impression material (with care not to scratch the stone cast during cutting).

6. Direct removal: when the teeth are in reasonably normal alignment, the tray and the impression material may be removed with a straight pull after first releasing the anterior portion by a slight downward and forward movement. When this method is used, do not apply lateral pressures or rock the tray back and forth, as it is easy to break the teeth by using such forces.

G. Trimming

Trimming is started promptly, or if delayed, the cast should be thoroughly soaked in water before trimming.

IV. Trimming the Casts

The exact proportions of the study casts, and the steps required to accomplish the trimming and finishing depend on several factors. These include the measurements of the patient's dental arches, the positions of the teeth, and the preferences of the dentist. Development of a routine, systematic procedure for trimming can lead to the production of consistent, attractive, and useful diagnostic casts.

The method described here is dependent on the use of a precision-type model trimmer. No specific directions are provided for the use of angulators which are available to fit on the table of the model trimmer to give average set angles for trimming the margins of the casts; when these are available, directions are usually supplied by the manufacturer.

When a mechanical model trimmer is not available, greater skill must be developed to produce well-proportioned and smooth casts. The use of the model-base formers or a boxing method can be developed to a higher degree of precision. Trimming with a plaster knife must be started as soon as the impression is separated. Plaster files are available to aid in cutting the borders of the base.

Before the step-by-step description of the trimming procedure, an outline of the characteristics of the finished casts is provided as an overall guide.

A. Objectives: Characteristics of the Finished Casts

1. *Overall Base Shape:* figure 10–5.
2. *Proportions:* approximately one third art

portion and two thirds anatomic (figur 10–6 A).

3. *Bases:* mean occlusal plane of the relate casts is parallel with both bases whic are parallel with each other (figure 10– A).

4. *Posterior Borders*
   a. At a right angle with the bases (figur 10–6 B).
   b. Maxillary and mandibular posterio borders are in the same plane: whe standing, the casts will rest togethe in natural intercuspation (figure 10– B).
   c. Perpendicular to the median lin from the incisors through the palat (maxillary) and the middle of th tongue (mandibular) (figure 10–7).

5. *Sides:* symmetrical angulation with pos terior border and heel cuts (figure 10–7) parallel with a line through the centra grooves of the premolars of the sam side.

6. *Heels:* $1/_2$ inch cuts parallel with the mes iodistal plane of the opposite canine (fig ure 10–7).

7. *Anterior:* mandibular is shaped in an arc maxillary in a point, with the cuts ex tending from the canine area (figur 10–7).

8. *Borders*
   a. Posterior: to include retromolar are and tuberosity (figure 10–7).
   b. Sides: $1/_4$ to $5/_{16}$ inch from bony pro tuberance over premolars and mo lars; anatomy of mucobuccal fold in cluded in the cast.
   c. Anterior: $1/_4$ to $5/_{16}$ inch from the mos protruded tooth or from the depth o

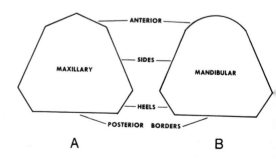

Figure 10–5. Base shapes for maxillary and mandibula study casts with designations of trimmed areas.

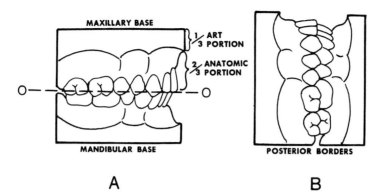

Figure 10–6. Finished study casts. **A.** Proportions and planes. The *art* portion is ¹/₃ and the *anatomic* portion ²/₃ of the total height of the cast. Note parallelism of the maxillary and mandibular bases with the mean occlusal plane (0–0). **B.** Posterior borders are at right angles to the bases. When the maxillary and mandibular casts are placed on their posterior borders, the teeth will intercuspate.

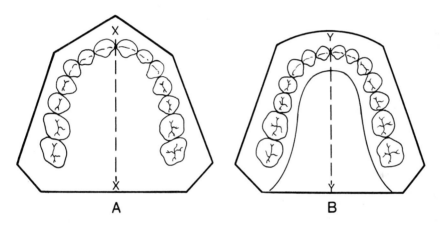

Figure 10–7. Occlusal views of finished casts, **A.** Maxillary, **B.** Mandibular. The posterior border is perpendicular to the median line from the incisors through the palate (X–X), and the middle of the tongue (Y–Y). The tuberosity areas of the maxillary arch and the retromolar areas of the mandibular arch are preserved.

the mucobuccal fold, whichever is most labial.

9. *Surfaces of the Cast:* smooth and polished with air bubbles removed or filled.

B. Preliminary Steps to Trimming the Cast

1. Casts must be wet: soak at least 5 minutes.
2. Remove bubbles of stone on or about the teeth with a small sharp instrument; use care not to scar the cast.
3. Level down excess stone which is distal to the retromolar area and tuberosity so that casts may be occluded. Do not shorten the cast anteriorly-posteriorly at this time.

4. Trim casts conservatively on the sides to make a smooth surface for marking.

C. Trimming the Bases

1. *Objectives*
   a. To make bases parallel with the mean occlusal plane and to each other.
   b. To make correct proportions for the height of the casts: art portion one third and anatomic portion two thirds (figure 10–6 A).
2. *Mandibular Cast Is Trimmed First*
   a. Measure the greatest height of the anatomic portion (usually this is from the tip of the canine to the depth of the vestibule) with a plastic ruler (figure 10–8).

b. Divide by two: this will be the height of the art portion.

c. Add the measured height of the anatomic portion to the height of the art portion for the total height of the cast. Set compass or dividers at this measurement.

d. Place the cast teeth down on a flat surface and mark a line around the art portion at the height calculated in part 2c. This line should be parallel with the occlusal plane (line 0–0 in figure 10–8). Trim the cast at the line.

3. *Maxillary Cast*

a. Measure the greatest depth of the anatomic portion (usually at the canine) and divide by two to obtain the height of the art portion.

b. Relate the two casts (use the wax bite if necessary) and place the mandibular base on the flat surface.

c. Measure from the base of the mandibular cast to the highest point of the maxillary anatomic portion (usually in the vestibule over the canine), and add this figure to the height of the maxillary art portion calculated in part *a* above.

d. Set the compass at this measurement and mark a line around the maxillary cast at the total height. The line must be parallel to the base of the mandibular cast and to the occlusal plane. Trim.

D. Posterior Borders

1. Select the longest cast to trim first by measuring from the incisors to points

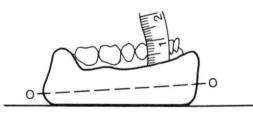

Figure 10–8. Preparation for trimming the base. The anatomic portion is measured at its greatest height which is usually from the tip of the canine to the depth of the vestibule. One-half of this measurement will be the height of the art portion. The trimming line (0–0) is parallel with the mean occlusal plane. See text for details.

distal to the retromolar and tuberosity areas.

2. On the longest cast, place the tip of the compass at the gingival border behind the midline anteriorly (usually this is between the central incisors) and mark an arc ¼ inch distal to the tuberosity (if the maxillary cast) or retromolar area (if the mandibular cast) on each side.

3. Intersect the arc with a line through the central grooves of the molars (figure 10–9 A).

4. Connect the two points across the back of the cast (0–0 in figure 10–9 A). Check that this line is perpendicular to the median line from the incisors through the palate or the tongue (X–Y in figure 10–9 B).

5. With the base of the cast flat on the model trimmer table, trim on the line marked for the posterior border.

6. For the shorter cast, relate the two casts with the wax bite and place flat on the base of the first trimmed cast. Bring them carefully to the cutting surface of the model trimmer, and trim until the two posterior borders are even and parallel.

7. Check by placing the casts on their posterior borders and bringing them together. They should relate in their natural intercuspation (figure 10–6 B).

E. Sides and Heels

1. Select the widest cast to trim first: casts are usually widest at the molar region.

2. Mark with ruler two symmetrical lines ¼ to ⁵/₁₆ inch buccal from the buccal bony prominence at the premolar regions and parallel with lines through the central grooves of the premolars (figure 10–10 A).

a. Check that the lines form equal angles with the posterior border.

b. Before trimming, make certain that the lines when cut would not remove any vestibular anatomy.

c. Trim the sides with the base flat on the model trimmer table.

3. Mark trimming lines for the heels: cuts are ½ inch wide and parallel with a line through the mesiodistal plane of the op

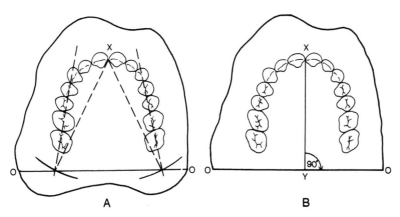

Figure 10–9. Trim line for the posterior borders. **A.** On the longest cast, use a compass to draw arcs from the anterior midline point (X) to ¼ inch distal to the tuberosity area (maxillary) or retromolar area (mandibular). Intersect the arc with line through the central grooves of the molars and connect the two points across the cast (0–0). **B.** Check that the 0–0 line is perpendicular to the median line from the incisors through the palate or tongue (X–Y) before trimming.

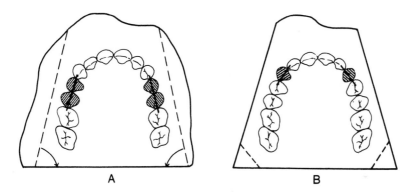

Figure 10–10. Trim lines for the sides and heels. **A.** On the widest cast, the trim lines for the sides are drawn parallel with lines through the central grooves of the premolars. The two symmetrical lines form equal angles with the posterior border of the cast. **B.** Mark trim lines for the heels ¼ inch wide and parallel with lines through the mesiodistal plane of the opposite canine. The lines are symmetrical with each other and form equal angles with the posterior border.

posite canine (figure 10–10 B). Trim with base flat on the model trimmer table.

4. Relate the opposite cast with the wax bite and trim the sides and heels to match the previously trimmed cast.

F. Anterior

The maxillary cast is trimmed to a point and the mandibular cast is rounded (figure 10–5).

1. *Maxillary*
   a. A ruler can be used to draw guidelines for trimming on each side of the midline to the canine areas. Note the dotted lines in figure 10–11 A. The lines should be ¼ to ⁵⁄₁₆ inch labial to the depth of the mucobuccal fold (vestibule) or to the most labially inclined tooth.
   b. Before trimming, check that both sides of the cast will be the same length from the intersection of the front cut to the heels.

2. *Mandibular*
   a. Sketch the shape of an arc from canine to canine to conform generally with the curvature of the anterior teeth and approximately ¼ to ⁵⁄₁₆ inch labial to the depth of the mucobuccal fold or the most labially inclined or positioned tooth (figure 10–11 B).
   b. Before trimming, check that both sides of the cast will be the same length from the intersection of the front cut to the heels.

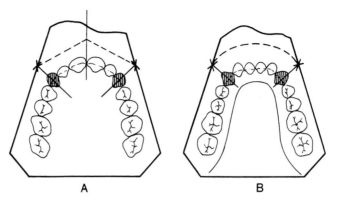

Figure 10–11. Trim lines for anterior. **A.** Maxillary lines are drawn from opposite the middle of each canine to meet in point at the midline and approximately ¼ inch labial to the most labially positioned tooth. **B.** Mandibular line forms an arc drawn from the middle of each canine approximately ¼ inch labial to the most labially positioned tooth.

G. Finishing and Polishing

1. Trim rough edges and margins of both casts and the lingual portion of the mandibular cast to even off irregularities and make the depth of the vestibule visible. Remaining bubbles are removed.
2. Use waterproof sandpaper and a plaster smoothing stone to remove marks left by the model trimmer on the art portion. Sandpaper is not used on the anatomic portion.
3. Fill any holes in the wet casts with stone applied with a spatula to the flat surfaces of the art portion or a camel's hair brush to the anatomic portion. Smooth off excess.
4. Finish and polish:
   a. Allow casts to dry thoroughly for 2 to 3 days.
   b. Smooth the art portion with fine sandpaper.
   c. Soak in heated soap solution for 30 to 60 minutes. Concentrated model gloss soap is available commercially.
   d. Rub with chamois, cotton, or a soft cloth.
   e. Talc or baby talcum powder with olive oil may be used, followed by rubbing with a chamois or soft cloth.

TECHNICAL HINTS

I. Safety Factors[12]
   A. Wear protective eyeglasses while handling powdered dental materials or using a model trimmer. Goggles are advised for laboratory procedures (figure 4–2, page 52).
   B. Do not agitate powders unnecessarily during mixing. Inhaled dust particles can cause serious irritation to the respiratory system.
II. Label each cast with the patient's name and the date. These may be inscribed into the posterior border of the cast before soaping and polishing.
III. Boxes of an appropriate size are available commercially for storage of one or more pairs of casts.
IV. Note in the patient's permanent record the size of impression tray used. When casts are made periodically for follow-up, time is saved both in the sterilization of all sizes for try-in and by preparing the wax rim in advance of the patient's appointment.
V. Make duplicate cast for the permanent record when the dentist uses the original for the design of prosthesis or fabrication of a secondary impression tray. The duplicate cast is made by taking a laboratory impression of the original and pouring it in the same manner as the original.
VI. To care for the model trimmer, following its use, allow motor to run until clear water is flowing through and all particles of stone or plaster have been washed away.
VII. Replace scratched mixing bowls.
VIII. Sterilize aluminum impression trays. Clean completely to prepare for sterilization.

FACTORS TO TEACH
THE PATIENT

I. Importance and purposes of study casts. Reasons for comparative casts following treatment or at a later date.

II. Use of the casts of other patients to show effects of treatment or what can happen if the prescribed treatment is not carried out.

II. Areas that present difficulty in the plaque control and oral physical therapy program: use of devices can be demonstrated on the patient's own study cast.

References

. Stankewitz, C.G., Carpenter, W.M., and Kate, W.: Bacteremia Associated With Irreversible Hydrocolloid Dental Impressions, *J. Prosthet. Dent.*, *44*, 251, September, 1980.

2. American Dental Association, Council on Dental Materials, Instruments and Equipment: *Dentist's Desk Reference: Materials, Instruments and Equipment*, 1st ed. Chicago, American Dental Association, 1981, pp. 180–182.

3. Craig, R.G., O'Brien, W.J., and Powers, J.M.: *Dental Materials, Properties and Manipulation*, 2nd ed. St. Louis, The C.V. Mosby Co., 1979, pp. 131–145.

4. Phillips, R.W.: *Elements of Dental Materials for Dental Hygienists and Assistants*, 3rd ed. Philadelphia, W.B. Saunders Co., 1977, pp. 96–103.

5. Phillips, R.W.: *Skinner's Science of Dental Materials*, 7th ed. Philadelphia, W.B. Saunders Co., 1973, pp. 114–123.

6. American Dental Association, Council on Dental Materials and Devices: Certification and Classification Programs for Dental Materials and Devices, *J. Am. Dent. Assoc.*, *98*, 272, February, 1979.

7. American Dental Association, Council on Dental Materials, Instruments and Equipment: Certification and Acceptance Programs for Dental Materials, Instruments, and Equipment, *J. Am. Dent. Assoc.*, *101*, 68, July, 1980.

8. American Dental Association, Council on Dental Materials, Instruments and Equipment: op. cit., pp. 199–201.

9. Craig, O'Brien, and Powers: op. cit., pp. 166–178.

10. Phillips: op. cit., pp. 48–69.

11. Phillips, R.W.: *Skinner's Science of Dental Materials*, 7th ed. Philadelphia, W.B. Saunders Co., 1973, pp. 55–82.

2. American Dental Association, Council on Dental Materials, Instruments and Equipment: op. cit., p. 29.

Suggested Readings

Chadha, J.M. and Rayson, J.H.: Diagnostic Casts, in Clark, J.W., ed.: *Clinical Dentistry, Volume 1*, Chapter 7. Hagerstown, Maryland, Harper & Row, 1981, pp. 1–4.

Graber, T.M.: *Orthodontics, Principles and Practice*, 3rd ed. Philadelphia, W.B. Saunders Co., 1972, pp. 403–413.

Hill, C.J. and Gellin, M.E.: Impression Making for the Young Child Who Gags, *J. Am. Dent. Assoc.*, *81*, 161, July, 1970.

LeCompte, E.J. and Whitford, G.M.: The Biologic Availability of Fluoride from Alginate Impressions and APF Gel Applications in Children, *J. Dent. Res.*, *60*, 776, April, 1981.

McGrath, J.: Role of the Auxiliary in Orthodontics, in Castano, F.A. and Alden, B.A., eds.: *Handbook of Expanded Dental Auxiliary Practice*, 2nd ed. Philadelphia, J.B. Lippincott Co., 1980, pp. 243–248.

Rigsby, B.E. and Wyss, H.E.: Pouring and Trimming Casts, in Peterson, S., ed.: *The Dentist and the Assistant*, 4th ed. St. Louis, The C.V. Mosby Co., 1977, pp. 217–232.

Rudd, K.D.: Making Diagnostic Casts is Not a Waste of Time, *J. Prosthet. Dent.*, *20*, 98, August, 1968.

Rudd, K.D. and Morrow, R.M.: A Simplified Method for Mixing Dental Stone, *J. Prosthet. Dent.*, *32*, 675, December, 1974.

Schwarzrock, S.P. and Jensen, J.R.: *Effective Dental Assisting*, 5th ed. Dubuque, Iowa, Wm. C. Brown Co., 1978, pp. 581–591.

Strang, R.H.W. and Thompson, W.M.: *A Textbook of Orthodontia*, 4th ed. Philadelphia, Lea & Febiger, 1958, pp. 786–798.

Thompson, E.O.: Constructing and Using Diagnostic Models, *Dent. Clin. North Am.*, p. 67, March, 1963.

Thurow, R.C.: *Atlas of Orthodontic Principles*, 2nd ed. St. Louis, The C.V. Mosby Co., 1977, pp. 239–247.

Woodall, I.R., Dafoe, B.R., Young, N.S., Weed-Fonner, L., and Yankell, S.L.: *Comprehensive Dental Hygiene Care*. St. Louis, The C.V. Mosby Co., 1980, pp. 154–174.

Safety Factors

Brune D. and Beltesbrekke, H.: Dust in Dental Laboratories. Part III: Efficiency of Ventilation Systems and Face Masks, *J. Prosthet. Dent.*, *44*, 211, August, 1980.

Brune, D. and Beltesbrekke, H.: Levels of Airborne Particles Resulting from Handling Alginate Impression Material, *Scand. J. Dent. Res.*, *86*, 206, May, 1978.

Firtell, D.N., Moore, D.J., and Pelleu, G.B.: Sterilization of Impression Materials for Use in the Surgical Operating Room, *J. Prosthet. Dent.*, *27*, 419, April, 1972.

Katberg, J.W.: Cross-contamination via the Prosthodontic Laboratory, *J. Prosthet. Dent.*, *32*, 412, October, 1974.

Mack, P.J.: Inhalation of Alginate Powder During Spatulation, *Br. Dent. J.*, *146*, 141, March 6, 1978.

Polan, M., Frommer, S., and Roistacher, S.: Incidence of Viable Mycobacteria Tuberculosis on Alginate Impressions in Patients with Positive Sputum, *J. Prosthet. Dent.*, *24*, 335, September, 1970.

Posti, J.J., Nakki, K., and Siirilä, H.S.: The Effect of Pre-impression Mouth Rinsing on the Viscosity of Saliva, *Proc. Finn. Dent. Soc.*, *74*, 31, Number 1–2, 1978.

Rowe, A.H.R. and Forrest, J.O.: Dental Impressions. The Probability of Contamination and a Method of Disinfection, *Br. Dent. J.*, *145*, 184, September 19, 1978.

11

The Gingiva

The true test of successful treatment, the real evaluation of the effects of scaling and related instrumentation, is the *health* of the gingival tissues. The objective of all treatment is to bring the diseased gingiva to a state of health that can be maintained by the patient. To do this, the first thing is to learn to recognize normal healthy tissue, to observe certain characteristics of color, texture, and form, to test for bleeding, and to apply this knowledge to the treatment and supervision of the patient's gingiva until health is attained.

An outline of the clinical features of the periodontal tissues in health and disease is included in this chapter. It is expected that complete information about the gross and microscopic anatomy of the periodontium and periodontal pathology will have been studied or will be studied in preparation for clinical practice. Textbooks and other references are listed in *Suggested Readings* at the end of the chapter for review.

OBJECTIVES

The ultimate objective is that the dental hygienist's knowledge and skill in examination and evaluation of the periodontal tissues will be applied in patient care so that each patient will attain and maintain optimum oral health. The dental hygienist will know when the treatment provided by dental hygiene services is definitive in restoring health and when additional treatment is needed. The patient can be properly informed so that complete treatment can be provided.

Specific objectives for the dental hygienist are to be able to

   I. Recognize normal periodontal tissues.
  II. Know the features of the periodontal tissues that must be examined for a complete assessment.
 III. Recognize the basic signs of periodontal diseases and classify them by type and degree of severity.
  IV. Identify the dental hygiene treatment and instruction needed.
   V. Outline the patient's preventive periodontal program (page 333).

THE FIELD OF OPERATION

The techniques of dental hygiene are applied directly to the teeth, the gingiva, and the gingival sulcus. Detailed knowledge and understanding of the anatomy and normal clinical appearance of the field of operation are prerequisite to meaningful examination and treatment.

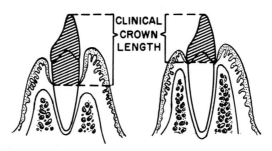

Figure 11–1. Diagram to show clinical crown. The clinical crown is the part of a tooth that is above the attached periodontal tissue. **Left,** when there is increased pocket depth, the clinical crown may extend to a position where the clinical crown length is longer than the clinical root length. The clinical root is that part of the tooth with attached periodontal tissues. **Right,** when the attachment is at the cementoenamel junction, the clinical crown and the anatomic crown are the same.

I. The Teeth

A. Clinical Crown

The part of the tooth above the attached periodontal tissues. It can be considered the part of the tooth where clinical techniques are applied (figure 11–1).

B. Clinical Root

The part of the tooth below the base of the gingival sulcus or periodontal pocket. It is the part of the root to which periodontal fibers are attached.

C. Anatomic Crown

The part of the tooth covered by enamel.

D. Anatomic Root

The part of the tooth covered by cementum.

II. Oral Mucosa

The lining of the oral cavity, the oral mucosa, is a mucous membrane composed of connective tissue covered with stratified squamous epithelium. There are three divisions or categories of oral mucosa.

A. Masticatory Mucosa

1. Covers the *gingiva* and the *hard palate*, the areas used most during the mastication of food.
2. Except for the free margin of the gingiva, the masticatory mucosa is firmly attached to underlying tissues.
3. The epithelial covering is generally keratinized.

B. Lining Mucosa

1. Covers the inner surfaces of the *lips and cheeks*, the *floor of the mouth*, the *under side of the tongue*, the *soft palate*, and the *alveolar mucosa*.
2. These tissues are not firmly attached to underlying tissue.
3. The epithelial covering is not generally keratinized.

C. Specialized Mucosa

1. Covers the *dorsum* (upper surface) *of the tongue*.
2. Anterior part is composed of many papillae; some contain tastebuds.

III. The Periodontium

The periodontium is the functional unit of tissues that surrounds and supports the tooth. There are four parts: the gingiva and the attachment apparatus made up of the periodontal ligament, cementum, and bone.

A. Gingiva

The part of the masticatory mucosa that surrounds the necks of the teeth and is attached to the teeth and the alveolar bone.

B. Periodontal Ligament

Connective tissue fibers that surround the root and connect the tooth and bone.

. **Cementum**

The calcified tissue that covers the root and attaches the fibers of the periodontal ligament to the tooth.

. **Alveolar Bone**

The bone of the mandible and the maxilla that surrounds the roots of the teeth to support them. Periodontal ligament fibers are attached to the bone.

THE GINGIVA AND RELATED STRUCTURES

The gingiva is made up of the free gingiva, the attached gingiva, and the interdental gingiva or interdental papilla.

. **Free Gingiva (Marginal Gingiva)**

The free gingiva is closely adapted around each tooth. It connects with the attached gingiva at the free gingival groove and attaches to the tooth at the coronal portion of the junctional epithelium (Figure 11–2).

. **Free Gingival Groove**

1. A shallow linear groove that demarcates the free from the attached gingiva. Generally, about one third of the teeth show a visible gingival groove when the gingiva is in health.[1]

2. In the absence of disease and pocket formation, the gingival groove runs somewhat parallel with and about 0.5 to 1.5 millimeters from the gingival margin,[2] and is approximately at the level of the bottom of the gingival sulcus.

B. **Oral Epithelium** (outer gingival epithelium, figure 11–3)
   1. Covers the free gingiva from the gingival groove over the gingival margin.
   2. It is composed of keratinized stratified squamous epithelium.

C. **Gingival Margin** (gingival crest, margin of the gingiva, or free margin)
   1. It is the edge of the gingiva nearest the incisal or occlusal.
   2. Marks the opening of the gingival sulcus.

D. **Gingival Sulcus** (crevice)
   1. It is the crevice or groove between the free gingiva and the tooth.
   2. Boundaries (figure 11–3)
      a. Inner: tooth surface. May be the enamel, cementum or part of each, depending on the position of the junctional epithelium.

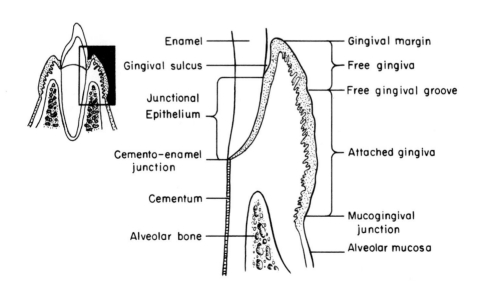

Enamel	Gingival margin
Gingival sulcus	Free gingiva
Junctional Epithelium	Free gingival groove
Cemento-enamel junction	Attached gingiva
Cementum	Mucogingival junction
Alveolar bone	Alveolar mucosa

Figure 11–2. Parts of the gingiva. Diagram to illustrate the parts of the gingiva and adjacent tissues of a partially erupted tooth. Note that the junctional epithelium is on the enamel.

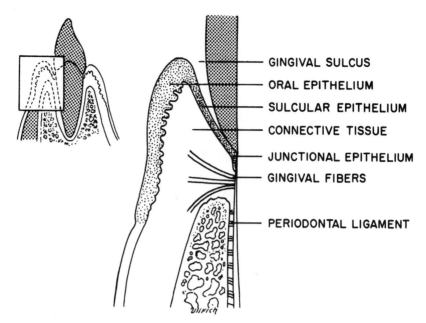

Figure 11–3. The gingival tissues. Cross section to show the histologic relationships of the oral, sulcular, and junctional epithelia, and the connective tissue of the gingiva.

b. Outer: sulcular epithelium.
c. Base: coronal margin of the attached tissues. The base of the sulcus or pocket is also called the "depth of the sulcus" or the "bottom of the pocket."
3. Sulcular epithelium: the continuation of the oral epithelium covering the free gingiva. Sulcular epithelium is not keratinized.
4. Depth of sulcus: approximately 1 to 2 millimeters. Healthy sulci are shallowest and may be only 0.5 millimeter. The average depth of the healthy sulcus is about 1.8 millimeters.[3]
5. Gingival sulcus fluid (sulcular fluid, crevicular fluid)[4,5]
a. A serum-like fluid secreted from the connective tissue through the epithelial lining of the sulcus or pocket.
b. Occurrence: slight to none in a normal sulcus; increased with inflammation; and considered part of the local defense mechanism.

II. Junctional Epithelium (Epithelial Attachment, Epithelial Cuff)

A. Description

The junctional epithelium is a cuff-like band of stratified squamous epithelium which is continuous with the sulcular epithelium and completely encircles the tooth. It is triangular in cross section, widest at the junction with the sulcular epithelium, and narrowing down to the width of a few cells at the apical end.

The *epithelial attachment* is the inner part of the junctional epithelium which is adjacent to the tooth.

B. Size

3 to 4 layers of cells thick in the young and up to 20 cells thick in later life. The length ranges from 0.25 to 1.35 millimeters.[6]

C. Position

1. As the tooth erupts, the attachment is on the enamel; during eruption, the epithelium migrates toward the cemento-enamel junction (figure 11–4).
2. At full eruption, the attachment is on the cementum where it becomes firmly attached.
3. With wear of the tooth on the incisal or occlusal surface and in disease, the at-

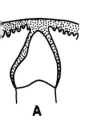
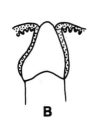
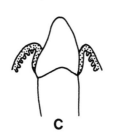
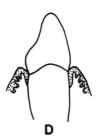
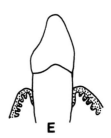

Figure 11–4. Position of junctional epithelium. **A.** Before eruption the oral epithelium covers the tooth. **B.** As the tooth merges, the reduced enamel epithelium joins the oral epithelium as the gingival sulcus is formed. **C.** Partial eruption with the junctional epithelium along the enamel (see also figure 11–2). **D.** Eruption complete, with junctional epithelium at the cementoenamel junction. **E.** When there is disease or other cause, the junctional epithelium migrates along the root.

tachment migrates along the root surface (figure 11–4 E).

D. Relation of Crest of Alveolar Bone to the Attached Gingival Tissue

The distance between the base of the attachment and the crest of the alveolar bone is approximately 1.0 to 1.5 millimeters. This distance is maintained in disease when the epithelium moves along the root surface during pocket formation.

C. Attachment of the Epithelium to the Tooth Surface

An adhesive, organic, mucopolysaccharide substance secreted by the epithelial cells provides a seal at the base of the sulcus and along the border of the junctional epithelium and the tooth surface.

II. Interdental Gingiva (Interdental Papilla)

A. Location

Between the teeth; it occupies the interproximal area. The tip and lateral borders are continuous with the free gingiva, while other parts are attached gingiva.

B. Shape

1. Varies with spacing or overlapping of the teeth: a papilla may be flat or saddle-shaped when there are wide spaces between the teeth, or tapered and narrow when the teeth are crowded or overlapped.

2. Between anterior teeth: pointed, pyramidal.
3. Between posterior teeth
   a. Flatter than anterior papillae, which is caused by wider teeth, wider contact areas, and flattened interdental bone.
   b. Two papillae, one facial and one lingual, connected by a col, are found when teeth are in contact.

C. Col

1. A depression between the lingual and facial papillae which conforms to the proximal contact area (figure 11–5).
2. The center of the col area is not usually keratinized, which makes it more susceptible to disease. Most periodontal disease begins in the col area.

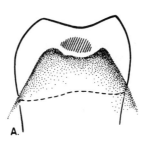
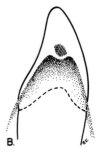

Figure 11–5. Col. The col is the depression between the lingual and facial papillae under the contact area. Contact area is represented by the striped line areas. **A.** Mesial of mandibular molar to show wide col area, and **B.** Mesial of mandibular lateral incisor shows narrow anterior col. The col deepens when there is gingival enlargement.

IV. Attached Gingiva

A. Dimensions

1. Continuous with the oral epithelium of the free gingiva and covered with keratinized stratified squamous epithelium.
2. Maxillary lingual: continuous with the palatal mucosa.
3. Mandibular facial and lingual, and maxillary facial: demarcated from the alveolar mucosa at the mucogingival junction by the mucogingival lines.

B. Attachment

Firmly bound to the underlying cementum and alveolar bone.

C. Shape

Follows the depressions between the eminences of the roots of the teeth.

D. Mucogingival Junction

1. *Appearance*

   The mucogingival junction appears as a scalloped line which marks the connection between the attached gingiva and the alveolar mucosa.

   A sharp contrast can be seen between the pink of the keratinized, stippled, attached gingiva and the darker alveolar mucosa.

2. *Location*

   A mucogingival line is found on the facial of all quadrants and on the lingual of the mandibular arch. There is no alveolar mucosa on the palate. The palatal tissue is firmly attached to the bone of the roof of the mouth. There are three mucogingival lines: facial and lingual mandibular, and facial maxillary. In figure 11–6 the facial maxillary and mandibular mucogingival lines are shown in relation to the attached gingiva and the alveolar mucosa.

V. Alveolar Mucosa

A. Description

Movable tissue loosely attached to the underlying bone. Has a smooth, shiny surface with nonkeratinized epithelium which thin. Underlying vessels may be see through the epithelium.

B. Frena (Singular: frenum or frenulum)

1. A frenum is a narrow fold of mucou membrane which passes from a mor fixed to a movable part; for example, fro the gingiva to the lip, cheek, or unde surface of the tongue. A frenum serve to check undue movement.
2. Locations
   a. Maxillary and mandibular anteri frena: at midlines between central i cisors. Figure 11–6 shows diagran matically the location of the anteri frena.
   b. Lingual frenum: from undersurfac of the tongue.
   c. Buccal frena: in the canine–premol: areas, both maxillary and mandibu lar.
3. Attachment of frena in relation to th attached gingiva
   a. May be closely associated with th mucogingival line.
   b. When the attached gingiva is narro or missing, the frena may pull on th free gingiva and displace it laterall

THE RECOGNITION OF GINGIVAL AND PERIODONTAL DISEASES

The recognition of normal gingiva, gingiv

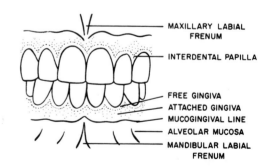

Figure 11–6. Parts of the gingiva, labial view. Maxillar and mandibular mucogingival lines are shown in relation t the attached gingiva, alveolar mucosa, and labial frenum Dots represent stippling of the attached gingiva. The fre gingiva is not stippled.

diseases, and deeper periodontal involvement depends on a disciplined, step-by-step examination. To recognize the signs of disease, a basic examination must include clinical observation for gingival tissue changes, bleeding, exudate, pockets, furcation involvement, mucogingival involvement, occlusion factors, tooth mobility, and a radiographic examination.

It is also necessary to know the extent of the disease. *Gingival diseases* are confined to the gingiva; whereas *periodontal diseases* include all parts of the periodontium, namely, the gingiva, periodontal ligament, bone, and cementum.

Patients may or may not have specific symptoms to report because periodontal diseases are insidious in development. Symptoms the patient notices or feels may include bleeding gingiva, sometimes only while brushing, sometimes with drooling at night, or sometimes spontaneously. Other possible symptoms are sensitivity to hot and cold, tenderness or discomfort while eating or some pain after eating, food retained between the teeth, unpleasant mouth odors, chronic bad taste, or a feeling that the teeth are loose. Most of these are symptoms of advanced disease.

I. Clinically Normal

The terms "clinically normal" or "clinically healthy" may be used to designate gingival tissue that is pale pink; has a knife-edged gingival margin which adapts closely around the tooth; is stippled; firm; has minimal sulcus depth with no bleeding when probed. Although "normal" will vary with anatomic, physiologic, and other factors, general characteristics form a baseline for a contrast in the recognition of disease.

II. Causes of Tissue Changes

Disease changes produce alterations in the color, size, position, shape, consistency, surface texture, bleeding readiness, and exudate production.

To understand the changes that take place in the gingival tissues during the transition from health to disease, it is necessary to have a clear picture of what plaque is, the role of plaque microorganisms in the development of disease, and the inflammatory response by the body.

When the products of the plaque microorganisms cause breakdown of the intercellular sub-stances of the sulcular epithelium, injurious agents can pass into the connective tissue where an inflammatory response is initiated. An inflammatory response means that there is increased blood flow, increased permeability of capillaries, and increased collection of defense cells and tissue fluid. It is these changes that produce the tissue alterations such as color, size, shape, and consistency that are described in the next section.

III. Descriptive Terminology

The degree of severity and distribution of a change should be noted when examining the gingiva. When a deviation from normal affects a single area, it can be designated by the number of the adjacent tooth and the surface of the tissue involved, namely, facial, lingual, mesial, or distal. Teeth numbering systems are described on pages 81–83.

A. Severity. Severity is expressed as slight, moderate, or severe.

B. Distribution. Terms used for describing distribution are
1. *Localized.* Localized means that the gingiva is involved only about a single tooth or a specific group of teeth.
2. *Generalized.* Generalized means that the gingiva is involved about all or nearly all of the teeth throughout the mouth. A condition may also be generalized throughout a single arch, the maxillary or mandibular.
3. *Marginal.* A change that involves the free or marginal gingiva. This is specified as either localized or generalized.
4. *Papillary.* A change that involves a papilla but not the rest of the free gingiva around a tooth. A papillary change may be localized or generalized.
5. *Diffuse.* When the attached gingiva is involved as well as the free gingiva, it is referred to as a diffuse change. A diffuse condition is most frequently localized, rarely generalized.

IV. Early Recognition of Tissue Changes

Marked changes, such as moderate to severe

generalized redness, enlargement, sponginess, deep pockets, and definite mobility, are relatively easy to detect even with limited experience, provided there is good light and accessibility for vision. In contrast, when changes are subtle, localized about one or a few teeth, and of a lesser degree of severity, more skillful application of knowledge is needed.

Early recognition of gingival and periodontal disease prevents neglect of conditions that can develop into severe disease. Treatment is less complicated, and the success of treatment and recovery to healthy tissue is predictable when early recognition makes early treatment possible.

THE GINGIVAL EXAMINATION

The examination of the gingiva includes evaluation of the color, size, shape, consistency, surface texture, position, mucogingival lines, bleeding, and exudate. These are summarized in table 11–1, which is a clinical reference chart.

I. Color

A. Normal

1. *Pale Pink:* darker in people with darker complexions.
2. *Factors Influencing Color*
   a. Vascular supply.
   b. Thickness of epithelium.
   c. Degree of keratinization.
   d. Physiologic pigmentation: melanin pigmentation occurs frequently in Negroes, Orientals, Indians, and Caucasians of Mediterranean countries.

B. Changes in Disease

1. *In Chronic Inflammation:* dark red, bluish red, magenta, or deep blue.
2. *In Acute Inflammation:* bright red.
3. *Extent:* deep involvement can be expected when color changes extend into the attached gingiva or from the marginal gingiva to the mucogingival line or over into alveolar mucosa.

II. Size

A. Normal

1. *Free Gingiva:* flat, not enlarged; fits snugly around the tooth.
2. *Attached Gingiva*
   a. Width of attached gingiva varies between patients and between teeth for an individual, from 1 to 9 millimeters.[7]
   b. Wider in maxilla than mandible: broadest zone related to incisors, narrowest at the canine and premolar regions.

B. Changes in Disease

1. *Free Gingiva and Papillae:* become enlarged, which may be localized or limited to specific areas or generalized throughout the entire gingiva. The col deepens as the papillae increase in size.
2. *Attached Gingiva:* decreases in amount as the pocket deepens. How to measure the amount of attached gingiva is described on page 218.

III. Position

The *actual* position of the gingiva is the level of the attached gingival tissue. It is not directly visible, but can be determined by probing.

The *apparent* position of the gingiva is the level of the gingival margin or crest of the free gingiva which is seen by direct observation.

A. Normal

In an adult, for the fully erupted tooth, the apparent position of the gingival margin is normally at the level of, or slightly below, the enamel contour or prominence of the cervical third of a tooth.

B. Changes in Disease

1. *Effect of Gingival Enlargement.* When the gingiva enlarges, the gingival margin may be high on the enamel, partly or nearly covering the anatomic crown.
2. *Effect of Gingival Recession*
   a. Definition: recession is the exposure of root surface which results from the apical migration of the junctional epithelium.

b. Types (figure 11–7)
   (1) Apparent, visible recession. Visible recession is evidenced by the position of the gingival margin. An area of root surface may be seen above the gingival margin.
   (2) Actual, hidden recession. Actual recession is shown by the position of the junctional epithelium on the root surface. The area of recession is covered by gingival tissue which forms the pocket wall.
c. Measurement. Both actual and apparent recession can be measured with a probe from the cementoenamel junction. Total recession is the actual and apparent added together.

IV. Shape (Form or Contour)

A. Normal

1. *Free Gingiva*
   a. Follows a curved line around each tooth; may be straighter along wide molar surfaces.

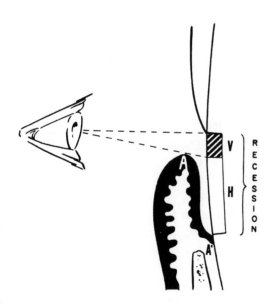

Figure 11–7. Gingival recession. Diagram to show *Apparent* position of the gingiva (A), *Actual* position (A'), *Visible recession* (V) with an area of the root of the tooth visible above the gingival margin, and *Hidden recession* (H) the tooth surface pocket wall. (From Carranza, F.A.: Glickman's Clinical Periodontology, 5th ed. Philadelphia, W.B. Saunders Co., 1979.)

   b. The margin is knife-edged or slightly rounded on facial and lingual; closely adapted to the tooth surface.
2. *Papillae*
   a. Teeth with contact area: facial and lingual pointed or slightly rounded papillae with col area under the contact (figure 11–5).
   b. Spaced teeth (with diastemas): interdental gingiva is flat or saddle-shaped.

B. Changes in Disease

1. *Free Gingiva:* rounded or rolled.
2. *Papillae:* blunted, flattened, bulbous, cratered (figure 11–8).
3. *Festoon ("McCall's Festoon"):* an enlargement of the marginal gingiva with the formation of a lifesaver-like gingival prominence. Frequently, the total gingiva is very narrow and there is associated apparent recession as shown in figure 11–8D.
4. *Clefts*
   a. Localized recession (figure 11–9A). A localized recession or cleft may be narrow or wide, deep or shallow. The root surface is denuded, and the cleft may extend to or through the mucogingival junction.
   b. "Stillman's Cleft" (figures 11–9B and C). A localized recession may be V-shaped, apostrophe-shaped, or form a slit-like indentation. It may extend several millimeters toward the mucogingival junction or even to or through the junction.

V. Consistency

A. Normal

1. Firm and resilient when palpated with the side of a blunt instrument (probe).
2. Attached gingiva is bound down firmly to the underlying bone.

B. Changes in Disease

1. *To Determine Consistency:* gently press side of probe on free gingiva. Soft,

spongy gingiva will dent readily; firm hard tissue resists.

2. *Soft Spongy Gingiva:* related to acute stages of inflammation with increased infiltration of fluid and inflammatory elements. The tissue appears red, may be smooth and shiny with loss of stippling, has marginal enlargement, and bleeds readily on probing.

3. *Firm, Hard Gingiva:* related to chronic inflammation with increased fibrosis. The tissue may appear pink and well stippled. Bleeding, when probed, usually will occur only in the deeper part of a pocket, not near the margin.

4. *Retraction of the Margin Away From the Tooth:* normally the free gingiva fits snugly about the tooth. When the margin tends to hang slightly away or is readily displaced with a light air blast, it means that the gingival fibers that support the margin have been destroyed.

VI. Surface Texture

A. Normal

1. *Free Gingiva:* smooth.
2. *Attached Gingiva:* stippled (minutely "pebbled" or "orange peel" surface).
3. *Interdental Gingiva:* the free gingiva is smooth; the center portion of each papilla is stippled.

B. Changes in Disease

1. *Inflammatory Changes:* may be loss of stippling, with smooth, shiny surface.
2. *Hyperkeratosis:* may result in a leathery, hard, or nodular surface.
3. *Chronic Disease:* tissue may be hard and fibrotic with a normal pink color, and have normal or deep stippling.

VII. Bleeding

A. Normal

1. *No Bleeding:* healthy tissue does not bleed.
2. *Gingival Index Score:* zero (page 299).

B. Changes in Disease

1. *Bleeding:* occurs spontaneously or when pockets are probed.
2. *Changes in Sulcular Epithelium* during the inflammatory process result in a thin, ulcerated pocket wall which bleeds readily. Development of inflammation and pocket formation are described on pages 202–203.
3. *Gingival Index Score:* 2 or 3, depending on the severity of the condition.

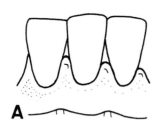

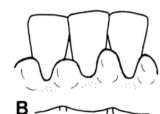

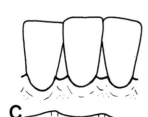

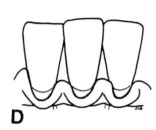

Figure 11–8. Gingival shape or contour. **A.** Blunted, **B.** Bulbous, **C.** Cratered papillae. **D.** Rolled, lifesaver-shaped "McCall's Festoon."

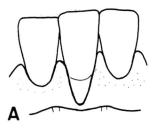 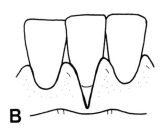 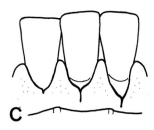

Figure 11–9. Gingival clefts. **A.** Localized recession showing a wide deep cleft. **B.** V-shaped Stillman's Cleft, and **C.** Slit-like clefts of varying degrees of severity in relation to the mucogingival junction.

VIII. Exudate

A. **Normal:** none, except slight gingival sulcus fluid (page 188). Gingival sulcus fluid could not be observed by direct observation.

B. **Changes in Disease**

1. *Suppuration:* Formation or secretion of pus.
2. *White Fluid:* may appear at the entrance to the pocket or may be squeezed out of the sulcus by light finger pressure on the external wall of the pocket. Pus is a semi-fluid creamy, yellow-white product of inflammation composed mainly of leukocytes and serum.
3. *Amount of Exudate:* is related to the severity of the acute inflammation, not to the depth of the pocket.

IX. The Gingiva of Young Children[8–10]

A. **Normal**

1. *Primary Dentition.*
   a. Color: pink or slightly red.
   b. Shape: thick, rounded, or rolled.
   c. Consistency: firm, but not tightly adapted to the teeth; it may be easily displaced with a light air jet.
   d. Surface texture: may or may not have stippling; high percentage have shiny gingiva.
   e. Width of attached gingiva ages 3 to 5: between 1 and 6 millimeters.[7]

   f. Interdental gingiva.
      (1) Anterior: diastemas are frequently present and the papillae are flat or saddle-shaped; when teeth are in contact, the usual pyramid or col is present.
      (2) Posterior: col between facial and lingual papillae when teeth are in contact (figure 11–5).
2. *Mixed Dentition*
   a. Constant state of change related to exfoliation and eruption.
   b. Free gingiva may appear rolled or rounded, slightly reddened, shiny, and with a lack of firmness.
   c. Position: the gingiva covers a varying portion of the anatomic crown, depending on the stage of eruption (figure 11–4).

B. **Changes in Disease**

Gingivitis affects over 80 percent of young children[11] and increases in prevalence until a high of over 90 percent can be found in the 9- to 14-year-old group. Periodontitis can occur in primary dentition as well as in a percentage of children of all ages.

Mucogingival problems occur in children.[12] The recognition of deficiencies of attached gingiva has particular significance for the child who will need orthodontic treatment.

Examination of the periodontal tissues for a child is not different from that of an adult. A complete examination is necessary, including probing around each tooth.

Table 11–1. Examination of the Gingiva. Clinical Reference Chart

	Normal Appearance	*Changes in Disease Clinical Appearance*	*Causes for Changes*

Color	Uniformly pale pink
	
	Variations in pigmentation related to complexion, race
		Acute: bright red	Inflammation:
			  capillary dilation
			  increased blood flow

		Chronic: bluish pink, bluish red	Vessels engorged Blood flow sluggish Venous return impaired Anoxemia
		pink	Increased fibrosis
		Attached gingiva: color change may extend to the mucogingival line	Deepening of pocket, muco-gingival involvement

Size	Flat, not enlarged
	
	Fits snugly around the tooth
		Enlarged	Edematous:
			  inflammatory fluid
			  cellular exudate
			  vascular enlargement
			  hemorrhage
			
			Fibrotic:
			  new collagen fibers

Shape	Marginal gingiva:
	  Knife-edged, flat
	  Follows a curved line about the tooth
	Papillae:
	  (1) Normal contact: papilla is pointed and pyramidal; fills the interproximal area
	  (2) Space (diastema) between teeth: gingiva is flat or saddle-shaped
		Marginal gingiva:
		  rounded
		  rolled
		  bulbous
		Papillae:
		  bulbous
		  flattened
		  blunted
		  cratered
			Inflammatory changes:
			  edema or fibrosis
			
			Bulbous with gingival enlargement
			
			Cratered in necrotizing ulcerative gingivitis

Consistency	Firm, resilient Attached gingiva firmly bound down	Soft, spongy: dents readily when pressed with probe Associated with red color, smooth shiny surface, loss of stippling, bleeding on probing	Edematous: fluid between cells in connective tissue
		Firm, hard: resists probe pressure Associated with pink color, stippling, bleeding only in depth of pocket	Fibrotic: collagen fibers

Table 11–1. *continued*

	Normal Appearance	*Changes in Disease Clinical Appearance*	*Causes for Changes*
Surface texture	Free gingiva: smooth Attached gingiva: stippled	Acute condition: loss of stippling, with smooth, shiny gingiva Chronic: hard, firm, with stippling, sometimes heavier than normal	Inflammatory changes in the connective tissue; edema, cellular infiltration Fibrosis
Position of Gingival Margin	Fully erupted tooth: margin is 1–2 mm. above cementoenamel junction, at or slightly below the enamel contour	Enlarged gingiva: margin is higher on the tooth, above normal, pocket deepened Recession: margin is more apical; root surface is exposed	Edematous or fibrotic Junctional epithelium has migrated along the root; gingival margin follows
Position of Junctional Epithelium	Fully erupted tooth: the junctional epithelium is at the cementoenamel junction During eruption: along the enamel surface	Position, determined by use of probe, is on the root surface	Apical migration of the epithelium along the root
Mucogingival Lines	Make clear demarcation between the pink, stippled, attached gingiva and the darker alveolar mucosa with smooth shiny surface	No attached gingiva: (1) color changes may extend full height of the gingiva; mucogingival line obliterated (2) Probing reveals that the bottom of the pocket extends into the alveolar mucosa (3) Frenal pull may displace the gingival margin from the tooth	Deepening of the pocket Apical migration of the junctional epithelium Attached gingiva decreases with pocket deepening Inflammation extends into alveolar mucosa
Bleeding	No spontaneous bleeding or upon probing	Spontaneous bleeding, Bleeding on probing: Bleeding near margin in acute condition; bleeding deep in pocket in chronic condition	Degeneration of the sulcular epithelium with ulceration Blood vessels engorged Tissue edematous
Exudate	No exudate on pressure	White fluid, pus, visible on digital pressure Amount not related to pocket depth	Inflammation in the connective tissue Excessive accumulation of white blood cells with serum and tissue fluid makes up the exudate (pus)

X. The Gingiva after Periodontal Treatment

The characteristics of "normal healthy gingiva" take on different dimensions for the patient who has completed the treatment for pockets, bone loss, and other signs of periodontal disease. The junctional epithelium will be apical to the cementoenamel junction, yet after healing, the sulcus depth will be within normal range and no bleeding should occur when probed.

Depending on the exact treatment performed, examination will show changes from the initial evaluation. For example, where the initial examination showed a deficiency of attached gingiva with frenal pull, mucogingival surgery was designed and treatment satisfactorily completed to create new attached gingiva. With each recall, a thorough, careful examination is necessary to control factors that may permit recurrence of disease.

FACTORS TO TEACH THE PATIENT

I. Characteristics of normal healthy gingiva.
II. The significance of bleeding: healthy tissue does not bleed.
III. Relationship of findings during a gingival examination to the personal daily care procedures for disease control.
IV. The special attention needed for an area of gingival recession to prevent abrasion, inflammation, and further involvement.
V. How the method of brushing, stiffness of toothbrush filaments, abrasiveness of a dentifrice, and pressure applied during brushing, can be factors in gingival recession.

References

1. Ainamo, J. and Löe, H.: Anatomical Characteristics of Gingiva. A Clinical and Microscopic Study of the Free and Attached Gingiva, *J. Periodontol.*, *37*, 5, January-February, 1966.
2. Bhaskar, S.N., ed.: *Orban's Oral Histology and Embryology*, 9th ed. St. Louis, The C.V. Mosby Co., 1980, p. 291.
3. Ibid., p. 324.
4. Goldman, H.M. and Cohen, D.W.: *Periodontal Therapy*, 6th ed. St. Louis, The C.V. Mosby Co., 1980, pp. 25–28.
5. Carranza, F.A.: *Glickman's Clinical Periodontology*, 5th ed. Philadelphia, W.B. Saunders Co., 1979, p. 13.
6. Ibid., p. 8.
7. Bowers, G.M.: A Study of the Width of Attached Gingiva, *J. Periodontol.*, *34*, 201, May, 1963.
8. Carranza: op. cit., pp. 303–309.
9. Baer, P.N. and Benjamin, S.D.: *Periodontal Disease in Children and Adolescents*. Philadelphia, J.B. Lippincott Co., 1974, pp. 1–35.
10. Kopczyk, R.A. and Lenox, J.A.: Periodontal Health and Disease in Children: Examination and Diagnosis, *Dent. Clin. North Am.*, *17*, 25, January, 1973.
11. World Health Organization: *Epidemiology, Etiology, and Prevention of Periodontal Diseases*. WHO Technical Report Series Number 621, Geneva, World Health Organization, 1978, 60 pp.
12. Maynard, J.G. and Ochsenbein, C.: Mucogingival Problems, Prevalence and Therapy in Children, *J. Periodontol.*, *46*, 543, September, 1975.

Suggested Readings

Allen, D.L., McFall, W.T., and Hunter, G.C.: *Periodontics for the Dental Hygienist*, 3rd ed. Philadelphia, Lea & Febiger, 1980, pp. 7–37.
Boyd, R.L.: Mucogingival Considerations and Their Relationship to Orthodontics, *J. Periodontol.*, *49*, 67, February, 1978.
Bral, M.M. and Stahl, S.S.: Keratinizing Potential of Human Crevicular Epithelium, *J. Periodontol.*, *48*, 381, July, 1977.
Carranza, F.A.: *Glickman's Clinical Periodontology*, 5th ed. Philadelphia, W.B. Saunders Co., 1979, pp. 3–28.
Dummett, C.O.: Normal and Locally Induced Oral Pigmentations, *Int. Dent. J.*, *26*, 152, June, 1976.
Dummett, C.O.: Systemic Significance of Oral Pigmentation and Discoloration, *Postgrad. Med.*, *49*, 78, January, 1971.
Glickman, I. and Smulow, J.B.: *Periodontal Disease: Clinical, Radiographic, and Histopathologic Features*. Philadelphia, W.B. Saunders Co., 1974, pp. 2–12, 38–48.
Goldman, H.M. and Cohen, D.W.: *Periodontal Therapy*, 6th ed. St. Louis, The C.V. Mosby Co., 1980, pp. 1–49.
Gordon, N.C., Brown, S., Khosla, V.M., and Hansen, L.S.: Lead Poisoning. A Comprehensive Review and Report of a Case, *Oral Surg.*, *47*, 500, June, 1979.
Grant, D.A., Stern, I.B., and Everett, F.G.: *Periodontics*, 5th ed. St. Louis, The C.V. Mosby Co., 1979, pp. 3–56.
Israel, H.: A Complication of Orthodontic Therapy: Localized Facial Recession and Loss of Attached Gingiva Treated by Grafting, *Angle Orthod.*, *48*, 149, April, 1978.
Maynard, J.G. and Wilson, R.D.K.: Physiologic Dimensions of the Periodontium Significant to the Restorative Dentist, *J. Periodontol.*, *50*, 170, April, 1979.
Meitner, S.W., Zander, H.A., Iker, H.P., and Polson, A.M.: Identification of Inflamed Gingival Surfaces, *J. Clin. Periodontol.*, *6*, 93, April, 1979.
Melfi, R.C.: *Permar's Oral Embryology and Microscopic Anatomy*, 7th ed. Philadelphia, Lea & Febiger, 1982, pp. 142–153.
Stoner, J.E. and Mazdyasna, S.: Gingival Recession in the Lower Incisor Region of 15-year-old Subjects, *J. Periodontol.*, *51*, 74, February, 1980.
Takei, H.H.: The Interdental Space, *Dent. Clin. North Am.*, *24*, 169, April, 1980.
Ten Cate, A.R.: The Dento-gingival Junction. An Interpretation of the Literature, *J. Periodontol.*, *46*, 475, August, 1975.

oigt, J.P., Goran, M.L., and Fleisher, R.M.: The Width of Lingual Mandibular Attached Gingiva, *J. Periodontol.*, *49*, 77, February, 1978.

Volchansky, A., Cleaton-Jones, P., and Fatti, L.P.: A 3-year Longitudinal Study of the Position of the Gingival Margin in Man, *J. Clin. Periodontol.*, *6*, 231, August, 1979.

12

Pockets

Early in the process of case assessment in preparation for treatment planning, the severity of periodontal disease must be determined. Is the patient's disease limited to the gingival tissue without loss of periodontal attachment? Or does the patient have bone loss, pocket formation, as well as other signs of periodontitis? Where is the attachment level? Is altered cementum exposed within the pockets?

When the disease is limited to the gingiva, the next question will be: can the disease be reversed by having the patient follow daily disease-control self-treatment methods supplemented by professional scaling? On the other hand, if there is apical positioning of the periodontal attachment, accompanied by other indications of periodontitis, will conservative procedures of scaling, root planing, and gingival curettage provide sufficient professional treatment or will more complex periodontal therapy be required?

For the dental hygienist an understanding is necessary of what can be accomplished by dental hygiene therapeutic procedures and when the patient will need more advanced therapy by a dentist or be referred to a periodontist in order to bring the oral tissues to a state of maximum health. It is not always possible to distinguish when additional therapy will be required until after the initial steps have been completed and a reevaluation has been made. When the initial treatment program is presented to the patient,

it should be made clear that a reevaluation will be necessary.

CLASSIFICATION OF PERIODONTAL DISEASE

A widely used system for classifying the severity of periodontal diseases is the one prepared by the American Academy of Periodontology.[1] The four divisions are as follows:

Type I GINGIVITIS
Inflammation of the gingiva characterized clinically by gingival hyperplasia, edema, retractability, gingival pocket formation and no bone loss.

Type II EARLY PERIODONTITIS
Progression of gingival inflammation into the alveolar bone crest and early bone loss resulting in moderate periodontal pocket formation.

Type III MODERATE PERIODONTITIS
A more advanced state of the above condition, with increased destruction of periodontal structures associated with moderate to deep pockets, moderate to severe bone loss and tooth mobility.

Type IV ADVANCED PERIODONTITIS
Further progression of periodontitis with severe destruction of the periodontal structures and increased tooth mobility.

Attachment levels and related pocket depths are major factors in the severity of periodontal diseases. Determinations are made with a probe and coordinated with other clinical and radiologic findings.

GINGIVAL AND PERIODONTAL POCKETS

A pocket is a diseased sulcus. It is the presence or absence of disease and the level of attachment on the tooth that distinguish a pocket from a sulcus, and not only the depth as measured with a probe. A pocket has an *inner wall, the tooth surface*, and an *outer wall, the sulcular epithelium* of the free gingiva. The two walls meet at the base of the pocket. The base of the pocket is the coronal margin of the attached periodontal tissues.

Histologically, the base of a healthy sulcus is the coronal border of the junctional epithelium, whereas the base of a pocket (diseased sulcus) may be at the coronal border of the connective tissue attachment. Research has shown that during probing of a healthy sulcus the end of the probe is near the level of the junctional epithelium. When periodontal disease is present, the position of the probe tip will vary depending on the degree of inflammation and adjacent connective tissue destruction.[2]

I. Types of Pockets

Pockets are divided into *gingival* and *periodontal* types to clarify the degree of anatomic involvement. They are then further categorized by their position in relation to the alveolar bone; that is, whether their pocket base is suprabony or intrabony (figure 12–1).

A. Gingival Pocket

1. Definition: a pocket formed by gingival enlargement without apical migration of the junctional epithelium (figure 12–1B).
2. Other names: pseudopocket, false pocket, relative pocket.
3. The margin of the gingiva has moved toward the incisal or occlusal without the deeper periodontal structures becoming involved.
4. The tooth wall is enamel.
5. During eruption, the base of the pocket is at various levels along the enamel. The base of the pocket of a fully erupted tooth is near the cementoenamel junction (figure 11–4, page 189).

6. All gingival pockets are suprabony; that is, the base of the pocket is coronal to the crest of the alveolar bone.

B. Periodontal Pocket

1. Definition: a pocket formed as a result of disease or degeneration which causes the junctional epithelium to migrate apically along the cementum.
2. Other names: true pocket, absolute pocket.
3. The periodontal deeper structures (attachment apparatus) are involved, that is, the cementum, periodontal ligament, and bone.
4. The tooth wall is cementum or partly cementum and partly enamel.
5. The base of the pocket is on cementum at the level of attached periodontal tissue.
6. Periodontal pockets may be suprabony or intrabony.
   a. Suprabony: pocket in which the base of the pocket is coronal to the crest of the alveolar bone (figure 12–1C).
   b. Intrabony: pocket in which the base of the pocket is below or apical to the crest of the alveolar bone (figure 12–1D).

II. Pocket Formation

A. Steps in the Development of a Gingival Pocket

1. Microorganisms of plaque produce harmful substances: enzymes and toxins.
   a. Plaque collects at and below the gingival margin.
   b. Bacterial products (enzymes and toxins) cause breakdown of epithelial intercellular substances, which leads to ulceration of the sulcular epithelium.
   c. Widening of intercellular spaces permits injurious agents to penetrate into the connective tissue beneath the epithelium.
2. Inflammatory reaction in the connective tissue
   a. Dilation and increased permeability of capillaries with increased blood flow results in redness of tissue and bleeding when probed.

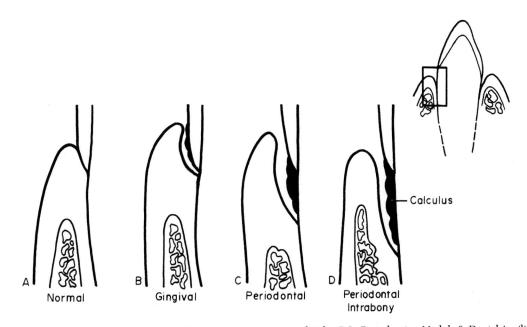

A — Normal B — Gingival C — Periodontal D — Periodontal Intrabony — Calculus

Figure 12–1. Diagram of types of pockets. (Adapted from Stone, S. and Kalis, P.J.: Periodontics. Module 6, Dental Auxiliary Practice; M. J. Dunn, Series Editor. Baltimore, The Williams & Wilkins Co., 1975.)

b. Increased numbers of inflammatory cells collect for defense: primarily lymphocytes, plasma cells, polymorphonuclear leukocytes, and macrophages. An exudate may be produced in an acute stage.

c. Edema from the leakage of fluid into the tissues results in an increase in size and alteration in shape of the gingival tissue.

3. Gingival pocket formation
   a. Junctional epithelium does not move at the base of the pocket.
   b. Increased depth is due to the enlarged gingiva.

4. Reversible: when plaque is controlled and calculus that is harboring plaque is removed, the number of microorganisms is reduced and the irritant is removed. The inflammation then subsides and the enlargement can decrease.

5. Continued exposure to plaque organisms means continued inflammatory reaction and increased pocket depth.

6. Chronic gingivitis develops.
   a. Destruction (inflammation) and healing (new collagen fibers and blood vessels produced) go on simultaneously.

b. Fibrosis may result which leads to the formation of firm hard gingiva.

B. **Steps in the Development of a Periodontal Pocket**

1. Extension of inflammation from the gingival pocket into the deeper structures.
   a. Plaque microorganisms collect in large numbers because plaque control procedures were ineffective in the depth of the gingival pocket.
   b. Plaque microorganisms continue to produce irritants: inflammation increases in severity and spreads.
   c. Inflammation spreads through the loose connective tissue along (beside) the blood vessels to the bone.[3]
   d. Most commonly, the inflammation enters the bone through small vessel channels in the alveolar crest.
   e. Inflammation spreads through the bone marrow and out into the periodontal ligament.

2. Progressive destruction of connective tissue fibers under the base of the sulcus at the apical border of the junctional epithelium.
   a. Undermining destruction: epithelium migrates along the root surface.

b. Coronal portion of the junctional epithelium becomes detached.

c. Since the epithelial cells must be living for migration, the junctional epithelium usually remains partially intact and does not have the severe ulcerations or other destructive changes that occur in the sulcular epithelium.

3. Exposed cementum where the fibers were attached becomes altered.[4] There are changes chemically and physically and in permeability. Bacterial and inflammatory products from the periodontal pocket become incorporated. The diseased cementum contains endotoxin.

4. Pocket becomes progressively deepened as the migration of epithelium continues toward the apex of the tooth.

a. Pocket retains plaque microorganisms and is not cleanable by the patient.

b. Plaque retention leads to calculus formation.

C. Systemic Influence on Pocket Formation

1. Pocket formation is not caused by or initiated by a systemic condition or disease.

2. Systemic condition can influence the *severity* and *rate* of development and the response to healing.

a. An altered, exaggerated response to plaque bacterial irritants can occur.

b. Alteration of healing capacity and lowered resistance to infection can influence outcome of treatment.

TOOTH SURFACE POCKET WALL

I. Tooth Structure Involved

A sulcus or a pocket has a gingival side, which is the sulcular epithelium, and a tooth side. In gingival pockets the tooth surface wall is enamel, while in periodontal pockets the tooth surface wall is either cementum, or a combination of cementum and enamel.

The positions of the junctional epithelium and gingival margin determine whether the tooth surface wall will be cementum or enamel. Pockets may be the same depth when measured with a probe, but because of the location of the junctional epithelium on the tooth surface, the tooth surface pocket wall varies.

II. Contents of a Pocket

A. Pocket Size

A pocket is narrow and the sulcular epithelial lining is adjacent to and follows closely the contour of the tooth. When there are calculus deposits, the pocket wall follows the contour of the calculus. The firmness of the free gingiva is influential in confining and shaping the subgingival calculus deposit.

Access of the opening of the pocket to the oral cavity provides an opportunity for bacterial plaque to collect. The deeper the pocket, the less it can be cleaned by toothbrushing or other plaque control devices.

B. Substances Found

The following may be inside a pocket in contact with the tooth surface on one side and on the surface of the sulcular epithelium on the other.

1. Microorganisms and their products: enzymes, endotoxins, and other metabolic products

2. Calculus deposits and other rough areas covered with dental plaque

3. Gingival sulcus fluid

4. Food remnants

5. Salivary mucin

6. Desquamated epithelial cells

7. Leukocytes

8. Purulent exudate made up of living and broken down leukocytes, living and dead microorganisms, and serum.

III. Nature of the Tooth Surface

Knowledge of the characteristics and quality of the tooth surface pocket wall is of prime importance in instrumentation. During the examination of the tooth surface with probe and explorer, differentiation needs to be made of the various irregularities that can occur. How the irregularities came into existence is important for interpretation and understanding.

A. Pocket Development Factors

1. The pocket deepens as a result of continuing action of the irritants and destructive agents from dental plaque.

2. The periodontal ligament fibers become detached and the junctional epithelium migrates apically.
3. The cementum becomes exposed to the open pocket and the oral fluids.
4. Cementum is altered and there are effects of physical, structural, and chemical changes.
5. Surface changes occur as a result of exchange of minerals with oral fluids and exposure to plaque bacteria and their products. On different surfaces of the same teeth or different teeth in the same mouth, any of the following can occur[5]:
   a. Hypermineralization of the surface cementum which increases with time
   b. Decalcification
   c. Calculus formation
   d. Plaque and debris collection

B. Tooth Surface Irregularities

Surface irregularities are detected supragingivally by drying the surface with air and observing under adequate direct or indirect light, followed by the use of an explorer as needed. Subgingivally, examination is dependent, for the most part, on tactile and auditory sensitivity transmitted by a probe and an explorer. Causes of surface roughness include the following:
1. *Enamel Surface*
   a. Structural defects: cracks, grooves
   b. Dental caries, decalcification
   c. Calculus deposits and heavy stain deposits
   d. Erosion, abrasion
   e. Pits and irregularities from hypoplasia
2. *Cementoenamel Junction.* Cementum overlaps enamel in 60 to 65 percent of teeth; cementum and enamel meet directly in 30 percent; or there may be a small zone of dentin between, in 5 to 10 percent.[6] The relationships of enamel and cementum at the cementoenamel junction are shown in figure 12–2.

   Despite the differences, the junction is usually smooth or with a slight groove, except when cementum is worn away by abrasion. Abrasion may undermine the enamel.
3. *Cemental Surface*
   a. Diseased altered cementum
   b. Cemental resorption
   c. Calculus
   d. Cemental caries
   e. Abrasion
   f. Deficient or overhanging filling
   g. Grooves from previous incomplete instrumentation
4. *The Cementum.* The cementum varies in thickness.[7,8] It is thickest around the apical third of the tooth where it may be 200 to 600 μ (0.2 to 0.6 mm.). It is thinnest at the cervical third next to the cementoenamel junction where it may be only 20 to 50 μ (0.02 to 0.05 mm.).

An objective of root planing is to remove the thin layer of diseased altered cementum, because the toxic materials in the altered cementum may prevent the adjacent gingival soft tissue from returning to health. The instrumentation for root planing is described in Chapter 33.

COMPLICATIONS OF POCKET FORMATION

I. Furcation Involvement

Furcation involvement means that the pocket

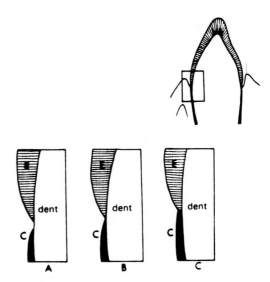

Figure 12–2. Possible relationships at the cementoenamel junction. **A.** Cementum (C) and enamel (E) do not contact and a small zone of dentin (dent) is exposed in 5 to 10 percent; **B.** cementum meets the enamel in approximately 30 percent; and **C.** cementum overlaps enamel in 60 to 65 percent. (From Stone, S. and Kalis, P.J.: Periodontics. Module 6, Dental Auxiliary Practice; M. J. Dunn, Series Editor. Baltimore, The Williams & Wilkins Co., 1975.)

and bone loss have extended into the furcation area, or furca, the area between the roots of a multirooted tooth.

A. Significance of Furcation Involvement

1. Furcation involvement, however incipient it may appear to be in a radiograph or by probing, indicates progressive periodontal disease.
2. Causes and steps in pocket formation in a furcation are the same as for other pockets (pages 202–203).

B. Clinical Observations

1. When the gingiva over the furcation has not receded, the following may be seen:
   a. The furcation is covered by the gingival tissue pocket wall.
   b. No differences in color, size, or other tissue changes may exist to differentiate the area from adjacent gingiva; but when color changes do exist, they provide clues to supplement probe examination.
2. When the gingiva over a molar buccal furcation is receded, the root division may be seen directly.

C. Detection

A suggested procedure for probing furcations is described on page 217. Radiographic examination of furcation areas may be studied on page 228.

II. Mucogingival Involvement

When a pocket extends to or beyond the mucogingival junction and into the alveolar mucosa, it is described as *mucogingival involvement*. There is no attached gingiva in the area, and a probe can be passed through the pocket and beyond the mucogingival junction into the alveolar mucosa (figure 13–8, page 218).

A. Significance of Attached Gingiva

1. *Functions of the Attached Gingiva*
   a. Give support to the marginal gingiva.
   b. Withstand the frictional stresses of mastication and toothbrushing.
   c. Provide attachment or a solid base for the movable alveolar mucosa for the action of the cheeks, lips, and tongue.

2. *Barrier to Passage of Inflammation* Without attachment, the inflammation from the pocket area can extend to the alveolar mucosa. The junctional epithelium (epithelial attachment) acts as a barrier to keep infection outside the body.

   With destruction of the connective tissue and periodontal ligament fibers under the junctional epithelium, the epithelium migrates along the root. A pocket is created.

   In mucogingival involvement the bottom of the pocket extends into the alveolar mucosa. There, the unconfined inflammation can spread more rapidly in the loose tissue.

B. Clinical Observations

Color changes, tension test, and probe measurements are used during assessment. These are described on pages 217–218.

1. *Width of Attached Gingiva.* A narrow zone of gingiva from gingival margin to mucogingival line, caused by recession or occurring naturally without recession, is more susceptible to developing mucogingival involvement because there is less attached gingiva at the start.
2. *Base of Pocket at Mucogingival Line.* When the probe measures only 1 to mm. and there is no bleeding on probing but the tip of the probe is at the mucogingival line, the area should be charted and called to the dentist's attention since surgery may be indicated. Such an area needs specific instruction in plaque control procedures for preventive maintenance.

   When an area of minimal attached gingiva (1 to 2 mm.) will be placed under stress by restorative, prosthetic, or orthodontic treatment procedures, an assessment should be made of the need for periodontal treatment to increase the zone of attached gingiva.

CLINICAL EXAMINATION

I. Identification of Pockets

A. Method

The use of a calibrated probe is the only

accurate, dependable way by which pockets can be located, measured, and the topography evaluated. Detailed technique and charting procedures are described on pages 213–220.

3. Signs and Symptoms That Suggest the Presence of Pockets

Although precise information about pockets is determined by the use of a probe, notice of clinical changes in the tissues can be of invaluable assistance while probing. All of the indicators of disease that were described with the gingival examination (pages 192–198) can provide clues to the presence of pockets.

Extended color changes, loss of stippling, margins that retract and do not fit snugly about a tooth, bleeding, exudate, and changes in form and size are all indicators of disease and pocket formation. It is the evidence of disease that determines the severity of a pocket, not only the depth. A shallow pocket can be severely involved with inflammation and degeneration.

II. Examination of the Tooth Surface

Examination of the tooth surface pocket wall is made with a probe and an explorer. The techniques are described on pages 213–216 and 222–225.

The distribution and amount of calculus, plaque, and other soft deposits are recorded with the periodontal charting and records.

FACTORS TO TEACH THE PATIENT

I. What a pocket is and how it forms.
II. How a pocket is measured with a probe and that, until the sulci and pockets are probed, it is not possible to tell whether disease is present and how far it has progressed. Pockets and sulci must be checked regularly all around every tooth to be sure nothing is developing insidiously.

References

1. American Academy of Periodontology: *Current Procedural Terminology for Periodontics*, 4th ed. Chicago, American Academy of Periodontology, 1977, p. 11.
2. Listgarten, M.A., Mao, R., and Robinson, P.J.: Periodontal Probing and the Relationship of the Probe Tip to Periodontal Tissues, *J. Periodontol.*, 47, 511, September, 1976.
3. Weinmann, J.P.: Progress of Gingival Inflammation into the Supporting Structures of the Teeth, *J. Periodontol.*, 12, 71, July, 1941.
4. Armitage, G.C.: *Biologic Basis of Periodontal Maintenance Therapy.* Berkeley, California, Praxis Publishing Co., 1980, pp. 88–94.
5. Selvig, K.A.: Biological Changes at the Tooth-saliva Interface in Periodontal Disease, *J. Dent. Res.*, 48, 846, September-October, 1969.
6. Bhaskar, S.N., ed.: *Orban's Oral Histology and Embryology*, 9th ed. St. Louis, The C.V. Mosby Co., 1980, p. 193.
7. Furseth, R. and Johansen, E.: A Microradiographic Comparison of Sound and Carious Human Dental Cementum, *Arch. Oral Biol.*, 13, 1197, October, 1968.
8. Bhaskar: op. cit., p. 185.

Suggested Readings

Caffesse, R.G. and Nasjleti, C.E.: Enzymatic Penetration Through Intact Sulcular Epithelium, *J. Periodontol.*, 47, 391, July, 1976.
Daryabegi, P., Pameijer, C.H., Ruben, M.P., and Ricchetti, P.A.: Root Surface–Soft Tissue Interface, *J. Periodontol.*, 51, 77, February, 1980.
Goldman, H.M. and Cohen, D.W.: *Periodontal Therapy*, 6th ed. St. Louis, The C.V. Mosby Co., 1980, pp. 105–146, 177–221.
Hurt, W.C.: Periodontal Diagnosis—1977, A Status Report, *J. Periodontol.*, 48, 533, September, 1977.
Ramfjord, S.P. and Ash, M.M.: *Periodontology and Periodontics.* Philadelphia, W.B. Saunders Co., 1979, pp. 112–137.
Ranney, R.R.: Pathogenesis of Periodontal Disease, in *International Conference on Research in the Biology of Periodontal Disease.* Chicago, College of Dentistry, University of Illinois, 1977, pp. 222–304.
Sabag, N., Saglie, R., and Mery, C.: Ultrastructure of the Normal Human Epithelial Attachment to the Cementum Root Surface, *J. Periodontol.*, 52, 94, February, 1981.

Altered Cementum

Adelson, L.J., Hanks, C.T., Ramfjord, S.P., and Caffesse, R.G.: *In vitro* Cytotoxicity of Periodontally Diseased Root Surfaces, *J. Periodontol.*, 51, 700, December, 1980.
Aleo, J.J. and Vandersall, D.C.: Cementum. Recent Concepts Related to Periodontal Disease Therapy, *Dent. Clin. North Am.*, 24, 627, October, 1980.
Daly, C.G., Kieser, J.B., Corbet, E.F., and Seymour, G.J.: Cementum Involved in Periodontal Disease: A Review of Its Features and Clinical Management, *J. Dent.*, 7, 185, September, 1979.
Emslie, R.D.: Some Considerations on the Role of Cementum in Periodontal Disease, *J. Clin. Periodontol.*, 5, 1, February, 1978.
Garrett, J.S.: Cementum in Periodontal Disease, *Periodont. Abstr.*, 23, 6, Spring, 1975.
Robinson, P.J.: Possible Roles of Diseased Cementum in Periodontitis, *J. Prev. Dent.*, 2, 3, May-June, 1975.
Ruben, M.P. and Shapiro, A.: An Analysis of Root Surface Changes in Periodontal Disease—A Review, *J. Periodontol.*, 49, 89, February, 1978.
Stahl, S.S.: The Nature of Healthy and Diseased Root Surfaces, *J. Periodontol.*, 46, 156, March, 1975.
Wirthlin, M.R., Pederson, E.D., Hancock, E.B., Lamberts, B.L., and Leonard, E.P.: The Hypermineralization of Diseased Root Surfaces, *J. Periodontol.*, 50, 125, March, 1979.

Predisposing Factors

Armitage, G.C.: *Biologic Basis of Periodontal Maintenance Therapy*. Berkeley, California, Praxis Publishing Co., 1980, pp. 204–216.

Buckley, L.A.: The Relationships Between Irregular Teeth, Plaque, Calculus and Gingival Disease, A Study of 300 Subjects, *Br. Dent. J.*, *148*, 67, February 5, 1980.

Buckley, L.A.: The Relationships Between Malocclusion, Gingival Inflammation, Plaque and Calculus, *J. Periodontol.*, *52*, 35, January, 1981.

Goldstein, A.R.: Enamel Pearls as a Contributing Factor in Periodontal Breakdown, *J. Am. Dent. Assoc.*, *99*, 210, August, 1979.

Hakkarainen, K. and Ainamo, J.: Influence of Overhanging Posterior Tooth Restorations on Alveolar Bone Height in Adults, *J. Clin. Periodontol.*, *7*, 114, April, 1980.

Hancock, E.B., Mayo, C.V., Schwab, R.R., and Wirthlin, M.R.: Influence of Interdental Contacts on Periodontal Status, *J. Periodontol.*, *51*, 445, August, 1980.

Ingervall, B., Jacobsson, U., and Nyman, S.: A Clinical Study of the Relationship Between Crowding of Teeth, Plaque and Gingival Condition, *J. Clin. Periodontol.* 4, 214, August, 1977.

Kepic, T.J. and O'Leary, T.J.: Role of Marginal Ridge Relationships as an Etiologic Factor in Periodontal Disease, *J. Periodontol.*, *49*, 570, November, 1978.

Pennel, B.M. and Keagle, J.G.: Predisposing Factors in the Etiology of Chronic Inflammatory Periodontal Disease, *J. Periodontol.*, *48*, 517, September, 1977.

Shiloah, J. and Kopczyk, R.A.: Developmental Variations in Tooth Morphology and Periodontal Disease, *J. Am. Dent. Assoc.*, *99*, 627, October, 1979.

Vogan, W.I.: The Effect of Bucco-lingual Crown Contour on Gingival Health, A Reappraisal, *J. Prev. Dent.*, 30, July-August, 1976.

13

Examination Procedures

Parts of the gingival and dental examinations are made by direct *visual* observation, while other parts require *tactile* examination using a probe and an explorer. These two types of instruments, assisted by a mouth mirror, are key instruments in patient evaluation. Considerable skill is required for accurate and efficient probing and exploring.

General principles of instrumentation are described in Chapter 31, pages 477–484. Study that chapter for basic descriptions of instrument parts, grasp, finger rests, and stroke.

I. Precaution

There are several reasons why a probe or an explorer should not be applied to the teeth and gingiva until an initial review of information from the patient history and oral examination has been made. The immediate application of information from the history was outlined on page 99. Of particular significance is knowledge of a patient's susceptibility to bacteremia. Patients at risk must receive prophylactic antibiotic premedication before instrumentation (page 100).

II. Basic Set-up

All tray arrangements need a basic set-up composed of a mouth mirror, probe, explorer, and cotton pliers. Wrapping these together for sterilizing increases efficiency. The packet should be labeled "basic set-up." When a complete ex- amination tray is assembled, the basic set-up may be included with other essentials (page 32).

THE MOUTH MIRROR

I. Description

A. Parts

The mirror has three parts: the handle, shank, and working end which is the mounted mirror or mirror head. Instrument parts are described on pages 477–478.

B. Mirror Surfaces

1. Plane (flat): may produce a double image.
2. Concave: magnifying.
3. Front surface: the reflecting surface is on the front of the lens rather than the back as with plane or magnifying mirrors. The front surface eliminates "ghost" images.

C. Diameters

Diameters vary from $5/8$ to $1 1/4$ inches. In addition, special examination mirrors are available in $1 1/2$- to 2-inch diameters.

D. Attachments

Mirrors may be threaded plain stem or cone socket to be joined to a handle. Since mirrors tend to become scratched, replacement of the working end is possible without purchasing new handles.

E. Handles

1. Thicker handles contribute to a more comfortable grasp and greater control.
2. Wider mirror handles are especially useful for mobility determination (page 225).

F. Disposable Mirrors

1. Plastic in one piece or a handle with replaceable head for professional use; may have front surface.
2. Take-home mirrors for patient instruction. Patient may observe lingual and posterior aspects. One type of mirror has a light attachment.

II. Purposes and Uses

The mouth mirror is used to provide:

A. Indirect Vision

This is particularly needed for distal surfaces of posterior teeth and lingual surfaces of anterior teeth.

B. Indirect Illumination

Reflection of light from the dental overhead light to any area of the oral cavity is accomplished by adapting the mirror.

C. Transillumination

Reflection of light through the teeth.
1. Mirror is held to reflect light from the lingual, while the teeth are examined from the facial.
2. Mirror is held for indirect vision on the lingual while light from the overhead dental light passes through the teeth. Translucency of enamel can be seen clearly while dental caries or calculus deposits appear opaque.

D. Retraction

The mirror is used to protect or prevent interference by the cheeks, tongue, or lips.

III. Technique for Use

A. Grasp

Use modified pen grasp with finger rest on a tooth surface.

B. Retraction

1. Use petrolatum or other lubricant on dr or cracked lips and corners of mouth.
2. Adjust the mirror position so that th angles of the mouth are protected fron undue pressure of shank of the mirror.
3. Insert and remove mirror carefully t avoid hitting the teeth, since this can b very disturbing to the patient.

C. Maintain Clear Vision

1. Warm mirror with water, rub along buc cal mucosa to coat mirror with thin trans parent film of saliva, and request patien to breathe through the nose, to preven condensation of moisture on mirror; use a detergent or other means for keeping a clear surface.
2. Discard scratched mirrors.

IV. Care of Mirrors

A. Dismantle mirror and handle for sterilization.
B. Examine carefully after scrubbing with brush prior to sterilization to assure removal of debris around back, shank, and rim of reflecting surface.
C. Handle carefully during sterilization procedures to prevent other instruments from scratching the reflecting surface.
D. Consult manufacturer's specifications for sterilizing or disinfecting procedures which may cloud the mirror, particularly the front surface type.

INSTRUMENTS FOR APPLICATION OF AIR

I. Purposes and Uses

With appropriate, timely application of air to clear saliva and debris and/or dry the tooth surfaces, the following can be accomplished:

A. Improve and Facilitate Examination Procedures

1. Make a thorough, more accurate examination.
2. Dry supragingival calculus to facilitate exploring and scaling. Small deposits may be light in color and not visible until they are dried. Dried calculus appears

chalky and presents a contrast to tooth color.

3. Deflect free gingival margin for observation into the subgingival area. Subgingival calculus usually appears dark.
4. Make identification of areas of decalcification and carious lesions easier.
5. Recognize location and condition of restorations, particularly tooth-color restorations.

B. Improve Visibility of the Field of Operation during Instrumentation

1. Dry area for finger rest to provide stability during instrumentation.
2. Facilitate positive scaling techniques.
3. Minimize operating time.
4. Evaluate complete removal of calculus after instrumentation.

C. Prepare Teeth and/or Gingiva for Certain Procedures

1. Dry tooth surfaces for application of caries-preventive agents.
2. Make impression for study cast.
3. Apply topical anesthetic.

II. Compressed Air Syringe

A. Description

1. *Air Source:* air compressor with tubing attachment to syringe.
2. *Air Tip:* with angled working end which can be turned for maxillary or mandibular application. Tip is removable for sterilization.

B. Technique for Use

1. Use palm grasp about the handle of the syringe; place thumb on release lever or on button on handle.
2. Test the air flow so that the strength of flow can be controlled.
3. Make controlled, relatively short, gentle applications of air.
4. Supplement air drying with use of saliva ejector and folded gauze sponge placed in vestibule.

C. Precautions

1. Avoid sharp blasts of air on sensitive cervical areas of teeth or open carious lesions. Such areas may be dried by blotting with a gauze sponge or cotton roll to avoid causing discomfort.
2. Avoid applying air directly into a pocket. Subgingival plaque may be forced into the tissues and a bacteremia created.
3. Forceful application of air may direct saliva and debris out of the oral cavity, contaminate the working area and operator, and create aerosols (pages 16–17). Air directed toward the posterior region of the patient's mouth may cause coughing.
4. Avoid silicate cement or other restorations which may be harmed by excessive drying.
5. Avoid startling the patient: forewarn when air is to be applied.

D. Care of Compressed Air Syringe

1. Clean inside of air tip with pipe cleaner or brush prior to sterilization.
2. Sanitize syringe that cannot be removed for sterilization by vigorous wiping with a gauze sponge moistened with disinfecting solution (pages 38–39, 60).

PROBE

Early in patient examination, the patient's periodontal disease status must be determined. Treatment planning will vary depending on whether the condition is gingivitis or whether it is periodontitis with periodontal pockets, bone loss, and root surface involvement.

The probe is used to make the initial assessment and to follow that with a detailed evaluation to determine the extent and degree of severity for specific treatment planning. During treatment, the probe is applied to assess progress, and after treatment, to determine completion of professional services. At each maintenance recall appointment, a reevaluation with the probe is needed to assure continued self-care by the patient and to identify early disease changes which require additional professional treatment.

I. Purposes and Uses

A probe is used to

A. Assess the Periodontal Status for Preparation of a Treatment Plan

1. Classify the disease as gingivitis or per-

iodontitis by determining whether there is bone loss and the pockets are gingival or periodontal (figure 12–1, page 203).

2. Determine the extent of inflammation in conjunction with the overall gingival examination. Bleeding on probing is an early sign of inflammation in the gingiva.

B. Make a Sulcus and Pocket Survey

1. Examine the shape, topography, and dimensions of sulci and pockets.
2. Measure and record pocket depths.
3. Evaluate tooth-surface pocket wall.
   a. Chart calculus location and severity.
   b. Record other irregularities discerned by the probe.

C. Make a Mucogingival Examination

1. Determine relationship of the gingival margin, attachment level, and the mucogingival junction.
2. Measure the width of the attached gingiva (figure 13–9, page 219).

D. Make Other Gingival Determinations

1. Evaluate gingival bleeding on probing and prepare a gingival bleeding index (pages 309–311).
2. Measure the extent of gingival recession.
3. Determine the consistency of the gingival tissue.

E. Guide to Instrumentation

1. Define depth of sulcus or pocket for application of instruments for scaling, root planing, and curettage and depth for use of an explorer for evaluation of these procedures.
2. Detect anatomic configuration of roots, subgingival deposits, and root irregularities that complicate instrumentation. For this, the probe is used in conjunction with the explorer.

F. Evaluate Success and Completeness of Treatment

1. Evaluate tissue response to professional treatment postoperatively on an immediate, short-term basis as well as at periodic recall appointments.

2. Evaluate patient's self-treatment throug disease control procedures.
3. Signs of health revealed by probing
   a. No bleeding: healthy tissue does n bleed.
   b. Reduced pocket depth: comparise of pre- and postoperative pock depths.
   c. Tissue is firm as shown by applicatic of the probe to the surface of the fr gingiva.

II. Description

A. Parts

There are three parts: the handle, the ai gled shank, and the working end which the probe itself.

B. Probe Characteristics

1. Slender, rod-like working end may l straight or tapered; round, flat, or re tangular in cross section with a smoot rounded end.
2. Marked in millimeters at intervals spe cific for each kind of probe.

C. Examples of Probes

In table 13–1 several probe markings ai listed with examples and descriptions. Fig ure 13–1 shows a comparison of types c probe markings and sizes.

III. Selection

The probe chosen for use by a dentist or dental hygienist is frequently the instrument firs used when a particular technique was learned or one that provides comfort and ease of manip ulation. Another reason for selection is that con sistency in reading can be accomplished.

Analysis of a probe and comparison with othe probes is recommended. Important features t be considered in probe selection are

A. Adaptability

The probe should be adaptable aroun the complete circumference of each tooth both posterior and anterior, so that no mil limeter of pocket depth can be neglected ✇Flat probes require more attention to ad aptation and are useful primarily on facia and lingual surfaces.

Table 13–1.   Types of Probes

Probe Markings (in mm.)	Examples	Description
...arks at 3–6–8	University of Michigan O Premier O Marquis M-1	Round, fine, narrow diameter
...arks at 1, 2, 3–5–7, 8, 9, 10	Williams Goldman-Fox University of Michigan with Williams markings Glickman Merritt A and B	Round Flat (rectangular) Fine, round, narrow diameter Round, with longer shank Round, single bend in shank
...arks at 1, 2, 3–5, 6, 7, 8, 9, 10	Nabers 3N	Flat, double-ended with ends at right angles to each other
...arks at 3–6–9–12 3–6–8–11	Color-coded	Round
...o marks	Gilmore Nabers 1N and 2N	Tapered, sharper than other probes Curved, with curved shank for adaptation in a furcation area

... Markings

Markings should be easy to read so that pocket depth can be readily identified and measured, and no disease area will be overlooked.

PROCEDURES FOR USE OF PROBE

The information in Chapters 11 and 12 concerning the gingival examination, the normal tissues, and the development and types of pockets, should be studied in conjunction with this outline of probing techniques.

A *pocket is a diseased gingival sulcus.* The use of a probe is the only accurate, dependable method to locate, assess, and measure sulci and pockets.

Strategic use of light, retraction, a mouth mirror, and air for drying surfaces is necessary for efficiency and accuracy during the examination and measurement of sulci and pockets.

I. Pocket Characteristics: Guide to Probing

A. A pocket is measured from the base of the pocket (top of attached periodontal tissue) to the gingival margin. Figure 13–2 shows two pockets of different depths beneath gingival margins which are at the same level.

B. The pocket (or sulcus) is continuous around the entire tooth, and the entire pocket or sulcus must be measured. "Spot" probing is inadequate.

C. The depth varies around an individual tooth: it is unusual for a pocket to measure the same all around a tooth or even around one side of a tooth.
   1. The level of attached tissue assumes a varying position around the tooth.
   2. The gingival margin varies in its position on the tooth.

D. Proximal surface pockets
   1. Gingival and periodontal disease begin in the col area more frequently than other areas (page 189).
   2. Pocket may be deepest directly under the contact area because of crater formation in the alveolar bone (figure 13–3).

E. Anatomic features of the tooth-surface wall of the pocket influence the direction of probing. Examples are concave surfaces, anomalies, shape of cervical third, and position of furcations.

II. Preparation for Probe Insertion

A. Grasp probe with modified pen grasp (pages 478–479).

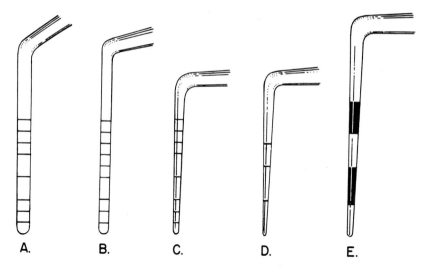

Figure 13–1.   Examples of probes. Names and calibrated markings for probes shown are **A.** Goldman-Fox (1-1-1-2-2-1-1-1, flat), **B.** Nabers (1-1-1-2-1-1-1-1-1, flat), **C.** Williams (1-1-1-2-2-1-1-1, round), **D.** Michigan O (3-3-2, round), **E.** Hu-Friedy or Marquis Color-coded (3-3-3-3 or 3-3-2-3 round). See Table 13–1 for additional data on probes.

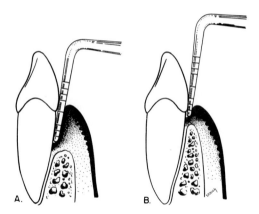

Figure 13–2.   Pocket depth. A pocket is measured from the top of the attached periodontal tissue to the gingival margin. Shown is the contrast of probe measurements of two pockets with gingival margins at the same level: **A.** Deep periodontal pocket (7 mm.) with apical migration of the attachment tissues. **B.** Shallow pocket (2 mm.) with attachment near the cementoenamel junction.

B. Establish finger rest on a neighboring tooth, preferably in the same dental arch.

C. Hold side of instrument tip flat against the tooth near the gingival margin with the probe approximately parallel with the long axis of the tooth for insertion. The cervical third of a primary tooth is more convex (figure 13–4).

D. Gently insert the tip under the gingival margin.

  1. Healthy or firm fibrotic tissue: insertion is more difficult because of the close adaptation of the tissue to the tooth surface;
underlying gingival fibers are strong and tight.

  2. Spongy, soft tissue: gingival margin is loose and flabby due to the destruction of underlying gingival fibers. Probe will insert readily and bleeding can be expected on gentle probing.

III. Advance Probe to Base of Pocket

A. Hold side of probe tip flat against the tooth surface. Widespread roots of primary molars may make this probe position difficult unless the tissue is unduly distended by the probe (figure 13–4).

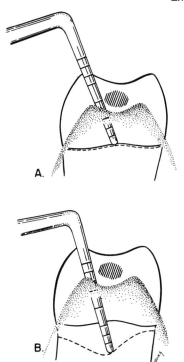

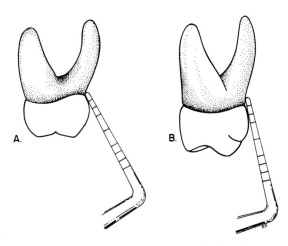

Figure 13–4. Probe placement on lingual of maxillary primary and permanent molars. **A.** Accentuated convexity of the cervical third and widespread roots of the primary tooth complicate probe placement. Probe may encounter the root. **B.** Permanent tooth with less convexity of the cervical third and roots that are less spread. Probe placement is easier than on primary tooth.

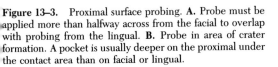

Figure 13–3. Proximal surface probing. **A.** Probe must be applied more than halfway across from the facial to overlap with probing from the lingual. **B.** Probe in area of crater formation. A pocket is usually deeper on the proximal under the contact area than on facial or lingual.

B. Slide the probe along the tooth surface vertically down to the base of the sulcus or pocket.
1. Maintain contact of the side of the tip of the probe with the tooth.
   a. Gingival pocket: side of probe is on enamel.
   b. Periodontal pocket: side of probe is on the cemental or dentinal surface when inserted to a level below the cementoenamel junction.
2. Interference: as the probe is passed down the side of the tooth, roughness may be felt. Evaluation of the topography and nature of the tooth surface is important to instrumentation.
3. Obstruction by hard bulky calculus deposit on tooth surface: lift the probe away from tooth and follow over the edge of the calculus until the probe can move vertically into the pocket again.
4. The bottom of the sulcus or pocket will feel soft and elastic (compared with tooth surface and calculus deposits which are

hard) and, with slight pressure, the tension of the attached periodontal tissue at the base of the pocket can be felt.
C. Position probe for reading.
1. Bring the probe to position as nearly parallel with the long axis of the tooth as possible for reading the depth.
2. Interference of the contact area does not permit placing the probe parallel for the measurement directly beneath the contact area. Hold the side of shank of the probe against the contact to minimize the angle.

IV. Read the Probe

A. Measurement is made from the gingival margin to the base of the pocket.
B. Count the millimeters that show on the probe above the gingival margin and subtract the number from the total number of millimeters marked on the particular probe being used. A comparison of pocket measurement using probes with different calibrations is shown in figure 13–5.
C. When the gingival margin appears at a level between probe marks, use the higher mark for the final reading.
D. Drying the area being probed improves visibility for specific reading.

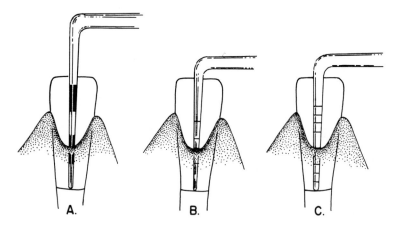

Figure 13–5.   Measurement of same 5 mm. pocket with three different probes. **A.** Color-coded, **B.** Michigan O. **C.** Williams.

V. Circumferential Probing

A. Probe Stroke

Maintain the probe in the sulcus or pocket of each tooth as the probe is moved in a walking stroke.

1. It is not correct to remove the probe and reinsert it to make individual readings.
2. Repeated withdrawal and reinsertion will cause unnecessary trauma to the gingival margin and hence increase postoperative discomfort.

B. Walking Stroke

1. Hold the side of the tip against the tooth at the base of the pocket.
2. Slide the probe up (coronally) about 1 to 2 mm. and back to the attachment in a

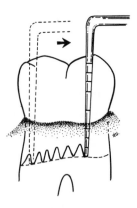

Figure 13–6.   Probe walking stroke. The side of the tip of the probe is held in contact with the tooth. From the base of the pocket the probe is moved up and down in 1 to 2 mm. strokes. The attached periodontal tissue is contacted on each down stroke to identify pocket depth in each area.

"touch . . . touch . . . touch . . ." rhythm (figure 13–6).

3. Observe probe measurement at the gingival margin at each touch.
4. Advance millimeter by millimeter along the facial and lingual surfaces into the proximal areas.

C. Horizontal Stroke

To test bleeding through the pocket epithelium, the probe is applied inside the pocket wall. The technique is shown for a gingival or bleeding index on pages 299 and 310 and figure 19–5, page 300.

VI. Probing Proximal Surfaces

A. Continue the walking stroke around each line angle and onto the proximal surfaces.
B. Roll the instrument handle between the fingers to keep the side of the probe tip adapted to the tooth surface at line angles and as the tooth contour varies.
C. Continue stroke under the contact area. Overlap strokes from facial with strokes from lingual to assure full coverage (figure 13–3). Make sure that the col area under each contact has been thoroughly examined.

VII. Evaluation of Tooth Surface

During the movement of the probe on the surface, irregularities can be felt and evaluated. Although the probe may not be as sensitive as a fine explorer, it can be of assistance especially during the preliminary examination.

FURCATIONS EXAMINATION

When a pocket extends into a furcation area, special adaptation of the probe must be made to determine the extent and topography of the furcation involvement.

I. Types of Furcations

Furcation involvement is usually classified by the amount of a furcation that has been exposed as a result of periodontal bone destruction. A description of the radiographic appearance may be found on page 228.

The three general classes are as follows:

Class I. Early, beginning involvement. The probe can enter the furcation area and the anatomy of the roots on either side can be felt by moving the probe from side to side. Figure 33–1C illustrates this on page 510.

Class II. Moderate involvement. Bone has been destroyed to an extent that permits the probe to enter the furcation area but not to pass through it.

Class III. Severe involvement. The probe can be passed between the roots through the entire furcation.

II. Anatomic Features

A. Bifurcation (teeth with two roots)

1. *Mandibular Molars.* The furcation area is accessible for probing from the facial and lingual (figure 13–7).
2. *Maxillary First Premolars.* The furcation area is accessible from the mesial and distal, under the contact area.
3. *Primary Mandibular Molars:* widespread roots.

B. Trifurcation (teeth with three roots)

1. *Maxillary Molars:* a palatal root and two buccal roots, the mesiobuccal and the distobuccal roots. Access for probing is from the mesial, buccal, and distal.
2. *Maxillary Primary Molars:* widespread roots (figure 13–4).

III. Examination Methods

A. Early Furcation

1. Probe to measure pocket depth.
2. Inspect the area by adapting the probe closely to the tooth surface and moving the end of the probe over the anatomic curvatures of the roots.
3. Check radiograph for early signs of furcation involvement.

B. Points of Access

Probe to measure pocket depths at points of access for each bifurcation or trifurcation area. Position of gingival margin will vary. Figure 13–7 shows apparent recession and 3-mm. pocket in bifurcation.

C. Probe Adaptation

Use probe in diagonal or horizontal position to examine between roots when there is gingival recession or a flexible, short, soft pocket wall which permits access.

D. Use of Curved Instrument

Use a curved instrument such as a curved probe (Nabers 1N or 2N) or a curet to examine advanced furcation.

E. Complications

Anatomic variations that complicate furcation examination: fused roots, anomalies such as extra roots, or low or high furcations.

MUCOGINGIVAL EXAMINATION

I. Tension Test[1]

A. Purposes

1. To detect adequacy of the width of the attached gingiva.

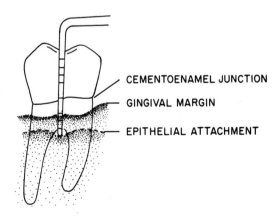

CEMENTOENAMEL JUNCTION

GINGIVAL MARGIN

EPITHELIAL ATTACHMENT

Figure 13–7. Furcation involvement. Probe inserted into bifurcation in area of gingival recession shows pocket of 3 mm. The probe is used to examine the topography of the furcation area.

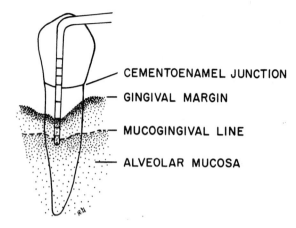

CEMENTOENAMEL JUNCTION

GINGIVAL MARGIN

MUCOGINGIVAL LINE

ALVEOLAR MUCOSA

Figure 13–8. Mucogingival involvement. Probe in position for measuring pocket depth where there is no attached gingiva. Absence of attached gingiva permits probe to pass through mucogingival line into alveolar mucosa.

2. To locate frenal attachments and their proximity to the free gingiva.
3. For prompt identification of the mucogingival junction.

B. Procedures

1. *Facial*
   a. Retract cheeks and lips laterally by grasping the lips with the thumbs and index fingers.
   b. Move the lips and cheeks up and down and across, creating tension at the mucogingival junction.
   c. Follow around from the molar areas on the right to molar areas on the left, both maxillary and mandibular.
2. *Lingual (Mandibular)*
   a. Hold a mouth mirror to tense the mucosa of the floor of the mouth, gently retracting the side of the tongue, so that the mucogingival junction is clearly visible.
   b. Request patient to move the tongue to the left, right, and lift up to touch the palate.

C. Observations

1. Blanching at the mucogingival junction.
2. Frenal attachments.
3. Area(s) of apparent recession where there is very little keratinized gingiva and the base of the sulcus or pocket is near the mucogingival junction.

4. Area where color, size, loss of stippling, smooth shininess or other characteristic indicates the need for careful probing to determine the amount of attached gingiva.
5. Area where tension pulls the free gingiva away from the tooth.

II. Gingival Tissue Examination

When inflammation is present and a pocket extends to or through the mucogingival junction, there may be a streak of color (red, bluish-red) which shows the inflammatory changes from the gingival margin to the mucogingival junction. When such an area does not pull away during a tension test or does not permit passage of a probe through the alveolar mucosa, the area should be noted in the record for future review.

III. Probing

When a pocket extends to or beyond the mucogingival junction, the probe may pass through the pocket directly into the alveolar mucosa (figure 13–8). Mucogingival involvement was described on page 206.

IV. Measure the Amount of Attached Gingiva

A. Place the probe on the external surface of the gingiva and measure from the mucogingival line to the gingival margin to determine the width of the total gingiva (figure 13–9A).
B. Insert the probe and measure pocket depth (figure 13–9B).
C. Subtract the pocket depth from the total gingival measurement to get the width of the attached gingiva.

PERIODONTAL CHARTING

Pocket charting is a part of the complete periodontal recordings. The summary of periodontal observations and records may be found on pages 320–321.

The procedure described here assumes the use of a chart form with outline drawings of teeth with both facial and lingual root drawings. The exact procedure and format is entirely the choice of an individual dentist. A composite chart to include dental as well as periodontal findings is frequently used.

In the preparation of the charting, colors used

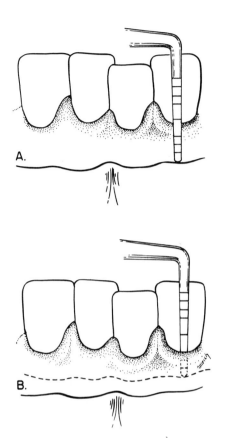

Figure 13–9. Measuring the width of the attached gingiva. **A.** Place the probe over the surface of the gingiva and measure from the mucogingival junction to the free gingival margin to determine the total width of the gingiva. **B.** Measure the pocket or sulcus depth. Dotted line represents the coronal border of the attached periodontal tissue at the bottom of the pocket. Subtract the pocket measurement (B) from the total width of the gingiva (A) to obtain the width of the attached gingiva. In the area illustrated there are two millimeters of attached gingiva.

should contrast with other colors on the chart. For example, when red is used to chart dental caries on a composite charting, red would not be a good color selection for drawing the gingival margin because of possible interference with a drawing of a Class V carious lesion. One procedure for a relatively simple charting system is described here.

I. Teeth Identification

Mark missing, unerupted, or impacted teeth. Prepare these markings in advance of the patient's appointment by reviewing and comparing the radiographs and the study casts.

II. Draw Gingival Lines

A. **Gingival Margin**

   1. Draw the outline of the position and contour of the gingival margin on the chart form as it appears in relation to the teeth both facial and lingual.
   2. Prepare in advance of the patient's appointment when study casts are available.

B. **Mucogingival Lines** (page 190)

   1. Use contrasting color to that used for drawing the gingival line.
   2. Draw on the facial for all quadrants; draw lingual only on mandibular.
   3. Study casts: when parts or all of the mucogingival lines show clearly on the casts, the drawing can be made in advance of the patient's appointment.

III. Record Pocket Measurements

A. Record all diseased pockets of any depth.
B. Record deepest millimeter measurement for each of the six areas around a tooth as shown in figure 13–10. Areas numbered 1, 3, 4, 6 extend from the line angle to under the contact area.
C. Supplement the six recordings with additional readings to show particular areas of unusually deep pockets, furcation involvement, or mucogingival involvement.
D. How to record on the charting form: figure 13–11 shows five possible methods for recording the millimeter depth.

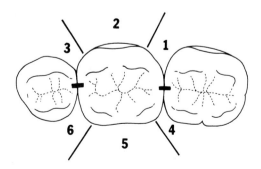

Figure 13–10. Charting pocket measurements. The pocket (sulcus) is measured completely around each tooth. Record the deepest measurement for each of the six areas around the tooth. Areas 1, 3, 4, 6 extend from the line angle to under the contact area.

IV. Record Special Disease Problems

Furcation involvement, mucogingival involvement, and frenal pull must be recorded either by a conspicuous symbol, or by writing directly on the chart or in the record. See previous section for methods of examination.

EXPLORERS

I. General Purposes and Uses

An explorer is used to
A. Detect, by tactile sense, the texture and character of the tooth surface.
B. Examine the supragingival tooth surfaces for calculus, decalcified and carious lesions, defects or irregularities in the surfaces and margins of restorations, and other irregularities that are not apparent to direct observation. An explorer is used to confirm direct observation.
C. Examine the subgingival tooth surfaces for calculus, decalcified and carious lesions, diseased altered cementum, and other cemental changes which can result from periodontal pocket formation.
D. Define the extent of instrumentation needed and guide techniques for
   1. Scaling and root planing.
   2. Finishing a restoration.
   3. Removal of an overhanging filling.
E. Evaluate the completeness of treatment as shown by the smooth, glassy tooth surface or the smooth restoration.

II. Description

The basic parts of an instrument are described on pages 477–478.

A. Working End
   1. Slender, wire-like, metal *tip* approximately 1 to 2 mm. in length, which is circular in cross section and tapers to a fine sharp *point*.
   2. Design
      a. Single: a single instrument may be universal and adaptable to any tooth surface, or it may be designed for specific groups of surfaces. In figure 13–12, Numbers 2 through 7, 17, 18, 20, and 23 are single instruments.
      b. Paired: paired instruments are mirror images of each other, curved to provide access to contralateral tooth surfaces. In figure 13–12, Numbers 9 and 10, 11 and 12, 13 and 14, and 21 and 22 are paired.
      c. Design of a balanced instrument: middle of working end (tip of an explorer) should be centered over the long axis of the handle (figure 13–13).

B. Shank
   1. *Straight, Curved, or Angulated.* Whether a shank is straight, curved or angulated depends on the use and adaptation for which the explorer was designed. In figure 13–12 compare the straight shanks of Numbers 2, 5, 6, 7,

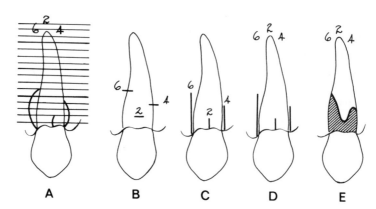

A   B   C   D   E

Figure 13–11. Methods for charting pocket measurements. **A.** Chart form with horizontal lines at millimeter intervals. Pocket measurements are written about the apex. Other chart forms do not have the millimeter markings, and may be used with **B.** horizontal lines, **C.** and **D.** vertical lines, or **E.** a continuous line to define the entire pocket area which can be shaded.

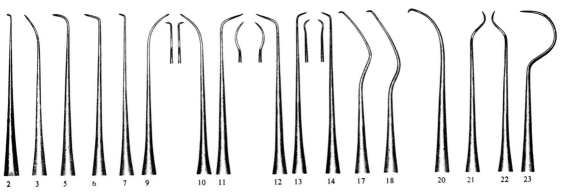

Figure 13–12. Explorers. This series from Numbers 2 through 23 shows standard shapes of explorer tips. Numbers 2 through 7, 17, 18, 20, and 23 are single instruments. Numbers 9 and 10, 11 and 12, 13 and 14, and 21 and 22 are paired instruments. (Courtesy of the S. S. White Company, Philadelphia, Pennsylvania.)

13, 14 with the others in the series which are not straight. A curved shank may facilitate application of the instrument to proximal surfaces, particularly of posterior teeth.

2. *Flexibility.* The slender, wire-like explorers have a degree of flexibility that contributes to increased sensitivity.

C. Handle

1. *Weight.* For increased acute tactile sensitivity, a lightweight handle is more effective.
2. *Diameter.* A wider diameter with serrations for friction while grasping can prevent finger cramping from too tight a grasp. With a lighter grasp, tactile sensitivity can be increased.

D. Construction

1. *Single-ended.* A single-ended instrument has one working end on a separate handle.
2. *Double-ended.* A double-ended instrument has two working ends, one on each end of a common handle. Most paired instruments are available double-ended. Other double-ended instruments combine two single instruments; for example, two unpaired explorers or an explorer with a probe.

III. Preparation of Explorers

Sharpen and retaper a dull explorer tip (page 503). With the explorer tip sharp and tapered, the following can be expected:

A. Increased tactile sensitivity with less pressure required.
B. Prevention of unnecessary trauma to the gingival tissue, because with less pressure there can be greater control.
C. Decreased operating time with increased patient comfort.

IV. Specific Explorers and Their Uses

A variety of explorers are available as shown by the examples in figure 13–12. The function of each type is related to its adaptability to specific surfaces of teeth at particular angulations. Certain explorers can be used effectively for detection of dental caries in pits and fissures and others are designed to be adapted to examine proximal surfaces for calculus or dental caries. By other criteria, some can be used subgingivally, while others cannot be adapted subgingivally without inflicting damage to the sulcular epithelium, and therefore are limited to supragingival adaptation only.

A. Subgingival Explorer (figure 13–13)

1. *Names and Numbers:* Orban Number 20, TU-17, pocket explorer.
2. *Shape.* The pocket explorer has an angulated shank with a short tip at a right-angle bend (figure 13–13). The tip should be measured to make sure that it is less than 2 millimeters, as a longer tip cannot be adapted to narrow roots, where a pocket narrows near the base.
3. *Use*
   a. Subgingival root examination
   b. Features

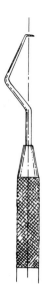

Figure 13–13. Balanced explorer design. With the middle of the tip centered over the long axis of the handle, the explorer can be positioned in a sulcus or pocket with ease and cause no trauma to the gingival tissue. Shown is the balanced Number 17 explorer (TU-17).

(1) Back of tip can be applied directly to the attached periodontal tissue at the base of the pocket without lacerating. When a straight or sickle explorer is directed toward the base of the pocket, the sharp tip can pass into the epithelium without resistance.

(2) The short tip can be adapted to rounded tooth surfaces and line angles. Long tips of other explorers have tangential relationship with the tooth, and cause distention and trauma to sulcular epithelium.

(3) Narrow short tip can be adapted at the base where the pocket narrows without undue displacement of the pocket soft tissue wall.

   c. Supragingival use of Number TU-17. It may be adapted to all surfaces and is especially useful for proximal surface examination. It is not readily adaptable to pits and fissures.

B. Sickle or Shepherd's Hook (Number 23 in figure 13–12)

   1. *Use:* examining pits and fissures and su-

pragingival smooth surfaces; examining surfaces and margins of restorations.

   2. *Adaptability*

      a. Difficult to apply to proximal surfaces, as the wide hook can contact an adjacent tooth and the straight long section of the tip can pass over a small proximal carious lesion.

      b. Not adaptable for deep subgingival exploration. When the point is directed to base of a pocket, there is danger of trauma to the attachment area. In the attempt to prevent such damage, the operator may not explore to the base of the pocket, thus providing incomplete service.

C. Pigtail or Cowhorn (Numbers 21 and 22 in figure 13–12)

   1. *Use:* proximal surfaces for calculus, dental caries, or margins of restorations.

   2. *Adaptability:* as paired, curved tips, they are applied to opposite tooth surfaces.

D. Straight (Numbers 2, 6, 7 in figure 13–12)

   1. *Use:* supragingival, for pits and fissures, tooth irregularities of smooth surfaces, and surfaces and margins of restorations.

   2. *Adaptability*

      a. For pit and fissure caries: the explorer tip is held parallel with the long axis of the tooth and applied straight into a pit.

      b. Not adaptable deep in subgingival area: straight shanked instruments or those with long tips cannot be adapted readily in the apical portion of the pocket near the attached tissue or on line angles.

BASIC TECHNIQUES FOR USE OF EXPLORERS

Development of ability to use an explorer and a probe is achieved first by learning the anatomic surface features of each tooth surface and the types of irregularities that may be encountered on the surfaces. The second step is repeated practice of careful and deliberate techniques for application of the instruments.

The objective is to adapt the instruments in a routine manner which will relay consistent

mparative information about the nature of the
oth surface. Concentration, patience, atten-
ɔn to detail, and alertness to each irregularity,
ɔwever small it may seem, are necessary.

Use of Sensory Stimuli

Both explorers and probes can transmit tactile
imuli from tooth surfaces to the fingers. A fine
xplorer usually gives a more acute reaction to
nall irregularities than a thicker explorer.
robes vary in diameter; the narrower types may
rovide greater sensitivity.

. Tooth Surface Irregularities

Three basic tactile sensations must be distinguished when probing or exploring. These
may be grouped as normal tooth surface,
irregularities created by excesses or elevations in the surface, and irregularities caused
by depressions in the tooth surface. Examples of these are listed here.

1. *Normal*
   a. Tooth structure: the smooth surface
      of enamel and root surface that has
      been planed; anatomic configura-
      tions such as cingula, furcations.
   b. Restored surfaces: smooth surfaces of
      metal (gold, amalgam) and the softer
      feeling of plastic; smooth margin of a
      restoration.
2. *Irregularities: Increases or Elevations in
   Tooth Surface*
   a. Deposits: calculus, and stain that is
      thick.
   b. Anomalies: enamel pearl; unusually
      pronounced cementoenamel junc-
      tion.
   c. Restorations: overcontoured, irreg-
      ular margins (overhang).
3. *Irregularities: Depressions, Grooves*
   a. Tooth surface: decalcified or carious
      lesion, abrasion, erosion, pits such as
      those caused by enamel hypoplasia,
      areas of cemental resorption on the
      root surface.
   b. Restorations: deficient margin, rough
      surface (figure 41–2, page 585).

⌐. Types of Stimuli

During exploring and probing, distinction
of irregularities can be made through auditory and tactile means.

1. *Tactile.* Tactile sensations pass through
   the instrument to the fingers and hand
   and to the brain for registration and action. Tactile sensations, for example, may
   be the result of catching on an overcontoured restoration, dropping into a carious lesion, hooking the edge of a restoration or lesion, encountering an
   elevated deposit, or simply passing over
   a rough surface.
2. *Auditory.* As an explorer or probe moves
   over the surface of enamel, cementum,
   a metallic restoration, a plastic restoration, or any irregularity of tooth structure or restoration, a particular surface
   texture is apparent. With each contact,
   sound may be created. The clean smooth
   enamel is quiet, the rough cementum or
   calculus is scratchy or noisy. Sometimes
   a metallic restoration may "squeak" or
   have a metallic "ring." With experience,
   differentiations can be made.

II. Procedures: Supragingival

A. Use of Vision

Supragingival exploration for defects of the
tooth surface differs from subgingival in that,
when a surface is dried, much of the actual
exploration is to confirm visual observation.
The exceptions are the proximal areas near
and around contact areas that cannot be directly observed.

Unnecessary exploring should be avoided.
With adequate light and a source of air,
proper retraction, and use of mouth mirror,
dried supragingival calculus can generally
be seen, since it is apt to be either chalky
white or brownish yellow and in contrast to
tooth color. A minimum of exploration can
confirm the finding.

B. Facial and Lingual Surfaces

1. Adapt the side of tip with the point always on the tooth surface.
2. Move the instrument in short walking
   strokes over the surface being examined,
   or direct the tip gently into a suspected
   carious lesion.
3. Cervical sensitivity: avoid deliberate exploration of cervical third areas where

there is recession or where the patient has previously exhibited sensitivity. If necessary to dry a sensitive area, avoid an air blast, and blot with a gauze sponge or a cotton roll. Methods for desensitization are described on pages 556–558.

C. Proximal Surfaces

1. Lead with the tip onto the proximal surface, rolling the handle between the fingers to assure adaptation around the line angle.
2. Explore under the proximal contact area when there is recession of the papilla and the area is exposed. Overlap strokes from facial and lingual to assure full coverage.

III. Procedures: Subgingival

A. Essentials for Detection of Tooth Surface Irregularities

1. Definite but light grasp.
2. Consistent finger rest with light pressure.
3. Definite contact of the instrument with the tooth.
4. Light touch as the instrument is moved over the tooth surface.

B. Steps

1. With the tip in contact with the tooth supragingivally, hold the part of the shank that is next to the tip parallel with the long axis of the tooth, and gently slide the tip under the gingival margin into the sulcus or pocket.
2. Keep the point in contact with the tooth at all times to prevent lacerations of the sulcular epithelium. Adapt the tip closely to the tooth surface on the side of the point.
3. Slide the explorer tip over the tooth surface to the base of the pocket until, with the back of the tip, the resistance of the soft tissue of the attached periodontal tissue is felt (figure 13–14). Calculus deposits may obstruct direct passage of the instrument to the base of the pocket. Lift the tip slightly away from the tooth surface and follow over the deposit to proceed to the base of the pocket.

4. Stroke: use a "walking" stroke, vertic or diagonal (oblique).
   a. Lead with the tip: move it ahead the instrument progresses (figu 13–15).
   b. Length of stroke depends on t depth of a pocket; for example,
      (1) Shallow pocket: the stroke m extend the entire depth, from th base of the pocket to just b neath the gingival margin.
      (2) Deep pocket: controlled strok 2 to 3 mm. long can provide mo acute sensitivity to the surfac and allow improved adaptatio of the instrument. It is advisab to divide a deep pocket and fir

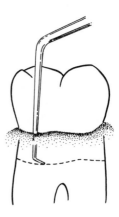

Figure 13–14. Use of subgingival explorer. The section the shank next to the working tip is held parallel with th long axis of the tooth. The sharp explorer tip is maintaine in contact with the tooth surface at all times. The explore is passed into the pocket and over the tooth surface unt the back of the working end meets resistance from the to of the attached periodontal tissue at the base of the pocke

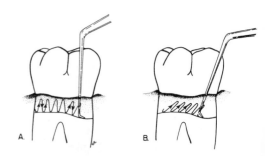

Figure 13–15. Explorer walking stroke. With the side o the tip of the explorer in contact with the tooth surface a all times, the explorer is moved over the surface in **A.** vertic walking stroke, or **B.** diagonal or oblique walking stroke Complete exploration of the tooth surface is needed; there fore groups of strokes are overlapped.

explore all of the apical section next to the base of the pocket, and then move up to explore another section, overlapping to assure full coverage.

  c. Do not remove the explorer from the pocket for each stroke on a particular surface because

    (1) Trauma to the gingival margin caused by repeated withdrawal and reinsertion can cause the patient postoperative discomfort.

    (2) Concentration on the texture of the tooth surface is interrupted.

    (3) More time is consumed.

  5. Proximal surface

    a. Lead with tip of instrument: do not "back into" an area.

    b. Continue the strokes around the line angle: roll the instrument handle between the fingers to keep the tip closely adapted as the tooth contour changes.

    c. Continue strokes under the contact area. Overlap stroke from facial and lingual to assure full coverage.

V. Record Findings

A. Supragingival Calculus

1. *Distribution.* Supragingival calculus is generally localized. It is most commonly confined to the lingual of the mandibular anterior teeth, and the buccal of the maxillary first and second molars, opposite the openings to the salivary ducts (page 275).
2. *Amount:* slight, moderate, heavy.

B. Subgingival Calculus

1. *Distribution:* Subgingival calculus can be either localized or generalized.
2. *Amount:* slight, moderate, heavy.

C. Other Irregularities of Tooth Surface

Note on the chart or in the record any other deviation from normal detected while using the explorer.

MOBILITY EXAMINATION

Because of the nature and function of the periodontal ligament, teeth have a slight normal mobility. Mobility can be considered abnormal or pathologic when it exceeds normal. Increased mobility can be an important clinical sign of disease.

I. Causes of Mobility

A. Inflammation

Inflammation in the periodontal ligament leads to degeneration or destruction of the fibers.

B. Loss of Support

Loss of sufficient support by alveolar bone and periodontal ligament (destroyed in periodontal disease) can increase the mobility.

C. Trauma from Occlusion

Injury to the periodontal tissues can result from occlusal forces (page 256).

II. Procedure for Determination of Mobility

A. Position the patient for clear visibility with maximum light and ready accessibility through convenient retraction.

B. Stabilize the head. Motion of the head, lips, or cheek can interfere with a true evaluation of tooth movement.

C. Use two single-ended metal instruments with wide blunt ends, held with a modified pen grasp. Using wooden tongue depressors or plastic mirror handles is not recommended because of their flexibility. Testing with the fingers without the metal instruments can be misleading since the soft tissue of the finger tips can move and give an illusion of tooth movement.

D. Apply specific, firm finger rests (fulcrums). A standardized finger rest pressure contributes increased consistency to the determinations. The teeth may be dried with air or sponge to prevent slipping of the instruments or the finger on the finger rest.

E. Apply the blunt ends of the instruments to opposite sides of a tooth, and rock the tooth to test horizontal mobility. Keep both instrument ends on the tooth as pressure is applied first from one side and then the other.

F. Test vertical mobility (depression of the tooth into its socket) by applying, on the occlusal or incisal surface, pressure with one of the mirror handles.

G. Test each primary abutment tooth of a fixed partial denture.

H. Move from tooth to tooth in a systematic order.

III. Record Degree of Movement

A. Scale

N, 1, 2, 3 or I, II, III are frequently used, sometimes with a + to indicate mobility between numbers.

B. Recording

Although subjective, interpretation may be considered as follows:[2]

N = Normal, physiologic

1 = slight mobility, greater than normal

2 = moderate mobility, greater than 1 mm. displacement

3 = severe mobility, may move in all directions, vertical as well as horizontal.

C. The Letter N Means *Normal* Mobility

All teeth that have a periodontal ligament have normal mobility. No tooth has zero mobility except in a condition such as ankylosis when there is no periodontal ligament.

D. Chart Form

A chart form should provide for a place to record mobility, and preferably more than one place so that comparative readings may be recorded at successive recall appointments.

FREMITUS

I. Definition

Fremitus means palpable vibration or movement. In dentistry it refers to the vibratory patterns of the teeth. When a tooth has fremitus it means there is excess contact and this may be related particularly to a premature contact. Usually, the tooth also demonstrates some degree of mobility because the excess contact forces the tooth to move. The test is used in conjunction with occlusal analysis and adjustment.

II. Procedure for Determination of Fremitus

A. Seat the patient upright.

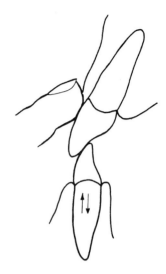

Figure 13–16. Fremitus determination. With the patie[nt] seated upright, an index finger is placed firmly over t[he] cervical third of each maxillary tooth in succession, starti[ng] with the most posterior tooth on one side and moving arou[nd] the arch. The patient is requested to click the posteri[or] teeth.

B. Press an index finger on each maxillary toot[h] at about the cervical third (figure 13–16).

C. Request the patient to "click the back teet[h] repeatedly.

D. Start with the most posterior maxillary toot[h] on one side and move the index finger toot[h] by tooth around the arch.

E. Record by tooth number the teeth wher[e] vibration is felt and those teeth where actu[al] movement is noted. The degree recorde[d] may be subjective, but the following rang[e] has been suggested[3]:

1. One-degree fremitus: when only sligh[t] movement can be felt.

2. Two-degree fremitus: when the tooth [is] clearly palpable but movement is barel[y] visible.

3. Three-degree fremitus: when move[-] ment is clearly observed visually.

RADIOGRAPHIC EXAMINATION

Radiographs provide essential information t[o] aid and supplement clinical findings. Durin[g] other phases of the examination, and especiall[y] during probing, the mounted radiographs shoul[d] be on a viewbox for viewing in conjunction wit[h] examination. When the radiographs have no[t] been processed at the time of probing, areas fo[r]

ecial confirmation can be marked on the re-
rd for review at the next appointment.

For observing evidence of periodontal in-
olvement, periapical radiographs are needed.
ite-wing radiographs do not show the complete
eriodontal tissues that extend around the roots.
hen there is moderate to severe bone loss, the
rest of the bone cannot be seen in a bite-wing
rvey.

Principles for use of radiographs were de-
ribed on pages 159 and 161. The need for
ounted radiographs free from errors of tech-
ique and viewed on an adequately lighted
ewbox cannot be overemphasized. A magni-
ing reading glass is of special assistance when
udying periodontal findings.

Radiographic Changes in Periodontal Diseases

Bone Level

1. *Normal Bone Level.* The crest of the interdental bone appears from 1.0 to 1.5
   mm. from the cementoenamel junction
   (figure 13–17).
2. *Bone Level in Periodontal Disease.* The
   height of the bone is lowered progressively as the inflammation is extended
   and bone is resorbed.

Shape of Remaining Bone

1. *Horizontal*
   a. When the crest of the bone is parallel
      with a line between the cementoen-
      amel junctions of two adjacent teeth,
      it is called "horizontal bone loss" (fig-
      ures 13–18 and 13–19).
   b. When inflammation is the sole de-
      structive factor, the bone loss usually
      appears horizontal.

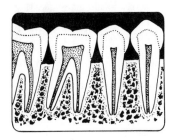

Figure 13–17. Drawing of a radiograph to show normal
one level, 1 to 1.5 mm. from the cementoenamel junction.

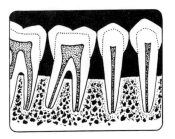

Figure 13–18. Horizontal bone loss. Bone level in periodontal disease is more than 1 to 1.5 mm. from the cementoenamel junction. When bone loss is horizontal the crest
of the alveolar bone is parallel with a line between the cementoenamel junctions of adjacent teeth. Note early furcation involvement in the second molar and moderate furcation involvement in the first molar.

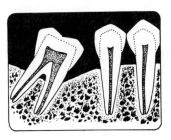

Figure 13–19. Horizontal bone loss. Second molar has
drifted mesially into the space created when the first molar
was removed. Note that the level of the crestal bone is
parallel with a line between the cementoenamel junctions
of the second premolar and the tipped second molar.

   c. Generalized: when the amount of re-
      maining bone is fairly evenly distrib-
      uted throughout the dentition, it is
      described as generalized horizontal
      bone loss. It may be designated either
      by millimeters from the position of
      the normal bone level or by per-
      centage. When making estimates,
      referral to the table of average root
      lengths can be helpful (Appendix, ta-
      bles A–3 and A–4).
   d. Localized: when bone loss is con-
      fined to specific areas.
2. *Angular or Vertical*
   a. Reduction in height of crestal bone
      that is irregular; the bone level is not
      parallel with a line joining the adja-
      cent cementoenamel junctions (fig-
      ure 13–20); and there is greater bone
      loss on the proximal surface of one
      tooth than on the adjacent tooth.
   b. Angular bone loss is more commonly
      localized than generalized.

c. When inflammation and trauma from occlusion are combined in causing the destruction and irregular shape of the bone, the bone appears with "angular defects" or with "vertical bone loss."

C. Crestal Lamina Dura

1. *Normal:* white, radiopaque; continuous with and connects the lamina dura about the roots of two adjacent teeth; covers the interdental bone.
2. *Evidence of Disease:* the crestal lamina dura is indistinct, irregular, radiolucent, fuzzy.

D. Furcation Involvement

1. *Normal:* bone fills the area between the roots (figure 13–17).
2. *Evidence of Disease:* radiolucent area in the furcation.
   a. Early: beginning furcation involvement may appear as a small radiolucent black dot or as a slight thickening of the periodontal ligament space. It can be confirmed by probing. Early furcation involvement is shown in the second molar in figure 13–18.
   b. Furcation involvement of maxillary molars may become advanced before radiographic evidence can be seen. Superimposition of the palatal root may mask a small area of involvement. When the proximal bone level in the radiograph appears at the level where the furcation is normally located, furcation involvement should

be suspected and probed for confirmation.
   c. Maxillary first premolar furcation furcation involvement cannot be seen in a radiograph except at an unusual angulation or unusual position of the tooth. With correct vertical and horizontal angulation the roots are superimposed.
   d. Furcations may show at one angulation but not at another; variation in technique can obscure a furcation involvement. All furcations must be carefully probed.

E. Periodontal Ligament Space

1. *Normal:* the periodontal ligament is connective tissue, hence appears radiolucent in a radiograph. It appears as a fine black radiolucent line next to the root surface. On its outer side is the lamina dura, the bone lining the tooth socket which appears radiopaque (figure 13–21).
2. *Evidence of Disease:* widening or thickening
   a. Angular thickening or triangulation the space is widened only near the coronal third, near the crest of the interdental bone.
   b. Complete periodontal ligament thickened along an entire side of a root to the apex, or around the root (figure 13–21). When viewed at different angulations (in the various radiographs of a complete survey), the ligament space may appear of varying thicknesses, which can show that the

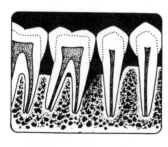

Figure 13–20. Angular or vertical bone loss, mesial of the first molar. The level of the crestal bone between the second premolar and the first molar is not parallel with a line between the cementoenamel junctions of the same teeth.

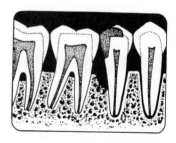

Figure 13–21. Periodontal ligament space. First and second molars have a normal periodontal ligament space which appears as a fine black line about the roots. The first premolar shows thickening of the ligament space about the entire root, and the second premolar has thickening about the mesial and periapical area.

disease involvement is not consistent around the entire root or that other structures are superimposed.

Early Periodontal Disease

The real preventive service a dental hygienist n perform is to recognize *early signs* of perdontal involvement so that treatment can be itiated to arrest the disease and prevent more vere involvement which could lead to tooth ss. To recognize severe bone loss, advanced rcation involvement, and marked thickening the periodontal ligament space is not difficult ter a basic understanding is gained. The difult part is to watch carefully for incipient, often olated indications of early periodontal disease. nese changes can be seen in all age groups, om young children to the elderly.

Earliest Signs

The early signs of periodontal involvement do not show in a radiograph. Only after the inflammation has extended from the soft tissue (gingivitis) to the supporting periodontal tissues and there is sufficient bone resorption will there be radiographic evidence.

Initial Bone Destruction

1. Pathway of inflammation: the usual interproximal pathway of inflammation from gingivitis to periodontitis is directly from the inflamed gingival connective tissue into the crest of the interdental bone (page 203).
2. Initial bone destruction takes place at the crest of the interdental bone in the crestal lamina dura.

Radiographic Evidence

1. Crestal lamina dura may appear slightly irregular, fuzzy, and radiolucent. At this stage it is best examined with a hand magnifying glass.
2. Angular thickening of the periodontal ligament space (triangulation) may also be apparent.

II. Other Radiographic Findings

Any other radiographic findings that may be lirectly or indirectly related to periodontal involvement and its contributing factors should be noted in the record for the attention of the dentist. Certain findings have a direct relation to dental hygiene care and instruction, particularly local factors that contribute to food impaction or plaque retention.

A. Calculus

Gross deposits, primarily those on proximal surfaces, may be seen in radiographs. Observing these may be helpful, but the probe and explorer are needed to define the exact location and extent.

The density and contrast of the radiograph influence whether or not calculus is seen. Since all deposits are not visible, the use of radiographs has limited value for specific calculus detection.

B. Overhanging Restorations

Some proximal overhanging margins may be seen in radiographs. The use of an explorer is necessary to detect irregular margins and to examine all proximal margins that do not reveal irregularities in the radiographs. Superimposition can mask an overhanging margin. Types of irregularities of restorations are described on page 585.

C. Dental Caries

Clinical and radiographic identification of carious lesions is described on pages 241–243. Certain findings should be noted for their relationship to the periodontal tissues.

1. Large carious lesions may leave open contact areas which permit food impaction and hence damage to the periodontal tissues.
2. Carious lesions, either enamel or cemental caries, hold plaque and provide a rough surface for retention of food debris and materia alba.
3. Cemental caries and decalcification may interfere with techniques of root planing (pages 205 and 510).

D. Relationship to Pockets

Radiographs do not show pockets; soft tissue does not show in a radiograph. Since a pocket is measured from the gingival margin to the base of the pocket, both of which are soft tissue, pockets cannot be seen in a radiograph. Probing is necessary to identify pockets.

TECHNICAL HINTS

I. Use topical anesthetic to help alleviate discomfort while probing.
II. The most common errors in probing are
   A. Not passing the probe to the full pocket depth.
   B. Not holding the probe as parallel with the long axis of a tooth as possible, and therefore obtaining a false reading.
   C. Not measuring around the entire tooth and therefore missing pockets. This most commonly applies to proximal pockets. The probe must be passed more than halfway across from the facial to overlap with the probe used on the lingual, which should also be passed more than halfway across.
III. Check the markings on a new probe by measuring on a standard millimeter ruler.
IV. When bleeding is readily elicited on probing or exploring and tooth surfaces are obscured so that examination is complicated, initiate toothbrushing and other appropriate disease control methods. Explain the problem to the patient and outline a specific home care routine designed to reduce gingival inflammation. Postpone the complete examination for one week when it would be expected that the gingival condition would be improved.
V. Replace mirror heads frequently. Scratched mirrors obscure vision and delay procedures.
VI. Handle explorers and probes carefully. Because the tips are pliable and relatively fragile, precautions must be taken against breakage, bending, or catching in a perforated tray of a sterilizing unit.

FACTORS TO TEACH THE PATIENT

I. The need for a careful, thorough examination if treatment is to be complete and effective.
II. Information about the instruments and techniques of examination and how their use makes the examination complete. Examples are the complete radiographic survey, probing 360 degrees around every

tooth, and exploring each subgingival tooth surface.
III. Why bleeding can occur when probing. Healthy tissue does not bleed.
IV. Relation of pocket measurements to normal sulci.
V. Significance of mobility.
VI. Signs of periodontal disease in radiographs.

References

1. Kopczyk, R.A. and Saxe, S.R.: Clinical Signs of Gingival Inadequacy: The Tension Test, *J. Dent. Child.*, 41, 35, September-October, 1974.
2. Miller, S.C.: *Textbook of Periodontia*, 3rd ed. Philadelphia, The Blakiston Co., 1950. p. 125.
3. Goldman, H.M. and Cohen, D.W.: *Periodontal Therapy*, 6th ed. St. Louis, The C.V. Mosby Co., 1980, p. 1092, 1107, 1110.

Suggested Readings

Chilton, N.W. and Miller, M.F.: Diagnostic Methods, *International Conference on Research in the Biology Periodontal Disease*, Chicago, University of Illinois, 1977, pp. 92–118.
Pattison, G.L. and Pattison, A.M.: *Periodontal Instrumentation*, Reston, Virginia, Reston Publishing Co., 1979, pp. 19–98, 104–136.
Ramfjord, S.P. and Ash, M.M.: *Periodontology and Periodontics*. Philadelphia, W.B. Saunders Co., 1979, 264–304.
Smith, M.P.: Periodontal Disease: Recognition and Examination, *Dent. Hyg.*, 54, 222, May, 1980.
Stone, J.S.: Abbreviated Periodontal Examination, *J. Am. Dent. Assoc.*, 92, 140, January, 1976.
Tibbetts, L.S. and Loughlin, D.M.: Expanded Periodontal Examination, in Clark, J.W., ed.: *Clinical Dentistry Volume 1*, Chapter 6, Addendum. Hagerstown, Maryland, Harper & Row, 1981, pp. 27–43.

Probing

Armitage, G.C, Svanberg, G.K., and Löe, H.: Microscopic Evaluation of Clinical Measurements of Connective Tissue Attachment Levels, *J. Clin. Periodontol.*, 4, 173, August, 1977.
Detsch, S.G.: A Periodontal Probe that Measures to One Tenth Millimeter, *J. Periodontol.*, 51, 298, May, 1980.
Garnick, J.J., Spray, J.R., Vernino, D.M., and Klawitter, J.J.: Demonstration of Probes in Human Periodontal Pockets, *J. Periodontol.*, 51, 563, October, 1980.
Hancock, E.B. and Wirthlin, M.R.: The Location of the Periodontal Probe Tip in Health and Disease, *J. Periodontol.*, 52, 124, March, 1981.
Hollister, L.P.: Periodontal Probing in the Clinical Detection of Periodontal Pockets, *Dent. Hyg.*, 53, 555, December, 1979.
Listgarten, M.A.: Periodontal Probing: What Does It Mean, *J. Clin. Periodontol.*, 7, 165, June, 1980.
Listgarten, M.A., Mao, R., and Robinson, P.J.: Periodontal Probing and the Relationship of the Probe Tip to Periodontal Tissues, *J. Periodontol.*, 47, 511, September, 1976.
Magnuson, I. and Listgarten, M.A.: Histological Evaluation of Probing Depth Following Periodontal Treatment, *J. Clin. Periodontol.*, 7, 26, February, 1980.

Parr, R.W.: *Examination and Diagnosis of Periodontal Disease.* DHEW Publication Number (HRA) 74–36, Washington, U.S. Government Printing Office, pp. 31–54, 70–76.

Polson, A.M., Caton, J.G., Yeaple, R.N., and Zander, H.A.: Histological Determination of Probe Tip Penetration into Gingival Sulcus of Humans Using an Electronic Pressure-sensitive Probe, *J. Clin. Periodontol.*, 7, 479, December, 1980.

Powell, B. and Garnick, J.J.: The use of Extracted Teeth to Evaluate Clinical Measurements of Periodontal Disease, *J. Periodontol.*, 49, 621, December, 1978.

Robinson, P.J. and Vitek, R.M.: The Relationship Between Gingival Inflammation and Resistance to Probe Penetration, *J. Periodont. Res.*, 14, 239, May, 1979.

Sivertson, J.F. and Burgett, F.G.: Probing of Pockets Related to the Attachment Level, *J. Periodontol.*, 47, 281, May, 1976.

Spray, J.R., Garnick, J.J., Doles, L.R., and Klawitter, J.J.: Microscopic Demonstration of the Position of Periodontal Probes, *J. Periodontol.*, 49, 148, March, 1978.

Tibbetts, L.S.: Use of Diagnostic Probes for Detection of Periodontal Disease, *J. Am. Dent. Assoc.*, 78, 549, March, 1969.

van der Velden, U.: Influence of Probing Force on the Reproducibility of Bleeding Tendency Measurements, *J. Clin. Periodontol.*, 7, 421, October, 1980.

van der Velden, U.: Influence of Periodontal Health on Probing Depth and Bleeding Tendency, *J. Clin. Periodontol.*, 7, 129, April, 1980.

van der Velden, U.: Probing Force and the Relationship of the Probe Tip to the Periodontal Tissues, *J. Clin. Periodontol.*, 6, 106, April, 1979.

van der Velden, U. and de Vries, J.H.: The Influence of Probing Force on the Reproducibility of Pocket Depth Measurements, *J. Clin. Periodontol.*, 7, 414, October, 1980.

van der Velden, U. and de Vries, J.H.: Introduction of a New Periodontal Probe: The Pressure Probe, *J. Clin. Periodontol.*, 5, 188, August, 1978.

Winter, A.A.: Measurement of the Millimeter Markings of Periodontal Probes, *J. Periodontol.*, 50, 483, September, 1979.

Mucogingival Examination

Boyd, R.L.: Mucogingival Considerations and Their Relationship to Orthodontics, *J. Periodontol.*, 49, 67, February, 1978.

Coatoam, G.W., Behrents, R.G., and Bissada, N.F.: The Width of Keratinized Gingiva During Orthodontic Treatment: Its Significance and Impact on Periodontal Status, *J. Periodontol.*, 52, 307, June, 1981.

Hall, W.B.: Present Status of Soft Tissue Grafting, *J. Periodontol.*, 48, 587, September, 1977.

Lang, N.P. and Löe, H.: The Relationship Between the Width of the Attached Gingiva and Gingival Health, *J. Periodontol.*, 43, 623, October, 1972.

Miyasato, M., Crigger, M., and Egelberg, J.: Gingival Condition in Areas of Minimal and Appreciable Width of Keratinized Gingiva, *J. Clin. Periodontol.*, 4, 200, August, 1977.

Stanford, T.W., Levin, M.P., and Payne, T.F.: A Comparison of the Mucogingival Junction in Dentulous and Edentulous Areas, *J. Periodontol.*, 47, 522, September, 1976.

Vincent, J.W., Machen, J.B., and Levin, M.P.: Assessment of Attached Gingiva Using the Tension Test and Clinical Measurements, *J. Periodontol.*, 47, 412, July, 1976.

Mobility

Carranza, F.A.: *Glickman's Clinical Periodontology*, 5th ed. Philadelphia, W.B. Saunders Co., 1979, pp. 294–302, 556–557.

Laster, L., Laudenbach, K.W., and Stoller, N.H.: An Evaluation of Clinical Tooth Mobility Measurements, *J. Periodontol.*, 46, 603, October, 1975.

Nyman, S. and Lindhe, J.: Persistent Tooth Hypermobility Following Completion of Periodontal Treatment, *J. Clin. Periodontol.*, 3, 81, May, 1976.

O'Leary, T.J.: Indices for Measurement of Tooth Mobility in Clinical Studies, *J. Periodont. Res.*, 9, Supplement 14, 94, 1974.

Persson, R.: Assessment of Tooth Mobility Using Small Loads. II. Effect of Oral Hygiene Procedures, *J. Clin. Periodontol.*, 7, 506, December, 1980.

Ryden, H., Bjelkhagen, H., and Sandström, U.: A Laser Instrument for Measuring Tooth Movements, *J. Periodontol.*, 50, 265, May, 1979.

Stoller, N.H. and Laudenbach, K.W.: Clinical Standardization of Horizontal Tooth Mobility, *J. Clin. Periodontol.*, 7, 242, June, 1980.

Vollmer, W.H. and Rateitschak, K.H.: Influence of Occlusal Adjustment by Grinding on Gingivitis and Mobility of Traumatized Teeth, *J. Clin. Periodontol.*, 2, 113, August, 1975.

Radiographs

Carranza, F.A.: *Glickman's Clinical Periodontology*, 5th ed. Philadelphia, W.B. Saunders Co., 1979, pp. 566–579.

Goldman, H.M. and Cohen, D.W.: *Periodontal Therapy*, 6th ed. St. Louis, The C.V. Mosby Co., 1980, pp. 350–359.

Lang, N.P. and Hill, R.W.: Radiographs in Periodontics, *J. Clin. Periodontol.*, 4, 16, February, 1977.

Wuehrmann, A.H. and Manson-Hing, L.R.: *Dental Radiology*, 5th ed. St. Louis, The C.V. Mosby Co., 1981, pp. 331–340.

14

The Teeth

Clinical examination of the teeth is essential prior to treatment to provide guidelines for treatment planning, instrumentation, instruction, and follow-up evaluation. In general, patients tend to be more concerned about their teeth than about their gingiva. The reasons may be related to personal appearance, degree of information, which is usually greater about teeth than gingiva, and the sensitivity and pain associated with ailments of the teeth.

Background study of histology, dental anatomy, and oral pathology is important to this phase of clinical practice. *Suggested Readings* at the end of this chapter have been selected for additional information, reference, and review.

I. Objectives

With information from the patient's personal dental history (table 6–3, page 97) and a thorough clinical and radiographic examination, the dental hygienist will be able to

A. Prepare a charting and provide a record of deviations from the normal teeth for the diagnostic work-up.
B. Identify the dental hygiene treatment and instruction needed in relation to the teeth for the particular patient.
C. Outline the patient's preventive dental program (page 333).
D. Utilize the specific data needed during treatment for instrument selection and adaptation.

II. Clinical Examination of the Teeth

Following is a list of major factors to observe when examining the teeth. A number of these are described in other chapters, for which page references are noted. Information about hypoplasia, attrition, erosion, abrasion, dental caries, and tooth vitality will be described in this chapter. Table 14–1 lists factors to observe during the examination of the teeth and suggests relationships to appointment procedures.

A. **General Characteristics**

1. Number of teeth; eruption pattern (Appendix, tables A–1 and A–2).
2. Anomalies of size, form, number.
3. Replacements: restorations for individual teeth and groups of teeth (fixed and removable).

B. **Deposits:** calculus, plaque, materia alba (table 16–1, page 262)

C. **Color**

1. Intrinsic stains (page 289)
2. Extrinsic stains (page 286)

D. **Developmental Defects**

1. Enamel hypoplasia
2. Amelogenesis Imperfecta; Dentinogenesis Imperfecta (page 290)

E. **Physical Injuries:** fractures

F. **Regressive changes**

1. Attrition
2. Erosion
3. Abrasion

Table 14—1. Examination of the Teeth

Feature	To Observe	Suggested Relationship to Appointment Procedures
Morphology	Number of teeth (missing teeth verified by radiographic examination) Size, shape Arch form Position of individual teeth	Selection and adaptation of instruments Areas prone to dental caries initiation, particularly the difficult-to-reach areas during plaque control
	Injuries; fractures of the crown (root fractures observed in radiographs)	Pulp test for vitality may be indicated
Development	Anomalies and developmental defects Pits and white spots	Distinguish hypoplasia and dental fluorosis from decalcification
Eruption	Sequence of eruption: normal, irregular Unerupted teeth observed in radiographs	Care in using floss in the col area where the epithelium is usually less mature in young children Procedures for preservation of primary teeth

Deposits
Food debris
Plaque
Calculus
  Supragingival
  Subgingival
	Overall evaluation of self-care and plaque control measures
	Relation of appearance of teeth to gingival health
	Extent and location of plaque, debris and calculus
	Calculus and the tooth surface pocket wall
		Need for instruction and guidance
		
		Frequency of follow-up and recall

Stains Extrinsic Intrinsic	Extrinsic: colors relate to causes Intrinsic: dark, grayish Tobacco stain	Need for test for pulp vitality Stain removal procedures; selection of polishing agent Dentifrice recommendation Plaque control emphasis for plaque-related stains Provide information concerning the oral effects of smoking
Regressive Changes	Attrition: primary and permanent Abrasion: physical agents which may be a cause Erosion	Evaluate causes and treat or counsel for prevention Dietary analysis: for finding foods that may be related Selection of non-abrasive dentifrice Habit evaluation

Table 14–1. *continued*

Feature	To Observe	Suggested Relationship to Appointment Procedures
Exposed Cementum	Relation to gingival recession, pocket formation	Special care areas where only slight attached gingiva remains Non-abrasive dentifrice advised Caries preventive measures to prevent cemental caries Care during instrumentation
	Hypersensitivity	Indication for application of desensitizing agent
Dental Caries	Areas of decalcification Carious lesions (proximal lesions observed in radiographs) Arrested caries	Charting Treatment plan Preventive program for caries control, fluoride, dietary factors Follow-up and frequency of recall
Restorations	Contour of restorations Proximal contact (see separate heading later in this table) Surface smoothness	Check for inadequate margins Chart and correct inadequate margins Selection of instruments and polishing agents
	Staining	Dentifrice selection to prevent discoloration
Factors Related to Occlusion Tooth Wear	Facets; worn-down cusp tips Health of supporting structures; observation of radiographs for signs of trauma from occlusion	Need for study of bruxism and other parafunctional habits
Proximal Contacts	Use of floss to find open contact areas Areas of food retention	Correction of inadequate contacts; chart Use of floss by patient
Mobility	Degree; comparison of chartings Possible causes	Need for reduction of inflammatory factors which may be related Dentist will identify and treat factors related to trauma from occlusion
Classification	Position of teeth Angle's classification	Relationship to orthodontic treatment needs
Habits	Nail or objects biting; lip or cheek biting Observe effects on lip, cheek, teeth Tongue thrust; reverse swallow	Guidance for habit correction when indicated
Edentulous Areas	Radiographic evaluation for impacted, unerupted teeth, retained root tips, other deviations from normal	Supplemental fulcrum selection during instrumentation Applied plaque control procedures for abutment teeth

Table 14–1. *continued*

Feature	*To Observe*	*Suggested Relationship to Appointment Procedures*
Replacement for Missing Teeth Dentures Partial dentures	Teeth and tissue which support an appliance Cleanliness of an appliance Factors which contribute to food and debris retention	Preventive measures for harm to supporting teeth and soft tissues Instruction in personal care of fixed and removable dentures; use of floss under fixed partial denture; other appropriate care
Saliva	Amount and consistency Dryness of mouth	Relation to instruction for prevention of dental caries: more caries can be expected in a dry mouth. Use of saliva substitute

G. **Occlusion** (pages 249–258)
  1. Proximal contact relation: areas of food impaction
  2. Mobility (page 225)

H. **Dental Caries and Decalcification**

I. **Vitality of Pulp**

ENAMEL HYPOPLASIA

I. Definition

Enamel hypoplasia is a defect that occurs as a result of a disturbance in the formation of the organic enamel matrix.

II. Types and Etiology

A. **Hereditary:** enamel is partly or wholly missing; an anomaly.

B. **Systemic** (environmental): factors that may contribute to enamel hypoplasia during tooth development include severe nutritional deficiency, particularly rickets; fever-producing diseases such as measles, chicken pox, and scarlet fever; congenital syphilis; hypoparathyroidism; birth injury; prematurity; Rh hemolytic disease; idiopathic.

C. **Local:** affecting a single tooth; caused by trauma or periapical inflammation about a primary tooth which can injure the adjacent developing permanent tooth.

III. Appearance

A. **Hereditary:** may appear brown (page 290).

B. **Systemic:** is also called "chronologic hypoplasia" because the lesions are found in areas of those teeth where the enamel was formed during the systemic disturbance.
  1. *Single Narrow Zone* (smooth or pitted): means the disturbance lasted a short period of time (figure 14–1).
  2. *Multiple:* disturbance to the ameloblast occurred over a period of time, or several times.
  3. *Teeth Most Frequently Affected:* first molars, incisors, canines, because the disturbances generally occur during the first year when those teeth are calcifying. A table of tooth development is available for reference in Appendix, tables A–1 and A–2.

C. **Hypoplasia of Congenital Syphilis**[1]

Transmission of syphilis from mother to fetus after the sixteenth week of pregnancy

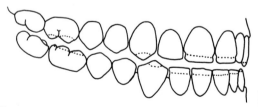

Figure 14–1. Enamel hypoplasia. Chronologic hypoplasia, usually in the form of grooves or pits, appears in the enamel at a level corresponding to the stage of development of the teeth. For this patient the disturbance in enamel development occurred at approximately 10 months of age.

may alter the development of the tooth germs. Figure 14–2 illustrates tooth forms that may result. There may be a reduction of mesiodistal width, and incisors are frequently narrowed at the incisal third.

Other conditions may also cause similar variations of tooth form. The cause of peg laterals is usually unknown.

D. Local: a single tooth with a yellow or brown intrinsic stain.

ATTRITION

I. Definition

Attrition is the wearing away of a tooth as a result of tooth-to-tooth contact.

II. Occurrence

A. Location: may be found on occlusal, incisal, and proximal surfaces.

B. Age Factor: increases with age, and more attrition is seen in men than women of comparable age.

III. Etiology

A. Bruxism

Predisposing factors may be psychologic, tension, or occlusal interferences.

B. Usage: wear of surfaces on each other. Predisposing factors may be coarse foods, chewing tobacco, or abrasive dusts associated with certain occupations.

IV. Appearance

A. Initial lesion: small polished facet on a cusp tip or ridge, or slight flattening of an incisal edge.

B. Advanced: gradual reduction in cusp height, flattening of occlusal plane (figure 14–3).

C. Staining of Exposed Dentin: may occur; usually brown.

D. Radiographic: the pulp chamber and canals may be narrowed and sometimes obliterated due to formation of secondary dentin.

EROSION

I. Definition

Erosion is the loss of tooth substance by a chemical process that does not involve known bacterial action.[2]

II. Occurrence

A. Location: facial surfaces of any teeth; most frequently, cervical third of anterior teeth.

B. Usually Involves Several Teeth

III. Etiology

The lesions are apparently due to some form of chemical dissolution.

A. May Be Idiopathic (unknown).

B. Intrinsic

Acid of chronic vomiting affects lingual surfaces, particularly anterior teeth.

C. Extrinsic

1. *Industrial:* workers' teeth can be exposed to atmospheric acids.
2. *Dietary:* labial surfaces most frequently affected
   a. Carbonated beverages or lemon juice used frequently.

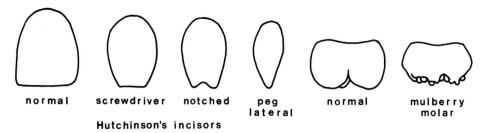

normal   screwdriver   notched   peg lateral   normal   mulberry molar

Hutchinson's incisors

Figure 14–2. Crown forms of enamel hypoplasia. Hutchinson's incisors and mulberry molars are typical crown forms which result from congenital syphilis.

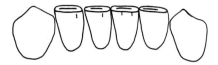

Figure 14–3. Attrition. Attrition of the incisal surfaces of mandibular anterior teeth which has extended to expose the dentin. Dentin usually appears as a brown line or ring.

    b. Lemons or other citrus fruit sucked frequently.

IV. Appearance

A. Smooth, shallow, hard, shiny (in contrast to dental caries, in which appearance is soft and discolored).

B. Shape: varies from shallow saucer-like depressions to deep wedge-shaped grooves; margins are not sharply demarcated.

C. May progress to involve the dentin and stimulate secondary dentin.

D. May occur in combination with dental caries, calculus, or dental restorations.[3]

ABRASION

I. Definition

Abrasion is the mechanical wearing away of tooth substance by forces other than mastication.

II. Occurrence

A. **Location:** exposed root surfaces, generally.

B. **Other Types:** at incisal edge.

III. Etiology

The lesion originates from a mechanical abrasive activity. The action of microorganisms is not essential for the development of abrasion. Dental caries may occur in the abraded area as a secondary lesion.

A. **Abrasive Agent**

    The most common cause is an abrasive dentifrice applied with vigorous horizontal toothbrushing (figure 14–4).

B. **Other Types**

    Abrasion may occur at the incisal or occlusal surfaces.

    1. Opening bobby pins may leave a small notch in one incisal edge. People with

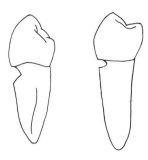

Figure 14–4. Abrasion. Profile view of facial surface of mandibular premolars to show shape of areas of abrasion on the cementum. Note that the area of abrasion undermines the enamel.

    this habit usually utilize the same tooth each time.

    2. Occupations: tacks held by carpenters, pins by dressmakers.

    3. Pipe held between teeth; usually held in the same place over many years.

IV. Appearance

A. Saucer-shaped or wedge-shaped with hard, smooth, shiny surface and clearly defined margins.

B. Except for incisal biting habits, the lesions occur initially on exposed cementum, then extend into the dentin.

DENTAL CARIES

Dental caries is a disease of the calcified structures of the teeth which is characterized by decalcification of the mineral components and dissolution of the organic matrix. As defined by the World Health Organization, dental caries is a "localized, post-eruptive, pathological process of external origin involving softening of the hard tooth tissue and proceeding to the formation of a cavity."[4]

I. Development of Dental Caries

Required for a carious lesion to develop are microorganisms, carbohydrate, primarily sucrose, and a susceptible tooth surface. Dental plaque contains numerous types of acid-forming bacteria, and *Streptococcus mutans* has been specifically implicated. The role of plaque and the factors in the initiation of caries are described in Chapter 16, pages 269–270.

A. **Enamel Caries**

    1. *Steps in the Formation of a Cavity*

a. Starts in pits or fissures or smooth surfaces that are not accessible for plaque removal.

b. Follows the general direction of the enamel rods.

c. Spreads at the dentinoenamel junction.

d. Continues along the dentinal tubules (figure 14–5).

2. *Types of Dental Caries:* described by location

a. *Pit and fissure.* Caries begins in a minute fault in the enamel.

(1) Occurs where three or more lobes of the developing tooth join; there is imperfect closure of the enamel plates. *Examples:* occlusal pits of molars and premolars.

(2) Occurs at the endings of grooves of the teeth. *Example:* the buccal groove of a mandibular molar.

b. *Smooth surface.* Caries begins in smooth surfaces where there is no pit, groove, or other fault. It occurs in areas where dental plaque collects, such as proximal tooth surfaces, cervical thirds of teeth, and other difficult-to-clean areas.

B. Cemental Caries (Root Caries)

1. *Steps in the Formation* of a cavity in the cementum

a. Rough root surfaces are conducive to the collection of plaque.

b. Microorganisms essential to root caries have been shown to differ from those responsible for enamel caries.[5]

c. Invasion of the cementum takes place either along Sharpey's fibers or between bundles of fibers.

d. Microorganisms tend to spread laterally between the concentric layers of cementum.[6]

2. *Incidence*

Cemental caries increases with age and with increased exposure of cementum. Therefore, the population who have had periodontitis show a higher incidence of cemental caries. A high percentage of teeth with root surface caries have not had previous enamel caries.[7]

3. *Location*

a. Above the attached periodontal tissue in the cementum.

b. May undermine the cervical enamel.

4. *Description*

a. Soft, shallow lesions, ill defined. They may have a broad or a narrow base.

b. Color: dark brown or deep yellowish brown.

II. Classification of Cavities

A. G.V. Black's Classification[8]

The standard method for classifying dental caries was developed by Dr. G. V. Black, a noted dental educator who divided the categories into five classes according to surfaces of the teeth; each class is represented by a Roman numeral. These categories are customarily used for carious lesions, cavity preparations, and finished restorations. See table 14–2 for definitions and illustrations.

B. Nomenclature by Surfaces

1. *Simple Cavity.* Involves one tooth surface. *Example:* occlusal cavity.

2. *Compound Cavity.* Involves two tooth surfaces. *Example:* mesio-occlusal cavity, referred to as an "M-O" cavity.

3. *Complex Cavity.* Involves more than two tooth surfaces. *Example:* mesio-occlusal-distal, referred to as an "M-O-D" cavity.

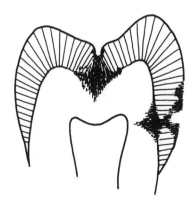

Figure 14–5. Cones of dental caries in a pit and fissure and on a smooth tooth surface. Dental caries follows the general direction of the enamel rods, spreads at the dentinoenamel junction, then continues along the dentinal tubules.

Table 14–2.   Dental Caries Charting: Classification of Cavities

Classification: Location	Appearance	Method of Examination
Class I. **Cavities in Pits or Fissures** a. Occlusal surfaces of premolars and molars. b. Facial and lingual surfaces of molars. c. Lingual surfaces of maxillary incisors		Direct or indirect visual Exploration Radiographs not useful
Class II. **Cavities in Proximal Surfaces of Premolars and Molars**		Early caries: by radiographs only Moderate caries not broken through from proximal to occlusal: (1) Visual by color changes in tooth and loss of translucency (2) Exploration from proximal. Extensive caries involving occlusal: direct visual
Class III. **Cavities in Proximal Surfaces of Incisors and Canines Which Do Not Involve the Incisal Angle**		Early caries: by radiographs or transillumination. Moderate caries not broken through to lingual or facial: (1) Visual by tooth color change (2) Exploration (3) Radiograph Extensive caries: direct visual.
Class IV. **Cavities in Proximal Surfaces of Incisors or Canines Which Involve the Incisal Angle**		Visual Transillumination
Class V. **Cavities in the Cervical 1/3 of Facial or Lingual Surfaces** (not Pit or Fissure)		Direct visual: dry surface for vision Exploration to distinguish decalcification: whether rough or hard and unbroken. Areas may be sensitive to touch

I. Other Descriptive Terminology

A. Primary Dental Caries

On a surface not previously affected; sometimes called initial or incipient dental caries.

B. Secondary Caries

On a surface that previously has been affected and has been restored.

C. Recurrent Caries (generally referred to as secondary)

On tooth surface adjacent to a restoration when the lesion may be a continuation of the previous carious lesion.

D. Rampant Caries

Widespread formation of chalky areas and incipient cavities in numerous teeth over a comparatively short time lapse. Most characteristically found in teen-aged patients.

E. Arrested Caries

Caries that becomes stationary and does not show a tendency to progress further is called arrested. It frequently takes on a dark brown or reddish brown color.[9]

F. Nursing Caries Syndrome

Nursing caries syndrome is a form of rampant caries found in very young children who routinely have been given a nursing bottle at times when they were going to sleep or have experienced prolonged at-will breast feeding. Other names for the same condition are nursing bottle caries, nursing bottle mouth, baby bottle syndrome, baby bottle caries, and prolonged nursing habit.

1. *Etiology*
    a. Nursing bottle: the bottle may contain sweetened milk or other fluid sweetened with sucrose.
    b. Pacifier dipped or filled with a sweet agent such as honey.
    c. Prolonged at-will breast feeding.
2. *Effects*
    Maxillary anterior teeth are the most severely affected. The pattern can be explained by the fact that as the baby falls asleep, pools of sweet liquid can collect about the teeth. While the sucking is active, the liquid passes beyond the teeth. The nipple covers the mandibular anterior teeth, hence they are rarely affected.
3. *Recognition*
    Children should be seen for a dental examination at age 1 year to 18 months. Decalcification may be noted along the cervical third of the maxillary anterior teeth. The source of the problem may be detected and preventive procedures initiated through parental counseling.
    At a later stage the lesions appear dark brown. Eventually, the crowns may be destroyed to the gum line, abscesses may develop, and the child may suffer severe pain and discomfort.

RECOGNITION OF CARIOUS LESIONS

Both visual and exploratory means are used to recognize dental caries.

I. Preparation

Dry each tooth or group of teeth with compressed air and carefully inspect each surface, first visually, and then with an explorer as necessary to confirm visual findings.

II. Visual Examination

Characteristic changes in the color and translucency of tooth structure may be observed which are either definite signs of dental caries progress, or lead the examiner to suspect dental caries which can then be followed by the use of an explorer. Variations in color and translucency include the following:

A. Chalky white areas of decalcification.
B. Grayish white discoloration of marginal ridges due to dental caries of the proximal surface underneath.
C. Grayish white color spreading from margins of restorations due to lesions of secondary dental caries.
D. In relation to an amalgam restoration, dental caries appears translucent in outer portion and white and opaque adjacent to the amalgam.
E. Open carious lesions may vary in color from yellowish brown to dark brown.

F. Less discoloration is generally present when dental caries progresses rapidly than when it progresses slowly.

G. Dull, flat white, opaque areas under direct light show loss of translucency, particularly of the enamel.

H. Dark shadow on a proximal surface may be shown by transillumination. This type of observation is especially useful for anterior teeth and unrestored posterior teeth.

III. Exploratory Examination

A. **Smooth Surface Caries**

1. *Technique.* Adapt the side of the tip of the explorer closely to the tooth surface as described on page 224. Examine for hardness versus softness, roughness versus smoothness, and continuity of tooth surface versus breaks in continuity.

2. *Restorations.* Follow the margins of all restorations around with an explorer. Overhanging margins may or may not appear in the radiographs, depending on superimposition. Types of overhangs are described on page 586. Chart all irregularities of existing restorations.

C. **Pit and Fissure Caries**

When a pit or fissure is discolored, it is not possible to determine visually whether dental caries is present except when a large obvious cavity can be seen. When a cavity is obvious, it should not be explored.

1. Direct the explorer tip so that it can pass straight into the pit or fissure. When it is not positioned correctly, caries in a small narrow pit can go undetected.

2. Explorer will catch when dental caries is present and there will be evidence of softening of tooth structure.

RADIOGRAPHIC EXAMINATION

During the clinical examination, information revealed by radiographs is utilized for supplementation and confirmation. Neither clinical nor radiographic examination is complete without the other. A few principal items to be seen in a radiographic examination of the teeth are:

Anomalies
Impactions
Fractures
Internal and root resorption
Dental caries
Periapical radiolucencies

I. Technique Principles

Periapical radiographs usually provide sufficient information concerning the teeth, but panoramic, extraoral, or occlusal radiographs may be needed for detecting or defining anomalies and pathologic lesions outside the scope of periapical radiographs. Bite-wing radiographs or periapical radiographs made by a paralleling technique with no overlapping are most satisfactory for dental caries detection.

Principles for examination were described on page 159. Mounted radiographs on an adequately lighted viewbox are a necessity during charting and treatment procedures. For the detection of early carious lesions a hand magnifying reading glass can be of invaluable assistance.

II. Detection of Dental Caries

Radiographs are not needed for facial, lingual, or occlusal carious lesions because they are accessible and best observed by exploration and direct vision. Because of superimposition of other parts of the tooth, facial, lingual, and occlusal carious lesions need to be fairly well advanced before they are definitely discernible in a radiograph.

A. **Proximal Caries**

Proximal surface lesions may be missed if radiographs are not used. However, clinical skills for caries discernment need to be perfected to prevent excess exposure of a patient to unnecessary radiation.

1. *Small Proximal Lesions.* Properly angulated radiographs with no overlapping are required for the detection of small lesions that involve the enamel or extend slightly into the dentin.

2. *Proximal Overhanging Restorations.* Because of superimposition, it is not necessarily true that there is no overhanging filling, or dental caries under that filling, if none can be seen in the radiograph. An explorer must be passed around the complete margin to confirm the condition.

B. **Cemental Caries**

1. *Location.* Although most cemental car-

ious lesions occur in the vicinity of and just beneath the cementoenamel junction, the lesions may also be found more apically located on the root. The use of an explorer subgingivally can sometimes locate a cavity that appeared indefinite in the radiograph.

2. *Appearance.* Cemental caries appears as a saucer-shaped lesion in a radiograph. It may appear to undermine the enamel or it may be located beneath an overhanging filling.

TESTING FOR PULPAL VITALITY

Any tooth suspected of being devital must be tested for pulpal vitality or degree of vitality. This is particularly significant prior to treatment involving periodontal surgery, any restorative procedures, and orthodontic appliance placement. Diagnosis of vitality cannot be made on a pulp test alone, but on consideration of all data from the patient history and clinical and radiographic examinations.

A tooth may become devital from bacterial causes, particularly invasion of the pulp from dental caries or periodontal disease. Physical causes may be mechanical or thermal injuries. Examples of mechanical injuries are trauma, such as a blow, or iatrogenic dental procedures, such as cavity preparation or too-rapid orthodontic movement.[10,11]

I. Observations That Suggest Loss of Vitality

A. Clinical

1. Discoloration of a tooth crown (intrinsic stains, page 289).
2. Fracture: part of the crown may be missing.
3. Large carious lesion or large restoration.
4. Fistula with opening into the oral cavity over the apical region of a tooth.

B. Radiographic

1. Apical radiolucency, which may indicate a granuloma, cyst, or abscess.
2. Bone loss with a thickened periodontal ligament space extending to the apex.
3. Fractured root.

4. Large carious lesion or restoration that appears closely related to the pulp chamber.

II. Response to Pulp Testing

A. Rationale

Electrical pulp testing is based on the knowledge that an electrical stimulus can create pain to which a patient can react. The pulp tester, therefore, determines the conduction of stimuli to the sensory receptors. The vitality of the pulp is dependent upon its blood supply and not on its nerve supply. For that reason, a positive or negative pulp test may not always show the true condition of the pulp.

B. Factors That Influence a Patient's Response to a Pulp Tester

1. *Degree of Pulpal Degeneration or Inflammation:* a necrotic pulp will give no response at all, while an acutely or chronically inflamed pulp will respond at varying degrees between no response and full normal response.
2. *Pain Perception Threshold:* the lowest perceptible intensity of pain caused by a threshold stimulus. A threshold stimulus is the minimum stimulus necessary to induce patient response.
3. *Reaction to Pain:* may vary with a patient's attitude, age, sex, emotional security, fatigue, drugs used, as well as the size of the pulp and thickness of the dentin, particularly the amount of secondary dentin.
4. *Nerve Transmission Blocks:* injuries or lesions of nerves, and anesthetics.
5. *Adjacent Metal:* restorations or continuous bridgework.

III. Electrical Pulp Testers

Although thermal tests using hot or cold applications have been used, the electrical pulp testers are considered more consistent and reliable.

A. Types

1. *Battery-operated*
   a. Advantages: hand held so operator can work alone; portable.

b. Disadvantage: battery can run down. Some types have a light to indicate current in circuit.

2. *Plug-in*

a. Advantage: more dependable than battery-operated.

b. Disadvantage: not self-contained; requires house-current plug.

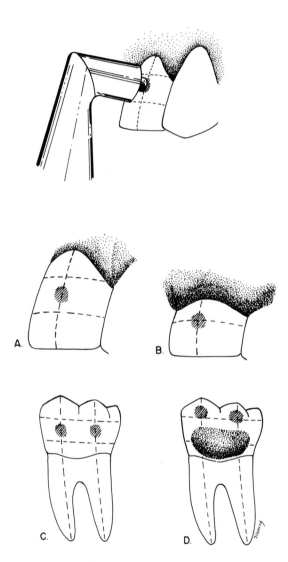

Figure 14–6. Pulp tester in position. **A.** Correct contact point for tip of pulp tester is within the middle third of the crown. Avoid contact with gingiva or restorations. **B.** Adjustment of position of the contact point because of gingival enlargement. **C.** Contact points on multirooted tooth. Place tip of pulp tester in middle third over each root. **D.** Adjustment of position of the contact points because of large Class V restoration.

B.   Precaution

The application of an electrical current to a patient with a cardiac pacemaker or any electronic life-support device by the use of a pulp tester, ultrasonic scaler, desensitizing equipment, or electrosurgical instrument can interfere with pacemaker function and may constitute a serious health hazard.[12,13] A review of the patient history is necessary prior to application of a pulp tester.

C.   Preparation and Use of Equipment

Manufacturer's instructions are provided for each tester and should be followed carefully. When the tester rheostat is separate from the applicator tip, an assistant is needed.

Consistency of procedures is essential in order to obtain consistent readings. The same pulp tester should be used for a particular patient at continuing comparative tests. If rubber gloves are worn, they should always be worn for that patient because readings taken when gloves are worn will be slightly higher than without gloves.[14] Notes in a patient's record can indicate specific directions for that patient.

D.   General Procedures

1. Assemble equipment and pretest current on the skin of finger of the operator to determine that current is passing through.

2. Explain briefly to the patient what is to be done, but avoid detailed description which could create anxiety or apprehension.

3. Dry the teeth to be tested to prevent the current from passing to the gingiva: isolate with cotton rolls and insert a saliva ejector, or use rubber dam.

4. Moisten the end of the tip of the tester with a small amount of toothpaste. Another electrolyte (conductor) may be used if the consistency allows it to remain where placed and not flow over the tooth surface.

5. Instruct the patient to signal when a sensation is felt: suggest raising a hand or making a sound.

6. Application of tester tip

a. Apply first to at least one tooth other than the one in question, preferably an adjacent tooth and the same tooth on the contralateral side, in order to determine a normal response for the patient.

b. Place without pressure but with definite contact on sound tooth structure in a consistent location on the middle or gingival third. The middle third of the crown of a single-rooted tooth and the middle third of each cusp of a multirooted tooth are frequently used (figure 14–6).

E. Readings

1. Prevent false readings
   a. Avoid contact with gingiva or other soft tissues. A low resistant circuit can be formed which allows the circuit to by-pass the tooth.
   b. Avoid contact with metallic restorations. The metal forms a more rapid conductor than tooth structure. When approximal restorations are in contact, the circuit can be transmitted across to the adjacent tooth. The reading obtained would not pertain to the tooth in question (figure 14–7).
2. Start with the rheostat at zero, advance slowly but steadily, stopping only momentarily after each number. Do not proceed with such regularity that the patient can count and anticipate.
3. Test each tooth at least twice. Average the readings.
4. Record on patient's record: the lowest number (average number) at which a minimal stimulus induced a response. Record for all teeth tested, not only the tooth in question.

FACTORS TO TEACH THE PATIENT

I. The cause and process of dental caries formation and development, and the route of attack through the enamel into the dentin.
II. About the hardness of the enamel and why a cavity is sometimes larger in the

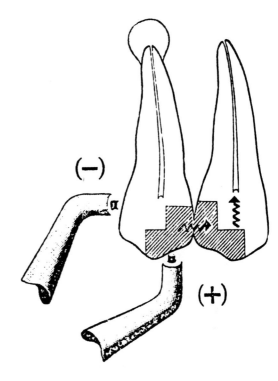

Figure 14–7. Use of pulp tester. False positive response can result when the tester is placed on a metallic restoration. The current can be transmitted across a contact area, to give a reading for the adjacent tooth rather than the tooth in question. (From Antel and Christie, Electical Pulp Testing, *Canadian Dental Association Journal,* 45, 597, November, 1979.)

dentin before there is evidence from the external surface.

III. Why radiographs may be used to detect proximal incipient caries.
IV. Reasons for preservation of primary teeth.
V. Frequency of complete oral examination in relation to a continuing preventive program.
VI. Methods for prevention of dental caries: fluorides, dietary sugar control, plaque prevention and control.
VII. Preventive measures for control and prevention of tooth abrasion: dentifrice selection and correction of brush selection and use.
VIII. Dietary factors related to erosion.
IX. When the patient asks specific questions about oral findings, explain why it is necessary for the dentist to observe and check before explanations can be made.

References

1. Giunta, J.: *Oral Pathology,* in Dunn, M.J., ed.: *Dental Auxiliary Practice,* Module 3. Baltimore, The Williams and Wilkins Co., 1975, p. 37.
2. Shafer, W.G., Hine, M.K., and Levy, B.M.: *A Textbook of Oral Pathology,* 3rd ed. Philadelphia, W.B. Saunders Co., 1974, pp. 285–290.
3. Sognnaes, R.F., Wolcott, R.B., and Xhonga, F.A.: Dental Erosion. 1. Erosion-like Patterns Occurring in Association With Other Dental Conditions, *J. Am. Dent. Assoc., 84,* 571, March, 1972.
4. World Health Organization: *The Etiology and Prevention of Dental Caries.* WHO Technical Report Series, Number 494, Geneva, World Health Organization, 1972, 19 pp.
5. Sumney, D.L. and Jordan, H.V.: Characterization of Bacteria Isolated from Human Root Surface Carious Lesions, *J. Dent. Res., 53,* 343, March-April, 1974.
6. Shafer, Hine, and Levy: op. cit., pp. 404–405.
7. Sumney, D.L., Jordan, H.V., and Englander, H.R.: The Prevalence of Root Surface Caries in Selected Populations, *J. Periodontol., 44,* 500, August, 1973.
8. Blackwell, R.E.: *G.V. Black's Operative Dentistry, Volume II,* 9th ed. Milwaukee, Medico-Dental Publishing Company, 1955, pp. 1–4.
9. Shafer, Hine, and Levy: op. cit., p. 394.
10. Grossman, L.I.: *Endodontic Practice,* 10th ed. Philadelphia, Lea & Febiger, 1981, pp. 48–56.
11. Ingle, J.I. and Beveridge, E.E.: *Endodontics,* 2nd ed. Philadelphia, Lea & Febiger, 1976, pp. 270–292, 416–419.
12. Wooley, L.H., Woodworth, J., and Dobbs, J.L.: A Preliminary Evaluation of the Effects of Electrical Pulp Testers on Dogs With Artificial Pacemakers, *J. Am. Dent. Assoc., 89,* 1099, November, 1974.
13. Ore, D.E. and Shriner, W.A.: Doctor: Don't Shut Off That Pacemaker, *Chicago Dent. Soc. Rev.,* pp. 22–23, August, 1974.
14. King, D.R. and King, A.C.: Use of the Vitalometer With Rubber Gloves, *Can. Dent. Assoc. J., 43,* 182, April, 1977.

Suggested Readings

Buchholz, R.E.: Histologic-radiographic Relation of Proximal Surface Carious Lesions, *J. Prev. Dent., 4,* 23, November-December, 1977.
Kerr, D.A., Ash, M.M., and Millard, H.D.: *Oral Diagnosis,* 5th ed. St. Louis, The C.V. Mosby Co., 1978, p. 199.
Massler, M. and Schour, I.: *Atlas of the Mouth,* 2nd ed. Chicago, American Dental Association, Plates 7–16.
Miller, M.F.: Odontologic Diseases, in Lynch, M.A., ed.: *Burket's Oral Medicine,* 7th ed. Philadelphia, J.B. Lippincott Co., 1977, pp. 283–301.
Mitchell, D.F., Standish, S.M., and Fast, T.B.: *Oral Diagnosis/Oral Medicine,* 3rd ed. Philadelphia, Lea & Febiger, 1978, pp. 147–159.
Rowe, N.H.: Dental Caries, in Steele, P.F., ed.: *Dimensions of Dental Hygiene,* 2nd ed. Philadelphia, Lea & Febiger, 1975, pp. 198–222.
Shafer, W.G., Hine, M.K., and Levy, B.M.: *A Textbook of Oral Pathology,* 3rd ed. Philadelphia, W.B. Saunders Co., 1974, pp. 34–66, 366–432, 490–493.

Hypoplasia, Attrition, Erosion

Berry, D.C. and Poole, D.F.G.: Attrition: Possible Mechanisms of Compensation, *J. Oral Rehabil., 3,* 201, July, 1976.
Boozer, C.H. and Richardson, D.J.: Attrition, Abrasion, and Erosion, in Clark, J.W., ed.: *Clinical Dentistry, Volume 1,* Chapter 6, Addendum. Hagerstown, Maryland, Harper & Row, 1981, pp. 19–21.
Brady, J.M. and Woody, R.D.: Scanning Microscopy of Cervical Erosion, *J. Am. Dent. Assoc., 94,* 726, April, 1977.
Eccles, J.D.: Dental Erosion of Nonindustrial Origin. Clinical Survey and Classification, *J. Prosthet. Dent. 42,* 649, December, 1979.
Fuller, J.L. and Johnson, W.W.: Citric Acid Consumption and the Human Dentition, *J. Am. Dent. Assoc., 95,* 80, July, 1977.
Hansen, B.F.: Clinical and Roentgenologic Caries Detection, *Dentomaxillofac. Radiol., 9,* 34, Number 1, 1980.
Johnson, C.G., Sayegh, F.S., and O'Toole, T.J.: Acid-etch Repair of Hereditary Type 4 Enamel Hypoplasia, *J. Am. Dent. Assoc., 97,* 223, August, 1978.
Radentz, W.H., Barnes, G.P., and Cutright, D.E.: A Survey of Factors Possibly Associated with Cervical Abrasion of Tooth Surfaces, *J. Periodontol., 47,* 148, March, 1976.
White, D.K.: Loss of Tooth Structure Associated with Chronic Regurgitation and Vomiting, *J. Am. Dent. Assoc., 97,* 833, November, 1978.
Winter, G.B. and Brook, A.H.: Enamel Hypoplasia and Anomalies of the Enamel, *Dent. Clin. North Am., 19,* 3, January, 1975.

Cemental Caries

Banting, D.W. and Ellen, R.P.: Carious Lesions on the Roots of Teeth: A Review for the General Practitioner, *Can. Dent. Assoc. J., 42,* 496, October, 1976.
Banting, D.W., Ellen, R.P., and Fillery, E.D.: Prevalence of Root Surface Caries Among Institutionalized Older Persons, *Community Dent. Oral Epidemiol., 8,* 84, April, 1980.
Glickman, I. and Smulow, J.B.: *Periodontal Disease: Clinical, Radiographic, and Histopathologic Features,* Philadelphia, W.B. Saunders Co., 1974, p. 102.
Hazen, S.P., Chilton, N.W., and Mumma, R.D.: The Problem of Root Caries. I. Literature Review and Clinical Description, *J. Am. Dent. Assoc., 86,* 137, January, 1973.
Jordan, H.V. and Sumney, D.L.: Root Surface Caries: Review of the Literature and Significance of the Problem, *J. Periodontol., 44,* 158, March, 1973.
Massler, M.: Geriatric Dentistry: Root Caries in the Elderly, *J. Prosthet. Dent., 44,* 147, August, 1980.
Shannon, I.L., Buchanan, W.E., and Mahan, C.J.: In Vitro Treatment of Human Root Surfaces with Fluorides, *J. Public Health Dent., 36,* 201, Summer, 1976.

Nursing Caries Syndrome

Barton, D.H. and Busch, K.: Communicate to Educate, *Dent. Surv., 54,* 42, February, 1978.
Dilley, G.J., Dilley, D.H., and Machen, J.B.: Prolonged Nursing Habit: A Profile of Patients and Their Families, *J. Dent. Child., 47,* 102, March-April, 1980.
Frigoletto, R.L.: Simplified Treatment of Bottle Baby Syndrome, *J. Dent. Child., 43,* 90, March-April, 1976.
Johnson, K.R.: Restorations for Bottle-mouth Syndrome and Fractured Anterior Teeth, *Dent. Surv., 56,* 30, January, 1980.
King, D.L. and Leimone, C.A.: Nursing Bottle Caries—A Preventive Dilemma, *Dent. Assist., 47,* 18, September-October, 1978.
Ripa, L.W.: Nursing Habits and Dental Decay in Infants "Bottle Caries," *Quintessence Journal, 1,* 37, October, 1979.

lver, D.H.: The Prevalence of Dental Caries in 3-year-old Children, *Brit. Dent. J.*, *137*, 123, August 20, 1974.

samtsouris, A. and White, G.E.: Nursing Caries, *J. Pedod.*, *1*, 198, Spring, 1977.

inter, G.B.: Problems Involved with the Use of Comforters, *Int. Dent. J.*, *30*, 29, March, 1980.

Pulp Vitality

merican Dental Association, Council on Dental Materials, Instruments and Equipment: *Dentist's Desk Reference: Materials, Instruments and Equipment*, 1st ed. Chicago, American Dental Association, 1981, pp. 269–272.

ntel, J. and Christie, W.J.: Electrical Pulp Testing, *Can. Dent. Assoc. J.*, *45*, 597, November, 1979.

ischoff, R.J. and Simon, W.J.: Vitality Testing, *Dent. Assist.*, *45*, 18, March, 1976.

ooley, R.L., White, J.H., and Barkmeier, W.W.: Thermal Pulp Testing, *Gen. Dent.*, *26*, 58, May-June, 1978.

url, M.D. and Prue, D.D.: Pulp Testing, in Boundy, S.S. and Reynolds, N.J., eds.: *Current Concepts in Dental Hygiene*. St. Louis, The C.V. Mosby Co., 1977, pp. 106–125.

Grayson, A.S.: A New Electric Pulp Vitality Tester, *Quintessence Int.*, *8*, 79, March, 1977.

Kerr, D.A., Ash, M.M., and Millard, H.D.: *Oral Diagnosis*, 5th ed. St. Louis, The C.V. Mosby Co., 1978, pp. 338–346.

Michaelson, R.E., Seidberg, B.H., and Guttuso, J.: An *in vivo* Evaluation of Interface Media Used with the Electric Pulp Tester, *J. Am. Dent. Assoc.*, *91*, 118, July, 1975.

Mitchell, D.F., Standish, S.M., and Fast, T.B.: *Oral Diagnosis/Oral Medicine*, 3rd ed. Philadelphia, Lea & Febiger, 1978, pp. 118–123.

Parris, L.: Endodontics, in Steele, P.F., ed.: *Dental Specialties for the Dental Hygienist*, 2nd ed. Philadelphia, Lea & Febiger, 1978, pp. 79–84.

15

The Occlusion

The occlusion is examined and recorded as part of the oral examination. The dental hygienist, by studying the occlusion of each patient, can contribute significantly to the complete dental care and instruction. Recognition of malocclusion assists the dentist in the referral of patients to the orthodontist, gives many valuable points of reference for patient instruction, and determines necessary adaptations in techniques.

. Objectives for Observing Occlusion

Recognizing a patient's occlusion and understanding the oral health problems of malocclusion can aid in accomplishing the following:

A. Provide information for the diagnostic work-up and planning dental hygiene care.

B. Plan personalized instruction in relation to such factors as oral habits, masticatory efficiency, personal oral care procedures, and predisposing factors to dental and periodontal disease.

C. Adapt techniques of instrumentation to malpositioned teeth or groups of teeth.

D. Plan the frequency of recall appointments for professional care on the basis of deposit retention areas, particularly those which are difficult to reach in routine personal care.

E. Assist by recording the general features of malocclusion for special consideration by the dentist who may wish to refer the patient to an orthodontist.

II. Definitions

A. Occlusion

The contact of the teeth in the mandibular arch with those in the maxillary arch.

B. Static Occlusion

The relationships of the teeth when the jaws are closed in centric occlusion is called static occlusion.

C. Functional Occlusion

Functional or dynamic occlusion refers to tooth contacts while the mandible is in action, such as during mastication and swallowing.

D. Centric Occlusion

The centric occlusion is the relation of opposing occlusal surfaces which provides the maximum contact and/or intercuspation.

E. Centric Relation

Centric relation is the most unstrained, retruded anatomic and functional position of the heads of the condyles of the mandible in the glenoid fossae of the temporomandibular joints.

STATIC OCCLUSION

Static occlusion relationships may be efficiently observed in occluded study casts, although they can be seen directly in the oral cavity when the lips and cheeks are retracted. Classification of malocclusion and the variations that occur with each category are described here.

I. Normal (Ideal) Occlusion

The ideal mechanical relationship between the teeth of the maxillary arch and the teeth of the mandibular arch.

A. All teeth in maxillary arch in maximum contact with all teeth in mandibular arch in a definite pattern.
B. Maxillary teeth slightly overlapping the mandibular teeth on the facial surfaces.

II. Malocclusion

Any deviation from the ideal relationship of the maxillary arch and/or teeth to the mandibular arch and/or teeth.

III. Types of Facial Profile (figure 15–1)

A. Mesognathic

Having slightly protruded jaws, which gives the facial outline a relatively flat appearance (straight profile).

B. Retrognathic

Having a prominent maxilla and a deficient, retruded mandible (convex profile).

C. Prognathic

Having a prominent, protruded mandible and normal (usually) maxilla (concave profile).

IV. Malrelations of Groups of Teeth

A. Crossbites

1. *Anterior:* maxillary incisors are lingual to the mandibular incisors (figure 15–10).

2. *Posterior:* maxillary or mandibular posterior teeth are either buccal or lingual to their normal position: this may occur bilaterally or unilaterally (figure 15–2).

B. Edge-to-Edge Bite

Incisal surfaces of maxillary teeth occlude with incisal surfaces of mandibular teeth instead of overlapping as in ideal occlusion (figure 15–3).

C. End-to-End Bite

Molars and premolars occlude cusp-to-cusp as viewed mesiodistally (figure 15–4).

D. Openbite

Lack of occlusal or incisal contact between maxillary and mandibular teeth because either or both have failed to reach the line of occlusion. The teeth cannot be brought together and a space remains due to the arching of the line of occlusion (figure 15–5).

E. Overjet

The horizontal distance between the labioincisal surfaces of the mandibular incisors and the linguoincisal surfaces of the maxillary incisors (figure 15–6). One way to measure the amount of overjet is to place the tip of a probe on the labial surface of the mandibular incisor and, holding it horizontally against the incisal edge of the maxillary tooth, read the distance in millimeters.

F. Underjet (maxillary teeth are lingual to mandibular teeth)

The horizontal distance between the la-

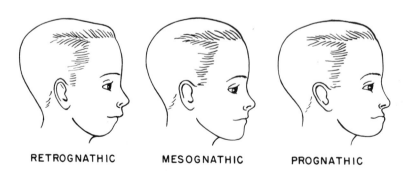

RETROGNATHIC   MESOGNATHIC   PROGNATHIC

Figure 15–1. Types of facial profiles.

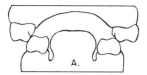 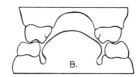 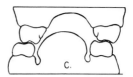

Figure 15–2. Posterior crossbite. **A.** Mandibular teeth lingual to normal position. **B.** Mandibular teeth buccal to normal position. **C.** Unilateral crossbite: right side normal; left side, mandibular teeth buccal to normal position.

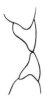

Figure 15–3. Edge-to-edge bite. Incisal surfaces occlude.

Figure 15–4. End-to-end bite. Molars in cusp-to-cusp occlusion as viewed from the buccal.

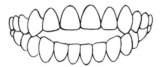

Figure 15–5. Openbite. Lack of incisal contact. Posterior teeth in their normal occlusion.

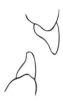

Figure 15–6. Overjet. Maxillary incisors are labial to the mandibular incisors. There is a measurable horizontal distance between the incisal edge of the maxillary incisors and the incisal edge of the mandibular incisors.

Figure 15–7. Underjet. Maxillary incisors are lingual to the mandibular incisors. There is a measurable horizontal distance between the incisal edges of the maxillary incisors and the incisal edges of the mandibular incisors.

Figure 15–8. Normal overbite. Profile view to show position of incisal edge of maxillary tooth within the incisal third of the facial surface of the mandibular incisor.

Figure 15–9. Severe anterior overbite. Incisal edge of maxillary tooth is at the level of the cervical third of the facial surface of the mandibular anterior tooth. See facial view in 15–11C.

Figure 15–10. Anterior crossbite. Maxillary anterior teeth are lingual to the mandibular anterior teeth. This occurs in Angle's Class III malocclusion.

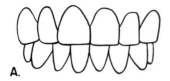

A.

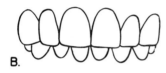

B.

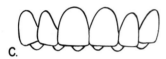

C.

Figure 15–11. Overbite, anterior view. **A.** Normal overbite; the incisal edges of the maxillary teeth are within the incisal third of the facial surfaces of the mandibular teeth. **B.** Moderate overbite: the incisal edges of the maxillary teeth are within the middle third of the facial surfaces of the mandibular teeth. **C.** Severe overbite: the incisal edges of the maxillary teeth are within the cervical third of the facial of the mandibular teeth. When the incisal edges of the mandibular teeth are in contact with the maxillary lingual gingival tissue, it is considered very severe overbite. See profile view figure 15–9.

bioincisal surfaces of the maxillary incisors and the linguoincisal surfaces of the mandibular incisors (figure 15–7).

G. **Overbite** (vertical overlap)

Overbite is the vertical distance by which the maxillary incisors overlap the mandibular incisors.
1. *Normal Overbite.* An overbite is considered normal when the incisal edges of the maxillary teeth are within the incisal third of the mandibular teeth as shown in figure 15–8 in side view and in figure 15–11A viewed from the anterior.
2. *Moderate Overbite.* When the incisal edges of the maxillary teeth appear within the middle third of the mandibular teeth, it is called moderate overbite (figure 15–11B).
3. *Severe Overbite.* When the incisal edges of the maxillary teeth are within the

cervical third of the mandibular teeth it is called severe overbite, and when in addition, the incisal edges of the mandibular teeth are in contact with the maxillary lingual gingival tissue, it is called very severe. A side view of very severe overbite is shown in figure 15–9.
4. *Anterior Crossbite.* The opposite situation occurs in anterior crossbite, when the maxillary anterior teeth are lingual to the mandibular anterior teeth (figure 15–10).
5. *Clinical Examination of Overbite.* Normal, moderate, and severe anterior overbite are observed directly when the teeth are closed in occlusion. With the posterior teeth closed together, the lips can be retracted and the teeth observed as in figure 15–11. The degree of anterior overbite is judged by the position of the incisal edge of the maxillary teeth: normal (slight) within the incisal third of the mandibular incisors; moderate overbite within the middle third; and severe overbite within the cervical third. By placing a mouth mirror under the incisal edge of the maxillary teeth, it is sometimes possible to see the mandibular teeth contact with the maxillary lingual gingiva. When this is not possible, an examination of the lingual gingiva may reveal teeth prints, or at least enlargement and redness from the contact.

V. **Malpositions of Individual Teeth**

A. **Labioversion.** A tooth that has assumed position labial to normal.

B. **Linguoversion.** Position lingual to normal.

C. **Buccoversion.** Position buccal to normal.

D. **Supraversion.** Elongated above the line of occlusion.

E. **Torsiversion.** Turned or rotated.

F. **Infraversion.** Depressed below the line of occlusion. (Example: primary tooth that is submerged or ankylosed.)

DETERMINATION OF THE CLASSIFICATION OF OCCLUSION

The determination of the classification of occlusion is based upon the principles of Edward I. Angle, which he presented in the early 1900s. He defined normal occlusion as "the normal relations of the occlusal inclined planes of the teeth when the jaws are closed"[1] and based his system of classification upon the relationship of the maxillary first permanent molars.

Although authorities have since agreed that the maxillary first permanent molars do not occupy a fixed position in the dental arch, Angle's system serves to provide an acceptable basis for a useful classification. A more comprehensive picture of malocclusion is made by the orthodontist who studies the relationships of the position of the teeth to the jaws, the face, and the skull.

Three general classes of malocclusion are described below. These are designated by Roman numerals. Since the mandible is movable and the maxilla is stationary, the classes describe the relationship of the mandible to the maxilla. For example, in Distoclusion (Class II) the mandible is distal, whereas in Mesioclusion (Class III) the mandible is mesial to the maxilla, as compared to the normal position.

Relative to the incidence of malocclusion, various surveys have been made that cannot be compared directly because of differences in methodology. Only between two and four percent of the population has normal or ideal occlusion. More than two-thirds of the population have been found to have malocclusion severe enough to require orthodontic treatment.

The prevalence of malocclusion is significantly less in communities where there is fluoride in the drinking water. Since there is less dental caries and fewer teeth are extracted, one factor that contributes to malocclusion is reduced or missing, namely, tooth loss with shifting of the positions of remaining teeth.

I. Normal (Ideal) Occlusion (figure 15–12)

A. Facial Profile

Mesognathic (figure 15–1).

B. Molar Relation

The mesiobuccal cusp of the maxillary first permanent molar occludes with the buccal groove of the mandibular first permanent molar.

C. Canine Relation

The maxillary permanent canine occludes with the distal half of the mandibular canine and the mesial half of the mandibular first premolar.

II. Malocclusion

A. Class I or Neutroclusion (figure 15–12)

1. *Facial Profile.* Same as Normal Occlusion (I, A, above).
2. *Molar Relation.* Same as Normal Occlusion (I, B, above).
3. *Canine Relation.* Same as Normal Occlusion (I, C, above).
4. *Malposition* of individual teeth or groups of teeth.
5. *General Types of Conditions That Frequently Occur in Class I.*
   a. Crowded maxillary or mandibular anterior teeth.
   b. Protruded or retruded maxillary incisors.
   c. Anterior crossbite.
   d. Posterior crossbite.
   e. Mesial drift of molars resulting from premature loss of teeth.

B. Class II or Distoclusion (figure 15–12)

1. *Description.* Mandibular teeth posterior to normal position in their relation to the maxillary teeth.
2. *Facial Profile.* Retrognathic; maxilla protrudes; lower lip is full and often rests between the maxillary and mandibular incisors; the mandible appears retruded or weak (figure 15–1, Retrognathic).
3. *Molar Relation*
   a. The buccal groove of the mandibular first permanent molar is distal to the mesiobuccal cusp of the maxillary first permanent molar by at least the width of a premolar.
   b. When the distance is less than the width of a premolar the relation should be classified as "tendency toward Class II."

Normal (Ideal) Occlusion

Molar relationship: mesiobuccal cusp of maxillary first permanent molar occludes with the buccal groove of the mandibular first permanent molar.

Malocclusion

Class I: Neutroclusion. Molar relationship same as Normal, with malposition of individual teeth or groups of teeth.

Class II: Distoclusion.

Molar relationship: buccal groove of the mandibular first permanent molar is distal to the mesiobuccal cusp of the maxillary first permanent molar by at least the width of a premolar.

Division 1: mandible is retruded and all maxillary incisors are protruded.

Division 2: mandible is retruded and one or more maxillary incisors are retruded.

Class III: Mesioclusion.

Molar relationship: buccal groove of the mandibular first permanent molar is mesial to the mesiobuccal cusp of the maxillary first permanent molar by at least the width of a premolar.

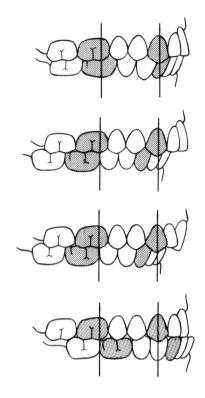

Figure 15–12.   Normal occlusion and classification of malocclusions.

4. *Canine Relation*
   a. The distal surface of the mandibular canine is distal to the mesial surface of the maxillary canine by at least the width of a premolar.
   b. When the distance is less than the width of a premolar the relation should be classified as "tendency toward Class II."
5. *Class II, Division 1*
   a. Description: the mandible is retruded and all maxillary incisors are protruded.
   b. General types of conditions that frequently occur in Class II, Division 1 malocclusion: deep overbite, excessive overjet, abnormal muscle function (lips), short mandible, or short upper lip.
6. *Class II, Division 2*
   a. Description: the mandible is retruded, and one or more maxillary incisors are retruded.
   b. General types of conditions that frequently occur in Class II, Division 2 malocclusion: maxillary lateral incisors protrude while both central in-

cisors retrude, crowded maxillary anterior teeth, or deep overbite.
7. *Subdivision.* One side is Class I, the other side is Class II (may be Division 1 or 2).

C. **Class III or Mesioclusion** (figure 15–12)

1. *Description.* Mandibular teeth are anterior to normal position in relation to maxillary teeth.
2. *Facial Profile.* Prognathic; lower lip and mandible are prominent (figure 15–1).
3. *Molar Relation*
   a. The buccal groove of the mandibular first permanent molar is mesial to the mesiobuccal cusp of the maxillary first permanent molar by at least the width of a premolar.
   b. When the distance is less than the width of a premolar the relation should be classified as "tendency toward Class III."
4. *Canine Relation*
   a. The distal surface of the mandibular canine is mesial to the mesial surface

of the maxillary canine by at least the width of a premolar.

b. When the distance is less than the width of a premolar the relation should be classified as "tendency toward Class III."

5. *General Types of Conditions That Frequently Occur in Class III Malocclusion*

a. True Class III: maxillary incisors are lingual to mandibular incisors in an anterior crossbite (figure 15–10).

b. Maxillary and mandibular incisors are in edge-to-edge occlusion.

c. Mandibular incisors are very crowded, but lingual to maxillary incisors.

OCCLUSION OF
THE PRIMARY TEETH[2]

I. Normal (Ideal)

A. Canine Relation

Same as permanent dentition.

1. *With Primate Spaces* (page 870 for definition).

a. Mandibular: between mandibular canine and first molar (figure 15–13A).

b. Maxillary: between maxillary lateral incisor and canine (figure 15–13B).

2. *Without Primate Spaces:* closed arches.

B. Second Molar Relation

The mesiobuccal cusp of the maxillary second primary molar occludes with the buccal groove of the mandibular second primary molar.

1. *Variations in Distal Surfaces Relationships:* terminal step.

a. The distal surface of the mandibular molar is mesial to that of the maxillary, thereby forming a mesial step (figure 15–14A).

b. Morphologic variation in molar size: maxillary and mandibular molars have approximately the same mesiodistal width.

2. *Variation:* terminal plane

a. The distal surfaces of the maxillary and mandibular molars are on same vertical plane (figure 15–14B).

b. The maxillary molar is narrower mesiodistally than the mandibular molar (occurs in high percentage of cases).

3. *Effects on Occlusion of First Permanent Molars*

a. Terminal step: first permanent molar erupts directly into proper occlusion (figure 15–14A).

b. Terminal plane: first permanent molars erupt end-to-end. With mandibular primate space there is early mesial shift of primary molars into the primate space and the permanent mandibular molar shifts into proper occlusion. Without primate spaces there is late mesial shift of permanent mandibular molar into proper occlusion, following exfoliation of

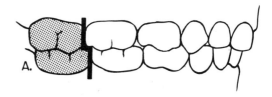

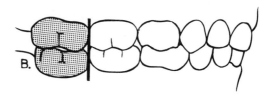

Figure 15–14. Eruption patterns of first permanent molars. **A.** Terminal step. Distal surface of mandibular second primary molar is mesial to the distal surface of the maxillary primary molar. **B.** Terminal plane. Distal surfaces of mandibular and maxillary second primary molars are on the same vertical plane. Permanent molars erupt in end-to-end occlusion.

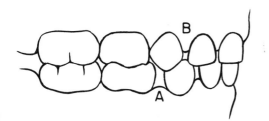

Figure 15–13. Primary teeth showing primate spaces. **A.** Mandibular primate space between canine and first molar. **B.** Maxillary primate space between lateral incisor and canine.

second primary molar (figure 15–14B).

II. Malocclusion of the Primary Teeth

Same as permanent dentition.

FUNCTIONAL OCCLUSION

In contrast to static occlusion, which pertains to the relationship of the teeth when the jaws are closed, functional occlusion consists of all contacts during chewing, swallowing, or other normal action. Functional occlusion is associated with performance.

The pressures or forces created by the muscles of mastication are transmitted from the teeth, after contact, to the periodontium. Such forces are necessary to maintain the occlusal relationship of the teeth and guide the teeth during eruption. The forces are also necessary to provide functional stimulation for the preservation of the health of the attachment apparatus, namely the periodontal ligament, the cementum, and the alveolar bone.

I. Types of Occlusal Contacts

A. Functional Contacts

Functional contacts are the normal contacts that are made between the maxillary teeth and the mandibular teeth during chewing and swallowing. Each contact is momentary, so the total contact time is only a few minutes each day.

B. Parafunctional Contacts

Parafunctional contacts are those made outside the normal range of function. They result from occlusal habits and neuroses, and are potentially injurious to the periodontal supporting structures. Parafunctional contacts can be divided into the following:
1. *Tooth-to-Tooth Contacts:* bruxism, clenching, tapping, doodling.
2. *Tooth-to-Hard Object Contacts:* nail biting, occupationally utilized objects such as tacks or pins, smoking equipment such as a pipe stem or hard cigarette holder.
3. *Tooth-and-Oral Tissues:* lip or cheek biting.

II. Proximal Contacts

Proximal contacts serve to stabilize the posi- tion of teeth in the dental arches and to prevent food impaction between the teeth. Attrition or wear of the teeth occurs at the proximal contacts.

A. Drifting

When proximal contact is lost, teeth can drift into spaces created by unreplaced missing teeth. There is also a natural tendency for mesial migration of teeth toward the midline. In the absence of disease, the surrounding periodontal tissues adapt to repositioned teeth (figure 13–19, page 227).

B. Pathologic Migration

With destruction of the supporting structures of a tooth due to periodontal disease and a force to move a tooth weakened by disease and bone loss, migration of the tooth can result. Pathologic migration occurs when disease is present, in contrast to drifting, which is migration with a healthy periodontium.

TRAUMA FROM OCCLUSION

Periodontal tissue injury caused by repeated occlusal forces which exceed the physiologic limits of tissue tolerance is called trauma from occlusion. Other names are periodontal traumatism, occlusal traumatism, and periodontal trauma.

I. Types of Trauma from Occlusion

A. Primary

When the excessive occlusal force is exerted on a tooth with normal bone support, it is called *primary trauma from occlusion.* An example is the effect of a restoration placed above the line of occlusion.

B. Secondary

When the excessive occlusal force is exerted on a tooth with bone loss and inadequate alveolar bone support, and the ability of the tooth to withstand occlusal forces is impaired, it is called *secondary trauma from occlusion.* It is possible that when a tooth has lost the support of the surrounding bone, even the pressures of what are usually considered normal occlusal forces can create lesions of trauma from occlusion.

I. Effects of Trauma from Occlusion

The attachment apparatus (periodontal ligament, cementum, and alveolar bone) has as its main purpose the maintenance of the tooth in the socket in a functional state. In a healthy situation, occlusal pressures and forces during chewing and swallowing are readily dispersed or absorbed and no unusual effects are produced.

A. Excess Forces

When the forces of occlusion are greater than can be taken care of by the attachment apparatus, damage can result. Circulatory disturbances, tissue destruction from crushing under pressure, bone resorption, and other pathologic processes are initiated.

B. Relation to Inflammatory Factors

1. *Trauma from occlusion does not cause gingivitis, periodontitis, or pocket formation.* The steps in the development of inflammatory disease and pockets were outlined on pages 203–204.
2. In the presence of inflammatory disease, the existing periodontal destruction may be aggravated or promoted by trauma from occlusion.

III. Methods of Application of Excess Pressure

To understand the nature of the occlusal forces that can cause periodontal trauma from occlusion, it is helpful to recognize types of tooth contacts that can overburden a tooth or group of teeth.[3]

A. Individual Teeth that Touch Before Full Closure

The contact is premature and may put excessive force on an individual tooth.

B. Two or Only a Few Teeth in Contact During Movement of the Jaw

The teeth involved receive a disproportionate amount of force.

C. Initial Contacts on Inclined Planes of Cusps

Following the initial contact, when the teeth are brought together in a closed position, there may be excess pressure on the teeth where initial contact was made.

D. Heavy Forces Not in a Vertical or Axial Direction

Normal occlusal relationships imply a direct cusp-to-fossa position during closure, with the force of occlusion in a vertical direction toward the tooth apex and parallel with the long axis. When pressures are exerted laterally or horizontally, excess force is placed on the periodontal attachment apparatus.

E. Increased Frequency, Intensity, and Duration of Contacts

When there are parafunctional habits such as bruxism, clenching, tapping, or biting objects, many more than usual tooth contacts are made each day, and the intensity and duration are altered.

IV. Recognition of Signs of Trauma from Occlusion

No one clinical or radiographic finding will clearly define the presence of trauma from occlusion. Diagnosis of the condition is complex. The possible observations listed below should be looked for specifically and recorded for evaluation and correlation with the patient history and all other clinical determinations.

A. Clinical Findings That May Occur in Trauma from Occlusion

1. Tooth mobility
2. Fremitus
3. Sensitivity of teeth to pressure and/or percussion.
4. Pathologic migration.
5. Wear facets or atypical occlusal wear.
6. Open contacts related to food impaction.
7. Neuromuscular disturbances in the muscles of mastication. In severe cases muscle spasm can occur.
8. Temporomandibular joint symptoms.

B. Radiographic Findings

Characteristics that may occur in trauma from occlusion include:
1. Widened periodontal ligament spaces, particularly angular thickening (triangulation). This finding frequently occurs in conjunction with tooth mobility.
2. Angular (vertical) bone loss in localized areas (figure 13–20, page 228).

3. Root resorption.
4. Furcation involvement.
5. Thickened lamina dura. Although related to occlusal forces, thickened lamina dura should not necessarily be considered a detrimental or destructive effect of trauma from occlusion. It may be a defense reaction to strengthen tooth support against occlusal forces. Thickened lamina dura is frequently associated with teeth that have undergone orthodontic treatment.

TECHNICAL HINTS

I. Observe the facial profile as the patient enters and is seated in the dental chair to estimate the classification of occlusion before examination of the teeth.

II. Avoid mention of a dentofacial deformity that would make the patient feel self-conscious.

III. Avoid suggesting to the patient or a parent the possible procedures the orthodontist may use in the treatment of the case, as complications of the case become known only after the complete diagnosis.

IV. To aid in closing to centric relation: instruct the patient to curl the tongue and try to hold the tip of tongue as far back as possible while closing.

V. When a small child has difficulty in occluding, the operator may firmly but gently press the cushions of the thumbs on the mucous membrane over the pterygomandibular raphe, holding the thumbs between the cheek and buccal surfaces of the teeth, as the patient is requested to close.

VI. Study the occlusion of the patient with removable dentures with the dentures in place in the mouth.

FACTORS TO TEACH THE PATIENT

I. Interpretation of the *general* purposes of orthodontic care (function and esthetics) to patients whom the dentist has referred to an orthodontist.

A. Dependence of masticatory efficiency on the occlusion of the teeth.

B. Influence of masticatory efficiency on food selection in the diet.

C. Influence of masticatory efficiency and diet on the nutritional status of the body and oral health.

II. Interpretation of the dentist's suggestions for the correction of oral habits.

III. The space-maintaining function of the primary teeth in prevention of malocclusion of permanent teeth.

IV. The role of malocclusion as a predisposing factor in the formation of dental caries and periodontal diseases.

V. Plaque removal methods for reducing dental calculus and soft deposit retention in areas where teeth are crowded, displaced, or otherwise not in normal occlusion.

VI. The relation of the occlusion and the position of the teeth to the patient's personal oral care procedures.

A. Selection of the proper type of toothbrush.

B. Application of thorough toothbrushing method or methods.

C. Use of dental floss.

VII. Specific reasons for frequency of recall when related to malocclusion.

References

1. Angle, E.H.: *Malocclusion of the Teeth*, 7th ed. Philadelphia, S. S. White, 1907.
2. Baume, L.J.: Physiological Tooth Migration and Its Significance for the Development of the Occlusion.
   I. The Biogenetic Course of the Deciduous Dentition, *J. Dent. Res.*, 29, 123, April, 1950.
   II. The Biogenesis of the Accessional Dentition, *J. Dent. Res.*, 29, 331, June, 1950.
   III. The Biogenesis of the Successional Dentition, *J. Dent. Res.*, 29, 338, June, 1950.
   IV. The Biogenesis of Overbite, *J. Dent. Res.*, 29, 440, August, 1950.
3. Allen, D.L., McFall, W.T., and Hunter, G.C.: *Periodontics for the Dental Hygienist*, 3rd ed. Philadelphia, Lea & Febiger, 1980, pp. 85–86.

Suggested Readings

Barber, T.K.: Prevention of Malocclusion and Minor Orthodontics, in Caldwell, R.C. and Stallard, R.E.: *A Textbook of Preventive Dentistry*. Philadelphia, W.B. Saunders Co., 1977, pp. 351–389.

Binder, R.E.: Orthodontic Evaluation for the Pediatric Dentist, in Forester, D.J., Wagner, M.L., and Fleming, J., eds.: *Pediatric Dental Medicine*. Philadelphia, Lea & Febiger, 1981, pp. 247–283.

Fisher, A.K.: Some Observations on the Use of the Term Prognathism, *J. Am. Dent. Assoc.*, 38, 611, May, 1949.

Graber, T.M.: *Orthodontics*, 3rd ed. Philadelphia, W.B. Saunders Co., 1972, pp. 204–254.

Herman, E.: Dental Considerations in the Playing of Musical Instruments, *J. Am. Dent. Assoc.*, 89, 611, September, 1974.

Lieberman, M.A. and Gazit, E.: Guides to Orthodontic Treatment Timing, *J. Am. Dent. Assoc.*, 88, 555, March, 1974.

Ma, H.-C. and Laracuente, J.M.: The Influence of Playing Musical Wind Instruments on Oral Tissues, *Gen. Dent.*, 27, 46, January-February, 1979.

Margolis, F.S.: Ordinary versus Orthodontic Pacifiers, *Dent. Surv.*, 56, 44, July, 1980.

Merow, W.W.: Orthodontics, in Steele, P.F., ed.: *Dental Specialties for the Dental Hygienist*, 2nd ed. Philadelphia, Lea & Febiger, 1978, pp. 199–237.

Oles, R.D.: Occlusal Examination, *Can. Dent. Assoc. J.*, 44, 28, January, 1978.

Pang, A.: Relation of Musical Wind Instruments to Malocclusion, *J. Am. Dent. Assoc.*, 92, 565, March, 1976.

Rubel, I.: Avulsion of Central Incisors by Elastic Bands with Subsequent Orthodontic Treatment, *J. Am. Dent. Assoc.*, 100, 211, February, 1980.

van der Linden, F.P.G.M.: Theoretical and Practical Aspects of Crowding in the Human Dentition, *J. Am. Dent. Assoc.*, 89, 139, July, 1974.

Wheeler, R.C.: *Dental Anatomy, Physiology, and Occlusion*, 5th ed. Philadelphia, W.B. Saunders Co., 1974, pp. 405–505.

Wirth, C.G.: Occlusion, in Boundy, S.S. and Reynolds, N.J., eds.: *Current Concepts in Dental Hygiene*. St. Louis, The C.V. Mosby Co., 1977, pp. 126–144.

Woerth, J.K.: Detecting Occlusal Dysfunction, *Dent. Hyg.*, 53, 456, October, 1979.

Trauma from Occlusion

Carranza, F.A.: *Glickman's Clinical Periodontology*, 5th ed. Philadelphia, W.B. Saunders Co., 1979, pp. 275–302, 455–488.

Glickman, I. and Smulow, J.B.: *Periodontal Disease: Clinical, Radiographic and Histopathologic Features*. Philadelphia, W.B. Saunders Co., 1974, pp. 136–146.

Goldman, H.M. and Cohen, D.W.: *Periodontal Therapy*, 6th ed. St. Louis, The C.V. Mosby Co., 1980, pp. 152–155, 244–259, 1065–1110.

Grant, D.A., Stern, I.B., and Everett, F.G.: *Periodontics*, 5th ed. St. Louis, The C.V. Mosby Co., 1979, pp. 400–425.

Ramfjord, S.P. and Ash, M.M.: *Periodontology and Periodontics*. Philadelphia, W.B. Saunders Co., 1979, pp. 175–193, 276–282.

Ratcliff, P.A. and Oliver, G.V.: Periodontics, in Steele, P.F., ed.: *Dimensions of Dental Hygiene*, 2nd ed. Philadelphia, Lea & Febiger, 1975, pp. 337–338, 363–365.

Schluger, S., Yuodelis, R.A., and Page, R.C.: *Periodontal Disease*. Philadelphia, Lea & Febiger, 1977, pp. 109–132, 611–616.

Stone, S. and Kalis, P.J.: Periodontics, in Dunn, M.J., ed.: *Dental Auxiliary Practice, Module 6*. Baltimore, The Williams and Wilkins Co., 1975, pp. 37–43, 86–88.

Bruxism

Ayer, W.A. and Levin, M.P.: Theoretical Basis and Application of Massed Practice Exercises for the Elimination of Tooth Grinding Habits, *J. Periodontol.*, 46, 306, May, 1975.

Buonomano, L. and Buonomano, V.D.: Biofeedback: The Emergence of a New Dental and Medical Perspective, *Gen. Dent.*, 27, 65, March-April, 1979.

Gallagher, S.J.: Diagnosis and Treatment of Bruxism: A Review of the Literature, *Gen. Dent.*, 28, 62, March-April, 1980.

Glaros, A.G. and Rao, S.M.: Effects of Bruxism: A Review of the Literature, *J. Prosthet. Dent.*, 38, 149, August, 1977.

Kardachi, B.J. and Clarke, N.G.: The Use of Biofeedback to Control Bruxism, *J. Periodontol.*, 48, 639, October, 1977.

Kardachi, B.J.R., Bailey, J.O., and Ash, M.M.: A Comparison of Biofeedback and Occlusal Adjustment on Bruxism, *J. Periodontol.*, 49, 367, July, 1978.

Love, R. and Clark, G.: Bruxism and Periodontal Disease: A Critical Review, *Periodont. Abstr.*, 26, 104, Number 4, 1978.

Mikami, D.B.: A Review of Psychogenic Aspects and Treatment of Bruxism, *J. Prosthet. Dent.*, 37, 411, April, 1977.

Suzuki, J.B.: Etiology of Parafunction: A Brief Review of Psychological and Occlusal Genesis, *Periodont. Abstr.*, 27, 48, Number 2, 1979.

Zeldow, L.L.: Treating Clenching and Bruxing by Habit Change, *J. Am. Dent. Assoc.*, 93, 31, July, 1976.

Habits

Barber, T.K. and Bonus, H.W.: Dental Relationships in Tongue-thrusting Children as Affected by Circumoral Myofunctional Exercise, *J. Am. Dent. Assoc.*, 90, 979, May, 1975.

Gellin, M.E.: Digital Sucking and Tongue Thrusting in Children, *Dent. Clin. North Am.*, 22, 603, October, 1978.

Graber, T.M.: *Orthodontics*, 3rd ed. Philadelphia, W.B. Saunders Co., 1972, pp. 292–328.

Lundeen, D.J., Kurtz, D.D., and Stanley, E.O.: Clinical Study of Dental Caries and Tongue Thrust, *J. Am. Dent. Assoc.*, 88, 1019, May, 1974.

Mason, R.M. and Proffit, W.R.: The Tongue Thrust Controversy: Background and Recommendations, *J. Speech and Hearing Disorders*, 39, 115, May, 1974.

Proffit, W.R. and Mason, R.M.: Myofunctional Therapy for Tongue-thrusting: Background and Recommendations, *J. Am. Dent. Assoc.*, 90, 403, February, 1975.

Shoaf, H.K.: Prevalence and Duration of Thumbsucking in Breast-fed and Bottle-fed Children, *J. Dent. Child.*, 46, 126, March-April, 1979.

16

Bacterial Plaque and Other Soft Deposits

During the examination of the teeth, it is necessary to recognize and assess the soft and hard deposits that accumulate on tooth surfaces. The soft deposits are acquired pellicle or cuticle, bacterial plaque, materia alba, and food debris, each of which is an entity, and the terms should not be interchanged. The hard, calcified deposit on teeth is dental calculus which is described in Chapter 17. A classification with definitions of the dental deposits is presented in table 16–1.[1]

ACQUIRED PELLICLE

The acquired pellicle is an amorphous, organic, tenacious membranous layer which forms over exposed tooth surfaces as well as restorations and dental calculus. Its thickness varies from 0.1 to several micra, usually thicker near the gingiva. Pellicles are acellular, that is, they are free from bacteria or other cell forms.

I. Development

A. Formation

Within minutes after all external material is removed by polishing with an abrasive, the acquired pellicle begins to form. It is composed primarily of glycoproteins which are selectively adsorbed by the hydroxyapatite of the tooth surface. The adsorbed material becomes a highly insoluble coating over the teeth, calculus deposits, restorations, and complete and partial dentures.

B. Source of Materials

Supragingival pellicle is derived from the saliva, and subgingival pellicle is from the gingival sulcus fluid.

II. Types of Pellicles[2]

A. Surface Pellicle, unstained

The unstained pellicle is clear, translucent, insoluble, and not readily visible until disclosing agent is applied. When stained with a disclosing agent, it appears thin, with a pale staining which contrasts with the thicker, darker staining of dental plaque.

B. Surface Pellicle, stained

Unstained pellicle can take on extrinsic stain and become brown, grayish, or other colors as described on page 288.

C. Subsurface Pellicle

Surface pellicle is continuous with pellicle that is embedded in tooth structure, particularly where the tooth surface is partially decalcified.[3]

Table 16–1. Tooth Deposits

Category	Tooth Deposit	Description	Derivation
Nonmineralized	Acquired Pellicle	Translucent, homogeneous, thin, unstructured film covering and adherent to the surfaces of the teeth, restorations, calculus, and other firm surfaces in the oral cavity	Supragingival: saliva Subgingival: gingival sulcus fluid
	Bacterial Plaques	Dense, organized bacterial systems embedded in an intermicrobial matrix which adhere closely to the teeth, calculus, and other firm surfaces in the oral cavity Water irrigation removes only the outer layer of loose organisms	Colonization of oral microorganisms
	Materia Alba	Loosely adherent, unstructured, white or grayish white mass of oral debris and bacteria which lies over dental plaque Vigorous rinsing and water irrigation can remove materia alba	Incidental accumulation
	Food Debris	Unstructured, loosely attached particulate matter Self-cleansing activity of tongue and saliva, and rinsing vigorously will remove debris	Food retention following eating
Mineralized	Calculus	Calcified dental plaque; hard, tenacious mass which forms on the clinical crowns of the natural teeth and on dentures and other appliances	Plaque mineralization
	a. Supragingival	Occurs coronal to the margin of the gingiva; is covered with dental plaque	Supragingival: source of the minerals is saliva
	b. Subgingival	Occurs apical to the margin of the gingiva; is covered with dental plaque	Subgingival: source of minerals is the gingival sulcus fluid

(Adapted from Schroeder, H.E.: *Formation and Inhibition of Dental Calculus.* Vienna, Hans Huber, 1969, pp. 14–15.)

III. Significance of Pellicle

A. Protective

Pellicle appears to provide a barrier against acids, thus it may aid in reducing dental caries attack.[3]

B. Nidus for Bacteria

Pellicle participates in plaque formation by serving as a nidus for the colonization of microorganisms.

C. Attachment of Calculus

One mode of calculus attachment is by the acquired pellicle (page 280).

BACTERIAL PLAQUE

Bacterial or dental plaque is a dense, noncalcified, complex mass of bacterial colonies in a gel-like intermicrobial matrix. It adheres firmly to the acquired pellicle and hence to the teeth, calculus, and fixed and removable restorations.

Supragingival and subgingival plaques have specific characteristics.

The microorganisms of dental plaque play a major role in the development of dental caries and inflammatory periodontal diseases. For that reason, the prevention, control, and removal of plaque has special significance in patient counseling and care. Instruction and supervision in plaque control methods are important parts of each patient's treatment plan.

I. Classification

A. By Location

1. Plaque on tooth surfaces may be divided into *coronal* plaque, which is on tooth surfaces not in contact with the gingiva; *gingival* or *cervical third* plaque, with reference to plaque in contact with the gingival margin; and *subgingival* plaque, which is found within the sulcus or pocket.[4]

2. It is more in general use to divide plaque into two categories demarcated by the gingival margin. Dental calculus is defined in the same manner.
   a. Supragingival plaque, coronal to the gingival margin.
   b. Subgingival plaque, located between the junctional epithelium and the gingival margin, within the sulcus or pocket.

3. Fissure plaque. Plaque also develops in pits and fissures and is referred to as *fissure* plaque.

4. Gingiva. Plaque forms on the external surfaces of the oral epithelium and attached gingiva.

B. By Pathogenic Effects

The role of plaque in the initiation and perpetuation of both dental caries and periodontal diseases has led to a realization that all dental plaque is not the same, but that the content and effects vary. The principal differences between plaques are brought about by microbial components. On the basis of their pathogenic effects, the three main categories of plaques are as follows:

1. *Cariogenic Plaque:* associated with the initiation of dental caries.

2. *Periodontal-Disease-Producing Plaque:* directly involved in promoting the inflammatory responses demonstrated by gingivitis, periodontitis, and other periodontal diseases.

3. *Calculus Plaque or Calculogenic Plaque:* invites mineralization of the plaque, leading to calculus formation.

II. Clinical Characteristics

Examination for dental plaque constitutes a specific part of the evaluation of the teeth and gingiva for patient instruction and treatment planning.

A. Distribution of Plaque

1. *During Formation*
   Supragingival plaque formation begins at the gingival margin, particularly on proximal surfaces, and increases rapidly when left undisturbed. It spreads over the gingival third and on towards the middle third of the crown.

2. *Tooth Surfaces Involved*
   a. Plaque occurs most frequently on proximal surfaces and around the gingival third, associated with protected areas (table 16–2).
   b. Least amounts occur on the palatal surfaces of maxillary teeth because of the activity of the tongue.
   c. Mandibular teeth accumulate more plaque than maxillary teeth.
   d. More rapid collection occurs on rough surfaces of teeth, restorations, and calculus.
   e. Thick, dense deposits usually collect in difficult-to-clean areas such as under overhanging margins of crowns or fillings, under ledges of calculus, and associated with carious lesions.
   f. Deposits may extend over an entire crown of a tooth which is unopposed, out of occlusion, or not used during mastication.

Table 16–2.   Characteristics of Dental Plaque and Materia Alba

Characteristic	Dental Plaque	Materia Alba
Clinical Appearance	Tooth: dull, dingy, slimy Thin, freshly deposited plaque: 　transparent (seen by application of 　disclosing agent) or stained light 　brown or gray from foods, tobacco, 　or chromogenic bacteria Heavy, older plaque: matted, fur-like 　surface, usually stained	Soft, cheese-like, mealy White or cream-colored Opaque May extend over the gingival margin Adjacent gingival margin frequently 　shows signs of irritation with redness 　and enlargement
Distribution	Supragingival plaque 　Initially on proximal surfaces and 　　cervical areas from which it creeps 　　over the tooth surfaces 　Heaviest deposits on: 　　Areas protected from cleaning 　　Proximal surfaces 　　Cervical third, particularly facial 　　　surfaces 　　Lingual mandibular molars Subgingival plaque on root surfaces Pit and fissure plaque External gingival surfaces 　oral epithelium 　attached gingiva	Surfaces not exposed to cleansing by 　brushing and flossing May cover entire crown of a tooth out 　of occlusion Collects in open interdental areas Heaviest deposits on: 　Facial cervical third 　Lingual mandibular molars 　Facial maxillary molars
Occurrence	All teeth and on removable appliances Always present before mineralization of 　calculus; occurs over the surface of 　calculus deposits	Associated with unclean areas of the 　mouth, and teeth out of occlusion
Method of Removal	Toothbrushing, flossing Not removed by rinsing or water spray	Toothbrushing Vigorous rinsing and water spray can 　remove the deposit
Recurrence	Pellicle forms within minutes Disclosable plaque forms within 12 to 　24 hours after complete removal	Readily when teeth are not cleaned 　regularly by toothbrushing
Composition and Structure	Gel-like mat of masses of microor- 　ganisms and intermicrobial matrix Early plaque: coccoid forms 　predominate, then filaments Older plaque: vibrios and spirochetes 　primarily Structured: filamentous organisms are 　arranged at right angles to the tooth 　surface Subgingival: more anaerobic forms	Unstructured accumulation of: masses 　of living and dead microorganisms 　(similar to types found in dental 　plaque); food debris particles; 　desquamated epithelial cells; 　disintegrated leukocytes
Source	Product of bacterial growth	Product of accumulation and bacterial 　growth

Table 16–2. *continued*

Characteristic	Dental Plaque	Materia Alba
Attachment	Firm: adheres closely to the acquired pellicle over the tooth surface and removable appliances Attaches to irregularities in the tooth surface	Loosely attached Adheres to dental plaque, teeth, restorations, and gingiva
Significance to Oral Health	Cariogenic plaque: harbors the strains of streptococci which form acid to decalcify tooth structure leading to dental caries Calculogenic plaque: provides matrix for mineralization of calculus Periodontal-disease-producing plaque: direct relation to the initiation of periodontal disease	Contributes to initiation and progress of dental caries, dental calculus, and gingivitis and periodontal diseases Unesthetic Contributes to halitosis: contains decomposing food debris

B. Detection

1. *Direct Vision*
   a. Thin plaque: may be translucent and therefore not visible.
   b. Stained plaque: may acquire stains that make it visible; for example, yellow, green, tobacco, as described on pages 286–288.
   c. Thick plaque: the tooth may appear dull, dingy, with a matted fur-like surface. Materia alba or food debris may collect over the plaque.

2. *Use of Explorer*
   a. Tactile examination. When calcification has started, plaque may feel slightly rough; otherwise the surface may feel only somewhat slippery due to the coating of soft, slimy plaque.
   b. Removal of plaque. When no plaque is visible, an explorer can be passed over the tooth surface, and if plaque is present, it will adhere to the explorer tip. This technique is used when evaluating for a Plaque Index (page 301).

3. *Use of Disclosing Agent.* When a disclosing agent is applied, plaque takes on the color and becomes readily visible. Disclosing agent should not be applied until after the evaluation of the oral mu-

cosa and gingival color has been recorded.

C. Clinical Record

1. Record plaque by location and extent (slight, moderate, or heavy). An index or plaque score may be used.
2. Plaque recordings and indices are kept for comparison in conjunction with the instructional plan for plaque control by the patient, both current and for recall appointments.
3. Plaque evaluation records are included with the complete charting and oral examination.

III. Formation of Plaque

A. Steps

   Plaque is formed in three basic steps, namely, pellicle formation, bacterial colonization, and plaque maturation (figure 16–1). Plaque formation does not occur randomly but involves a series of complex interactions, not all of which are completely researched.

1. *Formation of a Pellicle.* The pellicle forms on the tooth surface by rapid and selective adsorption of protein components from the saliva (page 261).
2. *Bacteria Attach to the Pellicle.* Initial attachment of bacteria to the pellicle is by

STAGE I Salivary glycoproteins are adsorbed onto dental enamel to form pellicle.

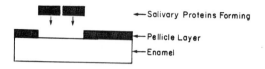

STAGE 2 Selective colonization of the pellicle by microorganisms.

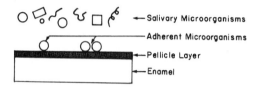

STAGE 3 Growth and maturation of plaque.

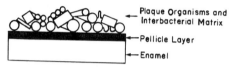

Figure 16–1. Diagrammatic representation of the three stages of plaque formation. (From Katz, McDonald, and Stookey: Preventive Dentistry. Upper Montclair, N.J., DCP Publishing, 1977.)

rapid and selective adsorption of specific bacteria from the oral environment. Innate characteristics of the bacteria and the pellicle determine the adhesive interactions that make a particular organism adsorb to a particular pellicle.

3. *Bacterial Multiplication.* Microcolonies form in layers as the bacteria multiply and grow. With increased size of colonies, they meet and coalesce to form a continuous bacterial mass.

4. *Plaque Growth and Maturation.* The increase in the mass and thickness of plaque results from
   a. Continued bacterial growth and multiplication.
   b. Continuous adsorption of bacteria to the plaque surface.

5. *Matrix Formation.* The carbohydrate-protein-lipid matrix material is derived mainly from saliva for supragingival plaque and from gingival sulcus fluid for subgingival plaque. Other materials are from the bacteria themselves.

B. Plaque Adhesion Interactions[5]

1. If plaque is to develop and adhere to the

teeth, mechanisms for adhesive interaction must be effective. The following interactions occur:
   a. Between cells and the pellicle and tooth.
   b. Cell-to-cell of the same species.
   c. Cell-to-cell between different species.

2. Agents or substances that provide adhesion.
   a. Surface components of the cells adsorb to the surface components of pellicle or other organisms.
   b. Extracellular polysaccharides, synthesized by the microorganisms, are sticky and aid in the aggregation of bacteria. The most profuse of these is dextran, produced by *Streptococcus mutans* from sucrose in the diet.

IV. Composition

Plaque is composed of microorganisms and intermicrobial matrix. Organic and inorganic solids constitute approximately 20 percent, and water 80 percent. Microorganisms make up at least 70 percent of the solid matter, which is higher in subgingival plaque than in supragingival.

Composition differs between individuals and between different tooth surfaces of an individual. As plaque ages, it changes.

A. Inorganic Elements[6,7]

1. *Calcium and Phosphorus.* The concentration of calcium, phosphorus, magnesium, and fluoride are higher in plaque than in saliva, which illustrates the ability of plaque to concentrate inorganic elements.

   Plaque on the lingual surfaces of the mandibular anterior teeth contains a higher concentration of calcium and phosphate than on the other teeth, and the amount is even higher on those same surfaces in heavy calculus formers.

2. *Fluoride.* Fluoride in plaque is higher when fluoridated water is used, and is increased following topical applications of fluoride or the use of dentifrices.[8,9] It has also been shown that the amount of

plaque was decreased following the use of a mouthrinse.[10]

B. Organic Components

In addition to the organic matrix and the microorganisms, plaque (particularly subgingival plaque) may have epithelial cells and leukocytes which contribute to the organic content. Materials contained within the matrix vary. Diet influences the available fermentable carbohydrate. Constituents of the matrix may include, or be derived from, the following:

1. Products of bacterial metabolism: acids, antigens, enzymes, toxins, and endotoxins.
2. Salivary constituents: proteins, carbohydrates, lipids.
3. Soluble food components, particularly fermentable carbohydrates.
4. Broken down cells of microorganisms.
5. Leukocytes and shed epithelial cells.
6. Extracellular polysaccharides synthesized from sucrose by bacteria. Dextran is a major carbohydrate component.
7. Subgingival plaque: contains components from the gingival sulcus fluid.

C. Plaque Microorganisms

Dental plaque consists of a complex mixture of microorganisms which occur primarily as microcolonies. The population density is very high and increases as plaque ages. The probability of the development of dental caries and gingivitis increases as the number of microorganisms increases.

Changes in the types of organisms occur within plaque as the plaque matures. When oral hygiene practices are discontinued, the numbers of bacteria increase rapidly. The changes in oral flora follow a pattern such as shown in figure 16–2. The changes may be described as follows:[11,12]

1. *Days 1 to 2.* Early plaque consists primarily of cocci. Streptococci, which dominate the bacterial population, include *Streptococcus mutans* and *Streptococcus sanguis.*
2. *Days 2 to 4.* The cocci still dominate, and increasing numbers of filamentous forms and slender rods may be seen on the surface of the cocci colonies. Grad-

ually, the filamentous forms grow into the cocci layer and replace most of the cocci. Slow plaque formers continue to form plaque comprised primarily of cocci for a longer time than fast plaque formers.

3. *Days 4 to 7.* Filaments increase in numbers, and a more mixed flora begins to appear with rods, filamentous forms, and fusobacteria. Plaque near the gingival margin is thicker and develops a more mature flora earlier, with spirochetes and vibrios. As plaque spreads coronally, the new plaque has the characteristic coccal forms.
4. *Days 7 to 14.* Vibrios and spirochetes appear and the number of white blood cells increases.

   As plaque matures and thickens, more gram-negative and anaerobic organisms appear. During the period when this is happening, signs of inflammation are beginning to be observable in the gingiva.
5. *Days 14 to 21.* Older plaque. Vibrios and spirochetes are prevalent, along with cocci and filamentous forms. The densely packed filamentous microorganisms arrange themselves perpendicular to the tooth surface in a palisade. Gingivitis is evident clinically.

D. Comparison of Supragingival and Subgingival Plaque

The sulcus or pocket provides a different environment for plaque than the supragingival areas. Almost the entire volume of pocket contents is microorganisms and leukocytes.

1. *Effect of Anatomic Form*[13]
   a. Shape. Plaque in a pocket is molded to the outline of the pocket wall. The shape of the pocket favors deposit retention.
   b. Cleaning limitations. A shallow sulcus can be cleaned by toothbrushing and other devices, but a deep pocket has a protected, deep, narrow base that cannot be reached by mechanical devices or by the saliva or tongue for self-cleansing.
2. *Microorganisms*[12,14]
   a. Types of organisms. Deep, closed

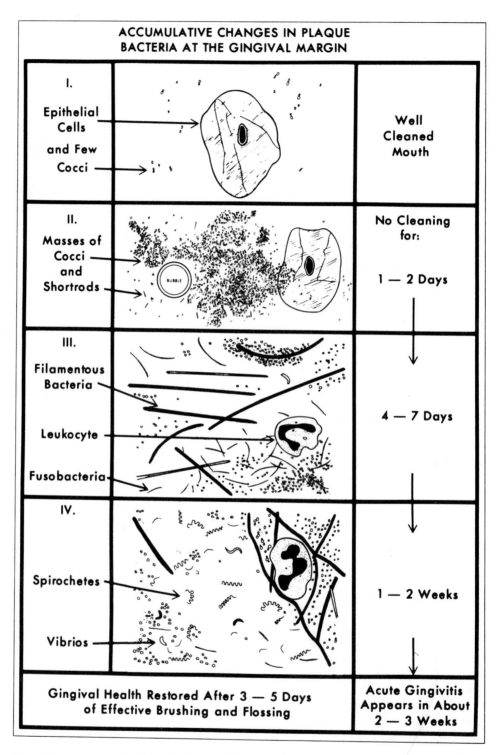

Figure 16–2.   Plaque microorganisms. Changes in plaque bacteria at the gingival margin as the plaque ages. (From Crawford, J.J., *In* Richardson and Barton: The Dental Assistant, 5th Ed. New York, McGraw-Hill Book Co., 1978.)

pockets create an environment favorable to the general growth of microorganisms and specifically to anaerobic growth.

  b. Flora. A more complex flora can be found in subgingival plaque earlier in development than is typical of supragingival plaque. Spirochetes, fusiforms, and *Bacteroides melaninogenicus* occur in greater numbers than in supragingival plaque. Specific organisms are related to specific periodontal diseases.

  c. Arrangement of microorganisms
    (1) External surface (the part next to the sulcular and junctional epithelia) has leukocytes, desquamated epithelial cells, and many spirochetes. Spirochetes tend to grow preferentially next to the gingival tissues.
    (2) Deep part of the pocket: the flora varies with the type of periodontal disease.

  d. Source of nutrients. Plaque matrix materials and nutrients for the bacteria are obtained from the gingival sulcus fluid.

V. Effect of Diet on Plaque

A. Content

1. Dental plaque is a product of bacterial growth and is not composed of food.
2. *Cariogenic Foods*
  a. Dental caries. The relationship of the cariogenic food content of the diet and its frequency of use to the development of dental caries is well defined in research and clinical application. Dental caries initiation is outlined in figure 16–3.
  b. Effect of sucrose on amount and pH of plaque. When a cariogenic diet is used, plaque forms and grows more profusely.[15] Patients fed sucrose by stomach tube had a less acidogenic plaque than patients who were fed by mouth.[16]

B. Food Intake

Food particles are not needed in the mouth for plaque to form. In one study, neither varying the number of meals nor feeding by stomach tube affected the development of plaque.[17] In another study, less plaque developed in a group of stomach-fed patients when compared with those fed by mouth.[16]

C. Texture of Diet

1. *Mechanical Removal of Plaque.* The friction of mastication has been shown to affect only the occlusal and incisal thirds of the crowns of teeth. Plaque on the gingival third collected in spite of a normal diet that included coarse bread and fresh fruit,[11] or chewing raw carrots three times daily as the only methods for personal care.[18] Chewing apples did not affect moderate amounts of plaque, but did tend to remove food debris in a group of 12-year-olds.[19]

2. *Soft Diet.* A soft diet tends to favor plaque accumulation. Although not well documented in the literature, clinical experience has shown the soft diet, especially one with excess fermentable carbohydrates, to lead to excess plaque formation. In one experiment using dogs, it was shown that more plaque developed when a soft diet was used.[20]

SIGNIFICANCE OF BACTERIAL PLAQUE

I. Plaque and Dental Caries

Dental caries is a disease of the dental calcified structures (enamel, dentin, and cementum) which is characterized by decalcification of the mineral components and dissolution of the organic matrix. Clinical characteristics and types of cavities were described on pages 238–242.

A. Essentials for Dental Caries

1. *Susceptible Tooth Surface.* A tooth with optimum fluoride content resists the process of dental caries.
2. *Specific Microorganisms.*[21] Dental plaque contains many acidogenic microorganisms, especially streptococci, which have been shown to be involved in the etiology of dental caries. *Streptococcus mutans* has particular cariogenic poten-

CARIOGENIC + FOODSTUFF	BACTERIAL PLAQUE	= ACID FORMATION
ACID +	SUSCEPTIBLE TOOTH SURFACE	= DECALCIFICATION (Initial Dental Caries)

Figure 16–3. Dental caries initiation.

tial in the development of smooth-surface caries.

3. *Cariogenic Foodstuff Source*

a. Cariogenic microorganisms have the ability to synthesize carbohydrates into extracellular polysaccharides (dextrans, levans, and other glucans and fructans) and intracellular polysaccharides which are stored. *Streptococcus mutans, Streptococcus sanguis,* and *Streptococcus mitis* are involved in enamel caries.

Other organisms, *Actinomyces viscosus* and *Actinomyces naeslundii,* are involved in root-surface caries. They do not produce glucans, but synthesize other surface constituents for aggregation and plaque formation.[22]

b. Dextran and other substances contribute to plaque formation and plaque adherence to the tooth; they may also serve as a barrier to the diffusion of buffers which might be available to neutralize the acids formed in plaque.

c. Acid is formed by the breakdown of the sucrose. The acid acts to dissolve or demineralize the tooth surface. With sufficient exposures (frequent use of cariogenic foods) tooth structure breaks down. At first, an area of decalcification (soft white spot) appears and then a definite carious lesion develops.

d. When cariogenic foods are not available in the diet, stored intracellular polysaccharides can be converted into acid. There are many more polysaccharide-storing organisms in

the plaque of a caries-active than the plaque of a caries-free person.

e. The dental caries process within the plaque and on the tooth surface outlined in figure 16–3.

B. **Contributing Factors**

1. *Time.* Acid formation begins *immediately* when the sucrose from food is taken into the plaque.

2. *The pH of the Plaque.* The plaque's pH is lowered promptly, and it takes from one to two hours for the pH to return to a normal level, assuming the plaque left undisturbed.

a. Plaque pH before eating ranges from 6.2 to 7.0; it is lower in the caries-susceptible person and higher in the caries-resistant.

b. Immediately following sucrose intake into plaque, a rapid drop in the pH of the plaque occurs.[23,24]

c. Critical pH for enamel decalcification averages about 5.0, below which the enamel will decalcify.

d. The amount of decalcification depends on the length of time and the frequency with which the acid with a pH below 5.0 is in contact with the tooth surface.

3. *Frequency of Carbohydrate Intake.* With each meal or snack, when sucrose is used, the pH of the plaque is lowered provided the specific streptococci are present. Large amounts of sucrose eaten at mealtimes can be expected to be less cariogenic than small amounts eaten at frequent intervals during the day.[2] These and other related facts can be presented to the patient when the diet is discussed as a part of the basic instruc-

tion or as part of a total dental caries control program with dietary analysis (pages 432–435).

I. Bacterial Plaque and Periodontal Diseases

Dental plaque is unquestionably the single most important etiologic factor in most periodontal diseases. The variations in clinical manifestations in different individuals can be accounted for by the differences in the bacterial activity within the plaque as well as by the tissue response and resistance to the microorganisms and their products.

A. Initiation of Gingival Disease

Microorganisms of the dental plaque at the gingival margin multiply and extend beneath the margin; the area of contact between the plaque and the soft tissue increases; and a high concentration of microorganisms is in contact with the sulcular epithelium. The irritation from the bacteria and their products leads to degeneration of the sulcular epithelium and inflammation in the adjacent connective tissue. The steps in the development of gingivitis and pocket formation are described on pages 202–204.

B. Experimental Gingivitis[11]

Gingivitis will develop in 2 to 3 weeks when plaque is left undisturbed on the tooth surfaces. The microbiologic changes were outlined on page 267. Acute gingivitis is reversible, and when the gingiva are treated by plaque removal procedures the gingiva will return to health in 5 to 7 days.

To demonstrate the effect of plaque, an experimental gingivitis program can be conducted as follows:
1. Observe and record characteristics of the healthy gingiva at the outset. Record a gingival index and a plaque index.
2. Withhold all plaque control procedures for a period of 3 weeks.
3. Repeat clinical observations of tissues and record indexes at least weekly during the test period. Note initial evidence of gingivitis.
4. Reinstate plaque removal measures after 3 weeks. Make daily observations rela-

tive to gingival bleeding and indications that healing is taking place. In one week, repeat gingival and plaque indexes.

C. Calculus Formation

Bacterial plaque forms a matrix for calculus formation (page 278). The significance of calculus is described on page 281.

MATERIA ALBA

Materia alba ("white material") distinguishes itself clinically by being a bulky, loosely connected, soft deposit that is clearly visible without application of a disclosing agent. It is white, or grayish-white, and characteristically may resemble cottage cheese. Other properties are compared with dental plaque in table 16–2.

Materia alba forms over dental plaque. It is a product of informal accumulation of living and dead bacteria, desquamated epithelial cells, disintegrating leukocytes, salivary proteins, and particles of food debris. Although the bacterial count is high, it has been shown that the bacterial counts of materia alba are significantly lower than for dental plaque, and there are fewer living organisms in materia alba.[26]

Surface bacteria in contact with the gingiva can contribute to gingival inflammation, but the degree of inflammation is less than from dental plaque.[27] Although clinically, tooth surface decalcification and dental caries are frequently seen under materia alba, the direct effect of the dental plaque under the materia alba is the significant action, and materia alba bacteria are not the specific etiologic agents.

Clinical distinction between materia alba, food debris, and dental plaque is necessary, but patient instruction for the removal of all three involves the same basic plaque control procedures. Materia alba can be removed with a water spray or oral irrigator whereas dental plaque cannot.

FOOD DEBRIS

Loose food particles following eating collect about the cervical third and proximal embrasures of the teeth.

When there are open contact areas, mobility of teeth, or irregularities of occlusion such as plunger cusps, food may be forced between the teeth during mastication and vertical food impaction result. Horizontal or lateral food impaction occurs in facial and lingual embrasures, particularly when the interdental papillae are reduced or missing.

The role of food in the oral cavity during plaque formation was described briefly on page 269. Food debris adds to a general unsanitary condition of the mouth. Cariogenic foods contribute to dental caries as liquified carbohydrate diffuses rapidly into the plaque and hence to the acid-forming bacteria.

Some self-cleansing through the action of the tongue, lips, saliva, and related factors takes place. Debris removal by toothbrushing, flossing, and other aids constitutes a total plaque control program. Cleansing of debris from about fixed prosthetic and orthodontic appliances is important to the plan for oral sanitation.

TECHNICAL HINTS

I. Check all surfaces of restorations and prosthetic appliances and remove rough areas and overhanging margins. Soft deposits accumulate on rough or irregular surfaces more rapidly and in greater quantity than on smooth surfaces.

II. Withhold the use of a disclosing agent until the intraoral mucosal and gingival examinations have been made. Coloring agents can disguise soft tissue changes and deviations from normal.

FACTORS TO TEACH THE PATIENT

I. Location, composition, and properties of dental plaque with emphasis on its role in dental caries and periodontal disease initiation.

II. The cause and prevention of dental caries.

III. Effects of personal oral care procedures in the prevention of dental plaque and materia alba.

IV. Plaque control procedures with special adaptations for individual needs.

V. Sources of cariogenic foodstuff in the diet with suggestions for control.

VI. Relationship of frequency of eating cariogenic foods to dental caries.

References

1. Schroeder, H.E.: *Formation and Inhibition of Dental Calculus.* Vienna, Hans Huber, 1969, pp. 14–15.
2. Meckel, A.H.: Formation and Properties of Organic Films on Teeth, *Arch. Oral Biol.*, *10*, 585, July–August 1965.
3. Meckel, A.H.: The Nature and Importance of Organic Deposits on Dental Enamel, *Caries Res.*, *2*, 104, Number 2, 1968.
4. Goldman, H.M. and Cohen, D.W.: *Periodontal Therapy*, 6th ed. St. Louis, The C.V. Mosby Co., 1980, pp. 78–85.
5. Gibbons, R.J. and van Houte, J.: On the Formation of Dental Plaques, *J. Periodontol.*, *44*, 347, June, 1973.
6. Mandel, I.D.: Relation of Saliva and Plaque to Caries, *J. Dent. Res.*, *53*, 246, March–April, 1974, Supplement.
7. Grøn, P., Yao, K., and Spinelli, M.: A Study of Inorganic Constituents in Dental Plaque, *J. Dent. Res.*, *48*, 799, September–October, 1969.
8. Jenkins, G.N., Edgar, W.M., and Ferguson, D.B.: The Distribution and Metabolic Effects of Human Plaque Fluorine, *Arch. Oral Biol.*, *14*, 105, January, 1969.
9. Birkeland, J.M.: Fluoride Content of Dental Plaque after Brushing with a Fluoride Dentifrice, *Scand. J. Dent. Res.*, *80*, 80, Number 1, 1972.
10. Birkeland, J.M.: Effect of Fluoride on the Amount of Dental Plaque in Children, *Scand. J. Dent. Res.*, *80*, 82, Number 1, 1972.
11. Löe, H., Theilade, E., and Jensen, S.B.: Experimental Gingivitis in Man, *J. Periodontol.*, *36*, 177, May–June 1965.
12. Listgarten, M.A., Mayo, H.E., and Tremblay, R.: Development of Dental Plaque on Epoxy Resin Crowns in Man, *J. Periodontol.*, *46*, 10, January, 1975.
13. Kelstrup, J. and Theilade, E.: Microbes and Periodontal Disease, *J. Clin. Periodontol.*, *1*, 15, Number 1, 1974.
14. Socransky, S.S.: Relationship of Bacteria to the Etiology of Periodontal Disease, *J. Dent. Res.*, *49*, 203, March–April, 1970 (Part 1).
15. Carlsson, J. and Egelberg, J.: Effect of Diet on Early Plaque Formation in Man, *Odont. Revy*, *16*, 112, Number 1, 1965.
16. Littleton, N.W., Carter, C.H., and Kelley, R.T.: Studies of Oral Health in Persons Nourished by Stomach Tube. I. Changes in pH of Plaque Material after the Addition of Sucrose, *J. Am. Dent. Assoc.*, *74*, 119, January, 1967.
17. Egelberg, J.: Local Effect of Diet on Plaque Formation and Development of Gingivitis in Dogs. III. Effect of Frequency of Meals and Tube Feeding, *Odont. Revy*, *16*, 50, Number 1, 1965.
18. Lindhe, J. and Wicén, P-O.: The Effects on the Gingivae of Chewing Fibrous Foods, *J. Periodont. Res.*, *4*, 193, Number 3, 1969.
19. Birkeland, J.M. and Jorkjend, L.: The Effect of Chewing Apples on Dental Plaque and Food Debris, *Community Dent. Oral Epidemiol.*, *2*, 161, Number 4, 1974.
20. Egelberg, J.: Local Effect of Diet on Plaque Formation and Development of Gingivitis in Dogs. I. Effect of Hard and Soft Diets, *Odont. Revy*, *16*, 31, Number 1, 1965.
21. Newbrun, E.: *Cariology*. Baltimore, The Williams and Wilkins Co., 1978, pp. 45–50.
22. Jordan, H.V. and Hammond, B.F.: Filamentous Bacteria Isolated from Human Root Surface Caries, *Arch. Oral Biol.*, *17*, 1333, September, 1972.
23. Stephan, R.M.: Intra-oral Hydrogen-Ion Concentrations Associated with Dental Caries Activity, *J. Dent. Res.*, *23*, 257, August, 1944.
24. Rosen, S. and Weisenstein, P.R.: The Effect of Sugar Solutions on pH of Dental Plaques from Caries-Susceptible and Caries-Free Individuals, *J. Dent. Res.*, *44*, 845, September–October, 1965.

5. Gustafsson, B.E., Quensel, C.E., Lanke, L.S., Lundquist, C., Grahnén, H., Bonow, B.E., and Krasse, B.: The Vipeholm Dental Caries Study. The Effect of Different Levels of Carbohydrate Intake on Caries Activity in 436 Individuals Observed for Five Years, *Acta Odont. Scand.*, 11, 232, Number 3–4, 1954.

6. Salkind, A., Oshrain, H.I., and Mandel, I.D.: Materia Alba and Dental Plaque, *J. Periodontol.*, 45, 489, July, 1974.

7. Schwartz, R.S., Massler, M., and LeBeau, L.J.: Gingival Reactions to Different Types of Tooth Accumulated Materials, *J. Periodontol.*, 42, 144, March, 1971.

Suggested Readings

Ashley, F.P. and Wilson, R.F.: Dental Plaque and Caries. A 3-year Longitudinal Study in Children, *Br. Dent. J.*, 142, 85, February 1, 1977.

Brown, A.T.: The Role of Dietary Carbohydrates in Plaque Formation and Oral Disease, *Nutrition Reviews*, 33, 353, December, 1975.

Carranza, F.A.: *Glickman's Clinical Periodontology*, 5th ed. Philadelphia, W.B. Saunders Co., 1979, pp. 374–404.

Crawford, J.J.: Microbiology, in Richardson, R.E. and Barton, R.E.: *The Dental Assistant*, 5th ed. New York, McGraw-Hill, 1978, pp. 117–134.

Grant, D.A., Stern, I.B., and Everett, F.G.: *Periodontics*, 5th ed., St. Louis, The C.V. Mosby Co., 1979, pp. 135–151.

Duke, S.A., Rees, D.A., and Forward, G.C.: Increased Plaque Calcium and Phosphorus Concentrations After Using a Calcium Carbonate Toothpaste Containing Calcium Glycerophosphate and Sodium Monofluorophosphate. Pilot Study, *Caries Res.*, 13, 57, Number 1, 1979.

Edgar, W.M.: The Role of Saliva in the Control of pH Changes in Human Dental Plaque, *Caries Res.*, 10, 241, Number 4, 1976.

Halhoul, N. and Colvin, J.R.: The Ultrastructure of Bacterial Plaque Attached to the Gingiva of Man, *Arch. Oral Biol.*, 20, 115, February, 1975.

Holm-Pedersen, P., Folke, L.E.A., and Gawronski, T.H.: Composition and Metabolic Activity of Dental Plaque from Healthy Young and Elderly Individuals, *J. Dent. Res.*, 59, 771, May, 1980.

Jenkins, G.N.: *The Physiology and Biochemistry of the Mouth*, 4th ed. Philadelphia, J.B. Lippincott Co., 1978, pp. 360–401.

Katz, S., McDonald, J.L., and Stookey, G.K.: *Preventive Dentistry*. Upper Montclair, New Jersey, D.C.P. Publishing, 1977, pp. 57–72.

Kelstrup, J., Theilade, J., and Fejerskov, O.: Surface Ultrastructure of Some Oral Bacteria, *Scand. J. Dent. Res.*, 87, 415, December, 1979.

Lie, T.: Morphologic Studies on Dental Plaque Formation, *Acta Odontol. Scand.*, 37, 73, Number 2, 1979.

Lie, T.: Ultrastructural Study of Early Dental Plaque Formation, *J. Periodont. Res.*, 13, 391, September, 1978.

Lie, T.: Scanning and Transmission Electron Microscope Study of Pellicle Morphogenesis, *Scand. J. Dent. Res.*, 85, 217, May, 1977.

Lie, T.: Early Dental Plaque Morphogenesis, *J. Periodont. Res.*, 12, 73, March, 1977.

Newbrun, E.: *Cariology*. Baltimore, Williams and Wilkins, 1978, pp. 129–191.

Newman, H.N.: Update on Plaque and Periodontal Disease, *J. Clin. Periodontol.*, 7, 251, August, 1980.

Newman, H.N.: The Approximal Apical Border of Plaque on Children's Teeth. 1. Morphology, Structure and Cell Content, *J. Periodontol.*, 50, 561, November, 1979.

Newman, H.N.: The Approximal Apical Border of Plaque on Children's Teeth. 2. Adhesion, Interbacterial Connections and Carbohydrate Metabolism, *J. Periodontol.*, 50, 568, November, 1979.

Ramfjord, S.P. and Ash, M.M: *Periodontology and Periodontics*. Philadelphia, W.B. Saunders Co., 1979, pp. 145–156.

Saglie, R., Johansen, J.R., and Flötra, L.: Scanning Electron Microscopic Study of Tooth Surfaces in Pathologic Pockets, *Scand. J. Dent. Res.*, 82, 579, Number 8, 1974.

Saglie, R., Johansen, J.R., and Tollefsen, T.: Plaque-free Zones on Human Teeth in Periodontitis, *J. Clin. Periodontol.*, 2, 190, November, 1975.

Satin, E., Apton, R., and Goldman, R.: Plaque pH: A New Frontier for the Dental Hygienist, *Dent. Hyg.*, 52, 119, March, 1978.

Saxton, C.A.: Scanning Electron Microscope Study of the Formation of Dental Plaque, *Caries Res.*, 7, 102, Number 2, 1973.

Smith, Q.T.: Acquired Pellicle: A Mediator of Enamel Demineralization and Remineralization, *Northwest Dent.*, 59, 152, May–June, 1980.

Theilade, J.: Development of Bacterial Plaque in the Oral Cavity, *J. Clin. Periodontol.*, 4, 1, December, 1977.

Tinanoff, N.: The Significance of the Acquired Pellicle in the Practice of Dentistry, *J. Dent. Child.*, 43, 20, January–February, 1976.

Tinanoff, N., Glick, P.L., and Weber, D.F.: Ultrastructure of Organic Films on the Enamel Surface, *Caries Res.*, 10, 19, Number 1, 1976.

Tinanoff, N., Gross, A., and Brady, J.M.: Development of Plaque on Enamel, Parallel Investigations, *J. Periodont. Res.*, 11, 197, July, 1976.

Tinanoff, N. and Tanzer, J.M.: Bacterial Pellicle-like Substances and Polyphosphate Formation by Enamel-adherent Oral Microorganisms, *Pediatric Dent.*, 1, 1, March, 1979.

Microbiologic Studies

Kelstrup, J. and Theilade, E.: Microbes and Periodontal Disease, *J. Clin. Periodontol.*, 1, 15, Number 1, 1974.

Listgarten, M.A.: Structure of Surface Coatings on Teeth. A Review, *J. Periodontol.*, 47, 139, March, 1976.

Listgarten, M.A.: Structure of the Microbial Flora Associated with Periodontal Health and Disease in Man, *J. Periodontol.*, 47, 1, January, 1976.

Listgarten, M.A. and Helldén, L.: Relative Distribution of Bacteria at Clinically Healthy and Periodontally Diseased Sites in Humans, *J. Clin. Periodontol.*, 5, 115, May, 1978.

Listgarten, M.A. and Levin, S.: Positive Correlation Between the Proportions of Subgingival Spirochetes and Motile Bacteria and Susceptibility of Human Subjects to Periodontal Deterioration, *J. Clin. Periodontol.*, 8, 122, April, 1981.

Loesche, W.J.: The Bacteriology of Dental Decay and Periodontal Disease, *Clin. Prev. Dent.*, 2, 18, May–June, 1980.

Newman, M.G., Grinenco, V., Weiner, M., Angel, I., Karge, H., and Nisengard, R.: Predominant Microbiota Associated with Periodontal Health in the Aged, *J. Periodontol.*, 49, 553, November, 1978.

Newman, M.G. and Socransky, S.S.: Predominant Cultivable Microbiota in Periodontosis, *J. Periodont. Res.*, 12, 120, March, 1977.

Newman, M.G., Socransky, S.S., Savitt, E.D., Propas, D.A., and Crawford, A.: Studies of the Microbiology of Periodontosis, *J. Periodontol.*, 47, 373, July, 1976.

Slots, J.: Microflora in the Healthy Gingival Sulcus in Man, *Scand. J. Dent. Res.*, 85, 247, May, 1977.

Slots, J.: The Predominant Cultivable Microflora of Advanced Periodontitis, *Scand. J. Dent. Res.*, *85*, 114, January–February, 1977.

Slots, J.: The Predominant Cultivable Organisms in Juvenile Periodontitis, *Scand. J. Dent. Res.*, *84*, 1, January, 1976.

Socransky, S.S.: Microbiology of Periodontal Disease—Present Status and Future Considerations, *J. Periodontol.*, *48*, 497, September, 1977.

Socransky, S.S. and Manganiello, A.D.: The Oral Microbiota of Man from Birth to Senility, *J. Periodontol.*, *42*, 485, August, 1971.

Socransky, S.S., Manganiello, A.D., Propas, D., Oram, V., and van Houte, J.: Bacteriological Studies of Developing Supragingival Dental Plaque, *J. Periodont. Res.*, *12*, 90, March, 1977.

Williams, B.L., Pantalone, R.M., and Sherris, J.C.: Subgingival Microflora and Periodontitis, *J. Periodont. Res.*, *11*, 1, February, 1976.

Experimental Gingivitis

Brecx, M., Theilade, J., and Attström, R.: Influence of Optimal and Excluded Oral Hygiene on Early Formation of Dental Plaque on Plastic Films, a Quantitative and Descriptive Light and Electron Microscopic Study, *J. Clin. Periodontol.*, 7, 361, October, 1980.

de la Rosa, M., Guerra, J.Z., Johnston, D.A., and Radike, A.W.: Plaque Growth and Removal with Daily Toothbrushing, *J. Periodontol.*, *50*, 661, December, 1979.

Holm-Pedersen, P.: Experimental Gingivitis in Young and Elderly Individuals, *J. Clin. Periodontol.*, *2*, 14, February, 1975.

Katayama, T., Suzuki, T., and Okada, S.: Clinical Observation of Dental Plaque Maturation, *J. Periodontol.*, *46*, 610, October, 1975.

Lang, N.P., Cumming, B.R., and Löe, H.: Toothbrushing Frequency as It Relates to Plaque Development and Gingival Health, *J. Periodontol.*, *44*, 396, July, 1973.

Löe, H.: Human Research Model for the Production and Prevention of Gingivitis, *J. Dent. Res.*, *50*, 256, Supplement to Number 2, 1971.

Matsson, L.: Development of Gingivitis in Pre-school Children and Young Adults, *J. Clin. Periodontol.*, *5*, 24, February, 1978.

von der Fehr, F.R., Löe, H., and Theilade, E.: Experimental Caries in Man, *Caries Res.*, *4*, 131, Number 2, 1970.

Smoking and Plaque

Bastiaan, R.J. and Waite, I.M.: Effects of Tobacco Smoking on Plaque Development and Gingivitis, *J. Periodontol.*, *49*, 480, September, 1978.

Kenney, E.B., Saxe, S.R., and Bowles, R.D.: The Effect of Cigarette Smoking on Anaerobiosis in the Oral Cavity, *J. Periodontol.*, *46*, 82, February, 1975.

Preber, H., Kant, T., and Bergström, J.: Cigarette Smoking, Oral Hygiene and Periodontal Health in Swedish Army Conscripts, *J. Clin. Periodontol.*, *7*, 106, April, 1980.

Sheiham, A.: Periodontal Disease and Oral Cleanliness in Tobacco Smokers, *J. Periodontol.*, *42*, 259, May, 1971.

Swenson, H.M.: The Effect of Cigarette Smoking on Plaque Formation, *J. Periodontol.*, *50*, 146, March, 1979.

Plaque Prevention

Addy, M., Griffiths, C., and Isaac, R.: The Effect of Povidone Iodine on Plaque and Salivary Bacteria. A Double-blind Crossover Trial, *J. Periodontol.*, *48*, 730, November, 1977.

Baker, P.J., Coburn, R.A., Genco, R.J., and Evans, R.T.: The *in vitro* Inhibition of Microbial Growth and Plaque Formation by Surfactant Drugs, *J. Periodont. Res.*, *13*, 474, September, 1978.

Esposito, E.J.: Effect of Daily Rinsing with Alexidine on Supragingival Plaque pH, *J. Periodontol.*, *45*, 833, November, 1974.

Johnson, R.H. and Rozanis, J.: A Review of Chemotherapeutic Plaque Control, *Oral Surg.*, *47*, 136, February, 1979.

Kaslick, R.S., Shapiro, W.B., and Chasens, A.I.: Studies on the Effects of a Urea Peroxide Gel on Plaque Formation and Gingivitis, *J. Periodontol.*, *46*, 230, April, 1975.

Keyes, P.H. and McCabe, R.M.: The Potential of Various Compounds to Suppress Microorganisms in Plaques Produced *in vitro* by a Streptococcus or an Actinomycete, *J. Am. Dent. Assoc.*, *86*, 396, February, 1973.

Kornman, K.S., Caffesse, R.G., and Nasjleti, C.E.: The Effect of Intensive Antibacterial Therapy on the Sulcular Environment in Monkeys. Part 1. Changes in the Bacteriology of the Gingival Sulcus, *J. Periodontol.*, *51*, 34, January, 1980.

Lobene, R.R.: Clinical Studies of Plaque Control Agents: An Overview, *J. Dent. Res.*, *58*, 2381, December, 1979.

Lobene, R.R.: Chemotherapeutics for the Prevention of Dental Plaque, *J. Prev. Dent.*, *3*, 32, July–August, 1976.

Lobene, R.R. and Soparkar, P.M.: A Clinical Study of Antiplaque Agents, *J. Periodontol.*, *45*, 561, August, 1974.

Löe, H.: Mechanical and Chemical Control of Dental Plaque, *J. Clin. Periodontol.*, *6*, 32, December, 1979.

Loesche, W.J.: Clinical and Microbiological Aspects of Chemotherapeutic Agents Used According to the Specific Plaque Hypothesis, *J. Dent. Res.*, *58*, 2404, December, 1979.

Lusk, S.S., Bowers, G.M., Tow, H.D., Watson, W.J., and Moffitt, W.C.: Effects of an Oral Rinse on Experimental Gingivitis, Plaque Formation, and Formed Plaque, *J. Am. Soc. Prev. Dent.*, *4*, 31, July–August, 1974.

Nagle, P.J. and Turnbull, R.S.: Chlorhexidine: An Ideal Plaque Inhibiting Agent? *Can. Dent. Assoc. J.*, *44*, 73, February, 1978.

Parsons, J.C.: Chemotherapy of Dental Plaque—A Review, *J. Periodontol.*, *45*, 177, March, 1974.

Reddy, J. and Salkin, L.M.: The Effect of a Urea Peroxide Rinse on Dental Plaque and Gingivitis, *J. Periodontol.*, *47*, 607, October, 1976.

Saxén, L., Harjola, O., and Ainamo, J.: The Effect of Two Commercial Antibacterial Mouthrinses on Plaque Growth *in vivo*, *J. Clin. Periodontol.*, *3*, 195, November, 1976.

Spolsky, V.W., Bhatia, H.L., Forsythe, A., and Levin, D.: The Effect of an Antimicrobial Mouthwash on Dental Plaque and Gingivitis in Young Adults, *J. Periodontol.*, *46*, 685, November, 1975.

Suppipat, N., Gjermo, P., and Johansen, J.R.: Gingival Fluid Flow after Gingivectomy Related to Mechanical or Chemical Plaque Control, *J. Periodontol.*, *49*, 542, October, 1978.

Turesky, S., Glickman, I., and Sandberg, R.: *In vitro* Chemical Inhibition of Plaque Formation, *J. Periodontol.*, *43*, 263, May, 1973.

Waerhaug, J.: Effect of Toothbrushing on Subgingival Plaque Formation, *J. Periodontol.*, *52*, 30, January, 1981.

17

Dental Calculus

Dental calculus, which is calcified bacterial plaque, is a hard, tenacious mass which forms on the clinical crowns of the natural teeth and on dentures and other dental appliances. Calculus is significant in the progression of inflammatory periodontal disease.

The control of plaque deposits by the patient, supplemented by complete calculus removal, can reduce or eliminate gingival inflammation. There is a close relationship between the amount of plaque and calculus on the teeth and the severity of most gingival and periodontal diseases.

Comprehensive understanding of the characteristics, origin, development, and methods of prevention of calculus is essential to patient examination, evaluation, treatment, and instruction. For successful treatment and prevention, the patient needs to know the interrelationship between plaque, calculus, and oral health, the need for complete removal of calculus, and the reasons for the painstaking manner in which scaling procedures must be carried out.

I. Classification and Distribution

Dental calculus is classified by its location on a tooth surface as related to the adjacent free gingival margin, that is, supragingival and subgingival (figure 17–1).

A. Supragingival Calculus

1. *Location:* on the clinical crown above the margin of the gingiva.

2. *Distribution*
   a. Most frequent sites: lingual of mandibular anterior teeth and buccal of maxillary first and second molars, opposite the openings of the ducts of the salivary glands.
   b. Crowns of teeth out of occlusion; nonfunctioning teeth; or teeth that are neglected during plaque removal (toothbrushing, flossing, or other personal care).
   c. Surfaces of dentures and dental appliances.

3. *Other Names for Supragingival Calculus*
   a. Supramarginal*
   b. Extragingival
   c. Coronal: indicating that the calculus is on the anatomic crown.
   d. Salivary: a term that indicates that the source of the calculus is the saliva.

B. Subgingival Calculus

1. *Location:* on the clinical crown beneath the margin of the gingiva. It extends nearly to the bottom of the pocket. As

---

*The terms supra- and subgingival are at present probably the most widely used. Supra- and submarginal are more specific in their definition since the margin of the free gingiva is the dividing line between the two categories. The gingiva includes free and attached.

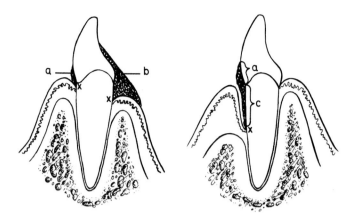

Figure 17–1. Location of dental calculus. **a.** Supragingival calculus. **b.** Extensive accumulation of supragingival calculus over crown, exposed root surface, and margin of the free gingiva. **c.** Subgingival calculus along root surface to bottom of periodontal pocket. **x.** Bottom of pocket. Note level of crest of alveolar bone in relation to bottom of the pocket.

the pocket is deepened by disease, calculus forms on the exposed root surface.

2. *Distribution*
   a. May be generalized or localized on single teeth or a group of teeth.
   b. Proximal surfaces have heaviest deposits.
3. *Other Names for Subgingival Calculus*
   a. Submarginal
   b. Serumal: term that indicates the source of the calculus materials is the blood serum.

II. Occurrence

A. Age

Calculus occurs at all ages and on both permanent and primary teeth. Incidence increases with age, and in some populations, 100 percent of the people over 30 have calculus, usually due to continuing accumulation, not an increased tendency to form new deposits as age advances.

B. Calculus in Children

In a survey of children ages 9 to 14, 56 to 85 percent had supragingival and 30 to 67 percent had subgingival calculus in the various age, sex, and racial–ethnic groups measured.[1] In another study in normal children, 9 percent of ages 4 to 6, 18 percent of ages 7 to 9, and 43 percent of ages 10 to 15 had calculus. In a group of children ages 10 to 15 with cystic fibrosis, 90 percent had calculus, and in a group of the same age with asthma, 100 percent had calculus.[2]

III. Clinical Characteristics

A. Appearance and Consistency

Identification of calculus prior to removal depends on knowledge of the appearance, consistency, and distribution. Appointment planning, selection of instruments, and techniques depend on understanding the texture, morphology, and mode of attachment of calculus. Table 17–1 provides a summary of clinical characteristics.

B. Supragingival Examination

1. *Direct Examination.* Supragingival deposits may be seen directly or indirectly, using a mouth mirror.
2. *Use of Compressed Air.* Small amounts of calculus that have not been stained are frequently invisible when they are wet with saliva. With a combination of retraction, light, and drying with air, small deposits usually can be seen. An explorer may be used when visual examination is not definite (page 223).

C. Subgingival Examination

1. *Visual Examination* of calculus within a pocket
   a. Dark edge of calculus may be seen at or just beneath the margin.

Table 17–1. Clinical Characteristics of Dental Calculus

Characteristic	Supragingival Calculus	Subgingival Calculus
Color	White, creamy-yellow, or gray May be stained by tobacco, food, or other pigments Slight deposits may be invisible until dried with compressed air	Light to dark brown, dark green, or black Stains derived from blood pigments from diseased pocket
Shape	Amorphous, bulky Gross deposits may: (1) Form interproximal bridge between adjacent teeth (2) Extend over the margin of the gingiva Shape of calculus mass is determined by the anatomy of the teeth, contour of gingival margin, and pressure of the tongue, lips, cheeks	Flattened to conform with pressure from the gingival pocket wall Combinations of the following calculus formations occur[3] (1) Crusty, spiny, or nodular (2) Ledge or ring-like formations (3) Thin, smooth veneers (4) Finger and fern-like formations (5) Individual calculus islands
Consistency and Texture	Moderately hard Newer deposits less dense and hard Porous Surface covered with plaque	Brittle, flint-like Harder and more dense than supragingival calculus Newest deposits near bottom of pocket are less dense and hard Surface covered with plaque
Size and Quantity	Quantity has direct relationship to: (1) Personal oral care procedures and plaque control measures (2) Physical character of diet (3) Individual tendencies (4) Function and use Increased amount in tobacco smokers	Related to pocket depth Increased amount with age because of accumulation Quantity is related to personal care, diet, and individual tendency as it is with supragingival. Subgingival is primarily related to the development and progression of periodontal disease
Distribution on Individual Tooth	Above margin of gingiva May cover a large portion of the visible clinical crown, or may form fine thin line near gingival margin	Below margin of gingiva Extends to bottom of the pocket and follows contour of soft tissue attachment With gingival recession, subgingival calculus may become supragingival and become covered with typical supragingival calculus
Distribution on Teeth	Symmetrical arrangement on teeth except when influenced by (1) Malpositioned teeth (2) Unilateral hypofunction (3) Inconsistent personal care (4) Abrasion from food Occurs with or without associated subgingival deposits Location related to openings of the salivary gland ducts: (1) Buccal of maxillary molars (2) Lingual mandibular anterior teeth	May be generalized or localized on a few teeth Heaviest on proximal surfaces, lightest on facials Occurs with or without associated supragingival deposits

b. Diseased gingival margin does not adapt closely to a tooth surface, thus permitting a view into the pocket where calculus can be seen.

c. Gentle air blast can deflect the margin from the tooth for observation into the pocket.

d. Transillumination: when light shines through anterior teeth, a dark opaque shadow-like area seen on a proximal tooth surface could be subgingival calculus. Supragingival calculus may also be found by this method. Without calculus, stain, or thick, soft deposit, the tooth is translucent.

2. *Gingival Tissue Color Change*. Dark calculus may reflect through a thin margin and suggest the presence of subgingival calculus.

3. *Tactile Examination*

a. Probe. While probing for sulcus/pocket depth, a rough subgingival tooth surface can be felt when calculus is present. Although there are other causes for roughness, subgingival calculus is the most frequent (page 205).

b. Explorer. The use of the subgingival explorer Number TU-17 was described on pages 223–224. Each subgingival area must be examined carefully to the bottom of the pocket, completely around each tooth.

D. Clinical Record

Calculus deposits are described in the examination record. The location of supra- and subgingival deposits and their extent (light, moderate, or heavy) need to be designated. A calculus index may be useful for patient evaluation and counseling at continuing maintenance recall appointments (page 298).

The calculus record is included with the complete charting and oral examination, page 320.

CALCULUS FORMATION

Calculus results from the deposition of minerals into a plaque organic matrix. Calculus formation occurs in three basic steps: pellicle formation, plaque formation, and mineralization. Formation of supra- and subgingival calculus is essentially the same, although the source of the elements for mineralization is not the same.

I. Pellicle Formation

The formation and characteristics of pellicle were described on page 261. The pellicle, or cuticle, is composed of mucoproteins from the saliva, and is an acellular material. Its thickness and contour vary on the tooth surface. It begins to form within minutes after a tooth is cleaned.

II. Plaque Maturation

A. Microorganisms settle in the pellicle layer.

B. Colonies are formed which originally consist primarily of cocci and rod-shaped organisms in a homogeneous ground substance (pages 265–266).

C. Colonies grow together to form a cohesive plaque layer (figure 16–1, page 266).

D. Mineralization centers or foci form. Within 24 to 72 hours, more and more mineralization centers develop close to the underlying tooth surface. Eventually the centers grow large enough to touch and unite.

III. Mineralization

Mineralization of dental plaque, and its transformation into calculus, proceeds rapidly, coincident with its growth. Mineralization may start as early as a few hours after plaque maturation.

A. Mineral Concentrations

Concentrations of calcium and phosphate increase daily. The mineral concentration varies in plaque of different areas. The amount of minerals is greatest on the lingual surfaces of the mandibular anterior teeth.[4]

B. Microorganisms

The microbial flora shifts from cocci and rods to primarily filamentous forms as mineralization continues beyond the initial stages.

C. Organic Matrix

The microorganisms serve as the matrix for the deposition of minerals. Many filamentous forms can be found.

A calculus-like deposit has been observed on the teeth of germ-free animals,[5–7] which may indicate that other organic substances may also serve as the matrix.

D. Source of Minerals

Saliva is the source of elements for supragingival calculus, and the gingival sulcus fluid supplies the material for the subgingival deposits.[8,9] Gingival sulcus fluid was described on page 188. Since the amount of gingival sulcus fluid increases in diseased pockets, more minerals are available for the deposition of more calculus.

E. Crystal Formation

Mineralization consists of crystal formation, namely, hydroxyapatite, octocalcium phosphate, whitlockite, and brushite, each with a characteristic developmental pattern. The crystals form in the intercellular matrix and on the surface of bacteria, and finally within the bacteria.[10-12]

F. Mechanism of Mineralization

The process by which minerals, mainly calcium and phosphate, become incorporated from the saliva or gingival sulcus fluid into the plaque matrix is still not completely understood. Current research studies point to the probability that calcification of calculus may involve the same phenomena as other ectopic calcifications (such as urinary or renal calculi) and with similarities to normal calcification of bone, cartilage, enamel, or dentin. For those wishing to read about this complex subject, a list of references is provided in the *Suggested Readings* at the end of this chapter.

IV. Formation Time

Formation time means the average number of days required for the primary soft deposit to change to the mature mineralized stage. The average time is about 12 days, with a range from 10 days for rapid calculus formers to 20 days for slow calculus formers.[13] Calcification can begin as early as 24 to 48 hours.

Formation time depends on individual tendency, but it is strongly influenced by the roughness of the tooth surface, and the care and character of personal plaque control measures. Determination of the approximate formation time for an individual is important to instruction and counseling, as well as treatment planning for professional care.

V. Structure of Calculus

A. Layers

Calculus forms in layers that are more or less parallel with the tooth surface. The layers are separated by a line which appears to be a pellicle that was deposited over the previously formed calculus, and, as mineralization progressed, the pellicle became imbedded.

The lines between the layers of calculus can be called incremental lines. They form around the tooth in supragingival calculus, but irregularly from crown to apex on the root surface in subgingival calculus. The lines are evidence that calculus grows or increases by apposition of new layers.

B. Surface

The surface of a calculus mass is rough and can be detected by use of an explorer. As observed by electron microscope, the surface roughness appears as peaks, valleys, and pits. When a section of a calculus mass was fractured off and the inner fractured surface examined by the electron microscope, the surface appeared granular, and the fracture followed through the intermicrobial matrix, leaving the calcified organisms visible.[14]

C. Outer Layer

The outer layer is partly calcified. On the surface there is a thick, mat-like soft layer of plaque and/or materia alba. It is the outer surface of the plaque on the subgingival calculus that is in contact with the diseased pocket epithelium.

VI. Attachment of Calculus

Calculus is more easily removed from some tooth surfaces than others. The ease or difficulty of removal can be related to the manner of attachment of the calculus to the tooth surface.

Several modes of attachment have been observed by conventional histologic techniques and by electron microscopy. On any one tooth and in any one area, more than one mode of attachment may be found. When studying the attachment types, the character of the hard, smooth enamel surface, and the rough, porous, cemental surface should be considered. Three general modes of attachment can be identified.[15]

A. Attachment by Means of an Acquired Pellicle or Cuticle

1. The pellicle is a thin, acellular, homogeneous layer positioned between the calculus and the tooth surface.
2. Calculus attachment is superficial since there is no interlocking or penetration.
3. It occurs most frequently on enamel and newly scaled and planed root surfaces.
4. Calculus may be removed readily because of the smooth attachment.

B. Attachment to Minute Irregularities in the Tooth Surface by Mechanical Locking into Undercuts

1. Enamel irregularities include cracks, lamellae, and carious defects.
2. Cemental irregularities include tiny spaces left at previous locations of Sharpey's fibers, resorption lacunae, scaling grooves, cemental tears or fragmentation.
3. Difficult to be certain all calculus is removed when it is attached by this method.

C. Attachment by Direct Contact Between Calcified Intercellular Matrix and the Tooth Surface

1. Remnants of microorganisms observed by electron microscope were near the root surface in the calculus but separated from it by the calcified intercellular matrix.
2. Cementum would be removed to assure removal of calculus that was attached by this method.

VII. Composition

Calculus is made up of inorganic and organic components and water. Although the percentage will vary depending on the age and hardness of a deposit, and the location from which the sample for analysis is taken, mature calculus usually contains between 75 and 85 percent inorganic components, and the rest is organic components and water. The chemical content of supra- and subgingival calculus is similar.[4,16,17]

A. Inorganic

1. *Inorganic Components.* The components are mainly salts of calcium, calcium phosphate primarily, with small amounts of magnesium phosphate and calcium carbonate.
2. *Trace Elements.* Various trace elements have been identified, including Na, Cl, Zn, Sr, Br, Cu, Mn, W, Au, Al, Si, Fe, and F.[18]
3. *Fluoride in Calculus*
   a. Concentration. The concentration of fluoride in calculus varies and is influenced by the amount of fluoride received from fluoride in the drinking water, topical application,[19] dentifrices,[20,21] or any form that is received by contact with the external surface of the calculus.
   b. Uptake. Fluoride uptake has been shown to be greater in calculus and silicate restorations than in intact enamel.[22] The surface of the cementum which is more permeable has a much higher content of fluoride than the enamel surface.

   Supragingival calculus has a much higher concentration than subgingival calculus, and supragingival calculus can have a higher fluoride content than the enamel surface,[23] since the calculus would be more porous than the enamel. The importance of the complete removal of calculus prior to a topical fluoride application can be explained by the need for the fluoride to be taken up by enamel not calculus.
4. *Crystalline Salts.* At least two thirds of the inorganic matter of calculus is crystalline, principally apatite. Predominating is hydroxyapatite, which is the same crystal present in enamel, dentin, cementum, and bone. Calculus also contains varying amounts of the crystalline salts brushite, whitlockite, and octocalcium phosphate.[24]
5. *Calculus Compared with Teeth and Bone.* Dental enamel is the most highly calcified tissue in the body and contains 96 percent inorganic salts as compared

with dentin, 65 percent, and cementum and bone at 45 to 50 percent.[25] Mature calculus has approximately 75 to 85 percent inorganic content. A comparison of calculus with the tooth parts provides insight into the effects of instrumentation, the difficulty of distinguishing calculus from cementum or dentin when scaling subgingivally, and the modes of attachment of calculus to the tooth surface.

B. Organic

The organic portion of calculus consists of various types of nonvital microorganisms, desquamated epithelial cells, leukocytes, and mucin from the saliva. Supra- and subgingival calculus, as well as calculus formed on artificial dentures, are all comparable in composition and similar to duct calculi.[26] Substances identified in the organic matrix include cholesterol, cholesterol esters, phospholipids, and fatty acids in the lipid fraction; reducing sugars and carbohydrate-protein complexes in the carbohydrate fraction; and keratins, nucleoproteins, amino acids in the protein portion.[27,28] Mucoprotein is the principal constituent.[26]

The microorganisms are predominantly filamentous. In early calculus, during the first 5 days cocci are found with some rods.[27,29] Most of the organisms within calculus are considered nonviable. The plaque on the calculus surface contains viable organisms.

SIGNIFICANCE OF DENTAL CALCULUS

Calculus has long been considered to have an important role in the development, promotion, and recurrence of gingival and periodontal conditions. With the newer knowledge of the role of dental plaque, and with understanding that dental calculus is mineralized plaque, the actual contribution of calculus to the disease process can be recognized.

Significant to the rationale for calculus removal and the production of a smooth tooth surface are the points listed here concerning the relationship of calculus to periodontal and gingival diseases.

I. Relation to Plaque

A. Calculus is mineralized plaque. Therefore calculus prevention depends on plaque prevention.
B. Calculus has a rough surface and provides a haven for plaque collection on its surface. Calculus increases the rate of plaque formation.

II. Relation to Pocket

A. Subgingival calculus is always covered by active plaque that is in direct contact with the sulcular epithelium. Plaque bacteria initiate gingivitis and periodontitis.
B. Subgingival calculus forms as a result of the calcification of the plaque on the subgingival tooth surface. Therefore, subgingival calculus is secondary to plaque, and its formation is secondary to pocket formation. Subgingival calculus is a *result* of pocket formation, not a cause.
C. With the perpetuation of inflammation in the pocket wall by the plaque on the calculus surface, the secretion of gingival sulcus fluid is promoted and increased. With more fluid come more minerals for calculus formation.

III. Relation to Plaque Control Techniques and Scaling

A. Plaque over a rough calculus surface is much more difficult to remove by toothbrushing, flossing, or other disease control procedures than from a smooth surface. The proximal surface calculus tears and shreds dental floss as it is passed over and under the deposit.
B. Removal and prevention of calculus leaves a smooth tooth surface which is possible for the patient to keep clean by toothbrushing and flossing, and which is resistant to plaque retention.

IV. Permeability of Calculus

With its rough surface and permeable structure, calculus can act as a reservoir for toxic microbial and tissue breakdown products. In a pocket, calculus holds the toxic products adjacent to the gingiva and inflammation can persist.

V. Drainage From Diseased Pocket

Calculus can reduce drainage from the pocket by helping to trap bacteria and debris. Healing is prevented and the advancement of disease encouraged. Gingival abscess formation may result (pages 540–541).

FACTORS TO TEACH THE PATIENT

I. What calculus is and how it forms from bacterial plaque.
II. The effect of calculus on the health of the periodontal tissues and therefore on the general health of the oral cavity.
III. Properties of calculus, which will explain the need for detailed, meticulous scaling procedures.
IV. Reasons for producing a smooth tooth surface during scaling and planing.
V. Plaque control measures which the patient may carry out to prevent calculus formation.

References

1. Suomi, J.D., Smith, L.W., McClendon, B.J., Spolsky, V.W., and Horowitz, H.S.: Oral Calculus in Children, *J. Periodontol.*, *42*, 341, June, 1971.
2. Wotman, S., Mercadante, J., Mandel, I.D., Goldman, R.S., and Denning, C.: The Occurrence of Calculus in Normal Children, Children with Cystic Fibrosis, and Children with Asthma, *J. Periodontol.*, *44*, 278, May, 1973.
3. Everett, F.G. and Potter, G.R.: Morphology of Submarginal Calculus, *J. Periodontol.*, *30*, 27, January, 1959.
4. Mandel, I.D.: Biochemical Aspects of Calculus Formation, *J. Periodont. Res.*, *9*, 10, Number 1, 1974.
5. Fitzgerald, R.J. and McDaniel, E.G.: Dental Calculus in the Germ-free Rat, *Arch. Oral Biol.*, *2*, 239, August, 1960.
6. Gustafsson, B.E. and Krasse, B.: Dental Calculus in Germfree Rats, *Acta Odont. Scand.*, *20*, 135, Number 2, 1962.
7. Theilade, J., Fitzgerald, R.J., Scott, D.B., and Nylen, M.U.: Electron Microscopic Observations of Dental Calculus in Germfree and Conventional Rats, *Arch. Oral Biol.*, *9*, 97, January–February, 1964.
8. Waerhaug, J.: The Source of Mineral Salts in Subgingival Calculus, *J. Dent. Res.*, *34*, 563, August, 1955.
9. Stewart, R.T. and Ratcliff, P.A.: The Source of Components of Subgingival Plaque and Calculus, *Periodont. Abstr.*, *14*, 102, September, 1966.
10. Gonzales, F. and Sognnaes, R.F.: Electron Microscopy of Dental Calculus, *Science*, *131*, 156, January 15, 1960.
11. Zander, H.A., Hazen, S.P., and Scott, D.B.: Mineralization of Dental Calculus, *Proc. Soc. Exp. Biol. and Med.*, *103*, 257, February, 1960.
12. McMillan, L., Hutchinson, A.C.W., and Fosdick, L.S.: Electron Microscopic Study of Dental Calculus, *Dental Prog.*, *1*, 188, April, 1961.
13. Schroeder, H.E.: *Formation and Inhibition of Dental Calculus*. Vienna, Hans Huber Publishers, 1969, pp. 73–74.
14. Baumhammers, A., Conway, J.C., Saltsberg, D., and Matta, R.K.: Scanning Electron Microscopy of Supra-

gingival Calculus, *J. Periodontol.*, *44*, 92, February, 1973.
15. Canis, M.F., Kramer, G.M., and Pameijer, C.M.: Calculus Attachment. Review of the Literature and New Findings, *J. Periodontol.*, *50*, 406, August, 1979.
16. Glock, G.E. and Murray, M.M.: Chemical Investigation of Salivary Calculus, *J. Dent. Res.*, *17*, 257, August, 1938.
17. Mandel, I.D. and Levy, B.M.: Studies on Salivary Calculus. I. Histochemical and Chemical Investigations of Supra- and Subgingival Calculus, *Oral Surg.*, *10*, 874, August, 1957.
18. Mukherjee, S.: Formation and Prevention of Supra-Gingival Calculus, *J. Periodont. Res.*, Supplementum 2, 1968, pp. 1–35.
19. Schait, A. and Mühlemann, H.R.: Fluoride Uptake by Calculus Following Topical Application of Fluorides, *Helv. Odont. Acta*, *15*, 132, October, 1971.
20. Kinoshita, S., Schait, A., Schroeder, H.E., and Mühlemann, H.R.: Origin of Fluoride in Early Dental Calculus, *Helv. Odont. Acta*, *9*, 141, October, 1965.
21. Mühlemann, H.R., Schait, A., and Schroeder, H.E.: Salivary Origin of Fluorine in Calcified Dental Plaques, *Helv. Odont. Acta*, *8*, 128, October, 1964.
22. Hellström, I.: Fluoride Uptake in Intact Enamel, Calculus Deposits, and Silicate Fillings, *Caries Res.*, *4*, 168, Number 2, 1970.
23. Yardeni, J., Gedalia, I., and Kohn, M.: Fluoride Concentration of Dental Calculus, Surface Enamel, and Cementum, *Arch. Oral Biol.*, *8*, 697, November–December, 1963.
24. Grøn, P., van Campen, G.J., and Lindstrom, I.: Human Dental Calculus. Inorganic Chemical and Crystallographic Composition, *Arch. Oral Biol.*, *12*, 829, July, 1967.
25. Bhaskar, S.N., ed.: *Orban's Oral Histology and Embryology*, 9th ed. St. Louis, The C.V. Mosby Co., 1980, pp. 47, 107, 180.
26. Stanford, J.W.: Analysis of the Organic Portion of Dental Calculus, *J. Dent. Res.*, *45*, 128, January–February, 1966.
27. Mandel, I.D., Levy, B.M., and Wasserman, B.H.: Histochemistry of Calculus Formation, *J. Periodontol.*, *28*, 132, April, 1957.
28. Mandel, I.D.: Histochemical and Biochemical Aspects of Calculus Formation, *Periodontics*, *1*, 43, March–April, 1963.
29. Turesky, S., Renstrup, G., and Glickman, I.: Histologic and Histochemical Observations Regarding Early Calculus Formation in Children and Adults, *J. Periodontol.*, *32*, 7, January, 1961.

Suggested Readings

Alexander, A.G.: The Relationship Between Tobacco Smoking, Calculus, and Plaque Accumulation and Gingivitis, *Dent. Health (Lond.)*, *9*, 6, January–March, 1970.
Alexander, A.G.: A Study of the Distribution of Supra and Subgingival Calculus, Bacterial Plaque and Gingival Inflammation in the Mouths of 400 Individuals, *J. Periodontol.*, *42*, 21, January, 1971.
Epstein, S.R., Mandel, I., and Scopp, I.W.: Salivary Composition and Calculus Formation in Patients Undergoing Hemodialysis, *J. Periodontol.*, *51*, 336, June, 1980.
Fischman, S.L., Cancro, L., Pader, M., and Picozzi, A.: Relationship of Dental Calculus and Periodontal Disease, *J. Prev. Dent.*, *2*, 24, January–February, 1975.
Friskopp, J. and Hammarström, L.: A Comparative, Scanning Electron Microscopic Study of Supragingival and

Subgingival Calculus, *J. Periodontol.*, *51*, 553, October, 1980.

Knuuttila, M., Lappalainen, R., and Kontturi-Närhi, V.: Concentrations of Ca, Mg, Mn, Sr and Zn in Supra- and Subgingival Calculus, *Scand. J. Dent. Res.*, *87*, 192, June, 1979.

Listgarten, M.A. and Ellegaard, B.: Electron Microscopic Evidence of a Cellular Attachment Between Junctional Epithelium and Dental Calculus, *J. Periodont. Res.*, *8*, 143, Number 3, 1973.

Mislowsky, W.J. and Mazzella, W.J.: Supragingival and Subgingival Plaque and Calculus Formation in Humans, *J. Periodontol.*, *45*, 822, November, 1974.

Oshrain, H.I., Salkind, A., and Mandel, I.D.: An Histologic Comparison of Supra and Subgingival Plaque and Calculus, *J. Periodontol.*, *42*, 31, January, 1971.

Sidaway, D.A.: A Microbiological Study of Dental Calculus. I. The Microbial Flora of Mature Calculus, *J. Periodont. Res.*, *13*, 349, July, 1978.

Sidaway, D.A.: A Microbiological Study of Dental Calculus. II. The *in vitro* Calcification of Microorganisms from Dental Calculus, *J. Periodont. Res.*, *13*, 360, July, 1978.

Sidaway, D.A.: A Microbiological Study of Dental Calculus. III. A Comparison of the *in vitro* Calcification of Viable and Non-viable Microorganisms, *J. Periodont. Res.*, *14*, 167, March, 1979.

Watts, T.L.P. and Combe, E.C.: An Estimation of the Strength of Attachment of Subgingival Calculus to Extracted Teeth, *J. Clin. Periodontol.*, *8*, 1, February, 1981.

Calculus Formation and Mineralization

Allen, D.L., McFall, W.T., and Hunter, G.C.: *Periodontics for the Dental Hygienist*, 3rd ed. Philadelphia, Lea & Febiger, 1980, pp. 72–74.

Carranza, F.A.: *Glickman's Clinical Periodontology*, 5th ed. Philadelphia, W.B. Saunders Co., 1979, pp. 411–424.

Dummett, C.O.: Microbiologic Calcification in the Formation of Calculus, *Q. Natl. Dent. Assoc.*, *33*, 79, April, 1975.

Ennever, J., Vogel, J.J., and Benson, L.A.: Lipid and Calculus Matrix Calcification *in vitro*, *J. Dent. Res.*, *52*, 1056, September–October, 1973.

Glimcher, M.J.: Specificity of the Molecular Structure of Organic Matrices in Mineralization, in Sognnaes, R.F., ed.: *Calcification in Biological Systems*. Washington, D.C., American Association for the Advancement of Science, 1960, p. 421 ff.

Grant, D.A., Stern, I.B., and Everett, F.G.: *Periodontics*, 5th ed. St. Louis, The C.V. Mosby Co., 1979, pp. 152–170.

Jenkins, G.N.: *The Physiology and Biochemistry of the Mouth*, 4th ed. Philadelphia, J.B. Lippincott Co., 1978, pp. 403–409.

Leung, S.W.: Calculus Formation. Salivary Factors, *Dent. Clin. North Am.*, p. 723, November, 1960.

Lustmann, J., Lewin-Epstein, J., and Shteyer, A.: Scanning Electron Microscopy of Dental Calculus, *Calcif. Tiss. Res.*, *21*, 47, Number 1, 1976.

Mandel, I.D.: Calculus Formation. The Role of Bacteria and Mucoprotein, *Dent. Clin. North Am.*, p. 731, November, 1960.

Mukherjee, S.: Formation and Prevention of Supra-gingival Calculus, *J. Periodont. Res.*, Supplementum 2, 1968, pp. 14–21.

Ramfjord, S.P. and Ash, M.M.: *Periodontology and Periodontics*. Philadelphia, W.B. Saunders Co., 1979, pp. 156–161.

Rizzo, A.A., Scott, D.B., and Bladen, H.A.: Calcification of Oral Bacteria, *Ann. New York Acad. Sci.*, *109*, 14, May 31, 1963.

Schroeder, H.E.: *Formation and Inhibition of Dental Calculus*. Vienna, Hans Huber, 1969, pp. 37–44, 94–108.

Calculus Attachment

Jones, S.J.: Morphology of Calculus Formation on the Human Tooth Surface, *Proc. R. Soc. Med.*, *65*, 903, October, 1972.

Kopczyk, R.A. and Conroy, C.W.: The Attachment of Calculus to Root Planed Surfaces, *Periodontics*, *6*, 78, April, 1968.

Moskow, B.S.: Calculus Attachment in Cemental Separations, *J. Periodontol.*, *40*, 125, March, 1969.

Selvig, K.A.: Attachment of Plaque and Calculus to Tooth Surfaces, *J. Periodont. Res.*, *5*, 8, Number 1, 1970.

Shroff, F.R.: An Observation on the Attachment of Calculus, *Oral Surg.*, *8*, 154, February, 1955.

Theilade, J.: Electron Microscopic Study of Calculus Attachment to Smooth Surfaces, *Acta Odontol. Scand.*, *22*, 379, Number 3, 1964.

Voreadis, E.G. and Zander, H.A.: Cuticular Calculus Attachment, *Oral Surg.*, *11*, 1120, October, 1958.

Zander, H.A.: Attachment of Calculus to Root Surfaces, *J. Periodontol.*, *24*, 16, January, 1953.

18

Tooth Stains and Discolorations

Discolorations of the teeth and restorations occur in three general ways: (1) stain adhering directly to the surfaces, (2) stain contained within calculus and soft deposits, and (3) stain incorporated within the tooth structure. Instructional and clinical techniques apply to all three. The first two may be removed by scaling or polishing. Certain stains may be prevented by the patient's routine personal care.

The significance of stains is primarily the appearance of the teeth. In general, any detrimental effect on the teeth or gingival tissues is related to the soft deposit or calculus in which the stain occurs. Thick, bulky deposits of stain can conceivably provide a rough surface on which bacterial plaque could collect and irritate the adjacent gingiva. Certain stains provide a means for evaluating oral cleanliness and the patient's habits of personal care.

I. Classification of Stains

A. Classified by Location

1. *Extrinsic*. Extrinsic stains occur on the external surface of the tooth and may be removed by techniques of toothbrushing, scaling, and/or polishing.
2. *Intrinsic*. Intrinsic stains occur within the tooth substance and cannot be removed by techniques of scaling or polishing.

B. Classified by Source

1. *Exogenous*. Exogenous stains develop or originate from sources outside the tooth. Exogenous stains may be extrinsic and stay on the outer surface of the tooth or intrinsic and become incorporated within the tooth structure.
2. *Endogenous*. Endogenous stains develop or originate from within the tooth. Endogenous stains are always intrinsic and usually are discolorations of the dentin reflected through the enamel.

II. Recognition and Identification

Accurately prepared medical and dental histories can provide information to supplement clinical observations when the need to identify a certain stain arises.

A food diary may aid in identifying certain contributing factors. The history of personal plaque removal with the type and frequency of use of toothbrush, floss, and other supplemental materials and devices, may help to explain the presence of certain stains. The state of oral hygiene and oral cleanliness is significant to the occurrence of dental stains.

More than one type of stain may occur and there may be more than one etiologic factor causing the stains of an individual's dentition. Making a differential diagnosis may be complicated.[1]

III. Application of Techniques to Stain Removal

A. Stains Occurring Directly on the Tooth Surface

1. Stains that are directly associated with the surface of the enamel or exposed cementum are removed as much as possible during toothbrushing by the patient. Some stains are removed by scaling while others will require polishing.

2. When stains are tenacious, excessive polishing should be avoided: precaution should be taken to prevent (1) abrasion of the tooth surface or gingival margin, (2) removal of a layer of fluoride-rich tooth surface, or (3) overheating with a power-driven polisher.

B. Stains Incorporated within Tooth Deposits

When stain is included within the substance of a soft deposit or calculus, it is removed with the deposit.

EXTRINSIC STAINS

The most frequently observed stains, yellow, green, black line, and tobacco will be described first; the less common orange, red, and metallic stains will follow.

I. Yellow Stain

A. Clinical Appearance

Dull, yellowish discoloration of dental plaque appears.

B. Distribution on Tooth Surfaces

Yellow stain is associated with presence of dental plaque. (Note distribution of dental plaque, table 16–2, page 264.)

C. Occurrence

1. Common to all ages.
2. More evident when personal oral care procedures are neglected.

D. Etiology

Usually food pigments.

II. Green Stain

A. Clinical Appearance

1. Light or yellowish green to very dark green.

2. Embedded in dental plaque.
3. Shape: occurs in three general forms.
   a. Small curved line following contour of labial gingival crest.
   b. Smeared irregularly, may even cover entire facial surface.
   c. Streaked, following grooves or lines in enamel.
4. The stain is frequently superimposed by soft yellow or gray debris (materia alba and food debris).
5. Dark green occasionally becomes embedded in surface enamel and may be observed as an exogenous intrinsic stain when superficial layers of deposit are removed.
6. Enamel under stain: sometimes decalcified as a result of cariogenic plaque or materia alba. The rough decalcified surface encourages plaque retention, decalcification, and recurrence of green stain.

B. Distribution on Tooth Surfaces

1. Primarily labial and buccal; may extend to proximal.
2. Most frequent: labial cervical third of maxillary anterior teeth.

C. Composition

1. Chromogenic bacteria and fungi.
2. Decomposed hemoglobin.
3. Inorganic elements: calcium, potassium, sodium, silicon, magnesium, phosphorus, and others in small amounts.[2]

D. Occurrence

1. May occur at any age; primarily found in childhood.
2. Collects on both permanent and primary teeth.
3. Green stain tends to occur without other stains (except yellow) in the same mouth.

E. Recurrence

Recurrence depends on fastidiousness of personal care procedures.

F. Etiology

Green stain results from oral uncleanliness, chromogenic bacteria, and gingival hemorrhage.

1. Chromogenic bacteria or fungi are retained and nourished in dental plaque where the green stain is produced.
2. Blood pigments from hemoglobin are decomposed by bacteria.
3. Predisposing factors. Means for retention and proliferation of chromogenic bacteria: dental plaque, materia alba, and food debris.

C. Other Green Stains

In addition to the clinical entity "Green Stain" described above, bacterial plaque and acquired pellicle may become stained by a variety of substances. Green discoloration may result from chlorophyl preparations, metallic dusts of industry, or certain drugs. Differential distinction may be determined by questioning or from items in the medical or dental histories.

II. Black Line Stain

Black line stain is a highly retentive black or dark brown calculus-like stain which forms along the gingival third near the gingival margin. It may occur on primary or permanent teeth.

A. Other Names

Mesenteric line, pigmented dental plaque, brown stain, black stain.

B. Clinical Features

1. Continuous or interrupted fine line, one mm. wide (average), no appreciable thickness.
2. May be a wider band or even occupy entire gingival third in severe cases (rare).
3. Follows contour of gingival crest about one mm. above crest.
4. Usually demarcated from gingival crest by clear white line of unstained enamel.
5. Appears black at bases of pits and fissures.
6. Heavy deposits slightly elevated from the tooth surface may be detected with an explorer.
7. Gingiva: firm, resilient, with little or no tendency to hemorrhage.

8. Teeth: frequently clean and shiny with a tendency to lower incidence of dental caries.

C. Distribution on Tooth Surfaces

1. Facial and lingual; follows contour of gingival crest onto proximal surfaces.
2. Rarely on labial of maxillary anterior.
3. Most frequently: lingual and proximal surfaces of maxillary posterior teeth.

D. Composition and Formation[3,4]

1. The composition is like plaque in that it is composed of microorganisms embedded in an intermicrobial substance.
2. The microorganisms are primarily gram-positive rods with other bacteria including cocci in smaller percentages.

   It is apparent that the composition of black stain is different than the composition of supragingival plaque, where cocci predominate. Attachment to the tooth of black line stain is by a pellicle-like structure.[5]

   Oral disease does not result from the presence of black line stain. In contrast, gingivitis is related to the formation of supragingival plaque, and in the presence of a cariogenic substrate, dental caries develops.

3. Calcification in black line stain occurs which is similar to the regular formation of calculus.

E. Occurrence

1. All ages; more common in childhood.
2. More common in females.
3. Frequently in clean mouths.

F. Recurrence

Black line stain tends to form again despite regular personal care, but quantity may be less when plaque control procedures are meticulous.

G. Predisposing Factors: none apparent, except a natural tendency.

IV. Tobacco Stain

A. Clinical Appearance

1. Light brown to dark leathery brown or black.

2. Shape
   a. Diffuse staining of dental plaque.
   b. Narrow band that follows contour of gingival crest, slightly above the crest.
   c. Wide, firm, tar-like band may cover cervical third and extend to central third of crown.
3. May be incorporated in calculus deposit.
4. Heavy deposits (particularly from chewing tobacco) may penetrate the enamel and become exogenous intrinsic.

B. Distribution on Tooth Surfaces

1. Cervical third, primarily.
2. Any surface, as well as pits and fissures.
3. Most frequent: lingual surfaces.

C. Composition

1. Tar products of combustion.
2. Brown pigment from chewing tobacco.

D. Predisposing Factors

1. Natural tendencies: quantity of stain not proportional to amount of tobacco used, which may indicate individual differences.
2. Personal oral care procedures: increased deposits occur with neglect.
3. Extent of dental plaque and calculus available for adherence.

V. Other Brown Stains

A. Brown Pellicle

The acquired pellicle is smooth and structureless and recurs readily after removal.[6] The pellicle can take on stains of various colors which result from chemical alteration of the pellicle.[7] A few of these are described next.

B. Stannous Fluoride[8,9]

Light brown, sometimes yellowish stain forms on the teeth in the pellicle after using a stannous fluoride dentifrice, mouthrinse, or having a topical fluoride application. The brown stain is the result of reactions of the tin ion to form stannous sulfide or a brown tin oxide.

C. Foodstuffs

Tea, coffee, and soy sauce are often in-

volved in the formation of a brownish stain pellicle. As with other brown pellicle stain there is less when the personal oral hygie and plaque control are excellent.

D. Anti-plaque Agents[10,11,12]

Chlorhexidine and alexidine have be used experimentally in a mouthrinse, g and dentifrice and shown effective again plaque formation. A brownish stain of too and silicate restorations results, usually mo pronounced on proximal and other surfac less accessible to routine plaque control pr cedures. The stain also tends to form mo rapidly on exposed roots than on ename Chlorhexidine or alexidine products have n been approved for general public use in t United States. Tooth staining has been co sidered a significant side effect.

E. Betel Leaf

Betel leaf chewing is common among pe ple of all ages in eastern countries. The di coloration imparted to the teeth is a da mahogany brown, sometimes almost blac It may become thick and hard, which i dicates that scaling is a better method f removal than the excessive amount of po ishing that would be required. Betel has caries-inhibiting effect.[13]

VI. Orange and Red Stains

A. Clinical Appearance

Orange or red stains appear at the cervic third.

B. Distribution on Tooth Surfaces

1. More frequently on anterior than po terior teeth.
2. Both labial and lingual of anterior teeth

C. Occurrence

Rare (red more rare than orange).

D. Etiology

Chromogenic bacteria.

VII. Metallic Stains

A. Metals or Metallic Salts from Metal-Containing Dust of Industry

1. *Clinical Appearance:* examples of color on teeth

a. Copper or brass: green or bluish-green.
b. Iron: brown to greenish-brown.
c. Nickel: green.
d. Cadmium: yellow or golden brown.

2. *Distribution on Tooth Surfaces*
a. Primarily anterior; may occur on any teeth.
b. Cervical third more commonly.

3. *Manner of Formation*
a. Industrial worker inhales dust through mouth, bringing metallic substance in contact with teeth.
b. Metal imparts color to dental plaque.
c. Occasionally, stain may penetrate tooth substance and become exogenous intrinsic stain.

Metallic Substances Contained in Drugs

1. *Clinical Appearance:* examples of colors on teeth
a. Iron: black (iron sulfide) or brown.
b. Manganese (from potassium permanganate): black.

2. *Distribution on Tooth Surfaces:* general, may occur on all.

3. *Manner of Formation*
a. Drug enters plaque substance, imparts color to plaque and calculus.
b. Pigment from drug may attach directly to tooth substance.

4. *Prevention:* Use a medication through a straw or in tablet or capsule form to prevent direct contact with the teeth.

INTRINSIC STAINS

Stains incorporated within the tooth structure may be related to the period of tooth development or may be acquired after eruption. An occasional patient, desiring an improvement in the appearance of the anterior teeth, may request removal of a discoloration. The dentist may employ one of two alternatives in the treatment of these teeth. Improvement in tooth color can be produced by bleaching in certain instances. In other cases, it is necessary to prepare a jacket crown to cover the discoloration.

. Pulpless Teeth

It should be realized that not all pulpless teeth

discolor. Improved endodontic procedures have contributed to the prevention of many discolorations formerly associated with that cause.

A. Clinical Appearance

A wide range of colors exists; they may be light yellow-brown, slate gray, reddish-brown, dark brown, bluish-black, or black. Others have an orange or greenish tinge.

B. Manner of Formation

1. Blood and other pulp tissue elements may be made available for breakdown as a result of hemorrhages in the pulp chamber, root canal operations, or necrosis and decomposition of the pulp tissue.

2. Pigments from the decomposed hemoglobin and pulp tissue penetrate into the dentinal tubules.

II. Drugs and Metals

A. Tetracycline[14]

1. Tetracycline antibiotics, used widely for combatting many types of infections, have an affinity for calcified tissues and are absorbed by the bones and teeth. They can be transferred through the placenta and enter fetal circulation.

2. Discoloration of the teeth of a child can result when the drug is administered during the third trimester of pregnancy or in infancy and early childhood.

3. Color of teeth: may be light green to dark yellow tones, or a gray-brown. The discoloration depends on the dosage, length of time the drug was used, and the type of tetracycline.

4. Teeth involved: may be generalized or limited to specific parts of individual teeth that were developing at the time of administration of the antibiotic; enamel hypoplasia has been noted in some patients. A lowered caries incidence is a common benefit.[15] Reference to the Table of Tooth Development can assist the identification of the source of an intrinsic stain (Appendix, tables A–1 and A–2).

B. Restorative Materials

1. Dental amalgam: silver amalgam can im-

part a gray to black discoloration to the tooth structure around a restoration.

a. Due to migration of metallic ions from the amalgam restoration into the enamel and dentin.

b. The silver, tin, and mercury ions eventually contact debris at the junction of the tooth and the restoration and form sulfides, which are products of corrosion.

2. Copper amalgam used for filling primary teeth may impart a bluish-green color.

3. Silver nitrate used in a cavity base under a restoration can produce black discoloration.

C. Endodontic Therapy and Restorative Materials

1. Silver nitrate: bluish-black.
2. Volatile oils: yellowish-brown.
3. Strong iodine: brown.
4. Aureomycin: yellow.
5. Silver-containing root canal sealer: black.

III. Imperfect Tooth Development

Defective tooth development may result from factors of genetic abnormality or environmental influences during tooth development.

A. Hereditary: Genetic[16]

1. *Amelogenesis Imperfecta.* The enamel is partially or completely missing due to a generalized disturbance of the ameloblasts. Teeth are yellowish-brown or gray-brown.

2. *Dentinogenesis Imperfecta ("Opalescent Dentin").* The dentin is abnormal as a result of disturbances in the odontoblastic layer during development. The teeth appear translucent or opalescent, and vary in color from gray to bluish-brown.

B. Enamel Hypoplasia[16]

1. *Systemic Hypoplasia* (chronologic hypoplasia resulting from ameloblastic disturbance of short duration). Teeth erupt with white spots or with pits. Over a long period of time, the white spots may become discolored from food pigments or other substances taken into the mouth.

Figure 14–1 (page 236) shows an example of chronologic hypoplasia.

2. *Local Hypoplasia* (affects single tooth) White spots may become stained as systemic hypoplasia.

C. Dental Fluorosis

Dental fluorosis was originally called "brown stain." Later, Dr. Frederick McKay, who studied the condition and described it in the dental literature, named "mottled enamel" (page 444).

1. *Manner of Formation*

a. Enamel hypocalcification resulting from ingestion of excessive fluoric ion content of the drinking water (more than two parts per million during the period of calcification. The enamel alterations are due to toxic damage to the ameloblasts.

b. When the teeth erupt, there are white spots or areas that later become discolored from oral pigment and appear light or dark brown.

c. Severe effects of excess fluoride during development may produce cracks or pitting; the discoloration concentrates in these. It was that condition and appearance that led to the name mottled enamel.

2. *Classification*[17,18]

Grade of Fluorosis	Description of Fluorosis
Normal	No irregularities present
Questionable	A few white flecks or white spots
Very Mild	Small opaque, paper-white areas involving less than 25 percent of the surface
Mild	White opacities are more extensive, but do not involve more than 50 percent of the surface
Moderate	Distinct brown stain; all enamel surfaces affected
Severe	Besides brown staining, the tooth is worn and hypoplastic. All enamel surfaces are affected and discrete or confluent pitting is present.

7. Other Systemic Causes

Several types of tooth discolorations may result from blood-borne pigments.

Pigments circulating in the blood are transmitted to the dentin from the capillaries of the pulp. *Example:* prolonged jaundice early in life can impart yellow or greenish discoloration to the teeth.

Erythroblastosis fetalis (Rh incompatibility) may leave a green, brown, or blue hue to the teeth.[19] A kidney disease patient who had uremia during tooth development may have hypoplasia with a brownish discoloration.[20]

B. Exogenous Intrinsic Stains

When intrinsic stains come from an outside source, not from within the tooth, the stain is called exogenous intrinsic. Extrinsic stains can provide stain that becomes intrinsic. Tobacco and green stains are examples of this.

1. Drugs

1. Stannous fluoride topical application[8]
   a. Light to dark brown staining from the formation of tin sulfide.
   b. Location: most frequently in occlusal pits and grooves of posterior teeth and cervical third facial surfaces of anterior; in carious and pre-carious lesions and margins of silicate and amalgam restorations.
   c. Staining may accompany dental caries arrestment.
2. Ammoniacal silver nitrate, used in treatment of sensitive areas such as exposed cementum or for inhibition of decalcification in dental caries prevention, imparts a dark brown to black discoloration.

2. Stain in Dentin

Example: discoloration resulting from a carious lesion.

TECHNICAL HINTS

I. Record color, type, extent, and location of stains with the patient's examination.

II. Make additions to the Dental History as information is gained concerning the origin of stains such as those related to tooth development, systemic disease, occupations, or medications.

III. Avoid making patient feel self-conscious by overemphasizing the appearance of stains, particularly those that may occur in spite of conscientious toothbrushing habits.

IV. Use tact when questioning patients with brown stain since nonsmokers do not appreciate having an assumption made concerning the etiology of the stain on the teeth.

V. Refer patient's questions concerning the removal of intrinsic stains to the dentist. Avoid expressing an opinion in terms of diagnosis or prognosis of treatment until the dentist has recommended a procedure.

FACTORS TO TEACH THE PATIENT

I. Predisposing factors that contribute to stain accumulation.

II. Personal care procedures that can aid in the prevention or reduction of stains.

III. Reasons for not using an abrasive dentifrice with vigorous brushing strokes to lessen or remove stain accumulation.

IV. The need to avoid tobacco, coffee, tea, and other beverages or foodstuffs that can stain, to prevent discoloration of new restorations.

V. Reasons for the difficulty in removal of certain extrinsic stains during scaling and polishing.

References

1. Giunta, J.L. and Tsamtsouris, A.: Case Review: Stains and Discolorations of Teeth: Review and Case Reports, *J. Pedod., 2,* 175, Winter, 1978.
2. Shay, D.E., Haddox, J.H., and Richmond, J.L.: An Inorganic Qualitative and Quantitative Analysis of Green Stain, *J. Am. Dent. Assoc., 50,* 156, February, 1955.
3. Theilade, J., Slots, J., and Fejerskov, O.: The Ultrastructure of Black Stain on Human Primary Teeth, *Scand. J. Dent. Res., 81,* 528, Number 7, 1973.
4. Slots, J.: The Microflora of Black Stain on Human Primary Teeth, *Scand. J. Dent. Res., 82,* 484, Number 7, 1974.
5. Theilade, J.: Development of Bacterial Plaque in the Oral Cavity, *J. Clin. Periodontol., 4,* 1, December, 1977.
6. Meckel, A.H.: The Formation and Properties of Organic Films on Teeth, *Arch. Oral Biol., 10,* 585, July–August, 1965.
7. Eriksen, H.M. and Nordbø, H.: Extrinsic Discoloration of Teeth, *J. Clin. Periodontol., 5,* 229, November, 1978.
8. Horowitz, H.S. and Chamberlin, S.R.: Pigmentation of Teeth following Topical Applications of Stannous Fluoride in a Nonfluoridated Area, *J. Public Health Dent., 31,* 32, Winter, 1971.
9. Shannon, I.L.: Stannous Fluoride: Does It Stain Teeth?

How Does It React with Tooth Surfaces? A Review, *Gen. Dent.*, *26*, 64, September–October, 1978.

10. Flotra, L., Gjermo, P., Rolla, G., and Waerhaug, J.: Side Effects of Chlorhexidine Mouthwashes, *Scand. J. Dent. Res.*, *79*, 119, 1971.

11. Weatherford, T.W., Finn, S.B., and Jamison, H.C.: Effects of an Alexidine Mouthwash on Dental Plaque and Gingivitis in Humans Over a Six-month Period, *J. Am. Dent. Assoc.*, *94*, 528, March, 1977.

12. Formicola, A.J., Deasy, M.J., Johnson, D.H., and Howe, E.E.: Tooth Staining Effects of an Alexidine Mouthwash, *J. Periodontol.*, *50*, 207, April, 1979.

13. Möller, I.J., Pindborg, J.J., and Effendi, I.: The Relation Between Betel Chewing and Dental Caries, *Scand. J. Dent. Res.*, *85*, 64, January, 1977.

14. American Dental Association, Council on Dental Therapeutics: *Accepted Dental Therapeutics*, 39th ed. Chicago, American Dental Association, 1982, p. 246–247.

15. Brearly, T.J. and Porteous, R.J.: Characteristics and Caries Experience of Tetracycline-affected Dentitions, *J. Dent. Res.*, *52*, 508, May–June, 1973.

16. Shafer, W.G., Hine, M.K., and Levy, B.M.: *A Textbook of Oral Pathology*, 3rd ed. Philadelphia, W.B. Saunders Co., 1974, pp. 47–57.

17. Dean, H.T.: Investigation of Physiological Effects by Epidemiological Method, in Moulton, F.R., ed.: *Fluorine and Dental Health*. Washington, American Association for the Advancement of Science, Number 19, 1942.

18. Newbrun, E., ed.: *Fluorides and Dental Caries*, 2nd ed. Springfield, Illinois, Charles C Thomas, 1975, p. 4.

19. Shafer, Hine, and Levy: op. cit., pp. 674–675.

20. Bottomley, W.K., Cioffi, R.F., and Martin, A.J.: Dental Management of the Patient Treated by Renal Transplantation: Preoperative and Postoperative Considerations, *J. Am. Dent. Assoc.*, *85*, 1330, December, 1972.

Suggested Readings

Burke, S.W.: Oral Physiology and Physiotherapy, in Steele, P.F., ed.: *Dimensions of Dental Hygiene*, 3rd ed. Philadelphia, Lea & Febiger, 1982, pp. 97–100.

Chan, K.C., Fuller, J.L., and Hormati, A.A.: The Ability of Foods to Stain Two Composite Resins, *J. Prosthet. Dent.*, *43*, 542, May, 1980.

Cianco, S.G. and Bourgault, P.C.: *Clinical Pharmacology for Dental Professionals*. New York, McGraw-Hill, 1980, pp. 183–186.

Dummett, C.O., Sakumura, J.S., and Barens, G.: The Relationship of Facial Skin Complexion to Oral Mucosa Pigmentation and Tooth Color, *J. Prosthet. Dent.*, *43*, 392, April, 1980.

Eisenberg, E. and Bernick, S.M.: Anomalies of the Teeth with Stains and Discolorations, *J. Prev. Dent.*, *2*, 7, January–February, 1975.

Jørgensen, K.D. and Asmussen, E.: Pseudo-discoloration of Plastic Fillings, *Acta Odontol. Scand.*, *29*, 649, Number 6, 1971.

Lökken, P. and Birkeland, J.M.: Dental Discolorations and Side Effects with Iron and Placebo Tablets, *Scand. J. Dent. Res.*, *87*, 275, August, 1979.

Massler, M. and Schour, I.: *Atlas of the Mouth*. Chicago, American Dental Association, Plate 12.

Ness, L., Rosekrans, D. de L., and Welford, J.F.: An Epidemiologic Study of Factors Affecting Extrinsic Staining of Teeth in an English Population, *Community Dent. Oral Epidemiol.*, *5*, 55, January, 1977.

Nordbø, H.: Discoloration of Dental Pellicle by Tannic Acid, *Acta Odontol. Scand.*, *35*, 305, Number 6, 1977.

Rakow, B. and Light, E.I.: A Preventive Oriented Classification of Tooth Discolorations, *J. Prev. Dent.*, *3*, 1, January–February, 1976.

Reid, J.S. and Beeley, J.A.: Biochemical Studies on the Composition of Gingival Debris from Children with Black Extrinsic Tooth Stain, *Caries Res.*, *10*, 363, Number 5, 1976.

Reid, J.S., Beeley, J.A., and MacDonald, D.G.: Investigations into Black Extrinsic Tooth Stain, *J. Dent. Res.*, *56*, 895, August, 1977.

Vogel, R.I.: Intrinsic and Extrinsic Discoloration of the Dentition (a Literature Review), *J. Oral Med.*, *30*, 99, October–December, 1975.

Tetracycline

Atkinson, D.: Tetracycline and Its Effect on Teeth, *Dent. Assist.*, *47*, 36, November/December, 1978.

Moffitt, J.M., Cooley, R.O., Olsen, N.H., and Hefferren, J.J.: Prediction of Tetracycline-induced Tooth Discoloration, *J. Am. Dent. Assoc.*, *88*, 547, March, 1974.

Ulvestad, H., Lökken, P., and Mjorud, F.: Discoloration of Permanent Front Teeth in 3,157 Norwegian Children Due to Tetracyclines and Other Factors, *Scand. J. Dent. Res.*, *86*, 147, May, 1978.

Zadik, D. and Eidelman, E.: Tetracycline-stained Teeth in Jerusalem Preschool Children, *Community Dent. Oral Epidemiol.*, *3*, 69, March, 1975.

Chemical Plaque Control Agents

Addy, M. and Prayitno, S.W.: Light Microscopic and Color Television Image Analysis of the Development of Staining on Chlorhexidine-treated Surfaces, *J. Periodontol.*, *51*, 39, January, 1980.

Addy, M., Prayitno, S., Taylor, L., and Cadogan, S.: An in vitro Study of the Role of Dietary Factors in the Aetiology of Tooth Staining Associated with the Use of Chlorhexidine, *J. Periodont. Res.*, *14*, 403, September, 1979.

Dolles, O.K., Eriksen, H.M., and Gjermo, P.: Tooth Stain During 2 Years' Use of Chlorhexidine- and Fluoride-containing Dentifrices, *Scand. J. Dent. Res.*, *87*, 268, August, 1979.

Prayitno, S. and Addy, M.: An in vitro Study of Factors Affecting the Development of Staining Associated with the Use of Chlorhexidine, *J. Periodont. Res.*, *14*, 397, November, 1979.

Prayitno, S., Taylor, L., Cadogan, S., and Addy, M.: An in vivo Study of Dietary Factors in the Aetiology of Tooth Staining Associated with the Use of Chlorhexidine, *J. Periodont. Res.*, *14*, 411, September, 1979.

Solheim, H., Eriksen, H.M., and Nordbø, H.: Chemical Plaque Control and Extrinsic Discoloration of Teeth, *Acta Odontol. Scand.*, *38*, 303, Number 5, 1980.

Hereditary Defects

Gertzman, G.B.R., Gaston, G., and Quinn, I.: Amelogenesis Imperfecta: Local Hypoplastic Type with Pulpal Calcification, *J. Am. Dent. Assoc.*, *99*, 637, October, 1979.

Giansanti, J.S. and Budnick, S.D.: Six Generations of Hereditary Opalescent Dentin: Report of Case, *J. Am. Dent. Assoc.*, *90*, 439, February, 1975.

Winter, G.B. and Brook, A.H.: Enamel Hypoplasia and Anomalies of the Enamel, *Dent. Clin. North Am.*, *19*, 3, January, 1975.

Witkop, C.J.: Hereditary Defects of Dentin, *Dent. Clin. North Am.*, *19*, 25, January, 1975.

19

Periodontal and Dental Indices and Scoring Methods

An index is an expression of clinical observations in numerical values. It is used to describe the status of the individual or group with respect to a condition being measured. By using a number scale and a standardized method for interpreting observations of a condition, an index score can be more consistent and less subjective than a word description of that condition.

Indices using various criteria have been developed to compare the extent and severity of disease. For example, dental caries is indexed by the number of teeth or surfaces with carious lesions and fillings. An index for dental fluorosis identifies very mild, mild, moderate, or severe involvement of the enamel, ranging respectively from white spots visible only when a tooth is dry to marked brown stains with pitting.

Various factors associated with gingivitis and periodontal diseases have been used in the development of indices. Measurement criteria include recession, bone loss, pocket formation, mobility of teeth, gingival inflammation, gingival bleeding, and the amount and distribution of plaque and calculus.

These measurements aid in the overall assessment of the oral health status.

I. Types of Indices

A distinction needs to be made between an epidemiologic survey, a clinical trial, and an individual clinical score. Indices designed for use in large populations for general epidemiologic surveys are not appropriate in clinical research studies planned for testing the effect of a preventive or treatment agent. In the third category, a personally adapted scoring system can serve to educate and motivate during individual treatment appointments, but would not supply appropriate data for group studies.

A. Epidemiologic Survey

The word epidemiology denotes the study of disease characteristics of populations. An example of an index designed for a survey of population groups is the DMF (Decayed, Missing, and Filled Teeth). It has been used with populations around the world to determine the extent of dental caries. Such a survey was not designed for evaluation of an individual patient.

B. Clinical Trial

A clinical trial is planned for the determination of the effect of an agent or procedure on the progression, control, or prevention of a disease. The trial would be conducted by comparing an experimental group with a control group which is similar to the experimental group in every way except for the variable being studied.

Examples of indices used for clinical trials are the Plaque Index (Pl I) of Silness and Löe[1] and the Patient Hygiene Performance (PHP) of Podshadley and Haley.[2] These and others are described in this chapter. They are used to assess dental plaque during the testing period.

C. Individual Clinical Score

In clinical practice, an index, plaque record, or scoring system for an individual patient can have significant value. The effects of personal disease control efforts, the progress of healing during professional treatments, and the maintenance of health over time, can be monitored. An example is the plaque-free score described on page 305 in which a patient is able to measure the effects of personal daily care efforts by the changes in the scores. This may prove to be a valuable motivating device.

D. Descriptive Categories of Indices

1. *General Categories*
   a. Simple index: one that measures the presence or absence of a condition. An example is an index that would measure the presence of dental plaque without an evaluation of its effect on the gingiva.
   b. Cumulative index: one that measures all the evidence of a condition, past and present. An example is the DMF Index for dental caries.
2. *Types of Simple and Cumulative Indices*
   a. Irreversible: one that measures conditions that will not change. An example is an index that measures dental caries.
   b. Reversible: one that measures conditions that can be changed. Examples are indices that measure dental plaque.
3. *Other Definitions*
   a. Incidence: the number of new cases of a specific disease or condition within a defined population over a period of time.
   b. Prevalence: the number of specific cases or lesions within a defined population at a single point in time or during a stated period of time.[3]

II. Purposes and Uses of an Index

A. For Individual Patients

An index can
1. Provide individual assessment to help patient recognize an oral problem.
2. Reveal the degree of effectiveness of present oral hygiene practices.
3. Motivate the person in preventive and professional care for the elimination and control of oral disease.
4. Evaluate the success of individual and professional treatment over a period of time by comparing index scores.
5. Provide a means for personal assessment by the dental hygienist of abilities to educate and motivate individual patients.

B. In Research

An index is used to
1. Determine baseline data before experimental factors are introduced.
2. Measure the effectiveness of specific agents for the prevention, control, or treatment of oral conditions.
3. Measure the effectiveness of mechanical devices for personal care, such as toothbrushes, interdental cleaning devices, or water irrigators.

C. In Community Health

An index can
1. Show the prevalence and trends of incidence of a particular condition occurring within a given population.
2. Provide baseline data to show existing dental health practices.
3. Assess the needs of a community.
4. Compare the effects of a community program and evaluate the results.

III. Characteristics of an Index

A useful and effective index will
A. Be simple to use and calculate.
B. Require minimal equipment and expense.
C. Have clear-cut criteria which are readily understandable.
D. Be as free as possible from subjective interpretation.
E. Be reproducible by the same examiner or different examiners.

ɤ. Be amenable to statistical analysis; have validity and reliability.

Ɔ. Not require an excessive amount of time to complete.

I. Not cause patient discomfort or be otherwise unacceptable to a patient.

GINGIVAL, PERIODONTAL, PLAQUE, AND CALCULUS INDICES

Several indices will be described in this chapter. The ones included have been selected because they are well known and widely used. The sequence of indices described follows a general outline in which periodontitis, gingivitis, dental plaque, and calculus indices are considered first, followed by plaque and bleeding scoring and recording systems. Dental caries indices for permanent and primary teeth are then outlined.

It should be realized that plaque indices are applicable for preventive instruction related to plaque control for dental caries as well as for gingival and periodontal disease. The *Suggested Readings* at the end of the chapter contain references to other indices. Familiarity with the various types may prove helpful when different evaluation criteria are needed.

THE PERIODONTAL INDEX (PI)

(Russell[4,5])

I. Purpose

To assess and score the periodontal disease status of populations in epidemiologic studies.

II. Procedure

A. Instruments

Each tooth present is examined using a mouth mirror and explorer with adequate illumination. In the original examinations[4] a Jacquette scaler and chip blower were used to define the presence of periodontal pockets. A periodontal probe would be the preferred instrument currently.

B. Calibration

When more than one examiner participates in a large survey, calibration between examiners is a necessity if the pooled findings are to be acceptable.

III. PI Computation

A. Criteria[5]

0 = Negative	There is neither overt inflammation in the investing tissues nor loss of function due to destruction of supporting tissue.
1 = Mild Gingivitis	There is an overt area of inflammation in the free gingiva which does not circumscribe the tooth.
2 = Gingivitis	Inflammation completely circumscribes the tooth, but there is no apparent break in the epithelial attachment.
6 = Gingivitis with Pocket Formation	The epithelial attachment has been broken and there is a pocket (not merely a deepened gingival crevice due to swelling in the free gingiva). There is no interference with normal masticatory function, the tooth is firm in its socket, and has not drifted.
8 = Advanced Destruction with loss of Masticatory Function	The tooth may be loose; may have drifted; may sound dull on percussion with a metallic instrument; may be depressible in its socket.

B. Scoring

1. Each tooth is assigned a score between 0 and 8: from no disease to severe disease with loss of function.

2. Add the scores for each tooth and divide by the number of teeth present and examined to obtain the individual's score.

3. Total the individuals' scores and divide by the number of people examined. The average ranges from 0 to 8.

4. Breakdown of scores: In a population group, scores may be averaged by specific age groups such as ages 1 to 9, 10 to 19, 20 to 29, and so forth. Scores may be calculated for each sex, or each sex within the various age groups. Data may also be used to calculate disease in relation to economic factors or educational background of the individuals.

THE PERIODONTAL DISEASE INDEX (PDI)

(Ramfjord[6,7])

I. Purpose

To assess the prevalence and severity of gingivitis and periodontitis and show the periodontal status of an individual or a group.

The Periodontal Index (PDI) combines the Gingivitis Index (GI) with measurements of the level of the periodontal attachment from the cementoenamel junction. Although not part of the PDI, a Calculus Index (CI) and a Plaque Index (PI) have usually been included when making a survey and will be described after the PDI.

II. Selection of Teeth and Surfaces

A. Areas Measured: Six teeth are used to represent the six segments of the dentition (figure 19–1).

Maxillary	Mandibular
#3 (1–6) right first molar	#19 (3–6) left first molar
#9 (2–1) left central incisor	#25 (4–1) right central incisor
#12 (2–4) left first premolar	#28 (4–4) right first premolar

B. Only fully erupted teeth are used.
C. Substitutions are not made for missing teeth; scores are derived from the teeth present.

III. Gingivitis Index (GI)

The gingiva around the six teeth is assessed

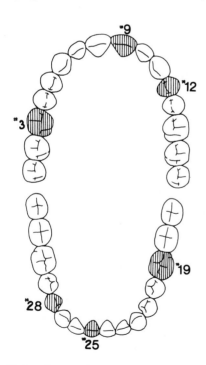

Figure 19–1. The Periodontal Disease Index (PDI). The six shaded teeth are scored. A gingivitis score is combined with measurements of the level of periodontal attachment.

for color, form, consistency, and bleeding tendency.

A. Procedure

1. Under consistent standardized light, dr the gingiva with cotton to observe colo and form.
2. Apply gentle pressure with the probe t determine consistency (density). Whe the color change definitely indicates th presence of inflammation, the consist ency is not checked.

B. Criteria

0 = Absence of signs of inflammation
1 = Mild to moderate inflammatory gingival changes not extending around the tooth
2 = Mild to moderately severe gingivitis extendin all around the tooth
3 = Severe gingivitis characterized by marked red ness, swelling, tendency to bleed, and ulcera tion, not necessarily extending around the tooth

C. Scoring

1. *Individual Teeth:* add the scores for each area and divide by the number of areas examined.
2. *Gingivitis Index:* add the scores for all o the examined teeth and divide by the total number of teeth examined. The Gingivitis Index ranges from 0 to 3.

IV. Crevice (Sulcus) Depth

The crevice or sulcus depth is measured from the cementoenamel junction.

A. Instrument

To obtain consistent readings, a probe is needed that has been calibrated for shape, thickness, angulation, and the placement and definition of reference marks. When the index was first used, a Michigan probe #0 was used (figure 13–1–D, page 214).

B. Locations of Measurements

1. *Two Measurements.* When two measurements are made, they are at the middle of the facial surface and at the facial aspect of the mesial contact area, with the side of the probe held touching both teeth (figure 19–2).
2. *Original PDI.* Four measurements were made for each tooth, on the facial,

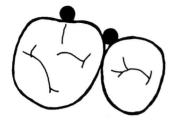

Figure 19–2. Probe positions for Periodontal Disease Index (PDI) shown by black dots beside tooth #3. Crevice (sulcus) depth is measured at the middle of the facial surface and at the facial aspect of the mesial contact area with the side of the probe held touching both teeth.

mesial, distal, and lingual. It was later found that no significant loss in accuracy resulted from using only two measurements. Four measurements are still used for certain types of research evaluations.

C. **Measurements**

1. Measure the distance from the gingival margin to the cementoenamel junction.
   a. Determine the location of the cementoenamel junction
      (1). By the difference in inclination of the enamel and cementum detected by the change in direction of the probe as it is moved apically (figure 19–3A).
      (2). By the change in surface texture from the smooth enamel surface to the rougher cemental surface.
   b. Scale to remove calculus when deposits interfere with detecting the location of the cementoenamel junction (figure 19–3B).
2. Measure from the gingival margin to the bottom of the crevice or pocket (figure 19–3C).
3. Subtract the distance (mm.) to the cementoenamel junction from the distance (mm.) to the bottom of the crevice or pocket.
4. Variations
   a. Junctional epithelium on the enamel: when the cementoenamel junction cannot be felt because it is not exposed, record the depth of the gingival crevice.
   b. Gingival margin on the cementum: record from the cementoenamel junction to the bottom of the crevice. The direct reading is used (figure 19–3D).

V. PDI Computation

A. Criteria

0 to 3 (Gingivitis Index)	= When the gingival crevice or pocket in none of the measured areas extends apical to the cementoenamel junction.

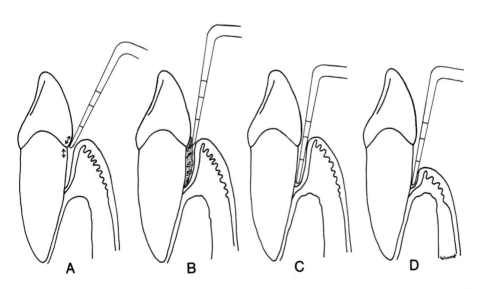

Figure 19–3. Periodontal Disease Index (PDI) crevice (sulcus) depth determination from the cementoenamel junction. **A.** Locating the cementoenamel junction with probe tip to measure the distance from the gingival margin to the cementoenamel junction. **B.** When calculus interferes with locating the cementoenamel junction, scaling is completed. **C.** Probe application to measure from gingival margin to bottom of the crevice or pocket; the distance to the cementoenamel junction is then subtracted. **D.** When there is apparent recession the direct reading from the cementoenamel junction to the bottom of the crevice is recorded. Note use of the Michigan 0 probe.

4 = When the crevices (pockets) of any two (or four) recorded areas extend apically to the cementoenamel junction not more than, but including, 3 mm. (The gingivitis score is then disregarded.)

5 = When the crevices (pockets) of any of the two (or four) recorded areas extend apically to the cementoenamel junction from 3 mm. to, and including, 6 mm. (The gingivitis score is disregarded.)

6 = When the crevices (pockets) extend more than 6 mm. apically to the cementoenamel junction in any of the two (or four) measured areas. (The gingivitis score is disregarded.)

B. PDI for an Individual

Add scores for individual teeth and divide by the number of teeth examined. The PDI will range from 0 to 6.

C. PDI Group Score

Total the individual PDI scores and divide by the number of people examined. The average ranges from 0 to 6.

D. Suggested Nominal Scale for Evaluation of Scores

1. *Gingivitis.* Numbers 0 to 3 indicate gingival involvement only, with increasing severity from 0 (no disease) through 3.9 (severe gingivitis).

2. *Periodontitis.* Numbers 4 through 6 indicate periodontal involvement with migration of the junctional epithelium and bone loss of increasing degree of severity from 4 (early disease) through 6 (advanced disease).

E. Calculation Example for an Individual

Tooth	Periodontal Disease Score
#3 (1–6)	4
#9 (2–1)	0
#12 (2–4)	5
#19 (3–6)	6
#25 (4–1)	4
#28 (4–4)	2
	Total 21

$$PDI = \frac{\text{Total scores}}{\text{Number of teeth}} = \frac{21}{6} = 3.5$$

Interpretation: For epidemiologic purposes using the average (mean) group score of 3.5 can be acceptable for showing overall characteristic of a large population. However, in the example above, the 3.5 PDI, which by the nominal score represents "severe gingivitis," would be misleading when reporting the condition of this individual. It is clear from the scores for each tooth that four of the six teeth examined have measurements that show loss of attachment and loss of bone typical of periodontitis. Care must be taken when interpreting the PDI on an individual basis.

CALCULUS INDEX (CI)

(Ramfjord[7])

The calculus index evaluates the presence and extent of calculus. This index is not an integral part of the PDI but was developed and used in conjunction with the PDI.

Because calculus may have to be removed to determine the location of the cementoenamel junction for crevice and pocket measurement in the PDI, calculus should be scored first, before its removal.

I. Instruments

A subgingival explorer (for example, the Number TU-17, figure 13–13, page 222) may be used to locate subgingival calculus and determine its extent. The probe (such as the Michigan 0) used for crevice and pocket determinations may provide sufficient sensitivity for calculus evaluation.

II. Surfaces Examined

Each of the four surfaces (facial, lingual, mesial, and distal) is given a score from 0 to 3.

III. Criteria

0 = No calculus.

1 = Supragingival calculus extending only slightly below the free gingival margin (not more than one mm.).

2 = Moderate amount of supra- and subgingival calculus, or subgingival calculus only.

3 = Abundance of supra- and subgingival calculus.

IV. Scoring

A. Individual Teeth

Add scores for each surface and divide by the number of surfaces (four).

Calculus Index for an Individual

Add the scores for the individual teeth and divide by the number of teeth. The Calculus Index ranges from 0 to 3.

DENTAL PLAQUE INDEX (PI)

(Ramfjord[7])

The plaque index aims to evaluate the extent f plaque on the basis of tooth surface coverage.

Procedure

. Apply disclosing agent, using two saturated pellets, one for the maxillary and one for the mandibular.
. Request patient to expectorate, then rinse with water.
C. Use direct or indirect (mirror) vision to observe specific surfaces with disclosed plaque.

I. Criteria

= No plaque.
= Plaque present on some but not all interproximal, facial, and lingual surfaces of the tooth.
= Plaque present on all interproximal, facial, and lingual surfaces, but covering less than one half of these surfaces.
= Plaque extending over all interproximal, facial, and lingual surfaces, and covering more than one half of these surfaces.

II. Criteria Modification

The original criteria listed above serve adequately for epidemiologic purposes. Criteria were developed later to refine the scoring for small differences in the distribution of dental plaque.[8] By the modified system, scores are recorded for the gingival half of the facial and lingual surfaces as shown in figure 19–4, and recorded as follows:

= No plaque on the gingival half.
= Plaque covering less than one third of the gingival half.
= Plaque covering one third or less than two thirds of the gingival half.
3 = Plaque covering two thirds or more of the facial or lingual of the gingival half.

IV. Scoring

Add the plaque scores for each tooth and divide by the number of teeth examined.

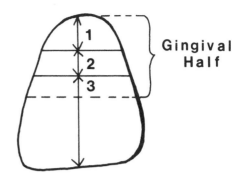

Figure 19–4. Ramfjord Dental Plaque Index (PI) criteria modification. Scores are recorded for the gingival half of the facial and lingual surfaces. See the text for scoring criteria.

GINGIVAL INDEX (GI)

(Löe and Silness[9,10])

I. Purpose

To assess the severity of gingivitis based on color, consistency, and bleeding on probing.

II. Selection of Teeth and Gingival Areas

A gingival index may be determined for selected teeth or for the entire dentition.

A. Areas Examined

Four gingival areas (distal, facial, mesial, lingual) are examined systematically for each tooth.

B. Modified Procedure

Omit the distal examination for each tooth. The score for the mesial is doubled and the total score for each tooth is divided by four.

III. Procedure

A. The teeth and gingiva are dried and, under adequate light, a mouth mirror and probe are used.
B. The probe is used to press on the gingiva to determine the degree of firmness.
C. The probe is used to run along the soft tissue wall near the entrance to the gingival sulcus to evaluate bleeding (figure 19–5).

IV. Criteria

0 = Normal gingiva.
1 = Mild inflammation—slight change in color, slight edema. *No bleeding on probing.*

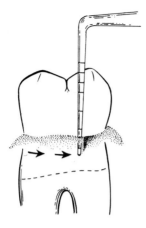

Figure 19–5. Gingival Index (GI) Löe and Silness. Probe stroke for bleeding evaluation. The broken line represents the junctional epithelium position. The probe is inserted a few millimeters and moved along the soft tissue pocket wall with light pressure in a circumferential direction. The probe stroke shown here is in contrast with the walking stroke used for pocket evaluation and measurement as described on page 216.

2 = Moderate inflammation—redness, edema and glazing. *Bleeding on probing.*

3 = Severe inflammation—marked redness and edema. Ulceration. *Tendency to spontaneous bleeding.*

V. Scoring

A. GI for Area

Each of the four gingival surfaces (distal, facial, mesial, lingual) is given a score of 0 to 3.

B. GI for a Tooth

Scores for each area are totalled and divided by four.

C. GI for Groups of Teeth

Scores for individual teeth may be grouped and totalled, and divided by the number of teeth. A Gingival Index may be determined for specific teeth, group of teeth, quadrant, or side of mouth.

D. GI for the Individual

By totalling scores and dividing by the number of teeth examined, the Gingival Index is determined. Indices range from 0 to 3.

E. Suggested Nominal Scale for Patient Reference

Rating	Scores
Excellent (healthy tissue)	0
Good	0.1–0.9
Fair	1.0–1.9
Poor	2.0–3.0

F. Calculation Example for an Individual

Gingival area

	M	F	D	L
3 (1–6)	3	1	3	1
9 (2–1)	1	0	1	1
12 (2–4)	2	1	2	0
19 (3–6)	3	1	3	3
25 (4–1)	1	1	1	1
28 (4–4)	2	1	2	0
Total	12 +	5 +	12 +	6 = 35

$$\text{Gingival Index} = \frac{\text{Total score}}{\text{Number of surfaces}}$$

$$= \frac{35}{24} = 1.45 \text{ GI}$$

Interpretation: According to the suggested nominal scale, the score for this individual (1.45) indicates only fair gingival health. The ratings for each gingival area or surface can be used during continuing patient instruction to help the patient compare scores at intervals as the gingival condition improves.

PLAQUE INDEX (Pl I)

(Silness and Löe[1,10])

I. Purpose

To assess the thickness of plaque at the gingival area.

II. Selection of Teeth

The entire dentition or selected teeth can be evaluated.

A. Areas Examined

Four gingival areas (distal, facial, mesial, lingual) are examined systematically for each tooth.

Plaque Evaluation

Only plaque of the cervical third is evaluated with no attention to plaque that has extended to the middle or incisal thirds.

II. Procedures

. The tooth is dried and examined visually for scores of 2 or 3 (see Criteria below).

. When no plaque is visible, an explorer is used to test the surface. The explorer is passed across the tooth surface in the cervical third and near the entrance to the sulcus. When no plaque adheres to the point of the explorer, the area is considered to have a 0 score. When plaque adheres, a score of 1 is assigned.

. Plaque that is on the surface of calculus deposits and on dental restorations of all types in the cervical third is evaluated and included.

. Modified Procedures
   1. Examine only the facial, mesial, and lingual. Assign double score to the mesial reading, and divide the total by four.
   2. Use a disclosing agent to assist evaluation for the 0 to 1 scores.

V. Criteria

= No plaque.

= A film of plaque adhering to the free gingival margin and adjacent area of the tooth. The plaque may be recognized only after application of disclosing agent or by running the explorer across the tooth surface.

= Moderate accumulation of soft deposits within the gingival pocket or on the tooth and gingival margin, which can be seen with the naked eye.

= Abundance of soft matter within the gingival pocket and/or on the tooth and gingival margin.

V. Scoring

A. Pl I for Area

Each area (mesial, distal, facial, lingual) is assigned a score from 0 to 3.

B. Pl I for a Tooth

Scores for each area are totalled and divided by four.

C. Pl I for Groups of Teeth

Scores for individual teeth may be grouped

and totalled and divided by the number of teeth. For instance, a Plaque Index may be determined for specific teeth or groups of teeth. The right side may be compared with the left.

D. Pl I for the Individual

Add the indices for each of the teeth and divide by the number of teeth examined. The Pl I ranges from 0 to 3.

E. Pl I for a Group

Add the indices for each member of a group and divide by the number of individuals to determine the population average score.

F. Suggested Nominal Scale for Patient Reference

Rating	Scores
Excellent	0
Good	0.1–0.9
Fair	1.0–1.9
Poor	2.0–3.0

SIMPLIFIED ORAL HYGIENE INDEX (OHI-S)

(Greene and Vermillion[11,12])

I. Purpose

To quantitate oral cleanliness by estimating the tooth surface area covered by debris or calculus.

The OHI-S has two components, the Debris Index and the Calculus Index. Each is based on numerical determinations which designate the amount of debris or calculus found on preselected tooth surfaces. The two scores may be useful singly or may be combined for the OHI-S.

II. Selection of Teeth and Surfaces
(figure 19–6)

A. Posterior. The first fully erupted tooth distal to each second premolar is examined. Facial surfaces of the two maxillary molars and lingual surfaces of the mandibular are used. Although usually a first molar, it may be a second or third.

B. Anterior. The facial surfaces of the maxillary right and the mandibular left central incisor are scored. When either is missing, the opposite central incisor is used.

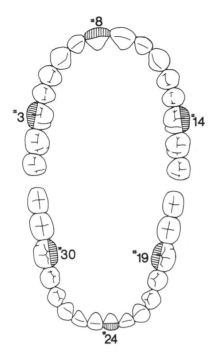

Figure 19–6. Simplified Oral Hygiene Index (OHI-S). Six tooth surfaces are scored as shown, namely the facial surfaces of maxillary molars and the maxillary and mandibular central incisors, and lingual surfaces of mandibular molars. The same tooth surfaces are used for a Patient Hygiene Performance (PHP).

C. A tooth is considered fully erupted when it has reached the occlusal plane.

D. Examination includes the proximal surfaces to the contact area, and therefore, the score is considered to represent half the circumference of each tooth examined.

E. An alternate tooth is selected when a tooth has a full crown restoration or is reduced in height by severe caries or trauma.

III. Simplified Debris Index (DI-S)

A. Definition of Oral Debris

Oral debris is the soft foreign matter attached to the teeth. It may consist of mucin, bacterial plaque, and food debris.

B. Procedure

The surface area covered by debris is estimated by running the side of the tip of an explorer across the tooth surface.

C. Criteria (figure 19–7)

0 = No debris or stain present.
1 = Soft debris covering not more than one third of

the tooth surface being examined, or the presence of extrinsic stains without debris, regardless of surface area covered.
2 = Soft debris covering more than one third but not more than two thirds of the exposed tooth surface.
3 = Soft debris covering more than two thirds of the exposed tooth surface.

D. Scoring

1. At least two of the six possible surfaces must have been examined for an individual score to be calculated.
2. Simplified Debris Index (DI-S): Add the scores for the individual teeth together and divide by the number of teeth examined.
3. The DI-S ranges from 0 to 3.

IV. Simplified Calculus Index (CI-S)

A. Procedure

An explorer is used similarly to the procedure for the DI-S previously described. The surface area covered by calculus is detected supragingivally, and subgingival calculus is explored.

B. Criteria (figure 19–8)

0 = No calculus present.
1 = Supragingival calculus covering not more than one third of the exposed tooth surface being examined.
2 = Supragingival calculus covering more than one third but not more than two thirds of the exposed tooth surface, or the presence of individual flecks of subgingival calculus around the cervical portion of the tooth.
3 = Supragingival calculus covering more than two thirds of the exposed tooth surface or a continuous heavy band of subgingival calculus around the cervical portion of the tooth.

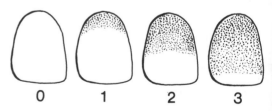

Figure 19–7. Simplified Debris Index (DI-S), a component of the OHI-S. Six teeth are scored according to figure 19–6. Scoring of 0 to 3 based on tooth surface covered by debris as shown.

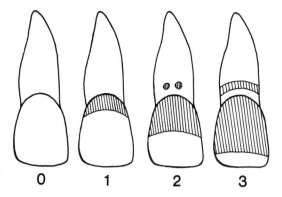

Figure 19–8. Simplified Calculus Index (CI-S), a component of the OHI-S. An explorer is used to detect the location of calculus on the six teeth designated by figure 19–6. Scoring of 0 to 3 is based on location and tooth surface area covered by calculus as shown.

C. Scoring

1. At least two of the six possible surfaces must have been examined for an individual score to be calculated.
2. Simplified Calculus Index (CI-S): Add the scores for the individual teeth and divide by the number of teeth examined.
3. The CI-S ranges from 0 to 3.

V. OHI-S Computation

A. OHI-S for an Individual

Add together the DI-S and the CI-S. The OHI-S value ranges from 0 to 6.

B. OHI-S Group Score

Compute the average of the individual scores by totalling the scores and dividing by the number of individuals.

C. Suggested Nominal Scale for Evaluation of Scores[12]

DI-S and CI-S

Rating	Scores
Excellent	0 (no plaque or calculus)
Good	0.1–0.6
Fair	0.7–1.8
Poor	1.9–3.0

OHI-S

Excellent	0
Good	0.1–1.2
Fair	1.3–3.0
Poor	3.1–6.0

D. Calculation Example for an Individual

Tooth	Individual Scores	
	DI-S	CI-S
#3 (1–6)	2	2
#8 (1–1)	1	0
#14 (2–6)	3	2
#19 (3–6)	3	2
#24 (3–1)	2	1
#30 (4–6)	2	2
Total	13	9

$$DI\text{-}S = \frac{\text{Total Debris Scored}}{\text{Number of Teeth Scored}} = \frac{13}{6} = 2.17$$

$$CI\text{-}S = \frac{\text{Total Calculus Scored}}{\text{Number of Teeth Scored}} = \frac{9}{6} = 1.5$$

$$OHI\text{-}S = DI\text{-}S + CI\text{-}S = 2.17 + 1.50 = 3.67$$

Interpretation: According to the suggested nominal scale the score for this individual (3.67) indicates a poor oral hygiene status.

VI. Comparison of OHI and OHI-S

Originally, the Oral Hygiene Index (OHI) was developed.[13] After experience with the Oral Hygiene Index, the need for simplification was recognized because of the length of time required to arrive at an evaluation of the debris and calculus, as well as the need for subjective decisions for tooth selection. The basic differences between the OHI and the OHI-S are as follows:

A. Number of Surfaces Evaluated

In the OHI there were 12 surfaces, both lingual and facial, whereas only 6 are used in the OHI-S.

B. Tooth Selection

In the OHI, the examiner had to select the tooth with the most debris or calculus in the segment. The lingual surface selected did not have to be of the same tooth as the facial surface.

C. Scoring

The OHI had a possible range from 0 to 12, whereas the OHI-S may range from 0 to 6.

PATIENT HYGIENE PERFORMANCE (PHP)

(Podshadley and Haley[2])

I. Purpose

To assess the extent of plaque and debris over a tooth surface. Debris is defined for the PHP as the soft foreign material consisting of mucin, bacteria, and food that is loosely attached to tooth surfaces.

II. Selection of Teeth and Surfaces

A. Teeth Examined

Maxillary	Mandibular
#3 (1–6) Right first molar	#19 (3–6) Left first molar
#8 (1–1) Right central incisor	#24 (3–1) Left central incisor
#14 (2–6) Left first molar	#30 (4–6) Right first molar

B. Substitutions

When a first molar is missing, less than three-fourths erupted, has a full crown, or is broken down, the second molar is used, or the third when the second is missing. The adjacent central incisor is used for a missing incisor.

C. Surfaces

The facial surfaces of incisors and maxillary molars and the lingual of mandibular molars are examined. These are the same surfaces as those used for the Simplified Oral Hygiene Index (figure 19–6).

III. Procedure

A. Apply disclosing agent. Instruct the patient to swish for 30 seconds and expectorate but not rinse.
B. Examination is made using a mouth mirror.
C. Each tooth surface to be evaluated is subdivided (mentally) into five sections (figure 19–9A) as follows:
   1. Vertically: three divisions, mesial, middle, and distal.
   2. Horizontally: the middle third is subdivided into gingival, middle, and occlusal or incisal thirds.

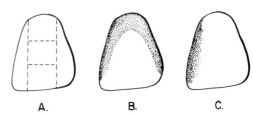

Figure 19–9. Patient Hygiene Performance (PHP). **A.** To assess oral debris, a tooth is divided into five subdivisions each of which is scored one (1) if debris is shown to be present after use of a disclosing agent. **B.** Example of Debris Score of 3. Shaded portion represents debris stained by disclosing agent. **C.** Example of Debris Score of 1. (Podshadley and Haley, Public Health Reports, 83, 259, 1968.)

IV. PHP Computation

A. Debris Score for Each Subdivision

Each of the five subdivisions is scored for the presence of stained debris as follows:

0 = No debris (or questionable).
1 = Debris definitely present.
Identify by M when all three molars or both incisors are missing.
Identify by S when a substitute tooth is used.

B. Debris Score for Individual Tooth

Add the scores for each of the five subdivisions. The scores range from 0 to 5.

C. PHP for the Individual

Total the scores for the individual teeth and divide by the number of teeth examined. The PHP ranges from 0 to 5.

D. PHP for a Group

To obtain the average PHP score for a group or population, total the individual scores and divide by the number of people examined.

E. Suggested Nominal Scale for Evaluation of Scores

Rating	Scores
Excellent	0 (no debris)
Good	0.1–1.7
Fair	1.8–3.4
Poor	3.5–5.0

F. Calculation Example for an Individual

Tooth	Debris Score
#3 (1–6)	5
#8 (1–1)	3
#14 (2–6)	4
#19 (3–6)	5
#24 (3–1)	2
#30 (4–6)	3
Total	22

$$PHP = \frac{\text{Total Debris Score}}{\text{Number of Teeth Scored}} = \frac{22}{6} = 3.66$$

Interpretation: According to the suggested nominal scale, this person with a PHP of 3.66 would be classified as having poor hygiene performance.

PLAQUE-FREE SCORE

(Grant, Stern, Everett[14])

I. Purpose

To determine the location, number, and percent of plaque-free surfaces for individual motivation and instruction. Interdental bleeding can also be documented.

II. Selection of Teeth and Surfaces

A. All erupted teeth are included. Missing teeth are identified on the record form by a single thick horizontal line through the box in the chart form.

B. Four surfaces are recorded for each tooth: facial, lingual, mesial, and distal.

III. Procedure

A. Plaque-free Score

1. Apply disclosing agent or give chewable tablet. Instruct patient to swish and rub the solution over the tooth surfaces with the tongue before rinsing.
2. Examine each tooth surface for evidence of plaque. Use adequate light and a mouth mirror for visualizing all surfaces. In patient instruction, the patient needs a hand mirror to see the location of the plaque that has been missed during personal hygiene techniques.
3. Record in red the surfaces showing plaque. Use an appropriate tooth chart form or a diagrammatic form such as shown in figure 19–10. Red for recording the plaque is suggested when a red dis-

closing agent is used to help the patient associate the location of the plaque in the mouth with the recording.

B. Papillary Bleeding on Probing

1. Note the small circles between the diagrammatic tooth blocks in figure 19–10. They are used to record proximal bleeding on probing.
2. Improvement in the gingival tissue health will be demonstrated over a period of time as fewer bleeding areas are noted.

IV. Calculations

A. Plaque-free Score

1. Total the number of teeth present.
2. Total the number of surfaces with plaque that appear red on the tooth diagram.
3. Consult table 19–1.
   a. Read across the top or bottom to locate the number of teeth and total surfaces.
   b. Read down the side to the number of surfaces with plaque.
   c. Find the intersect of the top and side numbers, which is the plaque-free score in percent.
4. To calculate without table 19–1 for reference
   a. Subtract the number of surfaces with plaque from the total available surfaces to find the number of plaque-free surfaces.
   b. Plaque-free score =

$$\frac{\text{Number of plaque-free surfaces} \times 100}{\text{Number of available surfaces}}$$

$$= \text{Percent plaque-free surfaces}$$

5. Evaluation of plaque-free score. Ideally, 100 percent is the goal. When a patient maintains a percent over 80, individual surfaces need to be checked to determine whether plaque is usually left in the same areas. To prevent the development of specific areas of periodontal disease, remedial instruction in the areas usually missed is indicated.

B. Papillary Bleeding on Probing

1. Total the number of small circles marked for bleeding. For a person with 32 teeth

Table 19–1. Plaque-Free Score

	32-128	31-124	30-120	29-116	28-112	27-108	26-104	25-100	24-96	23-92	22-88	21-84
1	99.2	99.2	99.2	99.2	99.2	99.1	99.1	99.0	99.0	99.0	98.9	98.9
4	96.9	96.8	96.7	97.6	96.5	96.3	96.2	96.0	95.9	95.7	95.5	95.3
7	94.6	95.4	94.2	94.0	93.8	93.6	93.3	93.0	92.8	92.4	92.1	91.7
10	92.2	92.0	91.7	91.4	91.1	90.8	90.4	90.0	89.6	89.2	88.7	88.1
13	89.9	89.6	89.2	88.8	88.4	88.0	87.5	87.0	86.5	85.9	85.3	84.5
16	87.5	87.1	86.7	86.3	85.8	85.2	84.7	84.0	83.4	82.7	81.9	81.0
19	85.2	84.7	84.2	83.7	83.1	82.5	81.8	81.0	80.3	79.4	78.5	77.4
22	83.9	82.3	81.7	81.1	80.4	79.7	78.9	78.0	77.1	76.1	75.0	73.9
25	80.4	79.9	79.2	78.5	77.7	76.9	76.0	75.0	74.0	72.9	71.6	70.3
28	78.2	77.5	76.7	75.9	75.0	74.1	73.1	72.0	70.9	69.6	68.2	66.4
31	75.8	75.0	74.2	73.3	72.4	71.3	70.2	69.0	67.8	66.4	64.8	63.1
34	73.5	72.6	71.7	70.7	69.7	68.6	67.4	66.0	64.6	63.1	61.4	59.6
37	71.1	70.2	69.2	68.2	67.0	65.8	64.5	63.0	61.5	59.8	58.0	56.0
40	68.8	67.8	66.7	65.6	64.3	63.0	61.6	60.0	58.4	56.6	54.6	52.4
43	66.5	65.4	64.2	63.0	61.7	60.2	58.7	57.0	55.3	53.3	51.2	48.9
46	64.1	63.0	61.7	60.4	59.0	57.5	55.8	54.0	52.1	50.0	47.8	45.3
49	61.8	60.5	59.2	57.8	56.3	54.7	52.9	51.0	49.0	46.8	44.4	41.7
52	59.4	58.1	56.7	55.2	53.6	51.9	50.0	48.0	45.9	43.5	41.0	38.1
55	57.1	55.7	54.2	52.6	50.9	49.1	47.2	45.0	42.8	40.3	37.5	34.6
58	54.7	53.3	51.7	50.0	48.3	46.3	44.3	42.0	39.6	37.0	34.1	31.0
61	52.4	50.9	49.2	47.5	45.6	43.6	41.4	39.0	36.4	33.7	30.7	27.4
64	50.0	48.4	46.7	44.9	42.9	40.8	38.5	36.0	33.4	30.5	27.3	23.9
67	47.7	46.0	44.2	42.3	40.2	38.0	35.6	33.0	30.3	27.2	23.9	20.3
70	45.4	43.6	41.7	39.7	37.5	35.2	32.7	30.0	27.1	24.0	20.5	16.7
73	43.0	41.2	39.2	37.1	34.9	32.5	29.9	27.0	24.0	20.7	17.1	13.1
76	40.7	38.8	36.7	34.5	32.2	29.7	27.0	24.0	20.9	17.4	13.7	9.6
79	38.3	36.3	34.2	31.9	29.5	26.9	24.1	21.0	17.8	14.2	10.3	6.0
82	36.0	33.9	31.7	29.4	26.8	24.1	21.2	18.0	14.6	10.9	6.9	2.4
85	33.6	31.5	29.2	26.8	24.2	21.3	18.3	15.0	11.5	7.7	3.3	–

Left	9-36	10-40	11-44	12-48	13-52	14-56	15-60	16-64	17-68	18-72	19-76	20-80	Right
88	31.3	29.1	26.7	24.2	21.5	18.6	15.4	12.0	8.4	4.4	0.0	—	79
91	29.0	26.7	24.2	21.6	18.8	15.8	12.5	9.0	5.3	1.1	—	1.3	78
94	27.6	24.2	21.7	19.0	16.1	13.0	9.7	6.0	2.1	—	0.0	5.0	78
97	24.3	21.8	19.2	16.4	13.4	10.2	6.8	3.0	—	2.8	4.0	8.8	73
100	21.9	19.4	16.7	13.8	10.8	7.5	3.9	0.0	1.5	7.0	7.9	12.5	70
103	19.9	17.0	14.2	11.3	8.1	4.7	1.0	—	5.9	11.2	11.9	16.3	67
106	17.2	14.6	11.7	8.7	5.4	1.9	—	0.0	10.3	15.3	15.8	20.0	64
109	14.9	12.1	9.2	6.1	2.7	—	3.4	4.7	14.8	19.5	19.8	23.8	61
112	12.5	9.7	6.7	3.5	0.0	1.8	8.4	9.4	19.2	23.7	23.7	27.5	58
115	11.2	7.3	4.2	.9	—	7.2	13.4	14.1	23.6	27.8	27.7	31.3	55
118	7.9	4.9	1.7	—	0.0	12.5	18.4	18.8	28.0	32.0	31.6	35.0	52
121	5.5	2.5	—	4.2	5.8	17.9	23.4	23.5	32.4	36.2	35.6	38.8	49
124	3.2	0.0	—	10.5	11.6	23.3	28.4	28.2	36.8	40.3	39.5	42.5	46
128	0.0	—	2.3	16.7	17.4	28.6	33.4	32.9	41.2	44.5	43.5	46.3	43
	—	0.0	9.1	23.0	23.1	34.0	38.4	37.5	45.6	48.7	47.4	50.0	40
	5.6	7.5	16.0	29.2	28.9	39.3	43.4	42.2	50.0	52.8	51.4	53.8	37
	13.9	15.0	22.8	35.5	34.7	44.7	48.4	46.9	54.5	57.0	55.3	57.5	34
	22.3	22.5	29.6	41.7	40.4	50.0	53.4	51.6	58.9	61.2	59.3	61.3	31
	30.6	30.0	36.4	48.0	46.2	55.4	58.4	56.3	63.3	65.3	63.2	65.0	28
	38.9	37.5	43.2	54.2	52.0	60.8	63.4	61.0	67.7	69.5	67.2	68.8	25
	47.3	45.0	50.0	60.5	57.7	66.1	68.4	65.7	72.1	73.7	71.1	72.5	22
	55.6	52.5	56.9	66.7	63.5	71.5	73.4	70.4	76.5	78.8	75.0	76.3	19
	63.9	60.0	63.7	73.0	69.3	76.8	78.4	75.0	80.9	82.0	79.0	80.0	16
	72.3	67.5	70.5	79.2	75.0	82.2	83.4	79.7	85.3	86.2	82.9	83.8	13
	80.6	75.0	77.3	85.5	80.8	87.5	88.4	84.4	89.8	90.3	86.9	87.5	10
	88.9	82.5	84.1	91.7	86.6	92.9	93.4	89.1	94.2	94.5	90.8	91.3	7
	97.3	90.0	91.0	98.0	92.4	98.3	98.4	93.8	98.6	98.7	94.8	95.0	4
		97.5	97.8		98.1			98.5			98.7	98.8	1

(From Grant, D.A., Stern, I.B., and Everett, F.G.: *Periodontics*, 5th ed. The C.V. Mosby Co., 1979.)

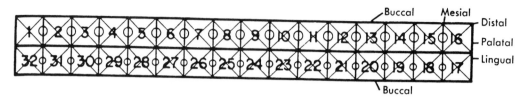

Figure 19–10.   Form for recording plaque-free score and papillary bleeding. (From Grant, D.A., Stern, I.B., and Everett F.G.: *Periodontics*, 5th ed., The C.V. Mosby Co. 1979.)

there are 30 interdental areas. The mesial or distal of a tooth adjacent to an edentulous area is probed and counted.

2. Evaluation of total interdental bleeding. In health there is no bleeding on probing.

C. **Calculation Example for Plaque-free Score**

Individual findings: 24 teeth scored
                     37 surfaces with plaque

1. Using table 19–1
   a. Locate the number of teeth across the top of table 19–1 (24–96): there are 96 total surfaces.
   b. Locate the number of surfaces with plaque down the side (37): find the intersect.
   c. The percent of plaque-free surfaces is 61.5.
2. Without reference table 19–1
   a. Multiply the number of teeth by four: 24 × 4 = 96 available surfaces
   b. Subtract the number of surfaces with plaque from total available surfaces: 96 − 37 = 59 plaque-free surfaces
   c. Percent plaque-free surfaces =

$$\frac{59 \times 100}{96} = 61.5$$

3. Interpretation: On the basis of the ideal 100 percent, 61.5 percent is very poor. More instruction is indicated.

PLAQUE CONTROL RECORD

(O'Leary[15])

I. Purpose

To record the presence of bacterial plaque on individual tooth surfaces to permit the patient to visualize progress while learning plaque control.

II. Selection of Teeth and Surfaces

A. All teeth are included. Missing teeth are identified on the record form by a single thick horizontal line.
B. Four surfaces are recorded: facial, lingual, mesial, and distal.

III. Procedure

A. Apply disclosing agent or give a chewable tablet. Instruct patient to swish and rub the solution over the tooth surfaces with the tongue before rinsing.
B. Examine each tooth surface for dental plaque at the gingival margin. No attempt is made to differentiate quantity of plaque.
C. Record by making a dash or coloring in the appropriate spaces on the diagram (figure 19–11) to indicate plaque on facial, lingual, mesial, and/or distal surfaces.
D. Modification: six areas recorded. The mesial and distal segments of the diagram may be divided to provide space to record proximal surfaces from the facial separately from the lingual.[16]

IV. Calculations

A. Total the number of teeth present; multiply by four (or six if modification is used) to obtain the number of available surfaces. Count the number of surfaces with plaque.
B. Multiply the number of plaque-containing surfaces by 100 and divide by the total number of available surfaces to derive the percent of surfaces.
C. Compare over subsequent appointments as the patient learns and practices plaque control. Ten percent or less can be considered a good goal, but if the plaque is regularly left in the same areas, special instruction is indicated to prevent the development of areas of pocket formation.

Plaque Control Record

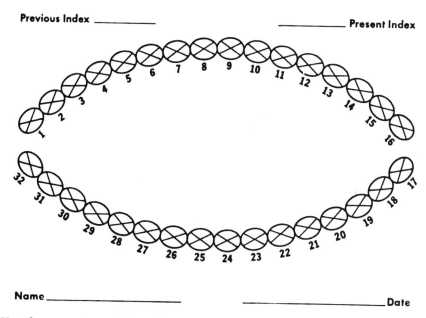

Previous Index _____   _____ **Present Index**

Name _____   _____ **Date**

Figure 19–11. Plaque control record form with diagrammatic representation of the teeth. Facial surfaces are on the outer, and lingual, on the inner, portion of the arches. (From O'Leary, T.J., Drake, R.B., and Naylor, J.E.: *J. Periodontol.*, 43, 38, 1972.)

D. Calculation example for plaque control record

Individual findings: 26 teeth scored

8 surfaces with plaque

1. Multiply the number of teeth by four:
   $26 \times 4 = 104$ surfaces
2. Percent with plaque =

$$\frac{\text{Number of surfaces with plaque} \times 100}{\text{Number of available tooth surfaces}}$$

$$= \frac{800}{104} = 7.6$$

Interpretation: Although 0 percent is ideal, less than 10 percent has been suggested as a guideline in periodontal therapy. After initial therapy and when the patient has reached a 10 percent level of plaque control or better, necessary additional periodontal and restorative procedures may be initiated.[15] In comparison, a similar evaluation using a plaque-free score would mean a goal of over 90 percent or better plaque-free before the surgical phase of treatment should be undertaken.

BLEEDING INDICES

Bleeding on gentle probing or flossing is an early sign of gingival inflammation and precedes color changes and enlargement of the gingival tissues.[17,18] Based on the principle that healthy tissue does not bleed, testing for bleeding has become a significant procedure for evaluation prior to treatment planning, after therapy to show the effects of treatment aimed to eliminate inflammation, and at recall appointments to assess maintenance.

For patient instruction and motivation, a variety of bleeding indices and scoring methods has been developed. The Gingival Index (GI) described on page 299 includes an estimate of bleeding on probing along with other clinical observations to arrive at a score to designate the severity of gingivitis. The GI has been used extensively in research as well as for patient instruction and motivation.

Another example is the record of bleeding following interdental probing which may accompany a plaque-free score as described on page 305. The form illustrated in figure 19–10 has small circles which can be colored in to illustrate interproximal bleeding. A series of diagrams over several weeks can show the patient's progress toward health, as less and less bleeding is charted.

In one system, a bleeding point determination is made by applying a probe just under the gingival margin at the distal aspect of the most posterior tooth and moving the probe in a continuous motion around the sulcus into the mesial aspect. The stroke is illustrated in figure 19–5. The probe is carried likewise around the sulci of all the teeth in both dental arches. Bleeding points are recorded on an appropriate chart and a percentage of total areas may be calculated.[19]

A papillary bleeding index has been used in which the probe is drawn with a light sweeping motion under the gingival margin from the line angle to the tip of the papilla on each side.[20] Each papilla around the mouth may be checked, or selected representative papillae may make up the index. A scoring on a scale of one to four has been used to designate the profuseness of bleeding. Instruction and participation of the patient, using a hand mirror to observe the proceedings, are essential if the objectives are to be attained. As with other indices, the purpose is to monitor the patient's progress toward oral health.

Two of the well-known bleeding indices will be described below. They are the Sulcus Bleeding Index developed by Mühlemann and the Gingival Bleeding Index of Carter and Barnes.

SULCUS BLEEDING INDEX (SBI)

(Mühlemann[17])

I. Purpose

To locate areas of gingival sulcus bleeding upon gentle probing and thus recognize and record the presence of early (initial) inflammatory gingival disease.

II. Areas Examined

Four gingival units are scored systematically for each tooth: the marginal gingiva, labial and lingual (M units), and the papillary gingiva, mesial and distal (P units).

III. Procedure

A. Use standardized lighting while probing each of the four areas with a probe.
B. Hold the probe parallel with the long axis of the tooth for M units, and direct the probe toward the col area for P units.

C. Wait 30 seconds after probing before scoring apparently healthy gingival units.
D. Dry the gingiva gently if necessary to observe color changes clearly.

IV. Criteria

0 = Healthy appearance of P and M, no bleeding on sulcus probing.
1 = Apparently healthy P and M showing no change in color and no swelling, but bleeding from sulcus on probing.
2 = Bleeding on probing *and* change of color due to inflammation. No swelling nor macroscopic edema.
3 = Bleeding on probing *and* change in color and slight edematous swelling.
4 = (1) Bleeding on probing *and* change in color *and* obvious swelling.
    (2) Bleeding on probing and obvious swelling.
5 = Bleeding on probing and spontaneous bleeding *and* change in color, marked swelling with or without ulceration.

V. Scoring

A. SBI for Area

Each of the four gingival units (M and P) is scored 0 to 5.

B. SBI for Tooth

Scores for the four units are totalled and divided by 4.

C. SBI for Individual

By totalling scores for individual teeth and dividing by the number of teeth, the SBI is determined. Indices will range from 0 to 6.

GINGIVAL BLEEDING INDEX (GBI)

(Carter and Barnes[21])

I. Purpose

To record the presence or absence of gingival inflammation as determined by bleeding from interproximal gingival sulci.

II. Areas Examined

Each interproximal area has two sulci which are scored as one interdental unit, or may be scored individually. Certain areas may be excluded from scoring because of accessibility, tooth position, diastemas, or other factors, and if exclusions are made, a consistent procedure should be followed for an individual and for a group if a study is to be made.

A full complement of teeth has 28 proximal areas. In the original studies, third molars were excluded, and 26 units were recorded.[21]

III. Procedure

A. Instrument

Unwaxed dental floss is used. The use of floss has the advantages of being readily available, disposable, and usable by the instructed patient.

B. Steps

1. Pass the floss interproximally first on one side of the papilla and then on the other.
2. Curve the floss around the adjacent tooth (figure 23–1 E and F, page 361), and bring the floss to the bottom of the sulcus.
3. Move the floss up and down for one stroke, with care not to lacerate the gingiva. Adapt finger rests to provide controlled, consistent pressure.
4. Use a new length of clean floss for each area.
5. Retract for visibility of hemorrhage from both facial and lingual.
6. Allow 30 seconds for reinspection of an area that does not show blood immediately either in the area or on the floss.

IV. Criteria

Bleeding indicates the presence of disease. No attempt is made to quantify the severity of bleeding because the important factor is no bleeding at all in health.

V. Scoring

The number of bleeding areas and the number of scorable units are recorded. Patient motivation can result when the patient participates in observing and recording over a series of appointments.

DENTAL CARIES INDICES

The most widely used indices are the DMFT (Decayed, Missing, Filled Teeth), DMFS (Decayed, Missing, Filled Surfaces) for permanent teeth,[22] and the counterparts deft (decayed, extracted, filled teeth) and defs (decayed, ex-

tracted, filled surfaces) for the primary teeth.[23] For a mixed dentition, two separate indices are used.

From the indices, information can be derived to show the number of persons affected by dental caries, the number of teeth that need treatment, the proportion of teeth that have been treated, and other statistical data useful in organizing and evaluating dental health program efforts.

When a survey is made, specific procedures must be carefully defined to fulfill the objectives of a specific study. The basic descriptions included in this section can be adapted in most situations.

DECAYED MISSING AND FILLED PERMANENT TEETH (DMFT)

I. Purpose

To determine total dental caries experience, past and present.

II. Selection of Teeth

A. DMF is based on 28 teeth.

B. Teeth Not Counted

1. Third molars
2. Unerupted teeth
   A tooth is considered erupted when any part projects through the gingiva. In certain types of research it may be necessary to differentiate clinical emergence, partial eruption, and full eruption.[24]
3. Congenitally missing and supernumerary teeth.
4. Teeth removed for reasons other than dental caries such as for an impaction or during orthodontic treatment.
5. Teeth restored for reasons other than dental caries such as trauma (fracture), cosmetic purposes, or for use as a bridge abutment.
6. Primary tooth retained with the permanent successor erupted. The permanent tooth is evaluated since a primary tooth is never included in this index.

III. Procedures

A. Instruments

Each tooth is examined in a systematic

sequence, using a mouth mirror and adequate light. Explorers of the same design and with standardized dimensions of the working ends are needed.

B. Examination

1. *Use of Explorer.* Teeth should be observed by visual means as much as possible. Unnecessary discomfort for the patient can be avoided by exploring only questionable small lesions.
2. *Criteria for Identification of Dental Caries.* A detailed description for clinical recognition of dental caries appears on page 241, and a review of that material is suggested. In brief, for a dental caries index, a tooth can be considered carious when
   a. the lesion is clinically visible and obvious
   b. the explorer tip can penetrate into soft yielding material
   c. there is discoloration or loss of translucency typical of undermined or demineralized enamel
   d. the explorer tip in a pit or fissure catches or resists removal after moderate to firm pressure on insertion, and when there is softness at the base of the area.

C. Recording Principles

1. *Each Tooth is Recorded Once.*
2. *"D" Recordings*
   a. When both dental caries and a restoration are present, the tooth is listed as D.
   b. When a crown is broken down due to dental caries, it may be counted as D, or in some surveys, delegated to an "I" component, which means *Indicated* for extraction. For each survey, objective criteria should be established and published.
3. *"M" Recordings.* A tooth is considered M when it has been extracted due to dental caries.
4. *"F" Recordings*
   a. Permanent and temporary fillings are recorded as F

b. A tooth with a defective filling but without evidence of dental caries is recorded as F.

IV. Calculation Examples

A. Individual DMFT

1. Total each component separately.
2. Total D + M + F = DMF
   Example:
   (1) D = 3, M = 2, F = 5.
   DMF = 3 + 2 + 5 = 10
   (2) A DMF of 10 may have different derivations. A person who had regular dental care may have a distribution: D = 0, M = 0, F = 10.

B. Group Average

1. Total the DMFs for each individual examined.
2. Divide the total DMFs by the number of individuals in the group.
   Example:
   30 people with a total DMF of 210.
   $$\frac{210}{30} = 7.0 \text{ average DMF for the group.}$$

C. Specific Treatment Needs of a Group

1. To calculate the percent of DMF teeth needing restorations, divide the total D component by the total DMFT.
   Example: D = 175, M = 55, F = 18.
   Total DMFT = 248
   $$\frac{D}{DMF} = \frac{175}{248} = .70 \text{ or } 70\% \text{ of the teeth need}$$
   restorations.
2. Tooth mortality in a group of 20 people.
   a. To calculate the percent of teeth lost by extraction, divide the total M component by the total DMFT.
   Example: D = 175, M = 55, F = 18.
   Total DMFT = 248
   $$\frac{M}{DMF} = \frac{55}{248} = .22 \text{ or } 22\% \text{ of the DMF}$$
   teeth are accounted for by extraction.
   b. To calculate the percent of *all* teeth lost by extraction because of dental caries. Twenty people have 32 × 20 = 640 permanent teeth.
   $$\frac{M}{total\ teeth} = \frac{55}{640} = .08 \text{ or } 8\% \text{ of all of}$$
   their teeth lost because of dental caries.

3. The same type of calculation can be used to determine the percent of filled teeth.

DECAYED MISSING AND FILLED PERMANENT TOOTH SURFACES (DMFS)

I. Purpose

To determine total dental caries experience, past and present, by recording tooth surfaces involved instead of teeth as in the DMFT previously described.

II. Selection of Teeth and Surfaces

A. Teeth not Counted: the same as listed for the DMFT (page 311)

B. Surfaces

1. *Posterior Teeth.* Each tooth has five surfaces examined and recorded: facial, lingual, mesial, distal, and occlusal.
2. *Anterior Teeth.* Each tooth has four surfaces for evaluation: facial, lingual, mesial, and distal.
3. *Total Surface Count for a DMFS:* 128 surfaces.

    Of 28 teeth, 16 are posterior (16 × 5 = 80) and 12 are anterior (12 × 4 = 48)

III. Procedures

The same criteria for instruments and examination apply as listed previously for DMFT. In all surveys, specific criteria must be predetermined.

IV. Calculation Examples

A. Individual DMFS

Teeth present = 24 (4 teeth have not yet erupted)
D (surfaces) = 3, M = 0, F (surfaces) = 8
DMFS = D + M + F = 3 + 0 + 8 = 11

B. Group DMFS

A group of 20 15- to 18-year old people live in an area of fluoridation. All have lived there continuously except 3 who moved there from a nonfluoridated town after reaching 12 years of age. The following data shows the distribution of DMFS:

	Total DMFS
10 individuals (each with 0 DMFS) ..	0
7 individuals (DMFS = 2,2,3,3,3,3,4)	20
3 individuals who had not lived continuously in the area (DMFS = 9,12,12)	33
Total DMFS	53

Average DMFS for the group $= \dfrac{53}{20} = 2.65$

Interpretation: The differences between those who had not lived with fluoridation is notable. The group average DMFS is 2.65 whereas the DMFS for those who lived in the fluoridated area all their lives is 1.18, and the DMFS for the other three is 11.0.

PRIMARY DENTITION

For primary teeth, lower case letters are used to designate the index *deft* (decayed, indicated for extraction because of dental caries, and *filled* teeth) and the index *defs* (decayed, indicated for extraction because of dental caries, and *filled* surfaces).

Because of the difficulty of deciding whether a missing primary tooth has been exfoliated or extracted because of dental caries, the *deft* and *defs* have been used in more than one way. The "observable dental caries prevalence," the "dft" and "dfs," and the possible use of "dmft" and "dmfs" for children over 7 years will all be described.

I. Observable Dental Caries Prevalence (deft and defs)[23]

A. Purpose

To determine the dental caries experience as shown by the primary teeth present in the oral cavity.

B. Criteria

d = number of primary teeth present that are carious and not restored.
e = number indicated for extraction because of dental caries.
f = number of filled primary teeth.

C. Teeth Not Counted

1. Missing teeth including unerupted and congenitally missing.
2. Supernumerary teeth.
3. Teeth restored for reasons other than dental caries are not counted as f.

II. Decayed, Filled Teeth or Surfaces (dft and dfs)

A. Description

In the deft and defs as described above, both "d" and "e" are used to describe teeth with dental caries. Because of that, d and e are sometimes combined and the index becomes the "dft" or "dfs."

B. Calculation Example

A 2½-year-old child with nursing caries syndrome (page 241) has 18 teeth. Teeth A (5-5) and J (6-5) are unerupted. There is no sign of dental caries in teeth M (7-3), N (7-2), 0 (7-1), P (8-1), Q (8-2), and R (8-3). All other teeth have two carious surfaces each except B (5-4), which is broken down to the gumline.

Summary:	Total teeth =	18
	Caries-free =	6
	"d" teeth =	12
	"f" teeth =	0
dft = d + f =	12 + 0 =	12

To calculate dfs

Total number of carious surfaces: $11 \times 2 = 22$
Tooth B (5-4) = $1 \times 5 = \underline{5}$
total $\overline{27}$ dfs

III. Decayed, Missing, and Filled Primary Teeth (dmf)[25]

For children over 7 years and up to 11 or 12, the decayed, missing, and filled primary molars and canines have been used to determine a *dmft* or dmfs when the surfaces are counted. A primary molar or canine is presumed missing because of dental caries when it is missing before the normal exfoliation time.

IV. Mixed Dentition

A DMFT or DMFS and a deft or defs are never added together. Each child is given a separate index for permanent teeth and another for primary teeth. The index for the permanent teeth is usually determined first, and then the index for the primary teeth separately.

TECHNICAL HINTS

I. Select an index or scoring method that best fits the needs of the situation or patient.
II. Calibrate criteria for each index used.
III. Implement an index at the beginning of an appointment series.

IV. Permit the patient to graph or chart the plaque or gingival index used and correlate the numeric values with the oral findings which may be seen.[26]
V. Keep a continuing record, graph, or chart for index recording in the patient's permanent file for observation and review at each recall appointment.

FACTORS TO TEACH THE PATIENT

I. How an index is used and calculated and what the scores mean.
II. Correlation of index scores with current oral health practices and procedures.
III. Procedures to follow to improve index scores and bring the oral tissues to health.

References

1. Silness, J. and Löe, H.: Periodontal Disease in Pregnancy. II. Correlation between Oral Hygiene and Periodontal Condition, *Acta Odontol. Scand.*, 22, 121, Number 1, 1964.
2. Podshadley, A.G. and Haley, J.V.: A Method for Evaluating Oral Hygiene Performance, *Public Health Rep.*, 83, 259, March, 1968.
3. Darby, M.L. and Bowen, D.M.: *Research Methods for Oral Health Professionals.* St. Louis, The C.V. Mosby Co., 1980, p. 11.
4. Russell, A.L.: A System of Classification and Scoring for Prevalence Surveys of Periodontal Disease. *J. Dent. Res.*, 35, 350, June, 1956.
5. Russell, A.L.: The Periodontal Index, *J. Periodontol.* 38, 585, November-December, 1967 (Part II).
6. Ramfjord, S.P.: Indices for Prevalence and Incidence of Periodontal Disease, *J. Periodontol.*, 30, 51, January 1959.
7. Ramfjord, S.P.: The Periodontal Disease Index (PDI), *J. Periodontol.*, 38, 602, November-December, 1967 (Part II).
8. Shick, R.A. and Ash, M.M.: Evaluation of the Vertical Method of Toothbrushing, *J. Periodontol.*, 32, 346, October, 1961.
9. Löe, H. and Silness, J.: Periodontal Disease in Pregnancy. I. Prevalence and Severity, *Acta Odontol. Scand.* 21, 533, Number 6, 1963.
10. Löe, H.: The Gingival Index, the Plaque Index and the Retention Index Systems, *J. Periodontol.*, 38, 610, November–December, 1967 (Part II).
11. Greene, J.C. and Vermillion, J.R.: The Simplified Oral Hygiene Index, *J. Am. Dent. Assoc.*, 68, 7, January, 1964.
12. Greene, J.C.: The Oral Hygiene Index—Development and Uses, *J. Periodontol.*, 38, 625, November–December, 1967 (Part II).
13. Greene, J.C. and Vermillion, J.R.: Oral Hygiene Index: A Method for Classifying Oral Hygiene Status, *J. Am. Dent. Assoc.*, 61, 172, August, 1960.
14. Grant, D.A., Stern, I.B., and Everett, F.G.: *Periodontics*, 5th ed. St. Louis, The C.V. Mosby Co., 1979, pp. 529–531.
15. O'Leary, T.J., Drake, R.B., and Naylor, J.E.: The Plaque Control Record, *J. Periodontol.*, 43, 38, January, 1972.

16. Ramfjord, S.P. and Ash, M.M.: *Periodontology and Periodontics.* Philadelphia, W.B. Saunders Co., 1979, p. 273.
17. Mühlemann, H.R. and Son, S.: Gingival Sulcus Bleeding—A Leading Symptom in Initial Gingivitis, *Helv. Odontol. Acta*, 15, 107, October, 1971.
18. Meitner, S.W., Zander, H.A., Iker, H.P., and Polson, A.M.: Identification of Inflamed Gingival Surfaces, *J. Clin. Periodontol.*, 6, 93, April, 1979.
19. Lenox, J.A. and Kopczyk, R.A.: A Clinical System for Scoring a Patient's Oral Hygiene Performance, *J. Am. Dent. Assoc.*, 86, 849, April, 1973.
20. Craig, D. and Duhamel, L.: The Papilla-Bleeding Index, A New Aspect in Motivation, Eighth International Symposium on Dental Hygiene, Brighton, England, 1981.
21. Carter, H.G. and Barnes, G.P.: The Gingival Bleeding Index, *J. Periodontol.*, 45, 801, November, 1974.
22. Klein, H. and Palmer, C.E.: Studies on Dental Caries. I. Dental Status and Dental Needs of Elementary School Children, *Public Health Rep.*, 53, 751, May 13, 1938.
23. Gruebbel, A.O.: A Measurement of Dental Caries Prevalence and Treatment Service for Deciduous Teeth, *J. Dent. Res.*, 23, 163, June, 1944.
24. Horowitz, H.S., Baume, L.J., Dirks, O.B., Davies, G.N., and Slack, G.L., eds.: Principal Requirements for Controlled Clinical Trials of Caries Preventive Agents and Procedures, *Int. Dent. J.*, 23, 506, September, 1973.
25. Young, W.O. and Striffler, D.F.: *The Dentist, His Practice, and His Community*, 2nd ed. Philadelphia, W.B. Saunders Co., 1969, p. 49.
26. Barrickman, R.W. and Penhall, O.J.: Graphing Indexes Reduces Plaque, *J. Am. Dent. Assoc.*, 87, 1404, December, 1973.

Suggested Readings

Ainamo, J. and Bay, I.: Problems and Proposals for Recording Gingivitis and Plaque, *Int. Dent. J.*, 25, 229, December, 1975.
Armitage, G.C.: *Biologic Basis of Periodontal Maintenance Therapy.* Berkeley, California, Praxis Publishing Co., 1980, pp. 8–20.

Federation Dentaire Internationale: FDI Technical Report: Principal Requirements for Controlled Clinical Trials in Periodontal Diseases, *Int. Dent. J.*, 27, 62, March, 1977.
Horowitz, H.S.: Some Thoughts on Epidemiologic Indexes for Assessing the Need for Treatment of Periodontal Diseases, *Int. Dent. J.*, 29, 230, September, 1979.
Llewelyn, J. and Addy, M.: A Photographic Method for the Assessment of Examiner Accuracy and Variability for the Scoring Criteria of the Debris Index, *J. Periodontol.*, 50, 84, February, 1979.
Love, W.D., Ramirez, J.M., and Fultz, R.P.: An Oral Hygiene Measurement System for Possible Research and Clinical Use, *J. Public Health Dent.*, 35, 227, Fall, 1975.
Odrich, J.: Problems in Epidemiological Research of Periodontal Disease, *Dent. Hyg.*, 54, 230, May, 1980.
Rubinson, L., Stone, D.B., and Mortimer, R.G.: Statistical Reliability of NPI Administered to a Sample of Sixth-Grade Children, *Dent. Hyg.*, 51, 109, March, 1977.
Saxer, U.P., Turconi, B., and Elsässer, Ch.: Patient Motivation With the Papillary Bleeding Index, *J. Prev. Dent.*, 4, 20, July–August, 1977.
World Health Organization: *Epidemiology, Etiology, and Prevention of Periodontal Diseases*, Report of a WHO Scientific Group. Technical Report Series Number 621, Geneva, 1978.

Other Indices

Grossman, F.D. and Fedi, P.F.: Navy Periodontal Screening Examination, *J. Am. Soc. Prev. Dent.*, 3, 41, November–December, 1973.
Hancock, E.B. and Wirthlin, M.R.: An Evaluation of the Navy Periodontal Screening Examination, *J. Periodontol.*, 48, 63, February, 1977.
Katz, R.V.: Assessing Root Caries in Populations: The Evolution of the Root Caries Index, *J. Public Health Dent.*, 40, 7, Winter, 1980.
Massler, M.: The P-M-A Index for the Assessment of Gingivitis, *J. Periodontol.*, 38, 592, November–December, 1967 (Part II).
Morgulis, J.R.: Indices of Periodontal Disease, *Periodont. Abstr.*, 23, 13, Spring, 1975.
Quigley, G.A. and Hein, J.W.: Comparative Cleansing Efficiency of Manual and Power Brushing, *J. Am. Dent. Assoc.*, 65, 26, July, 1962.

20

Records and Charting

Complete and accurate examinations with proper documentation by records and chartings are basic to all patient care. All findings of the diagnostic work-up are recorded. Some systems of recording involve the completion of forms with topics and spaces to check or fill in the information, while others call for a prose-style summary.

Radiographs, study casts, photographs, and all other materials collected during the initial examination and during continuing patient appointments, are official parts of the permanent records. A filing system which makes these records readily accessible is needed.

I. Purposes for Charting

The purpose of each type of charting is defined by its title: the dental charting includes diagrammatic representation of existing conditions of the teeth, whereas the periodontal charting indicates clinical features of the periodontium. Separate types of chart forms may be used to record the special features of each or the two may be combined on one chart. Neatness in the marking of symbols, drawings, and labels goes hand in hand with the accuracy of the examination itself.

A sense of responsibility to the patient and an earnest desire to be of the greatest possible assistance to the dentist are prerequisite. The dental hygienist does not diagnose: when the charting is prepared, a picture or diagram of observations is recorded. The charting would not be described specifically to a patient unless the dentist requested that certain aspects of the diagnosis and treatment plan be presented to the patient.

An accurate, detailed, and carefully recorded charting is used as follows:

A. For Treatment Planning

The charting is a graphic representation of the existing condition of the patient's teeth and periodontium from which needed dental procedures can be organized into a treatment plan.

B. For Treatment

During dental and dental hygiene appointments, the charting is useful for guiding specific techniques.

C. For Evaluation

Comparison can be made of existing conditions with future examinations and charting in order to evaluate the outcome of treatment.

D. For Protection

In the event of misunderstanding by a patient, or if legal questions should arise, the records and chartings are realistic evidence.

E. For Identification

In the event of emergency, accident, or disaster, a patient may be identified by the teeth for which a record has been maintained.

II. Materials for Charting

A. Instruments

1. Probe.
2. Sharp explorers.
3. Mouth mirror: clear and unscratched.
4. Dental floss.
5. Gauze sponges.
6. Airtip and saliva ejector.
7. Topical anesthetic if probing proves discomforting to the patient.

B. Study Casts

C. Radiographs

1. Advanced preparation: to facilitate coordination between clinical and radiographic examinations; the completely processed and dried radiographs provide greater assurance of a thorough analysis.
2. Bite-wing survey may be sufficient for the charting of dental caries, but a periapical survey is essential for periodontal evaluation.

D. Chart Form

Many variations of chart forms are in current use, some available commercially, some designed by the dentist to meet particular needs. Specifications for an adequate form include ample space to chart neatly, accurately, and completely; to label as needed for clarity; and to record in a manner that will be interpretable by all who use it. Three types of forms are described here.

1. Anatomic tooth drawings of the complete teeth: such a chart form lends itself to combined dental and periodontal charting. Figure 20–2 is an example of this type of chart form (page 321).
2. Anatomic, with the crowns of teeth only: difficult to chart adequately the periodontal findings; designed primarily for charting dental caries.

3. Geometric: a diagrammatic representation for each tooth with space for each surface; generally does not include the roots. Description: two circles, the inner circle representing the occlusal surface and the outer circle divided into four parts to represent the mesial, facial, distal, and lingual (figure 20–1).

E. Marking Pencils

1. Pens and pencils of various colors in keeping with the system of charting selected by the dentist are needed.
2. Sanitization. Sanitize pencils or pens to be used by rubbing vigorously with gauze sponge moistened in a chemical disinfectant.
3. Instrument arrangement. Particular care must be exercised when charting without an assistant to keep sterile dental instruments apart from materials that cannot be sterilized. Transmission of oral microorganisms to chart form, pencils, eraser, or radiographs presents a real problem in the maintenance of a clinically clean environment.

III. Clinic Procedures

A. Patient Position

Position for optimum visibility of and accessibility to the field of operation.

B. Illumination

Maximum illumination is important. Use direct or indirect (mirror) light or transillumination.

C. Sequence for Charting

The use of a set routine is prerequisite to accomplishing a complete and accurate charting. This is true not only for the tooth surface-to-surface pattern, but also for the parts of the charting itself.

It is suggested that to chart all of one kind of item for the entire mouth, rather than completely charting one tooth, helps in obtaining accuracy, since only one train of thought is required at a time. For example, in the dental charting, record all of the restorations and then start again at the first tooth and chart all of the deviations from

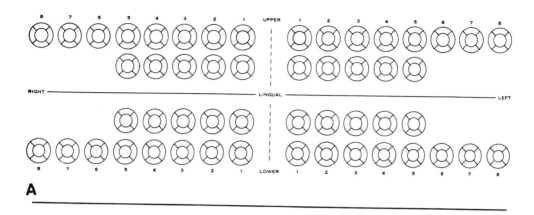

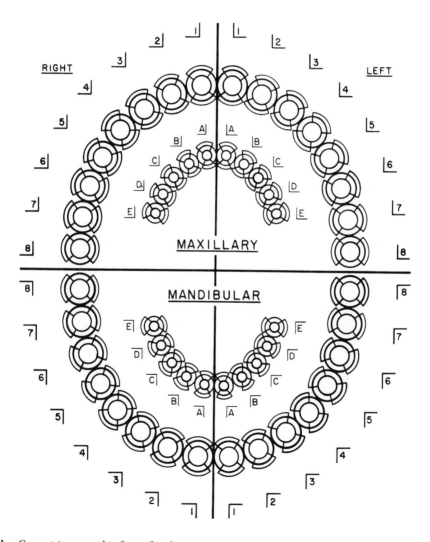

Figure 20–1. Geometric or graphic forms for charting. Type **A.** Linear format with primary teeth between permanent teeth. Type **B.** Permanent teeth in arch form with primary teeth inside. Teeth are numbered by Quadrant Numbers 1 through 8 (page 83).

normal rather than chart all restorations and deviations for each tooth separately.

PERIODONTAL RECORDS AND CHARTING

The patient's permanent records include the itemized findings of all the clinical and radiographic examinations. Material for the periodontal charting has been described on pages 218–220. Entries should be clear and easily understood by all who will read them and use them in continuing treatment.

Additions to the records are made to show the progress of treatment and comparative observations throughout the series of treatment appointments. After the mouth has been brought to a state of health the patient can maintain, a recall plan is outlined. At each recall appointment, new and comparative records and chartings are made.

Basic periodontal recordings are listed here. Frequently, the dentist prefers to do parts of the examination and assign other parts to the dental hygienist.

I. Clinical Observations of the Gingiva

A. **Describe Changes:** in color, size, position, shape, consistency, and surface texture; extent of bleeding when probed, and areas where exudate may be pressed from the pockets (page 195 and table 11–1, page 197).

B. **Describe Distribution:** localized or generalized, and specify the areas of severest involvement. Use tooth numbers to identify adjacent gingival tissue. Tooth numbering systems are described on pages 81–83.

C. **Describe Degree of Severity:** slight, moderate, severe.

II. Items to be Charted

A. Gingival line (margin) and mucogingival lines.
B. Pocket measurements.
C. Areas of suspected mucogingival involvement.
D. Furcation involvement.
E. Abnormal frenal attachments.
F. Mobility of teeth.

III. Deposits

A. **Stains**

1. *Extrinsic.* Record type of stain, color, distribution, specific location by tooth number, whether slight, moderate, or heavy.
2. *Intrinsic.* Record separately from extrinsic and identify by type when known.

B. **Calculus.** Record distribution and amount of supragingival and subgingival calculus separately for treatment planning purposes.

C. **Soft Deposits**

1. *Materia Alba and Food Debris:* distribution and amount. Record location by teeth when the plaque control instruction will require special area emphasis.
2. *Dental Plaque*
   a. Record direct observations with or without disclosing agent: distribution and degree or amount.
   b. Plaque index recorded.

IV. Factors Related to Occlusion

Clinical signs of trauma from occlusion were described on page 257. The following list is for consideration with other records for the treatment planning.

A. **Mobility of Teeth.** Record degree for each tooth (page 226). In figure 20–2, an example of a method for recording mobility is shown. The small box associated with each root apex and tooth number is to record mobility.

B. **Fremitus** (page 226)

C. **Possible Food Impaction Areas**

1. Inquire of patient where fibrous foods usually catch between the teeth.
2. Use dental floss to identify inadequate contact areas which may contribute to food impaction. An example of one method for recording an open contact is shown by the vertical parallel lines between teeth numbered 21 and 22 in figure 20–2.

D. **Occlusion-related Habits**

1. Observe for evidence of, and question patient concerning, parafunctional habits such as bruxism or clenching.

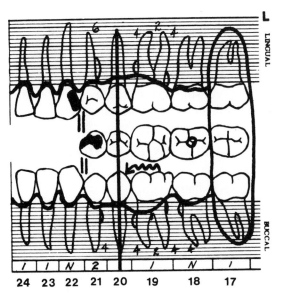

CODE FOR CHART

Missing tooth |

Caries — red

Restorations — blue

Encircle defective restorations in red

Fixed bridge ═

Partial denture ⁝⁝

Apparent gingival position ⌒

Bone line ⌒

Periodontal pocket ( )

Suppuration **S**

Drift and pathological migration ∿

Food impaction ↓

Mobility — N-1-2-3

Overhanging margins ▼

NV = non-vital

RCF = root filling

PT = Pulp treatment

Figure 20–2. Section of a charting (mandibular left quadrant) to show dental and periodontal charting combined. Dental caries and restorations are marked, usually with colored pencils such as red for caries and blue for restorations, on the anatomic crowns of the diagram. The gingival margin is clearly defined to show areas of recession and the points from which sulci and pockets are measured. Vertical parallel lines indicate open contact between teeth numbers 21 and 22. Encircled third molar (number 17) is unerupted, whereas the straight line through the second premolar (number 20) means the tooth has been removed. Numbers near the apices of the roots are millimeters of pocket measurement.

2. Note wear patterns and facets on study cast.

3. Note attrition.

E. **Tooth Migration** (page 256)

F. **Sensitivity to Percussion** (page 81)

G. **Radiographic Evidences:** related to trauma from occlusion (page 257).

V. **Radiographic Findings**

Specific notes should be made to correlate the radiographic findings with the clinical observations listed above. Details of radiographic findings in periodontal disease were described on pages 227–229. The following should be noted in particular:

A. **Bone Level:** height as related to the cementoenamel junction.

B. **Shape of Remaining Bone:** horizontal, angular.

C. **Crestal Lamina Dura:** intact, broken, or missing.

D. **Furcation Involvement**

E. **Periodontal Ligament Space:** thickening.

F. **Overhanging Fillings and Large Carious Lesions:** bacterial plaque-retention factors.

DENTAL RECORDS AND CHARTING

The patient's permanent records include the itemized findings of the clinical and radiographic examinations along with subjective symptoms reported by the patient. Material for the dental records has been included in Chapter 14, and occlusion in Chapter 15. Mobility of teeth has been charted with the periodontal examination because the causes of mobility are periodontally oriented. The outline here is for summary in anticipation of treatment planning.

After initial entries into the record, additions are made to show the progress of treatment. At each periodic recall, new and comparative records and chartings must be prepared.

The need for meticulous examination and recording cannot be overemphasized. Finding and recording a carious lesion may mean saving a tooth for the patient's lifetime; inadvertent neglect of a tooth may lead eventually to a need for endodontic therapy or even extraction.

I. Prior to Patient Appointment

When the radiographs and study casts have been prepared at an initial appointment prior to clinical examination for charting, they are useful for the preliminary charting. Conservation of patient chair time is important.

Supplemental and confirming observations and checks are made during the clinical examination with the patient. For example, when an overhanging restoration is noted but dental caries is not visible in the radiograph, examination by exploration is required since the restoration can be superimposed over the carious lesion.

Figure 20–2 is an example of a quadrant of dental charting using anatomic tooth drawings. Dental findings can also be charted on a geometric form such as is shown in figure 20–1.

A. Radiographic Charting

The following may be charted: missing, unerupted, impacted teeth, endodontic restorations, overhanging margins of existing restorations, proximal surface carious lesions, and any other deviation from normal evident from the radiographs.

B. Study Casts

Record the classification of occlusion (pages 253–255).

II. Patient Appointment

A. Chart existing restorations, including fixed and removable prostheses.
B. Chart apparent carious lesions and other deviations from normal.
C. Coordinate clinical and radiographic findings.
D. Use dental floss. Chart inadequate contact areas and observe proximal surface roughness. Fraying of dental floss when passing over a rough proximal surface may mean the defective margin of a restoration, a sharp cavity margin, or dental calculus.

E. Pulp vitality. Record numbers in the [p]ermanent record. Chart forms are someti[mes] prepared with a specific place for such [data] to be filled in. Procedures were descri[bed] on pages 243–245.
F. Tooth sensitivity. The patient may re[port] hypersensitive areas, or they may be [dis]covered during instrumentation. Record [the] tooth number and surface for reference d[ur]ing the treatment phase.

TECHNICAL HINTS

I. Use a record form with adequate space [for] recording details.
II. Prepare permanent records in ink.
III. Use abbreviations and symbols only wh[en] their meaning will be clear to all who r[ead] them.
IV. All records should be complete, accura[te,] clearly stated, readable, and neat.
V. Plan appointments, when possible, in [or]der that radiographs and study casts [will] be available prior to and at the time [of] clinical charting. By having an initial [ap]pointment when the medical and den[tal] history and the extraoral and intraoral [ex]aminations can be completed, time can [be] saved. Necessary consultations with a [pa]tient's physician, preparation with p[re]medication when indicated for the pati[ent] susceptible to bacteremia, or other spec[ial] adaptation can be made.
VI. When a patient asks specific questio[ns] about the charting or other recordings, [ex]plain why it is necessary for the dentist [to] observe and check before explanations c[an] be made.

FACTORS TO TEACH
THE PATIENT

I. The importance of making a complete stu[dy] of the patient's oral problems before b[e]ginning treatment.
II. Advantages of cooperation and patience [in] furnishing information that will help den[tal] personnel interpret observations acc[u]rately, in order that the correct diagno[sis] and appropriate treatment plan can [be] made.
III. All information received is completely co[n]fidential, and the records are locked wh[en] the office is closed.

Suggested Readings

Allen, D.L., McFall, W.T., and Hunter, G.C.: *Periodontics for the Dental Hygienist*, 3rd ed. Philadelphia, Lea & Febiger, 1980, pp. 104–131.

Boozer, C.H.: Clinical Examination, in Clark, J.W., ed.: *Clinical Dentistry, Volume 1*, Chapter 6. Hagerstown, Maryland, Harper & Row, 1981, pp. 7–16.

Carranza, F.A.: *Glickman's Clinical Periodontology*, 5th ed. Philadelphia, W.B. Saunders Co., 1979, pp. 555–566.

Castano, F.A. and Alden, B.A., eds.: *Handbook of Expanded Dental Auxiliary Practice*, 2nd ed. Philadelphia, J.B. Lippincott Co., 1980, pp. 5–25.

Grant, D.A., Stern, I.B., and Everett, F.G.: *Periodontics*, 5th ed. St. Louis, The C.V. Mosby Co., 1979, pp. 452–482.

Simon, W.J.: *Clinical Dental Assisting*. Hagerstown, Maryland, Harper & Row, 1973, pp. 79–82.

Woodall, I.R., Dafoe, B.R., Young, N.S., Weed-Fonner, L., and Yankell, S.L.: *Comprehensive Dental Hygiene Care*. St. Louis, The C.V. Mosby Co., 1980, pp. 110–125, 134–139.

21

The Dental Hygiene Treatment Plan

All of the information about the patient, collected as parts of the diagnostic work-up, is organized for evaluation. From the evaluation, before treatment is started, the dentist makes the diagnosis, and the treatment plan is prepared.

The *total treatment plan* is a sequential outline of the essential services and procedures which must be carried out by the dentist, the dental hygienist, and the patient to eliminate disease and restore the oral cavity to health and normal function. The *dental hygiene treatment plan*, which consists of those services to be performed by the dental hygienist with the patient, is formulated within the framework of the total treatment plan and is an integral part of it.

I. Objectives

The objectives of a treatment sequence as conducted by the dentist, patient, and the auxiliaries are:

A. To Eliminate and Control Etiologic and Predisposing Disease Factors

The principal etiologic agent in both dental caries and periodontal and gingival diseases is bacterial plaque. The goal should be to control the etiologic agent and thus prevent future recurrences of the same conditions.

B. To Eliminate the Signs and Symptoms of Disease

Treatment planning includes measures to eliminate signs of disease such as carious lesions, inflammation, and pockets.

C. To Restore Normal Function

This includes occlusal adjustment, restoration of teeth, replacement of missing teeth, orthodontic tooth movement, and recontouring of gingival form (gingivoplasty).

D. To Maintain Health and Prevent the Recurrence of Disease

Methods used are to counsel and supervise the patient in daily self-care and to provide regular follow-up professional supervision and care.

II. Preparation for the Treatment Plan

A. Diagnostic Work-up

The parts of a diagnostic work-up were listed on page 79 and described in Chapters 6 through 20. The histories, dental and periodontal chartings, radiographs, study casts, recorded information from the extraoral and intraoral examinations, indices, and all other available information are studied by the dentist. The key pertinent findings which point to the disease problems are selected and the diagnosis is made.

B. Diagnosis

The *diagnosis* is the identification of the

disease condition by recognition of characteristic signs and symptoms. A *differential diagnosis* means distinguishing the disease from other diseases that have similar manifestations.

Patients frequently have more than one disease condition. For example, dental caries and periodontal or gingival diseases commonly occur simultaneously. When the treatment plan is made, the treatment for each disease condition is outlined, and a coordinated treatment sequence is determined.

III. Parts of a Total Treatment Plan

A total treatment plan usually involves several interdependent areas of oral care based on an individual patient's diagnosis and disease symptoms. Divisions for a treatment plan are listed below with examples of services included in each.

A. Priority Treatment

1. Emergency care for pain or other acute condition.
2. Procedures such as biopsy of a lesion found during the extraoral and intraoral examinations, or a laboratory test for a suspected systemic condition.

B. Preventive Phase

1. Procedures for the patient's daily self-care, including plaque control.
2. Introduction to self-applied fluoride.

C. Preparatory Phase

1. Initial (Phase 1) periodontal therapy: plaque control, complete scaling and root planing.
2. Dental caries: excavation of large carious lesions; placement of sedative temporary fillings; pulp treatment as indicated.
3. Endodontic therapy.
4. Preparation for oral surgery: plaque control and scaling to reduce bacterial count and inflammation.
5. Removal of hopeless teeth which cannot be successfully treated.

D. Treatment Phase

1. Gingival and periodontal treatment: elimination of inflammation and pockets; surgical procedures; occlusal adjustment.
2. Restorative treatment.
3. Prosthetic treatment.
4. Orthodontic treatment.
5. Tissue maintenance during therapy (p. 327).

E. Maintenance Phase

1. Patient: specific daily plaque control and other preventive measures.
2. Professional recall at designated intervals.
   a. Complete reevaluation and update of records and all parts of the diagnostic work-up.
   b. Recall treatment plan: may include any service as a continuation, supplement, or addition to previous preventive, educational, or therapeutic measures. The recall appointment is described on pages 600–602.

PLANNING THE DENTAL HYGIENE TREATMENT PLAN

The dental hygienist's objective is to prepare a flexible, realistic, dental hygiene plan and sequence of procedures based on the plan for total care of the patient. As described on page 9, dental hygienist's services may be divided into preventive, educational, and therapeutic, all of which are applicable at various levels in the total treatment plan. Services to be performed are dependent on state or area practice acts, and any examples cited here are not intended to represent a specific location.

The treatment plan is recorded in the patient's record. The patient or parent of a young or mentally disabled patient needs to understand the treatment plan and be aware of the expected outcome of each appointment as well as of the total series. The role of the patient in treatment through self-care on a daily basis must be written into the treatment plan and explained to the patient.

An objective in planning dental hygiene care is to ensure the best possible sequence of procedures which will contribute to the restoration of the patient's oral health in the shortest possible time and pave the way to the long-range preventive program which will continue throughout the patient's lifetime. To achieve the goals of planned care, the dental hygienist must see the dental hygiene aspects within the total plan for the patient and contribute to the overall continuity of the corrective and maintenance phases.

I. Characteristics of a Well-planned Treatment Plan

An effective plan will be

A. Adapted to the needs of the patient's oral condition.
B. Orderly in sequence to allow for thoroughness in each procedure and to prevent duplication or repetition of efforts.
C. Composed of purposefully selected procedures which are
  1. Planned with a reasonable degree of predictability of outcome.
  2. Expected to resolve the condition and reach an optimum result in a minimum of time.
  3. Projected toward a state of health the patient can maintain with self-care procedures.

II. Steps in Planning

A. Review the patient's oral problems as described in the diagnosis and total treatment plan.
B. Identify objectives which may be attained.
  1. Overall objectives of the total treatment plan: anticipated outcome of treatment and anticipated state of oral health after treatment.
  2. Dental hygiene goals: short-term and long-term.
C. Select the preventive, educational, preparatory, and treatment procedures that can be expected to meet the objectives.
D. List in sequence, for the appointment series, the services to be performed for each phase of the total treatment plan.

No attempt is made here to list all possible dental hygiene services, but examples are given below for each treatment plan phase.
  1. *Preventive.* A typical program includes plaque control measures, self-applied and professionally applied fluorides, and diet counseling.
  2. *Preparatory.* Complete scaling, planing, and gingival curettage are major services in the preparation of a patient for per-

iodontal surgery. *Preparatory* treatment is in contrast to *definitive* treatment. By definitive is meant the complete treatment needed by a patient to bring the oral tissues to a state of health at that time.
  3. *Treatment*
    a. Periodontal: scaling, planing, and gingival curettage which were preparatory for one patient may be the definitive and curative treatment for another patient.
    b. Periodontal post-surgical procedures: suture removal, removal and placement of periodontal dressings, and other postoperative care and instruction are parts of the patient's treatment plan that are performed by the dental hygienist.
    c. Restorative. Finishing and polishing of restorations may best be scheduled in conjunction with topical fluoride application. After polishing restorations, it is recommended that a topical fluoride application be made in order to protect the enamel which has been highly polished adjacent to the restoration.
    d. Tissue maintenance during long-term therapy: when restorative, prosthetic, orthodontic, or other treatment continues over a long period, appointments are needed for gingival evaluation, supervision of plaque control measures, calculus removal, topical fluoride applications, and other procedures specific for the patient.
E. Estimate and allot time requirements for each preventive, educational, and therapeutic service.

III. Criteria for Determination of Sequence

Sequence planning involves first an outline of a series of appointments with the services to be performed. Secondly, sequence refers to the order in which the parts of an individual appointment are carried out. The sequence is influenced by numerous factors, including urgency of treatment, need for treating etiologic factors first, the severity and extent of the case, and certain special patient requirements. These are described here with examples.

A. Urgency

When discomfort or pain is present, the area involved requires first attention. In the dental hygiene treatment plan, this could apply to an area of the gingiva where the patient has particular difficulty, and either specially adapted plaque control instruction or scaling may be needed.

B. Etiologic Factors Should Be Treated First

It is necessary to arrest and control the factors that caused or contributed to the development of the existing disease. In patients with gingival or periodontal disease, the continued success of treatment is dependent on the removal of plaque.

Disease will recur when daily control measures for the removal of the etiologic agent, plaque, are not carried out. New dental caries also can develop unless continued attention is paid to preventive measures.

Pellicle forms within minutes after a tooth surface has been completely cleaned and disclosable plaque will be present within 24 hours or less. It is necessary, therefore, that plaque control measures be introduced in the treatment plan before scaling or root planing.

C. Special Patient Requirements: Items from the Patient History
1. Antibiotic premedication. A list of conditions that require antibiotic coverage may be found on page 99. For patients who need antibiotics, all instrumentation, including the examination procedures when instruments are used (probing, exploring), as well as tooth movement for mobility determination, must be done under antibiotic coverage.

    Bacteremias have been demonstrated during brushing, flossing, and other disease control measures. Instruction and practice of the plaque-removing procedures must be carried out while the patient is premedicated.

    It is important that appointments be planned and conducted efficiently to prevent the need for unnecessary pre-

medication. When a patient's physical health and strength do not contraindicate, appointments that are longer than customary may be reserved in order that more can be accomplished.
2. Chronic disease or physical disability may influence the content or length of appointments.
3. Disease transmission problems for patients with a history of a communicable disease may require postponement of all except urgent needs.

D. Severity and Extent of the Case

Findings that indicate the severity of gingival or periodontal involvement include changes in color, size, shape, consistency and bleeding of the gingiva, pocket measurements, mobility of teeth, and radiographic signs. To determine the length of appointments and sequence of procedures, consideration is given necessarily to the depth of pockets in relation to the distribution and hardness of dental calculus. The number of appointments and the length of appointments increase with severity.

A suggested division of cases graded by severity of disease involvement follows.
1. *Moderate to Severe Periodontal Disease.* For the patient who will require complicated periodontal, restorative, and prosthetic treatment, the dental hygiene treatment plan will include preventive and preparatory procedures as well as maintenance during therapy, postsurgical care, and follow-up.
2. *Moderate or Slight Periodontal Disease.* The dental hygiene treatment plan will include the preventive phase, complete scaling, planing, and gingival curettage as indicated. This treatment may be definitive, or the follow-up evaluation may show the need for surgical or other additional treatment.
3. *Gingivitis with Supra- and Subgingival Calculus.* The preventive phase and complete scaling are indicated and gingival pockets may require curettage. The treatment may be definitive or, upon reevaluation, gingivoplasty or other treatment may be needed.

4. *Gingivitis with Slight Supragingival Calculus or No Calculus.* Dental hygiene services usually constitute the definitive treatment. To eliminate gingival inflammation, plaque control measures may be the total treatment, which is supplemented by scaling when there is calculus or only polishing when stain is unsightly.

IV. Individual Appointment Sequence

A. Evaluation

Each appointment starts with an evaluation of the gingival tissues.
1. *Previously Treated Area.* The area is examined for progress towards health, the signs of inflammation which may still be present, and indications for additional treatment which is needed.
2. *Effects of Plaque Control Measures.* The self-treatment by the patient is evaluated. After the color, size, shape, consistency, and other characteristics of the gingiva are observed, a disclosing agent is used to evaluate the degree of plaque present on the teeth. This evaluates the patient's techniques and thoroughness in plaque removal.

B. Instruction

Instruction begins when evaluation starts, and continues throughout. Specific techniques for the use of plaque removal devices, such as toothbrush, floss, or other aid, are presented before instrumentation or other professional clinical services are performed. The reasons for this sequence are presented on pages 411 and 507–508.

C. Clinical Services

The questions of which area or quadrant should be scaled first and in which order the other areas and quadrants should follow can be answered for most patients by considering the following order of choices:
1. *Patient Selection:* when the patient indicates an area of discomfort, that area may be taken first.
2. *Apprehensive Patient:* to make the first scaling less complicated and help orient the patient to the procedures to be followed, the dental hygienist can select either the quadrant with the fewest teeth or the quadrant with the least deep periodontal disease.
3. *Need for Tissue Conditioning.* Preparation or conditioning of the gingival tissue for scaling can be of particular importance when there is spongy, soft tissue that bleeds on slight provocation, and when the area is generally septic from plaque, materia alba, and debris accumulation. Tissue conditioning is accomplished by initiating plaque control procedures and prescribing a concentrated daily program of plaque removal and hot salt water rinsing. A quadrant that needs tissue conditioning would not be selected for scaling until gingival healing and patient cooperation were apparent.

Objectives of such a program include:
a. Gingival healing: the tissue will become less edematous, bleeding will be minimized, and scaling procedures facilitated.
b. General oral cleanliness with lowered bacterial accumulation: there will be less likelihood that bacteremias will be produced during scaling, and there will be less contamination in aerosols produced.
c. Learning by the patient: the patient will be able to practice and see benefits of plaque removal.
4. *When Two Quadrants are to be Treated at the Same Appointment:* select a maxillary and mandibular of the same side.

SAMPLE DENTAL HYGIENE TREATMENT PLAN

It would be impossible to present sample treatment plans for each of the wide variety of patient problems or combinations of problems encountered in practice. Each case must be handled individually.

Examples of treatment sequences and plans are found in special areas of this book. An outline of a dental caries control study program may be found on page 433, a recall appointment on pages 601–602, and a treatment sequence for a patient with necrotizing ulcerative gingivitis on pages 538–540.

For the patient whose dental hygiene treatment plan is sketched below, the diagnostic work-up was completed by the dental hygienist. The dentist indicated a diagnosis of generalized moderate periodontal disease. The preliminary total treatment plan includes occlusal adjustment, restorative procedures, and the prosthetic replacement of two missing teeth. No emergency measures are required. None of the periodontal surgery or dental treatment will be started until the dental hygiene preventive and preparatory appointments have been completed and the patient's mouth has been reevaluated.

The examinations revealed slight localized supragingival calculus and generalized moderate-to-heavy subgingival calculus. Because the patient has enlarged, spongy marginal gingiva with generalized bleeding on probing and plaque on the cervical thirds of most teeth, scaling is not started on the first appointment. The rationale for introducing plaque control before scaling is described on page 411.

More detail is included in the treatment plan recorded below than probably would be written in practice. Abbreviations would be used which could be recognized by all personnel involved in using the patient's record. For example, "Plaque I," "Plaque II," "Plaque III" might be sufficient notation for the plaque control instruction series.

APPOINTMENT I
1. Record Gingival Index (GI) and Plaque Index (Pl I).
2. Give disease control instruction: *First Lesson*, page 412.
3. Introduce fluoride program.
   a. Dentifrice recommendation: reasons for frequent brushing to gain most benefit from fluoride in dentifrice.
   b. Mouthrinse. Demonstrate.

APPOINTMENT II
1. Disease control evaluation with the patient.
   a. Gingival tissue assessment (table 11–1, pages 196–197).
   b. Record indices.
2. Instruction: *Second Lesson,* page 414.
3. Scaling

   a. First quadrant scaling and root planing with anesthesia.
   b. Curettage as directed; dressing placed when needed.
   c. Postoperative instructions.

APPOINTMENT III
1. Remove dressing.
2. Evaluation
   a. Gingival tissue assessment; record Gingival Index.
   b. Specific examination for first quadrant scaled: note healing. Explore to check for residual calculus.
   c. Plaque evaluation: disclose and record Plaque Index.
3. Instruction: *Third Lesson*, page 414.
4. Scaling and root planing.
   a. Complete first quadrant when residual calculus is found.
   b. Second quadrant scaling with anesthesia.
   c. Gingival curettage as directed; dressing when needed.

APPOINTMENT IV
1. Remove dressing.
2. Evaluation
   a. Gingival tissue assessment: record Gingival Index.
   b. Specific examination for previously scaled quadrants; explore for residual calculus.
   c. Plaque evaluation: disclose and record Plaque Index.
3. Instruction: continue as needed.
4. Scaling and root planing.
   a. Complete first and second quadrants.
   b. Third quadrant scaling with anesthesia.
   c. Gingival curettage as directed; dressing when needed.

APPOINTMENT V
The same basic structure is followed as outlined for Appointments III and IV. Each time the previously treated quadrants must be checked and completed. Each time the instruc-

ion is continued if the patient is still not accomplishing disease control. The fourth quadrant is scaled under anesthesia and curettage performed as needed.

APPOINTMENT VI

1. Evaluation of four quadrants; additional scaling when indicated.
2. Reevaluation by the dentist; planning for the next phase of appointments when patient is ready as shown by the health of the gingival tissue.

APPOINTMENT VII: Maintenance During Therapy

When the restorative and prosthetic treatment extends over a period of time, periodic appointments are needed for monitoring the continued success of the patient's self-care. A gingival tissue evaluation, checks with a probe to determine bleeding, plaque checks with disclosing agents, additional instruction, particularly for the care of newly fixed or removable prosthetic appliances, and motivational encouragement are essential.

APPOINTMENT VIII: Recall

The recall frequency is determined. Components of the recall appointments are described on pages 600–602.

TECHNICAL HINTS

I. Treatment plans for minors or mentally disabled patients should be discussed with the parent or guardian. Permission should be obtained by signature, particularly when anesthesia will be used or prescriptions issued.

II. Complete records are essential. Misunderstandings can lead to legal involvements.

FACTORS TO TEACH THE PATIENT

I. Why a treatment plan is made.
II. Explanation of unclear parts of the total treatment plan.
III. Parts of the treatment plan carried out by the patient. Interrelation of roles of patient, dentist, and auxiliary personnel in eliminating the patient's oral disease.
IV. The long-term effects of comprehensive continuing care.
V. Why disease control measures must be learned before scaling and planing are done.
VI. Significance of the indices as guides to evaluating the health of the gingiva.
VII. What presurgical preparation means, what it consists of, and what the expected advantages are.

Suggested Readings

Bartlett, R.C. and Berry, T.G.: Treatment Planning, in Clark, J.W., ed.: *Clinical Dentistry, Volume 1*, Chapter 17, Hagerstown, Maryland, Harper & Row, 1981, pp. 1–15.

Carranza, F.A.: *Glickman's Clinical Periodontology*, 5th ed. Philadelphia, W. B. Saunders Co., 1979, pp. 603–605.

Chasens, A.I.: Treatment Planning for the Periodontal Patient, *N.Y.J. Dent.*, *48*, 79, March, 1978.

Cheney, H.G.: Effect of Patient Behavior and Personality on Treatment Planning, *Dent. Clin. North Am.*, *21*, 531, July, 1977.

Clark, J.D. and Morton, J.C.: Behavioral Assessment. An Appraisal of Beliefs and Behaviors, *Dent. Clin. North Am.*, *21*, 515, July, 1977.

Ekanayaka, A.N.I. and Sheiham, A.: Estimating the Time and Personnel Required to Treat Periodontal Disease, *J. Clin. Periodontol.*, *5*, 85, May, 1978.

Goldman, H.M. and Cohen, D.W.: *Periodontal Therapy*, 6th ed. St. Louis, The C.V. Mosby Co., 1980, pp. 412–438.

Grant, D.A., Stern, I.B., and Everett, F.G.: *Periodontics*, 5th ed. St. Louis, The C.V. Mosby Co., 1979, pp. 507–523.

Kerr, D.A., Ash, M.M., and Millard, H.O.: *Oral Diagnosis*, 5th ed. St. Louis, The C.V. Mosby Co., 1978, pp. 385–401.

Miller, P.L.: Treatment Planning for the Periodontal Patient, *Dent. Hyg.*, *54*, 331, July, 1980.

Pattison, G.L. and Pattison, A.M.: *Periodontal Instrumentation*. Reston, Virginia, Reston Publishing Co., 1979, pp. 337–344.

Simpson, E.F.: Treatment Planning Using a Plaque Index as a Baseline, *N.Z. Dent. J.*, *73*, 227, October, 1977.

IV

Prevention

INTRODUCTION

This section, *Prevention*, includes procedures for disease control, diet counseling, fluorides, sealants, and related preventive measures. In the sequence of treatment planning for the patient, initiation of preventive measures precedes dental and dental hygiene clinical services except in an emergency. The long-range success of treatment procedures is limited unless the causes of the condition being treated are removed.

Primary prevention, involving measures to prevent disease completely, is basic to continuing benefits of dental and dental hygiene treatment. The fluoridation of water supplies, and plaque and sucrose control for the prevention of dental caries, are examples of primary prevention.

Secondary preventive measures are those related to the early recognition and treatment of incipient disease before extensive lesions develop. The restoration of small carious lesions and the recognition and biopsy of a suspected lesion of the mucous membrane are examples of secondary prevention. The relationship of primary and secondary prevention to dental hygiene practice was introduced on page 9.

Tertiary preventive measures are represented in more complex and involved dental and periodontal therapy, even to the extent of the replacement of missing teeth. Prevention is still involved as long as complete breakdown and loss of function are prevented.

Preventive dentistry is the sum total of the efforts to promote, restore, and maintain the oral health of the individual. A *program for prevention* is composed of the cooperative steps taken by the patient, dentist, and dental auxiliary personnel to preserve the natural dentition and the supporting structures by preventing the onset, progress, and recurrence of oral diseases and other destructive or disfiguring conditions.

STEPS IN A PREVENTIVE PROGRAM

The dental hygienist prepares a *preventive treatment plan* for each patient. Planning and carrying out the preventive program may be divided into the six basic steps below. Details to describe each step are not included here, because the details were either part of the diagnostic work-up described in previous chapters or will be parts of the preventive section chapters to follow.

I. Assess Patient's Needs

A. Review all information from the diagnostic work-up; history, examinations, radiographs, chartings.
B. Identify the presence and severity of disease and predisposing factors.
C. Utilize indices to rate the extent of the needs and provide a baseline for continuing comparisons.

II. Select Applicable Preventive Methods

A. Apply information about the patient: educational level, occupation, socioeconomic background, and attitudes toward oral health.
B. Recognize the influence of physical or mental disabilities.

333

C. Determine the current personal oral care procedures carried out by the patient, and their frequency.

D. Outline the instruction recommended and the goals to be attained by the patient.

III. Provide Instruction for Self-care

A. Present information and demonstration for specific daily care techniques and self-applied fluoride.

B. Show methods for self-evaluation.

IV. Perform Clinical Preventive Services

A. Complete scaling and root planing.

B. Apply topical caries-prevention agents.

V. Evaluate Changes in the Patient's Oral Health

A. Evaluate gingival tissue, bleeding, plaque, and techniques performed by the patient.

B. Use successive indices to compare progress.

C. Provide preventive counseling for corrective action when initial goals are not met.

VI. Plan Long-Term Maintenance

A. Reevaluate periodically to monitor continuance of preventive practices.

B. Provide additional preventive measures when indicated, particularly following placement of new restorations or prosthetic devices.

PATIENT INSTRUCTION

Instruction is an essential part of the preventive program if goals for attaining a patient's oral health are to be reached. Personalized patient instruction contributes first to the knowledge, attitudes, and practices of the individual, then through the individual to the family and the community.

The outmoded concept that all teeth eventually must be removed has been replaced by current research findings. It is now known that periodontal diseases and dental caries can be prevented or controlled and therefore teeth can be preserved throughout the lifetime of the individual.

Dental health education is the provision of oral health information to people in such a way that they can apply it in everyday living.[1] To know and believe health facts is not enough; benefits result only when knowledge is put into action. Learning occurs when an individual changes behavior, and when changes are incorporated as a part of everyday living.

I. Motivation

Instruction is tailored to individual needs and motivations. An individual is motivated to practice behavior that leads to achievement of goals which are valued. Dental health instruction can be effective if the patient considers oral health a valuable asset or goal.

Stimulation of behavior, or motivation, stems from basic physiologic and social needs. Peer group approval and the need to conform to group standards, as well as the fear of disapproval or rejection when appearance of the teeth or odor of the breath is unacceptable, are frequently much higher motivating factors than a health reason such as freedom from infection or the ability to chew food for body cell maintenance.

The need for relief from pain can bring a patient to seek immediate dental care; however, additional motivation will be needed to help the patient realize that through a preventive care program, future pain can be avoided.

Motivation and what the patient will learn and practice are proportional to the sincerity and concern of the dental team members. A motivated dental professional develops patient-centered systems of instruction that are meaningful to the patient.

II. Patient-Centered Instruction

For most patients major emphasis needs to be placed on control of dental caries or periodontal disease. Attention should also be paid to oral accident prevention, particularly related to mouth protectors for contact sports, safety belts for automobiles, and children's accidents which lead to fractured anterior teeth.

Whereas patient instruction of the past connoted teaching a patient how and when to use a toothbrush, usually by means of a model, and in one short session, patient instruction now envelops a wide range of essential areas of learning aimed at developing a patient's knowledge, attitudes, and practices for continuing oral health. To be able to interpret and apply current dental research findings requires continuing review through reading and other educational efforts.

DISEASE CONTROL

Bacterial plaque is the most important etiologic factor in the development of dental caries and inflammatory periodontal diseases. A direct relationship exists between the degree of oral uncleanliness and the extent of periodontal disease.

Disease control in the individual is directly related to the measures employed for removing bacterial plaque from the teeth on a regular daily basis. The most effective means for plaque removal available at present are mechanical; that is, toothbrushing for tooth surfaces which can be reached with the brush, and dental floss or other devices for proximal surfaces.

Pellicle begins to form immediately and plaque forms again within a few to 24 hours following its removal. It is evident that self-care measures for control are necessary on a day-to-day basis.

Personal measures for disease control need supplementation by professional care. The removal of dental calculus, overhanging fillings, and other local plaque retainers is essential to create an environment that can be maintained effectively by the individual.

Continuing personal and professional care are mutually interdependent in a successful patient-centered plaque control program. Plaque control in combination with periodic scaling for complete calculus removal has been shown to arrest the progress of periodontal disease.

Oral physical therapy is accomplished by the use of physical agents in the prevention, management, and control of oral diseases. In physical medicine, physical therapy includes the use of various agents, particularly light, heat, water, electricity, and exercise. A few of the same agents are used in oral care, and many mechanical devices have been developed for specific application to the teeth and gingiva. The satisfactory use of an oral physical therapy device depends on the patient's understanding of the goals to be attained. Objectives may need reconsideration from time to time depending on new research findings relative to the cause and prevention of oral diseases.

OBJECTIVES

By way of introduction to subsequent chapters, primary objectives for disease control are listed below. The objectives apply from a pre-ventive or a treatment aspect depending on the status of the patient's health. For the patient undergoing definitive care for periodontal disease, bacterial plaque control and oral physical therapy are, first, essential parts of the treatment program. After treatment has been completed, plaque control becomes an essential part of the maintenance phase of care.

For all patients, fulfilling the goals of personal care contributes to prevention of disease. The patient becomes an active participant in obtaining and maintaining personal oral health, which is in itself the most important objective.

I. Primary Objective: Disease Control

A. Bacterial plaque control involves the following:
   1. Disorganization and reduction of the number of microorganisms through daily removal of plaque.
   2. Prevention of calculus formation by removing the components of calculus prior to calcification.
B. With effective removal of dental plaque from the tooth surfaces, the following benefits can be expected:
   1. Reduction and control of gingivitis and the development of periodontitis.
   2. Reduced incidence of dental caries.
   3. Reduction in sensitivity of exposed root surfaces.
   4. Lessened possibility of halitosis caused by oral uncleanliness.
   5. Improved oral comfort, sanitation, and appearance with a refreshed taste, smooth tooth surfaces, and general sense of well-being.

II. Plaque Control and Dental Caries

Control of acidogenic plaque microorganisms is necessary for dental caries prevention as part of a total dental caries control program. Toothbrushing with a dentifrice which contains fluoride combines plaque removal with fluoride application. The application of fluoride by way of a dentifrice is an important objective of toothbrushing.

III. Oral Physical Therapy and Gingival Massage

Gingival massage is the systematic application of a stroking or kneading pressure to the periodontium for the purpose of stimulating the blood circulation to these tissues. It should be realized that as stimulating as massage may seem to be, without plaque removal the benefits are not present or at least to a lesser degree.

Irritation to the gingiva will persist when plaque bacteria are present, and calculus will accumulate.

BACTEREMIA AND DISEASE CONTROL TECHNIQUES

Bacteria may enter the blood stream by way of the gingival sulcus or pocket during and following dental and dental hygiene procedures. Bacteremias have been demonstrated in relation to toothbrushing, flossing, irrigation, and other oral hygiene aids. A bibliography of references is included with the Suggested Readings at the end of this section.

Bacteremias occur more frequently when the gingiva are diseased. A high level of periodontal health has special significance for a patient with rheumatic heart disease, prosthetic heart valve, replacement joint such as a knee or hip, renal dialysis shunt, or a shunt for hydrocephalus drainage.

High risk patients, those who may develop bacterial endocarditis or other internal infection, are described on pages 99–100. Antibiotic premedication prior to all procedures that involve tissue manipulation is mandatory. This includes the appointments at which new plaque control procedures are introduced and practiced by the patient.

FACTORS TO TEACH THE PATIENT

I. The relationship between preventive measures and clinical services.

II. Why particular preventive measures were selected for the particular patient.

III. Self-evaluation methods for determining health of gingiva.

IV. Objectives of plaque disease control.

Reference

1. Young, W.O. and Striffler, D.F.: *The Dentist, His Practice, and His Community*, 2nd ed. Philadelphia, W.B. Saunders Co., 1969, p. 296.

Suggested Readings

Ainamo, J.: Relative Roles of Toothbrushing, Sucrose Consumption and Fluorides in the Maintenance of Oral Health in Children, *Int. Dent. J.*, *30*, 54, March, 1980.

Bye, F.L. and Caffesse, R.G.: The Process of Keratinization of the Gingival Epithelium, *Periodont. Abstr.*, *27*, 72, Number 3, 1979.

Henry, J.L. and Sinkford, J.C.: The Economic and Social Impact of Periodontal Disease, *Pub. Health Rep.*, *94*, 172, March–April, 1979.

Horowitz, A.M.: A Comparison of Available Strategies to Affect Children's Dental Health: Primary Preventive Procedures for Use in School-based Dental Programs, *J. Public Health Dent.*, *39*, 268, Fall, 1979.

Jenny, J. and Heifetz, S.B.: Prevention Update, *Dent. Hyg.*, *52*, 187, April, 1978.

Katz, S., McDonald, J.L., and Stookey, G.K.: *Preventive Dentistry*. Upper Montclair, New Jersey, D.C.P. Publishing, 1977, pp. 1–29.

Lavelle, C.L.B., Lewis, D.W., and Beagrie, G.S.: Summary of Symposium on Dental Perspectives—International Year of the Child, *J. Am. Dent. Assoc.*, *100*, 79, January, 1980.

Listgarten, M.A.: Prevention of Periodontal Disease in the Future, *J. Clin. Periodontol.*, *6*, 61, December, 1979.

Löe, H., Theilade, E., and Jensen, S.B.: Experimental Gingivitis in Man, *J. Periodontol.*, *36*, 177, May–June, 1965.

Mann, W.V.: Oral Hygiene Technics and Home Care, in Caldwell, R.C. and Stallard, R.E.: *A Textbook of Preventive Dentistry*. Philadelphia, W.B. Saunders Co., 1977, pp. 214–239.

Melcer, S. and Feldman, S.M.: Preventive Dentistry Teaching Methods and Improved Oral Hygiene—A Summary of Research, *Clin. Prev. Dent.*, *1*, 7, January–February, 1979.

Miller, C.K.: Preventive Dentistry: Where Are We and Where Are We Going? *Dent. Hyg.*, *54*, 432, September, 1980.

Mühlemann, H.R.: Psychological and Chemical Mediators of Gingival Health, *J. Prev. Dent.*, *4*, 6, July–August, 1977.

Silberman, S.L. and Yacovone, J.A.: Preventive Dentistry: A Conceptual Model for a Dental School, *Clin. Prev. Dent.*, *1*, 29, January–February, 1979.

Suomi, J.D.: Prevention and Control of Periodontal Disease, *J. Am. Dent. Assoc.*, *83*, 1271, December, 1971.

Tal, M.: Periodontal Disease and Oral Hygiene. Described by Antoni van Leeuwenhoek, *J. Periodontol.*, *51*, 668, November, 1980.

Dental Caries

Andlaw, R.J.: Oral Hygiene and Dental Caries—A Review, *Int. Dent. J.*, *28*, 1, March, 1978.

Clark, C.A., Fintz, J.B., and Taylor, R.: Effects of the Control of Plaque on the Progression of Dental Caries: Results After 19 Months, *J. Dent. Res.*, *53*, 1468, November–December, 1974.

Green, R.M.: Oral Hygiene and Caries Control, *Br. Dent. J.*, *150*, 117, March 3, 1981.

Rajala, M., Selkainaho, K., and Paunio, I.: Relationship Between Reported Toothbrushing and Dental Caries in Adults, *Community Dent. Oral Epidemiol.*, *8*, 128, June, 1980.

von der Fehr, F.R., Löe, H., and Theilade, E.: Experimental Caries in Man, *Caries Res.*, *4*, 131, Number 2, 1970.

Preventive Programs

Ashley, F.P. and Sainsbury, R.H.: The Effect of a School based Plaque Control Programme on Caries and Gingivitis, *Br. Dent. J.*, *150*, 41, January 20, 1981.

Axelsson, P. and Lindhe, J.: The Effect of a Preventive

Programme on Dental Plaque, Gingivitis and Caries in Schoolchildren. Results After One and Two Years, *J. Clin. Periodontol.*, 1, 126, Number 2, 1974.

xelsson, P. and Lindhe, J.: Effect of Fluoride on Gingivitis and Dental Caries in a Preventive Program Based on Plaque Control, *Community Dent. Oral Epidemiol.*, 3, 156, August, 1975.

amp, S.-E., Lindhe, J., Fornell, J., Johansson, L.-Å., and Karlsson, R.: Effect of a Field Program Based on Systematic Plaque Control on Caries and Gingivitis in Schoolchildren After 3 Years, *Community Dent. Oral Epidemiol.*, 6, 17, Number 1, 1978.

lorowitz, A.M., Suomi, J.D., Peterson, J.K., Mathews, B.I., Vogelsong, R.H., and Lyman, B.A.: Effects of Supervised Daily Dental Plaque Removal by Children After 3 Years, *Community Dent. Oral Epidemiol.*, 8, 171, August, 1980.

.ightner, L.M., O'Leary, T.J., Drake, R.B., Crump, P.P., and Allen, M.F.: Preventive Periodontic Treatment Procedures: Results Over 46 Months, *J. Periodontol.*, 42, 555, September, 1971.

indhe, J., Axelsson, P., and Tollskog, G.: Effect of Proper Oral Hygiene on Gingivitis and Dental Caries in Swedish Schoolchildren, *Community Dent. Oral Epidemiol.*, 3, 150, Number 4, 1975.

lcGuire, M.K., Sydney, S.B., Zink, F.J., Weber, M.B., and Fritz, M.E.: Evaluation of an Oral Disease Control Program Administered to a Clinic Population at a Suburban Dental School, *J. Periodontol.*, 51, 607, October, 1980.

)strom, C.A.: Effectiveness of a Preventive Dentistry Delivery System, *J. Am. Dent. Assoc.*, 97, 29, July, 1978.

uomi, J.D., Greene, J.C., Vermillion, J.R., Doyle, J., Chang, J.J., and Leatherwood, E.C.: The Effect of Controlled Oral Hygiene Procedures on the Progression of Periodontal Disease in Adults: Results After Third and Final Year, *J. Periodontol.*, 42, 152, March, 1971.

uomi, J.D., West, T.D., Chang, J.J., and McClendon, J.: The Effect of Controlled Oral Hygiene Procedures on the Progression of Periodontal Disease in Adults: Radiographic Findings, *J. Periodontol.*, 42, 562, September, 1971.

abita, P.V., Bissada, N.F., and Maybury, J.E.: Effectiveness of Supragingival Plaque Control on the Development of Subgingival Plaque and Gingival Inflammation in Patients with Moderate Pocket Depth, *J. Periodontol.*, 52, 88, February, 1981.

Bacteremia

3erger, S.A., Weitzman, S., Edberg, S.C., and Casey, J.I.: Bacteremia After the Use of an Oral Irrigation Device, *Ann. Int. Med.*, 80, 510, April, 1974.

Carroll, G.C. and Sebor, R.J.: Dental Flossing and Its Relationship to Transient Bacteremia, *J. Periodontol.*, 51, 691, December, 1980.

Cobe, H.M.: Transitory Bacteremia, *Oral Surg.*, 7, 609, June, 1954.

Drapkin, M.S.: Endocarditis After the Use of an Oral Irrigation Device, *Ann. Intern. Med.*, 87, 455, October, 1977.

Felix, J.E., Rosen, S., and App, G.R.: Detection of Bacteremia After the Use of an Oral Irrigation Device in Subjects with Periodontitis, *J. Periodontol.*, 42, 785, December, 1971.

Gillette, W.B. and van House, R.L.: Ill Effects of Improper Oral Hygiene Procedures, *J. Am. Dent. Assoc.*, 101, 476, September, 1980.

Lineberger, L.T. and DeMarco, T.J.: Evaluation of Transient Bacteremia Following Routine Periodontal Procedures, *J. Periodontol.*, 44, 757, December, 1973.

Madsen, K.L.: Effect of Chlorhexidine Mouthrinse and Periodontal Treatment Upon Bacteremia Produced by Oral Hygiene Procedures, *Scand. J. Dent. Res.*, 82, 1, Number 1, 1974.

Rise, E., Smith, J.F., and Bell, J.: Reduction of Bacteremia After Oral Manipulations, *Arch. Otolaryng.*, 90, 106, August, 1969.

Romans, A.R. and App, G.R.: Bacteremia, A Result from Oral Irrigation in Subjects with Gingivitis, *J. Periodontol.*, 42, 757, December, 1971.

Sconyers, J.R., Albers, D.D., and Kelly, R.: Relationship of Bacteremia to Toothbrushing in Clinically Healthy Patients, *Gen. Dent.*, 27, 51, May–June, 1979.

Sconyers, J.R., Crawford, J.J., and Moriarty, J.D.: Relationship of Bacteremia to Toothbrushing in Patients with Periodontitis, *J. Am. Dent. Assoc.*, 87, 616, September, 1973.

Silver, J.G., Martin, A.W., and McBride, B.C.: Experimental Transient Bacteraemias in Human Subjects with Varying Degrees of Plaque Accumulation and Gingival Inflammation, *J. Clin. Periodontol.*, 4, 92, May, 1977.

Silver, J.G., Martin, A.W., and McBride, B.C.: Experimental Transient Bacteremias in Human Subjects with Clinically Healthy Gingivae, *J. Clin. Periodontol.*, 6, 33, February, 1979.

Tamini, H.A., Thomassen, P.R., and Moser, E.H., Jr.: Bacteremia Study Using a Water Irrigation Device, *J. Periodontol.*, 40, 424, July, 1969.

Wank, H.A., Levison, M.E., Rose, L.F., and Cohen, D.W.: A Quantitative Measurement of Bacteremia and Its Relationship to Plaque Control, *J. Periodontol.*, 47, 683, December, 1976.

22

Oral Disease Control: Toothbrushes and Toothbrushing

The toothbrush is the principal instrument in general use for accomplishing plaque removal as a necessary part of disease control. Many different designs of toothbrushes and supplementary devices have been manufactured and promoted.

Patients who have not previously received professional advice concerning the best brush for their particular oral characteristics very likely have used brushes selected on the basis of cost, availability, advertising claims, family tradition, or habit. Because of the variety in shapes, sizes, textures, and other characteristics, the dental hygienist must become familiar with the many available products in order that patients be advised appropriately.

DEVELOPMENT OF TOOTHBRUSHES[1-4]

Crudely contrived toothpicks, presumably used for relief from food impaction, are believed to be the earliest implements devised for the care of the teeth. Excavations in Mesopotamia uncovered elaborate gold toothpicks used by the Sumerians about 3000 B.C.

The earliest record of the "chewstick," which has been considered the primitive toothbrush, dates back in the Chinese literature to about 1600 B.C. The care of the mouth was associated with religious training and ritual: the Buddhists had a "toothstick," and the Mohammedans used the "miswak." Chewsticks, made from various types of tasty woods by crushing an end and spreading the fibers in a brush-like manner, are still used by many Asiatic and African people.

The Ebers Papyrus, compiled about 1500 B.C. and dating probably at about 4000 B.C., contained reference to conditions similar to periodontal diseases and preparations to use as mouthwashes and dentifrices. The writings of Hippocrates (about 300 B.C.) include descriptions of diseased gums related to calculus and of complex preparations for the treatment of unhealthy mouths.

It is believed that the first bristled brush was that mentioned in the Chinese literature about 1600. Pierre Fauchard in 1728 in *Le Chirurgien Dentiste* described many aspects of oral health. He condemned the toothbrush made of horse's hair because it was rough and destructive to the teeth and advised the use of sponges or herb roots. Fauchard recommended scaling of teeth, and developed instruments and splints for loose teeth, as well as dentifrices and mouthwashes.

One of the earlier toothbrushes made in England was produced by William Addis around 1780. By the early nineteenth century, craftsmen in various European countries constructed handles of gold, ivory, or ebony, in which replaceable brush heads could be fitted. The first

339

patent for a toothbrush in the United States was issued to H. N. Wadsworth in the middle of the nineteenth century.

Many new varieties of toothbrushes were developed around 1900 when celluloid was available for the manufacture of toothbrush handles. In 1919, the American Academy of Periodontology defined specifications for toothbrush design and brushing methods in an attempt to standardize professional recommendations.[5]

Nylon came into use in toothbrush construction in 1938. World War II complications prevented Chinese export of wild boar bristles, and synthetic materials were substituted for natural bristles. Since then, synthetic materials have been improved and manufacturer's specifications standardized. Many current toothbrushes are made exclusively of synthetic materials. Powered toothbrushes had been developed earlier, but it was not until about 1960 that they were actively promoted.

MANUAL TOOTHBRUSHES

Although the American Dental Association does not evaluate and classify manual toothbrushes, certain recommendations have been made.[6] Desirable characteristics of a brush designed primarily to promote oral cleanliness are that it

1. Conform to individual patient requirements in size, shape, and texture.
2. Be easily and efficiently manipulated.
3. Be readily cleaned and aerated; impervious to moisture.
4. Be durable and inexpensive.
5. Have prime functional properties of flexibility, softness and diameter of the bristles or filaments; and strength, rigidity, and lightness in the handle.
6. Be designed for utility, efficiency, and cleanliness.

I. General Description

A. Parts (figure 22–1)

1. *Handle.* The part grasped in the hand during toothbrushing.
2. *Head.* The working end; that which holds the bristles or filaments.
   a. Tufts: clusters of bristles or filaments secured into the head.
   b. Brushing plane: the surface formed by the free ends of the bristles or filaments.
3. *Shank.* The section that connects the head and the handle.

B. Dimensions

1. *Total Brush Length:* about six inches; junior and child sizes are smaller.
2. *Head:* should be only large enough to accommodate the tufts.
   a. Length: 1 to $1\frac{1}{4}$ inches; width: $\frac{5}{16}$ to $\frac{3}{8}$ inch.
   b. Bristle or filament height: $\frac{7}{16}$ inch.

II. Handle

A. Composition

Nearly all current brush handles are plastics, which combine durability, imperviousness to moisture, pleasing appearance, low cost, sufficient rigidity, and smooth surface texture.

B. Shape

1. *Preferred.* Straight handle aligned on same plane as the head; with smooth form which is easy to grasp and may be

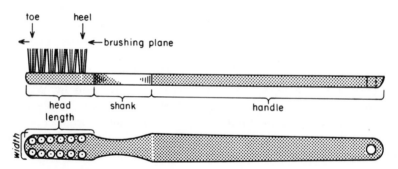

Figure 22–1. Parts of a toothbrush.

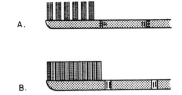

Figure 22–2. Toothbrush design. **A.** Tufted brush, five or six spaced tufts long and two or three rows wide. Tufted brushes are available with bristles or filaments in tapered lengths or all of equal lengths to form a smooth trim as shown. **B.** Multitufted brush, ten or twelve tufts long and three or four rows wide, spaced closely to provide a smooth brushing plane.

turned as needed but will not slip during manipulation.

   2. *Variations.* A twist, curve, offset, or angle in the shank may frequently be related to new ideas for advertising appeal. Slight deviations may not complicate manipulation or affect control of the brush placement and pressure.

      Bent or thickened handles can be helpful for use by handicapped patients (pages 700–702).

II. Head

A. Tufts (figure 22–2)

   1. *Tufted Design.* Five or six tufts long and two or three rows wide, spaced for easy cleaning of the brush.

   2. *Multitufted Design.* Ten or twelve tufts long and three or four rows wide, spaced closely to provide a smooth brushing plane and to allow the filaments to support each other for longer durability.

B. Brushing Plane

   1. *Preferred:* straight, with filaments all of equal length (figure 22–2); permits adaptability to all areas.

   2. *Uneven Planes.* Brushes are available with variously shaped planes, such as with high tufts in the middle or end position. These arrangements may be less efficient and may injure the gingiva or teeth since the longer filaments may be pressed too hard in the attempt to utilize the shorter filaments.

IV. Bristles and Filaments

A. Natural Bristles

   1. *Source.* Obtained from the hair of hog or wild boar.

   2. *Uniformity:* varies. The bristles are not consistent in texture, size, flexibility, or wearing properties.

   3. *Stiffness.* Variations are related to the following:

     a. Diameter of bristle: wider diameters are stiffer. They vary in size from .0035 to .0190 inch depending on the portion of the bristle and the age and life of the animal. Those between .007 and .010 were considered acceptable for use.

     b. Length of trim: shorter bristles are stiffer.

     c. Inherent resiliency: varies with the breed of animal as well as the geographic location and season in which the bristles were taken.

   4. *Properties*

     a. Water absorbent: become softened and stay softened longer.

     b. Bristles are hollow tubes that may harbor microorganisms.

B. Nylon Filaments

   1. *Source.* Manufactured according to federal specifications governing physical properties, composition, and diameter.

   2. *Uniformity:* controlled.

   3. *Stiffness*

     a. Diameter: thinner filaments are softer and more resilient.

     b. Diameter of soft nylon brushes: .006 to .007 inch.

     c. Diameter of regular nylon brushes: .008 inch = soft; .012 inch = medium; .014 inch = hard; .016 inch = extra hard. Note that what was considered "soft" in the regular nylon brushes (.008) is hard when compared with current standards for soft nylon brushes (.006 to .007).

   4. *Properties*

     a. Rinse clean and dry rapidly.

     b. Maintain form longer than natural bristles.

V. Toothbrush Selection for the Patient

A. Influencing Factors (see also pages 410–411)

Factors that influence the selection of the proper toothbrush for an individual patient include the following:

1. Ability of the patient to use the brush and remove plaque from all tooth surfaces without damage to the soft tissue or tooth structure.
2. Status of gingival or periodontal health.
3. Anatomic configurations of the gingiva.
4. Method of brushing to be recommended and instructed.
5. Position of teeth: displaced teeth require variations in brush placement.
6. Personal preferences
   a. Professional personnel preferences: dentist and dental hygienist may prefer to instruct certain methods and with certain brushes.
   b. Patient may have preferences and may resist change.
7. Manual dexterity of patient.
8. Motivation, ability, and willingness to follow the prescribed procedures.

B. Medium or Hard Brush: Tufted

Tufted medium or hard brushes were formerly used to a greater extent than currently. They are generally contraindicated because of potential damage to gingiva and teeth while removing plaque from the cervical thirds of the teeth, particularly if an abrasive dentifrice is used. Careful supervision by examination for evidences of trauma is needed, and corrections of technique made (pages 354–355).

C. Soft Nylon Brush: Tufted or Multitufted

The following are suggested as advantages for the use of a soft brush with rounded ends:

1. More effective in cleaning the cervical areas, both proximal and marginal.
2. Less traumatic to the gingival tissue, therefore patients can brush at the cervical area without fear of pain or lacerating the tissues.
3. Can be directed into the sulcus for sulcular brushing and into interproximal areas.
4. Applicable around fixed orthodontic appliances or fixation appliances required in fractured jaw treatment.
5. Tooth abrasion and/or gingival recession will be prevented or less severe in an over-vigorous brusher.
6. More effective use for sensitive gingiva in conditions such as necrotizing ulcerative gingivitis or desquamative gingivitis, or during healing stages following scaling and curettage or periodontal surgery.
7. Small size is ideal for a young child as a first brush on primary teeth.

TOOTHBRUSHING PROCEDURES

Complete toothbrushing instruction for a patient involves teaching many details related to why, what, when, where, and how. In addition to descriptions of specific toothbrushing methods, the succeeding sections will consider the grasp of the brush, the sequence and amount of brushing, the areas of limited access, supplementary brushing for the occlusal surfaces and the tongue, the possible detrimental effects from improper toothbrushing as well as contraindications, and the care of toothbrushes.

I. Grasp of Brush

A. Objectives

Manipulation of the brush for successful plaque removal can be related to the manner in which the brush is held. Most patients need specific instruction in how to hold and place the brush. When they start to brush to remove the dental plaque which has been colored with a disclosing agent, there is realization of the tenaciousness of the plaque and the need for controlled pressure. With a firm, comfortable grasp, the following can be expected:

1. Control of the brush during all movements.
2. Effective positioning at the beginning of each brushing stroke, follow-through during the complete stroke, and repositioning for the next stroke.
3. Sensitivity to the amount of pressure applied.

B. Procedure

1. Grasp toothbrush handle in the palm of the hand with thumb against the shank.
   a. Near enough to the head of the brush so that it can be controlled effectively.
   b. Not so close to the head of brush that manipulation of the brush is hindered or that fingers can touch the anterior teeth when reaching the brush head to molar regions.
2. Direct filaments in the direction needed for placement on the teeth; direction is dependent on the brushing method to be used.
3. Adapt grasp for the various positions of the brush head on the teeth throughout the procedure; adjust to permit unrestricted movement of the wrist and arm.

II. Sequence

A. The procedure in brushing, for any method used, should have a definite sequence.
B. To prevent omission of an area, it is recommended that brushing follow from the molar region of one arch around to the opposite side then back around the lingual or facial of the same quadrant.
C. Each brush placement must overlap the previous one for thorough coverage (figure 22–3).
D. Encourage the patient to begin by brushing one of the following which most meets the individual needs:
   1. Areas that are most frequently missed.
   2. Areas that are most difficult for brush placement and/or manipulation, such as the right side for the right-handed brusher or the left side for the left-handed brusher.
E. Suggest that the sequence be changed at least once each day so that the same areas are not always brushed last when the time may be limited and plaque removal may be less complete.

III. Amount of Brushing

A. The Count System

For thorough coverage with an even distribution of amount of brushing and to help the patient concentrate on the performance, a system of counting is useful.
1. Count six strokes in each area (or five or ten, whichever is most appropriate for the particular patient): for the rolling stroke, modified Stillman, or other method in which a stroke is used.
2. Count slowly to ten for each brush position while brush is vibrated and filament ends are held in position for the Bass, Charters', or other vibratory method.

B. The Clock System

Some patients brush thoroughly while watching a clock or an egg timer for three or four minutes. Timed procedures cannot assure thorough coverage, since single areas that are most accessible may get more time. Patients for whom this system is recommended must be selected carefully.

IV. Frequency of Brushing

Because of individual variations, one set rule for frequency cannot be applied. The emphasis in patient education should be placed on complete plaque removal rather than on number of brushings.

For the control of plaque, and for oral sanitation and halitosis prevention, more than one brushing and flossing each day is recommended. For patients who have difficulty in changing habits to make oral care a part of the daily routine, it may be better for them to have one thorough brushing than several incomplete attempts. When teeth are hastily and partially brushed, it

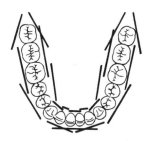

Figure 22–3. Brushing positions. A patient can be instructed to follow a specific order for brushing to prevent omissions. Each brush position, as indicated by a black line, should overlap the previous position. Note placement at canines where the distal of the canine is brushed with the premolars and the mesial is brushed with the incisors. Short lines on lingual anterior indicate brush placed the long narrow way. The maxillary teeth require a similar number of brushing positions.

is not unusual for the brusher to omit the same tooth surfaces each time.

Going to sleep with a clean mouth should be encouraged. For patients who will be using a chewable fluoride tablet, mouthrinse, or custom tray gel application before going to bed, plaque removal is completed before fluoride application.

Suggested recommendations for brushing frequency are as follows:[7]

A. Conscientious adult patients who demonstrate their ability to perform complete plaque control measures and who do not have gingival or periodontal disease or evidence of caries susceptibility: one brushing and flossing each day may be sufficient. Such patients usually prefer and are accustomed to more than one brushing, and no change of habits should be recommended.

B. Adult patients with gingival or periodontal involvement under treatment or who have been treated for periodontal disease: minimum of two brushings and one flossing with other aids as necessary. A fluoride dentifrice is particularly recommended when there is exposed cementum, as an aid in the prevention of root caries.

C. Young patients with gingival disease (or tendency towards gingival involvement): at least two and preferably three brushings, including at bedtime, after eating, and one flossing each day.

D. Patients of all ages who show susceptibility to dental caries: in conjunction with a total caries prevention program, thorough brushing after each meal and before going to bed to remove bacteria and sucrose left about the teeth. The patient should be reminded that more frequent application of fluoride dentifrice brings greater prevention and control benefits.

V. Methods

Most toothbrushing methods can be classified into one of seven groups based on the motion applied by the brush. Noted below beside certain categories are names of methods that utilize the designated motion as part or all of their particular procedure. Some of these methods are recorded for descriptive, comparative, or historic purposes only, and are not currently recommended. A few have even been proved detrimental.

A. **Roll:** Rolling stroke, modified Stillman.

B. **Vibratory:** Stillman, Charters', Bass.*

C. **Circular:** Fones'.

D. **Vertical:** Leonard's.

E. **Horizontal.**

F. **Physiological:** Smith's.

G. **Scrub-brush.**

THE ROLL or ROLLING STROKE METHOD

I. Purposes and Indications

A. Cleaning gingiva and removal of plaque, materia alba, and food debris from the teeth without emphasis on gingival sulcus.
   1. For children and adults with relatively healthy gingiva and normal tissue contour.
   2. For general cleaning in conjunction with the use of a vibratory technique (Charters', Stillman, or Bass).

B. Useful for preparatory instruction (first lesson) for modified Stillman's technique since the initial brush placement is the same. This can be particularly helpful when there is a question as to how complicated a technique the patient can master and practice.

II. Technique[5,8]

A. **Grasp Brush Handle**

   Direct filaments apically (up for maxillary, down for mandibular teeth).

B. **Place Side of Brush on the Attached Gingiva**

   The filaments are directed apically. When the plastic portion of the brush head is level with the occlusal or incisal plane, generally the brush will be at the proper height as shown in figure 22–4A.

---

*The Bass technique is not in the strictest sense a vibratory technique since a tiny back and forth stroke is used (pages 346–348).

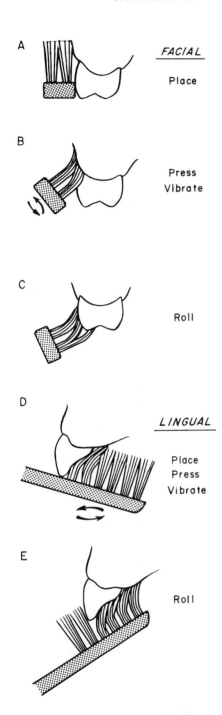

Figure 22–4. Modified Stillman method of brushing. **A.** Initial brush placement with sides of bristles or filaments against attached gingiva. **B.** The brush is pressed and angled, then vibrated, with sides of brush ends partly on the gingiva and partly on the tooth. **C.** Vibrating is continued as the brush is rolled over the crown to complete the stroke. **D.** Maxillary anterior lingual placement and activation. The brush is applied the long way. **E.** Vibrating continues as the brush is rolled over the crown and interdental areas. Placement for lingual of mandibular anterior is the same as for maxillary with the brush turned down.

C. Press to Flex the Filaments

The sides of the filaments are pressed against the gingiva. The gingiva will blanch.

D. Roll the Brush Slowly Over the Teeth

As the brush is rolled, the wrist is turned slightly. The filaments remain flexed and follow the contours of the teeth, thereby permitting the cleaning of the cervical areas. Some filaments will reach interdentally.

E. Replace and Repeat Five Times or More

The entire stroke (Parts A through D, above) is repeated at least five times for each tooth or group of teeth. When the brush is removed and repositioned, the wrist is rotated, the brush moved away from the teeth, and the cheek stretched buccally with the back of the plastic portion. Care must be taken not to drag the filament tips over the gingival margin when the brush is returned to the initial position (figure 22–4A).

F. Overlap Strokes

When moving the brush to an adjacent position, overlap the brush position as shown in figure 22–3.

G. Position Brush for Lingual Surfaces

1. Use the brush the long, narrow way.
2. Hook the heel of the brush on the incisal edge (figure 22–4D).
3. Press down for maxillary (up for mandibular) until the filaments lie flat against the teeth and gingiva.
4. Press and roll (curve up for mandibular, down for maxillary teeth).
5. Replace and repeat five times for each brush width. (Brush placement across the anterior lingual can be compared with the hands of a clock or spokes of a wheel.)

III. Problems

A. Brushing too high during initial placement can lacerate the alveolar mucosa.
B. Tendency to use quick, sweeping strokes results in no brushing for the cervical third of the tooth, since the brush tips pass over rather than into the area; and likewise for the interproximal areas.

C. Replacing brush with filament tips directed into the gingiva can produce punctate lesions (page 354).

THE MODIFIED STILLMAN METHOD

This method as originally described by Stillman[9] was designed for massage and stimulation as well as for cleaning the cervical areas. The brush ends were placed partly on the gingiva and partly on the cervical of the tooth, directed slightly apically, and pressure was applied to effect a blanching. The handle was given a slight rotary motion with the brush ends maintained in position on the tooth surface. After several applications, the brush was moved to the adjacent tooth.

In current use, a modified Stillman incorporates a rolling stroke after the vibratory (rotary) phase. The modifications minimize the possibility of gingival trauma and increase the cleaning effects.[10]

I. Purposes and Indications

A. Dental plaque removal from cervical areas below the height of contour of the enamel and from exposed proximal surfaces.
B. General application for cleaning tooth surfaces and massage of the gingiva.

II. Technique (figure 22–4)

A. Grasp Brush Handle

Direct filaments apically (up for maxillary, down for mandibular teeth).

B. Place Side of Brush on the Attached Gingiva

The filaments are directed apically. When the plastic portion of the brush head is level with the occlusal or incisal plane, generally the brush will be at the proper height as shown in figure 22–4A.

C. Press to Flex the Filaments

The sides of the filaments are pressed lightly against the gingiva. The gingiva will blanch.

D. Angle the Filaments

Turn the handle by rotating the wrist so that the filaments are directed at an angle of approximately 45 degrees with the long axis of the tooth.

E. Vibrate the Brush

Vibrate gently but firmly. Maintain light pressure on the filaments and keep the tips of the filaments in position with constant contact. Count to ten slowly as the brush is vibrated by a rotary motion of the handle.

F. Roll and Vibrate the Brush

Turn the wrist and work the vibrating brush slowly down over the gingiva and tooth. Make some of the filaments reach interdentally.

G. Replace Brush for Repeat Stroke

Reposition the brush by rotating the wrist. Avoid dragging the filaments back over the free gingival margin by holding the brush out, slightly away from the tooth.

H. Repeat Stroke Five Times or More

The entire stroke (Parts A through F, above) is repeated at least five times for each tooth or group of teeth. When moving the brush to an adjacent position, overlap the brush position as shown in figure 22–3.

I. Position Brush for Lingual Surfaces

1. Position the brush the long, narrow way for the anterior components as described for the rolling stroke technique and shown in figure 22–4 D and E.
2. Press and vibrate, roll, and repeat.

III. Problems

A. Without careful brush placement, tissue laceration can result when a hard brush is used. A soft brush used with lighter pressure is needed.
B. Patient may try to move the brush into the rolling stroke too quickly, and the vibratory aspect may be ineffective for plaque removal at the gingival margin.

THE BASS METHOD: SULCULAR BRUSHING

The Bass technique is widely accepted as the most effective method for dental plaque removal adjacent to and directly beneath the gingival margin. This area around the tooth is the most significant in the control of gingival and periodontal disease. Because of potential damage to the gingival tissue, only a soft nylon brush with rounded filament ends is indicated.

I. Purposes and Indications

A. For all patients for dental plaque removal adjacent to and directly beneath the gingival margin.

B. Particularly adaptable for open interproximal areas, cervical areas beneath the height of contour of the enamel, and exposed root surfaces.

C. Useful for the patient who has had periodontal surgery.

II. Technique[11]

A. Grasp Brush Handle

Direct the filaments apically (up for maxillary, down for mandibular teeth). Even though the brush placement calls for directing the filaments at a 45-degree angle, it is usually easier and safer for the patient to adjust the brush after first placing it parallel with the long axis of the tooth.

B. Angle the Filaments

Place the brush with the filament tips directed straight into the gingival sulcus. The filaments will be directed at approximately 45 degrees with the long axis of the tooth as shown in figure 22–5 A and B.

C. Press Lightly Without Flexing

Press lightly so the filament tips enter the gingival sulci and embrasures and cover the gingival margin. Do not bend the filaments.

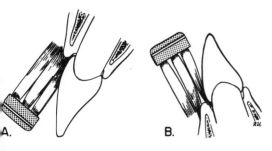

Figure 22–5. Sulcular method of brushing. Filament tips are directed into the gingival sulcus. The filaments are placed at approximately 45 degrees with the long axis of the tooth. **A.** Maxillary facial. **B.** Mandibular facial.

D. Vibrate the Brush

Vibrate the brush back and forth with very short strokes without disengaging the tips of the filaments from the sulci. Count at least ten vibrations.

E. Reposition the Brush

Apply the brush to the next group of two or three teeth. Take care to overlap placement as shown in figure 22–3.

F. Repeat Stroke

The entire stroke (Parts A through D, above) is repeated at each position around the maxillary and mandibular arches, both facially and lingually.

G. Position Brush for Lingual Anterior Surfaces (figure 22–6)

Hold the brush the long narrow way for the anterior components as described for the rolling stroke technique. The filaments are kept straight and directed into the sulci.

III. Problems

A. An over-eager brusher may convert the "very short strokes" (note II, D. above) into a scrub-brush technique and cause injury to the gingival margin.

B. Dexterity requirement is too high for certain patients.

C. Rolling stroke procedure may precede the sulcular brushing when a patient believes it helps to clean the teeth. It is recommended that the two techniques be performed separately rather than trying to combine them in what has been referred to as a "modified Bass."

The procedure of rolling the brush down over the crown after the vibratory part of the sulcular brush stroke has several disadvantages: (1) too often the brush is hastily and carelessly replaced into the sulcus position, or else the opposite is true and considerable time is consumed in the attempt to replace the brush carefully; (2) gingival margin injury by the constant replacement of the brush is common; and (3) concentration is not on the important objective, which is to remove the plaque at and under the gingival margin. Patients may tend to roll

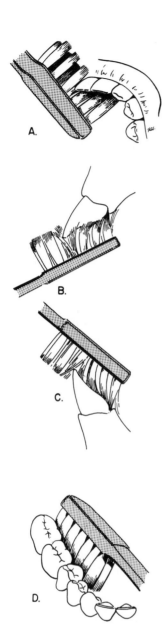

Figure 22–6. Sulcular brushing, lingual surfaces. **A.** Brush positioned for maxillary anterior. **B.** Filament tips are directed into the gingival sulcus. **C.** Lingual of mandibular anterior with filaments in sulcus. **D.** Brush positioned for lingual of posterior.

the brush down over the crown prematurely and very little sulcular brushing may be accomplished.

THE CHARTERS' METHOD

The original intent, as described by Charters,[12] was to use the toothbrush in a manner that would stimulate the gingival margin "all around each tooth, especially in the inter-dental spaces."

The method is generally not used when there are normal interdental papillae since other methods may be easier to teach.

I. Purposes and Indications

A. Loosening of debris and plaque.
B. Massage and stimulation for marginal and interdental gingiva.
C. Indicated to aid in plaque removal from proximal tooth surfaces when interproximal tissue is missing as, for example, following periodontal surgery.
D. Adaptable to cervical areas below the height of contour of the crown, and to exposed root surfaces.
E. Useful for cleaning abutment teeth and under the gingival border of a fixed partial denture (bridge), or the under-surface of a sanitary bridge.
F. Aids in cleansing orthodontic appliances (figure 24–6C, pages 383–384).

II. Technique[13]

A. Apply Rolling Stroke Technique

Instruct in a basic rolling stroke technique for general cleaning to be accomplished first.

B. Grasp Brush Handle

Hold brush (outside the oral cavity) with filaments directed toward the occlusal or incisal plane of the teeth that will be brushed. The tips are pointed down for application to the maxillary and pointed up for application to the mandibular arch. Insert the brush held in the direction it will be used.

C. Place the Brush

Place the sides of the filaments against the enamel with the brush tips toward the occlusal or incisal plane.

D. Angle the Filaments

Angle at approximately 45 degrees with the occlusal or incisal plane. Slide the brush to a position at the junction of the free gingival margin and the tooth surface (figure 22–7B).

E. Press Lightly

Press lightly to flex the filaments and force the tips between the teeth. The sides of the

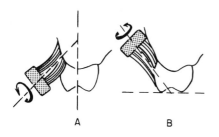

Figure 22–7. Comparison of brush positions for Stillman and Charters' methods. **A.** Stillman. The brush is angled at approximately 45 degrees with the long axis of the tooth. **B.** Charters'. The brush is angled at approximately 45 degrees with the occlusal plane, with brush tips directed toward the occlusal or incisal.

filaments are pressed against the gingival margin.

F. Vibrate the Brush

Vibrate gently but firmly, keeping the tips of the filaments in contact. Count to ten slowly as the brush is vibrated by a rotary motion of the handle.

G. Reposition the Brush and Repeat

Repeat Parts B through F, above, several times in each position around the dental arches.

H. Overlap Strokes

When moving the brush to an adjacent position, overlap the brush position as shown in figure 22–3.

I. Position Brush for Lingual Surfaces

Since Charters' brush positioning is difficult to accomplish on the lingual, a modified Stillman technique is frequently advised. When Charters' method is preferred, the positions are as follows:
1. Posterior
   a. With brush tips pointed toward the occlusal, extend the brush handle across the incisal of the canine of the side opposite that to be brushed.
   b. Place the sides of the toe-end filaments against the distal of the most posterior tooth and subsequently at each embrasure.
   c. Press and vibrate.
2. Anterior
   a. With brush handle parallel with the

long axis of the tooth, place the sides of the toe-end filaments over the interproximal embrasure.
   b. Press and vibrate.

J. Application of Brush for Fixed Partial Denture

When placing the brush, check that the filament tips are directed under the gingival border of the pontic.

III. Problems

A. Brush ends do not engage the gingival sulcus to remove subgingival bacterial accumulations.
B. In some areas, the correct brush placement is limited or impossible; therefore, modifications become necessary which add to the complexity of the procedure.
C. Requirements in digital dexterity are high.

OTHER TOOTHBRUSHING METHODS

The rolling stroke, modified Stillman, and Bass are probably the methods most used for patient instruction by dentists and dental hygienists. Other methods are and have been used, and a few of the well-known ones are included here. As these are reviewed, it will be realized that there is overlap in the technique and intent of some of the methods. Evaluation prior to special instruction generally reveals that a mixture of techniques may be in use by a patient.

I. Circular: The Fones' Method

It is likely that many people, especially school children, received instruction in this method since it was advocated by Fones who founded the first course for dental hygienists. He described the technique in the first dental hygiene text that was used for many years by dental hygiene students throughout the United States.

Although now considered a technique that could be detrimental for adults, particularly when used by a vigorous brusher, it may be recommended as an easy-to-learn first technique for young children. A soft brush with .006 to .008 inch filament diameter is selected. In abbreviated form, the technique described by Dr. Fones includes the following:[14]

A. With the teeth closed, place the brush inside the cheek with the brush tips lightly contacting the gingiva over the last maxillary molar.

B. Use a fast, wide, circular motion which sweeps from the maxillary gingiva to the mandibular gingiva with very little pressure (figure 22–8).

C. Bring anterior teeth in end-to-end contact, and hold lip out when necessary to make the continuous circular strokes.

D. Lingual: use an in-and-out stroke. Brush sweeps across palate on maxillary and back and forth to the molars on the mandibular.

II. Vertical: Leonard's Method

As described by Hirschfeld,[15] the up-and-down stroke was employed when teeth were cleaned with a primitive crude twig toothbrush. The true vertical stroke passes from the gingiva over the maxillary to the gingiva over the mandibular, with a vigorous sweeping motion.

Leonard described and advocated a vertical stroke in which maxillary and mandibular teeth are brushed separately. Paraphrased, he described his method as follows:[16]

A. With the teeth edge-to-edge, place the brush with the filaments against the teeth at right angles to the long axes of the teeth.

B. Brush vigorously, without great pressure, with a stroke that is mostly up and down on the tooth surfaces, with just a slight rotation or circular movement after striking the gingival margin with force.

C. Use enough pressure to force the filaments into the embrasure area, but not enough to injure the brush.

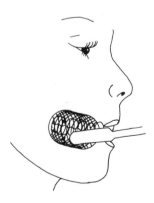

Figure 22–8. Fones' method of brushing. With the teeth closed, a circular motion extends from the maxillary gingiva to the mandibular gingiva, using a light pressure.

D. It is not intended that the upper and lower teeth shall be brushed in the same series of strokes: the teeth are placed edge-to-edge to keep the brush from slipping over the occlusal or incisal.

III. Horizontal

Horizontal or crosswise brushing is generally accepted as detrimental. An unlimited sweep with a scrubbing motion horizontally will bear pressure on teeth that are most facially inclined or prominent, and with an abrasive dentifrice, may produce tooth abrasion. Since the interdental areas are not touched by this method, various gingival and periodontal problems may ensue.

IV. Physiologic: Smith's Method

The physiologic method was described by Smith[17] and advocated later by Bell.[18] It was based on the principle that the toothbrush should follow the physiologic pathway that food does when it traverses over the tissues in a "natural" masticating act.

A soft brush with "small tufts of fine bristles arranged in four parallel rows and trimmed to an even length" was used in a brushing stroke directed down over the lower teeth onto the gingiva and upward over the teeth for the maxillary. Smith also suggested a few gentle horizontal strokes to clean the portion of the sulci directly over the bifurcations of the roots.

V. Scrub-Brush

It can be said that vigorously combined horizontal, vertical, and circular strokes with some vibratory motions for certain areas, comprise a scrub-brush technique. A soft brush with rounded brush ends, such as that recommended in particular for the Bass technique, can be used with a very short-stroked scrub-brush technique for plaque removal in the cervical area following periodontal surgery. However, without caution, vigorous scrubbing can encourage gingival recession, and with a dentifrice of sufficient abrasiveness, create areas of tooth abrasion.

SUPPLEMENTAL BRUSHING

I. Problem Areas

Each surface of each tooth must be brushed. Initial instruction may necessarily be limited to basic procedure, particularly when it varies from the patient's present procedures.

At succeeding lessons, the special hard-to-get areas are shown to the patient. Suggestions are made and demonstrated for brush adaptation for areas that were missed. Methods for cleaning the interdental areas and fixed and removable appliances are described in Chapters 23 and 24.

Attention in teaching should be given the following:

1. Facially displaced teeth, especially canines and premolars, where there may be a minimal zone of attached gingiva and where toothbrush abrasion frequently occurs.
2. Surfaces of teeth next to edentulous areas.
3. Inclined teeth; for example, lingual surfaces of mandibular molars that are inclined lingually.
4. Exposed root surfaces; cemental and dentinal surfaces may become abraded by extended application of an abrasive dentifrice.
5. Exposed furcation areas.
6. Right canine and lateral incisor, both maxillary and mandibular, are commonly missed by right-handed brushers; the opposite for left-handed.
7. Distal surfaces of most posterior teeth (figure 22–9).

II. Occlusal Brushing

A. Objectives

1. To loosen plaque microorganisms packed in pits and fissures.
2. To remove plaque deposits from occlusal surfaces of teeth out of occlusion or not used during mastication.

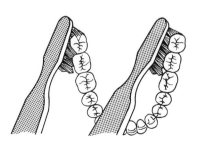

Figure 22–9. Brushing problems. Brush placement to clean the distal surfaces of the most posterior teeth. The distobuccal is approached by stretching the cheek; the distolingual by directing the brush across from the canine of the opposite side.

3. To remove plaque from the margins of restorations.
4. To apply fluoride from fluoride dentifrice.

B. Technique

1. Place brush on occlusal of molar teeth with filament tips pointed into the occlusal pits at a right angle. The handle should be parallel with the occlusal surface. The toe of the brush should cover the distal grooves of the most posterior tooth.
2. Two acceptable strokes are suggested
   a. Vibrate the brush in a slight circular movement while maintaining the filament tips on the occlusal surface throughout a count of ten. Press moderately so filaments do not bend but go straight into the pits and fissures (figure 22–10).
   b. Force the filaments against the occlusal surface with sharp, quick strokes; lift the brush off each time to dislodge debris; repeat about ten times.
3. Move brush to premolar area, overlapping previous brush position.

C. Precaution

Long scrubbing strokes from anterior to posterior on an occlusal surface may contact only the prominent parts of the cusps (figure 22–10B and -10C).

III. Tongue Brushing

Total mouth cleanliness includes tongue brushing.

A. Microorganisms of the Tongue

1. Main foci for oral microorganisms
   a. Dorsum of tongue.
   b. Gingival sulci and pockets.
   c. Dental plaque on all teeth.
2. Microorganisms in saliva are principally from the tongue.
3. Tongue organisms influence the flora of the entire oral cavity.

B. Effects of Cleaning the Tongue[19,20,21]

1. Reduction of oral debris.

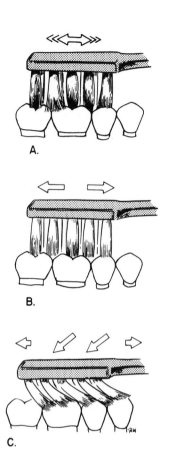

Figure 22–10. Occlusal brushing. **A.** Vibrating brush with light pressure while maintaining the filament tips on the occlusal surface to permit tips to work their way into the pits and fissures. **B.** Long horizontal strokes contact only the cusp tips. **C.** Excess pressure curves filament tips away from pits and fissures and damages the filaments.

   2. Retardation of plaque formation and total plaque accumulation.
   3. Reduction of number of microorganisms. When brushing of the tongue is discontinued, the number of organisms increases.
   4. Contribution to overall cleanliness.

C. Tongue Anatomy Conducive to Debris Retention

   1. *Surface Papillae.* Numerous filiform papillae extend as minute projections, while fungiform papillae are not as high and create elevations and depressions that entrap debris and microorganisms.
   2. *Fissured Tongue.* Fissures may be several millimeters deep and retain debris.

D. Brushing Procedure

   1. Hold the brush handle at a right angle to the midline of the tongue and direct the brush tips toward the throat.
   2. With the tongue extruded, the sides of the filaments are placed on the posterior part of the surface.
   3. With light pressure draw the brush forward and over the tip of the tongue. Repeat three or four times. Do not scrub the papillae.

POWERED TOOTHBRUSHES

Powered brushes are also known as automatic, mechanical, and electric brushes. The American Dental Association, Council on Dental Materials, Instruments and Equipment evaluates and classifies powered brushes as acceptable, provisionally acceptable, or unacceptable.[22]

Comparisons have been made in research between the powered and the manual brushes to determine the ability of each type to remove plaque, prevent calculus development, and reduce the incidence of gingivitis. Both types have been shown effective when used correctly.

I. Description

A. Head

The head, connected to the shank, is detachable from the handle and replaceable. In general, powered brush heads are smaller than manual brushes. They range in size from approximately $\frac{1}{4}$ to $\frac{1}{2}$ inch wide by $\frac{3}{4}$ inch long.

B. Filaments

Most powered brushes are multitufted with three or four rows of tufts. The diameters of the available filaments range from .005 to .007 inch to .010 or .012 inch.

C. Motion

The action on different models may be one of the following:
   1. Reciprocating: moves back and forth in a line.
   2. Arcuate: filament ends follow an arc as they move up and down.
   3. Orbital: circular.
   4. Vibratory.
   5. Elliptical: oval.

6. Dual motion: more than one of the above.

. Power Source

1. *Direct.* Cord from electrical outlet connects directly to the toothbrush handle.
2. *Replaceable Batteries.* Disadvantage in the nuisance and cost of repeatedly replacing or recharging batteries; also, as the batteries lose their power, the brush is slowed. Corrosion may be a problem if water gets into the case.
3. *Rechargeable.* The instrument is placed into a stand which contains the recharger and which is connected to the electrical outlet. A few models have a recharger built into the handle.
4. *Switches.* A few models require that the push button be held down during operation, which may present difficulties for some patients such as small children or persons with certain types of disabilities.

. Speeds

Speeds vary with the different models from low to high. Some have the speed coordinated with the filament texture; for example, a soft small brush with a fast vigorous action, or a larger, harder brush with a slower, more gentle motion. The number of strokes per minute varies from, for example, as low as 1000 cycles per minute for a replaceable battery type, to about 3600 oscillations per minute for an arcuate model. Between, the rechargeable battery types operate at approximately 2000 complete strokes per minute.

II. Purposes and Indications

A. General Application

For all patients for the removal of dental plaque, materia alba, and food debris. All of the general objectives that apply to plaque control measures and to manual brushes apply to powered brushes.

B. Patients with Disabilities

Powered brushes have been shown to be easily handled and manipulated by patients with certain handicaps (page 702).

C. Patients Unable to Brush

A powered brush may be readily handled by a parent, attendant, or other person who cares for the patient.

III. Instruction Compared with Manual

With a manual brush, an individual must learn to apply the brush tips in certain ways in order that each surface of each tooth be reached, slight pressure be applied for a thorough brushing effect, and the stroke be repeated a number of times. With a powered brush, the action is built in. The only muscle training required is turning the handle to apply the brush to each surface of each tooth and holding it there for a reasonable length of time in a correct position.

Not to underestimate the amount of instruction and practice needed for effective use of a powered brush, learning to use a manual brush usually requires more patience, time, and skill. A powered brush, on the other hand, tends to help overcome some of the learning difficulties.

IV. Methods for Use

The general suggestions presented here are basic and, as with all brushing techniques, need adaptations for an individual mouth. The dental hygienist should become familiar with the instructions provided by the manufacturers of the various powered brushes.

A. Select brush with extra-soft filaments. The tips included with a newly purchased brush handle are usually not extra-fine.
B. Select dentifrice with minimum abrasivity. The extra strokes made by a powered brush increase the effects of abrasion to the tooth surface.
C. Spread the dentifrice over the teeth and work some between the filaments of the brush to prevent splashing when the power is turned on.
D. Brush position: Nearly all brushing techniques can be applied for use with a powered brush. For vibratory techniques, wrist motion to change the brush position is not needed.
E. Vary the brush position for each tooth surface: brush each tooth separately.
   1. Apply the brush for sulcular brushing to the distal, facial, mesial surfaces of each tooth as the brush is moved from the

most posterior teeth toward the anterior, quadrant by quadrant.

2. Hold the brush in one location for a period of time, turn it or move it to reach adjacent areas while keeping the power on.

3. Angulate for access to surfaces of rotated, crowded, or otherwise displaced teeth.

4. Retract lip with fingers of other hand, to give access to and visibility of anterior facial surfaces, particularly including prominent canines.

5. Modify brush positions for application to proximal surfaces when there are missing interdental papillae: brush head may be positioned parallel with the long axis and inserted proximally for anterior teeth.

F. Strokes: make strokes slowly, with a slight steady pressure.

G. Precautions

1. Acrylic restorations should be avoided or treated without pressure, as they can wear down under repeated application of the fast-moving filaments with dentifrice.

2. Avoid pressure with abrasive dentifrice over exposed cementum or dentin.

EFFECTS OF IMPROPER TOOTHBRUSHING

I. Toothbrush Trauma: The Gingiva[23]

A. Acute Alterations (Lacerations)

1. *Appearance*
   a. Scuffed epithelial surface with denuded underlying connective tissue.
   b. Punctate lesions that appear as red, pinpoint spots.
   c. Diffuse redness and denuded attached gingiva.

2. *Precipitating Factors*
   a. Horizontal or vertical scrubbing toothbrushing method with pressure (either manual or powered).
   b. Overvigorous placement and application of the toothbrush.
   c. Penetration of gingiva by filament ends.
   d. Use of toothbrush with frayed, broken bristles or filaments.

e. Application of filaments beyond attached gingiva.

B. Chronic Alterations

1. *Location*
   a. Usually appear only on the facial gingiva, because of the vigor with which toothbrush is used.
   b. Frequently, inversely related to the right- or left-handedness of the patient.
   c. Areas most often involved are around canines or teeth in labio- or bucco version.

2. *Recession*
   a. Appearance: margin of gingiva has receded toward the apex, and the cementum is exposed.
   b. Predisposing anatomic factors.
      (1) Malposition of teeth: teeth in buccoversion usually have thin alveolar bone covering the buccal surface.
      (2) Narrow band of attached gingiva cannot withstand pressures of brushing.

3. *Changes in Gingival Contour*
   a. Rolled, bulbous, hard, firm marginal gingiva, in "piled up" or festoon shape (page 193).
   b. Gingival cleft: narrow groove or slit that extends from the crest of the gingiva to the attached gingiva ("Stillman's Cleft," figure 11–9, page 195).

4. *Precipitating Factors*
   a. Repeated use of a vigorous rotary, vertical, or horizontal toothbrushing method over a long period of time.
   b. Use of a long, brisk stroke with excessive pressure, over a long period of time.
   c. Habitual prolonged brushing in one area.
   d. Excessive pressure applied with a worn, nonresilient brush.

C. Suggested Corrective Measures

1. Recommend substitution of a softer toothbrush.

2. Correct the patient's toothbrushing technique; demonstrate a toothbrushing

method better suited to the oral condition.

. Abrasion of the Teeth

Abrasion is the loss of tooth substance produced by mechanical wear other than that by mastication, or it may be defined as the pathologic wearing away of tooth substance through some abnormal mechanical process.

. Contributing Factors

1. Hard toothbrush
2. Horizontal brushing
3. Excessive pressure during brushing
4. Abrasive agent in the dentifrice
5. Prominence of the tooth surface labially or buccally.

. Location of Abraded Areas

1. Primarily on facial surfaces especially of canines, premolars, and sometimes first molars, or any tooth in bucco- or labioversion, those most available to the pressure of the toothbrush. The canines are susceptible because of their prominence on the curvature of the dental arches.
2. Most abraded areas are on the cervical areas of exposed root surfaces, but occasionally may occur on the enamel. When adjacent teeth are involved, the lesions appear in line with each other.

C. Appearance

Saucer-shaped or wedge-shaped indentations with smooth, shiny surfaces (figure 14–4, page 238).

D. Corrective Measures

1. Explain the problem to the patient to assure full cooperation.
2. Advise a specific brush with soft-textured bristles or filaments.
3. Change the toothbrushing technique.
4. Recommend a less abrasive dentifrice.
5. Use a smaller amount of dentifrice
   a. Start brushing in the area of the dentition where the most plaque and calculus are noted at recall appointment.
   b. Avoid applying the dentifrice vigorously to the same tooth surfaces.[24]

CONTRAINDICATIONS FOR TOOTHBRUSHING

Even when an unusual oral condition develops, a patient must be encouraged to brush whenever possible to reduce the possibility of infection by decreasing the oral bacterial count. There are no indications for prolonged omission of techniques of plaque removal. Examples of conditions that may indicate a temporary departure from personal care routines are:

I. Acute Oral Inflammatory or Traumatic Lesions

When an acute oral condition precludes normal brushing, the patient should be instructed to brush all areas of the mouth that are not affected and resume regular plaque control measures on the affected area as soon as possible. When not otherwise contraindicated by instructions from the dentist, rinsing with a warm, mild saline solution can encourage healing and debris removal.

II. Following Periodontal Surgery

Patients will need to receive instructions concerning brushing. Since direct, vigorous brushing of a periodontal dressing could displace it, brushing of the occlusal surfaces and light strokes over the dressing may be advised. Other teeth and gingiva should be brushed as usual. Additional instructions appear in table 36–1, on page 548.

III. Acute Stage of Necrotizing Ulcerative Gingivitis

A major contributing factor in the development of this disease is a lack of oral cleanliness. During the acute stage, the oral tissues are sensitive to any touch, and toothbrushing will be neglected. Instructions for these patients are on pages 539 and 540. A very soft brush is indicated along with careful brush placement to avoid trauma.

IV. Following Dental Extraction

Instructions may be found on page 661 and include brushing all except the surgical wound area. Teeth adjacent to the extraction site need cleaning as soon as possible, to reduce bacterial collections and decrease the possibility of oral infection.

V. Following Dental Restorations

Patients will have a tendency to avoid a new crown, newly placed fixed partial denture, or other appliance. Specific instructions should be given at the time of insertion.

CARE OF TOOTHBRUSHES

When discussing the type and features of the brush selected for an individual patient, the number of brushes needed and the frequency of replacement should be included. Perhaps the ideal time to teach cleaning and daily care of brushes would be after a practice session when the brush has to be washed and cleaned for storage at the dental office.

That patients need instruction concerning the care and supply of their brushes is apparent from a survey of family toothbrush practices conducted by the American Dental Association.[25] From the questions asked the 751 participating families, about 40 percent believed that a toothbrush would last 6 months, 25 percent thought a brush would last only 3 months, while about 19 percent thought a brush should last up to 1 year.[25]

The condition of a brush is dependent on many factors, including the amount and manner of use, the type of care, as well as the quality of the brush at the start. Toothbrushes in current use were collected from the families in the survey mentioned above and evaluated. Only 55 percent were considered satisfactory for use. The unsatisfactory brushes were worn out, and dangerous for the gingiva because of marked splaying. Many were caked with dentifrice or unsightly deposits, and a few had broken plastic heads.[25]

I. Supply of Brushes

A. Advise at least two brushes for home use and a third in a portable container for use at work, school, or travel.
B. Brush purchase should be staggered so that all brushes are not new at the same time, but more important that they are not old at the same time so that the gingival condition is maintained at less than optimum.
C. Replace brushes before bristles or filaments become splayed, frayed, or lose resiliency. Worn brushes remove significantly less plaque than new brushes.

II. Cleaning Toothbrushes

A. Clean thoroughly after each use.
B. Hold brush head under strong stream warm water from faucet to force particle dentifrice, and bacteria from between th bristles.
C. Tap the handle on edge of sink to remov remaining particles.
D. Use another toothbrush to clean a brus bristles or filaments can be worked betwee those of the other brush to remove resistan debris.
E. Rinse completely and tap out excess wate

III. Brush Storage

A. Keep brush in open air with head in an up right position, apart from contact with othe brushes, particularly those of another pel son.
B. Portable brush container should have suf ficient holes to give air temporarily until th brush can be completely exposed for drying A closed container encourages bacteria growth.

References

1. Hirschfeld, I.: *The Toothbrush: Its Use and Abuse* Brooklyn, N.Y., Dental Items of Interest, 1939, pp 1–27.
2. Kimery, M.J. and Stallard, R.E.: The Evolutionary De velopment and Contemporary Utilization of Various Ora Hygiene Procedures, *Periodont. Abstr.*, *16*, 90, Sep tember, 1968.
3. McCauley, H.B.: Toothbrushes, Toothbrush Material and Design, *J. Am. Dent. Assoc.*, *33*, 283, March 1 1946.
4. Weinberger, B.W.: *An Introduction to the History o Dentistry.* St. Louis, The C.V. Mosby Co., 1948, pp 43, 140–144.
5. American Academy of Periodontology, Committee Re port: The Tooth Brush and Method of Cleaning th Teeth, *Dent. Items Int.*, *42*, 193, March, 1920.
6. American Dental Association, Council on Dental Ther apeutics: *Accepted Dental Therapeutics*, 39th ed. Chi cago, American Dental Association, 1982, p. 335.
7. Katz, S., McDonald, J.L., and Stookey, G.K.: *Preven tive Dentistry.* Upper Montclair, N.J., D.C.P. Publish ing, 1977, pp. 106–108.
8. Hard, D.: Oral Prophylaxis, in Bunting, R.W.: *Ora Hygiene*, 3rd ed. Philadelphia, Lea & Febiger, 1957 pp. 280–283.
9. Stillman, P.R.: A Philosophy of the Treatment of Per iodontal Disease, *Dent. Dig.*, *38*, 315, September, 1932
10. Hirschfeld: op. cit., p. 380.
11. Bass, C.C.: An Effective Method of Personal Oral Hy giene, *J. Louisiana State Med. Soc.*, *106*, 100, March 1954.
12. Charters, W.J.: Immunizing Both Hard and Soft Mouth Tissue to Infection by Correct Stimulation with the Toothbrush, *J. Am. Dent. Assoc.*, *15*, 87, January, 1928.

. Charters, W.J.: Home Care of the Mouth. I. Proper Home Care of the Mouth, *J. Periodontol.*, *19*, 136, October, 1948.

. Fones, A.C., ed.: *Mouth Hygiene*, 4th ed. Philadelphia, Lea & Febiger, 1934, pp. 299–306.

. Hirschfeld: op. cit., pp. 369–371.

. Leonard, H.J.: Conservative Treatment of Periodontoclasia, *J. Am. Dent. Assoc.*, *26*, 1308, August, 1939.

. Smith, T.S.: Anatomic and Physiologic Conditions Governing the Use of the Toothbrush, *J. Am. Dent. Assoc.*, *27*, 874, June, 1940.

. Bell, D.G.: Home Care of the Mouth. III. Teaching Home Care to the Patient, *J. Periodontol.*, *19*, 140, October, 1948.

. Gilmore, E.L., Gross, A., and Whitley, R.: Effect of Tongue Brushing on Plaque Bacteria, *Oral Surg.*, *36*, 201, August, 1973.

. Jacobson, S.E., Crawford, J.J., and McFall, W.R.: Oral Physiotherapy of the Tongue and Palate: Relationship to Plaque Control, *J. Am. Dent. Assoc.*, *87*, 134, July, 1973.

. Gross, A., Barnes, G.P., and Lyon, T.: Effects of Tongue Brushing on Tongue Coating and Dental Plaque Scores, *J. Dent. Res.*, *54*, 1236, November–December, 1975.

. American Dental Association, Council on Dental Materials, Instruments and Equipment: *Dentist's Desk Reference: Materials, Instruments and Equipment*, 1st ed. Chicago, American Dental Association, 1981, pp. xxxvii–xl, 340.

. Carranza, F.A.: *Glickman's Clinical Periodontology*, 5th ed. Philadelphia, W.B. Saunders Co., 1979, p. 449.

. Moore, W.F.: Oral Hygiene (Letter to Editor), *J. Am. Dent. Assoc.*, *101*, 896, December, 1980.

. Craig, T.T. and Montague, J.L.: Family Oral Health Survey, *J. Am. Dent. Assoc.*, *92*, 326, February, 1976.

Suggested Readings

naise, J.Z.: The Toothbrush in Plaque Removal, *J. Dent. Child.*, *42*, 186, May–June, 1975.

aer, C. and Baer, P.N.: A Story of the Toothpick, *J. Periodontol.*, *37*, 158, March–April, 1966.

arenie, J.T., Leske, G.S., and Ripa, L.W.: The Effect of Toothbrushing Frequency on Oral Hygiene and Gingival Health in Schoolchildren: Reassessment after Two and One-half years, *J. Public Health Dent.*, *36*, 9, Winter, 1976.

arenie, J.T., Ripa, L.W., and Leske, G.: The Relationship of Frequency of Toothbrushing, Oral Hygiene, Gingival Health, and Caries Experience in School Children, *J. Public Health Dent.*, *33*, 160, Summer, 1973.

Barnes, G.P., Radi, W.R., and Katz, R.V.: Clinical Effects of Varying the Numbers and Distribution Patterns of Toothbrush Bristle Tufts on Plaque Removal, *J. Prev. Dent.*, *3*, 12, July–August, 1976.

Berdon, J.K., Hornbrook, R.H., and Hayduk, S.E.: An Evaluation of Six Manual Toothbrushes by Comparing Their Effectiveness in Plaque Removal, *J. Periodontol.*, *45*, 496, July, 1974.

Elliott, J.R., Bowers, G.M., Clemmer, B.A., and Rovelstad, G.H.: II. A Comparison of Selected Oral Hygiene Devices in Dental Plaque Removal, *J. Periodontol.*, *43*, 217, April, 1972.

Frandsen, A.M., Barbano, J.P., Suomi, J.D., Chang, J.J., and Houston, R.: A Comparison of the Effectiveness of the Charters', Scrub, and Roll Methods of Toothbrushing in Removing Plaque, *Scand. J. Dent. Res.*, *80*, 267, Number 4, 1972.

Fry, H.R.: The Effect of Intrasulcular Toothbrushing on the Amount of Sulcular Fluid, *J. Periodontol.*, *49*, 538, October, 1978.

Fry, H.R. and App, G.R.: Histologic Evaluation of the Effects of Intrasulcular Toothbrushing on Human Sulcular Epithelium, *J. Periodontol.*, *49*, 163, April, 1978.

Galil, K.A.: Scanning and Transmission Electron Microscopic Examination of Occlusal Surface Plaque Following Tooth Brushing, *Can. Dent. Assoc. J.*, *41*, 499, September, 1975.

Gibson, J.A. and Wade, A.B.: Plaque Removal by the Bass and Roll Brushing Techniques, *J. Periodontol.*, *48*, 456, August, 1977.

Hall, A.W. and Conroy, C.W.: Comparison of Automatic and Hand Toothbrushes: Toothbrushing Effectiveness for Preschool Children, *J. Dent. Child.*, *38*, 309, September–October, 1971.

Hansen, F. and Gjermo, P.: The Plaque-removing Effect of Four Toothbrushing Methods, *Scand. J. Dent. Res.*, *79*, 502, Number 7, 1971.

Horowitz, A.M. and Suomi, J.D.: A Comparison of Plaque-removal With a Standard or an Unconventional Toothbrush Used by Youngsters, *J. Periodontol.*, *45*, 760, October, 1974.

International Conference on Research in the Biology of Periodontal Disease. Chicago, University of Illinois, College of Dentistry, 1977, pp. 323–325, 371, 388.

Kelner, R.M., Wohl, B.R., Deasy, M.J., and Formicola, A.J.: Gingival Inflammation as Related to Frequency of Plaque Removal, *J. Periodontol.*, *45*, 303, May, 1974.

Lang, N.P., Cumming, B.R., and Löe, H.: Toothbrushing Frequency as it Relates to Plaque Development and Gingival Health, *J. Periodontol.*, *44*, 396, July, 1973.

Love, W.D., Ramirez, J.M., and Fultz, R.P.: Comparative Toothbrush Efficiency Utilizing a New Oral Hygiene Index, *J. Public Health Dent.*, *35*, 231, Fall, 1975.

McAllan, L.H., Murray, J.J., Brook, A.H., and Crawford, A.N.: Oral Hygiene Instruction in Children Using Manual and Electric Toothbrushes, Benefits after Six Months, *Br. Dent. J.*, *140*, 51, January, 20, 1976.

MacGregor, I.D.M. and Rugg-Gunn, A.J.: Survey of Toothbrushing Duration in 85 Uninstructed English Schoolchildren, *Community Dent. Oral Epidemiol.*, *7*, 297, October, 1979.

MacGregor, I.D.M. and Rugg-Gunn, A.J.: A Survey of Toothbrushing Sequence in Children and Young Adults, *J. Periodont. Res.*, *14*, 225, May, 1979.

Nygaard-Østby, P., Edvardsen, S., and Spydevold, B.: Access to Interproximal Tooth Surfaces by Different Bristle Designs and Stiffnesses of Toothbrushes, *Scand. J. Dent. Res.*, *87*, 424, December, 1979.

Nygaard-Østby, P., Spydevold, B., and Edvardsen, S.: Suggestion for a Definition, Measuring Method and Classification of Bristle Stiffness of Toothbrushes, *Scand. J. Dent. Res.*, *87*, 159, June, 1979.

O'Connor, N.J.: Brands, Bristles, and Tufts. A Toothbrush Survey, *Dent. Assist.*, *46*, 22, October, 1977.

Owen, T.L.: A Clinical Evaluation of Electric and Manual Toothbrushing by Children with Primary Dentitions, *J. Dent. Child.*, *39*, 15, January–February, 1972.

Richardson, J.L.: Mechanical Plaque Control, a Review of the Literature, *J. Am. Soc. Prev. Dent.*, *5*, 24, March–April, 1975.

Robinson, E.: A Comparative Evaluation of the Scrub and Bass Methods of Toothbrushing With Flossing as an Adjunct (in Fifth and Sixth Graders), *Am. J. Pub. Health*, *66*, 1078, November, 1976.

Rugg-Gunn, A.J. and MacGregor, I.D.M.: A Survey of Toothbrushing Behaviour in Children and Young Adults, *J. Periodont. Res.*, *13*, 382, July, 1978.

Rugg-Gunn, A.J., MacGregor, I.D.M., Edgar, W.M., and Ferguson, M.W.: Toothbrushing Behaviour in Relation to Plaque and Gingivitis in Adolescent Schoolchildren, *J. Periodont. Res.*, 14, 231, May, 1979.

Sangnes, G., Zachrisson, B., and Gjermo, P.: Effectiveness of Vertical and Horizontal Brushing Techniques in Plaque Removal, *J. Dent. Child.*, 39, 94, March–April, 1972.

Scopp, I.W., Cohen, G., Cancro, L.P., and Bolton, S.: Clinical Evaluation of a Newly Designed Contoured Toothbrush, *J. Periodontol.*, 47, 87, February, 1976.

Updike, J.R.: A New Handle for a Child's Toothbrush, *J. Dent. Child.*, 46, 123, March–April, 1979.

Updike, J.R. and Terrell, M.E.: Toothbrush Selection of a Young Child, *J. Pedod.*, 4, 295, Summer, 1980.

Vowles, A.D. and Wade, A.B.: Importance of Filament Diameter When Using Bass Brushing Technique, *J. Periodontol.*, 48, 460, August, 1977.

Waerhaug, J.: Effect of Toothbrushing on Subgingival Plaque Formation, *J. Periodontol.*, 52, 30, January, 1981.

Effects of Improper Brushing

Aker, D.A., Aker, J.R., and Sorensen, S.E.: Toothbrush Abrasion of Color-corrective Porcelain Stains Applied to Porcelain-fused-to-metal Restoration, *J. Prosthet. Dent.*, 44, 161, August, 1980.

Bergstrom, J. and Lavstedt, S.: An Epidemiologic Approach to Toothbrushing and Dental Abrasion, *Commun Dent. Oral Epidemiol.*, 7, 57, February, 1979.

Breitenmoser, J., Mörmann, W., and Mühlemann, H.: Damaging Effects of Toothbrush Bristle End Form Gingiva, *J. Periodontol.*, 50, 212, April, 1979.

Burgett, F.G. and Ash, M.M.: Comparative Study of t Pressure of Brushing with Three Types of Toothbrushe *J. Periodontol.*, 45, 410, June, 1974.

Gillette, W.B. and Van House, R.L.: Ill Effects of Improp Oral Hygiene Procedures, *J. Am. Dent. Assoc.*, 1(476, September, 1980.

Heath, J.R. and Wilson, H.J.: Abrasion of Restorative M terial by Toothpaste, *J. Oral Rehabil.*, 3, 121, Apr 1976.

Padbury, A.D. and Ash, M.M.: Abrasion Caused by Thr Methods of Toothbrushing, *J. Periodontol.*, 45, 43 June, 1974.

Radentz, W.H., Barnes, G.P., and Cutright, D.E.: A Su vey of Factors Possibly Associated with Cervical Abr sion of Tooth Surfaces, *J. Periodontol.*, 47, 148, Marc 1976.

Sangnes, G.: Traumatization of Teeth and Gingiva Relate to Habitual Tooth Cleaning Procedures, *J. Clin. Pe iodontol.*, 3, 94, May, 1976.

Sangnes, G. and Gjermo, P.: Prevalence of Oral Soft ar Hard Tissue Lesions Related to Mechanical Toothclea sing Procedures, *Community Dent. Oral Epidemiol.*, 77, March, 1976.

23

Auxiliary Plaque Control Measures

Auxiliary measures are selected to complement toothbrushing. Since plaque on proximal tooth surfaces is not totally accessible to usual brushing, a means for proximal plaque removal is necessary in complete preventive care. Other objectives and uses are outlined as each auxiliary aid is described in this chapter. Following, in Chapter 24, particular applications are given for care of teeth and tissues related to dental appliances. In Chapter 25, necessary adaptations are described for a mouth with complete rehabilitation.

When the plaque control and oral physical therapy regimen is outlined for an individual patient, the first consideration is given to the specific oral condition and how it can be improved or maintained in health. Next, it is necessary to consider which goals of oral health can be reached by the use of particular implements. For example, certain devices can be expected to remove plaque, whereas others will not remove plaque, but are efficient at removing debris, materia alba, and superficial layers of less tenaciously attached microorganisms over the surface of the plaque.

After matching the available devices with the goals for health of the individual oral condition, teaching, learning, and time must be considered. The simplest possible procedures are selected for the patient's convenience and ease of learning as well as for keeping the daily oral care regimen at a realistic level with respect to the time the patient is able and willing to spend.

INTERDENTAL PLAQUE CONTROL

Normally, the interdental gingiva fills the gingival embrasure between two teeth and beneath their contact area. Between posterior teeth there are two papillae, one facial and one lingual, connected by a col which is a depressed concave area (figure 11–5, page 189). Between anterior teeth interdental papillae are generally single, with a pyramidal shape. The epithelium covering the col is thin and less resistant to disease.

The interdental col area is generally inaccessible for toothbrushing. It is a protected area when the teeth are in normal position. Because of its shape, it tends to harbor microorganisms. Most gingival disease starts in the interdental areas and the incidence of gingivitis is highest in the interdental col gingiva.

When interdental papillae are reduced in height or missing, the proximal tooth surfaces are exposed and the gingiva takes on a different shape, sometimes craterlike. Dental plaque collects on the tooth surfaces and retention of debris in the interproximal area can occur. Irregularities of tooth position, such as rotation or alterations related to malocclusion or tooth loss, contribute to differences in the shape of the gingival embrasure, and further complicate the plan for plaque control.

359

I. Objectives of Interdental Care

The interdental papillae may be missing or reduced in height because of (1) disease such as necrotizing ulcerative gingivitis, (2) surgical procedures essential in the treatment of periodontal diseases, or (3) habitual pressure atrophy caused by the use of interdental tips or other devices which are contraindicated when interdental gingiva fill the embrasure. As a result of the exposure of the tooth surfaces, the changes in shape of the interdental tissue, and the general trapping of debris in the unnatural spaces, specific care is needed.

The general objectives for plaque control and oral physical therapy apply to this area (page 335). With the judicious use of the various methods and devices available, disease control of the interdental area can be accomplished by a motivated patient.

II. Role of Toothbrushing

Interproximal vibratory and sulcular brushing such as Charters', Stillman, and the Bass techniques using a soft brush, can be successful to some degree in removing dental plaque from the proximal surfaces of the teeth. However, all of the proximal plaque is rarely removed by toothbrushing alone.

For complete plaque and debris removal from proximal tooth surfaces, more than the toothbrush is generally needed. Various materials and devices are described in the sections following.

Removal of all calculus and smoothing of the tooth surface increases the effectiveness of devices. Rough tooth surfaces retain plaque which initiates inflammation. Large deposits of calculus and overhanging restorations interfere with the use of devices; for example, dental floss catches and shreds when applied to overhanging margins of restorations or calculus deposits.

It is not generally recommended that instruments that are used to apply pressure for massage or stimulation be used without first removing subgingival calculus. Rubbing the inflamed gingival wall of the pocket over calculus may aggravate the inflammatory reaction.

DENTAL FLOSS AND TAPE

When dental floss is applied with firm pressure to a flat or convex proximal tooth surface, plaque can be removed. A concave tooth surface would escape contact with the floss. Figure 23–9A (page 365) illustrates this for the mesial of the maxillary first premolar.

I. Types of Floss

A. Unwaxed

Frequently recommended because it is thinner and slips through close contacts with ease, and because it may be more absorbent and hold plaque as it is removed.

B. Waxed

May be particularly indicated during the initial period of patient care before restorative work is completed and tooth surfaces are completely scaled and root planed, because the unwaxed floss shreds and tears more easily. The tearing may aggravate the patient and discourage continued use.

II. Indications

For most patients dental floss can best be used before toothbrushing. Not only does this assure that caries-susceptible proximal surfaces will be de-plaqued, but also that the fluoride from the dentifrice used during brushing will be able to reach the proximal surfaces for caries prevention.

In addition to plaque removal from proximal tooth surfaces, flossing removes food debris and materia alba from interproximal areas. This contributes to general oral sanitation and the control of halitosis.

When there is inadequate contact and the patient indicates that floss or toothpicks are required to relieve pressure from impacted food, dental attention may be needed. The area should be charted or otherwise brought to the attention of the dentist.

III. Procedure

A. Floss Preparation

1. Hold a 12- to 15-inch length of floss with the thumb and index finger of each hand; grasp firmly with one-half inch of floss between the finger tips. The ends of the floss may be tucked into the palm and held by the ring and little finger, or the floss may be wrapped around the middle fingers (figure 23–1A, B, and C).

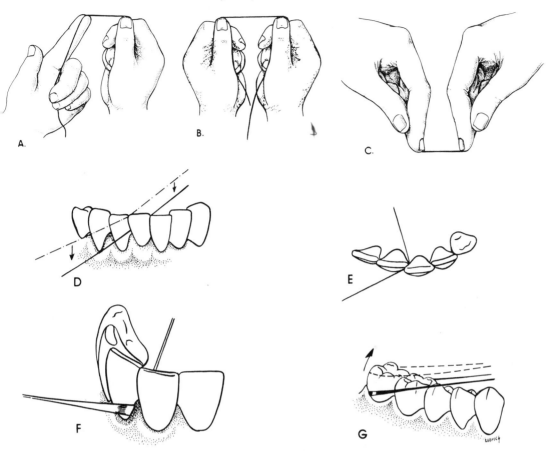

Figure 23–1. Directions for use of floss. **A.** For maxillary insertion hold the floss between the thumb and index finger or **B.** between thumbs. Grasp the floss firmly. Allow one-half to one inch between fingers. **C.** For mandibular teeth, direct the floss down, guided by the index fingers. **D.** Work the floss slowly between the teeth in a short sawing motion. Avoid snapping through the contact area. **E.** Curve the floss around the tooth in a C-shape. Hold the floss toward the mesial for cleaning the distal surfaces, and toward the distal for cleaning mesial surfaces. **F.** Press the floss firmly against the tooth. Move gently beneath the gingiva until tissue resistance is felt. Slide the floss horizontally and vertically with pressure to remove plaque. **G.** Begin flossing with the distal of the most posterior tooth and work systematically around the arch.

2. A circle of floss may be made by tying the ends together; the circle may be rotated around as the floss is used (figure 23–2).

B. Application

1. *Mandibular Teeth.* Direct the floss down by holding the two index fingers on top of the strand. One index finger holds the floss on the lingual and the other on the facial. The side of the finger on the lingual is held on the teeth of the opposite side of the mouth to serve as a fulcrum or rest.

2. *Maxillary Teeth.* Direct the floss up by holding the floss over two thumbs or a thumb and and index finger as shown in figure 23–1A, B, C. Rest a side of a finger on teeth of opposite side of the maxillary arch to provide balance and a fulcrum.

C. Insertion

1. Hold floss in a diagonal or oblique position (figure 23–3).
2. Ease the floss past each contact area with a gentle sawing motion.
3. Control floss to prevent snapping through the contact area onto the gingival tissue.

D. Cleaning Stroke

1. Clean adjacent teeth separately: for the distal aspect curve the floss mesially, and for the mesial aspect curve the floss dis-

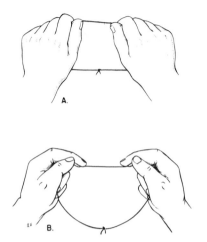

Figure 23–2. Circle of floss. The ends of the floss are tied together for convenient holding. A child may be able to manage floss better with this technique. **A.** Held for maxillary. **B.** Mandibular.

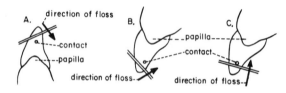

Figure 23–3. Insertion of floss. Hold floss in a diagonal or oblique position. Arrows indicate direction of movement of floss. **A.** Mandibular. **B.** Maxillary. **C.** Incorrect. When floss is held horizontally there is greater possibility for damage to the papilla.

tally, around the tooth (figure 23–1E, F, and G).

2. Pass the floss below the gingival margin, press to adapt the floss around the tooth, and slide up the tooth surface. Repeat.

E. Additional Suggestions

1. When a dentifrice is used, dental tape may retain the dentifrice against the tooth better than floss.
2. Slide the floss to a new, unused portion for succeeding proximal tooth surfaces.
3. Floss may be used double to provide a wider rubbing surface.

IV. Precautions

A. Pressure in Col Area

The col area is not keratinized and is vulnerable to disease. Plaque control of the area

is of great importance since most gingival and periodontal disease begins in the col area. Too great pressure with floss one or more times daily, particularly very fine floss that tends to cut more easily than thicker floss, can be destructive to the attachment. This may be of particular significance in children while teeth are in the process of eruption.

B. Prevention of Floss Cuts

1. *Location.* Floss cuts occur primarily on facial or lingual surfaces directly beside or in the middle of an interdental papilla. They appear as straight line cuts from the gingival margin toward the mucogingival junction.
2. *Causes of Floss Cuts*
   a. Too long a piece of floss between the fingers when held for insertion.
   b. Snapping the floss through the contact area.
   c. Not curving the floss about the teeth; floss held straight across the papilla.
   d. Not using a rest to prevent undue pressure.

V. Use of Floss Holder

A. Types

Several types of plastic floss holders are available (figure 23–4).

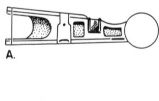

A.

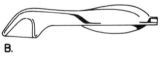

B.

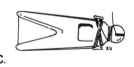

C.

Figure 23–4. Examples of floss holders. **A.** has replaceable floss container. **B.** has replaceable floss cartridge and thin edge for cleaning the tongue. **C.** has threading mechanism which requires a 24-inch length of floss applied at each use.

Use

Careful instruction should be provided and supervision given periodically to prevent tissue damage. As threaded into a holder, the floss is in a straight line (23–5A).

To avoid cutting the papilla when applied interproximally:

. Use a rest or fulcrum to prevent snapping through the contact.

.. Pull the floss mesially (to clean the distal of a tooth) or push distally (to clean mesial surface) to allow floss to be positioned on the side of the papilla (figure 23–5).

KNITTING YARN

. **Indications for Use**

A. For tooth surfaces adjacent to wide proximal spaces, dental floss is narrow and does not remove plaque efficiently.

B. For mesial and distal abutments of fixed partial dentures and under pontic, using a floss threader (page 381).

C. For isolated teeth, teeth separated by a diastema, and distal surfaces of most posterior teeth.

II. Technique

A. Preparation of yarn: fold double about 8 inches of three- or four-ply smooth synthetic yarn and loop through about 8 inches of dental floss; tie floss with one overhand knot.

B. Insert floss through the contact area: draw the yarn into the embrasure (figure 23–6).

C. Clean adjacent teeth separately with a bucco-lingual back-and-forth stroke: hold the ends of the yarn distally and then around mesially.

D. For specific areas where a papilla may be high or access not otherwise sufficient for the wide yarn, the dental floss end of the combination can be used.

E. Dentifrice may be used.

F. For closed contacts, use a floss threader (figure 24–3, page 381).

GAUZE STRIP

I. Indications for Use

To clean proximal surfaces of teeth that are widely spaced or adjacent to edentulous areas. Gauze is too thick to pass through contact areas.

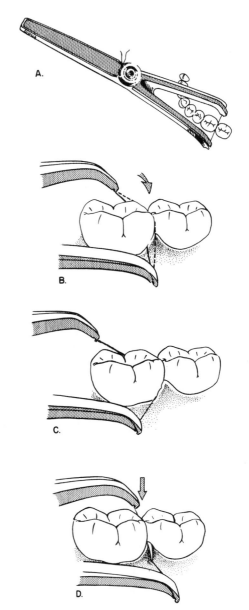

Figure 23–5. Use of floss holder. **A.** Applied interproximally. **B.** As floss is drawn through the contact area, the holder should be pulled mesially when the floss is to be applied to a distal surface (and pushed distally when applied to a mesial surface). **C.** Floss is lowered into sulcus. **D.** Floss cut in papilla resulting from incorrect use.

II. Technique

A. Prepare strip: cut 1-inch gauze bandage into a 6-inch length and fold in thirds or down the center.

B. Position the fold of the gauze on the cervical area next to the gingival crest and work back and forth several times; hold ends toward

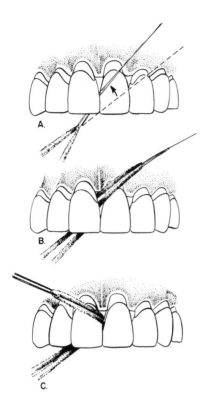

Figure 23–6. Use of knitting yarn in open gingival embrasure. **A.** Yarn is looped through dental floss, and dental floss is drawn through the contact area in usual manner, as shown by arrow. **B.** Yarn is drawn through the embrasure. **C.** Yarn is positioned against the surface of the tooth for plaque removal.

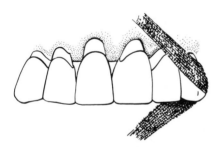

Figure 23–7. Use of gauze strip for surfaces without contact with an adjacent tooth. A 6-inch length of 1-inch gauze bandage is folded in thirds and placed around the tooth with the folded edge over the cervical third of the tooth. A "shoeshine" stroke is used to clean the surface.

distal to clean a mesial surface, and mesial to clean a distal surface (figure 23–7).

PIPE CLEANER

I. Indications for Use

Proximal surfaces when interdental gingiva is missing; furcation areas.

II. Technique

A. One third of a regular length pipe cleaner is adequate at a time. Check wire end to prevent damaging the gingiva or scratching the cemental surface.

B. Carefully work the end of the cleaner through the space with care not to press wire end into the gingiva.

C. Work back and forth pressing toward one surface and then the other.

D. Furcation: slide pipe cleaner through between exposed roots of a furcation. Work back and forth (figure 23–8).

TOOTHPICK HOLDER (PERIO-AID)

I. Indications for Use

A. **Patient with Periodontitis:** plaque removal at and just under the gingival margin; interdental cleaning particularly for concave proximal tooth surfaces (figure 23–9); exposed furcation area.

B. **Orthodontic Patient:** plaque removal at gingival margin above appliance; cleaning around fixed appliances (figure 24–7, page 384).

II. Technique

A. **Prepare Instrument**

1. Insert round tapered toothpick into the end of the holder. One type has angulated ends for use in various positions.

2. Twist the toothpick firmly into place. Break off the long end cleanly so that sharp edges cannot scratch the inner cheek or the tongue during use.

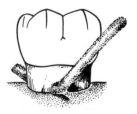

Figure 23–8. Use of pipe cleaner in area between roots where furcation has been exposed.

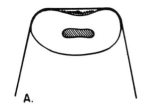

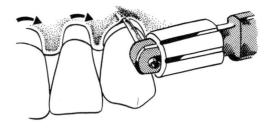

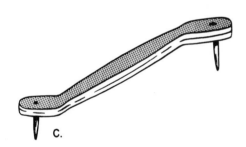

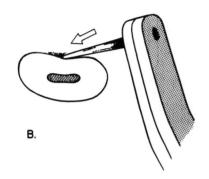

Figure 23–9. Cross section of maxillary first premolar at the cementoenamel junction to show use of Perio-aid on the concave tooth surface. **A.** Note inability of floss to remove plaque from the concavity. **B.** Perio-aid is applied for plaque removal from facial and lingual. **C.** Perio-aid handle angulated for adaptation of one end on facial and the other on lingual.

B. Application

1. Apply toothpick at the gingival margin. At a right-angle application, with moderate pressure, trace the gingival margin around each tooth.
2. To remove plaque just below the gingival margin, apply the end at less than 45 degrees, maintain the tip on the tooth surface, and follow around the sulcus or pocket (figure 23–10).

Figure 23–10. Perio-aid applied subgingivally. Tip is placed on the tooth surface just below the gingival margin, and plaque is removed by moving the toothpick over the surface around the tooth. The toothpick tip should be moistened in water before use.

3. After the tip becomes frayed from use, it can be used as a small cleaning "brush" to rub on tooth surfaces where plaque has collected. It should be checked for loose bits of wood which might become deposited in the sulcus or gingiva.
4. For hypersensitive spots, usually at the cervical third of a tooth, the patient can use the tip daily to massage fluoride dentifrice for desensitization.

BALSA WOOD WEDGE

I. Description

The balsa wood wedge is a 2-inch long, wooden "toothpick," known commercially as the Stim-U-Dent. It is triangular in cross section.

II. Indications for Use

A. Application

For cleaning interdental areas where there are exposed tooth surfaces and missing interdental gingiva. There must be space, otherwise the gingival tissue can be traumatized and the teeth forced apart.

B. Limitation

As with most interdental devices, it is advised only for the patient who will follow instructions carefully, since tissue injury is possible and the use of the implement after the wood has splayed may force splinters into the gingiva.

III. Technique

A. Fulcrum (Rest)

First teach the patient to use the hand as a rest by placing it on the cheek or chin, or

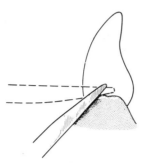

Figure 23–11. Balsa wood wedge. The wedge is used only when there are exposed proximal tooth surfaces and reduced interdental papillae. It is applied at an angle toward the occlusal or incisal to follow the contour of the interdental papilla. The broken line drawing shows horizontal positioning which could flatten the interdental papilla if used regularly.

placing a finger on the gingiva convenient to the place where the tip will be applied. This will help to prevent inserting the wedge with too much pressure.

B. Preparation

Soften the wood: place the pointed end in the mouth and moisten with saliva.

C. Procedure

1. Apply base of the triangular wedge to the gingival border of the interdental area and insert with the tip pointed slightly toward the occlusal or incisal to follow the contour of the interdental gingiva (figure 23–11). When the wedge is held horizontally, the interdental tissue can be flattened.
2. Clean the tooth surfaces by moving the wedge in and out while applying a burnishing stroke with moderate pressure first to one side of the embrasure and then the other, about 10 or 12 strokes each.
3. Discard wedge after a few embrasures have been treated or as soon as the first signs of splaying are evident.

INTERDENTAL BRUSHES

I. Types

A. Small Insert Brushes with Reusable Handle

1. Soft nylon filaments are twisted into a

fine stainless steel wire for insertion into a handle with an angulated shank (figure 23–12D).
2. The small tapered or cylindrical brush heads are of varying sizes approximately 12 to 15 mm. ($\frac{1}{2}$ inch) in length, with a diameter of 3 to 5 mm. ($\frac{1}{8}$ to $\frac{1}{4}$ inch).

B. Brush with Wire Handle

1. Soft nylon filaments are twisted into a fine stainless steel wire. The wire continues to make the handle, which is approximately 35 to 45 mm. ($1\frac{1}{2}$ to $1\frac{3}{4}$ inches) in length (figure 23–12C).
2. The filaments form a narrow brush approximately 30 to 35 mm. ($1\frac{1}{4}$ to $1\frac{1}{2}$ inches) in length with a diameter 5 to 8 mm. ($\frac{1}{4}$ to $\frac{5}{16}$ inches).

II. Indications for Use

A. Open interproximal areas.
B. Exposed bifurcations or trifurcations.
C. Plaque removal to supplement toothbrushing.

III. Technique

A. Select brush of appropriate diameter.
B. Moisten the brush and insert into interdental area or furcation at an angle in keeping with gingival form; brush in and out (figure 23–13).

IV. Care of Brushes

A. Clean brush during use to remove debris and plaque by holding under actively running water.
B. Clean thoroughly after use and dry in open air.
C. Discard when filaments become loose or deformed.

SINGLE-TUFT BRUSH (END-TUFT, UNITUFT)

I. Description

The single tuft, or group of small tufts, may be from 3 to 6 mm. in diameter and may be flat or tapered (figure 23–12A and B). The handle may be straight or contra-angled.

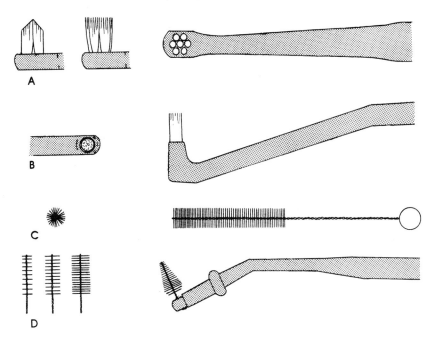

Figure 23–12. Interdental and single-tuft brushes. **A.** Single-tuft brush showing tapered and flat-shaped groups of filaments. **B.** Single-tuft brush on handle with angulated shank. **C.** Interdental brush with filaments twisted into a fine wire which continues to make the handle. **D.** Insert brushes for a reusable handle with a contra-angled shank.

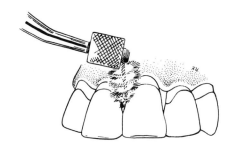

Figure 23–13. Use of interdental brush. Small soft nylon brush is applied for plaque removal from the facial, and may be applied from the lingual in open embrasures.

II. Indications for Use

A. Open Interproximal Areas

B. Fixed Dental Appliances

The single-tuft brush may be adaptable around and under a fixed partial denture, pontic, orthodontic appliance, and precision attachment.

C. Difficult-to-Reach Areas

The lingual surfaces of the mandibular molars, abutment teeth, the distals of the most posterior teeth, and teeth that are crowded are examples of where an end-tuft brush may prove of value.

III. Technique

A. Direct the end of the tuft into the interproximal area along the gingival margin.

B. Combine a rotating motion with intermittent pressure.

C. Use a sulcular brushing stroke.

INTERDENTAL TIP

I. Composition and Design

Conical or pyramidal flexible rubber or plastic tip attached to the end of the handle of a toothbrush, or on a special plastic handle. The soft, pliable rubber tip is preferred to the hard, more rigid plastic tip because it can be adapted to the interdental area more easily, and because there is less pain or discomfort for the patient when the instrument is pressed on the tissue.

II. Indications for Use

A. Cleaning debris and materia alba from the interdental area; by rubbing the exposed tooth surfaces, possible removal of some plaque.

B. May contribute to reshaping of gingiva following periodontal surgery.

C. Adaptation to areas where toothbrushing is difficult; for example, exposed furcation areas, mesial of mesially inclined teeth, or abutment teeth.

D. Contraindicated in clinically healthy gingiva with intact interdental papillae. Interdental devices are usually unnecessary and can be harmful.

III. Technique

The interdental tip is a difficult instrument to use correctly. Learning to use it may require more patience and time than the average patient will care to give. A mirror should be used to show the placement of the tip and the patient should use a mirror for home practice.

A. Prepare for application: outside the mouth, hold the handle of the instrument firmly (a palm grasp may give best control), with the tip angled up for application to the mandibular and down for the maxillary arch.

B. Insert the tip interdentally, diagonally toward the occlusal or the incisal to follow the contour of the interdental gingiva (figure 23–14).

C. The tip is inserted until it fits the embrasure and touches the sides of the teeth, but it is never pressed forcefully. If forced repeatedly in a horizontal direction, the interdental tissue can be blunted or flattened by pressure, thus increasing the size of the interdental space.

D. Press the side of the tip against the attached gingiva and apply a gentle rotary motion, which provides intermittent pressure against the gingival tissue (figure 23–15). The rotary motion is continued to a slow count of ten.

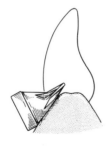

Figure 23–14. Interdental tip. The conical, flexible rubber tip is angled diagonally toward the occlusal or incisal to follow the contour of the interdental gingiva.

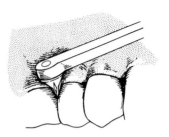

Figure 23–15. Interdental tip. The rubber tip may be indicated when interdental papillae are missing or reduced in height. The tip is inserted until it fits the embrasure and touches the sides of the teeth, but it is not forced interdentally. The side of the tip is then pressed against the attached gingiva and a gentle but firm rotary motion is used to apply intermittent pressure against the gingival tissue.

E. When the interdental area is wide, press the tip against one tooth and the attached gingiva for a count of ten, and then slide it over to the side of the adjacent tooth.

F. Repeat at next embrasure and on around the arch; apply to lingual when access and visibility permit.

G. For additional cleaning of the proximal surfaces of the teeth, the tip may be rubbed against the teeth as it is moved in and out of the embrasure, and directed toward the part of the tooth surface under the contact area.

H. Rinse the tip as indicated during use to remove debris, and wash thoroughly at the finish.

MOUTH RINSING

Vigorous rinsing to dislodge debris may contribute to general oral cleanliness. Rinsing with clear water has been suggested for after meals and after snacks, particularly "sweet" snacks, when toothbrushing is not possible.

I. Indications for Use

The limitations of rinsing should be recognized, for although it can aid in removing gross debris, plaque is not disturbed. The rinse passes over the surface of plaque rather than removing it.

Use of a saline solution at home can be a helpful postoperative procedure following scaling and root planing (page 524). Rinsing is also frequently advised the day following oral surgery, including tooth removal and periodontal surgery.

er dressing removal. Mouthrinses are consid-
ed on pages 373–375, and fluoride rinses on
ge 456.

. Procedure for Rinsing

Many patients, particularly children, should
: shown very specifically how to rinse, and the
ethod should be practiced under supervision.
ninstructed, many patients will hold water in
eir mouths and bow the head from side to side,
: other action which cannot force the water
out and between the teeth.

A small amount of fluid is taken into the
mouth; lips are closed.

With the teeth kept slightly apart, the fluid
is forced through the interdental areas with
as much pressure as possible to loosen debris.

. A combination of lip, tongue, and cheek action is used as the fluid is forced back and
forth between the teeth while the cheeks
are ballooned and sucked in alternately.

. The mouth is divided into three sections and
the rinsing should be concentrated on first
the anterior, then on one side followed by
the other.

. Expectorate or swallow.

ORAL IRRIGATION

The use of a forced intermittent or steady
ream of water in oral physical therapy is some-
mes called hydrotherapy. It has proven to be
useful adjunct to toothbrushing but must not
: considered a substitute for brushing or other
laque removal devices since it is not effective
the complete removal of dental plaque.

Oral irrigating devices are evaluated by the
merican Dental Association, Council on Den-
l Materials, Instruments and Equipment. They
re classified as acceptable, provisionally ac-
eptable, or unacceptable.[1]

. Objectives

Water irrigation devices have been shown to
: aids in maintaining the cleanliness of the oral
avity. From reported research (see bibliog-
aphy in *Suggested Readings* at the end of this
hapter) benefits which may be derived from the
se of irrigation include the following:

. Effective removal of unattached debris from
about the teeth and interdental areas. At-

tached deposits (dental plaque or calculus)
are not removed.

B. Reduction in numbers of microorganisms.

II. Types and Description of Irrigators

A. Power-driven

Power-driven pump unit which generates
an intermittent jet of water.

1. Adjustable dial to regulate water pressure and a reservoir to maintain a steady
flow.
2. Hand-held, interchangeable, adjustable
tip which can be turned a complete 360
degrees for application at various angulations.

B. Water Faucet Attachment

Single line type which attaches directly
to the water faucet.

1. Delivers a continuous stream of water
which is adjustable by varying the line
pressure.
2. Hand-held interchangeable tip which
rotates a complete 360 degrees for application to all areas.

III. Technique and Operational Factors

A. Instruction of Patient

For most patients, it can be recommended that the irrigator be used before
toothbrushing and other plaque-removal
procedures.

1. Debris can be removed by irrigation,
thus leaving tooth surfaces available for
plaque removal and for fluoride from the
dentifrice.
2. Precaution: Since water irrigation tends
to impart a feeling of oral cleanliness,
the patient may not realize the need for
complete plaque removal and may neglect toothbrushing or other necessary
procedures.

B. Procedure

The user turns on and adjusts the water
jet stream, leans over the washbowl, and
directs the tip interproximally in a horizontal direction and along the gingival margins.
The stream should not be directed into the
sulcus or pocket (figure 23–16).

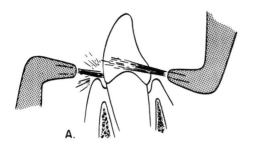

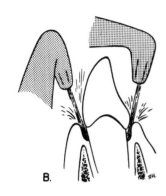

Figure 23–16. Water irrigator. **A.** The water jet stream must be directed horizontally across the gingival margin and through the gingival embrasure. **B.** Incorrect use. Water is directed into the gingival sulcus or pocket and can damage the junctional epithelium and cause periodontal abscess formation. Note correctly positioned horizontally held tip on lingual of **A** compared with vertically downward positioned tip in **B**.

C. Operational Factors

    1. Pressure need only be great enough to flush out the interdental area.

    2. Avoid high pressure or prolonged application to a limited or single area. Although adverse effects are uncommon, periodontal abscess formation from water being forced below the junctional epithelium is possible.

IV. Indications

Patients for whom particular benefit can be derived include those with potential food retentive areas:

A. Missing or reduced interdental papillae.

B. Fixed orthodontic appliances.

C. Restorative rehabilitative appliances: fixed partial dentures, splints, precision attachments.

V. Contraindications

A. Patients who require antibiotic premedica-

tion (see list on pages 99–100). Bacteremi can occur following the use of oral irriga tion,[2,3] particularly in patients with un treated gingivitis and periodontitis.

B. Deep periodontal pockets or tissue flap covering unerupted or partially erupte third molars. Abscesses or pericoronal in fections can be induced.

C. Patients with acute conditions, for example necrotizing ulcerative gingivitis or perio dontal abscess.

D. Clinically healthy gingiva, with minimum o normal sulcus depths, no bleeding on prob ing, and a patient who is capable of doing satisfactory plaque removal and cleaning with a toothbrush and dental floss. The pa tient who does not need an irrigating devic for a particular reason should not be en couraged to purchase and use one. Constan pressure of the water stream over an inter dental papilla and col area may act to reduc the height of the papilla. Repeated pressur of other interdental devices such as the in terdental tip and balsa wood wedge may als result in flattened papillae.

DENTIFRICES

A dentifrice is a substance used with a tooth brush for the purposes of removing denta plaque, materia alba, and debris, and for apply ing specific agents to the tooth surfaces for pre ventive or therapeutic purposes. As a result o research, the dentist and dental hygienist ca apply current knowledge to aid the patient i the selection of an appropriate dentifrice whicl will benefit or prevent harm to the teeth an gingiva.

For a few patients, dentifrice selection can b based on individual preference for flavor an cleaning ability, provided the dentifrice is no excessively abrasive. For most patients, denta caries control is an important factor, and a den tifrice containing fluoride is essential.

I. Basic Components[4,5,6]

Powder dentifrices contain abrasives, deter gents, flavoring, and sweetener. Paste denti frices contain the same plus binders, humec tants, preservative, and water. Either may have a coloring agent. The range of content of the various ingredients in commercially available dentifrices is as follows:

Detergent	1–2%
Abrasive	25–60%
Binder (thickener)	1–2%
Humectant	20–40%
Flavoring	1–1.5%
Water	15–50%
Preservative, Sweetener, and Coloring Agent	2–3%

A therapeutic dentifrice has a drug or chemical agent added for a specific preventive or treatment action. In manufacturing products, a major problem is to combine agents that are compatible with each other.

A. Detergents (Foaming Agents or Surfactants)

1. *Purposes:* to lower surface tension, penetrate and loosen surface deposits and stains, emulsify debris for easy removal by the toothbrush, and contribute to the foaming action which many people like.
2. *Criteria for Use:* nontoxic, neutral in reaction, active in acid or alkaline media, stable, compatible with other dentifrice ingredients, no distinctive flavor, and foaming characteristics.
3. *Substances Used:* synthetic detergents

    Sodium lauryl sulfate USP
    Sodium n-lauryl sarcosinate
    Sodium cocomonoglyceride sulfonate

B. Abrasives and/or Polishing Agents

1. *Purposes:* an abrasive for cleaning, and a polishing agent to produce a smooth, shiny tooth surface which will resist discoloration and bacterial accumulation and retention. Properties of abrasive agents are described on pages 565–566.
2. *Criteria for Use:* the ideal abrasive is one that cleans well with no damage to the tooth surface and provides a high polish that can prevent or delay the reaccumulation of stains and deposits.
3. *Abrasives Used*

    Calcium carbonate
    Calcium sulfate
    Calcium pyrophosphate
    Calcium orthophosphate
    Dicalcium phosphate, dihydrate
    Insoluble sodium metaphosphate (IMP)

Hydrated aluminum oxide
Magnesium carbonates and phosphates
Silica, Silicates, and dehydrated silica gels

C. Binders (Thickeners)

1. *Purpose:* to prevent separation of the solid and liquid ingredients during storage.
2. *Criteria:* stable, nontoxic, compatible with other ingredients.
3. *Types Used:* organic hydrophilic colloids

    Alginates
    Synthetic derivatives of cellulose
    Gum Tragacanth USP

    Organic colloids require a preservative to prevent microbial growth.

D. Humectants

1. *Purposes:* to retain moisture and prevent hardening on exposure to air.
2. *Criteria:* stable, nontoxic.
3. *Substances Used*

    Glycerol
    Sorbitol
    Propylene glycol

    These agents require a preservative to prevent microbial growth.

E. Preservatives

1. *Purpose:* to prevent bacterial growth.
2. *Criteria:* compatible with other ingredients.
3. *Substances Used*

    Alcohols
    Benzoates
    Formaldehyde
    Dichlorinated phenols

F. Sweetening Agents

1. *Purpose:* to impart a pleasant flavor.
2. *Criteria:* must be nonfermentable sugar.
3. *Substances Used*

    Artificial non-cariogenic sweetener
    Sorbitol and glycerin, used as humectants, contribute to sweet flavor

G. Flavoring Agents

1. *Purpose:* to make the dentifrice desirable; to mask other ingredients that may have a less pleasant flavor.

2. *Criteria:* remain unchanged during manufacturing and storage; compatible with other ingredients.

3. *Substances Used*

> Essential oils (peppermint, cinnamon, wintergreen, clove)
> Menthol
> Artificial non-cariogenic sweetener

H. Coloring Agents

1. *Purpose:* attractiveness
2. *Criteria:* does not stain teeth or discolor other oral tissues.
3. *Types:* vegetable dyes.

II. Prophylactic or Therapeutic Dentifrices

The American Dental Association, Council on Dental Therapeutics evaluates only those dentifrices that claim therapeutic value. Categories of acceptance are described under *Technical Hints* at the end of this chapter.

Over the years research on chlorophyll dentifrices, ammoniated dentifrices, dentifrices containing enzyme inhibitors such as sodium-n-lauryl sarcosinate and sodium dehydroacetate, and antibiotics, penicillin and tyrothricin, contributed to the search for a major break into dental caries prevention.[5,7] The fluoride dentifrice research has been shown to contribute the greatest benefits at the present time.

Problems with the fluoride dentifrices primarily have been related to finding compatible constituents to be combined with the fluoride in the dentifrice formula. The lack of caries prevention by early sodium fluoride dentifrices has been attributed to the use of abrasives containing calcium which combined with the fluoride and rendered it inactive. This problem has been overcome and compatible fluoride and abrasive systems have been developed.[8]

Stannous fluoride suffered similar problems since its instability in paste combination decreased its effectiveness in a relatively short time. Additional research was required to find variations in the constituents that could overcome the problem. The benefits derived from fluoride dentifrices are described in the chapter on fluorides, page 457.

III. Dentifrice Selection

The dentifrice that has been used by a patient should be recorded with other information about self-care habits when the dental history is prepared. Later the dentifrice must be evaluated and a change recommended when necessary in accord with the individual oral condition and treatment objectives.

There are specific reasons for recommending particular dentifrices and for discouraging the use of others. The patient looks to the dentist and dental hygienist for professional advice and expects it to be in keeping with current research. The factors described below should be considered in dentifrice selection.

A. Dental Caries Control

The use of a fluoride-containing dentifrice is generally recommended for all age groups and is mandatory for children and caries prone adults. Fluoride for prevention of cemental caries is necessary after gingival recession and root exposure after periodontal therapy.

B. Abrasiveness

The degree of abrasiveness of a dentifrice is influenced by several factors including dentifrice concentration, hardness of toothbrush used, and brushing force or pressure. The greater the dilution of the abrasive agent, the less abrasive the preparation. The harder the toothbrush, the more abrasion of tooth structure. The more force used with a brush, the greater abrasiveness of the agent. Even the temperature can alter the abrasive effect since the toothbrush filaments are softer in a warmer environment. Ranking of dentifrices by their abrasiveness should be relative and subject to several variables.[9,10]

Reference tables for the comparative abrasiveness of commercial dentifrices to dentin and enamel are available.[5,6,11] Dentifrice abrasion is described on page 355.

A patient with exposed cementum or dentin must be advised to use an exceptionally mild abrasive dentifrice. It may be advantageous for a patient with marked recession to use plain water with a soft toothbrush dipped in a fluoride gel for a part of the time, since that would be the least abrasive of all.

C. Desensitization

Dentifrices designated specifically for desensitization are within the scope of the acceptance program of the Council on Dental Therapeutics. Potassium nitrate has been shown to be an effective agent. Desensitizing effects of sodium monofluorophosphate dentifrice have been demonstrated (page 556).

Since most tooth sensitivity is related to areas of exposed dentin and cementum, careful attention must be paid the abrasiveness of a dentifrice with desensitizing claims.

D. Cleaning Ability

Selection of a dentifrice on its cleaning ability alone assumes that none of the problems of caries prevention, susceptibility to dentifrice abrasion, or hypersensitivity is present, otherwise the dentifrice must meet dual or triple goals. The cleansing dentifrice is for general oral health and comfort, to improve the appearance, to aid in temporary reduction of mouth odors, to lower the bacterial count, and to aid in the control of dental plaque. However, the ultimate beneficial effect depends on the frequency and thoroughness of brushing, flossing, and other plaque removal devices.

MOUTHRINSES

Mouthrinses may be classified as cosmetic or therapeutic. When claims for therapeutic value have not been scientifically substantiated, there may be harm in repeated use of a product.

Mouthrinses that claim no therapeutic or disease preventive value are not included in the acceptance program of the American Dental Association, Council on Dental Therapeutics.[12] At present, the unsupervised use of medicated mouthrinses by the public cannot be considered to contribute to oral health. Medicated mouthrinses that claim pain relief or elimination of halitosis should be considered with reservation.[4] Several fluoride solutions have been accepted as effective agents for use as mouthrinses for reducing the incidence of dental caries.[13]

When recording information about the oral health practices of a patient as part of the medical and dental history, it is advisable to determine whether a particular mouthrinse is used, how frequently, and what the patient believes to be the benefit from its use. If any detrimental effects are suspected after the oral examination, or if adverse effects are known to be possible, the patient can be informed and alternate procedures for rinsing can be recommended.

Rinsing as an aid in plaque control and suggestions for teaching a patient how to rinse were described on pages 368–369.

I. Purposes and Uses

A. Dental Office or Clinic

1. Preoperative rinse to reduce incidence of bacteremia following instrumentation (page 508).[14,15]
2. Preoperative rinse to reduce air contamination during use of handpiece and ultrasonic scaler (pages 17, 63, 520).
3. Facilitate impression procedures (page 169).
4. Rinse and refresh the mouth during film placement for radiography and following a dental or dental hygiene procedure.

B. Patient at Home

1. *Postoperative Care*
   a. After oral surgery as directed (pages 660–661).
   b. After periodontal surgery: while the dressing is in place, a flavored mouthrinse aids in removing debris and freshening the breath.
   c. After subgingival instrumentation: mild hypertonic salt solution may be advised for cleaning the area and encouraging healing.
2. *Treatment.* During pathologic conditions, for example, necrotizing ulcerative gingivitis, to remove debris, encourage healing, and soothe tender gingiva (pages 539–540).
3. *Cosmetic Purposes.* Advertising claims can be misleading and patients need assistance in interpreting what they read and hear. Without advice, people may select a mouthrinse on the basis of advertising promises or flavor. Purposes and effects that may be expected from the use of a cosmetic mouthrinse are:
   a. Removes loose debris when rinsing is vigorous.

b. Gives temporary benefit through mechanical reduction in numbers of oral microorganisms.

c. Imparts a pleasant taste, odor, and stimulating sensation to the oral cavity.

d. Contributes to a temporary suppression of halitosis when causes are local.

4. *Dental Caries Prevention.* The use of sodium fluoride and stannous fluoride mouthrinses for dental caries control is included in the chapter on fluoride application (pages 456–457).

II. Self-Prepared Mouthrinses

Plain water, saline solutions, or solutions of bicarbonate of soda may be considered the most practical mouthrinses from the point of view of availability, cost, and effectiveness for debris removal and general oral cleanliness. Frequently prescribed or recommended by dentists, they may be helpful in postoperative care following dental and dental hygiene procedures.

When a salt solution is of greater strength than the physiologic salt solution concentration of body cells, by osmotic force fluid is drawn out of the cells to balance the pressure. This may act to produce a reduction of edema and related benefits. The patient history must be checked, as a patient on a low salt or sodium-free diet should not use a saline rinse.

A. Water

B. Isotonic Sodium Chloride Solution

1. Isotonic is normal or physiologic salt solution which is 0.9% aqueous solution; same concentration as cellular fluids.

2. Preparation (household measurements): level $1/2$ teaspoonful salt added to one cup (8 ounces) of warm water.

C. Hypertonic Sodium Chloride Solution

1. A salt solution the osmotic pressure of which is greater than that of physiologic salt solution is hypertonic.

2. Preparation (household measurements): $1/2$ teaspoonful salt added to $1/2$ cup (4 ounces) of warm water.

D. Sodium Bicarbonate Solution

Level $1/2$ teaspoonful "soda" added to an 8-ounce glass of water.

E. Sodium Chloride—Sodium Bicarbonate Solution (flavored)

Sodium chloride	2.0 g. ($1/2$ teaspoonful)
Sodium bicarbonate	1.0 g. ($1/4$ teaspoonful)
Amaranth solution	2.0 ml. ($1/2$ teaspoonful)
Peppermint water to make	240.0 ml. (8 oz. glass)

III. Commercial Mouthrinse Ingredients[16,17]

Basic ingredients for both cosmetic and therapeutic types include surface active agents, flavoring, alcohol, water, and coloring.

A. Surface Active Agents

To facilitate cleaning and aid in the solubility of other ingredients.

B. Flavoring

Essential oils and their derivatives (eucalyptus oil, oil of wintergreen) or aromatic waters (peppermint, spearmint, wintergreen, or others).

C. Alcohol

Ethyl alcohol is used to increase the solubility of the essential oils. The concentration should not exceed 10 percent because of irritation to the tissues. Alcohol acts to lower surface tension, is mildly astringent but is not antibacterial at 10 percent.

D. Water

Makes up the largest percent by volume.

E. Sweetening Agent

Artificial non-cariogenic sweetener.

F. Coloring

Which will not discolor oral tissues.

IV. Active Ingredients[16,17]

Commercial mouthrinses generally contain more than one active ingredient and therefore may advertise more than one claim for useful-ess. A number of factors influence how effective an agent may be, including the dilution by the saliva, the length of time the agent may be in contact with the tissue or bacteria, and the effect that contact with the organic matter of the mouth may have in changing the action. Agents and products listed below are for information only and should not be considered recommendations.

A. **Antibacterial Agents**

1. *Purposes*
   a. To reduce the oral microbacterial count. Although a partial effect is possible, inadequate evidence exists to show that there is any specific benefit from a nonspecific change in the oral flora.
   b. Current research points to the possibility of an antibacterial mouthrinse that will reduce the amount or inhibit the formation of dental plaque and calculus.
2. *Limitations of Agents to Use:* many have disagreeable flavors or high cost, or their activity decreases when contact is made with organic matter in the mouth.
3. *Active Ingredients*

   Phenolic Compounds
   Hexylresorcinol, thymol, and other phenol derivatives (Chloraseptic, ST 37)
   Quaternary Ammonium Compounds
       Benzethonium chloride (Colgate 100)
       Cetylpyridinium chloride (Scope, Cepacol, Micrin, Reef)
   Boric and Benzoic acid (Listerine, Mi 31)
   Chlorine-liberating compounds (Chlorpactic WCS 60, Kasdenol)
   Hexetidine (Sterisol)

B. **Oxygenating Agents**[4]

1. *Purposes:* their effervescence makes them effective in debridement, and they are active against anaerobic microorganisms.
2. *Uses:* particularly in the treatment of necrotizing ulcerative gingivitis.
3. *Active Ingredients*

   Hydrogen peroxide (Hydrogen peroxide USP diluted with water)
   Sodium Perborate (Amosan, Vince)
4. *Precaution:* continued use of hydrogen peroxide solution, as well as most other oxygen-liberating drugs after the treatment of a disease, can lead to sponginess of the gingiva, formation of black hairy tongue, hypersensitivity of exposed root surfaces, and because an acid is produced when water is added, decalcification of tooth surfaces.

C. **Astringents**

1. *Purpose:* shrinkage of tissues.
2. *Uses:* during impression making.
3. *Active Ingredients*

   Zinc chloride (Lavoris)
   Zinc acetate
   Alum
   Tannic, acetic, and citric acids
4. *Precaution:* the agents are acid in water solution and can cause tooth decalcification and tissue irritation with repeated use.

D. **Anodynes**

1. *Purposes:* alleviate pain, soothe sore spots.
2. *Uses:* temporary pain relief for lesions of mucous membranes; during radiographic film exposure; aid in impression making.
3. *Active Ingredients*

   Phenol derivatives (Chloraseptic)
   Essential oils

E. **Buffering Agents**

1. *Purpose and Uses:* reduce oral acidity created by the fermentation of food debris; dissolve mucinous films; give relief for soreness of soft tissues.
2. *Active Ingredients*

   Sodium borate solution NF
   Sodium perborate NF
   Sodium bicarbonate USP

F. **Deodorizing Agents**

1. *Purpose:* neutralize odors from decomposed oral debris.
2. *Uses:* lessen possibility of halitosis from local causes.
3. *Active Ingredients*

   Chlorophyll and other deodorizing agents (Green Mint)

TECHNICAL HINTS

I. Inquire and record while preparing the patient's dental history, specific devices, dentifrices, mouthrinses, or other auxiliary aids used, in anticipation of evaluation for professional advice needed.

II. Request that a patient bring for demonstration a plaque control device used, to assure that no harm is being done which, though not producing symptoms currently, could cause problems after long-term use.

III. Classification of Products Evaluated by the Council on Dental Therapeutics, American Dental Association[12]

Commercial products are examined either upon the request of the manufacturer or distributor or upon the initiative of the Council. Products are usually accepted for 3 years. After consideration of a product has been completed, the Council will classify the product as "accepted," "provisionally accepted," or "unaccepted."

Accepted products include those for which there is adequate evidence for safety and effectiveness. They will be listed in *Accepted Dental Therapeutics* and may use the Seal of Acceptance or an authorized statement, unless otherwise provided.

Provisionally accepted will include those products for which there is reasonable evidence of usefulness and safety, but which lack sufficient evidence of dental usefulness to justify being "accepted." These products meet the other qualifications and standards established by the Council on Dental Therapeutics. The Council may authorize the use of a suitable statement to define specifically the area of usefulness of a product classified as "provisionally accepted." It is the policy of the Council to reconsider these products each year on the basis of new evidence which may be produced in their support. Classification in this category is not ordinarily continued for more than 3 years.

Unaccepted products will include those for which the Council has determined that there is no substantial evidence of usefulness or that a question of safety exists.

References

1. American Dental Association, Council on Dental Materials, Instruments and Equipment: *Dentist's Desk Reference: Materials, Instruments and Equipment*, 1st ed. Chicago, American Dental Association, 1981, pp. xxxviii, 342–343.
2. Romans, A.R. and App, G.R.: Bacteremia, a Result from Oral Irrigation in Subjects with Gingivitis, *J. Periodontol.*, 42, 757, December, 1971.
3. Felix, J.E., Rosen, S., and App, G.R.: Detection of Bacteremia after the Use of an Oral Irrigation Device in Subjects with Periodontitis, *J. Periodontol.*, 42, 785, December, 1971.
4. American Dental Association, Council on Dental Therapeutics: *Accepted Dental Therapeutics*, 39th ed. Chicago, American Dental Association, 1982, pp. 369–378.
5. Volpe, A.R.: Dentifrices and Mouth Rinses, in Caldwell, R.C. and Stallard, R.E., eds.: *A Textbook of Preventive Dentistry*. Philadelphia, W.B. Saunders Co., 1977, pp. 173–197.
6. Ciancio, S.G. and Bourgeault, P.C.: *Clinical Pharmacology for Dental Professionals*. New York, McGraw Hill, 1980, pp. 141–146.
7. Hine, J.W.: The Industrial Contribution to Safe and Effective Dentifrices, *Community Dent. Oral Epidemiol.*, 8, 230, Extra Issue, 1980.
8. Forward, G.C.: Action and Interaction of Fluoride in Dentifrices, *Community Dent. Oral Epidemiol.*, 8, 257, Extra Issue, 1980.
9. Harte, D.B. and Manly, R.S.: Effect of Toothbrush Variables on Wear of Dentin Produced by Four Abrasives, *J. Dent. Res.*, 54, 993, September–October, 1975.
10. Harte, D.B. and Manly, R.S.: Four Variables Affecting Magnitude of Dentifrice Abrasiveness, *J. Dent. Res.* 55, 322, May–June, 1976.
11. Hembree, M.E. and Hembree, J.H.: Relative Abrasiveness of Dentifrices, *Dent. Hyg.*, 51, 253, June, 1977.
12. American Dental Association, Council on Dental Therapeutics: op cit., p. xviii.
13. American Dental Association, Council on Dental Therapeutics: op. cit., pp. 352–353.
14. Scopp, I.W. and Orvieto, L.D.: Gingival Degerming by Povidone-iodine Irrigation: Bacteremia Reduction in Extraction Procedures, *J. Am. Dent. Assoc.*, 83, 1294, December, 1971.
15. Brennan, H.S. and Randall, E.: Local Degerming with Povidone-iodine. II. Prior to Gingivectomy, *J. Periodontol.*, 45, 870, December, 1974.
16. Volpe: op. cit., pp. 197–213.
17. Rosenthal, M.W.: Mouthwashes, in Balsam, M.S. and Sagarin, E., eds.: *Cosmetics, Science and Technology*, 2nd ed., *Volume 1*. New York, Wiley-Interscience, 1972, pp. 533–563.

Suggested Readings

Anaise, J.Z.: Plaque-removing Effect of Dental Floss and Toothpicks in Children 12–13 Years of Age, *Community Dent. Oral Epidemiol.*, 4, 137, July, 1976.

Balshi, T.J. and Mingledorff, E.B.: Maintenance Procedures for Patients After Complete Fixed Prosthodontics, *J. Prosthet. Dent.*, 37, 420, April, 1977.

Barton, R.F. and Diamond, B.: Evaluation and Patient Acceptance of a Mechanical Dental Flossing Device Compared to Hand-held Floss, *Clin. Prev. Dent.*, 2, 10, May–June, 1980.

Bass, C.C.: The Optimum Characteristics of Dental Floss for Personal Oral Hygiene, *Dent. Items Int.*, 70, 921, September, 1948.

Bassiouny, M.A. and Grant, A.A.: Oral Hygiene for the Partially Edentulous, *J. Periodontol.*, 52, 214, April, 1981.

Bergenholtz, A., Bjorne, A., and Vikström, B.: The Plaque-removing Ability of Some Common Interdental Aids. An Intraindividual Study, *J. Clin. Periodontol.*, 1, 160, Number 3, 1974.

Bergenholtz, A., Bjorne, A., Glantz, P.-O., and Vikström, B.: Plaque Removal by Various Triangular Toothpicks, *J. Clin. Periodontol.*, 7, 121, April, 1980.

rgenholtz, A. and Brithon, J.: Plaque Removal by Dental Floss or Toothpicks, An Intra-individual Comparative Study, *J. Clin. Periodontol.*, 7, 516, December, 1980.

yer, E.M. and Field, H.M.: Tissue Response to Initial Performance of Flossing and Sulcular Toothbrushing, *Dent. Hyg.*, 54, 370, August, 1980.

Ghamrawy, E.: A Toothbrush Designed for Proximal Surfaces Adjacent to Toothless Spaces in the Partially Edentulous Patient, *J. Oral Rehabil.*, 6, 323, October, 1979.

nkelstein, P. and Grossman, E.: The Effectiveness of Dental Floss in Reducing Gingival Inflammation, *J. Dent. Res.*, 58, 1034, March, 1979.

andsen, A., ed.: *Oral Hygiene*. Copenhagen, Munksgaard, 1972, pp. 39–62.

ermo, P. and Flötra, L.: The Effect of Different Methods of Interdental Cleaning, *J. Periodont. Res.*, 5, 230, Number 3, 1970.

anath, L.-E., Martinsson, T., Matsson, L., Nilsson, G., Schröder, U., and Söderholm, B.: Intraindividual Effect of Daily Supervised Flossing on Caries in Schoolchildren, *Community Dent. Oral Epidemiol.*, 7, 147, June, 1979.

ill, H.C., Levi, P.A., and Glickman, I.: The Effects of Waxed and Unwaxed Dental Floss on Interdental Plaque Accumulation and Interdental Gingival Health, *J. Periodontol.*, 44, 411, July, 1973.

rman, A.C. and Christen, A.G.: Floss Holders: What Do Periodontists Think of Them? *Clin. Prev. Dent.*, 3, 5, January–February, 1981.

ayak, R.P. and Wade, A.B.: The Relative Effectiveness of Plaque Removal by the Proxabrush and Rubber Cone Stimulator, *J. Clin. Periodontol.*, 4, 128, May, 1977.

ewbrun, E., Heiblum, R., and Mayeda, A.: Effect of Flossing, With and Without Iodine, on Human Interproximal Plaque Flora, *Caries Res.*, 14, 75, Number 2, 1980.

adentz, W.H., Barnes, G.P., Carter, H.G., Ailor, J.E., and Johnson, R.M.: An Evaluation of Two Techniques of Teaching Proper Dental Flossing Procedures, *J. Periodontol.*, 44, 177, March, 1973.

eitman, W.R., Whiteley, R.T., and Robertson, P.B.: Proximal Surface Cleaning by Dental Floss, *Clin. Prev. Dent.*, 2, 7, May–June, 1980.

chmid, M.O., Balmelli, O.P., and Saxer, U.P.: Plaqueremoving Effect of a Toothbrush, Dental Floss, and a Toothpick, *J. Clin. Periodontol.*, 3, 157, August, 1976.

tevens, A.W.: A Comparison of the Effectiveness of Variable Diameter vs. Unwaxed Floss, *J. Periodontol.*, 51, 666, November, 1980.

erhune, J.A.: Predicting the Readiness of Elementary School Children to Learn an Effective Dental Flossing Technique, *J. Am. Dent. Assoc.*, 86, 1332, June, 1973.

an Swol, R.L., Carter, H.G., and Barnes, G.P.: Effectiveness of Interproximal Dental Hygiene Aids for Troop Field Use, *Military Med.*, 142, 391, May, 1977.

ogel, R.I., Sullivan, A.J., Pascuzzi, J.N., and Deasy, M.J.: Evaluation of Cleansing Devices in the Maintenance of Interproximal Gingival Health, *J. Periodontol.*, 46, 745, December, 1975.

Waerhaug, J.: The Interdental Brush and Its Place in Operative and Crown and Bridge Dentistry, *J. Oral Rehabil.*, 3, 107, April, 1976.

Wolffe, G.N.: An Evaluation of Proximal Surface Cleansing Agents, *J. Clin. Periodontol.*, 3, 148, August, 1976.

Wright, G.Z., Banting, D.W., and Feasby, W.H.: Dorchester Dental Flossing Study, *Caries Res.*, 10, 379, Number 5, 1976.

Wright, G.Z., Banting, D.W., and Feasby, W.H.: The Dorchester Dental Flossing Study: Final Report, *Clin. Prev. Dent.*, 1, 23, May–June, 1979.

Wright, G.Z., Feasby, W.H., and Banting, D.B.: The Effectiveness of Interdental Flossing With and Without a Fluoride Dentifrice, *Pediatr. Dent.*, 2, 105, Number 2, 1980.

Zarkowski, P.: Effectiveness of Dental Floss in Oral Hygiene Practice, *Dent. Hyg.*, 53, 67, February, 1979.

Oral Irrigation

Astwood, L.A.S.: Oral Irrigating Devices; An Appraisal of Current Information, *J. Public Health Dent.*, 35, 2, Winter, 1975.

Brady, J.M., Gray, W.A., and Bhaskar, S.N.: Electron Microscopic Study of the Effect of Water Jet Lavage Devices on Dental Plaque, *J. Dent. Res.*, 52, 1310, November–December, 1973.

Cantor, M.T. and Stahl, S.S.: Interdental Col Tissue Responses to the Use of a Water Pressure Cleansing Device, *J. Periodontol.*, 40, 292, May, 1969.

Clynes, J.T. and Wilderman, M.N.: Effectiveness of a Waterpressure Device in Removing Debris from Teeth, *J. Public Health Dent.*, 30, 2, Winter, 1970.

Covin, N.R., Lainson, P.A., Belding, J.H., and Fraleigh, C.M.: The Effects of Stimulating the Gingiva by a Pulsating Water Device, *J. Periodontol.*, 44, 286, May, 1973.

Cutright, D.E., Bhaskar, S.N., and Larson, W.J.: Variable Tissue Forces Produced by Water Jet Devices, *J. Periodontol.*, 43, 765, December, 1972.

Elliot, J.R., Bowers, G.M., Clemmer, B.A., and Rovelstad, G.H.: II. A Comparison of Selected Oral Hygiene Devices in Dental Plaque Removal, *J. Periodontol.*, 43, 217, April, 1972.

Fine, D.H. and Baumhammers, A.: Effect of Water Pressure Irrigation on Stainable Material on the Teeth, *J. Periodontol.*, 41, 468, August, 1970.

Gupta, O.P., O'Toole, E.T., and Hammermeister, R.O.: Effects of a Water Pressure Device on Oral Hygiene and Gingival Inflammation, *J. Periodontol.*, 44, 294, May, 1973.

Hoover, D.R. and Robinson, H.B.G.: The Comparative Effectiveness of a Pulsating Oral Irrigator as an Adjunct in Maintaining Oral Health, *J. Periodontol.*, 42, 37, January, 1971.

Hugoson, A.: Effect of the Water Pik Device on Plaque Accumulation and Development of Gingivitis, *J. Clin. Periodontol.*, 5, 95, May, 1978.

Jann, R.: Water Irrigating Devices, *Periodont. Abstr.*, 18, 6, March, 1970.

Lainson, P.A., Bergquist, J.J., and Fraleigh, C.M.: A Longitudinal Study of Pulsating Water Pressure Cleansing Devices, *J. Periodontol.*, 43, 444, July, 1972.

Lainson, P.A., Bergquist, J.J., and Fraleigh, C.M.: Clinical Evaluation of Pulsar, a New Pulsating Water Pressure Cleansing Device, *J. Periodontol.*, 41, 401, July, 1970.

Lobene, R.R.: A Study of the Force of Water Jets in Relation to Pain and Damage to Gingival Tissues, *J. Periodontol.*, 42, 166, March, 1971.

Lobene, R.R., Soparkar, P.M., Hein, J.W., and Quigley, G.A.: A Study of the Effects of Antiseptic Agents and a Pulsating Irrigating Device on Plaque and Gingivitis, *J. Periodontol.*, 43, 564, September, 1972.

Manhold, J.H., Vogel, R.I., and Manhold, E.A.: Carbon Penetration of Gingival Tissue by Oral Irrigating Devices, *J. Prev. Dent.*, 5, 3, September–October, 1978.

O'Leary, T.J., Shafer, W.G., Swenson, H.M., Nesler, D.C., and Van Dorn, P.R.: Possible Penetration of Crevicular Tissue from Oral Hygiene Procedures: I. Use of Oral Irrigating Devices, *J. Periodontol.*, 41, 158, March, 1970.

Wheatcroft, M.G. and Sciantarelli, E.: The Effect of Oral Water Irrigation on the Prevention of Gingival Inflammation, *J. Am. Soc. Prev. Dent.*, *4*, 38, July–August, 1974.

Dentifrices

Allen, A.L., Hawley, C.E., Cutright, D.E., and Seibert, J.S.: An Investigation of the Clinical and Histologic Effects of Selected Dentifrices on Human Palatal Mucosa, *J. Periodontol.*, *46*, 102, February, 1975.

Baxter, P.M., Davis, W.B., and Jackson, J.: Toothpaste Abrasive Requirements to Control Naturally Stained Pellicle, *J. Oral Rehabil.*, *8*, 19, January, 1981.

Beiswanger, B.B., Gish, C.W., and Mallatt, M.E.: Effect of a Sodium Fluoride-silica Abrasive Dentifrice Upon Caries, *J. Dent. Res.*, *60*, 577, Abstract 1072, Special Issue A, March, 1981.

Bogle, G.C.: Abrasivity of Dentifrices and Toothbrushes, *Periodont. Abstr.*, *22*, 7, Spring, 1974.

Dowell, T.B.: The Use of Toothpaste in Infancy, *Br. Dent. J.*, *150*, 247, May 5, 1981.

Gershon, S.D. and Pader, M.: Dentifrices, in Balsam, M.S. and Sagarin, E., eds.: *Cosmetics Science and Technology*, 2nd ed., *Volume 1*. New York, Wiley-Interscience, 1972, pp. 423–531.

Heath, J.R. and Wilson, H.J.: The Effect of Dentifrices on Restorative Materials, *J. Oral Rehabil.*, *1*, 47, Number 1, 1974.

Naylor, M.N. and Pindborg, J.J., eds.: The Contribution of Dentifrices to Oral Health, *Community Dent. Oral Epidemiol.*, *8*, 217–285, Extra Issue, 1980.

O'Connor, B.S.: Consumer-oriented Aspects of Dentifrices, *Dent. Hyg.*, *54*, 121, March, 1980.

Phillips, R.W.: *Elements of Dental Materials for Dental Hygienists and Assistants*, 3rd ed. Philadelphia, W.B. Saunders Co., 1977, pp. 354–361.

Reisstein, J.: Abrasion of Enamel and Cementum in Human Teeth Due to Toothbrushing Estimated by SEM, *J. Dent. Res.*, *57*, 42, January, 1978.

Rubright, W.C., Walker, J.A., Karlsson, U.L., and Diehl, D.L.: Oral Slough Caused By Dentifrice Detergents and Aggravated by Drugs With Antisialic Activity, *J. Am. Dent. Assoc.*, *97*, 215, August, 1978.

Saxton, C.A. and Cowell, C.R.: Clinical Investigation of the Effects of Dentifrices on Dentin Wear at the Cementoenamel Junction, *J. Am. Dent. Assoc.*, *102*, 38, January, 1981.

Sjöblom, M., Ainamo, A., and Ainamo, J.: Antimicrobial Effect of Four Different Toothpastes, *Scand. J. Dent. Res.*, *84*, 377, November, 1976.

Suömi, J.D., Horowitz, H.S., Barbano, J.P., Spolsky, V.W., and Heifetz, S.B.: A Clinical Trial of a Calculus-inhibitory Dentifrice, *J. Periodontol.*, *45*, 139, March, 1974.

Toto, P.D. and Rapp, G.W.: A Clinical Comparison of a New Low Abrasive Dentifrice With Intermediate and High Abrasive Dentifrices, *J. Periodontol.*, *43*, 492, August, 1972.

Volpe, A.R., Mooney, R., Zumbrunnen, C., Stahl, D., and Goldman, H.M.: A Long Term Clinical Study Evaluating the Effect of Two Dentifrices on Oral Tissues, *J. Periodontol.*, *46*, 113, February, 1975.

Zacherl, W.A.: Clinical Evaluation of a Sodium Fluoride-silica Abrasive Dentifrice, *J. Dent. Res.*, *60*, 577, Abstract 1071, Special Issue A, March, 1981.

Mouthwashes

Barnes, G.P., Roberts, D.W., Katz, R.V., and Woolridge, E.D.: Effects of Two Cetylpyridinium Chloride-containing Mouthwashes on Bacterial Plaque, *J. Periodontol.*, *47*, 419, July, 1976.

Bernstein, M.L.: Oral Mucosal White Lesions Associated with Excessive Use of Listerine Mouthwash, *Oral Surg.*, *46*, 781, December, 1978.

Carter, H.G. and Barnes, G.P.: Effects of Three Mouthwashes on Existing Dental Plaque Accumulations, *J. Prev. Dent.*, *2*, 6, May–June, 1975.

Compton, F.H. and Beagrie, G.S.: Inhibitory Effect of Benzethonium and Zinc Chloride Mouthrinses on Human Dental Plaque and Gingivitis, *J. Clin. Periodontol.*, *2*, 33, February, 1975.

De La Rosa R., M. and Sturzenberger, O.P.: Clinical Reduction of Gingivitis Through the Use of a Mouthwash Containing Two Quaternary Ammonium Compounds, *J. Periodontol.*, *47*, 535, September, 1976.

Derdivanis, J.P., Bushmaker, S., and Dagenais, F.: Effect of a Mouthwash in an Irrigating Device on Accumulation and Maturation of Dental Plaque, *J. Periodontol.*, *49*, 81, February, 1978.

Duany, L.F., Fitzgerald, R.J., Llorente, M., and Zinner, D.D.: Effects of Povidone-iodine and Isotonic Saline on the Oral Health of Children, *J. Prev. Dent.*, *2*, 22, May–June, 1975.

Gjermo, P.: Chlorhexidine in Dental Practice, *J. Clin. Periodontol.*, *1*, 143, Number 3, 1974.

Hull, P.S.: Chemical Inhibition of Plaque, *J. Clin. Periodontol.*, *7*, 431, December, 1980.

24

Care of Dental Appliances

Total cleanliness of the oral cavity for the health of the teeth and supporting structures involves specific procedures for the care of the natural teeth and all appliances, both fixed and removable. A dental *appliance* is a device used to provide function or for therapeutic purposes. A *prosthesis* is an appliance for the replacement of a missing part of the body by an artificial part.

From the dentist's viewpoint, the success of a dental appliance depends to a large degree on the cooperation of the patient in daily cleaning of the appliance and plaque control and oral physical therapy for the remaining natural teeth. Likewise, the orthodontist is concerned that appliances be kept clean and periodontal health be maintained by the control of bacterial plaque.

The patient's cooperation depends on the motivation, information, and sense of appreciation and concern imparted by the dentist and the dental auxiliaries. For the natural teeth involved, instruction begins early, before construction of the partial denture or placement of orthodontic appliances. Instruction is supplemented when an appliance is inserted to demonstrate specific techniques for daily care. Continuing supervision and review of procedures at succeeding appointments and recall appointments are required.

Fixed appliances include fixed partial dentures, space maintainers, periodontal splints, and orthodontic appliances. Examples of removable types are complete and partial dentures, space maintainers, and orthodontic appliances, as well as obturators for closure of palatal defects.

A patient may have more than one prosthesis. For example, there may be a complete maxillary denture and both fixed and removable partial dentures in the mandibular arch. For this patient, the regimen for personal care involves the natural teeth as well as the fixed and removable dentures. A program of instruction must be worked out for each patient, depending on individual needs.

FIXED PARTIAL DENTURES

A partial denture replaces one or more but less than all of the natural teeth.* The fixed partial denture, otherwise called a fixed bridge, is one that cannot be removed, but is permanently attached to natural teeth or roots which furnish support to the appliance.

I. Components of a Fixed Partial Denture (figure 24–1)

A. Abutment

A tooth used for the support or anchorage of a fixed prosthesis is called an abutment tooth.

---

*All definitions in this chapter that pertain to prosthetic appliances are taken from or adapted from and are in accord with the *Glossary of Prosthetic Terms*, 4th ed. *J. Prosthet. Dent.*, 38, 70, July, 1977.

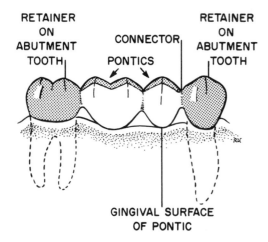

RETAINER ON ABUTMENT TOOTH CONNECTOR PONTICS RETAINER ON ABUTMENT TOOTH

GINGIVAL SURFACE OF PONTIC

Figure 24–1. Parts of a fixed partial denture. Mandibular four unit fixed partial denture to show characteristic parts. Cast gold crowns on abutment teeth serve as the retainers for this bridge.

B. Retainer

An inlay, onlay, or crown that restores an abutment tooth and is used for fixation and support of the fixed partial denture is called a retainer.

C. Pontic

A pontic is an artificial tooth that replaces a lost natural tooth, restores its function, and usually occupies the space previously occupied by the natural crown.

D. Connector

A connector unites the retainer to the pontic or joins two individual pontics. In a fixed partial denture, the connector may be a solder joint or, when the entire bridge is cast as a single unit, the connector may be continuous with the retainer.

E. Surfaces

1. *Occlusal:* the surface that occludes with opposing teeth.
2. *Gingival:* the portion or side of the pontic that is adjacent to the edentulous gingiva beneath it.

II. Care Procedures

A. Debris Removal

When suggesting a procedure to follow for cleaning the oral cavity when a fixed partial denture is present, debris removal with an oral irrigator may be recommended as first step. By removing food and debris, access of the toothbrush and other aids for plaque removal is facilitated. The patient must understand the function of the irrigator and be aware that the bacterial plaque has not been removed. Procedure for use of an oral irrigator is described on page 369–370.

B. Plaque Removal from Abutment Teeth

Nearly all of the methods proposed for plaque control and oral physical therapy in the two previous chapters may be applicable to abutment teeth. The proximal surface and gingiva of an abutment tooth adjacent to a pontic usually require special attention.

1. *Toothbrushing.* Sulcular brushing is generally indicated. The area of the tooth surface adjacent to and beneath the gingival margin must be kept meticulously free of dental plaque.
2. *Dentifrice Selection.* A nonabrasive dentifrice is indicated to prevent the possibility of abrasion when pontic or crown facings are made of acrylic, when the gold of the partial denture is highly polished and could be scratched, and when there are areas of root exposure on abutment teeth.

   A fluoride-containing dentifrice is important for protection of remaining tooth surfaces, particularly exposed cementum.
3. *Additional Interdental Care.* An interdental plaque removal method is indicated. This is selected on the basis of the individual patient or the appliance. The interdental cleaning device is adapted specifically to the distal of the mesial abutment and the mesial of the distal abutment, and from both facial and lingual. The same interdental cleaning procedure can usually be applied to the gingival surface of the fixed partial denture. Interdental cleaning methods and devices are described on pages 359–368.

C. The Appliance

1. *Areas Requiring Emphasis.* The gingival surfaces of the pontics and beneath the connectors are particularly prone to plaque retention.

2. *Toothbrushing.* A toothbrush in the Charters' position may be helpful for cleaning the gingival surface of the pontic from the facial aspect. The filaments can be directed under the pontic to clean the gingival surface. Charters' brush position is shown in figure 22–7, page 349.

3. *Dental Floss*

   a. Thread a 12- to 15-inch length between an abutment and pontic, or under the pontic if space permits. The floss may be rigid enough if folded on the end and pressed together, or a plastic or metal floss threader may be more conveniently used. Several types are available (figure 24–2).

   b. Draw the floss through and, using single or double thickness, remove loose debris (figure 24–3).

   c. Apply a new section of the floss with moderate pressure and dentifrice to the undersurface (gingival surface) of the pontic and then to the proximal surfaces of the abutment teeth to remove dental plaque. Remove floss and rinse.

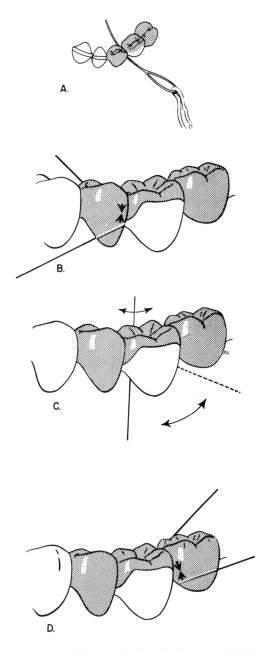

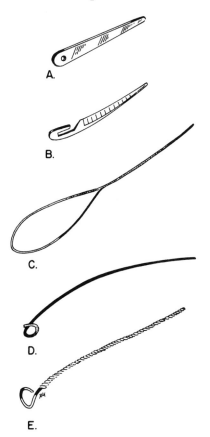

Figure 24–2. Examples of floss threaders. **A.** Clear plastic with closed eye. **B.** Tinted plastic with open eye. **C.** Soft plastic loop. **D.** Flexible wire. **E.** Twisted wire.

Figure 24–3. Cleaning a fixed partial denture. **A.** Use floss threader to draw floss (or yarn when space permits) between an abutment and a pontic. **B.** Apply floss to the distal surface of the mesial abutment. **C.** Slide floss under pontic. Move back and forth several times as shown by the arrows to remove plaque from the gingival surface of the pontic. **D.** Apply new section of floss to the mesial surface of the distal abutment tooth.

4. *Knitting Yarn.* Put length of yarn in floss threader and pull through under the appliance for a thicker cleaning device than floss alone (page 363).

5. *Other Interdental Devices.* A pipe cleaner, interdental brush, a single tufted brush, or an interdental tip should be recommended and demonstrated as indicated by the needs of the individual appliance.

ORTHODONTIC APPLIANCES

A high dental caries rate has been associated with teeth with orthodontic appliances, and severe gingival and periodontal diseases during and following treatment are not unusual. A rigid preventive program for the patient with orthodontic appliances along with a specific plan of instruction, motivation, and supervision are essential.

The dental hygienist who works with an orthodontist is in a position to perform a highly specialized service. Since the patient will be under care with regular appointments for a long period, frequently over a few years, periodic communication between the patient's referring dentist and dental hygienist is necessary in order that instruction be coordinated along with other necessary dental and dental hygiene care.

I. Complicating Factors

A. Age

Most orthodontic patients are preteen and teen-age.

1. The incidence of gingivitis is high in this age group. The incidence of periodontal disease increases from early childhood to late teenage.

2. There is a tendency for the gingival tissue to show deviations from normal when plaque increases because of lack of attention to oral health needs.

B. Gingival Enlargement

Puberty is occasionally accompanied by an exaggerated response of the gingiva to local irritation.[1] With orthodontic appliances, the reaction may be compounded, the degree varying from slight to severe enlargement particularly of the interdental pa-

pillae. The tissue may greatly enlarge and cover the bands.

C. Position of Teeth

Teeth that are irregularly positioned are naturally more susceptible to the retention of deposits and are more difficult to clean. With the severe malocclusions of orthodontic patients, this factor becomes even more significant.

D. Increased Oral Microbial Flora

The greater the number of bands on the teeth, the greater increase in bacterial plaque retention.[2]

E. Problems with Appliances

1. Plaque, debris, and materia alba are retained.

2. Accidents may cause wires to bend adversely and become imbedded in the gingiva. A loosened band may be forced under the gingiva.

3. Removable appliances or their clasps may press excessively against the gingiva.

4. Rubber bands may slip under the gingiva and detach the junctional epithelium.

F. Effects on the Periodontium[3,4]

1. Increased plaque retention leads to increased gingival and periodontal pocket formation.

2. Excessive forces during too rapid tooth movement may produce necrosis in the periodontal ligament and resorption of alveolar bone.

G. Self-care is Difficult

Even the patient who tries to maintain oral cleanliness has difficulty because the appliances are in the way and interfere with the application of the toothbrush and other devices used for plaque control and oral physical therapy.

II. Plaque Control

With such a variety of appliances utilized for orthodontic treatment,[5] it is not possible to specify a single type of brush, the brushing method, or the auxiliary aids that should be selected for

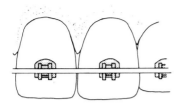

Figure 24–4. Direct bond orthodontic appliance. The bracket is attached to the tooth surface by an acid etch technique.

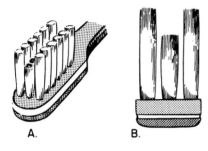

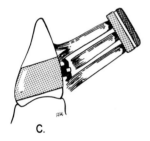

Figure 24–5. Orthodontic toothbrush. **A.** Middle row of filaments trimmed short to fit over fixed appliance. **B.** Cross section. **C.** Illustration of incorrect position of brush. Note that the tipped brush prevents full use of filament tips in cleaning plaque and debris from around bracket and wire.

A. General Instructions

1. Perform brushing before a mirror so that brush application is accurate and brushing is thorough.
2. Use a disclosing solution rinse to assist in self-evaluation. Orthodontic patients may find it difficult to chew disclosing wafers without discomfort or pain.[6]
3. Dentifrice: an approved fluoride dentifrice is recommended to aid in dental caries control.
4. Emphasis in brushing should be placed on sulcular brushing and cleaning the area between the orthodontic bands and brackets and the gingiva.

B. Toothbrushing

1. *Brush Selection*
   a. A soft nylon brush with rounded filaments is generally recommended.
   b. Special orthodontic brush designed with two spaced rows of soft nylon

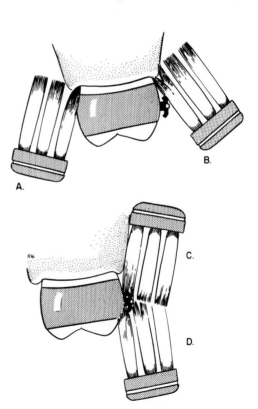

Figure 24–6. Toothbrushing for the patient with fixed orthodontic appliances. Sulcular brushing is advised. **A.** Lingual. **B.** Facial. **C.** Cleaning the appliance: brush in Charters' brushing position for the gingival side, and **D.** in Stillman's position for occlusal side of bracket and wire.

each individual patient. Fixed orthodontic appliances may consist of brackets bonded directly to the tooth surfaces after an acid etch procedure as shown in figure 24–4. Other appliances are bands cemented around each tooth with brackets attached to the bands to support an archwire. Figure 24–6 shows teeth with complete bands.

The selection of plaque control procedures for an individual patient is determined by the severity of the gingivitis or periodontitis, the anatomic features of the gingiva, the position of the teeth, as well as the type and position of the orthodontic appliance. Several variations of brush positioning are suggested below.

filaments with a third middle row which is shorter can be applied directly over the fixed appliance and used with a short horizontal stroke (figure 24–5).

2. *Brushing Procedure*
   a. A sulcular method is needed by most patients for cleaning the appliances and maintaining the gingiva.
   b. Special adaptation for facial surface: place the brush in the Charters' position for over the wire and bracket (or under for mandibular); and Stillman's position for the opposite side (figure 24–6).
   c. To assure cleanliness, the appliances should be brushed in any way that the filaments can be manipulated: insert the brush from below, over, and above the arch wire, rotate and vibrate to remove plaque and debris.
   d. Lingual: appropriate method which is similar to the basic strokes used on the facial surfaces.

III. Additional Measures

A. Interdental Aids

The previously described applications of the interdental tip and Perio-aid (pages 364, 367) also apply for care of the orthodontic patient (figure 24–7). A floss threader is needed for plaque removal from proximal tooth surfaces when the appliance prevents passage of floss from the occlusal.

An interdental brush and a single-tuft brush can be particularly beneficial around individual teeth. The entire system should be kept as simple as possible.

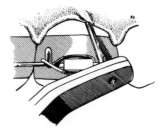

Figure 24–7. Perio-aid for the orthodontic patient. Moistened toothpick end can be applied to clean about appliances and in the subgingival area of gingival sulci and pockets. Directions for use of the Perio-aid are on page 364.

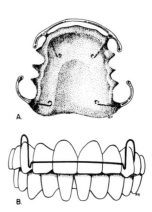

Figure 24–8. Hawley appliance. **A.** Removable acrylic retainer with labial retaining wire and clasps of type worn by orthodontic patient following removal of fixed appliance. **B.** Anterior view of patient showing Hawley appliance in position. Cleaning instructions are the same as for a removable denture (pages 392–393).

B. Oral Irrigation

Most orthodontic patients can benefit from the regular use of an irrigator.[6,7]

C. Care of Removable Appliance or Hawley Retainer (figure 24–8)

1. Clean the appliance after each meal and before retiring. Instructions for cleaning procedures and agents for removable appliances are described with the care of the removable denture (pages 392–393).
2. Brush and rinse teeth and gingival tissue under the appliance each time the appliance is removed. Unless absolutely necessary as directed by the orthodontist, it is best for the health of the underlying tissues if the appliance is not kept in the mouth continuously.
3. Brushing the mucosa under the appliance is advisable. Methods are described on page 389.
4. Keep appliance in a container with water when it is out of the mouth.

D. Self-applied Fluoride

A patient with an orthodontic appliance has an increased risk of enamel decalcification and dental caries because of bacterial plaque retention. A daily fluoride program is mandatory to supplement mechanical daily plaque removal and periodic professional topical applications of fluoride solution or gel.

Self-applied fluorides are described on pages 456–458. A fluoride dentifrice is recommended, along with a daily mouthrinse, gel tray, or brush-on gel. Encouragement, repetition, reinforcement, and motivation are needed to achieve continuing interest and cooperation of an orthodontic patient in both the plaque control and the self-applied fluoride programs.

COMPLETE DENTURES

It should not be assumed that the patient who is new to the dental office and is wearing dentures or a denture knows the proper techniques for caring for the appliances. During questioning for the patient history, information about the method and frequency of denture care is recorded. Later the dentures are examined and the current method of care is reviewed. Alternate cleaning agents, devices, or procedures are recommended and demonstrated as indicated.

Instruction may be for the patient receiving a maxillary and mandibular denture for the first time, for the patient whose dentures have been remade or relined, or for the patient with a single denture which opposes natural teeth. Another patient may be receiving an immediate denture, that is, a denture inserted immediately following removal of natural teeth. Types of dentures and characteristics of the edentulous mouth are described on pages 637–638.

The need for individual instruction in care of the denture was brought out in a survey of nearly one thousand patients. Of these, only 17.5 percent considered their cleaning methods inefficient, but nearly 70 percent exhibited unclean, stained dentures.[8]

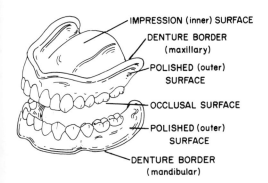

Figure 24–9. Parts of a complete denture.

I. Components of a Complete Denture
(figure 24–9)

To understand the effects of various cleaning agents and devices, information about the structure and material of the parts of a denture is pertinent.

A. Denture Base

That part of a denture which rests on the oral mucosa and to which the teeth are attached. Most denture bases are of plastic resin. Others may be metal, for example, chrome-cobalt or gold in combination with a plastic resin.

B. Surfaces

1. *Impression Surface.* Also called the tissue or inner surface, it is the part that lies adjacent to the mucous membrane of the alveolar ridge and immediately associated parts; in the maxillary the tissue surface is adjacent to the hard palate.
2. *Polished Surface.* The external or outer surface is highly polished and includes everything except the occlusal surface.
3. *Occlusal Surface.* That portion of the surface of a denture that makes contact or near contact with the corresponding surface of the opposing denture or natural teeth.

C. Teeth

The denture teeth may be made of plastic resin or porcelain. Anterior porcelain teeth have metal pins for retention.

II. Purposes for Cleaning

Inadequate oral and denture hygiene practices are major causes of oral lesions under dentures (page 641).

A. Prevent Irritation to the Oral Tissues

1. *Mechanical Irritants:* rough deposits of plaque, calculus, thick stains.
2. *Chemical Irritants:* products of putrefaction of food debris and bacterial metabolic products.

B. Control Infection

There may be reactions to microbial denture plaque and/or secondary infections by way of traumatic lesions.[9,10]

C. Prevent Mouth Odors

D. Maintain Appearance

III. Denture Deposits

Accumulation of stains and deposits on dentures varies between individuals in a manner similar to that on natural teeth. The phases of deposit formation may be divided as follows:

A. Mucin and Food Debris on the Denture Surface

Readily removed by rinsing or brushing.

B. Denture Pellicle and Denture Plaque

Denture pellicle forms readily after a denture is cleaned. Denture plaque is composed of bacteria with a predominance of gram positive cocci and rods in an intermicrobial substance.[11]

Plaque serves as a matrix for calculus formation and stain accumulation when the denture is not cleaned. Plaque, particularly older plaque, is tenacious and less easily removed than other soft deposits.

C. Calculus

Hard and fixed to the denture surface, generally located on the buccal of the maxillary molars and lingual of mandibular anterior region.

IV. Methods for Cleaning

A. Rinsing under Running Water

Although it would be unusual if a denture could be kept clean by this method only, the use of rinsing after meals when other methods are not possible is necessary.

B. Brushing

With water, soap, or other mild cleansing agent. Coarse abrasives produce scratches.

C. Immersion

The denture is soaked in a solvent or detergent where chemical action removes or loosens stains and deposits which can then be rinsed or brushed away.

D. Mechanical Denture Cleaners[12]

Commercially available devices include ultrasonic, sonic, magnetic, and agitating mechanisms which can be combined with an immersion agent. The action of the mechanical cleaning device appears to make the solution more efficient than when the solution is used alone. Ultrasonic cleaning during a professional appointment is described on pages 580–581.

V. Types of Denture Cleaners[13,14,15]

A. Chemical Solution Cleaners (Immersion)

1. *Alkaline Hypochlorite*
   a. Active ingredient: dilute sodium hypochlorite with bleaching properties.
   b. Action: loosen debris and light stains; dissolve mucin; dissolve plaque matrix.
   c. Example: household bleach
   d. Disadvantages: odor; tarnish; surface pitting
2. *Alkaline Peroxide*
   a. Active ingredient: alkaline peroxide with oxygen-liberating agent.
   b. Action: loosen debris and light stains; a preventive cleaner which should be used regularly from the day a denture has been cleaned professionally.
   c. Examples: most proprietary cleaners.
   d. Disadvantage: will not remove heavy stains or calculus.
3. *Dilute Acids*
   a. Active ingredient: organic or inorganic acids.
   b. Action: dissolve inorganic deposits.
   c. Examples: vinegar, 5% hydrochloric acid; commercially prepared ultrasonic solutions.
   d. Disadvantage: corrosion of chrome alloys (hydrochloric acid).
4. *Enzymes*. The enzymes act to break down plaque mucoproteins, glycoproteins, and mucoproteins to less adhesive molecules.

B. Abrasive Cleaners

1. *Denture Pastes and Powders*, toothpastes and powders.
   a. Active ingredient: an abrasive (see Dentifrices, page 371).

b. Examples: various commercial products.

c. Disadvantage: can abrade the plastic resin denture base and acrylic teeth. A paste with low abrasiveness should be selected.

2. *Household Agents*

a. Active ingredient: detergent and/or abrasive agent.

b. Examples: salt, bicarbonate of soda, are mildly abrasive; hand soap is cleansing and not particularly abrasive. Scouring powders or other excessively abrasive cleaners should not be used.

VI. General Cleaning Procedures

A. When to Clean

1. Regularly after each meal and before retiring.

2. Chemical immersion: daily or twice weekly, depending on the rate of formation of calculus and stain and the type of solution used.

a. May be at one of the regular cleanings.

b. Suggested: while bathing.

c. Overnight when denture is removed as instructed by the dentist.

B. Selection of Method for Cleaning

Most people use immersion, brushing, or a combination of the two. When unable to clean, rinsing after eating is advised.

C. Preparation for Cleaning

For all denture care methods, denture adherent material must be carefully and thoroughly removed with a brush and the denture rinsed. The material should be cleaned from the denture-bearing oral mucosa twice daily and rinsed.[12]

VII. Cleaning by Immersion

A. Advantages

1. The solution reaches all areas of the denture for a complete cleaning.

2. Minimizes danger of dropping the appliance: prevents need for handling which is required during brushing.

3. Safe storage when dentures are out of the mouth.

4. Abrasion of the denture material is not possible.

5. Aid to person with limited ability to manage a brush.

6. When cleaning is distasteful, immersion involves the least handling and observation. This is an advantage particularly for an attendant or nurse who must clean the denture of a helpless patient.

B. Procedure

1. Rinse the denture when it is taken from the mouth to remove saliva and loose debris; place in a plastic container with fitted cover which is maintained specifically for this purpose.*

2. Use only warm water for rinsing and for mixing the solution: warm water promotes the action of the cleaner, whereas hot water should never be used because it can distort plastic resin.

3. Cover the denture with solution; cover the container.

4. When the denture is removed, rinse under running water and brush to remove loosened debris and chemicals before placing in the mouth.

C. Solutions

1. *Proprietary.* Purchasable in powder or tablet form.

a. Preparation: add measured warm water as directed by the manufacturer.

b. Length of immersion: usually 10 to 15 minutes or as suggested by the manufacturer. Since the action is dependent on the mechanical bubbling effect of released oxygen, the solution has little value after the available oxygen has been released.

c. Effect: these solutions are only effective against loose debris; denture cleanliness is dependent on regular daily immersion supplemented by brushing.

2. *Hypochlorite Solution.* Household bleach (5% sodium hypochlorite) and

---

*Procedure for removal of a denture for a patient is described on page 580.

Calgon. Calgon acts to improve the penetrating and detaching power of the bleach.

a. Proportions

1 tablespoon household bleach
2 teaspoons Calgon
$\frac{1}{2}$ glass (4 ounces) warm water

b. Length of immersion: usually 10 to 15 minutes. When stains or calculus form, it may be suggested that the patient soak the denture overnight provided there are no metal parts that can become corroded.

3. *White Household Vinegar*
   a. Indication for use: only when calculus is observed on the denture; not routinely.
   b. Proportion: one or two teaspoonfuls in one cup of warm water.
   c. Length of immersion: the denture may be immersed overnight when necessary for complete cleaning.

VIII. Cleaning by Brushing

A. Type of Brush

1. *Denture Brush.* A good quality denture brush with rounded filaments is preferable because it is designed for the purpose with two arrangements of filaments: one group in a large round arrangement of tufts permits access to the inner, curved impression surface of the denture. The second group of tufts is arranged to form a rectangular brush for convenient adaptation to the polished and occlusal denture surfaces (figure 24–10).

2. *Other Brushes.* A few patients prefer not to have a denture brush for personal reasons. A hand brush can be used, provided the filaments are long enough to reach into the deeper portions of the impression surfaces. Prerequisite is that each area of each surface of the denture must be reached by the brush if dental plaque formation is to be controlled.

   If a patient prefers to use an ordinary toothbrush, a multitufted soft nylon brush with end-rounded filaments should be acceptable if access to all of the inner curvatures is possible without undue

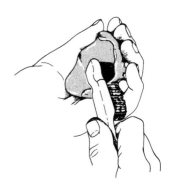

Figure 24–10. Brushing to clean a complete denture. The denture is held securely in the palm of the hand but without a squeezing pressure. A specially designed denture brush is preferred because one group of tufts is arranged to provide access to the inner impression surface of the denture as shown.

pressure on certain parts in the attempt to clean others. When the patient wears a single denture, it is advisable to keep separate brushes for the natural teeth and the denture in order that the brush for the natural teeth be in the best condition possible.

B. Procedure

1. Grasp denture in palm of hand securely, but without a squeezing pressure because dentures can be broken (figure 24–10).
2. Hold the denture low in a sink in which has been placed a towel, wash cloth, or rubber mat spread over the bottom to serve as a cushion should the denture be dropped. The sink should be partially filled with water.
3. Apply warm water, nonabrasive soap, and brush to all areas of the denture. Particular attention should be paid the impression surfaces where configurations of the surface correspond with those of the oral topography. Rinse thoroughly.

C. Precautions Related to Brushing

1. Overzealous brushing with an abrasive cleaning agent on the impression surface could alter the fit of the denture.
2. Plastic resin is easily abraded. Scratches make a rough surface; the denture may become more subject to the collection of debris and calculus.

3. Possibility of incomplete coverage during cleaning, particularly in the more inaccessible areas.
4. Uneven pressure: brush applied more vigorously to accessible areas.
5. Danger of dropping and breaking the denture is increased when it is soaped, wet, and therefore slippery.
6. Patient who requires eyeglasses should be advised to wear them when brushing: to watch the procedure and to observe the cleanliness of the denture after brushing.

X. Additional Instructions

A. Care of Plastic Resin

An appliance made with plastic resin should be immersed in water or cleaning solution when it is not in the mouth.

B. Prevention of Denture Deposits

When the denture is kept clean by regular procedures from the time of insertion, accumulation of heavy stains and calculus can be prevented.

C. Professional Recall

A denture should never be scraped with a sharp instrument in the attempt to remove calculus deposits. When the cleaning methods recommended in this chapter do not remove deposits, the denture should be taken to the dental hygienist and dentist for professional cleaning. A regular recall plan is arranged.

D. Paste Cleaners

Paste cleaners (dentifrices or denture pastes) may be too abrasive for dentures, but also it is difficult to rinse all traces of the pastes from the denture. Residual chemical agents such as essential oils may cause inflammatory or allergic reactions of the oral mucosa, and phenolic agents can have deleterious effects on plastic resin.

E. Soft Lining Materials

Temporary soft conditioning lining material may be sensitive to proprietary cleansers. Washing with cold water and a soft cloth, cotton, or soft brush (gently) can be used,

provided the denture plaque is removed several times each day. Outer, polished surfaces should be thoroughly brushed in the usual manner. When the denture is placed in water overnight, it is suggested that the teeth be placed down so that the soft material at the denture border cannot become deformed.[16]

X. The Underlying Mucosa

A. Rinsing

Each time the denture is removed, the mouth should be rinsed thoroughly with warm water or a mild salt solution (pages 568–569).

B. Cleaning

It is recommended that the edentulous mucosa be brushed at least once daily. A soft brush with end-rounded filaments is applied in long, straight strokes from posterior to anterior.

C. Massage

For stimulation of circulation and increased resistance to trauma, frequent massage is recommended. Methods for massage that may be suggested to the patient are:
1. *Digital.* Place thumb and index finger over the ridge and apply massage with a press and release stroke. The palate may be rubbed with the ball of the thumb.
2. *Multitufted Soft Toothbrush.* Apply sides of filaments and vibratory motion to each area. Prevent trauma to the tissue by placing the brush carefully and avoiding scrubbing with undue pressure.
3. *Powered Brush.* Apply to each area with smooth, even strokes.

COMPLETE OVERDENTURE

An overdenture is a complete denture supported by both retained natural teeth and the soft tissue of the residual alveolar ridge. It is also known as an overlay denture, coping denture, and tooth-mucosa-supported denture.

I. Purposes[17]

The advantages of an overdenture when compared with a denture in a completely edentulous mouth are that having natural teeth present

A. Helps preserve bone.
B. Allows the remaining teeth to bear occlusal pressures, which reduces the pressures placed on the edentulous areas.
C. Improves stability and retention of the denture.
D. Improves the patient's tactile and proprioceptive senses by having the periodontal ligament present.
E. Increases the patient's psychological acceptance of the denture. The patient does not feel that all natural teeth have been lost.

II. Criteria

The overdenture should be considered for any patient whose treatment plan calls for extraction of all teeth. Teeth to be preserved must meet certain standards of health.

A. Periodontal Condition

Since wearing the overdenture brings stress to the periodontium, the tissues must have, or be treatable to obtain, the following:
1. Healthy sulci. There must be no bleeding or other signs of inflammation; minimal sulci depth; and all requirements of health (Table 11–1, page 196).
2. A band of attached gingiva (page 190).

B. Bone Support

The bone level following tooth preparation must be adequate to withstand occlusal forces.

C. Teeth

Teeth must have minimal mobility. Teeth selected are frequently the mandibular canines and premolars, and maxillary canines.

III. Preparation of the Teeth

A. Endodontics

Most preserved teeth need endodontic therapy because the crown will be reduced.

B. Periodontics

Treatment procedures depend on clinical findings, but may include measures to eliminate inflammation and pockets, to increase the zone of attached gingiva, or to reshape the architecture of the bone or gingival tissue.

C. Restorative

1. Tooth crowns are reduced to short rounded preparations or in some cases to the level and contour of the gingival margin.
2. There may be only an amalgam restoration to cover the root canals, or the teeth may be protected by a gold coping (figure 24–11). A coping is a cast thin metal covering or cap.
3. The gold coping may be used as a retainer for a retentive attachment.

IV. Dental Hygiene Care and Instruction

The patient must be well informed concerning the problems of care of the retained teeth and gingiva. A high degree of motivation to want to save the remaining teeth is needed. Supervision by frequent recall appointments for scaling and planing, topical fluoride applications, and motivation and instruction for plaque control will be essential.

A. Denture Care

The impression surface of the denture must be kept meticulously free from plaque collection. Denture care is outlined on pages 386–389.

B. Gingival Tissue and Natural Teeth

1. Complete plaque control procedures

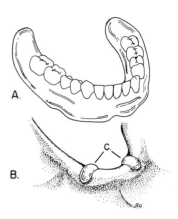

Figure 24–11. Overdenture. **A.** Complete mandibular denture supported by **B.** both mucosa and prepared roots of natural teeth which have been endodontically treated and restored with gold copings (**C**).

using a soft nylon brush with round ends or a powered toothbrush (pages 342, 352). Massage of the edentulous gingiva is also recommended.

2. Interdental tip or a Perio-aid should be used daily to trace around each natural tooth to clean subgingivally (page 364).

C. **Fluoride**

A specific fluoride application plan must be included. The requirements depend partly on the past history of dental caries. When the teeth have been extracted because of dental caries, caries control measures take on special significance, particularly if dietary habits remain the same. Current dietary habits need to be checked by asking the patient to keep a daily food diary (page 425). Sucrose intake limitations can be recommended accordingly.

1. *Fluoride Self-application.* All patients need to use a fluoride dentifrice. In addition, either a mouthrinse or a gel-tray can be recommended. After cleaning, the patient's denture can be used for a custom tray, and the gel drops can be placed inside at the locations of the natural teeth. Pressure of the denture as it is seated will force the gel about the teeth.

2. *Professional Topical Applications.* When daily mouthrinse or gel-tray is not carried out by the patient or when additional fluoride is indicated, professional topical applications are made. Since frequent recall is needed to check the health of the gingival tissues, an application can be made at each recall. Benefit is derived from the fluoride in direct proportion to the frequency of application: the more frequent the application of fluoride, the greater the benefit derived from it.

REMOVABLE PARTIAL DENTURES

The removable partial denture replaces one or more but less than all of the natural teeth and associated structures, and can be removed from the mouth and replaced at will. Depending on the location and number of remaining natural teeth, a partial denture may receive all of its support from the teeth, or it may be partly tooth-borne and partly tissue-borne.

Self-care procedures for the patient with a removable appliance involve much more than cleaning the appliance. The abutment teeth, the gingival tissue, and the mucosa of edentulous areas require regular attention. Gingival health is unfavorably affected by removable partial dentures because bacterial plaque accumulates more readily and in greater quantities. Plaque control is a major factor in the long-term effectiveness of a partial removable denture.

Procedures suggested here for care of the removable partial denture apply also to various other removable appliances. Examples of these are removable space maintainers, appliances for orthodontic purposes such as a Hawley biteplate or retainer (figure 24–8), obturators for closure of palatal openings as for cleft palate (page 652) or for replacement of tissue removed in the treatment of oral cancer.

I. **Components of a Removable Partial Denture** (figure 24–12)

The selection of cleaning agents and the procedures for cleaning are complicated by the intricacy of the metallic parts and their relation to the natural teeth as well as by the dental materials used in construction.

A. **Abutment Teeth**

Natural teeth used for the support or anchorage of the appliance.

B. **Denture Base**

The part that rests on the oral mucosa and carries the artificial teeth. The base may be made of plastic resin or alloys of gold or chrome.

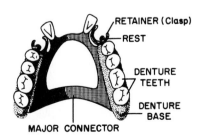

Figure 24–12. Parts of a partial removable denture. A maxillary denture is shown.

C. Denture Teeth

Are made of porcelain, plastic resin, or metal.

D. Major Connectors

Bars of rigid metal which unite the parts of the denture. In the maxillary there can be one or two *palatal bars;* in the mandibular, the *lingual bar.* Minor connectors are between the major connectors and the other units such as clasps and occlusal rests.

E. Retainer

Any type of clasp, attachment, or device used for the fixation or stabilization of a prosthesis.

F. Precision Attachment

A type of retainer which consists of a metal receptacle and a close-fitting part. The former (the metal receptacle) is usually included within the restoration of an abutment tooth, and the latter is attached to a pontic or denture framework. The precision attachments are used for removable partial dentures, and occasionally for fixed partial and overdentures. A wide variety of attachments is available.[18]

G. Rest

A rigid, stabilizing extension of a fixed or removable partial denture which contacts a remaining tooth or teeth for the dissipation of vertical or horizontal forces.

II. Objectives

A. The Appliance

Because natural teeth are adjacent to the appliance, objectives for cleaning the appliance take on added significance. The same basic objectives applied to the complete denture apply to the removable: remove irritants to the oral tissues, prevent mouth odors, and improve appearance.

B. The Natural Teeth

The objective is to control plaque for the prevention of dental caries and periodontal disease. Other objectives may be found on page 335.

III. Cleaning A Removable Appliance

Rinsing, immersion, and brushing methods, as well as the cleaning agents described for the complete denture on pages 387–388, apply alike to the partial appliance, with the few additions noted below.

A. Rinsing

After each meal the denture and the natural teeth should be brushed. When regular cleaning facilities are not available, rinsing is important for both the natural teeth and the removable appliance. While the appliance is out, the tongue can be used to rub the sides of abutment teeth.

B. Immersion

An agent known to discolor metal can be avoided. Procedures for immersion cleaning are described on page 387.

C. Brushing
1. *Recommended Brushes*
   a. *Toothbrush:* one or more should be reserved for the natural teeth. Although using a regular toothbrush for partial care of a removable appliance is not recommended, when a patient does so, a separate brush is definitely indicated. Brushing the clasps and other metal parts can be destructive to fine toothbrushes.
   b. *Powered brush:* a powered toothbrush is sometimes appropriate for the natural teeth of the partial denture patient. However, the powered brush should not be used in and about the intricate clasps and other parts of a removable appliance because of the danger of catching the brush and damaging the appliance.
   c. *Clasp brush:* a specially designed narrow, tapered, cylindrical brush about 2 to 3 inches long which can be adapted to the inner surfaces of clasps is recommended (figure 24–13). Clasps and their connectors are closely adapted to the supporting teeth, and the protected internal surfaces are prone to plaque formation. These difficult-to-clean areas require special care.

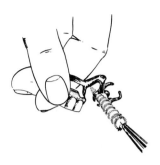

Figure 24–13. Use of a clasp brush for cleaning the inside of a clasp of a partial removable denture. A denture brush is used to clean other surfaces.

  d. *Denture brush:* this was described for the complete denture (figure 24–10) and is an excellent brush for cleaning all of the smooth surfaces and the metal bars of the partial denture.

  2. *Precautions During Brushing.* Too tight a grasp of a partial appliance can result in bending or fracture of clasps or bars. Filaments of a brush can inadvertently catch the appliance and cause it to drop. A liner for the sink is mandatory (pages 388–389).

IV. The Natural Teeth

A. Plaque Control

Toothbrushing and interdental cleaning methods selected for the particular needs of the patient must be followed meticulously. The longevity of the removable appliance is dependent on the health of the supporting teeth, and in turn, the natural teeth are dependent on the cleanliness of the appliance.

B. Dental Caries Control

The topical application of fluoride, the use of a fluoride dentifrice, and other self-applied fluoride measures such as a daily mouthrinse or custom tray, and the control of refined sugars in the diet must be definite parts of the complete program of oral care for the patient with a removable appliance.

The patient must be constantly alert to the control of plaque retention by the appliance and the need for rinsing immediately after eating when brushing is not possible. For the patient who has been caries-susceptible, and whose teeth are missing because of dental caries, a dietary analysis and specific dental caries control program may increase a patient's motivation.

TECHNICAL HINTS

I. Review instructions for each patient with a fixed or removable prosthesis. Do not assume that, because a denture has been in use for a long time, the patient knows how to clean it properly or how to care for the soft tissue adjacent to it.

II. To prevent cross-contamination when receiving a denture from a patient:
  A. Offer a container or disposable napkin in which the patient can place the denture. When the denture is removed by the dental hygienist, rubber gloves should be worn.
  B. Scrub the denture with surgical soap using a disposable scrub brush or one that can be resterilized. Wear rubber gloves and a mask while cleaning the appliance as well as when demonstrating care procedures for patient education.

III. Acrylic restorations, crowns, and pontics are subject to toothbrush attrition and dentifrice abrasion. Select soft brush and nonabrasive cleaning material.

IV. Provide printed instructions for each patient. Personalize the instructions with notations related to particular problem areas of the patient.

V. Sources of educational materials for patients:
  A. American Dental Association, Order Department, 211 East Chicago Avenue, Chicago, Illinois 60611. Request current catalog. Samples of the following booklets are available on request:
  Orthodontics: Questions and Answers (P11)
  Removable Partial Dentures (G6)
  B. American Association of Orthodontists, 747 Delmar Boulevard, St. Louis, Missouri 63130. Request the pamphlet *Orthodontic Tooth Brushing.*
  C. Materials for the edentulous patient are listed on page 645.

References

1. Carranza, F.A.: *Glickman's Clinical Periodontology*, 5th

ed. Philadelphia, W.B. Saunders Co., 1979, pp. 120–121, 515.

2. Balenseifen, J.W. and Madonia, J.V.: Study of Dental Plaque in Orthodontic Patients, *J. Dent. Res.*, 49, 320, March–April, 1970.

3. Carranza: op. cit., pp. 1036–1039.

4. Schluger, S., Yuodelis, R.A., and Page, R.C.: *Periodontal Disease*. Philadelphia, Lea & Febiger, 1977, pp. 611–616.

5. Stibbs, G.D.: Treatment—Clinical Procedures, in Morrey, L.W. and Nelson, R.J., eds.: *Dental Science Handbook*. Superintendent of Documents, U.S. Government Printing Office, Washington, D.C., 1970, pp. 190–197.

6. York, T.A. and Dunkin, R.T.: Control of Periodontal Problems in Orthodontics by Use of Water Irrigation, *Am. J. Orthod.*, 53, 639, September, 1967.

7. Hurst, J.E. and Madonia, J.V.: The Effect of an Oral Irrigating Device on the Oral Hygiene of Orthodontic Patients, *J. Am. Dent. Assoc.*, 81, 678, September, 1970.

8. MacCallum, M., Stafford, G.D., MacCulloch, W.T., and Combe, E.C.: Which Cleanser? A Report on a Survey of Denture Cleansing Routine and the Development of a New Denture Cleanser, *Dent. Pract. Dent. Rec.*, 19, 83, November, 1968.

9. Burket, L.W.: Oral Medicine in the Edentulous Patient, in Lynch, M.A., ed.: *Burket's Oral Medicine*, 7th ed. Philadelphia, J.B. Lippincott Co., 1977, pp. 568–576.

10. Budtz-Jorgensen, E.: Oral Mucosal Lesions Associated with the Wearing of Removable Dentures, *J. Oral Path.*, 10, 65, April, 1981.

11. Theilade, J.: Development of Bacterial Plaque in the Oral Cavity, *J. Clin. Periodontol.*, 4, 1, December, 1977.

12. American Dental Association, Council on Dental Materials, Instruments and Equipment: *Dentist's Desk Reference: Materials, Instruments and Equipment*, 1st ed. Chicago, American Dental Association, 1981, pp. 343–348.

13. Gallagher, J.B., Jr.: *Handbook for Complete Dentures*. Boston, Tufts University, School of Dental Medicine, 1981.

14. Budtz-Jorgensen, E.: Materials and Methods for Cleaning Dentures, *J. Prosthet. Dent.*, 42, 619, December, 1979.

15. Abere, D.J.: Post-placement Care of Complete and Removable Partial Dentures, *Dent. Clin. North Am.*, 23, 143, January, 1979.

16. Ortman, L.F.: Patient Education and Complete Denture Maintenance, in Winkler, S.: *Essentials of Complete Denture Prosthodontics*. Philadelphia, W.B. Saunders Co., 1979, p. 477.

17. Zamikoff, I.I.: Overdentures—Theory and Technique, *J. Am. Dent. Assoc.*, 86, 853, April, 1973.

18. American Dental Association, Council on Dental Materials, Instruments and Equipment: op. cit., pp. 102–128.

Suggested Readings

Borjian, H.: Removable Prostheses in Preschool Children, *J. Pedod.*, 2, 246, Spring, 1978.

House, J.E.: Prosthodontics, in Steele, P.F., ed.: *Dental Specialties for the Dental Hygienist*, 2nd ed. Philadelphia, Lea & Febiger, 1978, pp. 307–339.

Skyberg, R.L.: Stabilization of Avulsed Teeth in Children with the Flexible Mouthguard Splint, *J. Am. Dent. Assoc.*, 96, 797, May, 1978.

Orthodontic Appliances

Alexander, C.M., Jacobs, J.D., and Turpin, D.L.: Disease Control in an Orthodontic Practice, *Am. J. Orthod.*, 71, 79, January, 1977.

Gold, S.L.: Plaque-control Motivation in Orthodontic Practice, *Am. J. Orthod.*, 68, 8, July, 1975.

Gwinnett, A.J. and Ceen, R.F.: Plaque Distribution on Bonded Brackets: A Scanning Microscopic Study, *Am. J. Orthod.*, 75, 667, June, 1979.

Gwinnett, A.J. and Ceen, R.F.: An Ultraviolet Photographic Technique for Monitoring Plaque During Direct Bonding Procedures, *Am. J. Orthod.*, 73, 178, February, 1978.

Hickory, W. and Nanda, R.: Nutritional Considerations in Orthodontics, *Dent. Clin. North Am.*, 25, 195, January, 1981.

Kessler, M.: Interrelationships Between Orthodontics and Periodontics, *Am. J. Orthod.*, 70, 154, August, 1976.

Lundström, F. and Hamp, S-E.: Effect of Oral Hygiene Education on Children With or Without Subsequent Orthodontic Treatment, *Scand. J. Dent. Res.*, 88, 53, February, 1980.

Magness, W.S., Shannon, I.L., and West, D.C.: Office Applied Fluoride Treatments for Orthodontic Patients, *J. Dent. Res.*, 58, 1427, April, 1979.

Merow, W.W.: Orthodontics, in Steele, P.F., ed.: *Dental Specialties for the Dental Hygienist*, 2nd ed. Philadelphia, Lea & Febiger, 1978, pp. 199–237.

Ogaard, B., Gjermo, P., and Rølla, G.: Plaque-inhibiting Effect in Orthodontic Patients of a Dentifrice Containing Stannous Fluoride, *Am. J. Orthod.*, 78, 266, September, 1980.

Prichard, J.F.: The Effect of Bicuspid Extraction Orthodontics on the Periodontium, *J. Periodontol.*, 46, 534, September, 1975.

Rich, S.K.: Behavior Modification for Orthodontic Patients: An Exploratory Approach to Patient Education, *Am. J. Orthod.*, 78, 426, October, 1980.

Robertson, P.B., Schultz, L.D., and Levy, B.M.: Occurrence and Distribution of Interdental Gingival Clefts Following Orthodontic Movement into Bicuspid Extraction Sites, *J. Periodontol.*, 48, 232, April, 1977.

Shannon, I.L. and Miller, J.T.: Caries Risk in Teeth with Orthodontic Bands: A Review, *Gen. Dent.*, 20, 24, May, 1972.

Shannon, I.L. and Tarin, D.: Fluoride Mouthrinsing by Orthodontic Patients, *Int. J. Orthod.*, 18, 15, March, 1980.

Shaw, W.C., Addy, M., and Ray, C.: Dental and Social Effects of Malocclusion and Effectiveness of Orthodontic Treatment: A Review, *Community Dent. Oral Epidemiol.*, 8, 36, February, 1980.

Tersin, J.: Studies on Gingival Conditions in Relation to Orthodontic Treatment. IV. The Effect of Oral Hygiene Measures on Gingival Exudation During the Course of Orthodontic Treatment, *Swed. Dent. J.*, 2, 131, Number 4, 1978.

Tillery, T.J., Hembree, J.H., and Weber, F.N.: Preventing Enamel Decalcification During Orthodontic Treatment, *Am. J. Orthod.*, 70, 435, October, 1976.

Trossello, V.K. and Gianelly, A.A.: Orthodontic Treatment and Periodontal Status, *J. Periodontol.*, 50, 665, December, 1979.

Vandersall, D.C. and Varble, D.L.: The Missing Orthodontic Elastic Band, a Periodontic-orthodontic Dilemma, *J. Am. Dent. Assoc.*, 97, 661, October, 1978.

White, L.W.: A Behavioristic Approach to Oral Hygiene, *Am. J. Orthod.*, 72, 406, October, 1977.

White, L.W.: Behavioristic Technique for Oral Hygiene—An Update, *Am. J. Orthod.*, 77, 568, May, 1980.

Wisth, P.J. and Nord, A.: Caries Experience in Orthodontically Treated Individuals, *Angle Orthod.*, 47, 59, January, 1977.

Zachrisson, B.U. and Årthun, J.: Enamel Surface Appearance After Various Debonding Techniques, *Am. J. Orthod.*, 75, 121, February, 1979.

Zachrisson, B.U. and Brobakken, B.O.: Clinical Comparison of Direct Versus Indirect Bonding With Different Bracket Types and Adhesives, *Am. J. Orthod.*, 74, 62, July, 1978.

Zager, N.I. and Barnett, M.L.: Severe Bone Loss in a Child Initiated by Multiple Orthodontic Rubber Bands: Case Report, *J. Periodontol.*, 45, 701, September, 1974.

Denture Cleansing

Abelson, D.C.: Denture Plaque and Denture Cleansers, *J. Prosthet. Dent.*, 45, 376, April, 1981.

Altman, M.D., Yost, K.G., and Pitts, G.: A Spectrofluorometric Protein Assay of Plaque on Dentures and of Denture Cleaning Efficacy, *J. Prosthet. Dent.*, 42, 502, November, 1979.

Backenstose, W.M. and Wells, J.G.: Side Effects of Immersion-type Cleansers on the Metal Components of Dentures, *J. Prosthet. Dent.*, 37, 615, June, 1977.

Budtz-Jorgensen, E.: A 3-months' Study of Enzymes as Denture Cleansers, *J. Oral Rehabil.*, 5, 35, January, 1978.

Budtz-Jorgensen, E. and Kelstrup, J.: Enzymes as Denture Cleansers, *Scand. J. Dent. Res.*, 85, 209, March, 1977.

Budtz-Jorgensen, E. and Knudsen, A.M.: Chlorhexidine Gel and Steradent Employed in Cleaning Dentures, *Acta Odontol. Scand.*, 36, 83, Number 2, 1978.

Connor, J.N.E., Schoenfeld, C.M., and Taylor, R.L.: An Evaluation of an Enzyme Denture Cleanser, *J. Prosthet. Dent.*, 37, 147, February, 1977.

Gwinnett, A.J. and Caputo, L.: The Effectiveness of Ultrasonic Denture Cleaning, *J. Dent. Res.*, 60, 649, Abstract 1361, Special Issue A, March, 1981.

Mueller, H.J. and Greener, E.H.: Characterization of Some Denture Cleansers, *J. Prosthet. Dent.*, 43, 491, May, 1980.

Muenchinger, F.S.: Evaluation of an Electrosonic Denture Cleaner, *J. Prosthet. Dent.*, 33, 610, June, 1975.

Myers, H.M. and Krol, A.J.: Effectiveness of a Sonic-action Denture Cleaning Program, *J. Prosthet. Dent.*, 32, 613, December, 1974.

Nicholson, R.J., Stark, M.M., and Scott, H.E.: Calculus and Stain Removal from Acrylic Resin Dentures, *J. Prosthet. Dent.*, 20, 326, October, 1968.

Shannon, I.L., McCrary, B.R., and Starcke, E.N.: Removal of Salivary Deposits by Commercial Denture Cleansers, *Gen. Dent.*, 24, 30, November–December, 1976.

Shannon, I.L. and Starcke, E.N.: Higher Performance Denture Cleansers, *N.Y.J. Dent.*, 48, 246, October, 1978.

Overdentures

Cooper, T.M. and Ellinger, C.W.: The Overdenture, in Ellinger, C.W., Rayson, J.H., Terry, J.M., and Rahn, A.O.: *Synopsis of Complete Dentures.* Philadelphia, Lea & Febiger, 1975, pp. 309–319.

Davis, R.K., Renner, R.P., Antos, E.W., Schlissel, E.R., and Baer, P.N.: A Two-Year Longitudinal Study of the Periodontal Health Status of Overdenture Patients, *J. Prosthet. Dent.*, 45, 358, April, 1981.

Feldstein, S. and Teitel, M.: The Immediate Overdenture, *J. Am. Dent. Assoc.*, 93, 775, October, 1976.

Fenton, A.H. and Hahn, N.: Tissue Response to Overdenture Therapy, *J. Prosthet. Dent.*, 40, 492, November, 1978.

Key, M.C.: Topical Fluoride Treatment of Overdenture Abutments, *Gen. Dent.*, 28, 58, May–June, 1980.

Licht, W.S. and Leveton, E.E.: Overdentures for Treatment of Severe Attrition, *J. Prosthet. Dent.*, 43, 497, May, 1980.

Lord, J.L. and Teel, S.: The Overdenture: Patient Selection, Use of Copings, and Follow-up Evaluation, *J. Prosthet. Dent.*, 32, 41, July, 1974.

Reitz, P.V., Weiner, M.G., and Levin, B.: An Overdenture Survey: Preliminary Report, *J. Prosthet. Dent.*, 37, 246, March, 1977.

Reitz, P.V., Weiner, M.G., and Levin, B.: An Overdenture Survey: Second Report, *J. Prosthet. Dent.*, 43, 457, April, 1980.

Renner, R.P., Foerth, D., and Pesserillo, E.: Maintenance of Root Integrity and Periodontal Health Under Overdentures: a Pilot Study, *Gen. Dent.*, 26, 42, January–February, 1978.

Robbins, J.W.: Success of Overdentures and Prevention of Failure, *J. Am. Dent. Assoc.*, 100, 858, June, 1980.

Thayer, H.H.: Overdentures and the Periodontium, *Dent. Clin. North Am.*, 24, 369, April, 1980.

Toolson, L.B. and Smith, D.E.: A 2-year Longitudinal Study of Overdenture Patients. Part I: Incidence and Control of Caries on Overdenture Abutments, *J. Prosthet. Dent.*, 40, 486, November, 1978.

Partial Dentures

Addy, M. and Bates, J.F.: The Effect of Partial Dentures and Chlorhexidine Gluconate Gel on Plaque Accumulation in the Absence of Oral Hygiene, *J. Clin. Periodontol.*, 4, 41, February, 1977.

Addy, M. and Bates, J.F.: Plaque Accumulation Following the Wearing of Different Types of Removable Partial Dentures, *J. Oral Rehabil.*, 6, 111, April, 1979.

Bates, J.F. and Addy, M.: Partial Dentures and Plaque Accumulation, *J. Dent.*, 6, 285, December, 1978.

Bissada, N.F., Ibrahim, S.I., and Barsoum, W.M.: Gingival Response to Various Types of Removable Partial Dentures, *J. Periodontol.*, 45, 651, September, 1974.

Brill, N., Tryde, G., Stoltze, K., and El Ghamrawy, E.A.: Ecologic Changes in the Oral Cavity Caused by Removable Partial Dentures, *J. Prosthet. Dent.*, 38, 138, August, 1977.

Dail, R.A. and Kopczyk, R.A.: Removable Partial Dentures and Oral Health: A Literature Review, *Periodont. Abstr.*, 25, 122, Number 3, 1977.

El Ghamrawy, E.: Qualitative Changes in Dental Plaque Formation Related to Removable Partial Dentures, *J. Oral Rehabil.*, 6, 183, April, 1979.

El Ghamrawy, E. and Runov, J.: Offsetting the Increased Plaque Formation in Partial Denture Wearers by Tooth Brushing, *J. Oral Rehabil.*, 6, 399, October, 1979.

Gomes, B.C., Renner, R.P., and Baer, P.N.: Periodontal Considerations in Removable Partial Dentures, *J. Am. Dent. Assoc.*, 101, 496, September, 1980.

Rantanen, T., Siirilä, H.S., and Lehvilä, P.: Effect of Instruction and Motivation on Dental Knowledge and Behavior Among Wearers of Partial Dentures, *Acta Odontol. Scand.*, 38, 9, Number 1, 1980.

Rissin, L., House, J.E., Conway, C., Loftus, E.R., and Chauncey, H.H.: Effect of Age and Removable Partial Dentures on Gingivitis and Periodontal Disease, *J. Prosthet. Dent.*, 42, 217, August, 1979.

Stipho, H.D.K., Murphy, W.M., and Adams, D.: Effect of Oral Prostheses on Plaque Accumulation, *Br. Dent. J.*, 145, 47, July 18, 1978.

Schwalm, C.A., Smith, D.E., and Erickson, J.D.: A Clinical Study of Patients 1 to 2 Years After Placement of Removable Partial Dentures, *J. Prosthet Dent.*, 38, 380, October, 1977.

25

The Patient With Complete Rehabilitation

Complete oral rehabilitation refers to the combined treatment of the teeth and periodontium to restore health, function, and physical form. As generally used, *oral rehabilitation* applies to involved extensive restorative procedures in a mouth that cannot be treated with routine dental care. It is also known as *mouth rehabilitation, occlusal rehabilitation, occlusorehabilitation, complete reconstruction,* or *periodontal prosthesis.*

The term *periodontal prosthesis* is used to designate restorative and prosthetic treatment that is necessary for the treatment of advanced periodontal disease. The prosthesis used may be a splint for immobilization or stabilization of a group of teeth or an entire arch, maxillary or mandibular.

Periodontal, restorative, and prosthetic treatments are interdependent. The function and duration of all restorative and prosthetic treatment depend directly on the health of the periodontium which provides the attachment and support necessary for the restored tooth. Likewise, periodontal health is influenced by restorative and prosthetic treatment. Many predisposing factors which contribute to the initiation, development, and progress of periodontal disease are a direct result of untreated dental caries, incomplete or inadequate restorations, unreplaced missing teeth, and inadequate occlusal relationships built into restorations or prostheses.

I. Objectives of Complete Rehabilitation

Objectives for complete rehabilitation involve the same principles as for all oral care and include the need to
A. Restore optimal functional occlusion.
B. Maintain the health of the periodontium.
C. Produce biologically contoured restorations in harmony with normal oral physiology.
D. Replace missing teeth.
E. Provide support to teeth with advanced bone loss and marked mobility.
F. Provide desirable esthetics.
G. Establish acceptable phonetics.

II. Components of Treatment

Complete oral reconstruction means total mouth involvement, which brings in many phases of dentistry, often accomplished by individual specialists. The overall treatment plan may include some or all of the following:
A. Extensive periodontal therapy involving various surgical procedures.
B. Occlusal adjustment.
C. Endodontic therapy.
D. Correction of oral habits.
E. Orthodontic tooth movement.
F. Splinting of teeth temporarily or permanently.

G. Restorations involving individual teeth: crowns, inlays, onlays.

H. Replacement of teeth by fixed and/or removable prostheses.

III. Accomplishment of Treatment

Treatment is usually long and involved for the patient who undergoes complete oral rehabilitation. It requires patience, persistence, and dedication of the patient, dental hygienist, and the dentist.

The dental hygiene treatment plan overlaps into every phase of the total treatment, beginning with the initial preparation of the patient's mouth. Maintenance and supervision of the patient's self-care program is essential throughout restorative and prosthetic therapy, and continuing into the recall phase.

Specific measures for self-care in terms of plaque removal and dental caries prevention must be selected and supervised. The patient is shown how to self-evaluate, so that minor deviations from normal can be recognized and called to the attention of the dentist.

IV. Characteristics of the Rehabilitated Mouth

To select the appropriate methods for plaque control and caries prevention, existing conditions must be identified, such as contour and position of the gingiva, contour of restorations, and problem areas adjacent to fixed prostheses. When these are known, the variety of possible techniques and devices for plaque removal can be reviewed and a plan for care outlined.

A patient who has undergone extensive periodontal therapy and restorative and prosthetic rehabilitation may have some or all of the characteristics listed here. Each condition may require specially selected or adapted plaque control measures. Fixed and removable appliances can provide many areas for plaque and debris retention.

A. Periodontal Findings

1. Gingival recession.
2. Exposed root surfaces.
3. Exposed furcation areas.
4. Alterations of gingival contour: the gingival margins may be rolled or rounded.
5. Changes in size and shape of the gingival embrasures.

a. Missing interdental papillae: wide embrasures with gingival recession and increased root exposure (figure 25–1).

b. Narrowed embrasures: created by overcontoured restorations or variously shaped pontics (figure 25–2).

B. Fixed Partial Denture

The parts of a fixed prosthesis are described on pages 379–380 and in figure 24–1.

A patient may have:

1. Fixed splinting around long segments of, or an entire, arch (figure 25–3).
2. Abutment teeth with difficult access areas adjacent to a pontic.
3. Closed contacts between teeth involved in a multitooth prosthesis.
4. Gingival surfaces of pontics.
5. Embrasures created by pontics may be wide and triangular, or narrow, unnatural, non-self-cleansing areas created by

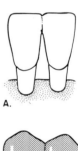

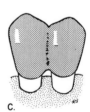

Figure 25–1. Gingival embrasures. **A.** Wide embrasure between two central incisors with missing interdental papilla and gingival recession which resulted from periodontal disease. **B.** Double abutment with closed contact area to show open embrasure which gives access for plaque removal. **C.** Overcontoured crowns of a double abutment showing narrowed embrasure with limited access for cleaning.

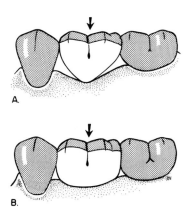

Figure 25–2. Shape of pontics. Mandibular three-unit fixed partial denture to show **A.** "bullet" shape giving wide triangular embrasures for access for cleaning and plaque removal, and **B.** improperly shaped pontic with closed embrasures and wide gingival surface for plaque retention. Arrows indicate pontics.

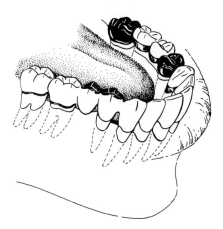

Figure 25–3. Complete arch fixed splint. A continuous therapeutic fixed appliance to stabilize periodontally involved teeth and replace missing components to provide appropriate occlusal relationships. Numerous problem areas for plaque removal exist.

improperly shaped pontics (figure 25–2B).

C. Removable Prostheses

1. *Complete Denture:* may be used in one dental arch opposing natural teeth and partial dentures, fixed or removable.
2. *Removable Partial Denture*
   a. Creation of potential areas of plaque and debris retention.
      (1) Alteration of tooth form by clasp, rest, or precision attachment.

   (2) Improperly contoured edge of partial at the junction of the partial and the abutment tooth.
   b. Partial denture may impinge on the gingiva surrounding the abutment tooth.
   c. Double abutment (two natural teeth with crowns that are soldered or cast together): closed contact requiring lateral (from facial or lingual) access to the gingival embrasure (figure 25–1B and C).
   d. Mucosa under partial denture may be susceptible to plaque retention.

D. Single Tooth Restorations

1. Crowns: gingival margin may appear bluish or bluish/red when the crown margin is below the gingival margin.
2. Various restorations.

V. Self-care of the Rehabilitated Mouth

These special patients require greater than average attention, patience, and teaching skill in order to obtain a favorable result which will assure continuing health of the patient's periodontal tissues. Total commitment on the part of the patient is necessary if the selected plan is to meet the requirements for daily care.

Research has shown that when patients with fixed partial dentures had received special instruction and therefore had been influenced to change their tooth cleansing habits, the periodontal condition about the denture was no different from other parts of the same mouth used as a control. On the other hand, patients in the same study who did not receive instruction showed greater periodontal deterioration about the fixed partial dentures than about their control teeth.[1]

A. Planning the Control Program[2]

The control program should be planned as a concentrated effort to maintain gingival tissue, the tooth structure that is exposed, and hence, the underlying supporting periodontium, as well as the restorations and prostheses. There are two parts to the instructions: first, before the surgical, restorative, and prosthetic treatment; and, second, after reconstruction.

1. *Part 1.* Basic plaque control measures are learned and practiced by the patient during the preparatory phase. The same treatment plan outlined on page 329 is typical of the procedure that can be used in conjunction with scaling appointments. During these lessons, principles for self-evaluation can be presented.

2. *Part 2.* After therapy is completed, another set of self-care procedures is required in order to meet the needs of the rehabilitated mouth. Special devices and techniques are selected and tried until the most efficient and thorough procedures are determined.

3. *Dietary Survey.* Whether the need for the rehabilitation was related to extensive dental caries or periodontal disease, dietary counseling is indicated. Every possible means must be taken to prevent carious lesions of the exposed root surfaces about the restorations. Overall diet factors should be checked to assure support from a nutritional standpoint. Procedures for obtaining the Food Diary and conducting the counseling session are described on pages 425–432.

4. *Fluorides*
   a. Dentifrices: A fluoride dentifrice is needed to strengthen exposed tooth surfaces adjacent to restorations.

      A dentifrice containing monofluorophosphate would generally be selected because of its desensitizing properties (page 556), and because exposed cementum and tooth color restorations could be discolored by stannous fluoride.

   b. Self-application: A daily mouthrinse or custom-tray gel application would be advised to prevent the development of root caries. The use of an overdenture as a fluoride tray was described on page 391.

   c. Topical applications in the dental office: When self-treatment methods are not used on a regular basis, professional topical applications are recommended for each recall appointment.

B. **Plaque Control: Selection of Methods**

Any of the methods and techniques described in Chapters 22, 23, and 24 may be needed in the care of the oral soft tissues, tooth surfaces, restorations, and fixed and removable prostheses. Methods selected must accomplish complete daily plaque removal from each area around every tooth or replacement. A summary of devices and methods is provided in table 25–1.

Most patients need a method for each of the following:

1. Debris removal, particularly from interproximal areas and around fixed prostheses.

2. Sulcular brushing.

3. Interdental plaque removal.
   a. Proximal surfaces of natural and restored teeth including exposed roots where there is access from the incisal or occlusal.
   b. Proximal surfaces of abutment teeth under closed contact areas (figure 25–4).
   c. Mesial and/or distal surfaces of teeth without proximal contact.

4. Fixed partial denture: cleaning and plaque removal.
   a. Gingival surfaces of pontics.
   b. Proximal surfaces of pontics.

5. Removable prosthesis: cleaning.

C. **Procedure**

No fixed procedure can be stated that will apply to every patient. A personalized sequence must be worked out, often by trial and error.

1. Outline a possible sequence.
   a. Select methods and devices that can meet the requirements of the individual oral characteristics (IV, above
   b. Demonstrate the use of the method and have the patient practice under supervision. Avoid presenting too many procedures in one lesson which can confuse and discourage the patient.
   c. Provide step-by-step written directions for home reference.

2. Recheck successes within a few days and at least by one week.

Table 25–1.   Care of the Rehabilitated Mouth

Problem	Device/Method	Special Adaptations
Debris Removal	Water irrigation Toothbrush	Wide embrasures Under fixed partial dentures
Sulcular Brushing	Toothbrush with soft nylon filaments with rounded tips	Facial and lingual surfaces Distals of most-posterior teeth, particularly terminal abutment
Proximal Surfaces plaque removal	Floss Floss with threader Yarn with floss and/or threader Perio-aid Pipe cleaner Interdental brush Single-tufted brush	Abutment teeth Proximal root surfaces Pontic surfaces Narrowed embrasures
Proximal Surfaces without contact with adjacent tooth	Gauze strip Yarn	Terminal abutment of removable partial denture Distals of most-posterior teeth in the dental arch
Exposed Furcation of molars	Pipe cleaner Floss/yarn in threader Interdental brush Interdental rubber tip	Rotated tooth
Exposed Furcation of maxillary first premolar	Perio-aid Interdental rubber tip	Fused root with groove
Exposed Root Surfaces	Perio-aid with dentifrice containing desensitizing agent Nonabrasive dentifrice	Desensitization Prevent abrasion of cementum or dentin
Fixed Partial Denture	Toothbrush (soft nylon) Floss threader with floss/yarn Any other proximal surface procedures as applicable	Gingival surfaces of pontics Proximal surfaces of pontics and retainers
Edentulous Gingiva under removable denture	Toothbrush (soft nylon) (manual or powered)	Stimulation and plaque removal
Tongue Brushing	Toothbrush (soft nylon)	Fissures
Removable Denture	Denture brush Clasp brush Chemical cleanser for immersion	Clasps

a. Evaluate gingival tissue (table 11–1, page 196).
b. Evaluate plaque. Use a disclosing agent to provide the patient with an evaluation of areas that need additional attention.
c. Evaluate technique performance
   (1) Observe patient's dexterity in managing the techniques
   (2) Note relationship of techniques to areas where disclosing agent revealed plaque retention.
d. Make necessary adjustments to simplify, clarify, and assure that all areas are completely deplaqued daily.
3. Reevaluate weekly or as frequently as needed to maintain the patient's motivation, to follow the health of the gin-

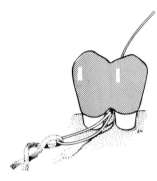

Figure 25–4. Use of floss threader to pull yarn through embrasure created by double abutment. Narrowed embrasure from overcontoured crowns increases plaque and debris retention and makes cleaning difficult. Procedures for use of yarn are on pages 363 and 382.

gival tissues, and to recognize a need for changes in the procedure used.

D. Sample Procedure

The patient described below has a complete maxillary fixed partial denture (splint), which has several natural teeth as abutments and four areas of double pontics; a mandibular removable partial denture with double abutments connecting mandibular canines and first premolars on each side; and wide embrasures between mandibular incisors caused by previous periodontal disease which has since been treated with periodontal surgery.

The patient might use the following procedure:

1. *Morning After Eating*
   a. Complete brushing with powered brush (containing softest filaments available), applying the brush to proximal surfaces.
   b. Brush partial removable denture and rinse thoroughly.
2. *Noon After Eating (away from home)*
   a. Rinse partial under running water.
   b. Use manual toothbrush, covering all surfaces as thoroughly as possible.
   c. Rinse carefully, forcing the water under fixed partial denture areas.
3. *Evening, After All Eating*
   a. Remove partial denture, rinse under running water, and place in cleansing solution. (Complete procedure for

partial removable denture is described on page 392).
   b. Use water irrigator to remove debris from all parts of fixed splint and from all proximal surfaces of mandibular teeth.
   c. Use toothbrush for facial and lingual sulcular brushing, applying the brush interdentally as much as possible. Use fluoride dentifrice.
   d. Brush tongue and edentulous gingiva under removable dentures.
   e. Use dental floss and/or yarn for proximal surfaces accessible from incisal
   f. Clean all gingival and proximal surfaces of fixed partial denture. Use floss and yarn with floss threader for all proximal and gingival surfaces not accessible from incisal or occlusal. Interdental brush may be needed for certain wide embrasures.
   g. Use yarn or gauze strip for distals of the abutment teeth for the mandibular removable denture (mandibular premolars).
   h. Use Perio-aid with dentifrice containing monofluorophosphate or other desensitizing agent to massage hypersensitive areas of exposed roots.
   i. Rinse with fluoride mouthrinse, vigorously forcing the solution between the teeth and under fixed appliances.
   j. Clean partial denture using denture brush and clasp brush, and rinse the denture thoroughly.

VI. Recall

Continuing supervision of the patient with oral rehabilitation is an absolute essential. The well-informed and conscientious patient who devotes up to an hour each day on personal care procedures expects a recall review appointment that thoroughly evaluates the gingival tissue, the rehabilitation appliances, and the completeness of plaque control efforts.

Everything listed on pages 601–602 for inclusion in the recall examination applies with special meaning and emphasis to the rehabilitated patient. What could seem like a minute area of gingival bleeding on probing, whether the pocket is shallow or has started to deepen, should be a warning signal that an area may not be covered by present self-care procedures and needs some form of treatment. *Each millimeter of sulcus-pocket must be probed carefully to detect incipient changes.*

FACTORS TO TEACH THE PATIENT

I. Importance of Daily Care

The health of the periodontal tissues and the duration of the restorations and prostheses depend on the daily self-care by the patient.

II. Need for Concentration

More thought and concentration are required to maintain the mouth with advanced restorative dentistry or periodontal prosthesis than are needed for an average mouth.

III. Time Requirement

It takes longer to clean a mouth with complex restorations. Time must be allotted in the daily schedule for complete cleaning and plaque removal once each day, supplemented by cleaning at least three times each day, or after each meal.

IV. Diligence and Thoroughness

Do not go easy with the brush and other devices in the attempt to protect the restorations from breakage. *Protection* is for the gingival tissues and the preservation of the periodontium, and is accomplished only by thorough plaque removal about every tooth.

V. Recall Importance

The need for frequent, regular recall appointments for professional supervision and cooperative care.

References

1. Silness, J. and Ohm, E.: Periodontal Conditions in Patients Treated with Dental Bridges, V. Effects of Splinting Adjacent Abutment Teeth, *J. Periodont. Res.*, 9, 121, No. 2, 1974.
2. Bradbury, E.: Harvard University School of Dental Medicine, Boston, Massachusetts, personal communication.

Suggested Readings

Balshi, T.J. and Mingledorff, E.B.: Maintenance Procedures for Patients after Complete Fixed Prosthodontics, *J. Prosthet. Dent.*, 37, 420, April, 1977.

Burch, J.G.: Periodontal Considerations in Operative Dentistry, *J. Prosthet. Dent.*, 34, 156, August, 1975.

Carranza, F.A.: *Glickman's Clinical Periodontology*, 5th ed. Philadelphia, W.B. Saunders Co., 1979, pp. 989–1027.

Goldman, H.M. and Cohen, D.W.: *Periodontal Therapy*, 6th ed. St. Louis, The C.V. Mosby Co., 1980, pp. 1112–1154.

Grant, D.A., Stern, I.B., and Everett, F.G.: *Periodontics*, 5th ed. St. Louis, The C.V. Mosby Co., 1979, pp. 886–914.

Moloff, R.L., Stein, S., and Small, S.A.: A Team Effort from Oral Hygiene Instruction to Staple Implant in a Perioprosthetic Case (I), *Quintessence Int.*, 8, 33, August, 1977.

Palomo, F. and Peden, J.: Periodontal Considerations of Restorative Procedures, *J. Prosthet. Dent.*, 36, 387, October, 1976.

Ramfjord, S.P. and Ash, M.M.: *Periodontology and Periodontics*. Philadelphia, W.B. Saunders Co., 1979, pp. 675–690.

Sackett, B.P. and Gildenhuys, R.R.: The Effect of Axial Crown Overcontour on Adolescents, *J. Periodontol.*, 47, 320, June, 1976.

Saltzberg, D.S., Ceravolo, F.J., Holstein, F., Groom, G., and Gottsegen, R.: Scanning Electron Microscope Study of the Junction Between Restorations and Gingival Cavosurface Margins, *J. Prosthet. Dent.*, 36, 517, November, 1976.

Schluger, S., Yuodelis, R.A., and Page, R.C.: *Periodontal Disease*. Philadelphia, Lea & Febiger, 1977, pp. 408–422, 586–611, 620–699.

Silness, J.: Periodontal Conditions in Patients Treated with Dental Bridges. IV. The Relationship Between the Pontic and the Periodontal Condition of the Abutment Teeth, *J. Periodont. Res.*, 9, 50, Number 1, 1974.

Valderhaug, J. and Birkeland, J.M.: Periodontal Conditions in Patients 5 Years Following Insertion of Fixed Prostheses. Pocket Depth and Loss of Attachment, *J. Oral Rehabil.*, 3, 237, July, 1976.

Valderhaug, J. and Heløe, L.A.: Oral Hygiene in a Group of Supervised Patients with Fixed Prostheses, *J. Periodontol.*, 48, 221, April, 1977.

26

Disclosing Agents

A disclosing agent is a preparation in liquid, tablet, or lozenge form which contains a dye or other coloring agent. In dentistry a disclosing agent is used for the identification of soft deposits for instruction, evaluation, and research.

When applied to the teeth, the agent imparts its color to soft deposits but can be rinsed readily from clean tooth surfaces. After staining, the deposits that can be distinctly seen provide a valuable visual aid in patient instruction. Such a procedure can demonstrate dramatically to the patient the presence of deposits and the areas that need special attention during personal oral care.

I. Purposes

A disclosing agent clearly demarcates soft deposits which might otherwise be invisible, and therefore facilitates

A. Personalized patient instruction in the location of soft deposits and the techniques for removal.
B. Self-evaluation by the patient on a daily basis during initial instruction and periodic checks thereafter.
C. Continuing evaluation of the effectiveness of the instruction for the patient
   1. To determine the need for revisions of the plaque control procedures.
   2. To study the long-term effects over successive recall appointments.
D. Preparation of plaque indices.

E. Research studies to gain new information about the incidence and formation of deposits on the teeth, the effectiveness of specific devices for plaque control, antiplaque agents, and to evaluate clinical and instructional group health programs.

II. Properties of an Acceptable Disclosing Agent

A. Intensity of Color

A distinct staining of deposits should be evident. The color should contrast with normal colors of the oral cavity.

B. Duration of Intensity

The color should not rinse off with ordinary rinsing methods, or be removable by the saliva for the period of time required to complete the instruction or clinical service. It is desirable for the color to be removed from the gingival tissue and lips by the completion of the appointment, as the patient may have a personal reaction to color retained for a long period of time.

C. Taste

The patient should not be made uncomfortable by an unpleasant or highly flavored substance. The main reason for using the disclosant is to motivate the patient; therefore the use of the agent should be pleasant and encourage cooperation.

D. Irritation to the Mucous Membrane

The patient should be questioned concerning the possibility of an idiosyncrasy to an ingredient. When this information is obtained, it should be entered on the patient's permanent history record. Because of the possibility of allergy, more than one type of disclosing agent should be available for use.

E. Diffusibility

A solution should be thin enough so it can be applied readily to the exposed surfaces of the teeth, yet thick enough to impart an intensive color to bacterial plaque.

F. Astringent and Antiseptic Properties

These properties may be highly desirable in that the disclosing agent may contribute other factors to the techniques. It is frequently recommended that an antiseptic be applied prior to scaling, and if an antiseptic disclosing agent is used, one solution serves a dual purpose.

A disclosant may inhibit the growth of microorganisms. In quantitative plaque research studies, therefore, it would be necessary to use disclosing agents lacking antibacterial properties.

III. Formulae

A wide variety of disclosing agents has been used. Skinner's Iodine Solution was formerly the most classic and widely used. In general, iodine solutions are less desirable because of their unpleasant flavor.

Aniline dyes have been shown to have carcinogenic potential. Therefore, the use of basic fuchsin and beta rose (flavored basic fuchsin) has been discouraged.

The formulae of a few disclosing agents are included in this chapter. Other well-known ones are Buckley's, Berwick's, Talbot's Iodo-glycerol, and Metaphen solutions.

A. Iodine Preparations

1. Skinner's Solution

Iodine crystals	3.3	g.
Potassium iodide	1.0	g.
Zinc iodide	1.0	g.
Water (distilled)	16.0	ml.
Glycerin	16.0	ml.

2. Diluted Tincture of Iodine

Tincture of iodine	21.0	ml.
Water (distilled)	15.0	ml.

B. Mercurochrome Preparations

1. Mercurochrome Solution (5%)

Mercurochrome	1.5	g.
Water (distilled) to make	30.0	ml.

2. Flavored Mercurochrome Disclosing Solution

Mercurochrome	13.5	g.
Water (distilled)	3.0	L.
Oil of peppermint	3	drops
Artificial noncariogenic sweetener		

C. Bismarck Brown (Easlick's Disclosing Solution)

Bismarck Brown	3.0	g.
Ethyl alcohol	10.0	ml.
Glycerin	120.0	ml.
Anise (flavoring)	1	drop

D. Merbromin

Merbromin, N.F.	450.0	mg.
Oil of peppermint	1	drop
Distilled water to make	100.0	ml.

E. Erythrosin

1. Concentrate for Application by Rinsing

F.D.C. Red No. 3	6.0	g.
Water to make	100.0	ml.

2. For Direct Topical Application

Erythrosin	0.8	g.
Water (distilled)	100.0	ml.
Alcohol (95%)	10.0	ml.
Oil of peppermint	2	drops

3. Tablet[1]

F.D.C. Red No. 3	15.0 mg.
Sodium chloride	.747%
Sodium sucaryl	.747%
Calcium stearate	.995%
Soluble saccharin	.186%
White oil	.124%
Flavoring	2.239%

Sorbitol to make a 7 grain tablet

F. Fast Green

F.D.C. Green No. 3.	5% or 2.5%

G. Fluorescein[2]

F.D.C. Yellow No. 8 (used with a special ultraviolet light source to make the agent visible)

I. **Two-tone**[3]

　　F.D.C. Green No. 3
　　F.D.C. Red No. 3

IV. **Technique for Application**

A. **Solution for Direct Application**

1. Dry the teeth with compressed air, retracting cheek or tongue.
2. Use very small cotton pellet with cotton pliers to carry the solution to the teeth.
3. Apply solution to the crowns of the teeth only.
4. Direct the patient to spread the agent over all surfaces of the teeth with the tongue.
5. Examine the distribution of agent and request the patient to rinse if indicated.

B. **Rinsing**

A few drops of a concentrated preparation are placed in a paper cup and water is added for the appropriate dilution. Instruct the patient to rinse and swish the solution over all tooth surfaces.

C. **Tablet or Wafer**

The patient chews the wafer (one half may be sufficient for some patients), swishes it around for 30 to 60 seconds, and rinses.

D. **Effect**

Clean tooth surfaces do not absorb the coloring agent; when pellicle and dental plaque are present they absorb the agent and are disclosed. Pellicle stains as a thin, relatively clear covering, whereas dental plaque appears darker, thicker, and more opaque.

The oral mucous membrane and lips may retain the color from certain disclosing agents. Application of petrolatum or other coating substance may prevent absorption of the color by the lips.

V. **Patient Instruction**

Since plaque and pellicle are frequently invisible to a patient, a disclosing agent can provide a method for patient instruction.

A. **Explain Plaque**

The patient needs to be informed about the composition and effect of plaque in the production of gingival and periodontal diseases, with particular reference to the individual mouth.

B. **Show Location and Distribution of Plaque**

With a hand mirror the patient can observe the teeth and the disclosed bacterial plaque. A small mouth mirror is needed to show the lingual surfaces and posterior facial areas.

C. **Demonstrate Methods for Daily Plaque Removal**

A plan of instruction is outlined in Chapter 27. The techniques for toothbrushing and associated procedures were described in the previous chapters.

TECHNICAL HINTS

I. Avoid using disclosing or antiseptic solutions on teeth that have silicate cement or resin restorations as these materials may be stained by coloring agents.

II. Purchase solutions in small quantities. Do not keep solutions containing alcohol longer than 2 or 3 months since the alcohol will evaporate and render the solution too highly concentrated.

III. Use small bottles with dropper caps for solutions. Transfer solution to a dappen dish for use. Do not contaminate the solution by dipping cotton pliers with pellet directly into the container bottle.

IV. Use only small, unsaturated cotton pellets with adequate retraction of cheeks and tongue to aid in the control of staining of tongue and alveolar mucosa.

V. Maintain a list of methods for spot removal in case the dye-containing solutions are inadvertently spilled.

VI. Request local druggists to stock disclosing tablets for patients to purchase. Advise patients of the stores where the agents may be purchased.

FACTORS TO TEACH THE PATIENT

I. Purposes for use of disclosing agents: the appearance of stained dental plaque and the methods of daily care necessary to keep plaque controlled.

II. Self-evaluation of plaque control methods by using a disclosing agent.

III. For the parent: method of application of a disclosing agent to a small child's teeth to evaluate the presence of plaque.

References

1. Arnim, S.S.: Use of Disclosing Agents for Measuring Tooth Cleanliness, *J. Periodontol.*, 34, 227, May, 1963.
2. Lang, N.P., Østergaard, E., and Löe, H.: A Fluorescent Plaque Disclosing Agent, *J. Periodont. Res.*, 7, 59, Number 1, 1972.
3. Block, P.L., Lobene, R.R., and Derdivanis, J.P.: A Two-tone Dye Test for Dental Plaque, *J. Periodontol.*, 43, 423, July, 1972.

Suggested Readings

American Dental Association, Council on Dental Therapeutics: *Accepted Dental Therapeutics*, 39th ed. Chicago, American Dental Association, 1982, p. 338.

American Dental Association, Council on Dental Materials, Instruments and Equipment: *Dentist's Desk Reference: Materials, Instruments and Equipment*, 1st ed. Chicago, American Dental Association, 1981, pp. 339–340.

Barton, J.E.: Disclosants: Their Role in Dentistry, *Dent. Hyg.*, 55, 31, January, 1981.

Begue, W.J., Bard, R.C., and Koehne, G.W.: Microbial Inhibition by Erythrosin, *J. Dent. Res.*, 45, 1464, September–October, 1966.

Caldwell, R.C. and Hunt, D.E.: A Comparison of the Antimicrobial Activity of Disclosing Agents, *J. Dent. Res.*, 48, 913, September–October, 1969.

Cohen, D.W., Stoller, N.H., Chace, R., and Laster, L.: A Comparison of Bacterial Plaque Disclosants in Periodontal Disease, *J. Periodontol.*, 43, 333, June, 1972.

Gallagher, I.H.C., Fussell, S.J., and Cutress, T.W.: Mechanism of Action of a Two-tone Plaque Disclosing Agent, *J. Periodontol.*, 48, 395, July, 1977.

Gillings, B.R.D.: Recent Developments in Dental Plaque Disclosants, *Aust. Dent. J.*, 22, 260, August, 1977.

Katayama, T., Suzuki, T., and Okada, S.: Clinical Observation of Dental Plaque Maturation. Application of Oxidation-reduction Indicator Dyes, *J. Periodontol.*, 46, 610, October, 1975.

Kieser, J.B. and Wade, A.B.: Use of Food Colourants as Plaque Disclosing Agents, *J. Clin. Periodontol.*, 3, 200, November, 1976.

Pitcher, G.R., Newman, H.N., and Strahan, J.D.: Access to Subgingival Plaque by Disclosing Agents Using Mouthrinsing and Direct Irrigation, *J. Clin. Periodontol.*, 7, 300, August, 1980.

Squillaro, R.C., Cohen, D.W., and Laster, L.: A Comparison of Microbial Plaque Disclosants After Personal Oral Hygiene Instruction and Prophylaxis, *J. Prev. Dent.*, 2, 3, March–April, 1975.

Tan, A.E.S. and Wade, A.B.: The Role of Visual Feedback by a Disclosing Agent in Plaque Control, *J. Clin. Periodontol.*, 7, 140, April, 1980.

27

Plaque Control: Instruction Procedures

People will learn and adhere to the principles and details of methods for the prevention and control of dental caries and periodontal diseases in proportion to the concern and professional enthusiasm shown for their future oral health by members of the dental team. Specialized knowledge of dental and periodontal diseases and skill in teaching foster confidence, but of greatest importance is *conviction* that careful treatment and teaching for the particular patient is worthwhile.

An effective teaching program provides both detailed information and principles to guide and motivate the patient to cooperate in optimal personal management. The overall teaching objective is to assist the patient to acquire knowledge, attitudes, and practices that will aid in attaining and maintaining oral health.

I. Planned Instruction

Instruction needs to be planned if it is to stay directed toward goals, utilize available time efficiently, and help the patient to learn sequentially, from the simpler to the more complex. The design of instruction may be divided into certain basic steps.

A. Objectives

What knowledge and skills will be expected of the learner-patient after instruction?

B. Presentation

What knowledge-content must be in-cluded? How will the patient be oriented to the overall requirements for reaching the goals? Which instructional methods can be most helpful? What teaching aids will be most efficient?

C. Demonstration

What mode of demonstration will be most meaningful to this patient? What is the sequence of steps in the procedures to be learned? How can the steps be shown for sequential learning?

D. Practice

How will the procedures be practiced? How much practice will be needed? How can knowledge and skill-practice be integrated?

E. Evaluation

Can the patient demonstrate the procedures for self-care? Do the teeth and gingiva show the benefits of learning? Does the patient show basic understanding and motivation for continuing care?

The suggested procedure for patient instruction outlined in this chapter will follow these five steps. There are numerous modes of presentation, demonstration, motivation, and practice that can be used.

Each dental hygienist will develop patient-centered systems of instruction which prove effective, and which are in accord with the policies and beliefs of the dentist. The important considerations for the methods used are that they are based on current, sound, scientific knowledge, and that they are applied efficiently so that the patient acquires the skill and know-how for adequate daily self-care.

II. Principles of Learning[1]

A. Learning is more effective when an individual is physiologically and psychologically ready to learn.
B. Individual differences must be considered if effective learning is to take place.
C. Motivation is essential for learning.
D. What an individual learns in a given situation depends upon what is recognized and understood.
E. Transfer of learning is facilitated by recognition of similarities and dissimilarities between past experiences and the present situation.
F. An individual learns what is actually used.
G. Learning take place more effectively in situations from which the individual derives feelings of satisfaction.
H. Evaluation of the results of instruction is essential to determine whether or not learning is taking place.

INDIVIDUAL PATIENT PROGRAM

Each patient has personal requirements for self-care, and objectives to fulfill these requirements must be related realistically to individual needs, interests, and ability level. If the patient is to participate effectively in the learning process, there must be active involvement in setting goals.

The general objectives for disease control and oral physical therapy described on page 335 provide the basis for the goals of an individual patient. The primary goal is plaque control, and the objectives for action are selected to accomplish this.

I. Selection of Objectives

From the patient history, oral examination, radiographs, study casts, all other data collected during the initial evaluation, and the diagnosis, details of the self-care program are evolved. The factors considered for toothbrush selection (page 342) are included in the total program.

The items listed below summarize factors that must be considered.

A. **The Gingiva**
   1. *Current Status of Gingival Health:* as evidenced by the color, size, contour, consistency, surface texture, and tendency to bleed.
   2. *Treatment Plan:* whether to be treated by scaling and root planing, or whether the condition will require more complicated periodontal therapy.
   3. *Specific Anatomic Features*
      a. Open interdental areas or intact interdental gingiva.
      b. Recession with root exposure.
      c. Evidence of previous detrimental practices.

B. **The Teeth**
   1. *Position*
      a. Malrelations, such as crowding, overbite, crossbite; malpositions of individual teeth; normal alignment.
      b. Teeth adjacent to edentulous areas.
   2. *Abutment Teeth.*
   3. *Dental Appliances:* fixed, removable, orthodontic.

C. **General Health**
   1. *Chronic Disease:* or other systemic condition which may limit the ability to perform certain tasks or which may cause an exaggerated response of the gingiva to local irritants and require more intensive care.
   2. *Ability of Patient for Self-care:* physical and mental handicaps that require that another person perform plaque control procedures.

D. **Age**
   1. Preschool child requires parental assistance.
   2. Motivation varies with age.

E. **Dexterity**
   1. Occupation which requires manual or digital dexterity may contribute to in-

creased facility in the manipulation of oral care devices.

2. For most patients, dexterity cannot be detected until after instruction has begun.

F. **Motivational Factors**

1. *Immediate Evaluation.* Previous oral health habits can reveal present attitudes and motivation, but frequently a lack of oral cleanliness can be attributed to a lack of knowledge. Many people have had little or no instruction in how to care for their mouths.

2. *Long-range Motivation.* Prejudging a patient's motivation and willingness to carry out prescribed procedures is rarely possible. Some people show tremendous enthusiasm which may be short-lived; other reveal little interest at first, but prove to be highly conscientious.

3. *Motivation Related to Attitude.* Motivation is directly related to the concern and enthusiasm of the members of the dental health team.

II. **Program Outline**

A. **Program Planning**

All of the above factors which apply to an individual patient are matched with the available plaque control and oral physical therapy procedures. These include the selection of a toothbrush, toothbrushing method, interdental care devices and methods, dentifrice, and applied techniques for fixed and removable dental appliances.

With a clear definition of the needs of a patient, a recommended regimen or program can be outlined. The patient is shown the oral condition, changes and benefits which can be expected are explained, and cooperation is solicited. In this framework, the patient helps to formulate the goals that must be accomplished.

B. **Immediate and Long-Range Programs**

Immediate and long-range programs are usually indicated. The immediate program is related to the treatment phase, whereas the long-range program is related to the maintenance phase of care.

The immediate program may be more complicated and intensified than the long-range program. It may seem more complicated to the patient because of the anxieties generally associated with learning new procedures and changing former habits.

The new habits and attitudes acquired during the immediate program phase may aid the transition to the long-range program. With continuing reinforcement of instruction and encouragement, plaque control measures become a part of the daily routine and the health of the oral cavity can be maintained.

C. **When to Teach**

Unless a patient has an unusual amount of calculus, the initial instruction is best given *first*, before any clinical treatment. Reasons related to the educational aspects are as follows:

1. *Emphasis on Importance of Self-care.* Clinical professional services have only short-term effectiveness if the patient does not maintain the plaque control program. If considered first, and first in succeeding appointments, the degree of importance placed on self-care procedures by the dental team will become apparent to the patient.

2. *Teaching Is More Effective.* If instruction is delayed until after the clinical procedures in an appointment,
   a. Time may be limited.
   b. The gingival margin may be sensitive from instrumentation.
   c. Blood clots forming in sulci after scaling and curettage should not be disturbed.
   d. Patient may be tired, anxious to leave, and less receptive to instruction.

3. *Plaque on Patient's Teeth.* With removal of tooth deposits during scaling, the opportunity to utilize the patient's plaque as a demonstrative educational aid is missed. Instruction is more effective when it is specifically concerned with the patient's own oral condition.

PRESENTATION, DEMONSTRATION, PRACTICE

With the use of a disclosing agent, a method

of instruction is available that can clearly and dramatically show the patient what is to be accomplished. Dental plaque is not visible on most teeth without staining. Words fail to impress upon patients that there are bacterial colonies on their teeth and these multitudes of microorganisms, also called microcosms,[2] are the responsible agents for dental and periodontal diseases.

Because of the need for the light and rinsing facilities during the demonstration, instruction may best be given at the dental chair. Without an extensive display of instruments and other equipment to distract the patient, and with the dental hygienist seated beside the dental chair at the patient's eye level, an atmosphere conducive to learning can be created.

A specific area may be set aside and furnished for plaque control instruction in a dental office or clinic. Such an area should be planned with mirrors for the patient to use to observe the stained plaque on posterior teeth and distal surfaces. The patient should also be able to see placement of the toothbrush and floss in all areas of the mouth. Requirements for such a facility for a patient in a wheel chair are described on page 690 and in figure 50–2.

A suggested outline for conducting the plaque control program follows. Various adaptations can be made to adjust the plan to individual patients. A Gingival Index (GI), Plaque Index (P1 I), or other plaque control record can be educational and motivating for patients.[3-5] Indices are described in Chapter 19.

I. First Lesson

A. Objective

Orientation to dental plaque removal.

B. Describe

The formation and composition of dental plaque, its relationship to oral disease, and specifically its relationship to the patient's present condition. Present an overview of the plaque control program, what it can accomplish, and its purposes in relation to professional treatment.

C. Illustrate

Sketch on a pad of paper or use prepared materials. Show a tooth and gingiva and point out where the bacterial masses collect to form plaque. Explain how inflammation develops in the gingiva. The complete description should be divided over more than one instruction period. Too long a "lecture" with too many facts and details at one time may mean the patient cannot absorb any of them.

1. *Patient with Gingivitis.* Show and explain the formation of dental calculus and how periodontal disease can develop if gingivitis is left untreated.
2. *Patient with Periodontitis.* Introduce pocket formation and the reasons for pocket elimination.
3. *Patient Whose Most Severe Problem is Dental Caries.* When a dietary survey will be made, orientation to the preparation of the survey precludes discussion of plaque, sucrose, and dental caries, until the dietary record is obtained (page 425).

D. Demonstrate

1. While the patient observes in a hand mirror, a healthy area of gingiva and an inflamed area can be compared.
2. A probe is used to show the gingival sulcus and increased pocket depth related to periodontal involvement. Bleeding on probing is an important indicator of disease and should be recorded.
3. Remove a sample of plaque with a curet to demonstrate the thickness and consistency of plaque, to use in a test for acid formation (Methyl Red Spot Plate Test, or Snyder Test, pages 435–436) and to use for a phase microscope demonstration.[6,7]

E. The Disclosing Agent

1. *Explain Its Purpose.* Discoloration of plaque shows where the masses of bacteria accumulate.
2. *Apply Disclosing Agent.* Use a topical application, provide diluted concentrate for a rinse, or request the patient to chew a tablet, swish for approximately one minute, and rinse (pages 368–369, 407).
3. *Examine the Teeth with the Patient.* Point out the stained plaque and explain how these areas (generally the proximal sur-

faces and cervical third of the teeth) are adjacent to the gingiva, and therefore the bacteria must be removed to control inflammation.

4. *Record Plaque Score or Index (pages 300–309)*. Explain the score to the patient and use it to compare at future evaluations.

5. *Observe Location*. Observation of the location of disclosed plaque will guide the instruction for plaque removal.

Plaque Removal Instruction

1. *Keep Instruction Simple*. It is usually better not to teach both flossing and brushing during the first control lesson.

2. *Floss First*
   a. Review objective.
   b. Show manner of holding the floss, inserting proximally, pressing around the tooth, and activating for plaque removal (figure 23–1, page 361).
   c. Examine in mirror to observe proximal areas where plaque has been removed.

3. *Brush*. Give a soft brush and ask the patient to remove the stained plaque. No specific brushing instructions should be given at this time so that the patient can concentrate on the single objective related to plaque removal.

4. *After Brushing, Examine the Teeth with the Patient*. The patient will see that accessible plaque was removed.

5. *Explain:* that the use of a toothbrush is the most effective means for plaque control for facial and lingual surfaces and floss for proximal surfaces.

G. Summary of Lesson I

1. Review the basic objectives: to learn about plaque composition, occurrence, and relationship to oral disease; to learn about the use of a disclosing agent to aid in plaque detection and removal.

2. At the first lesson, a specific toothbrushing method is not necessarily presented. The basic objectives should not be obscured by inclusion of excess information or diversion of the patient's thinking by concentration on details of brush position. There are exceptions; for example:

   a. The patient who demonstrates an acceptable brushing technique, whose mouth has been kept reasonably clean and shows no signs of detrimental brushing, may only need to be shown a few special adaptations for the difficult-to-reach areas or other improvements.

   b. The patient who demonstrates a brushing method that is detrimental such as a vigorous horizontal stroke or a haphazard scrub-brush method, and whose teeth and/or gingiva show the effects of harmful brushing, will need an introduction to a less destructive method.

H. Continuation of Appointment

Usually instruction and practice in plaque removal should occupy the first appointment, and clinical services should not be started until the gingival inflammatory clinical signs have been lessened and the patient shows good progress in learning self-care. When calculus removal is initiated, the relation of clinical procedures to plaque control should be made clear to the patient. The satisfactory long-range outcome of scaling, curettage, and other professional treatment is dependent on complete daily plaque removal.

I. End of Appointment Instruction

1. Use of disclosing agent at home: provide patient with tablets or instructions for purchasing. Suggest using a tablet for daily plaque checks.

2. Emphasize the need for cleaning regularly for complete daily plaque removal. Discuss carrying a toothbrush for use when not at home.

3. When extra brushes cannot be supplied, explain that the toothbrush that has been used that day will be kept in the office for use during future appointments. Write down the specific name (number) of the brush for the patient to purchase for home use.

J. Patient Records

Methods, procedures, and patient progress and problems should be recorded following each appointment. The documented record can be reviewed prior to each appointment as a guide to continuing instruction.

II. Second Lesson

A. Objectives

To evaluate patient's success to date and to review and expand the knowledge-content of the previous lesson.

B. Evaluation

1. *Examine the Gingival Tissue with the Patient.* Evaluate and compare with notes recorded from previous examination. Changes in color, size, and bleeding on probing should be noted and recorded.
2. *Apply the Disclosing Agent.* Evaluate the plaque as the patient self-evaluates, using a hand mirror. Chart plaque index or other record and compare, with the patient, with previous scores or indices.

C. Review and Expand Knowledge

1. Invite questions from patient concerning plaque formation and gingival and periodontal diseases to determine how clearly information from the previous lesson was understood and retained.
2. Discuss dentifrice recommendation when information from the dental history and the oral examination indicates the need for a change.
3. Explain why the patient needs a more scientific brushing method (or how a few alterations in the previous method can improve the oral condition).
4. Relate brushing to the treatment phase of oral care.

D. Demonstrate

When not previously done, demonstrate the brushing technique of choice for this particular patient.

1. Show the basic stroke on the anterior teeth where the patient can observe brush position and activation. Explain each step.
2. For certain patients, only the facial aspects are demonstrated and practiced and the lingual is presented in a separate

lesson. Instruction is divided appropriately to permit the patient to learn at a comfortable pace. When a patient has a power-driven brush, it is recommended that initial instruction be given with the manual brush so that proficiency can be attained with both. The patient should be asked to bring the power-driven brush to the next appointment for demonstration and instruction.

E. Practice

1. Each position around each arch must be practiced because of the variations in grasp of brush and hand positions, the difficulty of access, and the individual tooth positions, particularly malpositions.
2. A recommended sequence for brushing which will include all areas and the tongue is discussed with the patient.

F. Instructions for Home Procedures

Use disclosing agent after flossing and brushing to test completeness of plaque removal. A mouth mirror for the patient to use at home can be helpful. Inexpensive plastic mirrors are available specifically for this purpose.

III. Third Lesson

A. Objectives

1. Patients with reasonable mastery of the flossing and brushing methods and who need auxiliary plaque control and oral physical therapy measures (interdental, dental appliances, or other) will begin the third phase of their instruction.
2. When a patient is not ready and the plaque score or index still shows a lack of reasonable skill and motivation, introduction of new material may be postponed and previous instruction reviewed and practiced.
3. Many dentists will postpone therapy until the patient shows that an effective plaque control program can be carried out and an acceptable level of oral cleanliness can be maintained.

B. Evaluation and Review

1. *Evaluate Gingiva.* Inspect with the pa-

tient for color, size, bleeding, and other characteristics of disease. Review the features of normal gingiva and commend improvements. Quadrants that have been scaled and root planed can be compared with other quadrants so that the effect of healing can be shown.

Question the patient relative to changes observed during the past week or since the previous appointment, such as less bleeding when brushing and an overall feeling of cleanliness. Emphasize the role of self-care in accomplishing the improvements rather than the effects of professional treatment.

2. *Evaluate Plaque.* Apply disclosing agent and inspect for areas that need additional instruction. Relate areas of persistent gingival redness to areas inadequately flossed and brushed.
3. *Evaluate Brushing.* Patient demonstrates with emphasis on the areas missed as revealed by gingival and disclosing agent examinations. Help the patient to evaluate and make corrections. Supplement as needed with demonstration.

C. Introduce New Material

Demonstrate auxiliary interdental or other methods; explain the purposes and procedures for each method selected for this patient.

D. Practice

Continued instruction is usually needed for most interdental methods. A specific appointment to check the method of use is particularly important by at least the end of the first week, since incorrect habits may become permanent if allowed to persist.

IV. Continuous Instruction

A. Number of Lessons

It is not possible to predict in advance the number of specific teaching sessions a patient will need to demonstrate mastery of the recommended procedures and to show by the appearance of the teeth and gingiva that the practices have been carried out daily. When additional supervision is indi-

cated after dental hygiene professional treatment has been completed, short appointments may be scheduled in conjunction with dental appointments.

One teaching-learning experience is rarely adequate. When a patient has been able to maintain relatively clean teeth and clinically healthy gingiva and can demonstrate an acceptable toothbrushing method, a review of difficult-to-reach areas can be made and reevaluated at a follow-up appointment.

B. Relationship to Gingival Health

When areas of gingival marginal redness and sponginess persist, tooth surfaces are checked carefully for residual calculus and scaling and planing are completed as indicated. When the patient consistently fails to remove dental plaque in certain areas, a reevaluation of the program is made. Perhaps the selected procedures are too difficult for the patient to accomplish or perhaps supplementary measures are needed.

C. Recall

The first recall after the initial instruction series is best scheduled after a shorter interval than may be used for succeeding recall appointments. It is necessary to evaluate the patient's ability to continue adequate self-care and to determine whether true learning has resulted and new habits have been adopted. Learning means that a change in behavior has occurred.

At each recall appointment, a plaque score or index is recorded, and the patient can evaluate the progress made. The complete procedures for the recall appointment are described on pages 601–602.

V. Instruction Adaptability

The methods for presentation, demonstration, practice, and evaluation described in the previous pages can be adapted readily to various age levels. Awareness of the changing motivation and interests from the young to the elderly, and adaptations of terminology with respect for the patient's level of understanding, ease the transition from patient to patient.

Others for whom instruction is provided are the nurses or family members who attend patients who are unable to care for themselves. In

Section VI, the various chapters that pertain to patients with disabilities include suggestions for patient care. Aids and devices are described on pages 699–702.

THE PRESCHOOL CHILD

The establishment of positive health habits and attitudes in the adult has its beginnings in childhood. Even before birth and during the first year after birth, the parent's education for prevention of dental caries and gingival disease should begin.

After birth, regular daily systemic fluoride in the absence of fluoridation, as well as attention to the control of dietary sucrose, can mean a great deal to the future oral health of the child. Nursing caries syndrome was described on page 241. Information about plaque control for gingival health has application while the child's primary teeth are erupting.

I. Early Plaque Control

Conditioning a child to associate cleaning of the oral cavity with total body cleanliness can begin when the first teeth erupt. A small, soft toothbrush may be used or, at first, the parent can rub the teeth and gingiva with a cloth wrapped over a finger.

As time goes on, the child will want to use the brush, particularly if given the opportunity to watch the parents brush their teeth. At first a tiny child may only chew on the brush, but eventually may try to imitate the parents. Gradually, an actual brushing procedure can be encouraged, which frequently may resemble a scrub-brush technique (page 350).

For several years the parents will have the responsibility for brushing after meals and before the child retires. The age varies with the individual child relative to when the child can take on the responsibility. It has been suggested that when a child attends to bathing, all personal toothbrushing may also be done. Parental supervision and encouragement must continue for a few more years for most children.

II. Professional Instruction

A. The First Dental Appointment

Early visits to the dental office for orientation and getting acquainted are to be encouraged. If the child has not had a dental emergency and therefore visited the dental office earlier, oral examination and necessary treatment are indicated by 2 or, at the latest, 3 years of age. It is recommended that the first appointment be reserved for instruction in plaque control for child and parent.

B. Effect of Age[8,9]

There is a great deal of difference with each year of age of preschoolers. The child at 2 years may be cooperative and well-behaved; at about $2\frac{1}{2}$, contrary and difficult; by 3, amiable and in good control, yet at 4 be difficult and dogmatic. The general suggestions made below should be applied to the individual child, and are presented only as a basis from which instruction can be planned.

C. Instruction for the Child

1. *Toothbrush Selection.* A child-sized, soft nylon brush is recommended. When possible, let the child select the brush from assorted colors.
2. *Method.* Control of dental plaque at the gingival margin and on proximal tooth surfaces requires the same emphasis for the very young as at other ages. Although the very young child will have a short interest span for specific instruction, the mother can be coached to assist with supplementary home instruction. Many dentists favor instruction in a scrub-brush method for preschool children.

III. Instruction for the Parent

The parent who is a patient in the same dental practice may be already familiar with the teaching methods used and well-oriented to the importance of plaque control. Transfer of knowledge and skills to care of the child can be relatively easy. When the child is a patient in a pedodontic specialty practice or the parent is a patient elsewhere, orientation will be needed in accord with the parent's present knowledge.

A. Disclosing Agent

1. When the child will chew a tablet, it is preferable so that the tablets can be used at home for the parent to evaluate. One-

half tablet is sufficient. When a young child cannot understand about chewing the tablet, disclosing solution can be applied.

2. Examination: the child is given a mirror to "watch" the teeth. The plaque deposits are pointed out and discussed with the parent, and a little plaque removed with a probe to illustrate.

B. Demonstration

The brushing method of choice is shown to the parent while the child is in the dental chair under the light.

C. Procedure and Practice

1. *Provide Natural Setting.* Demonstration is given with the child and parent to simulate the home setting. Several positions are possible and are shown in figure 50–6 on page 705.

2. *Demonstrate Head Support.* Show the parent how, if the child's teeth are brushed from the front, the child's head falls back, unsupported, and seeing into the mouth is difficult.

3. *Suggested Standing Position.* Child stands in front of parent and leans back against the parent. Parent cradles the child's head with the nondominant arm and brings the hand around to hold the chin in the palm of the hand and to retract the lips and cheek with the fingers.

4. *Brush Mandibular Teeth.* Retract lip for anterior and cheek for posterior. The back of the brush head will retract the tongue.

5. *Maxillary Teeth.* Child is asked to tip the head back so that the parent can look in the mouth while fingers retract the upper lip for anterior and the cheek for posterior.

6. *Dental Floss.* With the child's head supported as described above for brushing, the parent can be shown how finger and hand rests (fulcrums) can be maintained while floss is applied. When primary teeth are widely spaced, brushing may be adapted to remove plaque from all surfaces without a need for flossing. If necessary, the parent can use nylon yarn for proximal surfaces. Flossing may not

be recommended for all children (page 362).

7. *Dentifrice Recommendation.* A fluoride dentifrice is preferred, even when there is fluoride in the drinking water. When a child has a dental caries problem, brushing the child's teeth with a fluoride gel by the parent may be recommended. As the child matures and rinsing is possible, a daily fluoride rinse can be used.

D. Summary

Instructions include brushing after each meal, using the disclosing test before one of the brushings, and complete plaque removal followed by fluoride supplement (mouthrinse or chewable tablet, page 447) before going to bed.

E. Second Appointment

Procedure follows that of an adult. The gingiva are examined and bleeding on probing evaluated, plaque is disclosed and areas with stain are discovered; the child demonstrates brushing, and then the parent. Suggestions for improvement are offered.

As needed, calculus and stain are removed professionally. Brushing demonstration precedes each succeeding restorative appointment until proficiency is demonstrated.

IV. Recall

Instruction continues with each 4 to 6 months' recall appointment.

THE TEACHING SYSTEM

A simple, direct approach such as has been described, with specific content and unembellished with excess distracting material, focuses the attention of the patient-learner on the central theme: disease control. The more practical, realistic, and goal-centered the components of instruction can be, the more effective the outcomes will be in terms of treatment and prevention of recurrence of disease. An *informed*, knowledgeable patient will have reasons for *practicing* appropriate, scientifically based, self-care measures.

A teaching system must be reevaluated from time to time, particularly as new research reveals new aspects of prevention and treatment.

New devices for plaque removal and gingival care may become available and these need study before recommendations to patients can be made.

The teaching system presented in this chapter has a built-in evaluation of patient learning. The outcomes of learning are shown by examination and demonstration: examination for the gingival characteristics consistent with health, demonstration of disclosable plaque, and the demonstration of the patient's ability to use floss and brush for plaque removal without harm to the oral tissues.

Since the ultimate objective of plaque control is to prevent dental caries and periodontal diseases, the oral health history of the patient over several years will document a true evaluation. The teaching system must involve development of the patient's attitudes relative to continuing professional supervision and regular appointments for examination and treatment.

EVALUATION OF TEACHING AIDS

I. General Characteristics

Evaluation of teaching aids involves consideration of the following:

A. Simplicity

Ease of management, ready obtainability, ease of understanding by the patient.

B. Content

Practical, scientifically sound, meaningful.

C. Level of Orientation

Appropriate to the individual patient.

D. Durability

If reusable, they must maintain their cleanliness and freshness.

E. Cost

Reasonable. Cost relates to their essential value in reaching goals.

F. Objectives

1. Objective of a teaching aid must be clear and readily understood by the patient.

2. In teaching, activities should be reality-centered not fantasy-centered. A well-intentioned visual aid may provide entertainment rather than education and have no transfer value, in terms of the actual oral health lesson, to the behavioral pattern of the patient.

II. Reading Material for the Patient

Effectively presented, informational books and leaflets can supplement and reinforce individually presented instruction. Selected with a purpose, a booklet or other printed material may be presented to the patient to read while at the dental office or it may be given for "homework." The booklet's contents must be reviewed with the patient and particular sections may be marked to personalize the instruction and encourage reading. Indiscriminate distribution of printed materials is pointless.

Obtaining copies and reviewing newly available materials are essential parts of a dental hygienist's work, even as a teacher reviews new textbooks and materials for possible use in a classroom.

Instruction sheets and leaflets can be custommade by the dental hygienist with the cooperation and recommendations of the dentist. It is especially helpful to have postoperative instructions, plaque control, and oral physical therapy procedures outlined so that the patient will have a reference for home use. Materials can be personalized by writing the patient's name and special procedures or reminders.

III. Use of Models

A. Patient's Study Cast

The cast can be useful to explain oral conditions or restorations such as the need to replace missing teeth. With certain patients, aspects of plaque control and oral physical therapy can be demonstrated, provided the patient is properly oriented to associate the cast with the teeth in the mouth.

B. Commercially Available Models

Although plastic models (dentoforms) have been used extensively for teaching toothbrushing methods, their meaningfulness to the patient has not been demonstrated. When a toothbrush is to be available for the patient to practice brushing in his mouth, the usefulness of the time spent to demonstrate on a model first may be questioned. When teaching is by means of the model and brush only, and particularly when the oversized model will be used, the patient's learning should be carefully evaluated. It is suggested that all three of the patient evaluation methods described in this chapter (gingival status, disclosed plaque, and ability of patient to brush) be utilized.

It is probable that the model and the toothbrush do not represent a problem to the patient and that most patients can imitate the movements of the toothbrush on the model accurately when asked. The difficulty comes in transferring the motions to the mouth, and the more complex the technique, the greater the difficulty of transfer.

TECHNICAL HINTS

Sources of Educational Materials

1. American Dental Association, Order Department, 211 East Chicago Avenue, Chicago, Illinois 60611. (Request current year's catalog)
2. American Academy of Periodontology, Public and Professional Relations Committee, 211 East Chicago Avenue, Chicago, Illinois 60611. (Request list of materials)
3. Information Office, National Institute of Dental Research, National Institutes of Health, Bethesda, Maryland 20014. (Request sample copies of Plaque and Periodontal Disease leaflets)

References

1. Sand, O.: *Curriculum Study in Basic Nursing Education.* New York, Putnam's, 1955, pp. 53–60.
2. Arnim, S.S. and Williams, Q.E.: How to Educate Patients in Oral Hygiene, *Dent. Radiogr. Photogr.*, 32, 61, Number 4, 1959.
3. O'Leary, T.J., Drake, R.B., and Naylor, J.E.: The Plaque Control Record, *J. Periodontol.*, 43, 38, January, 1972.
4. Barrickman, R.W. and Penhall, O.J.: Graphing Indexes Reduces Plaque, *J. Am. Dent. Assoc.*, 87, 1404, December, 1973.
5. Garnick, J.J.: Use of Indexes for Plaque Control, *J. Am. Dent. Assoc.*, 86, 1325, June, 1973.
6. Katz, S., McDonald, J.L., and Stookey, G.K.: *Preventive Dentistry.* Upper Montclair, N.J., D.C.P. Publishing, 1977, pp. 119–123.
7. Wren, L.A. and Corrington, J.D.: *Understanding and Using the Phase Microscope.* Unitron Instrument Company, 66 Needham Street, Newton Highlands, Massachusetts, 59 pp.
8. Routh, D.K.: The Preschool Child, in Gabel, S. and Erickson, M.T., eds.: *Child Development and Developmental Disabilities.* Boston, Little, Brown and Company, 1980, pp. 21–42.
9. Wagner, M.: The Child's Introduction to the Dentist, in Forrester, D.J., Wagner, M.L., and Fleming, J., eds.: *Pediatric Dental Medicine.* Philadelphia, Lea & Febiger, 1981, pp. 209–216.

Suggested Readings

Bakdash, M.B. and Keenan, K.M.: An Evaluation of the Effectiveness of Community Preventive Periodontal Education, *J. Periodontol.*, 49, 362, July, 1978.

Barnes, G.P. and Perkins, B.E.: Plaque Control and Oral Hygiene Status of Dental Auxiliary Personnel, *Dent. Hyg.*, 49, 63, February, 1975.

Beedle, G.L., Henderson, W.G., Field, H.M., and Karagan, N.J.: Psychosocial Variables as Predictors of an Improved Oral Health State, *J. Prev. Dent.*, 3, 17, July–August, 1976.

Berk, G.: The Effectiveness of a Dental Hygiene Education Program on Oral Hygiene, *Dent. Hyg.*, 49, 161, April, 1975.

Bowen, D.M. and Darby, M.L.: Effectiveness of the Phase Contrast Microscope, *Dent. Hyg.*, 55, 26, February, 1981.

Chambers, D.W.: Patient Susceptibility Limits to the Effectiveness of Preventive Oral Health Education, *J. Am. Dent. Assoc.*, 95, 1159, December, 1977.

Conte, T.G.: Realistic Dental Care in Jails and Prisons: Summary of Proceedings, *J. Am. Dent. Assoc.*, 102, 343, March, 1981.

Durlak, J.A. and Levine, J.: Seeing Oral Health Patients in Groups, *J. Am. Dent. Assoc.*, 90, 426, February, 1975.

Gift, H., Muller, T., and Newman, J.: Characteristics of Dental Oral Hygiene Education in Private Practice, *J. Prev. Dent.*, 2, 37, January–February, 1975.

Glavind, L. and Attström, R.: Periodontal Self-examination. A Motivational Tool in Periodontics, *J. Clin. Periodontol.*, 6, 238, August, 1979.

Heifetz, S.B., Bagramian, R.A., and Suomi, J.D.: Programs for the Mass Control of Plaque: An Appraisal, *J. Public Health Dent.*, 33, 91, Spring, 1973.

Heløe, L.A. and König, K.G.: Oral Hygiene and Educational Programs for Caries Prevention, *Caries Res.*, 12, 83, Supplement 1, 1978.

Rayant, G.A.: Relationship between Dental Knowledge and Tooth Cleaning Behavior, *Community Dent. Oral Epidemiol.*, 7, 191, August, 1979.

Rogalin, J.A.T.: Designing a Plaque Control Program for General Dentistry Practices, *Dent. Hyg.*, 53, 274, June, 1979.

Young, M.A.C.: Dental Health Education. An Overview of Selected Concepts and Principles Relevant to Programme Planning, *Int. J. Health Educ.*, 13, 2, January–March, 1970.

Communication and Motivation

Barton, D.H. and Busch, K.: Communicate to Educate, *Dent. Surv.*, 54, 42, February, 1978.

Baseheart, J.R.: Nonverbal Communication in the Dentist-patient Relationship, *J. Prosthet. Dent.*, 34, 4, July, 1975.

Emler, B.F., Windchy, A.M., Zaino, S.W., Feldman, S.M., and Scheetz, J.P.: The Value of Repetition and Reinforcement in Improving Oral Hygiene Performance, *J. Periodontol.*, 51, 228, April, 1980.

Gold, S.L.: Establishing Motivating Relations in Preventive

Dentistry, *J. Am. Soc. Prev. Dent.*, 4, 17, November–December, 1974.

Huntley, D.E.: Five Principles of Patient Education, *Dent. Hyg.*, 53, 420, September, 1979.

Jackson, E.: Effective Persuasion in Dental Practice, *J. Am. Soc. Prev. Dent.*, 5, 15, May–June, 1975.

Kaplis, N., Drolette, M., Boffa, J., and Kress, G.: A Longitudinal Study of Multiple Approaches to Dental Health Education, *Community Dent. Oral Epidemiol.*, 7, 133, June, 1979.

Levy, R.L., Weinstein, P., and Milgrom, P.: Behavioral Guidelines for Plaque Control Programs, *Dent. Hyg.*, 51, 13, January, 1977.

MacDonald, K.: Affective Patient Education, in Boundy, S.S. and Reynolds, N.J., eds.: *Current Concepts in Dental Hygiene*, Volume 2. St. Louis, The C.V. Mosby Co., 1979, pp. 199–206.

Rayant, G.A. and Sheiham, A.: An Analysis of Factors Affecting Compliance with Tooth-cleaning Recommendations, *J. Clin. Periodontol.*, 7, 289, August, 1980.

Shulman, J.: Current Concepts of Patient Motivation Toward Long Term Oral Hygiene: A Literature Review, *J. Am. Soc. Prev. Dent.*, 4, 7, November–December, 1974.

Siewert, J.: A Review of the Preventive Dentistry Counseling Approach, *Dent. Hyg.*, 53, 262, June, 1979.

Children

Albino, J.E., Tedesco, L.A., and Lee, C.Z.: Peer Leadership and Health Status: Factors Moderating Response to a Children's Dental Health Program, *Clin. Prev. Dent.*, 2, 18, January–February, 1980.

Bird, W.F. and Hazel, D.R.: Parental Dental Health Education, Non-effect on Oral Hygiene Among American Indian Pre-school (Headstart) Children, *J. Prev. Dent.*, 3, 5, July–August, 1976.

Blinkhorn, A.S.: Influence of Social Norms on Toothbrushing Behavior of Preschool Children, *Community Dent. Oral Epidemiol.*, 6, 222, September, 1978.

Chambers, D.W.: Communicating with the Young Dental Patient, *J. Am. Dent. Assoc.*, 93, 793, October, 1976.

Claus, J. and Alexander, K.: Dental Health Programs in Preschools, *Dent. Hyg.*, 55, 21, February, 1981.

Englander, H.R.: Supervised Deplaquing and Improved Gingival Health in a School Program, *J. Periodontol.*, 50, 394, August, 1979.

Fanning, E.A. and Leppard, P.I.: Oral Hygiene Home Care Kits: Effects on the Dental Behaviour of Kindergarten Children, *Aust. Dent. J.*, 20, 39, February, 1975.

Frazier, P.J.: School-based Instruction for Improving Oral Health: Closing the Knowledge Gap, *Int. Dent. J.*, 30, 257, September, 1980.

Gill, S. and Jorstad, M.E.: A Public School Preventive Dental Health Program, *Dent. Hyg.*, 54, 281, June, 1980.

Horowitz, A.M., Suomi, J.D., Peterson, J.K., Vogelsong, R.H., and Mathews, B.L.: Effects of Supervised Daily Dental Plaque Removal by Children: First-year Results, *J. Public Health Dent.*, 36, 193, Summer, 1976.

Horowitz, A.M., Suomi, J.D., Peterson, J.K., and Lyman, B.A.: Effects of Supervised Plaque Removal by Children: II. 24 Months' Results, *J. Public Health Dent.*, 37, 180, Summer, 1977.

Hudson, L.C.: A School Plaque Control Program for First Grade, *Dent. Hyg.*, 48, 299, September–October, 1974.

Huntley, D.E.: A Dental Health Program for Fifth Graders: Results After Three Months, *Dent. Hyg.*, 53, 380, August, 1979.

Keith, K.D., Wentz, F.M., and Wood, R.M.: A Practical Behavior-based Oral Hygiene Program for Elementary School Children, *J. Am. Dent. Assoc.*, 94, 1183, June, 1977.

Linn, E.L.: Mother's Involvement in Children's Oral Hygiene, *J. Am. Dent. Assoc.*, 92, 398, February, 1976.

Mescher, K.D., Brine, P., and Biller, I.: Ability of Elementary School Children to Perform Sulcular Tooth-brushing as Related to Their Hand Function Ability, *Pediatr. Dent.*, 2, 31, March, 1980.

Sangnes, G.: Effectiveness of Vertical and Horizontal Toothbrushing Techniques in the Removal of Plaque, II Comparison of Brushing by Six-year-old Children and Their Parents, *J. Dent. Child.*, 41, 119, March–April, 1974.

Shaw, O.: Dental Anxiety in Children, *Br. Dent. J.*, 139, 134, August 19, 1975.

Sutcliffe, P., Wishart, W.A., and Clemson, N.: Supervised Toothbrushing in a Nursery School, *Br. Dent. J.*, 142, 192, March 15, 1977.

Telford, A.B. and Murray, J.J.: The Effect of Systematic Chairside Oral Hygiene Instruction on Gingivitis and Oral Cleanliness in Children, *Community Dent. Oral Epidemiol.*, 2, 50, Number 2, 1974.

Terhune, J.A.: Predicting the Readiness of Elementary School Children to Learn an Effective Dental Flossing Technique, *J. Am. Dent. Assoc.*, 86, 1332, June, 1973.

Tsamtsouris, A., White, G.E., and Clark, E.R.: The Effect of Instruction and Supervised Toothbrushing on the Reduction of Dental Plaque in Kindergarten Children, *J. Dent. Child.*, 46, 204, May–June, 1979.

28

Nutrition, Diet, and Dietary Analysis

Planning for a total preventive program for an individual patient involves consideration of dietary and nutritional factors. The status of oral health can be affected by nutrition, diet, and food habits. Since proper nutrition improves general health, it follows that improved general health can contribute to a higher degree of oral health.

Instruction relating to diet is coordinated with other phases of teaching. To give information about a diet conducive to oral health is a responsibility, and to help motivate a patient to adopt new eating patterns, a challenge.

Food selection by an individual is influenced by age, sex, geographic location, economic status, available foods, family traditions, religion, cultural habits, prejudices, fallacies, and advertising, as well as emotional and social factors. Instruction must be made practical and possible to apply if it is to have impact on such forceful influences.

I. Definitions

A. Nutrition

The term nutrition refers to the combination of processes by which the living organism receives and utilizes the materials (food) necessary for the maintenance of its functions and for the growth and renewal of its components.

B. Diet

The diet is the total food and drink regularly consumed.

C. Nutrients

Nutrients are those chemical substances in food that are needed by the body. They are divided into six classes: proteins and amino acids, fats and fatty acids, carbohydrates, mineral elements, vitamins, and water.

D. Nutritional Deficiency

A nutritional deficiency means there is an inadequacy of nutrients in the tissues. A deficiency may be the result of inadequate dietary intake, or impairment in digestion, absorption, transport metabolism, or excretion.

II. Periodontal Tissues[1,2,3]

A. Nutritional Deficiencies

1. Protein, vitamins, and other nutrients are essential to the health of the periodontal tissues, just as they are for the tissues throughout the body.
2. A nutritional deficiency has never been shown to be the specific cause of periodontal pocket formation, gingivitis, or periodontal disease. For these condi-

tions to develop, local irritants must be present, particularly plaque.

3. Certain nutritional deficiencies (notably protein, ascorbic acid, and vitamin B complex) modify gingival tissue resistance so that an inflammatory condition (initiated by plaque bacteria) may be accelerated or increased in intensity.
4. The effects of periodontal disease can alter the capacity of the tissues to utilize available nutrients; therefore, the potential for repair is modified.

B. Consistency of Food

1. Soft sticky foods cling to the teeth and gingiva and encourage food and debris accumulation, increased dental plaque, and calculus formation.
2. Firm fibrous foods may stimulate the tissues and improve circulation. Fibrous foods (particularly uncooked fruits and vegetables) tend to clear away loose debris and impart a generally clean sensation. They do not remove plaque from the cervical area.[4]

C. Dietary Analysis

Patients with acute gingival disease, necrotizing ulcerative gingivitis, and most patients undergoing periodontal therapy need specific instruction in diet selection. A dietary survey with analysis is important if a true idea of the patient's diet is to be available for study. Procedures for the survey and analysis are described later in this chapter.

III. Mucous Membranes

A. Nutritional Deficiencies

Severe nutritional deficiencies are rare except in underdeveloped areas of the world. Deficiencies tend to produce symptoms of mixed clinical entities, but infrequently of a severe acute disease. When certain oral symptoms suggest nutritional deficiencies, the patient would most likely be suffering from multiple deficiencies.

Ordinarily, the effects of a deficiency would be chronic in nature and run a slow, gradual course. The clinical manifestations are influenced by trauma, local irritation, or

systemic factors, such as a chronic disease, which act on tissue resistance.

B. Oral Lesions

Types of oral lesions that suggest the possibility of an underlying nutritional deficiency are stomatitis, glossitis, cheilitis, and localized ulcerations and areas of atrophic change.[5] Definitive diagnosis by the dentist is difficult or impossible even with the patient history, a dietary analysis, and laboratory tests. Nutrients that are considered particularly associated with the health of the oral mucosa are iron, ascorbic acid, and various B vitamins.

C. Instruction

Assistance to patients through recommendations for an adequate diet for general health will contribute to preserving the integrity of the oral mucosa.

IV. Dental Caries[3,6]

A. Prevention

The nutrient fluoride is the essential tooth component for dental caries prevention. A deficiency of fluoride during the years of tooth formation results in an increase in carious lesions when exposed to a cariogenic diet.

B. Role of Cariogenic Foods

Dental caries is the result of action on the external surface of the tooth. Instead of being a deficiency disease, it can be considered the result of an excess of cariogenic foods. Dietary sugars produce acids when acted upon by specific plaque bacteria. These factors were discussed in connection with dental plaque, pages 269–271.

C. Dietary Analysis

The use of a dietary analysis in the instruction of patients and their parents relative to dental caries control has proven helpful to many people. The dental caries control study is described later in this chapter.

DAILY FOOD REQUIREMENTS

Patient instruction centers around helping paients learn which foods make up an adequate diet and improve their food selection. Poor food habits, such as missed meals, omission of essential foods, regular use of non-nutritious snacks, or illogical, unsupervised dieting, frequently are important to recommendations related to nutritional practices for oral health. Generalities may be useful to a degree; but for daily application, specific suggestions for meal planning and food selection are needed.

The information in this chapter and the suggestions for application assume that there has been an opportunity to study the science of nutrition comprehensively. It is also expected that reference books and other materials are available. Knowledge of sources of informational leaflets which can be made available to provide patients with useful, practical facts about diet and meal planning is necessary. Continued review of new materials constitutes an important phase of teaching.

I. Recommended Dietary Allowances[7]

A standard of dietary adequacy was prepared by the United States National Research Council for certain nutrients. The daily allowances specified are considered adequate to meet the known nutritional needs of healthy persons.

Recommended daily dietary allowances are not the same for all, are not recommended as an ideal diet, and do not include special needs such as during illness. The figures are intended as a guide. The designations of the amounts of nutrients are impractical for patient instruction. To be meaningful, nutrients must be expressed in terms of the foods that contain them and how much of each of these foods must be used daily to meet the requirements.

II. The Food Groups

To fulfill minimum requirements of nutrients for the maintenance of health and resistance to disease is not a problem when a wide variety of foods is included in the diet each day. The foods that contain the essential nutrients, called foundation or protective foods, have been divided into four food groups: the milk group, the meat group, the vegetable-fruit group, and the bread-cereal group.

Table 28–1 provides a summary of the groups, examples of foods included in each, the rec-

ommended daily servings, and the major nutrients each group contributes to the diet.

III. Applications

The size of the servings of the protective foods (table 28–1, middle column) varies with age and physiologic states. Servings for children will be smaller, for teen-agers extra large or increased in number. Nutritional requirements for teenage boys are higher than at any other time in their lives, and for girls the only time they will be higher will be during pregnancy or lactation. Dietary requirements for pregnancy are summarized in the chapter on prenatal care, pages 611–612.

With old age, total requirements decrease, but the components of the daily requirements remain the same. Tissue building and repair continue throughout life, and nutrients must be supplied accordingly. Problems of the diet of aging persons are summarized on pages 631–633.

THE DIETARY ANALYSIS

A dietary analysis is used as a guide for instruction of the patient.* Whether the analysis is made to help a patient whose major oral health problem is dental caries or periodontal disease, the same general procedures can be followed.

The type of dietary analysis made is sometimes referred to as *qualitative*. It takes into consideration the general food groups essential or detrimental to good oral health and does not pretend to show precise mathematical calculations of the chemical constituents as does the *quantitative* type of dietary analysis. The nutritionist is skilled in making detailed quantitative diet analyses and works under the direction of the physician to provide specific therapeutic diets for physiologic and pathologic conditions.

I. Objectives of a Dietary Analysis

A. To provide an opportunity for a patient to study, objectively, personal dietary habits.
B. To obtain an overall picture of the types of food in the patient's diet, food preferences, and quantity of food eaten.
C. To study the food habits with particular reference to frequency and regularity of eating and the order in which food is taken.

---

*The word "patient" is used to mean the patient and the parent when the patient is a child.

Table 28–1. Food for an Adequate Diet

Food Group	Recommended Daily Amount		Contribution to Diet
Milk Group	Servings*		
Milk: whole, evaporated, skim, dry, buttermilk **Cheese** and other milk products	Children under 9 Children 9 to 12 Teen-age Adults Pregnant women Nursing mothers	2 to 3 3 or more 4 or more 2 or more 3 or more 4 or more	Calcium Protein Riboflavin Vitamin A (whole milk) Vitamin D (when fortified) Thiamine
Meat Group			
Meats, fish, poultry **Eggs** **Alternates:** vegetable protein (dry beans, dry peas, lentils, nuts)	2 or more servings to include 3 to 5 eggs weekly		Protein Iron Thiamine Riboflavin Niacin Vitamin A (egg yolk, liver)
Vegetables—Fruit Group			

All vegetables and fruits
 	
Divided between
  Dark green or yellow
    vegetables and
  Citrus fruits
Includes potato
	4 or more servings		Vitamin A (deep yellow and green vegetables)
			
			Ascorbic acid (citrus fruits)
			
			Other minerals and vitamins

Bread—Cereal Group			
All breads and cereals that are whole grain, enriched or restored	4 or more servings		Protein Iron B vitamins Food energy
Other Foods			
Butter, margarine Other fats	To round out meals and meet energy needs		

*Servings: *Milk group:* one serving is one 8-ounce glass of fluid milk or its calcium equivalent in cheese and other milk products.

      Meat group: one serving is 2 to 3 ounces of lean meat, fish, poultry, two eggs, or one cup cooked dried beans or peas.

      Vegetables—Fruits group: one serving is one-half cup or portion normally used such as one apple, orange, potato.

      Bread—Cereal group: one serving is one slice of bread, one-half cup cooked cereal, rice, pasta.

D. To record for study and future comparison the types and frequency of use of potentially cariogenic food.

E. To determine the overall consistency of the diet and which fibrous foods are regularly included.

F. To compare the frequency of cariogenic exposures with clinical and radiologic findings and the results of caries activity tests.

G. To provide a basis for making individual recommendations for changes in the diet important to the health of the oral mucosa and the periodontium and to the prevention of dental caries.

II. The Food Diary

A. Types

1. *Short.* A record of the food eaten by the patient over the previous 24 hours can be obtained by interview. Although of assistance for discussion during instruction, a truer picture of the patient's usual diet can be obtained from a food diary kept for a week or at least five days.

2. *Week-long.* The week or series of consecutive days selected should be typical of ordinary daily living uncomplicated by illness, holidays, fasting, or other unusual events.

B. Characteristics of Forms to Use

1. Simple, with ample spacing.
2. Space indicated for patient's name, the day, and the date on each page.
3. Blocked off areas for each meal and between-meal.
4. Space to indicate time of eating.
5. Column to record food item and amount (figure 28–1).
6. Cover page with sample procedure for entering items (figure 28–2).

III. Presentation to Patient

Result obtained can be expected to be directly proportional to the care taken in presentation.

A. Explain the Purpose

Avoid mention of specific foods and their relationships to oral health: the patient may not provide a true diary if what will be checked is known.

B. Explain the Form

Discuss the cover page suggestions for listing various foods and the use of household measurements for indicating quantity.

C. Complete the Current Day's Diary with the Patient

To illustrate how to itemize and how to list the foods in the order in which they are eaten.

D. General Directions

1. Emphasize importance of completing each meal's record as soon after eating as possible to avoid forgetting.
2. Explain need for recording what was actually eaten in contrast to recording everything served.
3. Review details of recording the component parts of a combination dish such as a salad, sandwich, casserole.
4. Indicate need for recording vitamin concentrates, prescribed medicines, water.
5. Request that meals eaten other than at home be identified by writing "restaurant," "guest at friend's home," or "party."

IV. Receiving the Completed Food Diary

The appointment for receiving the food diary should follow soon after its completion.

A. Obtain Supplemental Data

Question the patient and record additional information.

1. Whether the diary represents that of a typical week.
2. Appetite.
3. Food likes and dislikes; preferences.
4. Allergies.
5. Specially prescribed diets for the patient or other members of the family.

B. Review Patient's Food Diary

Review with the patient each day's recorded food list and supplement details that have been omitted.

1. Identify additions by using ink if the diary has been kept in pencil or vice versa.
2. Common omissions
   a. Garnishes: frosting, whipped cream, butter or oleomargarine on vegetables, salad dressings?
   b. Size of drinking glass: 4-ounce, 8-ounce?
   c. Bread or toast: white, enriched, wheat?
   d. Chewing gum: sugarless, amount?
   e. Canned fruit: packed in water or heavy or light syrup?
   f. Fruit salad: canned, fresh?

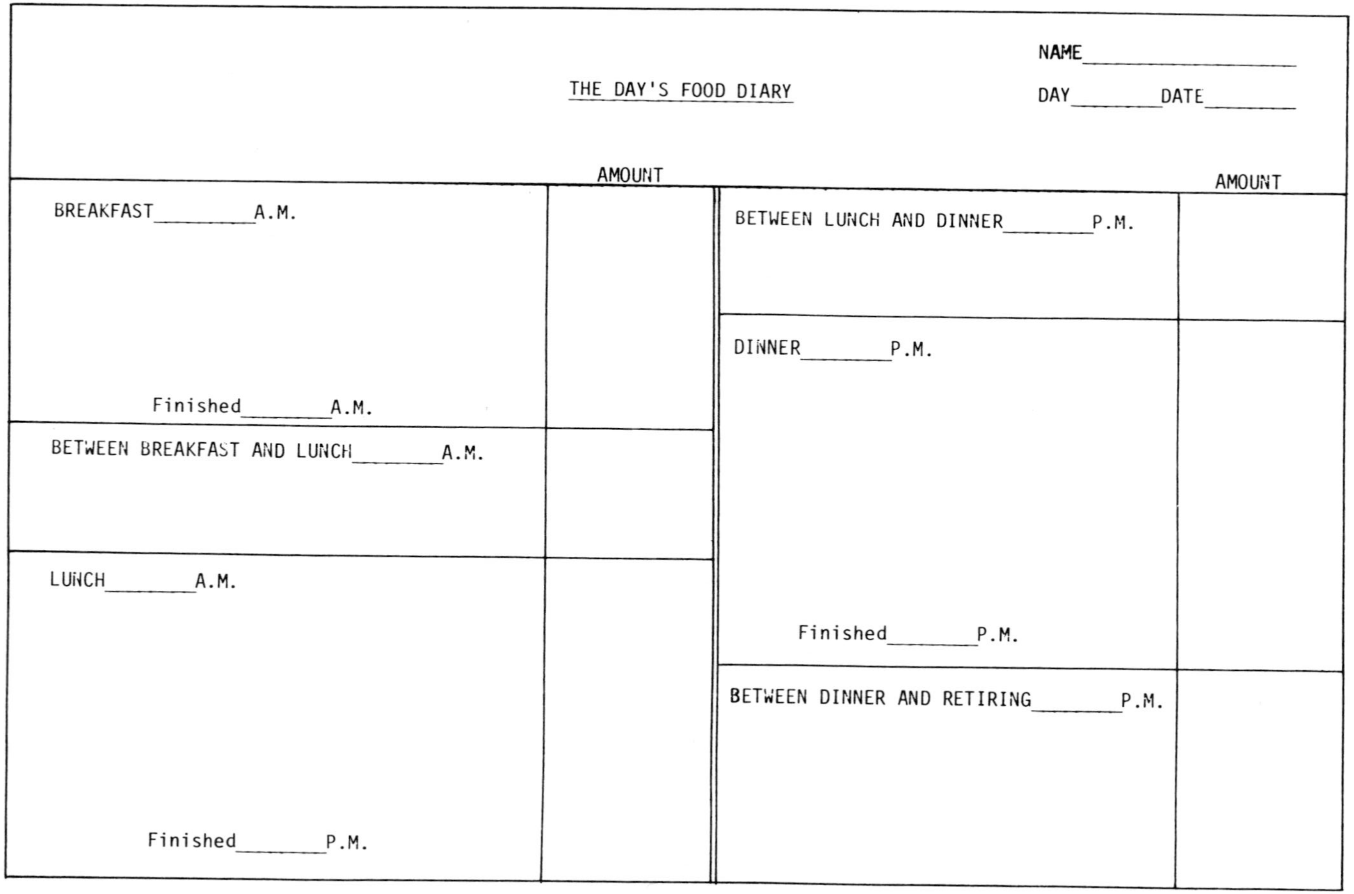

THE DAY'S FOOD DIARY

NAME________

DAY______ DATE______

	AMOUNT		AMOUNT
BREAKFAST______A.M. Finished______A.M.		BETWEEN LUNCH AND DINNER______P.M.	
BETWEEN BREAKFAST AND LUNCH______A.M.		DINNER______P.M. Finished______P.M.	
LUNCH______A.M. Finished______P.M.		BETWEEN DINNER AND RETIRING______P.M.	

Figure 28–1. Food diary: example of form used by patient to record daily diet. A booklet for a week's record is made by fastening seven of these forms together. The cover for the booklet is shown in figure 28–2.

FOOD DIARY

EXAMPLE OF HOW FOODS SHOULD BE LISTED

BREAKFAST 7:30 A.M.

Oatmeal	1 cup
with milk	½ cup
with brown sugar	2 teasp.
Milk	1-8 oz. glass
Toast - whole wheat bread	2 slices
with butter	generous
Egg - boiled	1
with butter	½ teasp.
Prunes - stewed -- with syrup	6 large

Finished 7:45 A.M.

BETWEEN BREAKFAST AND LUNCH 10:00 A.M.

Coffee	1 cup
with cream	1 teasp.
with sugar	2 teasp.
Water (around 11:00)	1 paper cup

Food eaten at lunch and dinner should be listed just as carefully as the breakfast shown above. If sandwiches are eaten, list the contents of the filling, such as egg, beef, lettuce, dressing.

Please show the approximate amounts of every kind of food that you ate. Do not mention any food that is served unless you ate it.

Please record all candy, cough drops, milk shakes, soft drinks, ice cream cones, popcorn, fruit (kinds), or cookies that you ate between meals. Also record vitamin concentrates or medicaments related to diet.

NAME _____

AGE ____ WEEK OF _____

SUMMARY

Figure 28-2. Food diary: cover page for patient's dietary record. Examples of how to list foods and indicate household measurements are provided on the left. The blank space on the right is for summary. The cover is fastened with seven copies of the form for recording a day's food diary as shown in figure 28-1.

g. Cereal: kind, milk, cream, sugar, quantity?

h. Potato: baked, buttered, fried?

i. Doughnut: sugared, glazed, plain?

V. Summary and Analysis

The three principal parts to analyze are foods from the four food groups, texture and consistency of foods, and the cariogenic foods. For convenience, check sheets should be devised for recording the frequency of use of each of the three.

A. Protective Foods

1. Analysis of overall content of the diet.
   a. Comparison with four food groups (table 28–1).
   b. Approximate proportion of foods that are cariogenic compared with proportion of protective foods.
2. Suggested procedure: use check sheet to mark daily portions of each food group (figure 28–3).
   a. Total for the week may be summarized for each category.
   b. Gross excesses and deficiencies can be identified readily.

B. Cariogenic Foods

1. Types of sugar-containing foods included.
2. Frequency of use
   a. Daily or occasionally.
   b. Number of between-meal snacks and how many of these include sweets.
3. Time of use.
4. Consistency of sugar-containing foods: related to probable length of time food might remain on the tooth surfaces.
5. Quantity: related to frequency more than size of individual serving (page 270).
6. Water taken at times when it could aid in rinsing sugars from the tooth surfaces.
7. Underline in red on the food diary the foods that contain sugar, or during the counseling appointment ask the patient to underline them to help learn more about the extent of the problem. The experience can be impressive to the patient, since people usually do not realize how many of the foods they are eating are cariogenic.

C. Consistency of Diet

1. Types of fibrous foods used: primarily uncooked, crisp, juicy fruits and vegetables.
2. Frequency of use: daily or occasionally.
3. Time of use
   a. During meal, end of meal, or between-meals.
   b. Relationship to providing cleansing mechanism for sugar contained in other foods.

D. Analysis

1. The patient can identify desirable and undesirable practices.
2. Compare findings with clinical findings and the patient's oral health problems.

PREPARATION FOR COUNSELING OF PATIENT

I. Define Objectives

A. To help the patient study the individual oral problems and understand the need for changing habits.

B. To explain specific changes in the diet necessary for improved general and oral health.

C. For dental caries control, to promote the elimination of sugar-containing foods, particularly those between meals, and to substitute protective foods.

II. Planning Factors

A. Patient Attitude

Consider patient's willingness and ability to cooperate in relation to other demonstrations, such as conscientiousness in keeping appointments and following personal oral care procedures.

B. Problem Areas

Identify problems that arise in presenting changes in the diet as they apply to this particular patient.

1. Difficulty in change of any habit.
2. Patient may feel dissatisfied without the usual or customary foods.
3. Lack of appreciation of need for change because of limited knowledge concerning diet, nutrition, and their relationship to oral health.

DIETARY ANALYSIS

Name _____

Age _____ Date _____

FOOD GROUPS	Day 1	2	3	4	5	6	7	Daily Average	Recommended Daily Amounts	Ade-quate	Inade-quate
MILK GROUP Milk									Child Adol. Adult 2-4 4+more 2+more		
Milk Products											
MEAT GROUP Meat, Fish Poultry									2 or more servings		
Eggs									(Eggs: 3-5 per week)		
VEGETABLE { Yellow & Dark Green									4 or more servings		
Other									including 1 yellow or dark green vegetable 1 citrus fruit		
& { Potato											
FRUIT { Raw- Citrus											
Other											
Cooked											
BREAD & CEREALS GROUP									4 or more servings		
SWEETS								Total			
Liquid { With Meal											
End of Meal											
Between Meal									NOTES AND RECOMMENDATIONS		
Soft (Sticky Retentive) { With Meal											
End of Meal											
Between Meal											
Hard (Sucked-Long-Lasting) { End of Meal											
Between Meal											

Figure 28-3. Dietary analysis: form used with patient to summarize the diet. From the food diary kept by the patient (figures 28-1 and 28-2), each item is indicated by a check in the space beside the appropriate food group. These are totaled, averaged, and compared with the recommended daily amounts on the right. The lower section provides space to categorize and count foods that are cariogenic.

4. Common misconception that concentrated sugar is an indispensable source of energy.
5. Degree of emphasis: dental disease does not kill anyone and nothing drastic is going to happen if minor deviations from the recommended diet occur.
6. Social prejudices against coarse, raw, or unrefined foods.
7. Cultural patterns.
8. Financial considerations.
9. Emotional disturbances which have led to or contributed to a craving for sweets.
10. Parental attitude that removal of sweets from the diet would deprive the child of normal childhood pleasures.

III. Select Appropriate Teaching Aids

A. Patient's radiographs, charting, and food diary.
B. Diagrams, models, or charts applicable to material to be presented.
C. Instructive leaflets to illustrate patient's special dietary or oral health needs.
D. Printed outline of diet plan with specific suggestions for food substitutes.
E. Printed list of snack suggestions.

IV. Review

Review data and recommendations with dentist for additions and suggestions.

CONFERENCE PROCEDURES

I. Setting

The conference should be held in a setting free from interruptions and distracting background sounds. Participants seated comfortably in a group will contribute to an atmosphere conducive to learning.

For the child patient, both parents should be encouraged to be present since both may supervise the child's eating and plaque control activities. For any age, it is particularly important for the person who plans and prepares the family meals to be present. To emphasize the importance of the conference and the concern of the entire dental group for the patient's problem, the dentist should participate by opening the conference and reviewing factors related to the treatment plan.

II. Pointers for Success

A. Be prepared—on time.
B. Plan for only a few simple visual aids.
C. Encourage parents to exclude small children (other than patient) from the conference, as they create distraction.
D. Develop a permissive atmosphere.
E. Take care not to follow a written outline of recommendations so rigidly that the conference lacks informality.
F. Include all people present in the discussion.
G. Use a conversational tone of voice.
H. Make certain that all questions from patient or parent are discussed adequately.
I. Avoid note taking during the conference as much as possible.

III. Presentation

A. Review of Purposes

Extent of detail included depends on whether parents attending conference have already participated in previous appointments. A teen-age patient may have been coming for appointments unattended, hence the need for clear review for understanding of all details by the parents.

B. Examine the Patient's Food Diary and Summary

Discuss deficiencies and excesses, defining the role of the various food groups, fibrous foods, and carbohydrates in dental caries initiation or prevention.

To make major changes in food habits is difficult, if not traumatic, for any individual. Application of the knowledge of the principles of learning (page 410) and the skills of a counselor are essential. The attempt must be made to retain as many as possible of the patient's present food habits, and to make recommendations that can be adapted into the patient's pattern of living.

1. Discuss foods from each food group that are liked by the patient and can be added to the diet or substituted for less desirable foods used.
2. Guide the patient to select those items from the present diet that need changing, and to make suggestions for appropriate substitutes.

Follow-up

All teaching needs review and reinforcement. A single learning experience is rarely effective in producing lasting change. With each appointment and recall, continued efforts to help the patient can be made.

DIET CONTROL PROGRAM

For the caries-susceptible patient, control of the cariogenic foods in the diet is essential. The plan for the patient is to make immediate changes which will remove all excess sucrose-containing foods, particularly those ordinarily consumed between meals, and to substitute foods from the four food groups. It is expected that the appetite will be satisfied, and cravings for sweet foods will diminish gradually over the first 3 weeks of the program so that the new eating pattern will continue indefinitely.

A suggested plan for presenting the problem and initiating discussion with the patient or parents to motivate interest in changing the diet is outlined below.

Dental Caries and Cariogenic Foods

It should be obvious that the patient cannot be told simply to "cut out the sweets in the diet." The meaning of "sweets" must be made clear, and specific suggestions provided for "cutting them out."

Clarify "Cariogenic" Foods

Define what is meant by a cariogenic food and use specific examples from the patient's dietary survey.

Describe Dental Caries Initiation

Discuss principles for understanding the role of sucrose in dental caries initiation.
1. Sugar on the tooth surface is changed to acid within 5 minutes.
2. Acid left undisturbed is not cleared from the mouth for $1\frac{1}{2}$ to 2 hours.
3. *Amount* of sugar consumed is not as important as *when* it is consumed; large amounts of sweet foods with a meal are not as detrimental as small amounts at intervals between meals.
4. Natural sugars are just as detrimental as refined ones (examples: maple syrup, honey).

C. Discuss the Significance of Length of Time Food is Retained in the Mouth

1. Sugar in liquid form is retained in the mouth for less time than solid.
2. Texture of the food that contains the sugar influences the length of time it will stay in the mouth (whether sticky or combined with a sticky substance).
3. Vigorous rinsing after eating a concentrated sweet helps to remove it from the mouth.
4. Sweet food taken before going to bed is not cleared readily from the mouth since salivary flow decreases during sleep.

II. Presentation of Specific Dietary Recommendations

The suggestions listed below represent basic principles to be applied. More specific recommendations should be added as they relate to an individual family. Directions must be simple and specific as the interpretation of many new ideas is difficult for the patient.

A. Incorporate foods from the basic groups to complete the patient's diet. A diet high in protective foods frequently may imply a diet low in fermentable carbohydrate.

B. Limit the use of fermentable carbohydrates to mealtimes. Pay particular attention to the final food used in the meal which may remain on the teeth if immediate toothbrushing is not possible.

C. Omit sweet foods even at mealtime when a very high dental caries rate is evident, and limit the diet to foods from the meat, milk, and vegetable-fruit groups (table 28–1). Selections from the bread and cereals groups should be limited to dark bread and whole grain and enriched cereals.

D. Select between-meal snacks from protective noncariogenic foods such as plain milk, fresh fruits, and raw vegetables.

E. Use as little concentrated sweet in the preparation of foods as possible, and observe care in the purchase of prepared foods. Examples: unsweetened fruit juice, dietetically prepared canned fruits, and sugar-free ice cream.

F. Eat well at mealtime to lessen desire for between-meal snacks. Protein and fat-containing foods digest more slowly and need to be included at each meal to prevent between-meal hunger.

G. Emphasize need for rigid adherence to the diet features: even occasional deviations can affect the results.

III. Summary

At the end of dietary counseling, the entire study needs to be reviewed and the parts correlated into a meaningful program for the patient. Exactly how a particular patient (and/or parent) will learn to apply the principles of dietary control of sugar, which can influence the incidence of dental caries, cannot be predicted. Frequently, a variety of teaching methods needs to be tried over a period of time.

Patient participation is very important. Using the patient's own food diary as a pattern, the patient can provide suggested substitutes for foods containing sugar, particularly the retentive foods—those that will cling to the teeth. Substitutes selected from the basic food groups are needed, and as the patient makes the suggestions, they can be written down for the patient to take home for reference. When time permits, it may be possible to compose a full week's diary of the foods known to be liked by the patient. Additional meal plan suggestions in printed form can be provided by the dental hygienist.

A snack list can also be discussed and prepared. When a snack list has been prepared and printed in advance, it must be discussed, and additions made at the patient's suggestion. If a patient responds with foods that are cariogenic, it may be evident that the principle has not been understood and further interpretation of which foods are to be avoided must be made.

DENTAL CARIES CONTROL STUDY

Patients who are subject to marked dental caries activity are a particular responsibility of the members of the dental profession. These patients, and their parents when the patient is a child, need special help in coping with the problem which, if left unattended, may well lead to an extensive and premature loss of teeth. To instigate a program of dental caries control requires thought, effort, and patience on the part of the dental team in determining the method of approach.

A dental caries control study may be described as a planned effort to help the patient analyze the problem and initiate an effective preventive program. This educational effort includes in part much of the same information provided for all patients. In a caries control study the instruction becomes more intensified as the patient is counseled to put into effect a specific program for diet and personal care.

To the pertinent information obtained through patient history, oral examination, radiographic survey, charting, and other initial evaluation procedures, is added a study of the diet made through use of a week-long diary kept by the patient. A dental caries activity test may be used as an instructional device to monitor the progress made.

A critical review of all information obtained leads to the preparation of a plan for the elimination of foods with high sucrose content and for the limitation of all cariogenic foods, in the attempt to curb the process of dental caries. Meticulous procedures for the patient's personal oral care are emphasized. Through dental health instruction, the patient comes to learn the purposes of each step in the study and to accept responsibility in carrying out the program of action.

The success of dental caries control measures is dependent on the patient's clear understanding and appreciation of the procedures, as well as the ability and willingness to cooperate. In turn, the dental hygienist applies knowledge of the physical and emotional problems at various age levels to try to understand and motivate the patient.

I. Patient Selection

The study can be proposed as a result of the initial diagnosis and treatment planning by the dentist, or preferably, at a recall appointment when the patient has shown real concern for the problem and has demonstrated a cooperative attitude in having necessary restorations completed. Interest in participation in a study can and should be developed in patients who need help.

A patient of any age who has dental caries activity can benefit from the study. A number of factors are involved in determining the probability of success.

A. **Acceptance of Responsibility**

1. *Dentist and Dental Hygienist:* must sincerely demonstrate their desire for better oral health for the patient.
2. *Patient*
   a. Young children: parents bear weight of responsibility.
   b. Intermediate children: child will have certain responsibilities along with the parents.
   c. Teen-agers: patient will have responsibility, but parent cooperation is essential, particularly in relation to food preparation.
   d. Adult: has own responsibility, but family cooperation will contribute.

B. **Patient Evaluation**

It is difficult to determine whether interest and enthusiasm evidenced at the beginning will carry on throughout a study. Continued acceptance and enthusiasm of dental personnel contribute much to patient motivation.

II. Preparation for the Study

A. Review physical and emotional characteristics of the patient's age group.
B. Plan the approach to the patient in accord with the appraisal of the individual characteristics.
C. Outline objectives for the patient in terms of the basic oral health needs.

APPOINTMENT PLANNING

There is no standard or uniform procedure that can be applied for all patients. A number of factors will enter into the determination of the number and length of appointments, particularly the patient's capacity for learning. Overcrowded, hurried appointments with too much material presented at one time will make it difficult for the patient to absorb the material and follow instructions.

A series of appointments permits time to review and to encourage the patient to ask questions. A suggested procedure is presented here.

. **First Appointment**

. **Explanation of Procedures**

The final outcome frequently depends on the preliminary understanding by the patient of the objectives and expected effects. A well-informed patient is more cooperative and appreciative. At the outset, at least the four factors listed below should be described, discussed, and clarified by encouraging patient (and parent) questions.

1. Purposes and general objectives in terms of better oral health and the social and economic advantages.
2. An outline of the procedures involved.
3. Description of the time involved and suggestions concerning appointment planning.
4. Need for mutual cooperation.

B. **Obtain Saliva Sample for Dental Caries Activity Test** (Described on pages 435–437).

C. **Explain and Record Indices To Be Used:** Gingival Index (GI), Plaque Index (Pl I), or a plaque-free score may be selected. These are described on pages 299–308.

D. **Take Plaque Sample:** when a plaque pH test, Methyl Red-Plaque-Sugar test, or a phase microscope can be used.

E. **Introduce Plaque Control Procedures**

1. Follow *First Lesson* as described on page 412.
2. Omit reference to diet control for dental caries so the patient will be unprejudiced while preparing the food diary.

F. **Introduce the Food Diary**

G. **Make Impressions for Study Casts:** if the use of custom-trays for daily application of fluoride is to be recommended.

H. **Complete the Case History Record:** Following dismissal of the patient, enter material for case history record in the patient's permanent record. Following each appointment, additions are made.

II. Second Appointment

A. **Receive and Review the Food Diary**

Discuss the entries and record additional information where needed (page 425).

B. Counseling the Patient

1. Follow Summary and Analysis Procedures, page 428.
2. Guide patient to complete the analysis form, figure 28–3.
3. Explain dental caries and the diet control program (page 431). Tie in the results of the caries tests made at the previous appointment.
4. Assist patient in preparing suggestions for the new diet that must be followed.

C. Continue Plaque Control Instruction

1. Follow *Second Lesson* as described on page 414.
2. Relate plaque control with diet procedures previously described.

D. Describe and Give Instructions for Self-applied Fluoride: dentifrice and mouthrinse or custom-tray.

E. Complete the Written Record

1. Make entries in the case history.
2. Discuss case with the dentist.
3. Telephone patient in 3 or 4 days to give encouragement and to clarify questions about the expected procedures.

III. Third Appointment

A. Make Inquiries

Inquire concerning all procedures, particularly the sugar-control diet. Commend and encourage. Provide informal question-references to the instruction given to determine any misconceptions.

B. Continue Plaque Control Instruction

1. Follow *Third Lesson*, page 414.
2. Explain the relation of professional treatment to plaque control and diet control.

C. Scaling

The extent of the calculus and the depth of the pockets will determine the time needed. When there is extensive scaling to be done by quadrants and under anesthesia, four appointments are planned, each to be preceded by an evaluation of gingiva, plaque, bleeding, and, as needed, demonstration of toothbrushing, flossing, or other aids. As the condition of the gingival tissue continues to improve, other parts of the treatment plan are undertaken.

IV. Fourth Appointment (3 to 4 weeks after start of special diet)

A. Obtain Saliva Sample for Caries Activity Test

In a mouth with many large carious lesions, this is not done until restorative dentistry has been initiated and, in some instances, completed. Since there are many acid-forming organisms held within a carious lesion, a positive test response can always be expected when the lesions are present.

B. Evaluation of Personal Care Procedures

Gingival tissue, plaque, and plaque removal techniques.

C. Give Encouragement

Encourage continuation of sugar-control diet and personal oral care measures.

D. Plan the Recall in 3 to 4 Months

E. Follow Up the Appointment

Telephone to tell the patient the results of the dental caries activity test.

CASE HISTORY RECORD

The written history of the dental caries control study relates and integrates the events that have occurred with observations made during the study. Interpretation of the facts should be done as objectively as possible.

The case history becomes a part of the patient's permanent record. Careful and complete recording is important in order that the text of the report will be meaningful and clear for follow-up reference.

I. General Instructions

A. Date Each Recorded Entry

B. Record Events As Soon As Possible After They Occur

1. Make brief notes during the appointments as an aid to writing the case history. Note taking should be done incon

spicuously so it does not distract the patient.

2. Record in the history all contacts with the patient during the study, including telephone conversations.
3. Include specific quotes from conversations if they reflect attitudes, habits, or acquired knowledge.

I. Observations of Patient's Personality and Development

The study provides an excellent opportunity to gain insight into the personality and development of the patient. Knowledge acquired can greatly augment understanding of the young patient and the parental influences.

DENTAL CARIES ACTIVITY TESTS

A dental caries activity test may be used as an instructional and motivational aid to guide the patient toward practicing habits conducive to the prevention of dental caries. The use of test results for a visual aid can be helpful since changes in results of a series of tests can show dramatically the effects of the patient's personal efforts in carrying out dietary and oral care preventive procedures.

A caries activity test can be used to monitor the progress of diet therapy; therefore, it is important that plaque control and various treatment procedures be done. The acid-forming organisms will be present in carious lesions, and only a drastic, rigid, sucrose-free diet will make a difference in a successive caries activity test. Control of dental caries by diet should follow and supplement plaque control procedures and the restoration of carious lesions.[8]

Caries activity tests provide information about the current oral environment. The tests are not "susceptibility" tests to predict what may occur at some future time. Various types of tests have been devised to detect dental caries activity. Evaluation may be made by counting the numbers of acid-forming bacteria or determining the acid produced or other specialized activity of the microorganisms.

Studies of the oral bacteria show that they are not distributed evenly. Microorganisms in the dental plaque on tooth surfaces contribute very little to the pool of bacteria obtained when a saliva sample is collected. A large part of the organisms in the saliva is from the tongue. Such findings provide at least a partial explanation for the inconsistencies of dental caries activity tests.

I. Snyder Colorimetric Test[9]

The Snyder Test Agar contains the indicator brom-cresol-green and is adjusted to a pH of 5.0. Acid formation by bacteria from the saliva sample added to the medium lowers the pH. At the lowered pH, the brom-cresol-green changes from green to yellow. It is the rapidity of color change that indicates the caries activity at that time.

A. Obtain Saliva Sample

The patient chews a piece of paraffin for 3 minutes and expectorates into a sterile bottle.

B. Laboratory Procedures

1. Place tube of Snyder Test Agar in boiling water until agar melts; cool until it can be held comfortably against the cheek.
2. Shake the saliva sample well to distribute bacteria, and pipette 0.2 ml. into the agar. Mix by gentle rotation.
3. Allow to solidify and incubate at 37° C.
4. Examine daily for 3 days and record changes in color compared with uninoculated control. Hold tubes against a white background when making observations.

C. Interpretation of Results

The rate of color change from green to yellow is related to the degree of caries activity. In the process of changing color, the agar will appear light green, then greenish-yellow, and finally appear a definite yellow.

No change in color indicates little or no caries activity, whereas a prompt change to yellow within 24 hours indicates marked acid formation or caries activity. The significance of the color changes is summarized in table 28–2.

II. Modified Snyder Test[10]

A miniature version of the standard Snyder test has been used which is simpler, less expensive, and occupies less space, particularly during incubation.

Table 28–2. Color Changes in the Snyder Test

Color of Snyder Test Agar after Incubation			Suggested Degree of Caries Susceptibility
24 hours	*48 hours*	*72 hours*	
Green	Green	Green	Little or none
Green	Light green	Yellow	Slight
Green	Yellow		Moderate
Yellow			Marked or rampant

A. Obtain Saliva Sample (I.A. above)

B. Laboratory Procedures

1. Shake specimen of saliva and use wire loop (flamed for sterility) to withdraw saliva (loop holds about .0113 ml.). Stab loop into the agar for inoculation.
2. Culture medium: Snyder test agar with the concentration of brom-cresol-green increased to facilitate the observation of the color change in the small amount of agar (0.2 ml.).
3. Incubate at 37° C for 24, 48, and 72 hours.
4. Examine daily.

C. Interpretation of Results

See table 28–2. The results are easier to read than the standard Snyder because the whole of the small amount of agar changes color.

III. Swab Test[11]

The Swab test is also a modified Snyder test. Time is saved in that a saliva sample is not obtained, and the test results are evaluated after 48 hours.

A. Obtain Sample

Stroke the buccal gingival areas of the teeth in each of the four quadrants with a sterile cotton applicator.

B. Laboratory Procedures

1. Remove cap from a vial of the special medium, insert the applicator to the bottom, and rotate it about five times. Raise the applicator and break off the stick against the lip of the vial, let it drop down, and replace the cap firmly.
2. Incubate at 37° C for 48 hours.
3. Make pH reading by a color comparator or electric pH meter.

C. Interpretation of Results

1. Color comparator: the brom-cresol-green changes from green to yellow as the pH declines.
2. Measurement and significance of pH (meter method).

Rampant:	pH below 4.1
Active:	pH 4.2 to 4.4
Slightly active:	pH 4.5 to 4.6
Inactive:	pH over 4.6

IV. Salivary Reductase Test[12]

This test measures the activity of the reductase enzyme present in salivary bacteria.

A. Obtain Saliva Sample (I.A. above)

B. Laboratory Procedures

1. Saliva sample is mixed with the dye diazoresorcinol (Resazurin reagent) and allowed to stand 15 minutes.
2. The color changes as the dye is reduced, and the caries conduciveness is interpreted after 15 minutes at room temperature.

C. Interpretation of Results

See table 28–3.

V. Methyl Red-Plaque-Sugar Test[13]

This test is also known as the Spot Plate Colorimetric Test. A dramatic change in color of the methyl red from yellow to red occurs as the pH changes from about 6.3 to 4.2. Lowering of the

Table 28–3. Color Changes in the Salivary Reductase Test

Color	Caries Conduciveness
Blue in 15 minutes	Nonconducive
Orchid in 15 minutes	Slightly conducive
Red in 15 minutes	Moderately conducive
Red immediately on mixing	Highly conducive
Colorless in 15 minutes	Extremely conducive

H is accomplished by the acid-producing bac-ria in the plaque acting on sucrose.

Obtain Plaque Sample

With a curet, scrape plaque from the distobuccal of maxillary molars, lingual of mandibular molars, or other surfaces with thick plaque. Collect enough plaque to cover the working end of the curet.

Test Procedure

1. Arrange the plaque sample in a small circle (about $1/4$ inch diameter) on a white porcelain tile.
2. Cover with two to three drops of methyl red indicator. Sprinkle a few crystals of sugar (sucrose) into the center of the circle. A second method for accomplishing the same result is to use a 2% sucrose sodium salt methyl red solution. Explain to the patient that it contains sucrose.
3. Wait 10 to 30 minutes for the color change.

Interpretation

1. The following criteria for scoring the color change may be used. The amount of red present determines the degree of acid production.
   0 = Yellow
   +1 = Yellow with a small red circle
   +2 = Yellow with a red circle one half of the area
   +3 = Yellow with a red circle covering all but the edges
   +2 and +3 indicate the presence of a significant number of plaque bacteria that are acid producing
2. Record results in patient's record.

I. Streptococcus Mutans Count[14]

Dental caries incidence and *Streptococcus mutans* infection have been correlated and there evidence to show that an increased count may recede the development of carious lesions.

Obtain Saliva Sample

Insert wooden tongue depressor into the mouth and turn it several times to cover it with saliva.

Laboratory Procedures

1. Press the wooden depressor against the selective agar plate.

2. Incubate anaerobically or in a sealed plastic bag containing expired air for 48 hours.
3. Count colony-forming units.

C. Interpretation

Highly infected patients may be readily detected because of the density of colonies. In a similar method using plaque samples, numbers of colonies were graded 1, 2, or 3, with Group 3 being the high colony counts.[15]

EVALUATION OF PROGRESS

The success of the dental caries control study is dependent upon learning by the patient. Learning implies a change of behavior and progress toward goals that are clearly understood by the learner.

I. Immediate Evaluation

A. A lowered caries activity test result at the end of the 3- to 4-week test period of restricted diet may indicate success to that date.
B. The patient's expressed interest and demonstration of cooperation in the caries control program indicate that at least temporarily the patient is motivated.

II. Overall Evaluation

A. Consistent reduction in dental caries rate in the years following the study shows sustained change in habits.
B. Patient's and parents' attitudes toward maintaining adequate oral health habits of personal care, diet containing minimum cariogenic foods, and routine professional dental care indicate application of learning.

RECALL

I. 3-Months' Follow-up

A. Obtain saliva sample for caries activity test.
B. Request patient to keep a 5- to 7-day food diary for analysis and evaluation.
C. Review plaque control procedures and provide suggestions as needed.
D. Recommend return to restricted diet when indicated.

II. 6-Months' Recall

A. Obtain saliva sample for caries activity test.

B. Examination and clinical procedures
1. Scaling when needed.
2. Topical application of fluoride, depending on self-applied fluoride program.
3. Charting.
C. Compare dental caries incidence with previous chartings and completed restorative dentistry.
D. Make dietary recommendations in accord with results from the test.

References

1. Carranza, F.A.: *Glickman's Clinical Periodontology*, 5th ed. Philadelphia, W.B. Saunders Co., 1979, pp. 489–505.
2. Grant, D.A., Stern, I.B., and Everett, F.G.: *Periodontics*, 5th ed. St. Louis, The C.V. Mosby Co., 1979, pp. 171–197.
3. *Preventive Dental Services, Practices, Guidelines and Recommendations.* Report of the Working Group on Preventive Dental Services, Health and Welfare, Canada, September, 1979, pp. 142–171.
4. Arnim, S.S.: The Use of Disclosing Agents for Measuring Tooth Cleanliness, *J. Periodontol.*, 34, 227, May, 1963.
5. McCarthy, P.L. and Shklar, G.: *Diseases of the Oral Mucosa*, 2nd ed. Philadelphia, Lea & Febiger, 1980, pp. 376–388.
6. Newbrun, E.: *Cariology*. Baltimore, The Williams & Wilkins Co., 1978, pp. 76–96.
7. National Research Council, Committee on Dietary Allowances, Food and Nutrition Board: *Recommended Dietary Allowances*, 9th ed. Washington, D.C., National Academy of Sciences, Office of Publications, 1980.
8. Sims, W.: The Interpretation and Use of Snyder Tests and Lactobacillus Counts, *J. Am. Dent. Assoc.*, 80, 1315, June, 1970.
9. Snyder, M.L.: A Simple Colorimetric Method for the Estimation of Relative Numbers of Lactobacilli in the Saliva, *J. Dent. Res.*, 19, 349, August, 1940.
10. Sims, W.: A Modified Snyder Test for Caries-activity in Humans, *Arch. Oral Biol.*, 13, 853, August, 1968.
11. Grainger, R.M., Jarrett, M., and Honey, S.L.: Swab Test for Dental Caries Activity: an Epidemiological Study, *Can. Dent. Assoc. J.*, 31, 515, August, 1965.
12. Rapp, G.W.: Fifteen Minute Caries Test, *Ill. Dent. J.*, 31, 290, May, 1962.
13. Arnim, S.S. and Sweet, A.P.: Acid Production by Mouth Organisms. Use of Aqueous Methyl Red for Patient Education, *Dent. Radiogr. Photogr.*, 29, 1, Number 1, 1956.
14. Köhler, B. and Bratthall, D.: Practical Method to Facilitate Estimation of Streptococcus Mutans Levels in Saliva, *J. Clin. Microbiol.*, 9, 584, May, 1979.
15. Woods, R.: A Dental Caries Susceptibility Test Based on the Occurrence of Streptococcus Mutans in Plaque Material, *Aust. Dent. J.*, 16, 116, April, 1971.

Suggested Readings

Alfano, M.C.: Controversies, Perspectives, and Clinical Implications of Nutrition in Periodontal Disease, *Dent. Clin. North Am.*, 20, 519, July, 1976.
American Dental Association, Council on Dental Therapeutics: *Accepted Dental Therapeutics*, 39th ed. Chicago, American Dental Association, 1982, pp. 117–142.

Bakdash, M.B. and Zaki, H.A.: The Impact of Diet and Nutrition on Periodontal Health, *Northwest Dent.*, 57, 5, January–February, 1978.
Bibby, B.G.: Diet and Nutrition and Dental Caries, *Can. Dent. Assoc. J.*, 46, 47, January, 1980.
Clark, J.W.: Nutrition in Dental Therapy, in Clark, J.W. ed.: *Clinical Dentistry, Volume 1*, Chapter 22. Hagerstown, Maryland, Harper & Row, 1981, pp. 1–103.
Dennis, D.A., Gawronski, T.H., Sudo, S.Z., Harris, R.S. and Folke, L.E.A.: Variations in Microbial and Biochemical Components of Four-day Plaque During a Four-week Controlled Diet Period, *J. Dent. Res.*, 54, 716, July–August, 1975.
Hix, J.O. and O'Leary, T.J.: The Relationship Between Cemental Caries, Oral Hygiene Status and Fermentable Carbohydrate Intake, *J. Periodontol.*, 47, 398, July, 1976.
Hsu, S.C., Pollack, R.L., Hsu, A.-F.C., and Going, R.E.: Sugars Present in Tobacco Extracts, *J. Am. Dent. Assoc.*, 101, 915, December, 1980.
Modrow, C.L., DePaola, D.P., and Alfano, M.C.: Nutrition Counseling in a Preventive Practice, in DePaola, D.P. and Cheney, H.G., eds.: *Preventive Dentistry.* Preventive Dental Handbook Series, Volume 2. Littleton, Massachusetts, P.S.G. Publishing, 1979, pp. 103–155.
Newman, H.N.: Diet, Attrition, Plaque and Dental Disease, *Br. Dent. J.*, 136, 491, June 18, 1974.
Osborn, M.O., Hornbuckle, C., and Stumbo, P.: Nutritional Evaluation of Food Intake Records of Periodontal Patients, *J. Periodontol.*, 48, 659, October, 1977.
Palmer, C.A.: The Human Touch in the Dental Office, *Dent. Assist.*, 44, 28, March, 1975.
Randolph, P.: The Continuing Vitamin C Controversy, *J. Prev. Dent.*, 2, 18, May–June, 1975.
Randolph, P.M.: Sociological, Cultural, and Psychological Influences on Food Selection Patterns, in Boundy, S.S. and Reynolds, N.J., eds.: *Current Concepts in Dental Hygiene, Volume 2*. St. Louis, The C.V. Mosby Co., 1979, pp. 169–178.
Richardson, E.R.: Effects of Nutrition on the Development of Teeth and Dental Caries: A Review, *Q. Natl. Dent. Assoc.*, 36, 81, April, 1978.
Sander, P.P. and Anderson, N.F.: *Developing Skills for Dietary Counseling for Prevention and Control of Dental Caries.* Minneapolis, University of Minnesota, 1981, 98 pp.
Shulman, J.S.: Nutrition and Dental Health of Children, in Forrester, D.J., Wagner, M.L., and Fleming, J., eds.: *Pediatric Dental Medicine.* Philadelphia, Lea & Febiger, 1981, pp. 353–376.
Weiss, R.L. and Trithart, A.H.: Between-meal Eating Habits and Dental Caries Experience in Preschool Children, *Am. J. Public Health*, 50, 1097, August, 1960.
Woolfe, S.N., Hume, W.R., and Kenney, E.B.: Ascorbic Acid and Periodontal Disease: A Review of the Literature, *Periodont. Abstr.*, 28, 44, Number 2, 1980.

Diet Counseling

Alban, A.L.: Dental Office Nutrition Counseling, *J. Am. Soc. Prev. Dent.*, 5, 27, May–June, 1975.
Alfano, M.C. and DePaola, D.P.: Role for Auxiliaries in Assessing Nutritional Status of Patients, *Quintessence Journal*, 1, 29, May, 1979.
Cline, A.: The Role of the Dental Hygienist as a Nutritional Counselor, *Dent. Hyg.*, 49, 555, December, 1975.
DePaola, D.P.: Dietary Counseling, in American Academy of Pedodontics: *Changing Perspectives in Nutrition and Caries Research.* New York, Medcom, 1979, pp. 30–37.
DePaola, D.P. and Alfano, M.C.: Triphasic Nutritional Analysis and Dietary Counseling, *Dent. Clin. North Am.*, 20, 613, July, 1976.

Hart, D.: Nutrition Counseling for Patients Should Be Basic, Realistic, *Quintessence Journal*, 1, 41, October, 1979.

Katz, S., McDonald, J.L., and Stookey, G.K.: *Preventive Dentistry*. Upper Montclair, N.J., D.C.P. Publishing, 1977, pp. 179–240.

Nizel, A.E.: *Nutrition in Preventive Dentistry: Science and Practice*, 2nd ed. Philadelphia, W.B. Saunders Co., 1981, pp. 417–506.

Poplin, L.E.: Cautions in Nutritional Counseling, *Dent. Hyg.*, 55, 40, February, 1981.

Randolph, P.M.: Dietary Counseling, in Boundy, S.S. and Reynolds, N.J., eds.: *Current Concepts in Dental Hygiene*, St. Louis, The C.V. Mosby Co., 1977, pp. 81–105.

Scanlan, D. and Wyatt, M.: Tools for Nutrition and Preventive Dental Counselling for South East Asian Refugees, *Can. Dent. Hyg.*, 14, 60, Fall, 1980.

Shank, S.E. and Guthrie, H.A.: Nutritional Counseling for Prevention of Dental Caries in Adolescents, *J. Am. Dent. Assoc.*, 92, 378, February, 1976.

Steel, J.E.: Nutrition Counselling in Oral Disease, *Aust. Dent. J.*, 23, 471, November, 1978.

Strieff, M., Seglins, B., Marshall, G., Finstad, S., and Borgendale, G.: The Caries Control Study, *J. Am. Dent. Hyg. Assoc.*, 29, 143, October, 1955.

Wittemann, J.K.: Behavioral Implications in Successful Dietary Counseling, *Dent. Clin. North Am.*, 20, 601, July, 1976.

Cariogenic Foods

Bibby, B.G.: The Cariogenicity of Snack Foods and Confections, *J. Am. Dent. Assoc.*, 90, 121, January, 1975.

Bowen, W.H., Amsbaugh, S.M., Monell-Torrens, S., Brunelle, J., Kuzmiak-Jones, H., and Cole, M.F.: A Method to Assess Cariogenic Potential of Foodstuffs, *J. Am. Dent. Assoc.*, 100, 677, May, 1980.

Catalanotto, F.A., Wrobel, W.R., and Epstein, D.W.: Sucrose Taste Thresholds and Dental Caries: Implications for Dietary Counseling, *Clin. Prev. Dent.*, 1, 14, March–April, 1979.

Clancy, K.L., Bibby, B.G., Goldberg, H.J.V., Ripa, L.W., and Barenie, J.: Snack Food Intake of Adolescents and Caries Development, *J. Dent. Res.*, 56, 568, June, 1977.

Dennison, C.I. and Randolph, P.M.: Diet and Dental Caries, in Randolph, P.M. and Dennison, C.I.: *Diet, Nutrition, and Dentistry*. St. Louis, The C.V. Mosby Co., 1981, pp. 200–223.

Edgar, W.M., Bibby, B.G., Mundorff, S., and Rowley, J.: Acid Production in Plaques after Eating Snacks: Modifying Factors in Foods, *J. Am. Dent. Assoc.*, 90, 418, February, 1975.

Feigal, R.J.: Cariogenicity Testing of Foods, *Northwest Dent.*, 59, 91, March–April, 1980.

Hartlmaier, K.M.: Cariogenic Sweets: Not All Fruit is a Suitable Substitute, *Quintessence Journal*, 1, 33, July/August, 1979.

Kreitzman, S.N.: Carbohydrates and Dental Caries: An Examination of the Evidence, *J. Prev. Dent.*, 6, 11, February, 1980.

Newbrun, E., Hoover, C., Mettraux, G., and Graf, H.: Comparison of Dietary Habits and Dental Health of Subjects with Hereditary Fructose Intolerance and Control Subjects, *J. Am. Dent. Assoc.*, 101, 619, October, 1980.

Rugg-Gunn, A.J., Edgar, W.M., and Jenkins, G.N.: The Effect of Eating Some British Snacks Upon the pH of Human Dental Plaque, *Br. Dent. J.*, 145, 95, August 15, 1978.

Shannon, I.L. and Edmonds, E.J.: Dietary Sucrose: Dental Dilemma, *Dent. Hyg.*, 49, 257, June, 1975.

Vogel, R.I. and Wechsler, S.M.: Nutritional Intake of a Dental School Population, *Clin. Prev. Dent.*, 1, 12, July–August, 1979.

Wilson, C.J.: Ready-to-eat Cereals and Dental Caries in Children: a Three-year Study, *J. Dent. Res.*, 58, 1853, September, 1979.

Fibrous and Non-retentive Foods

Birkeland, J.M. and Jorkjend, L.: The Effect of Chewing Apples on Dental Plaque and Food Debris, *Community Dent. Oral Epidemiol.*, 2, 161, Number 4, 1974.

Geddes, D.A.M., Edgar, W.M., Jenkins, G.N., and Rugg-Gunn, A.J.: Apples, Salted Peanuts and Plaque pH, *Br. Dent. J.*, 142, 317, May 17, 1977.

Lindhe, J. and Wicén, P.-O.: The Effects on the Gingivae of Chewing Fibrous Foods, *J. Periodont. Res.*, 4, 193, Number 3, 1969.

Longhurst, P.: Apples and Gingival Health, *Br. Dent. J.*, 134, 475, June 5, 1973.

Reece, J.A. and Swallow, J.N.: Carrots and Dental Health, *Br. Dent. J.*, 128, 535, June 2, 1970.

Wade, A.B.: Effect on Dental Plaque of Chewing Apples, *Dent. Pract. Dent. Rec.*, 21, 194, February, 1971.

Caries Activity Tests

Alban, A.: An Improved Snyder Test, *J. Dent. Res.*, 49, 641, May–June, 1970.

Ellen, R.P.: Microbiological Assays for Dental Caries and Periodontal Disease Susceptibility, *Oral Sciences Reviews*, 8, 3, 1976.

Jedrychowski, J.R., Luke, L.S., and Therrell, R.E.: Caries Susceptibility Testing: An Evaluation of Three Methods, *J. Pedod.*, 1, 281, Summer, 1977.

Katz, S., McDonald, J.L., and Stookey, G.K.: *Preventive Dentistry*. Upper Montclair, N.J., D.C.P. Publishing, 1977, pp. 127–138.

Krasse, B. and Klock, B.: Tests for Prediction of Caries, in American Academy of Pedodontics: *Changing Perspectives in Nutrition and Caries Research*. New York, Medcom, 1979, pp. 21–23.

Newbrun, E.: *Cariology*. Baltimore, The Williams & Wilkins Co., 1978, pp. 212–226.

Stolpe, J.R.: Chemical and Bacteriological Tests for Determining Susceptibility to and Activity of Dental Caries: A Review, *J. Public Health Dent.*, 30, 141, Summer, 1970.

29

Fluorides

The use of fluorides in preventive dental care is based on the knowledge that when the fluoride content of the teeth, particularly of the surface enamel, is increased to an optimum level, there is marked resistance to dental caries. Fluoride is a nutrient essential to the formation of sound teeth and bones, just as are calcium, phosphorus, and other elements obtained from food and water.

Fluoride is made available to the tooth structure by two general means: *systemically*, by way of the circulation to developing teeth, and *topically*, directly to the exposed surfaces of erupted teeth. Fluoride as a systemic nutrient is available from the community drinking water, either naturally or by fluoridation, from prescribed dietary supplements, or in small amounts from certain foods.

Fluoride can be made available for uptake at the surface of the erupted tooth by professional applications of fluoride solutions or gels, as well as by self-application, including mouthrinses, chewable tablets, and dentifrices. Fluoride is also taken up at the tooth surface from the drinking water as it passes over the teeth.

Fluorides have had a significant impact on the clinical practice of dentistry and dental hygiene. With less dental caries, fewer extractions, and more complete dental service possible for more patients, increased emphasis can be placed on preventive care.

FLUORIDE ACTION

Two basic factors are believed responsible for the remarkable action of fluoride against dental caries. These are related to the amount of fluoride contained in the surface of the tooth and the antibacterial or enzyme-inhibiting effects of the fluoride within dental plaque.

Resistance to dental caries is proportional to the amount of fluoride in the tooth surface present as fluorapatite.

I. Fluoride and Tooth Development

The teeth can acquire fluoride during three periods: during the *calcification stage* of tooth development, *after calcification* and before eruption, and *after eruption*. At this point of study, a review of the histology of tooth development and calcification can be helpful to supplement the information included here.[1,2]

A. Pre-eruptive: Calcification Stage

1. Fluoride is deposited during the formation of the enamel crystals, starting at the dentinoenamel junction, after the enamel matrix is laid down by the ameloblasts (figure 29–1A).
2. Fluoride is incorporated as fluorapatite during calcification.
3. Fluoride is available to the developing teeth by way of the blood stream to the tissues surrounding the tooth buds.

441

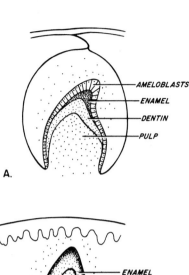

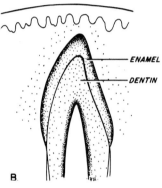

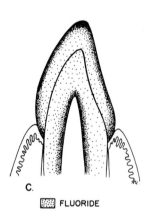

FLUORIDE

Figure 29–1. Systemic fluoride. Dots represent fluoride ions in the tissues and distribution throughout the tooth. **A.** Developing tooth during calcification to show fluoride from drinking water and other systemic sources deposited throughout the enamel and dentin. **B.** Maturation stage prior to eruption when fluoride is taken up from the tissue fluids surrounding the crown. **C.** Erupted tooth continues to take up fluoride on the surface from external sources. Note that the fluoride deposition is concentrated on the surface of the enamel and on the pulpal surface of the dentin.

4. Source of fluoride: drinking water and other ingested fluoride such as from tablets or drops.

5. During calcification, when there is excess fluoride, the normal activity of the ameloblasts may be inhibited and a defective enamel matrix can form. This is the fundamental mechanism of dental fluorosis.

B. Pre-eruptive: Maturation Stage

1. After calcification is complete and before eruption, fluoride deposition continues in the surface of the enamel (figure 29–1B).

2. Fluoride is taken up from the nutrient tissue fluids surrounding the tooth crown. Much more fluoride is acquired by the outer surface during this period than in the underlying layers of enamel during calcification. Children who are exposed to fluoride for the first time within the two years prior to eruption benefit from fluoride acquired during this pre-eruptive stage.

C. Posteruptive

1. After eruption and throughout the life span of the teeth, fluoride is taken up from the drinking water, food, and saliva (figure 29–2).

2. Uptake is rapid on the enamel surface during the first years after eruption, and is greater at high than at low levels of fluoride in the diet, including supplements and the drinking water.

3. Fluoride concentration decreases from the enamel surface to the dentinoenamel junction.[3] The fluoride concentration then increases from the dentinoenamel junction to the pulpal surface, where fluoride can still be added from the systemic source.

II. Tooth Surface Fluoride

A. Fluoride Deposition

Fluoride associated with caries prevention is deposited in the enamel, dentin, cementum, and bone as fluorapatite.

B. Fluoride Composition

The unit crystal is hydroxyapatite. The

fluoride ions substitute for the hydroxy radical of the hydroxyapatite and fluorapatite is formed. Fluoride is confined to the surface of the crystals.

C. Fluoride Uptake

Uptake of fluoride depends on the amount of fluoride ingested and the length of time of exposure.

D. Amount of Fluoride in the Enamel Surface

Extracted teeth have been analyzed from people who had used water with fluoride all their lives. The parts per million (ppm) fluoride in the enamel surface are shown by the following:[4]

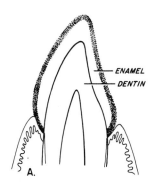

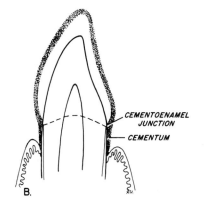

Figure 29–2. Fluoride acquisition after eruption without the benefit of systemic fluoride during tooth development. **A.** Fluoride on surface taken up from topical application, chewable tablets, mouthrinse, and other external sources. **B.** When there is recession, exposed cementum benefits by acquiring surface fluoride to aid in the prevention of root caries and sensitivity.

Fluoride in Water	Fluoride in Enamel Under Age 20	Over Age 50
0.1 ppm	571 ppm	1247 ppm
1.0 ppm	889 ppm	1552 ppm
3.0 ppm	1930 ppm	2290 ppm

Fluoride is a natural constituent of enamel; even at mininal fluoride exposure (0.1 ppm) there is 500 to 1200 ppm fluoride in the enamel.

E. Decalcified White Areas

When fluoride is applied to the surface, it diffuses deeper into decalcified areas than on intact enamel. The caries process is slowed because the fluoride encourages remineralization.

III. Topical Agents

A. Effectiveness

Effectiveness of topical agents depends on their ability to deposit fluoride as fluorapatite in the tooth surface.[5]

B. Reaction to Application

Calcium fluoride and fluorapatite are formed on the tooth surface immediately after application. Calcium fluoride and any unused fluoride which did not react during the application are gradually leached away, but fluorapatite remains. The loss of fluoride may occur over several days.[5] These factors explain why the patient should be instructed not to rinse, eat, or brush for as long as possible after an application.

C. Fluoride Uptake

The most fluoride is taken up from topical preparations applied soon after eruption.

IV. Plaque Fluoride

A. Dental plaque contains variable concentrations of fluoride which varies with the amount of fluoride in the drinking water and the use of fluoride dentifrice and mouthrinse.[6]

B. Less than five percent of the fluoride in plaque is in a free form (ions) and it is believed that most of the plaque fluoride is bound within the cells of plaque bacteria.[7]

C. Antibacterial effects of fluoride probably relate to inhibition of enzymes involved in acid production. The acid is part of the process of dental caries initiation (pages 269–270).

FLUORIDATION

Fluoridation is the adjustment of the fluoride ion content of a domestic water supply to the optimum physiologic concentration which will provide maximum protection against dental caries and enhance the appearance of the teeth with a minimum possibility of producing objectionable enamel fluorosis.[8] Fluoridation has been established as the most efficient, effective, reliable, and inexpensive means for improving oral health.

I. Historical Aspects[9,10]

A. Mottled Enamel and Dental Caries

Early in this century Dr. Frederick S. McKay began his extensive studies to find the cause of "brown stain," which later was called mottled enamel and now is known as dental fluorosis. He observed that people with mottled enamel had much less dental caries.[11] He associated the condition with the drinking water, but tests were inconclusive until 1931 when Churchill pinpointed fluorine as the specific element related to the tooth changes.[12]

B. Background for Fluoridation

Epidemiologic studies of the 1930s sponsored by the United States Public Health Service and directed by Dr. H. Trendley Dean led to the conclusion that the level of fluoride in the water optimum for dental caries prevention is 1 ppm. Clinically objectionable dental fluorosis is associated with levels well over 2 ppm.[13]

From this knowledge and the fact that many healthy people had lived long lives in communities where the fluoride content of the water was much greater than 1 ppm, the concept of adding fluoride to the water developed. It was still necessary, however, to show that the benefits from controlled fluoridation could parallel those of natural fluoride.

C. Fluoridation—1945

The first communities were fluoridated in 1945. Research in the communities began before fluoridation was started to obtain base-line information, and continued over the years with detailed examinations and reports in the following communities and their scientific controls:

Fluoridation	Control City
Grand Rapids, Michigan (January, 1945)	Muskegon, Michigan
Newburgh, New York (May, 1945)	Kingston, New York
Brantford, Ontario (June, 1945)	Sarnia, Ontario
Evanston, Illinois (February, 1947)	Oak Park, Illinois

Aurora, Illinois, where the natural fluoride level is optimum (1.2 ppm), was used to compare the benefits of natural fluoride in the water supply with those of fluoridation, as well as with a fluoride-free city, Rockford, Illinois.

The research conducted in the above cities, as well as other research throughout the world, has documented the influence of fluoride on oral health. The effects and benefits itemized below summarize important features of fluoridation; examples of research findings are given for illustration.

II. Fluoride Level

One part per million is considered the optimum fluoride level for water in temperate climates. For warmer and colder climates, the amount can be adjusted from approximately 0.6 ppm to 1.2 ppm, adapted in accord with the amount of water consumed.[8]

In the United States, close to 10,700,000 people live in 2600 communities where natural fluoride occurs in the drinking water at 0.7 ppm or more,[14] a level that is sufficient to prevent dental caries.

III. Effects and Benefits

A. Appearance of Teeth[15,16]

Teeth exposed to an optimum or slightly higher level of fluoride frequently are clear white, shining, opaque, and without blemishes. When there is slightly more than optimum level for the individual, there may be white areas, such as bands or flecks, which can be seen professionally by drying the teeth and observing under a dental light. Without such close scrutiny, such spots may blend with the overall appearance. Dental fluorosis associated with higher than optimum fluoride levels has been classified on page 290.

B. Dental Caries: Permanent Teeth

Continuous use of fluoridated water from birth results in an average of 60 to 70 percent fewer carious lesions. The effects are similar to those found in communities with optimum level natural fluoride in the water. Many more individuals are completely caries-free when there is fluoride in the water.
1. *Distribution.* Anterior teeth, particularly maxillary, have more protection from fluoride than do posterior teeth.[13] The anterior teeth are contacted by the drinking water as it passes into the mouth. Fluoride is added to the enamel after eruption.
2. *Posteruption.* Although maximum benefits are derived when fluoridated water is consumed through the entire pre-eruptive period, there are also significant benefits to teeth that have erupted prior to exposure to fluoride.[17,18,19]
3. *Progression.* Not only are there fewer carious lesions, but the rate of decay is slowed. Caries progression is also reduced in the surfaces that receive fluoride for the first time after eruption.[20]

C. Dental Caries: Primary Teeth

With fluoridation from birth, caries incidence is reduced in the primary teeth up to 50 percent.[17] For example, the children ages 6 to 9 in Newburgh had five times as many primary teeth present and caries-free as the children of Kingston where there was no fluoride.[21]

D. Prenatal Fluoride

There has been no clear clinical evidence that prenatal fluoride ingestion (from drinking water or prescription) by the mother has an effect on the calcification of the baby's primary teeth.[22,23,24] A major portion of the calcification of primary teeth takes place after birth: the crowns of primary incisors are not fully completed until approximately 3 months, canines at 9 months, and second molars at 11 months, average. The outermost layers of the enamel are formed last, so that fluoride ingested after birth has the most influence on the primary teeth.

E. Tooth Loss

Both primary and permanent tooth loss is much greater in teeth without fluoride[21] because of increased dental caries which progresses more rapidly.

F. Malocclusion

With fewer extractions, particularly less premature loss of primary molars, there is less malocclusion from local causes.[25]

G. Adults

When a person resides in a fluoride area throughout life, benefits continue. Colorado Springs adults ages 20 to 44 who had used water with natural fluoride showed 60 percent less caries experience than adults in fluoride-deficient Boulder. In Boulder, adults also had had three to four times as many permanent teeth extracted.[26] In a survey of adults in Rockford, Illinois (no fluoride), there were about seven times as many edentulous persons as there were in a comparable group in Aurora (natural fluoride).[27]

H. Bone

There is evidence that fluoride is important to the maintenance of normal bone and the improvement of calcium metabolism. Studies have shown that there are fewer bone fractures, and when they occur they heal more quickly; less osteoporosis, especially in women; and less calcification of the aorta, especially in men, when there is increased exposure to fluoride in the water over the years.[28,29,30] Fluoride has been used to improve the bone in the treatment of osteoporosis.[31]

I. Periodontal Diseases

Favorable effects of fluoride previously mentioned have indirect effects on periodontal health. Improved bone density resulting from fluoride can affect the alveolar bone along with all bones and may have an effect on bone resorption and resistance to local factors.

Dental caries favors plaque retention and therefore irritation to gingival tissues, particularly lesions adjacent to the gingival margin and proximal lesions which favor food impaction. With dental caries, tooth loss, and malocclusion decreased, a difference can be expected in the severity of periodontal conditions.

The incidence of periodontal diseases increases with age because of the cumulative effects of etiologic factors and the disease processes. With the use of fluorides, particularly fluoridation, fewer teeth are lost because of dental caries at younger ages. Therefore there is need for emphasis on periodontal disease prevention and control in communities with fluoride in the drinking water.

J. Cemental Caries

The incidence of root caries is approximately 50 percent less in life-long residents of a fluoridated community.[32]

IV. Partial Defluoridation

As noted earlier, approximately 400 communities use water that contains more than twice optimal level fluoride. With excess fluoride, the water does not meet the requirements of the United States Public Health Service. Defluoridation can be accomplished by one of several chemical systems.

The efficacy of the methods has been shown. The water supply in Britton, South Dakota, has been reduced from almost 7 ppm to 1.5 ppm since 1948, and in Bartlett, Texas, from 8 ppm to 1.8 ppm since 1952. Examinations have shown a dramatic reduction in incidence of objectionable fluorosis in children born since defluoridation.[33,34]

V. School Fluoridation

To bring the benefits of fluoridation to children living where there is no central water system, fluoridation of a school water supply has been shown to be a satisfactory method. Because of the intermittent use of the water (only part of each day for 5 days each week during the school year) the amount of fluoride added is increased over the usual 1 ppm.

Although children are 5 or 6 years old befor they go to school, definite benefits have bee shown. The effect is about twice as great on lat erupting teeth since they receive the benefit of systemic fluoride and topical exposure, wherea early erupting teeth have only topical benefits.[3]

After 12 years of fluoride at 5 ppm in th school drinking water of Elk Lake, Pennsylva nia, children who had attended that school reg ularly had 39 percent fewer decayed, missing and filled teeth than the control group. Th greatest benefits were found on proximal toot surfaces.[35]

The benefits increase with increased fluorid levels. In Elk Lake after 4 years at 5 ppm ther was 23 percent benefit. In the schools of Sea grove, North Carolina, after 8 years with fluo ride level at 6.3 ppm, there was a 40 percen decrease in decayed, missing, and filled surface when compared with the control.[36]

VI. Discontinued Fluoridation

The control of dental caries by fluorides ca be clearly shown in a community when fluorid is removed. For example, in Antigo, Wisconsin the action of antifluoridationists in 1960 brough about the discontinuance of fluoridation whic had been installed in 1949. Examinations in th years following revealed the marked drop in th number of children who were caries-free, an the steep increases in caries rates. For exampl from 1960 to 1966 there was a 67 percent de crease in the number of caries-free children i the second grade.[37] Fluoridation was reinstate in 1966 by popular demand.

VII. Economic Benefits

A. Cost of Fluoridation

In the United States, costs after installa tion have been estimated to average be tween 7 and 14 cents per person per year When the benefits are considered, and th fact that ALL children are reached, not jus those whose parents make the effort to see preventive professional care, there is littl question about the need for fluoridation i all possible domestic water supplies.

No other method for the administratio of fluorides has consistently shown equa benefits. All other methods require mor professional time, more effort on the part of the individual, and/or more financial outlay.

B. Cost of Professional Care

1. *Influence of Fluoridation.* Individual, family, and community costs of dental care can be reduced markedly. In addition, the quantity of dental care, number of dental appointments, the extent of individual restorations, and the number of dental extractions are all reduced.

2. *Newburgh-Kingston Study.*[38] Newburgh, New York, and the control city, Kingston (without fluoridation), have been used to demonstrate a specific program of dental care. After 6 years of dental clinic operation for the 5- and 6-year-old lifelong residents of the poorest socioeconomic areas of the cities, the cost for care of the children exposed to fluoridation has been shown to be less than half that required for the Kingston children.

    At the initial examinations, 41 percent of the Newburgh children were caries-free, whereas only 17 percent of the Kingston children were. Of the needed restorations, about 75 percent of those for the Kingston children were compound; in Newburgh only about 55 percent involved more than one surface. At the annual recall, the Kingston children consistently required more restorative services; the Newburgh children required only about one half as many appointments. These findings have marked significance for all types of dental programs for all ages.

DIETARY SUPPLEMENTS

Approximately 23 percent of the population of the United States live in areas that do not have central water systems. Without fluoride in the drinking water, individuals and communities must resort to other means for making fluoride available. Other methods are not substitutes for fluoridation but are needed as follows:

A. For people who use a private water supply that does not have natural fluoride and that is not practical to fluoridate.

B. For those whose community water supply has not yet been fluoridated.

C. At the start of fluoridation, fluoride applications and other methods are used to protect the teeth of children too old to receive the full benefits from fluoridation.

D. As a supplement to fluoridation, multiple use of fluorides has been shown to provide added benefits.

I. Foods

Certain foods contain fluoride but not enough to constitute a significant part of the day's need for caries prevention. Meat, eggs, vegetables, cereals, and fruits have very small but measurable amounts, while tea and fish have larger amounts.

Fluoridated salt has been used, particularly in Switzerland, and although reduced incidence of dental caries has been shown, effects comparable to fluoridation have not been attained. It has been estimated that by the use of salt as it is currently available (in Switzerland 90 mg. fluoride per kg. of salt is specified by governmental regulation), the amount of fluoride ingested daily is about one third to one half that obtained from one ppm fluoridated water, when average amounts of water used by individuals are compared.

II. Fluoride Supplements

A fluoride supplement can be administered as a pill, chewable tablet, lozenge, drop, or mouthrinse for swallowing after rinsing. The supplement may be prescribed on an individual patient basis for daily use at home, or it may be administered to school classroom groups as part of a total public health program.

By chewing and rinsing a supplement before swallowing, there is dual action: first, locally on the tooth surface, and second, systemically in teeth that have not erupted (figures 29–1 and 29–2, pages 442, 443). After chewing, the mixture should be swished over and between the teeth for one minute in order that optimal benefit can be obtained. The person should not eat, drink, or brush the teeth for 30 minutes after chewing the tablet. The maximum topical effect occurs on newly erupted teeth.

Studies using preschool children have shown caries incidence reduced by 50 to 80 percent in primary teeth. The benefit was greater for those children who started earlier and continued longer.[39] Studies in permanent teeth have been summarized to show a caries incidence reduction of 20 to 40 percent when the tablets were used over a 2- to 4-year period.[39]

For maximum possible effect, fluoride must be administered at least during the period of tooth development, from birth until 12 to 14 years of age or longer for the maturation of the crown of the third permanent molar.

The American Dental Association has classified a number of the proprietary fluoride preparations as *Accepted.** Prescriptions are advised only when the fluoride concentration in the drinking water used by the child is known to have a fluoride ion concentration no higher than 70 percent of the optimal level recommended for water fluoridation in that community.[40]†

A. **Available Forms**

  1. *Tablets and Lozenges.* Scored or unscored; may be chewed, rinsed, and swallowed, or dissolved slowly in the mouth as a lozenge. The resulting mix with saliva should be swished over and between the teeth for one minute.
  2. *Mouthrinse.* Measured amount of rinse contains prescribed daily fluoride. The rinse is swished for at least one minute before swallowing.
  3. *Liquid.* Prepared in a concentrate with directions that specify the number of drops for the prescription equivalent. The liquid form has its primary use for preparing 1.0 ppm water for the child from birth to 2 years. For other children, the tooth contact of the chewable tablet or mouthrinse is important to provide the enamel surface with protective fluoride.

B. **Prescription**

  1. *Adjust For No Fluoride in the Drinking Water*[40]
     a. *Over 3 years:* 1.0 mg (prescription: 2.2 mg. sodium fluoride. A 2.2 mg. tablet contains 1.0 mg. fluoride).

     b. *Between 2 and 3 years:* 0.5 mg. (one-half of a 2.2 mg. tablet).
     c. *Birth to 2 years:* dissolve a 2.2 mg. tablet or appropriate number of liquid drops in one quart of water. Bottled 1.0 ppm fluoridated water for drinking and preparation of formula and other foods may be purchased.
  2. *Adjust For Fluoride in The Water System Up to 0.7 ppm.* Table 29–1 shows the fluoride dosage necessary to supplement at the different levels of fluoride in the drinking water.
  3. *Limitation on Total Prescription.* No more than 264 mg. of sodium fluoride should be prescribed at one time, which is sufficient for 4 months when 2.2 mg. are used daily. The amount (264 mg.) is below the toxic or lethal doses and therefore eliminates the hazard of storing large amounts in the home.
  4. *Storage.* Tablets should be kept out of the reach of children.
  5. *Vitamins with Fluoride*
     a. Preparations are available in liquid and tablet form.
     b. The American Dental Association has not considered for acceptance vitamin fluoride combinations for several reasons: it is more difficult to adjust the prescribed fluoride to the amount already received through the water supply (table 29–1) since the preparation contains a fixed amount; there is no evidence that the vitamins enhance the effectiveness of the fluo-

Table 29–1. Supplemental Fluoride Dosage Schedule (in mg. F/day*) According to Fluoride Concentration of Drinking Water

Age (Years)	Concentration of Fluoride in Water (ppm)		
	Less Than 0.3	0.3 to 0.7	Greater Than 0.7
Birth to 2	0.25	0	0
2 to 3	0.50	0.25	0
3 to 13	1.00	0.50	0

*2.2 mg sodium fluoride contain 1 mg. fluoride.
(From American Dental Association, *Accepted Dental Therapeutics*)

---

*Consult *Accepted Dental Therapeutics* for current list of fluoride preparations. For a description of the American Dental Association classification of products see page 376.
†For list of communities and the amount of fluoride in the water supply, consult the local or state department of dental health.

ride; and the unnecessary expense of buying vitamins that are not needed or prescribed.[40]

C. Group Administration

Administration of fluoride supplements to groups of children as part of a school health program has been shown to be beneficial.[41,42] They should be started early, when the child enters kindergarten. Supervised group administration can be carried out by school personnel and adult volunteers under the supervision of a dental hygienist.

There are several advantages in the use of tablet administration as part of a school health program especially when compared with prescription on an individual basis. A minimum of professional service time is needed, and no special effort is required by the individual or his parents. It is a difficult undertaking to supervise use of a daily supplement until the child is 13 to 15 years of age.

D. Role of Dental Hygienist

1. *Patient Instruction.* The dental hygienist in private practice participates in instruction, motivation, and supervision for those patients who receive a prescription for fluoride tablets. When prescribed on an individual basis, problems arise in the continued administration of the tablets over the years of childhood, apparently even when parents are conscientious and highly motivated.

2. *Patient Recall.* It is generally advisable to plan recall appointments at the time when the patient's prescription will be in need of renewal so that encouragement and supervision can be provided.

TOPICAL FLUORIDE APPLICATION

Topical application of fluoride preparations may frequently be an essential part of a total preventive program particularly when fluoridation is not available. Although a number of fluoride preparations have been tried and caries-preventive effects shown, those most generally used have been sodium fluoride, acidulated phosphate-fluoride, and stannous fluoride.

Research has continued since the early 1940s when Bibby[43] conducted the initial topical sodium fluoride study using Brockton, Massachusetts, school children and demonstrated better than one third fewer new carious lesions at the end of a 2-year study. Since then, research has involved several fluoride compounds and a variety of preparations including solutions, gels, pastes, and dentifrices. These have been tried as agents to be applied professionally in the dental office, individually for home treatment, and for group preventive efforts such as in school dental health or the armed services preventive dentistry programs.

PROFESSIONAL TOPICAL FLUORIDE APPLICATION

Benefits and characteristics of sodium fluoride, acidulated phosphate-fluoride, and stannous fluoride solutions will be described first. Directions for specific clinical procedures for topical application follow. Other modes for dispensing topical fluorides such as gels, sprays, rinses, brushing with solution, prophylaxis pastes, and dentifrices will then be considered.

I. Sodium Fluoride

The original applications by Bibby in 1942 utilized a 0.1% aqueous sodium fluoride solution applied for 7 to 8 minutes on teeth thoroughly cleaned by oral prophylaxis at 4-month intervals.[43] Extensive studies by Knutson and others were sponsored by the United States Public Health Service in the 1940s. They were designed to determine the most effective concentration of sodium fluoride, the minimum time required for application, and procedural details.[44,45]

The effectiveness of sodium fluoride as a topical agent has been demonstrated in numerous studies. A 30 to 40 percent reduction in caries incidence can be expected in permanent teeth and 20 to 30 percent in primary teeth from a controlled, carefully performed topical application. Greatest protection is afforded newly erupted teeth, which is true of all topical applications.

A. Solution

2% aqueous sodium fluoride (neutral pH 7.0).

B. Frequency of Application

As originally planned, a series of four applications, two days to a week apart, were given at intervals throughout childhood in accord with the tooth eruption pattern of the individual child, so that teeth may receive protection as soon after eruption as possible. Ages 3, 7, 10, and 13 were considered average and used for applications in public health programs. In addition, a single application is recommended at 4- to 6-month intervals between the series of four in accord with routine dental and dental hygiene recall for the individual.

C. Advantages

1. Solution is relatively stable when kept in a polyethylene bottle.
2. Patient acceptance is favorable: solution tastes salty but is not objectionable.
3. No tooth staining or adverse gingival reactions occur.
4. Patient education: although the series of appointments required for four treatments has been considered a disadvantage, it is a distinct advantage for instruction of the patient in plaque control procedures. A series of appointments is usually necessary for a patient to gain proficiency in methods of plaque removal (toothbrushing, flossing, and other indicated procedures). The fluoride appointment series gives the opportunity for continuing instruction and review. Toothbrushing practice precedes each fluoride application and thus serves to prepare the teeth by removing plaque and debris.

II. Acidulated Phosphate-Fluoride (APF)

For the first clinical study, reported in 1963, a 1.23% fluoride with orthophosphoric acid was used for a single annual 4-minute application. In this research, caries incidence was reduced by 70 percent after 2 years.[46]

A succeeding study, which resulted in an average of 50 percent fewer new carious lesions, showed that the caries-reducing effect was greater in the children with cleaner mouths. Those with inadequate personal daily care had only 44 percent reduction, whereas in the cleaner mouths there was 60 percent.[47] APF is available for preventive treatment in three forms, a solution, a gel, and a thixotropic agent. A thixotropic agent is a type of gel that sets in a gel-like state, but under stress becomes fluid-like. Gels of this type can flow into interdental areas. In the gel form they may adhere to tooth surfaces.

Use of acidulated phosphate-fluoride in the form of a gel is described on pages 454–456. Laboratory studies using extracted teeth have shown that the amount of fluoride taken up by the enamel is the same whether the solution or the gel is applied, assuming the fluoride content, pH, and other factors are similar. Longer exposure and more treatments increase the fluoride concentration in the enamel.[48] In clinical research the gel and solution showed comparable effectiveness. Caries incidence was reduced 28 percent by solution and 24 percent by gel.[49]

A. Solution

A 1.23% sodium fluoride with 0.1 M orthophosphoric acid (pH between 3.0 and 3.5). Variations of this formula have been used.

B. Frequency of Application

At least twice annually, at recall appointments. More frequently will permit more fluoride uptake by the enamel, and therefore greater protection, which applies particularly to patients with rampant caries.

C. Advantages

1. Stable solution when kept in a polyethylene bottle.
2. No staining of the tooth structure.
3. Patient acceptance favorable: taste not objectionable.

III. Stannous Fluoride

The initial clinical study was reported in 1955.[50] Annually, four applications of 2% stannous fluoride were made with a cotton applicator or by a 4-minute spray. Under the conditions of the study, caries reductions were 59 percent and 65 percent respectively. Many studies have been conducted since and caries incidence reductions have ranged from 30 to 40 percent.

A 4% solution has also been used,[51] and single

application techniques with 8 and 10%.[52,53] The appeal of a single application to save appointment time led to generalized use of the 8% solution as well as the 10%, which was shown to be beneficial for adult teeth.

A. Solutions and Frequency

1. *The 2% and 4% Solutions:* used the same as 2% sodium fluoride with four applications spaced 2 days to a week apart repeated at 3-year intervals in accord with the tooth eruption pattern of the individual child to provide protection for new teeth soon after eruption.

2. *The 8% or 10% Solutions:* single applications at 4- or 6-month intervals beginning at approximately age 3.

B. Preparation of Solution[54,55]

A fresh solution of stannous fluoride must be used for each patient and prepared after the teeth are prepared, just prior to application. The solution quickly undergoes hydrolysis and oxidation to form stannous hydroxide and stannic ion, therefore decreasing in effectiveness.

1. Obtain from a pharmacist Lilly No. 0 gelatin capsules containing stannous fluoride powder: 0.2 g. for 2%; 0.4 g. for 4%; 0.8 g. for 8%; and 1.0 g. for 10%.

2. Keep capsules in a tightly sealed container.

3. Immediately before use add the contents of one capsule to 10.0 ml. distilled water and shake. Use a 25 ml. graduated cylinder for measuring the water and a 25 ml. polyethylene bottle for mixing the solution.

4. Do not add flavoring or coloring agents.

5. When contents have dissolved, apply immediately to clean, dry, isolated teeth (pages 452–454).

6. Discard excess solution.

C. Adverse Effects

1. *Gingival Reactions.* The occasional reactions that occur range from a mild irritation with blanching to a severe reaction comparable to a chemical burn followed by sloughing.[56,57] They are reversible and the tissue returns to normal within a few days to a week. Severe re-

actions have not generally been demonstrated except with higher concentrations and when the solution was applied to inflamed gingival tissues or tissues markedly irritated during polishing with a rubber cup (page 564).

2. *Pigmentation of Teeth.* Brown staining occurs primarily in areas of decalcification, dental caries, hypocalcification, pits, grooves, and margins of restorations.[56,58] The reaction causing the pigmentation results from the deposition of tin (stannous ion), probably in the form of tin sulfate. Tin phosphates are also formed and deposited on the enamel, which may retard the deposition of fluoride.

D. Precautions for Use

1. *Prevent Gingival Tissue Reactions*
   a. When a patient presents with moderate or severe gingivitis, begin toothbrushing and other plaque control instruction, complete the scaling with careful check for complete removal of local irritants, and postpone fluoride application until a future appointment when the tissue is healed.
   b. Other suggestions for tissue protection: use a rubber dam isolation technique, or coat the gingiva with lubricant (petrolatum) and use the 30-second application.[59,60] Many tissue reactions can also be prevented by using weaker solutions (2 or 4% stannous fluoride).

2. *Protect the Patient's Clothing.* Use a coverall to protect a patient's clothing in case the solution is inadvertently spilled. Stannous fluoride reacts to discolor certain materials.

3. *Make Necessary Radiographs Prior to Stannous Fluoride Application.* This avoids film contamination by stannous ions in the patient's mouth or on the fingers of the operator. Once contaminated, the ions may remain on the fingers for several hours, even following routine handwashing. Cleaning with citric acid followed by thorough rinsing has been recommended for removing the stannous ions.[61]

4. *Prevent Clogging of Saliva Ejector.* Run at least a cupful of water through after application on one side of the mouth, and again at the completion of the entire treatment.

5. *Provide Particular Care for Equipment that Contacts the Stannous Fluoride Solution.* A grayish-white deposit collects when the solution is left for a short time. Sterilizing equipment and disinfecting solution can become contaminated if instruments and dishes are not thoroughly precleaned. Disposable containers are recommended.

E. Disadvantages of Stannous Fluoride

1. Unstable solution: mixing fresh solution for each application is required.
2. Patient acceptance limited: astringent quality and unpleasant taste.
3. Staining of teeth (page 288).
4. Gingival reactions.

CLINICAL PROCEDURES FOR TOPICAL FLUORIDE APPLICATIONS

I. Principles of Application

Maximum benefits derived from topical fluoride preparations can be expected in proportion to the care taken for a well-defined, exacting application procedure. Essentials include the factors listed here.

A. Preparation of the Teeth

Prior to application, a decision must be made concerning the extent of preparation needed for the teeth of each patient. It is not always necessary to polish the teeth before a topical fluoride application.[62] When teeth are polished with an abrasive agent such as pumice, as much as 2 to 4 microns of enamel surface are removed.[63] The surface layer of enamel has the greatest concentration of fluoride and is therefore more protective against dental caries than underlying layers.

It has been shown that dental caries prevention was comparable in two groups of children who received a sodium fluoride topical application, which for one group was immediately preceded by a pumice clean-

ing.[64] In another research study, the fluoride content of the enamel was measured 3 days after a topical fluoride application on teeth that were brushed only and teeth that were pumiced. The fluoride content of the enamel of the two groups was similar, which means that the uptake of fluoride was not interrupted by the presence of pellicle left after toothbrushing.[65]

Therefore, a patient with clean teeth or one participating in a plaque control program should only brush with a commercial fluoride dentifrice and use dental floss to remove all possible dental plaque prior to topical application of fluoride. Appointments for scaling should be completed prior to the application. Only when polishing is required for stain removal should pumicing before a fluoride be needed.

When it is planned that polishing with a rubber cup will be done, a fluoride-containing prophylaxis paste should definitely be used. Although only a small amount of fluoride is added to the tooth from the paste, it has been suggested that the fluoride paste may replace, at least in part, the fluoride removed by the polishing abrasive.[63]

B. Solution

Exacting preparation and care of the solution in accord with its physical and chemical properties.

C. Isolation of Teeth

Drying of the teeth and isolation during the required length of time to permit fluoride to contact tooth surfaces without dilution or contamination by saliva.

D. Clock-timed Procedure

Continuous application to provide constant availability of fluoride ions for formation of fluorapatite.

E. Instructions for Patient

Use of foods or liquids should be avoided during at least 30 minutes following the application. This permits an extended contact of the fluoride with the tooth for additional benefit.

F. Repetition

Applications are made at intervals in accord with the eruption pattern and dental caries susceptibility of the individual. More frequent applications increase the fluoride content of the enamel. A minimum of two treatments annually should be recommended.

II. Supplies and Preparations

A. Cotton roll holders of appropriate size.
B. Cotton rolls of proper lengths attached to holders (see Section III, D and E following).
C. Cotton pellets (six to eight medium size) and cotton pliers. Cotton applicators may be used.
D. Container for fluoride solution.
E. Saliva ejector connected and water control adjusted.
F. Air tip connected to compressed air outlet.
G. Timer for 4 minutes (egg timer or a darkroom alarm).
H. Equipment for stannous fluoride solution (page 451).

III. Cotton Roll Preparation

A. Prepare in Advance

Sterilize cotton rolls on preprepared tray or in separate packages.

B. Objectives

To isolate the teeth in comfort for the patient and prevent absorption of the fluoride by the cotton rolls. For stannous fluoride, cotton rolls prevent the bitter-tasting solution from dispersing around the mouth. Cotton rolls that are too long are easily displaced by action of the tongue and cheek.

C. Supply

1. Use No. 2 cotton rolls except for small mouths or very shallow vestibules, when a No. 1 may be fitted and maintained more effectively.
2. Bevel ends at 45 degrees to facilitate placement and retention in the mucobuccal fold and under the tongue.

D. Lengths: Continuous Cotton Roll Technique

1. *Facial* (5- to 6-inch cotton roll)

   a. Attach to facial prong of cotton roll holder.
   b. To extend (in the mucobuccal fold) from the mandibular labial frenum to the maxillary labial frenum.
2. *Lingual* ($1\frac{1}{4}$- to 2-inch cotton roll)
   a. Attach to lingual prong of holder.
   b. To extend from canine area to just distal to the most posterior tooth.
   c. Extra cotton roll (1 to $1\frac{1}{4}$ inches): for most patients a short cotton roll is needed under the side of the tongue (before the cotton roll holder is placed) for balance. The vestibule is more shallow than the floor of the mouth, which permits the cotton roll holder to tip toward the lingual if not supported by an extra cotton roll.

E. Lengths: Discontinuous Cotton Roll Technique

1. *Indications.* The continuous method can only be used when retraction of the cotton roll from the distobuccal surfaces of the most posterior teeth can be assured during the application. Usually, when second permanent molars (and always the third) have erupted, separate facial cotton rolls are needed for the maxillary and mandibular teeth.
2. *Facial Maxillary* (3 inches)
   a. Finger-held.
   b. To extend from labial frenum to area distal to most posterior tooth and the opening to Stensen's duct.
3. *Facial Mandibular* (3 inches)
   a. Attach to facial prong of holder.
   b. To extend from mandibular labial frenum to the distal of the most posterior tooth. Prevent dislodgment by activity of muscles of throat or cheeks by not extending the cotton roll over the retromolar area.
4. *Lingual Mandibular.* Same as for continuous technique (D,2 previously).

IV. Patient Preparation

A. Preparation of the Teeth (see I,A, page 452).

B. Patient Position

The patient should be positioned upright

to prevent fluoride solution and excess saliva from passing into the throat.

V. Isolation Procedure

A. Place single cotton roll beneath the edge of the tongue.
B. Insert holder with attached cotton rolls over the mandibular teeth: adjust to proper position.
   1. Lingual cotton roll is placed beside and under the lateral margin of the tongue but not so it presses the tongue down.
   2. Check that the cotton rolls are positioned to protect the oral tissues from contact with the metal holder.
   3. Hold the holder with nondominant hand while adjusting the chin clamp; fasten securely.
C. Insert saliva ejector gently in the region of the canine of the side opposite the holder.
D. Adjust maxillary: the continuous cotton roll curves up, distal to the most posterior tooth.
   1. Retract the cheek and twist the cotton roll slightly (toward the gingiva) as it is brought into position in the mucobuccal fold.
   2. Adapt the end in position beside the labial frenum.
E. Hold maxillary section of the cotton roll with the fingers of the nondominant hand. When the discontinuous procedure is used, the maxillary facial cotton roll is held as described here.
   1. Hold the cotton roll away from the distal of the most posterior tooth to assure access of molar surfaces to fluoride.
   2. Maintain retraction throughout application.
F. Make a final check before application
   1. Cotton is not on the teeth.
   2. Oral tissues are protected from metal parts of the holder.
   3. Cotton rolls are not extended too far distally so they can be easily displaced.

VI. Application Procedure

A. Dry Teeth

Dry teeth thoroughly with compressed air: maxillary first, then mandibular. Direct the air to each surface and proximal area, as complete dryness contributes to the effectiveness of fluoride.

B. Apply Fluoride Preparation

Apply quickly to moisten all teeth: mandibular teeth first, then maxillary.

C. Start the Timer

The patient may be instructed to do this so that retraction is not interrupted.

D. Keep Tooth Surfaces Wet

Maintain wet tooth surfaces by continuous application of the solution throughout the 4-minute period.

E. Completion of Application

1. Remove saliva ejector.
2. Release cotton roll holder clamp and remove holder with cotton rolls attached.
3. Remove remaining cotton rolls with cotton pliers.

F. Proceed to Opposite Side of Mouth

The patient does not rinse either between sides or at completion of both sides.

G. Instruct Patient

Instruct patient not to rinse, eat, drink, or brush the teeth for at least 30 minutes, preferably longer.

FLUORIDE GEL PREPARATIONS

Tests to determine the effectiveness of fluoride gel applied by tray or mouthpiece have varied in their findings, which may be related to the difference in procedures used during the research. By far the most significant research has been that in which custom-fitted polyvinyl mouthpieces were used to apply an acidulated phosphate-fluoride (APF) gel and a plain neutral sodium fluoride gel. Both contained 1.1% sodium fluoride. Research statistics showed dental caries prevention to be 75 percent for the neutral and 80 percent for the acidulated after supervised daily 6-minute applications by the children for nearly two school years.[66] Two years after the final application, reexamination showed close to 70 percent retained effect.[67]

When the gel is self-applied in trays once or a few times per year, the caries prevention ranges from 25 to 45 percent fewer new carious lesions.[68-71] Stannous fluoride has been prepared in a water-free stable gel.[72] Its effectiveness when applied by toothbrush or rubber cup has been described.[73]

I. Principles for Professional Application

Some of the same factors that influence the benefits obtained from use of a solution also apply to application of a gel. Additional factors that may influence results should be considered. A gel preparation may not disperse as readily as a solution does about the teeth. Tray selection may make a difference. Soft wax trays may not be firm enough to force the gel into the inaccessible but strategic pits, fissures, and proximal areas. It is also possible that in the warmth of the mouth, the wax softens and by becoming flexible permits salivary contamination or dilution. Such problems may not arise when custom-fitted polyvinyl trays are used.

A. Gel Content

1. Fluoride 1.23% in 0.1 M orthophosphoric acid at pH 3.0 (same as the acidulated phosphate solution).
2. Gelling agent: hydroxyethyl cellulose.
3. Flavoring agent.

B. Modes of Application

1. Cotton roll isolation procedure with application using cotton pellets and cotton pliers (page 454). Other isolation procedures may also be used (page 458).
2. Trays: custom-fitted polyvinyl, or foam rubber; wax trays with or without cotton lining also have been used.

C. Procedure for Tray System

1. Preparation of teeth (see I,A).
2. Tray preparation
   a. Custom-fitted vinyl tray can be prepared for an individual patient and kept in a labeled box for use at continuing appointments.
   b. Wax tray: trimmed to the general size and contour of the mouth: check in the mouth for proper molding and length to cover distal surfaces of most-posterior teeth.
3. Place three to five drops of gel in the base of the tray and spread around. A thin layer is sufficient for a well-fitted tray. When excess gel is applied, it can be forced out from under the edge of the tray and may pass into the throat.

D. Application: Single Arch

1. Dry maxillary teeth: place tray over teeth and immediately insert saliva ejector.
2. Mold wax tray firmly around the teeth, starting over the occlusal and press horizontally to force the gel into the interproximal areas. A well-adapted tray can help exclude saliva.
3. Place a cotton roll over each side in the premolar area and request patient to close gently, without excess pressure, to hold the tray in position. The slight pressure can aid by forcing the gel into the pits, fissures and other inaccessible areas; with too much pressure on a soft wax tray, the sides of the tray may spread, thus encouraging contamination by saliva.
4. Start the timer: leave tray in position for at least 4 minutes; 6 preferred.
5. Remove tray with cotton pliers.
6. Patient does not rinse.
7. Dry mandibular teeth and place the tray; mold carefully over the teeth, as before, to press the gel between the teeth.
8. Insert saliva ejector and a cotton roll on each premolar-molar region before requesting patient to close gently.
9. Procedure is timed as before, and tray removed. Wipe excess gel from the teeth.
10. Instruct patient not to eat, drink, rinse, or brush the teeth for at least 30 minutes, preferably longer.

E. Additional Technique Suggestions

1. Acidulated phosphate-fluoride gels are stable when kept in polyethylene containers.
2. Relation to gingiva: an occasional reaction may occur in the form of a white color change within about 15 minutes after application. It can be wiped off, or if left untouched, will disappear within an hour or two. No postoperative effects occur, and no subjective symptoms have

been reported. Suggestions for prevention of a gingival reaction:

    a. Provide plaque control instruction and postpone application when gingiva is inflamed. The reaction rarely occurs except when there is moderate to severe inflammation.

    b. Use minimum amount of gel and confine it as much as possible to the base of the tray. When a wax tray is used, hold with horizontal pressure to force small excesses between the teeth rather than over the gingiva.

  3. Use of a double-arch technique in which both trays are inserted and timed simultaneously is not recommended for routine use, particularly when soft wax trays are used because of difficulty of control and adaptation.

II. Self-applied: Custom Tray

Fluoride gels (0.5% APF with a pH 4.5 to 7.0 or 0.4% stannous fluoride[74]) may be used in a custom-made tray (mouthguard type which covers the cervical third) for home use on a daily or weekly basis.

A. Directions

  1. Use toothbrush and floss: thoroughly remove all plaque.

  2. Dry mouth by swallowing several times.

  3. Apply a few drops or a small ribbon to the inside of each tray. Do not overload so that gel squeezes out excessively when applied.

  4. Apply trays over the teeth. Close with pressure to hold them in place. The slight pressure will force the gel to the proximal areas.

  5. Retain for 4 minutes.

B. Indications for Special Patients

Tray application on a daily basis is particularly applicable to patients with a high risk of dental caries. Examples are patients who have

  1. Rampant caries.

  2. Xerostomia.

  3. Exposure to radiation therapy (page 680).

  4. An overdenture (page 391).

  5. Gingival recession and, therefore, susceptibility to cemental caries.

APPLICATION BY SPRAY

A spray technique has not been used extensively, but reports have shown moderate effectiveness in prevention of dental caries. For examples, one study showed sodium fluoride (2%) to be equally effective when applied by spray as by cotton applicator;[45] and in another study stannous fluoride (2%) was somewhat more effective by spray than by cotton applicator.[50]

Without oral prophylaxis, an acidulated phosphate-fluoride solution was used as a spray three times, spaced during each of three school years as a research study, but with implications useful in a school dental health program. There was reduction in new carious lesions, with greatest benefit to those children with cleaner mouths who practiced regular daily brushing.[75]

In another study, an acidulated phosphate-fluoride spray was applied for rinsing during and following the use of a prophylaxis paste containing acidulated phosphate-fluoride.[76] Caries reductions from these procedures were not as great as from conventional topical fluoride application and generally should be considered a supplement rather than a substitute for more effective applications when made on an individual basis.

Based on these studies, for patients who do not or cannot cooperate by maintaining oral cleanliness even with repeated instruction, clinical procedures can be planned to include frequent applications by spray. The spray may also be used for rinsing following operative procedures.

FLUORIDE MOUTHRINSES

Self-applied fluoride by use of a mouthrinse provides a practical and effective means for dental caries prevention and desensitization. A summary of research studies using various concentrations shows that reductions in dental caries incidence range from 20 to 50 percent.[77,78]

The caries-preventing effects of fluoride solutions are related to frequency of use, whether daily, weekly, or once every two weeks. More frequent use has been shown to be more beneficial.

Rinsing is a more efficient method for fluoride use than professionally-applied techniques, and the benefits can be greater. It has definite advantages when applied in a school health preventive program since materials are not complicated or expensive and it does not take children out of the classroom. Minimal instruction is needed for teachers and adult volunteers to carry out the classroom procedures. Overall supervision can be provided by dental hygienists.

On an individual basis, home use of a fluoride mouthrinse is convenient for all ages. The rinses are important for prevention of dental caries, enamel remineralization, and dentinal desensitization.

Instruction and motivation to parents for supervision of children is provided by the dental hygienist as part of the dental hygiene treatment plan.

When fluoride supplements are indicated, the rinse supplement, which is actively swished over and between the teeth before swallowing, may be easier for certain patients than use of a chewable tablet and contains the same amount of ingestible fluoride.[41] In a community with fluoridation of the drinking water, mouthrinse should not be swallowed. Therefore it cannot be recommended for small children or others who cannot rinse without swallowing.

I. Mouthrinses[79]

A. Sodium Fluoride

1. *Solutions and Frequency*
   a. Aqueous solution of sodium fluoride 0.2%, pH 7.0 (neutral), used weekly or once every two weeks.
   b. Aqueous solution of sodium fluoride 0.05%, pH 7.0 (neutral), used daily.
   c. Aqueous solution of acidulated phosphate sodium fluoride 0.044%, pH approximately 4.0, used daily.
2. *Directions.* One teaspoonful (5 ml.) should be swished vigorously for not less than one minute. Rinsing directions are on page 369.

B. Stannous Fluoride

Stannous fluoride 0.1% to be dissolved in measured tap water as directed; for daily use.

II. Brush With Solution

Brushing with a fluoride solution has been shown to produce significant reductions in dental caries incidence. Periodic supervised brushing with sodium fluoride, sodium monofluorophosphate, and acidulated phosphate-fluoride has demonstrated beneficial results. These have been summarized in the literature.[80]

Despite a small increase in time and supervision, use of toothbrushing with the solution may be preferred over rinsing because of the importance of brushing to the removal of dental plaque. The procedure may be of help to parents and attendants of disabled persons who cannot carry out their own oral care and prevention techniques.

FLUORIDE DENTIFRICES

The principal fluoride compounds currently utilized in dentifrices are stannous fluoride, sodium fluoride, and sodium monofluorophosphate. A few of these dentifrices have been accepted by the American Dental Association.[40]*

I. Benefits

Various reductions in caries incidence have been shown by the reported research findings. Direct comparisons cannot be made between the studies because of the differences in research procedures. The overall range is 20 to 30 percent caries inhibition.

Greater benefits have been demonstrated for newly erupted teeth; a finding in keeping with the usual effect of topically applied fluoride. Added benefits have been shown for children who have used drinking water with fluoride at optimum level. Reviews of the literature are available.[81,82]

II. Dentifrice Components

The first sodium fluoride dentifrice study did not show statistically significant caries reduction.[83] It has been demonstrated that other ingredients of a dentifrice must be compatible with the fluoride ions. When the abrasive agent contains calcium, fluoride and calcium can react, thus rendering the fluoride inactive.

Components of dentifrices are described on pages 370–372. Fluoride dentifrices are made with the basic essential ingredients, a compatible abrasive agent, and a source of fluoride ions. Specific formulae for the dentifrices approved by the American Dental Association are included in *Accepted Dental Therapeutics.*[40]

---

* For description of American Dental Association classification, see page 376.

III. Recommendation

A fluoride dentifrice should be recommended for all patients as part of the complete preventive program. Certain fluoride dentifrices may also have desensitizing properties (page 556).

Since stannous fluoride dentifrices can stain teeth a light to moderate brown, they would not be recommended for use on exposed cementum.

FLUORIDE PROPHYLAXIS PASTES

Application of fluoride by pastes cannot be considered a substitute for conventional topical application on the basis of present-day research. Reviews of the research show that while moderate caries-preventive effects have been demonstrated, other studies have had minimal or no statistically significant results.

Incompatibility of the fluoride agent with the abrasive or other paste ingredients has been a problem with certain combinations. It is not merely a question of adding a fluoride solution to a cleaning paste. When mixed, agents may react, and the effect of the fluoride can be neutralized or at least the shelf-life may be limited.

Another limitation of the paste preparations is that certain abrasives can remove a thin layer of enamel during polishing. With the removal of the enamel, the outer layer of fluoride is also removed, possibly as fast as it is added from the paste, but this concept has not been researched.

In order to be able to evaluate fluoride preparations which become available on the market, a continuing review of the new research will be needed as additional studies are reported. Because the caries prevention that can be expected from the use of prophylaxis pastes is minimal, other means for applying fluoride must be used if the patient is to receive optimum protection by fluorides.

COMBINED FLUORIDE PROGRAM

Most patients can benefit from more than one method of use of fluorides. When the preventive program is planned for an individual patient, the fluoride preparations and modes of application selected should provide the greatest possible protection against dental caries.

When self-administered methods are chosen, patient cooperation is a significant factor. For example, a daily application of fluoride gel in a custom-made tray may be ideal for a patient, but cooperation may be difficult to obtain even when the patient has well-meaning parents. A single daily chewable tablet or daily mouthrinse may not be as difficult for some patients.

Age and eruption pattern influence the method selected, as it is particularly important to apply fluorides as soon after eruption as possible. Recall appointments can be scheduled for frequent topical applications and for continuing instruction and motivation. All methods are supplemented by the use of a dentifrice with fluoride.

TECHNICAL HINTS

I. Alternate Isolation Procedures for Topical Application

The procedure described on page 454 was for isolation of one half of the dentition at one time. Objectives are to conserve time, but also to maintain as dry a field as possible and to keep the fluoride solution from being absorbed by cotton rolls or the saliva from contaminating or diluting the solution. Other systems that may be applied include:

A. Rubber Dam

1. *Use.* For application of fluoride following operative procedures.
2. *Preparation.* When the rubber dam has not been fitted to include the entire quadrant, additional holes may be made in the dam with an explorer.
3. *Advantages*
   a. Better control of the patient during the application, particularly a small child or handicapped patient with special problems.
   b. Time saving: dry teeth can be maintained.
   c. Helpful when general anesthesia is used, particularly for a hospitalized patient.
   d. Stannous fluoride: the solution is confined and the patient does not experience the unpleasant taste.

B. Single Quadrant

Each quadrant can be done separately by holding the cotton rolls with the fingers. In a very small mouth it may be possible to hold a Number 1 continuous cotton roll around the entire maxillary arch to make the entire application in one timing. This can be particularly useful for a small child when cotton roll holders may not stay in place.

I. Appointment Planning

Because of the postapplication ruling concerning no eating for at least one-half hour, avoid scheduling topical fluoride procedures just before the mealtime hours. This would be particularly important for patients on special diets, such as diabetics.

III. Fluoride Application Following Polishing of Restorations

Since abrasive stones and polishing agents remove a layer of surface enamel and polishing procedures extend over the margins of the restoration, a topical application of fluoride can be particularly important (pages 592–593). The removal of surface fluoride about the margin weakens the enamel and may render it more susceptible to dental caries if precautions are not taken.

FACTORS TO TEACH THE PATIENT

I. Personal Use of Fluorides

A. Purposes, action, and expected benefits relative to the specific forms of fluoride treatment the patient will receive.

B. Specific instruction concerning self-applied techniques that will be performed at home. Prepared printed instruction materials can be especially useful.

C. Chewable tablets: avoid eating, drinking, or toothbrushing for one-half hour following use. The preferred time for use is after toothbrushing before going to bed.

D. Relate brushing technique to need for fluoride in dentifrice to reach all tooth surfaces.

II. Preparation for Topical Fluoride Application

When the teeth are free from plaque and the gingival tissue is firm and healthy, there is greater uptake of fluoride by the teeth and less possibility of a slight tissue reaction. When the gingiva is inflamed, the patient will need instruction in order to understand why the topical application is postponed until the tissue has healed.

III. Fluorides Are Part of the Total Preventive Program

Control of cariogenic foods in the diet, particularly between-meals, and professional care are still necessary to supplement fluoride treatment for caries control.

IV. Recall

There is a need for continuing applications of topical agents. Frequent applications increase the fluoride content of the enamel and provide greater resistance to dental caries.

V. Fluoridation

In a nonfluoridated community, information concerning the significance of fluoridation to the entire community and its benefits and operation should be available and disseminated.

VI. Stannous Fluoride

When topical stannous fluoride preparations are used, the patient (or parent) should be informed about the possibility of tooth staining.

References

1. Bhaskar, S.N., ed.: *Orban's Oral Histology and Embryology*, 9th ed. St. Louis, The C.V. Mosby Co., 1980, pp. 24–45, 75–106.
2. Melfi, R.C.: *Permar's Oral Embryology and Microscopic Anatomy*, 7th ed. Philadelphia, Lea & Febiger, 1982, pp. 154–171.
3. Brudevold, F., Gardner, D.E., and Smith, F.A.: The Distribution of Fluoride in Human Enamel, *J. Dent. Res.*, 35, 420, June, 1956.
4. Brudevold, F., Steadman, L.T., and Smith, F.A.: Inorganic and Organic Components of Tooth Structure, *Ann. New York Acad. Sci.*, 85, 110, March 29, 1960.
5. Brudevold, F., McCann, H.G., Nilsson, R., Richardson, B., and Coklica, V.: The Chemistry of Caries Inhibition Problems and Challenges in Topical Treatments, *J. Dent. Res.*, 46, 37, January–February, 1967.
6. Dawes, C., Jenkins, G.N., Hardwick, J.L., and Leach, S.A.: The Relation Between the Fluoride Concentrations in the Dental Plaque and in Drinking Water, *Br. Dent. J.*, 119, 164, August 17, 1965.
7. Jenkins, G.N., Edgar, W.M., and Ferguson, D.B.: The Distribution and Metabolic Effects of Human Plaque Fluorine, *Arch. Oral Biol.*, 14, 105, January, 1969.
8. Richards, L.F., Westmoreland, W.W., Tashiro, M., McKay, C.H., and Morrison, J.T.: Determining Optimum Fluoride Levels for Community Water Supplies in Relation to Temperature, *J. Am. Dent. Assoc.*, 74, 389, February, 1967.
9. McNeil, D.R.: *The Fight for Fluoridation*. New York, Oxford University Press, 1957, pp. 3–43.
10. Russell, A.L.: Epidemiology and the Rational Bases of Dental Public Health and Dental Practice, in Young,

W.O. and Striffler, D.F.: *The Dentist, His Practice, and His Community*, 2nd ed. Philadelphia, W.B. Saunders Co., 1969, pp. 37–42.

11. McKay, F.S.: The Relation of Mottled Enamel to Caries, *J. Am. Dent. Assoc.*, 15, 1429, August, 1928.

12. Churchill, H.V.: Occurrence of Fluorides in Some Waters of United States, *J. Indust. & Engin. Chem.*, 23, 996, 1931.

13. Dean, H.T., Arnold, F.A., Jr., and Elvove, E.: Domestic Water and Dental Caries. V. Additional Studies of the Relation of Fluoride Domestic Waters to Dental Caries Experience in 4425 White Children, Aged 12 to 14 Years, of 13 Cities in 4 States, *Pub. Health Rep.*, 57, 1155, August 7, 1942.

14. *Fluoridation Census 1975*. United States Department of Health, Education, and Welfare, Public Health Service, Center for Disease Control, Bureau of State Services, Atlanta, Georgia, April, 1977.

15. Forrest, J.R.: Caries Incidence and Enamel Defects in Areas with Different Levels of Fluoride in the Drinking Water, *Br. Dent. J.*, 100, 195, April 17, 1956.

16. Diefenbach, V.L., Nevitt, G.A., and Frankel, J.M.: Fluoridation and the Appearance of Teeth, *J. Am. Dent. Assoc.*, 71, 1129, November, 1965.

17. Arnold, F.A., Dean, H.T., Jay, P., and Knutson, J.W.: Effect of Fluoridated Public Water Supplies on Dental Caries Prevalence. Tenth Year of the Grand Rapids—Muskegon Study, *Pub. Health Rep.*, 71, 652, July, 1956.

18. Hayes, R.L., Littleton, N.W., and White, C.L.: Posteruptive Effects of Fluoridation on First Permanent Molars of Children in Grand Rapids, Michigan, *Am. J. Public Health*, 47, 192, February, 1957.

19. Russell, A.L. and Hamilton, P.M.: Dental Caries in Permanent First Molars after Eight Years of Fluoridation, *Arch. Oral Biol.*, 6, 50, July, 1961.

20. Backer Dirks, O., Houwink, B., and Kwant, G.W.: Some Special Features of the Caries Preventive Effect of Water Fluoridation, *Arch. Oral Biol.*, 4, 187, August, 1961.

21. Ast, D.B. and Fitzgerald, B.: Effectiveness of Water Fluoridation, *J. Am. Dent. Assoc.*, 65, 581, November, 1962.

22. Carlos, J.P., Gittelsohn, A.M., and Haddon, W., Jr.: Caries in Deciduous Teeth in Relation to Maternal Ingestion of Fluoride, *Pub. Health Rep.*, 77, 658, August, 1962.

23. Horowitz, H.S. and Heifetz, S.B.: Effects of Prenatal Exposure to Fluoridation on Dental Caries, *Pub. Health Rep.*, 82, 297, April, 1967.

24. Katz, S. and Muhler, J.C.: Prenatal and Postnatal Fluoride and Dental Caries Experience in Deciduous Teeth, *J. Am. Dent. Assoc.*, 76, 305, February, 1968.

25. Salzmann, J.A.: The Effects of Fluoride on the Prevalence of Malocclusion, *J. Am. Coll. Dent.*, 35, 82, January, 1968.

26. Russell, A.L. and Elvove, E.: Domestic Water and Dental Caries. VII. A Study of the Fluoride-Dental Caries Relationship in an Adult Population, *Pub. Health Rep.*, 66, 1389, October 26, 1951.

27. Englander, H.R. and Wallace, D.A.: Effects of Naturally Fluoridated Water on Dental Caries in Adults, *Pub. Health Rep.*, 77, 887, October, 1962.

28. Sognnaes, R.F.: Fluoride Protection of Bones and Teeth, *Science*, 150, 989, November 19, 1965.

29. Bernstein, D.S., Sadowsky, N., Hegsted, D.M., Guri, C.D., and Stare, F.J.: Prevalence of Osteoporosis in High- and Low-fluoride Areas in North Dakota, *J. Am. Med. Assoc.*, 198, 499, October 31, 1966.

30. Fluoride, Bony Structure, and Aortic Calcification, *Nutrition Rev.*, 25, 100, April, 1967.

31. Grøn, P., McCann, H.G., and Bernstein, D.: Effect of Fluoride on Human Osteoporotic Bone Mineral, *J. Bone & Joint Surg.*, 48A, 892, July, 1966.

32. Stamm, J.W. and Banting, D.W.: Comparison of Root Caries Prevalence in Adults with Life-long Residence in Fluoridated and Non-fluoridated Communities, *J. Dent. Res.*, 59, 405, Abstract 552, Special Issue A, March, 1980.

33. Horowitz, H.S., Maier, F.J., and Law, F.E.: Partial Defluoridation of a Community Water Supply and Dental Fluorosis, *Pub. Health Rep.*, 82, 965, November, 1967.

34. Horowitz, H.S. and Heifetz, S.B.: The Effect of Partial Defluoridation of a Water Supply on Dental Fluorosis—Final Results in Bartlett, Texas, After 17 Years, *Am. J. Public Health*, 62, 767, June, 1972.

35. Horowitz, H.S.: School Fluoridation for the Prevention of Dental Caries, *Int. Dent. J.*, 23, 346, June, 1973.

36. Heifetz, S.B., Horowitz, H.S., and Driscoll, W.S.: Effect of School Water Fluoridation on Dental Caries: Results in Seagrove, N.C. after Eight Years, *J. Am. Dent. Assoc.*, 97, 193, August, 1978.

37. Lemke, C.W., Doherty, J.M., and Arra, M.C.: Controlled Fluoridation: The Dental Effects of Discontinuation in Antigo, Wisconsin, *J. Am. Dent. Assoc.*, 80, 782, April, 1970.

38. Ast, D.B., Cons, N.C., Pollard, S.T., and Garfinkel, J.: Time and Cost Factors to Provide Regular Periodic Dental Care for Children in a Fluoridated and Nonfluoridated Area: Final Report, *J. Am. Dent. Assoc.*, 80, 770, April, 1970.

39. Driscoll, W.S.: The Use of Fluoride Tablets for the Prevention of Dental Caries, in Forrester, D.J. and Schulz, E.M., eds.: *International Workshop on Fluorides and Dental Caries Reductions*. Baltimore, Maryland, 1974, pp. 25–111.

40. American Dental Association, Council on Dental Therapeutics: *Accepted Dental Therapeutics*, 39th ed. Chicago, American Dental Association, 1982, pp. 344–368.

41. Aasenden, R., DePaola, P.F., and Brudevold, F.: Effects of Daily Rinsing and Ingestion of Fluoride Solutions Upon Dental Caries and Enamel Fluoride, *Arch. Oral Biol.*, 17, 1705, December, 1972.

42. Driscoll, W.S., Heifetz, S.B., and Brunelle, J.A.: Treatment and Posttreatment Effects of Chewable Fluoride Tablets on Dental Caries: Findings After 7½ Years, *J. Am. Dent. Assoc.*, 99, 817, November, 1979.

43. Bibby, B.G.: Use of Fluorine in the Prevention of Dental Caries. II. The Effects of Sodium Fluoride Applications, *J. Am. Dent. Assoc.*, 31, 317, March 1, 1944.

44. Knutson, J.W.: Sodium Fluoride Solutions: Technic for Application to the Teeth, *J. Am. Dent. Assoc.*, 36, 37, January, 1948.

45. Galagan, D.J. and Knutson, J.W.: The Effect of Topically Applied Fluorides on Dental Caries Experience. VI. Experiments with Sodium Fluoride and Calcium Chloride . . . Widely Spaced Applications . . . Use of Different Solution Concentrations, *Pub. Health Rep.*, 63, 1215, September 17, 1948.

46. Wellock, W.D. and Brudevold, F.: A Study of Acidulated Fluoride Solutions—II. The Caries Inhibiting Effect of Single Annual Topical Applications of an Acidic Fluoride and Phosphate Solution. A Two Year Experience, *Arch. Oral Biol.*, 8, 179, March–April, 1963.

47. Wellock, W.D., Maitland, A., and Brudevold, F.: Caries Increments, Tooth Discoloration, and State of Oral Hygiene in Children Given Single Annual Applications of Acid Phosphate-Fluoride and Stannous Fluoride, *Arch. Oral Biol.*, 10, 453, May–June, 1965.

48. Wei, S.H.Y.: Fluoride Uptake by Enamel from Topical Solutions and Gels: an *In Vitro* Study, *J. Dent. Child.*, *40*, 299, July–August, 1973.

49. Horowitz, H.S. and Doyle, J.: The Effect on Dental Caries of Topically Applied Acidulated Phosphate-fluorides: Results After Three Years, *J. Am. Dent. Assoc.*, *82*, 359, February, 1971.

50. Howell, C.L., Gish, C.W., Smiley, R.D., and Muhler, J.C.: Effect of Topically Applied Stannous Fluoride on Dental Caries Experience in Children, *J. Am. Dent. Assoc.*, *50*, 14, January, 1955.

51. McDonald, R.E. and Muhler, J.C.: Superiority of Topical Application of Stannous Fluoride on Primary Teeth, *J. Dent. Child.*, *24*, 84, 2nd Quarter, 1957.

52. Gish, C.W., Howell, C.L., and Muhler, J.C.: A New Approach to the Topical Application of Fluorides for the Reduction of Dental Caries in Children, *J. Dent. Res.*, *36*, 784, October, 1957.

53. Muhler, J.C.: The Effect of a Single Topical Application of Stannous Fluoride on the Incidence of Dental Caries in Adults, *J. Dent. Res.*, *37*, 415, June, 1958.

54. Muhler, J.C.: Topical Application of Stannous Fluoride, *J. Am. Dent. Assoc.*, *54*, 352, March, 1957.

55. Dudding, N.J. and Muhler, J.C.: Technique of Application of Stannous Fluoride in a Compatible Prophylactic Paste and as a Topical Agent, *J. Dent. Child.*, *29*, 219, 4th Quarter, 1962.

56. Muhler, J.C.: Effect on Gingiva and Occurrence of Pigmentation on Teeth Following the Topical Application of Stannous Fluoride or Stannous Chlorofluoride, *J. Periodontol.*, *28*, 281, October, 1957.

57. Swieterman, R.P., Muhler, J.C., and Swenson, H.M.: The Effect of Highly Concentrated Solutions of Stannous Fluoride on Human Gingival Tissue, *J. Periodontol.*, *32*, 131, April, 1961.

58. Hine, J.F., Swartz, M.L., and Phillips, R.W.: Staining of Resin and Silicate Restorations by Topically Applied Solutions of Stannous Fluoride, *J. Periodontol.*, *28*, 138, April, 1957.

59. McDonald, R.E.: Gingival Tissue Reaction to Topical Application of Stannous Fluoride for the General Anesthesia Patient, *J. Dent. Child.*, *31*, 100, 2nd Quarter, 1964.

60. Mercer, V. and Muhler, J.C.: The Effect of a 30-second Topical SnF_2 Treatment on Dental Caries Reductions in Children, *J. Oral Thera. and Pharm.*, *1*, 141, September, 1964.

61. Yamane, G.M., Meskin, L.H., and Mehaffey, P.: Stannous Ion Contamination of Radiographic Films. Etiology and Prevention, *J. Am. Dent. Hyg. Assoc.*, *42*, 147, 3rd Quarter, 1968.

62. Wei, S.H.Y.: The Potential Benefits To Be Derived from Topical Fluorides in Fluoridated Communities, in Forrester, D.J. and Schulz, E.M., eds.: *International Workshop on Fluorides and Dental Caries Reductions.* Baltimore, Maryland, 1974, pp. 193–196.

63. Vrbic, V., Brudevold, F., and McCann, H.G.: Acquisition of Fluoride by Enamel from Fluoride Pumice Pastes, *Helv. Odontol. Acta*, *11*, 21, April, 1967.

64. Chrietzberg, J.E.: Toothbrushing as a Substitute for Quick Cleansing in the Topical Fluoride Technic, *J. Am. Dent. Assoc.*, *42*, 435, April, 1951.

65. Tinanoff, N., Wei, S.H.Y., and Parkins, F.M.: Effect of a Pumice Prophylaxis on Fluoride Uptake in Tooth Enamel, *J. Am. Dent. Assoc.*, *88*, 384, February, 1974.

66. Englander, H.R., Keyes, P.H., and Gestwicki, M.: Clinical Anticaries Effect of Repeated Topical Sodium Fluoride Applications by Mouthpieces, *J. Am. Dent. Assoc.*, *75*, 638, September, 1967.

67. Englander, H.R., Carlos, J.P., Senning, R.S., and Mellberg, J.R.: Residual Anticaries Effect of Repeated Topical Sodium Fluoride Applications by Mouthpieces, *J. Am. Dent. Assoc.*, *78*, 783, April, 1969.

68. Bryan, E.T. and Williams, J.E.: The Cariostatic Effectiveness of a Phosphate-fluoride Gel Administered Annually to School Children: Final Results, *J. Public Health Dent.*, *30*, 13, Winter, 1970.

69. Englander, H.R., Sherrill, L.T., Miller, B.G., Carlos, J.P., Mellberg, J.R., and Senning, R.S.: Incremental Rates of Dental Caries After Repeated Topical Sodium Fluoride Applications in Children with Lifelong Consumption of Fluoridated Water, *J. Am. Dent. Assoc.*, *82*, 354, February, 1971.

70. Horowitz, H.S. and Kau, M.C.W.: Retained Anticaries Protection from Topically Applied Acidulated Phosphate-fluoride: 30- and 36-month Post-treatment Effects, *J. Prev. Dent.*, *1*, 22, May–June, 1974.

71. Trubman, A. and Crellin, J.A.: Effect on Dental Caries of Self-application of Acidulated Phosphate Fluoride Paste and Gel, *J. Am. Dent. Assoc.*, *86*, 153, January, 1973.

72. Shannon, I.L.: Preventive Dental Services in the Veterans' Administration Hospital, *J. Public Health Dent.*, *30*, 156, Summer, 1970.

73. Cowan, R.D. and Shannon, I.L.: Protective Effectiveness of a Stannous Fluoride Gel, *Aust. Dent. J.*, *17*, 293, August, 1972.

74. Shannon, I.L., Wescott, W.B., and Feller, R.P.: Use of Fluorides, in Clark, J.W., ed.: *Clinical Dentistry*, Volume 2, Chapter 7, Hagerstown, Maryland, Harper & Row, 1981, pp. 1–11.

75. DePaola, P.F., Wellock, W.D., Maitland, A., and Brudevold, F.: The Relationship of Cariostasis, Oral Hygiene, and Past Caries Experience in Children Receiving Three Sprays Annually with Acidulated Phosphate-fluoride: Three-year Results, *J. Am. Dent. Assoc.*, *77*, 91, July, 1968.

76. DePaola, P.F.: Combined Use of a Sodium Fluoride Prophylaxis Paste and a Spray Containing Acidulated Sodium Fluoride Solution, *J. Am. Dent. Assoc.*, *75*, 1407, December, 1967.

77. Torell, P. and Ericsson, Y.: The Potential Benefits Derived from Fluoride Mouth Rinses, in Forrester, D.J. and Schulz, E.M., eds.: *International Workshop on Fluorides and Dental Caries Reductions.* Baltimore, Maryland, 1974, pp. 114–176.

78. Birkeland, J.M. and Torell, P.: Caries-preventive Fluoride Mouthrinses, *Caries Res.*, *12*, 38, Supplement 1, 1978.

79. Ripa, L.W.: Fluoride Rinsing: What Dentists Should Know, *J. Am. Dent. Assoc.*, *102*, 477, April, 1981.

80. McConchie, J.M.: The Potential Benefits of "Brush-in" Programmes as Regards Prevention of Dental Caries, Dental Health Education and Public Relations, in Forrester, D.J. and Schulz, E.M., eds.: *International Workshop on Fluorides and Dental Caries Reductions.* Baltimore, Maryland, 1974, pp. 273–277.

81. von der Fehr, F.R. and Møller, I.J.: Caries-preventive Fluoride Dentifrices, *Caries Res.*, *12*, 31, Supplement 1, 1978.

82. Forrester, D.J. and Horowitz, H.S.: Individual Topical Fluoride Therapy, in Forrester, D.J., Wagner, M.L., and Fleming, J., eds.: *Pediatric Dental Medicine.* Philadelphia, Lea & Febiger, 1981, pp. 326–328.

83. Bibby, B.G.: A Test of the Effect of Fluoride-containing Dentifrices on Dental Caries, *J. Dent. Res.*, *24*, 297, December, 1945.

84. Horowitz, H.S. and Heifetz, S.B.: The Current Status

of Topically Applied Fluorides in Preventive Dentistry, in Newbrun, E., ed.: *Fluorides and Dental Caries,* 2nd ed. Springfield, Illinois, Charles C Thomas, 1975, pp. 56–59.

Suggested Readings

Aasenden, R.: Post-eruptive Changes in the Fluoride Concentrations of Human Tooth Surface Enamel, *Arch. Oral Biol.,* 20, 359, May/June, 1975.

Banting, D.W.: Effect of Age and Length of Residence in a Fluoridated Area on Root Surface Fluoride Concentration, *Clin. Prev. Dent.,* 1, 7, September–October, 1979.

Brudevold, F. and Naujoks, R.: Caries-preventive Fluoride Treatment of the Individual, *Caries Res.,* 12, 52, Supplement 1, 1978.

Bruun, C. and Givskov, H.: Release of Fluoride from Fluoride-containing Chewing Gum, *Community Dent. Oral Epidemiol.,* 6, 27, January, 1978.

Chaet, R. and Wei, S.H.Y.: The Effect of Fluoride Impregnated Dental Floss on Enamel Fluoride Uptake *in vitro* and *Streptococcus mutans* Colonization *in vivo, J. Dent. Child.,* 44, 122, March–April, 1977.

Congleton, J.B., Crenshaw, M.A., and Bawden, J.W.: The Diffusion of Fluoride Ion from Acidulated Phosphate Fluoride Topical Products, *J. Dent. Child.,* 45, 133, March–April, 1978.

Craig, G.G. and Powell, K.R.: Dental Caries in Susceptible Fissures After Prolonged Fluoride Application, *Community Dent. Oral Epidemiol.,* 7, 158, June, 1979.

Golinsky, A.: Fatal Incidents of Fluoride Intoxication, *Can. Dent. Hyg.,* 15, 14, Spring, 1981.

Going, R.E., Loehman, R.E., and Chan, M.S.: Mouthguard Materials: Their Physical and Mechanical Properties, *J. Am. Dent. Assoc.,* 89, 132, July, 1974.

Hirschfield, R.E.: Control of Decalcification by Use of Fluoride Mouthrinse, *J. Dent. Child.,* 45, 458, December, 1978.

Holland, R.I.: Cytotoxicity of Fluoride, *Acta Odontol. Scand.,* 38, 69, Number 2, 1980.

Horowitz, H.S.: Review of Topical Applications, Fluorides and Fissure Sealants, *Can. Dent. Assoc. J.,* 46, 38, January, 1980.

Keyes, P. and Englander, H.R.: Fluoride Therapy in the Treatment of Dentomicrobial Plaque Diseases, *J. Am. Soc. Prev. Dent.,* 5, 16, January–February, 1975.

Magness, W.S., Shannon, I.L., and West, D.C.: Office-applied Fluoride Treatments for Orthodontic Patients, *J. Dent. Res.,* 58, 1427, April, 1979.

Mellberg, J.R.: Enamel Fluoride and Its Anti-caries Effects, *J. Prev. Dent.,* 4, 8, January–February, 1977.

Mellberg, J.R.: Penetration of Fluorine from Sodium Monofluorophosphate into Artificially Produced Incipient Enamel Lesions, *Caries Res.,* 14, 115, Number 2, 1980.

Obersztyn, A., Kolwinski, K., Trykowski, J., and Starosciak, S.: Effects of Stannous Fluoride and Amine Fluorides on Caries Incidence and Enamel Solubility in Adults, *Aust. Dent. J.,* 24, 395, December, 1979.

Parkins, F.M.: Prescribing Low Potency Fluorides for Frequent Use, *J. Prev. Dent.,* 4, 30, November–December, 1977.

Poulsen, S. and Larsen, M.J.: Dental Caries in Relation to Fluoride Content of Enamel in the Primary Dentition, *Caries Res.,* 9, 59, Number 1, 1975.

Rotilie, J.A., McDaniel, T., and Rosen, S.: Root Surface Caries in the Molar Teeth of Rice Rats. III. Inhibition of Root Surface Caries by Fluoride, *J. Dent. Res.,* 56, 1408, November, 1977.

Schrotenboer, G.H.: Fluoride Benefits–After 36 Years, *J. Am. Dent. Assoc.,* 102, 473, April, 1981.

Seaman, F. and Shannon, I.L.: Fluoride Treatment and Microhardness of Dentin, *J. Prosthet. Dent.,* 41, 528, May, 1979.

Strach, E.P., Fan, P.L., and O'Brien, W.J.: Penetrativity and Wetting of Topical Fluoride Preparations: An *in vitro* Study, *Clin. Prev. Dent.,* 1, 11, November–December, 1979.

Thornton, C.B. and Stewart, G.P.: Effect of Waxed versus Unwaxed Floss on Fluoride Uptake by Enamel, *J. Dent. Child.,* 45, 203, May–June, 1978.

Weatherall, J.A., Robinson, C., and Patterson, C.: The Uptake and Action of Fluoride in Dental Enamel, *J. Clin. Periodontol.,* 6, 53, December, 1979.

Wei, S.H.Y. and Wefel, J.S.: Topical Fluorides in Dental Practice, *J. Prev. Dent.,* 4, 25, July–August, 1977.

Plaque Fluoride

Edgar, W.M., Jenkins, G.N., and Tatevossian, A.: The Inhibitory Action of Fluoride on Plaque Bacteria, *Br. Dent. J.,* 128, 129, February 3, 1970.

Ellingsen, J.E., Svatun, B., and Rolla, G.: The Effects of Stannous and Stannic Ions on the Formation and Acidogenicity of Dental Plaque *in vivo, Acta Odontol. Scand.,* 38, 220, Number 4, 1980.

Frostell, G. and Ericsson, Y.: Antiplaque Therapeutics in Caries Prevention, *Caries Res.,* 12, 74, Supplement 1, 1978.

Gross, A. and Tinanoff, N.: Effect of SnF_2 Mouthrinse on Initial Bacterial Colonization of Tooth Enamel, *J. Dent. Res.,* 56, 1179, October, 1977.

Jenkins, G.N. and Edgar, W.M.: Distribution and Forms of F in Saliva and Plaque, *Caries Res.,* 11, 226, Supplement 1, 1977.

Keene, H.J., Shklair, I.L., and Mickel, G.J.: Effect of Multiple Dental Floss–SnF_2 Treatment on *Streptococcus mutans* in Interproximal Plaque, *J. Dent. Res.,* 56, 21, January, 1977.

Loesche, W.J., Syed, S.A., Murray, R.J., and Mellberg, J.R.: Effect of Topical Acidulated Phosphate Fluoride on Percentage of *Streptococcus mutans* and *Streptococcus sanguis* in Plaque, *Caries Res.,* 9, 139, Number 2, 1975.

Rolla, G.: Effects of Fluoride on Initiation of Plaque Formation, *Caries Res.,* 11, 243, Supplement 1, 1977.

Svatun, B. and Attramadal, A.: The Effect of Stannous Fluoride on Human Plaque Acidogenicity in situ (Stephan Curve), *Acta Odontol. Scand.,* 36, 211, Number 4, 1978.

Svatun, B., Gjermo, P., Eriksen, H.M., and Rolla, G.: A Comparison of the Plaque-inhibiting Effect of Stannous Fluoride and Chlorhexidine, *Acta Odontol. Scand.,* 35, 247, Number 5, 1977.

Tinanoff, N. and Camosci, D.A.: Microbiological, Ultrastructural and Spectroscopic Analyses of the Anti-toothplaque Properties of Fluoride Compounds *in vitro, Arch. Oral Biol.,* 25, 531, Number 8/9, 1980.

White, S.T. and Taylor, P.P.: The Effect of Stannous Fluoride on Plaque Scores, *J. Dent. Res.,* 58, 1850, September, 1979.

Fluoridation

Al-Alousi, W., Jackson, D., Crompton, G., and Jenkins, O.C.: Enamel Mottling in a Fluoride and in a Non-fluoride Community (Part I), *Brit. Dent. J.,* 138, 9, January 7, 1975; (Part II), *Brit. Dent. J.,* 138, 56, January 21, 1975.

Doherty, N. and Powell, E.: Effects of Age and Years of Exposure on the Economic Benefits of Fluoridation, *J. Dent. Res.,* 53, 912, July–August, 1974.

Douglas, B.L., Wallace, D.A., Lerner, M., and Coppersmith, S.B.: Impact of Water Fluoridation on Dental

Practice and Dental Manpower, *J. Am. Dent. Assoc.*, *84*, 355, February, 1972.

Englander, H.R. and DePaola, P.F.: Enhanced Anticaries Action From Drinking Water Containing 5 ppm Fluoride, *J. Am. Dent. Assoc.*, *98*, 35, January, 1979.

Frazier, P.J.: Fluoridation: A Review of Social Research, *J. Public Health Dent.*, *40*, 214, Summer, 1980.

Fuller, J.F.: Cost-benefit and Cost-effectiveness Analysis, *New Zeal. Dent. J.*, *70*, 282, October, 1974.

Granados, E.A.: A Synoptic Review of Fluorosis, *Dent. Hyg.*, *55*, 17, June, 1981.

Künzel, W.: Effect of an Interruption in Water Fluoridation on the Caries Prevalence of the Primary and Secondary Dentition, *Caries Res.*, *14*, 304, Number 5, 1980.

Künzel, W.: The Cost and Economic Consequences of Water Fluoridation, *Caries Res.*, *8*, 28, Supplement 1, 1974.

Marthaler, T.M., Mejía, R., Tóth, K., and Vines, J.J.: Caries-preventive Salt Fluoridation, *Caries Res.*, *12*, 15, Supplement 1, 1978.

Myers, H.M., ed.: *Fluorides and Dental Fluorosis.* Monographs in Oral Science, Volume 7. Basel, New York, Karger, 1978, 76 pp.

Newbrun, E.: The Safety of Water Fluoridation, *J. Am. Dent. Assoc.*, *94*, 301, February, 1977.

Spears, N.D.: Reconsidering the 1975 Census of U.S. Communities Which Provide Naturally Fluoridated Waters, *J. Public Health Dent.*, *39*, 102, Spring, 1979.

Thylstrup, A.: Distribution of Dental Fluorosis in the Primary Dentition, *Community Dent. Oral Epidemiol.*, *6*, 329, Number 6, 1978.

Supplements

Aasenden, R. and Peebles, T.C.: Effects of Fluoride Supplementation from Birth on Dental Caries and Fluorosis in Teenaged Children, *Arch. Oral Biol.*, *23*, 111, Number 2, 1978.

Aasenden, R. and Peebles, T.C.: Effects of Fluoride Supplementation from Birth on Human Deciduous and Permanent Teeth, *Arch. Oral Biol.*, *19*, 321, April, 1974.

Adair, S.M. and Wei, S.H.Y.: Supplemental Fluoride Recommendations for Infants Based on Dietary Fluoride Intake, *Caries Res.*, *12*, 76, Number 2, 1978.

Arnold, F.A., McClure, F.J., and White, C.L.: Sodium Fluoride Tablets for Children, *Dent. Prog.*, *1*, 8, October, 1960.

Binder, K., Driscoll, W.S., and Schützmannsky, G.: Caries-preventive Fluoride Tablet Programs, *Caries Res.*, *12*, 22, Supplement 1, 1978.

Bruun, C. and Givskov, H.: Fluoride Concentrations in Saliva in Relation to Chewing of Various Supplementary Fluoride Preparations, *Scand. J. Dent. Res.*, *87*, 1, February, 1979.

Driscoll, W.S.: Dietary Fluoride Supplements, in Forrester, D.J., Wagner, M.L., and Fleming, J., eds.: *Pediatric Dental Medicine.* Philadelphia, Lea & Febiger, 1981, pp. 312–319.

Driscoll, W.S., Heifetz, S.B., and Korts, D.C.: Effect of Chewable Fluoride Tablets on Dental Caries in School-children: Results After Six Years of Use, *J. Am. Dent. Assoc.*, *97*, 820, November, 1978.

Fanning, E.A., Cellier, K.M., Leadbeater, M.M., and Somerville, C.M.: South Australian Kindergarten Children: Fluoride Tablet Supplements and Dental Caries, *Aust. Dent. J.*, *20*, 7, February, 1975.

Granath, L.E., Rootzén, H., Liljegren, E., Holst, K., and Köhler, L.: Variation in Caries Prevalence Related to Combinations of Dietary and Oral Hygiene Habits and Chewing Fluoride Tablets in 4-year-old Children, *Caries Res.*, *12*, 83, Number 2, 1978.

Lennon, D.K., Stookey, G.K., and Beiswanger, B.B.:

Fluoride-vitamin Supplements: Effects on Dental Caries and Fluorosis When Used in Areas With Suboptimum Fluoride in the Water Supply, *J. Am. Dent. Assoc.*, *95*, 965, November, 1977.

Shern, R.J., Driscoll, W.S., and Korts, D.C.: Enamel Biopsy Results of Children Receiving Fluoride Tablets, *J. Am. Dent. Assoc.*, *95*, 310, August, 1977.

Stephen, K.W. and Campbell, D.: Caries Reduction and Cost Benefit After 3 Years of Sucking Fluoride Tablets Daily at School, *Br. Dent. J.*, *144*, 202, April 4, 1978.

Wei, S.H.Y., Wefel, J.S., and Parkins, F.M.: Fluoride Supplements for Infants and Preschool Children, *J. Prev. Dent.*, *4*, 28, May–June, 1977.

Topical Applications: Gels and Solutions

Abrahams, L.J., Yonese, M., Higuchi, W.I., Fox, J.L., and Charbeneau, G.T.: *In vivo* Remineralization Using a Sustained Topical Fluoride Delivery System, *J. Dent. Res.*, *59*, 583, March, 1980.

Beal, J.F. and Rock, W.P.: Fluoride Gels, *Br. Dent. J.*, *140*, 307, May 4, 1976.

Beiswanger, B.B., Mercer, V.H., Billings, R.J., and Stookey, G.K.: A Clinical Caries Evaluation of a Stannous Fluoride Prophylactic Paste and Topical Solution, *J. Dent. Res.*, *59*, 1386, August, 1980.

Englander, H.R., Mellberg, J.R., and Engler, W.O.: Observations on Dental Caries in Primary Teeth After Frequent Fluoride Toplications in a Program Involving Other Preventives, *J. Dent. Res.*, *57*, 855, September–October, 1978.

Feller, R.P.: Reduction of Enamel Solubility by Daily Use of a 0.4% Stannous Fluoride Gel, *J. Dent. Res.*, *53*, 1280, September–October, 1974.

Friedman, M.: Fluoride Prolonged Release Preparations for Topical Use, *J. Dent. Res.*, *59*, 1392, August, 1980.

Heifetz, S.B., Franchi, G.J., Mosley, G.W., MacDougall, O., and Brunelle, J.: Combined Anticariogenic Effect of Fluoride Gel-trays and Fluoride Mouthrinsing in an Optimally Fluoridated Community, *Clin. Prev. Dent.*, *1*, 21, January–February, 1979.

Hock, J. and Tinanoff, N.: Resolution of Gingivitis in Dogs Following Topical Applications of 0.4% Stannous Fluoride and Toothbrushing, *J. Dent. Res.*, *58*, 1652, June, 1979.

Hoffman, S., Tow, H.D., and Cole, J.S.: Antiplaque Potential of Topical Stannous Fluoride, *J. Dent. Res.*, *56*, 709, July, 1977.

Krell, K.V., Logan, H.L., Peterson, L.C., Hall, D.L., and Scriven, C.L.: Time Requirements for Five APF Gel Application Techniques, *J. Am. Soc. Prev. Dent.*, *7*, 17, March/April, 1977.

Loesche, W.J.: Topical Fluorides as an Antibacterial Agent, *J. Prev. Dent.*, *4*, 21, January–February, 1977.

Mellberg, J.R., Nicholson, C.R., Franchi, G.J., Englander, H.R., and Mosley, G.W.: Enamel Fluoride Uptake and Retention from Intensive APF Gel Applications *in vivo*, *J. Dent. Res.*, *56*, 716, July, 1977.

Spears, N.D., Goldstein, C., Gordinier, N., and Crysler, C.: Effects of a Thrice Yearly Application of Fluoride Gel, *Dent. Hyg.*, *52*, 569, December, 1978.

Wefel, J.S. and Wei, S.H.Y.: *In vitro* Evaluation of Fluoride Uptake from a Thixotropic Gel, *Pediatr. Dent.*, *1*, 97, Number 2, 1979.

Wei, S.H.Y.: The Potential Benefits to be Derived from Topical Fluorides in Fluoridated Communities, in Forrester, D.J. and Schulz, E.M., eds.: *International Workshop on Fluorides and Dental Caries Reductions.* Baltimore, University of Maryland, 1974, pp. 179–240.

Williams, H.J., Shannon, I.L., and Stevens, F.D.: The Treatment of Intact Root Surfaces With Combinations of Fluoride, *J. Am. Soc. Prev. Dent.*, *4*, 40, July–August, 1974.

Yaffe, A. and Zalkind, M.: The Effect of Topical Application of Fluoride on Composite Resin Restorations, *J. Prosthet. Dent.*, *45*, 59, January, 1981.

Mouthrinses

Ashley, F.P., Mainwaring, P.J., Emslie, R.D., and Naylor, M.N.: Clinical Testing of a Mouthrinse and a Dentifrice Containing Fluoride. A Two-year Supervised Study in School Children, *Br. Dent. J.*, *143*, 333, November 15, 1977.

Ayers, C., Kolthoff, C., and Durr, D.: Fluoride Mouthrinses, *Dent. Hyg.*, *55*, 23, June, 1981.

Bissell, G.D., O'Shea, R.M., and Mann, J.: Recruitment and Participation in a School Mouthrinse Program, *J. Public Health Dent.*, *40*, 57, Winter, 1980.

DePaola, P.F., Soparkar, P., Foley, S., Bookstein, F., and Bakhos, Y.: Effect of High-concentration Ammonium and Sodium Fluoride Rinses on Dental Caries in Schoolchildren, *Community Dent. Oral Epidemiol.*, *5*, 7, January, 1977.

Gallagher, S.J., Glasgow, I., and Caldwell, R.: Self-application of Fluoride by Rinsing, *J. Public Health Dent.*, *34*, 13, Winter, 1974.

Heifetz, S.B., Driscoll, W.S., and Creighton, W.E.: The Effect on Dental Caries of Weekly Rinsing With a Neutral Sodium Fluoride or an Acidulated Phosphate-fluoride Mouthwash, *J. Am. Dent. Assoc.*, *87*, 364, August, 1973.

Helldén, L., Camosci, D., Hock, J., and Tinanoff, N.: Clinical Study to Compare the Effect of Stannous Fluoride and Chlorhexidine Mouthrinses on Plaque Formation, *J. Clin. Periodontol.*, *8*, 12, February, 1981.

Horowitz, H.S., Heifetz, S.B., Meyers, R.J., Driscoll, W.S., and Li, S.-H.: A Program of Self-administered Fluorides in a Rural School System, *Community Dent. Oral Epidemiol.*, *8*, 177, August, 1980.

Leske, G.S., Ripa, L.S., Levinson, A., and Koulourides, T.I.: Posttreatment Benefits from Participation in a School-based Fluoride Mouthrinsing Program, *J. Public Health Dent.*, *41*, 103, Spring, 1981.

Leverett, D.H., McHugh, W.D., and Jensen, Ø.E.: The Effect of Daily Mouthrinsing With Stannous Fluoride on Dental Plaque and Gingivitis—Four-month Results, *J. Dent. Res.*, *60*, 781, April, 1981.

McConchie, J.M., Richardson, A.S., Hole, L.W., McCombie, F., and Kolthammer, J.: Caries-preventive Effect of Two Concentrations of Stannous Fluoride Mouthrinse, *Community Dent. Oral Epidemiol.*, *5*, 278, November, 1977.

Radike, A.W., Gish, C.W., Peterson, J.K., King, J.D., and Segreto, V.A.: Clinical Evaluation of Stannous Fluoride as an Anticaries Mouthrinse, *J. Am. Dent. Assoc.*, *86*, 404, February, 1973.

Ripa, L.W. and Leske, G.S.: Two Years' Effect on the Primary Dentition of Mouthrinsing With a 0.2% Neutral NaF Solution, *Community Dent. Oral Epidemiol.*, *7*, 151, June, 1979.

Ripa, L.W., Leske, G.S., and Lowey, W.G.: Fluoride Rinsing: A School-based Dental Preventive Program, *J. Prev. Dent.*, *4*, 25, September–October, 1977.

Ripa, L.W., Leske, G.S., Sposato, A.L., and Rebich, T.: Supervised Weekly Rinsing With a 0.2% Neutral NaF Solution: Results of a Demonstration Program After Four School Years, *J. Am. Dent. Assoc.*, *102*, 482, April, 1981.

Shannon, I.L.: Responses of Enamel, Dentin, and Root Surfaces to Mouthrinse Concentrations of Sodium Fluoride and Stannous Fluoride, *J. Dent. Child.*, *47*, 17, January, 1980.

Shannon, I.L.: Mouthrinsing With Fluoride: A Review of Clinical Studies, *Dent. Hyg.*, *50*, 448, October, 1976.

Tinanoff, N., Brady, J.M., and Gross, A.: The Effect of NaF and SnF_2 Mouthrinses on Bacterial Colonization of Tooth Enamel: TEM and SEM Studies, *Caries Res.*, *10*, 415, Number 6, 1976.

Tinanoff, N., Hock, J., Camosci, D., and Helldén, L.: Effect of Stannous Fluoride Mouthrinse on Dental Plaque Formation, *J. Clin. Periodontol.*, *7*, 232, June, 1980.

Zahradnik, R.T.: Effect of Fluoride Rinses Upon *in vitro* Enamel Remineralization, *J. Dent. Res.*, *59*, 1065, June, 1980.

Dentifrices

Abrams, R.G. and Chambers, D.W.: Caries-inhibiting Effect of a Stannous Fluoride Silica Gel Dentifrice: A Three-year Clinical Study, *Clin. Prev. Dent.*, *2*, 22, January–February, 1980.

Beiswanger, B.B., Billings, R.J., Sturzenberger, O.P., and Bollmer, B.W.: Effect of an SnF_2-$Ca_2P_2O_7$ Dentifrice and APF Topical Applications, *J. Dent. Child.*, *45*, 137, March–April, 1978.

Beiswanger, B.B., Gish, C.W., and Mallatt, M.E.: Effect of a Sodium Fluoride–Silica Abrasive Dentifrice Upon Caries, *J. Dent. Res.*, *60*, 577, Abstract 1072, Special Issue A, March, 1981.

Ennever, J., Peterson, J.K., Hester, W.R., Segretto, V.A., and Radike, A.W.: Influence of Alkaline pH on the Effectiveness of Sodium Fluoride Dentifrice, *J. Dent. Res.*, *59*, 658, April, 1980.

Fogels, H.R., Alman, J.E., Meade, J.J., and O'Donnell, J.P.: The Relative Caries-inhibiting Effects of a Stannous Fluoride Dentifrice in a Silica Gel Base, *J. Am. Dent. Assoc.*, *99*, 456, September, 1979.

Goldstein, M. and Gedalia, I.: F Uptake and F Release by Root Dentin After Brushing with F-containing and F-free Dentifrice *in vitro*, *J. Dent. Res.*, *55*, 912, September–October, 1976.

Hope, T.: Results of 10 Years of Supervised Fluoride Toothbrushing in Rygge, Norway, *Community Dent. Oral Epidemiol.*, *7*, 330, December, 1979.

Kirkegaard, E.: *In vitro* Fluoride Uptake in Human Dental Enamel From Four Different Dentifrices, *Caries Res.*, *11*, 24, Number 1, 1977.

Mainwaring, P.J. and Naylor, M.N.: A Three-year Clinical Study to Determine the Separate and Combined Caries-inhibiting Effects of Sodium Monofluorophosphate Toothpaste and an Acidulated Phosphate-fluoride Gel, *Caries Res.*, *12*, 202, Number 4, 1978.

Murray, J.J. and Shaw, L.: A 3-year Clinical Trial Into the Effect of Fluoride Content and Toothpaste Abrasivity on the Caries Inhibitory Properties of a Dentifrice, *Community Dent. Oral Epidemiol.*, *8*, 46, February, 1980.

Peterson, J.K.: A Supervised Brushing Trial of Sodium Monofluorophosphate Dentifrices in a Fluoridated Area, *Caries Res.*, *13*, 68, Number 2, 1979.

Svatun, B.: Plaque-inhibiting Effect of Dentifrices Containing Stannous Fluoride, *Acta Odontol. Scand.*, *36*, 205, Number 4, 1978.

Zacherl, W.A.: Clinical Evaluation of a Sodium Fluoride–Silica Abrasive Dentifrice, *J. Dent. Res.*, *60*, 577, Abstract 1071, Special Issue A, March, 1981.

Fluoride for Infants and Small Children

Ericsson, Y. and Wei, S.H.Y.: Fluoride Supply and Effect in Infants and Young Children, *Pediatr. Dent.*, *1*, 44, March, 1979.

Holm, A.-K.: Effect of a Fluoride Varnish (Duraphat) i

Preschool Children, *Community Dent. Oral Epidemiol.*, 7, 241, October, 1979.

ouwink, B. and Wagg, B.J.: Effect of Fluoride Dentifrice Usage During Infancy Upon Enamel Mottling of the Permanent Teeth, *Caries Res.*, 13, 231, Number 4, 1979.

irkegaard, E., Christiansen, P.F., and Buch, J.: Children's Response to Various Local Fluoride Treatments, *Acta Odontol. Scand.*, 38, 236, Number 4, 1980.

phaug, R.H., Singer, L., and Harland, B.F.: Estimated Fluoride Intake of Average Two-year-old Children in Four Dietary Regions of the United States, *J. Dent. Res.*, 59, 777, May, 1980.

inger, L. and Ophaug, R.: Total Fluoride Intake of Infants, *Pediatrics*, 63, 460, March, 1979.

hylstrup, A.: Distribution of Dental Fluorosis in the Primary Dentition, *Community Dent. Oral Epidemiol.*, 6, 329, Number 6, 1978.

inanoff, N. and Mueller, B.: Fluoride Content in Milk and Formula for Infants, *J. Dent. Child.*, 45, 53, January–February, 1978.

Amine Fluorides

Dolan, M.M., Kavanagh, B.J., and Yankell, S.L.: Artificial Plaque Prevention With Organic Fluorides, *J. Periodontol.*, 43, 561, September, 1972.

Ringelberg, M.L. and Webster, D.B.: Effects of an Amine Fluoride Mouthrinse and Dentifrice on the Gingival Health and the Extent of Plaque of School Children, *J. Periodontol.*, 48, 350, June, 1977.

Ringelberg, M.L., Webster, D.B., Dixon, D.O., and LeZotte, D.C.: The Caries-preventive Effect of Amine Fluorides and Inorganic Fluorides in a Mouthrinse or Dentifrice After 30 Months of Use, *J. Am. Dent. Assoc.*, 98, 202, February, 1979.

Shern, R., Swing, K.W., and Crawford, J.J.: Prevention of Plaque Formation by Organic Fluorides, *J. Oral Med.*, 25, 93, July–September, 1970.

Stoller, N.H., Cohen, D.W., and Yankell, S.L.: Clinical Evaluations of an Amine Fluoride Mouthrinse on Gingival Inflammation and Plaque Accumulation, *J. Periodontol.*, 48, 650, October, 1977.

30

Sealants

As part of a complete preventive program, the use of pit and fissure sealants may be indicated for selected patients. Since fluorides protect smooth tooth surfaces more than occlusal surfaces, a method to reduce the incidence of occlusal dental caries is needed. Research studies have shown that the incidence of occlusal caries can be reduced significantly by the application of an adhesive sealant to the occlusal surfaces of caries-free molars and premolars.[1-4]

I. Definition and Action

A pit and fissure resin sealant is an organic polymer which bonds to the enamel surface mainly by mechanical retention. It acts as a physical barrier to prevent oral bacteria and their nutrients from collecting within a pit or fissure and creating the acid environment essential to the initiation of dental caries.

Before the sealant is applied, the enamel surface is treated with an acid etch process to increase the adhesion of the sealant. The acid etch creates micropores in the enamel. When the resin sealant is applied, it penetrates into the tiny pores and creates a bond or mechanical interlocking.

Currently, most sealants in clinical use are made of Bis-GMA (a reaction product of bisphenol A and glycidyl methacrylate). The techniques of application vary slightly among available products. Different products are designed to be activated in different ways, namely chemical autopolymerization, ultraviolet light activation, or visible light activation.

The American Dental Association Council on Dental Materials, Instruments, and Equipment has a program for evaluation and acceptance of pit and fissure sealants.[5] A list of the reports and review articles is provided in the *Suggested Readings* at the end of this chapter.

II. Selection of Teeth for Sealant Application

All caries-free pits and fissures are not necessarily indicated for sealant application. When evaluation is made and teeth for sealant are chosen selectively, consideration is given the patient's overall caries susceptibility, existing restorations and carious lesions, occlusal anatomy, as well as the other preventive measures used for and by the patient.

Factors to be considered are as follows:
A. Sealants are indicated for occlusal pits and fissures, buccal pits, and cingulum pits of primary and permanent teeth with no dental caries in the surfaces to be treated.
B. Applications should be made as soon as possible following eruption. When there is a delay, caries may start, and the surface no longer can be considered for sealant. When possible, sealant can be applied before full eruption, provided there is no tissue flap over the occlusal to interfere with application procedures.

C. Overall caries susceptibility is significant. When there are current carious lesions and previous restorations, newly erupted teeth should be treated with sealants promptly.

D. Sealant is not indicated when there are proximal carious lesions of the same tooth. When the proximal caries is restored, tooth preparation involves the occlusal surface, and the sealant would be removed.

E. Teeth with deep, narrow pits and fissures are indicated more than teeth in which the pits and fissures are shallow and well-coalesced. The latter are less likely to become carious.

F. The age of the patient may have particular significance. However, when teeth have been erupted several years and have not become carious, it should not necessarily follow that they are less susceptible indefinitely. Habits may change. For example, application of a sealant to caries-free occlusal surfaces during early teenage years when caries rates are high may prove to be very important to the individual.

G. Other preventive measures being used for and by the patient are necessary. Sealant application should be part of a complete prevention program, not an isolated procedure. As an isolated procedure, there can be patient (and parent) misunderstanding of the selected area of prevention which this measure represents. Other surfaces and other teeth need other methods of preventive protection.

III. Detection of Pit and Fissure Caries

When selecting a tooth for which a sealant application may be indicated, recognition of a gross carious lesion when the tooth structure is clearly broken down and discolored is not difficult. The more difficult lesions to discriminate are those that are small and do not have classic observable characteristics.

Criteria that have been defined for the determination of pit and fissure lesions of facial, occlusal, and lingual surfaces are as follows:[6]

A. Area is carious when the explorer "catches" or resists removal after the insertion into a pit or fissure with moderate to firm pressure and when this is accompanied by one or more of the following signs of caries:
1. A softness at the base of the area.

2. Opacity adjacent to the pit or fissure as evidence of undermining or demineralization.
3. Softened enamel adjacent to the pit or fissure which may be scraped away with an explorer.

B. Area is carious if there is loss of the normal translucency of the enamel, adjacent to a pit, which is in contrast to the surrounding tooth structure. The condition is considered to be reliable evidence of undermining. In some of these cases, the explorer may not catch or penetrate the pit.

APPLICATION OF SEALANT[1]

Each quadrant should be treated separately. Isolation to prevent contamination and moisture can then be controlled. The precise technique requires that two dental team members work together.[7]

The manufacturer's directions must be followed carefully for each specific product. Although the basic techniques are similar, there are characteristic steps unique to each product.

General directions are described here in sequence, with brief explanations of the purposes of each step. The main steps are cleaning and drying the tooth surfaces, conditioning (enamel etching), applying the sealant, and polymerization. The success of treatment is dependent on precision in the techniques of application.

I. Clean the Tooth Surface

A. Purposes
1. Remove deposits and debris completely.
2. Permit the chemicals of the sealant procedures to have maximum contact with the enamel surface.

B. Cleaning Agent

Fine pumice and water. It is important that there be no oil and no fluoride present. Commercial polishing pastes frequently contain ingredients with glycerin or oil, such as flavoring agents.

Apply the moistened pumice with a rotating pointed bristle brush. "Jab" the bristle ends into the pits and fissures in the attempt to remove as much of the bacterial debris as possible.

C. Rinse

Use water only, not mouthrinse.

D. Use Explorer

Use a fine Number 23 explorer to loosen debris and pumice from the pits and fissures. Rinse thoroughly.

II. Isolate the Tooth

A. Purposes

1. Keep the tooth clean and dry for optimal action and bonding of the sealant.
2. Eliminate the possible contact of saliva and moisture from the breath.
3. Keep the materials from contacting the oral tissues, being swallowed accidentally, or being unpleasant to the patient because of flavor.

B. Rubber Dam

1. Rubber dam application is the method of choice because the most complete isolation is obtained.
2. It is essential when profuse saliva flow and overactive tongue and oral muscles make retraction and consistent maintenance of a dry, clean field impossible.
3. Combined treatment should be planned. When a quadrant will have a rubber dam and anesthesia for restoration of other teeth, teeth indicated for sealant may be treated.
4. Rubber dam is not possible when
   a. Without anesthesia, application of the clamp could not be tolerated by the patient.
   b. Teeth are not fully erupted and may not hold the rubber dam clamp.

C. Cotton Rolls

When rubber dam is not feasible, cotton roll holders are placed, and saliva ejector positioned. Cotton roll isolation procedures are described on pages 453–454.

Great care that saliva does not enter the etched area is necessary. Increased stability of cotton rolls may be achieved by holding them with the fingers rather than using a cotton roll holder.[1]

III. Dry the Tooth

A. Purposes

1. Prepare the tooth for the conditioner.
2. Prevent dilution and contamination of the conditioner.

B. Use Only Dry, Clean Air

Many syringes, particularly the multi-purpose types, emit a combination of air and water spray. Some syringes may emit oil.
1. Clear the air by releasing the spray into a sink before directing it onto the tooth.
2. Test the air for water content by blowing on the back of the hand or on a mirror surface.

IV. Apply Conditioner for Enamel Etching

A. Purposes

To increase the adherence of the sealant, the conditioner is used to
1. Create surface irregularities to increase the area for retention.
2. Increase the size of the microspaces between prisms so they are accessible to the adhesive.

B. Conditioner

1. Apply the phosphoric acid (30 to 50%) with a brush, cotton pellet, or plastic sponge over the occlusal surface and the buccal and/or lingual when sealant is indicated.
2. Note the time or start timer. Total application time is 60 seconds.
3. Use a continuous dabbing, not a rubbing, motion. Gentle dabbing will not damage the fragile enamel latticework formed during the etching process.

V. Rinse Thoroughly

A. Purposes

1. Remove all excess acid and complexes formed from the action of the minerals of the tooth and the acid.
2. Prevent saliva from reaching the etched surface. It will reduce the bonding strength of the sealant by depositing the salivary constituents on the surface.

B. Procedure

1. Do not permit the patient to rinse and expectorate. Contaminants must be kept from the etched area.
2. Clear the water in the tubing by releasing the water into a sink.
3. Rinse thoroughly for 20 seconds for each tooth. Direct the water stream across the etched surfaces and then combine air and water so that each portion of the surface is washed. The assistant holds the wide-mouth evacuator tip adjacent to the tooth surface to prevent excess fluid from collecting in the floor of the mouth.
4. Evacuate excess water from the entire area immediately after rinsing.
5. When rubber dam is not used, change the cotton rolls by placing a dry roll over each wet cotton roll. The wet one may then be slid out from under the dry one. It is very important that no saliva contaminate the etched enamel.

C. Examine the Surface

The etched surface should be a dull, chalky white. When it is not, repeat the application of the conditioner, step by step. Primary teeth or older permanent teeth may require a repeat application.

VI. Dry the Tooth Thoroughly Again

A. Purposes

1. Prepare the tooth for the sealant application.
2. Prevent moisture from reducing the affinity of the adhesive for the enamel surface and preventing penetration of the adhesive into the microspaces created by etching.
3. Dry the tooth thoroughly for 15 to 30 seconds per tooth. Use only clean, dry air (see III above). Drying is continued while the assistant prepares the sealant resin.

VII. Apply the Sealant

There are three types of preparations in current use: one is polymerized by chemical means, one by ultraviolet light, and the third by visible light. Only general instructions are provided here. The manufacturer's instructions should be followed for specific applications.

A. Chemical Polymerization

The catalyst and the sealant are mixed and applied to the tooth with a small disposable sponge, brush, or specific applicator provided by the manufacturer. Cover all surfaces to be sealed quickly and then go over to add thickness. Thickness gives strength to the sealant. Time according to manufacturer (1 to 3 minutes).

B. Ultraviolet

The sealant is prepared and applied to the tooth. The ultraviolet light is directed over the sealant. Some lights require a 5- to 8-minute activation period before use. Care must be taken that each portion of the sealant receives the light for a specified length of time.

C. Visible Light

Composite systems have been introduced that are activated by an incandescent light in the visible spectrum. The sealants (unfilled resins) included with the composite systems can be used for pit and fissure sealing. The light is operated in a manner similar to ultraviolet light. In general, visible light has a significantly better penetration than ultraviolet light and requires less exposure time (10 to 20 seconds) for complete polymerization.[8]

VIII. Rinse

A. Examine the surfaces for complete coverage. An explorer will move smoothly over the shiny surface.
B. Remove cotton rolls or rubber dam.

PENETRATION OF SEALANT

The penetration of a sealant depends on the configuration of the pit or fissure, the presence of deposits and debris within the pit or fissure, and the properties of the sealant itself.[9]

I. Pit and Fissure Anatomy

A review of the anatomy of pits and fissures may be helpful in understanding the effects of sealants in the prevention of dental caries. The shape and depth of pits and fissures vary considerably even within one tooth.

There are *long narrow pits* and grooves which reach to, or nearly to, the dentinoenamel junction. Others are *wide V-shaped* or *narrow V-shaped*, while still others may have a *long constricted form* with a *bulbous terminal portion* (figure 30–1). The pit or fissure may take a wavy course so that it does not lead directly from the outer surface to the dentinoenamel junction.

II. Contents of a Pit or Fissure

A pit or fissure contains dental plaque, pel-

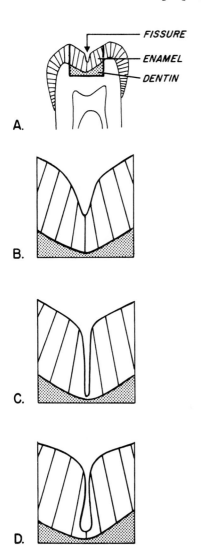

Figure 30–1. Occlusal fissures. Drawings made from microscopic slides to show variations in the shape and depth of fissures. **A.** Tooth showing section enlarged for B, C, and D. **B.** Wide V-shaped fissure. **C.** Long narrow groove which reaches nearly to the dentinoenamel junction. **D.** Long constricted form with a bulbous terminal portion.

licle, debris, and sometimes relatively intact remnants of tooth development.

III. Effect of Cleaning

When a tooth is cleaned and the conditioner is applied, it is not possible to clean out the narrow, long fissures, nor for the conditioner to reach the deeper portions. Retained cleaning material can block the sealant from filling the fissure. It can also become mixed with the sealant. Removal of pumice used for cleaning and thorough washing is necessary to the success of the sealant.

IV. Amount of Penetration

Wide V and shallow fissures are more apt to be filled by sealant (figure 30–2B). Although ideally the sealant should penetrate to the bottom of a pit or fissure, this is frequently impossible because of the debris. Microscopic examination of pits and fissures after sealant application has shown that the sealant does not penetrate to the bottom because residual debris, cleaning agents, and trapped air prevent passage of the material (figure 30–2C and D).

V. Caries Prevention

Although access of sealant to the bottom of a fissure or pit is limited, caries prevention by sealants is high. The sealant closes the opening to the pit or fissure, and there is no access for additional microorganisms, cariogenic food materials, and oxygen for aerobic bacteria.

When dental caries in a pit or fissure is inadvertently covered, the number of viable microorganisms decreases with time.[10,11] No progress in cavity development has been observed by depth changes or by radiographs.[12,13] The placement of sealant over known carious lesions is not recommended. However, sealing and so arresting caries in a questionable or suspected pit or fissure may be better than waiting for a future examination when the cavity has enlarged and deepened.[11]

FLUORIDE AND SEALANT

I. Topical Application in Conjunction with Sealant

When fluoride is used, it must be applied before the conditioner or after the sealant. It should not be applied between because the bond

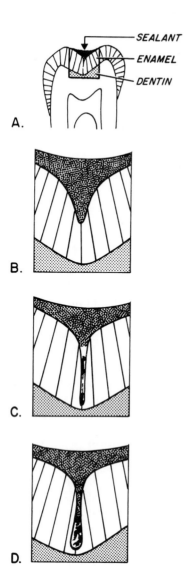

Figure 30–2. Pit and fissure sealant in fissures. Drawings made from microscopic slides to show extent of a fissure filled by sealant. **A.** Tooth showing section enlarged for B, C, and D. **B.** Sealant fills wide V-shaped fissure. **C.** and **D.** Partially filled fissures due to narrow constriction of the groove and blockage by trapped debris.

strength may be reduced between the sealant and the etched enamel surface.

Fluoride in the enamel surface and in a pit or fissure from previous topical professional or self-applications will be retained and sealed-in during placement of the pit and fissure sealant.[14] Continued protection is supplementary to the sealant. The feasibility of adding fluoride to the sealant has also been investigated.[15]

II. Combined Preventive Program

Sealants must be considered a part of a total preventive program. While sealant is applicable for certain occlusal surfaces, fluoride applications and other fluoride sources for self-administration are still necessary for all other surfaces.

RETENTION AND REPLACEMENT

Length of time of retention depends almost entirely on the precision of technique. Although surface sealant may be lost, sealant in the pits and fissures and that which penetrated into the microspaces of the enamel still remains and provides protection.[14]

I. Factors That Influence Retention Time

A. Precision of Technique

Each step in the preparation of the tooth and the application of the sealant must be carefully performed. It is generally believed that improper technique is the major cause of early loss of sealant from the tooth surface.

B. Effect of Contamination

Any contact of the etched enamel surface either by saliva, water, or any other contaminant before application of the sealant will markedly decrease the effectiveness of the sealant.

II. Reexamination

At each recall, or at least every 6 months, the sealant should be examined for deficiencies that may have developed.

III. Replacement

Consult the manufacturer's instructions. Tooth preparation is the same as for an original application. Re-etching the tooth surface is always essential.

TECHNICAL HINTS

I. Eye Protection

The patient must wear safety protective glasses during the etching process. Phosphoric acid could cause loss of sight if a drop inadvertently fell into an eye.[16]

II. Occlusion

The occlusion should be checked for interferences after thick sealants are placed. An occlusal wax or an articulating paper can be used to identify high spots, and a fine stone or finishing-type bur used to reshape.[17]

FACTORS TO TEACH THE PATIENT

I. Sealants as a part of a total preventive program. There should be a clear understanding of the teeth and surfaces involved.

II. What a sealant is and why such a meticulous application procedure is required.

III. What can be expected from a sealant: how long it will last, how it prevents dental caries.

IV. Preventive measures for other tooth surfaces. Sealants are not substitutes for other preventive measures including limitations of dietary sucrose, fluorides, and plaque control.

V. Need for examination of the sealant at frequent, scheduled appointments and replacement when indicated.

References

1. Simonsen, R.J.: *Clinical Applications of the Acid Etch Technique.* Chicago, Quintessence, 1978, pp. 19–42.
2. Ripa, L.W.: Occlusal Sealants: Rationale and Review of Clinical Trials, *Int. Dent. J.*, 30, 127, June, 1980.
3. Horowitz, H.S., Heifetz, S.B., and Poulsen, S.: Retention and Effectiveness of a Single Application of an Adhesive Sealant in Preventing Occlusal Caries: Final Report After Five Years of a Study in Kalispell, Montana, *J. Am. Dent. Assoc.*, 95, 1133, December, 1977.
4. Simonsen, R.J.: The Clinical Effectiveness of a Colored Pit and Fissure Sealant at 36 Months, *J. Am. Dent. Assoc.*, 102, 323, March, 1981.
5. American Dental Association, Council on Dental Materials, Instruments and Equipment: *Dentist's Desk Reference: Materials, Instruments and Equipment,* 1st ed. Chicago, American Dental Association, pp. 50–51.
6. Radike, A.W.: Criteria for Diagnosis of Dental Caries, in American Dental Association, Council on Dental Research and Council on Dental Therapeutics: *Clinical Testing of Cariostatic Agents.* Chicago, American Dental Association, 1968, pp. 87–88.
7. Stombaugh, E.F. and Simonsen, R.J.: The Four-handed Application of Pit and Fissure Sealants, *Quintessence Journal*, 2, 13, July/August, 1980.
8. Nathanson, D.: Tufts University School of Dental Medicine, Boston, Massachusetts, personal communication, 1982.
9. Taylor, C.L. and Gwinnett, A.J.: A Study of the Penetration of Sealants into Pits and Fissures, *J. Am. Dent. Assoc.*, 87, 1181, November, 1973.
10. Handelman, S.L., Washburn, F., and Wopperer, P.: Two-year Report of Sealant Effect on Bacteria in Dental Caries, *J. Am. Dent. Assoc.*, 93, 967, November, 1976.
11. Going, R.E., Loesche, W.J., Grainger, D.A., and Syed, S.A.: The Viability of Microorganisms in Carious Lesions Five Years After Covering With a Fissure Sealant, *J. Am. Dent. Assoc.*, 97, 455, September, 1978.
12. Mertz-Fairhurst, E.J., Schuster, G.S., Williams, J.E., and Fairhurst, C.W.: Clinical Progress of Sealed and Unsealed Caries. Part I. Depth Changes and Bacterial Counts, *J. Prosthet. Dent.*, 42, 521, November, 1979.
13. Mertz-Fairhurst, E.J., Schuster, G.S., Williams, J.E., and Fairhurst, C.W.: Clinical Progress of Sealed and Unsealed Caries. Part II. Standardized Radiographs and Clinical Observations, *J. Prosthet. Dent.*, 42, 633, December, 1979.
14. Buonocore, M.G.: Pit and Fissure Sealing, *Dent. Clin. North Am.*, 19, 367, April, 1975.
15. Swartz, M.L., Phillips, R.W., Norman, R.D., Elliason, S., Rhodes, B.F., and Clark, H.E.: Addition of Fluoride to Pit and Fissure Sealants—A Feasibility Study, *J. Dent. Res.*, 55, 757, September–October, 1976.
16. Colvin, J.: Eye Injuries and the Dentist, *Aust. Dent. J.*, 23, 453, December, 1978.
17. Spohn, E.E. and Berry, T.G.: Pit and Fissure Sealants, in Boundy, S.S. and Reynolds, N.J., eds.: *Current Concepts in Dental Hygiene*, Volume 2. St. Louis, The C.V. Mosby Co., 1979, pp. 115–129.

Suggested Readings

American Dental Association, Council on Dental Materials and Devices: Guidelines on the Use of Ultraviolet Radiation in Dentistry, *J. Am. Dent. Assoc.*, 92, 775, April, 1976.

Bohrer, J. and Gedalia, I.: Fluoride Concentration in Enamel Treated With 50% Phosphoric Acid and NaF With Subsequent Decalcification in "Acid-gel," *J. Dent. Res.*, 59, 1022, June, 1980.

Boudreau, G.E. and Jerge, C.R.: The Efficacy of Sealant Treatment in the Prevention of Pit and Fissure Dental Caries: A Review and Interpretation of the Literature, *J. Am. Dent. Assoc.*, 92, 383, February, 1976.

Breakspere, R.J. and Wilton, A.: Factors Affecting the Structure of a Fissure Sealant at the Enamel/Sealant Interface, *Aust. Dent. J.*, 22,199, June, 1977.

Dietz, E.R.: Application of Pit and Fissure Sealant—The Role of the Dental Assistant, *Dent. Assist.*, 44, 1x, November, 1975.

Katz, S., McDonald, J.L., and Stookey, G.K.: *Preventive Dentistry.* Upper Montclair, New Jersey, D.C.P. Publishing, 1977, pp. 241–250.

Low, T. and von Fraunhofer, J.A.: The Shelf Life of Activated Nuva Seal, *Br. Dent. J.*, 139, 280, October 7, 1975.

Newbrun, E.: *Cariology.* Baltimore, The Williams & Wilkins Co., 1978, pp. 241–254.

Retief, D.H.: Effect of Conditioning the Enamel With Phosphoric Acid, *J. Dent. Res.*, 52, 333, March–April, 1973.

Ripa, L.W.: Sealant Retention on Primary Teeth: A Critique of Clinical and Laboratory Studies, *J. Pedod.*, 3, 275, Summer, 1979.

Silverstone, L.M.: Fissure Sealants: The Susceptibility to Dissolution of Acid-etched and Subsequently Abraded Enamel *in vitro*, *Caries Res.*, 11, 46, Number 1, 1977.

Silverstone, L.M.: Should I Be Using Pit and Fissure Sealants or Amalgam? *Int. Dent. J.*, 26, 29, March, 1976.

Silverstone, L.M.: Fissure Sealants. Laboratory Studies, *Caries Res.*, 8, 2, Number 1, 1974.

Silverstone, L.M. and Dogon, I.L., eds.: *Proceedings of an International Symposium on the Acid Etch Technique.* St. Paul, Minnesota, North Central Publishing, 1975, pp. 13–39.

Silverstone, L.M., Saxton, C.A., Dogan, I.L., and Fejerskov, O.: Variation in the Pattern of Acid Etching of Human Dental Enamel Examined by Scanning Electron Microscopy, *Caries Res.*, 9, 373, Number 5, 1975.

Simonsen, R.J.: Acid Etch as a Preventive Technique in Dentistry, in Caldwell, R.C. and Stallard, R.E.: *A Textbook of Preventive Dentistry.* Philadelphia, W.B. Saunders Co., 1977, pp. 325–332.

Verity, S.: Fissure Sealants and Dental Auxiliaries, in Silverstone, L.M. and Dogon, I.L., eds.: *Proceedings of an International Symposium on the Acid Etch Technique.* St. Paul, Minnesota, North Central Publishing, 1975, pp. 190–194, 206–208.

Viewpoints on Preventive Dentistry, The Role of Pit and Fissure Sealants. Johnson and Johnson Dental Products Company, Woodbridge, New Jersey, Medical Education Dynamics, 1978, 20 pp.

Wei, S.H.Y.: Effect of Topical Fluoride Solutions on the Enamel Surface as Studied by Electron Microscopy, *Caries Res.*, 9, 445, Number 6, 1975.

Programs

Bagramian, R.A., Srivastava, S., and Graves, R.C.: Pattern of Sealant Retention in Children Receiving a Combination of Caries-preventive Methods: Three-year Results, *J. Am. Dent. Assoc.*, 98, 46, January, 1979.

Brooks, J.D., Mertz-Fairhurst, E.J., Della-Giustina, V.E., Williams, J.E., and Fairhurst, C.W.: A Comparative Study of Two Pit and Fissure Sealants: Three-year Results in Augusta, Ga., *J. Am. Dent. Assoc.*, 99, 42, July, 1979.

Burt, B.A.: Tentative Analysis of the Efficiency of Fissure Sealant in a Public Program in London, *Community Dent. Oral Epidemiol.*, 5, 73, March, 1977.

Charbeneau, G.T. and Dennison, J.B.: Clinical Success and Potential Failure After Single Application of a Pit and Fissure Sealant: A Four-year Report, *J. Am. Dent. Assoc.*, 98, 559, April, 1979.

Cline, J.T. and Messer, L.B.: Long Term Retention of Sealants Applied by Inexperienced Operators in Minneapolis, *Community Dent. Oral Epidemiol.*, 7, 206, August, 1979.

Douglas, W.H. and Tranter, T.C.: Fissure Sealant Treatment. An Assessment and Follow-up, *Br. Dent. J.*, 139, 140, August 19, 1975.

Ferguson, F.S. and Ripa, L.W.: Evaluation of the Retention of Two Sealants Applied by Dental Students, *J. Dent. Educ.*, 44, 494, August, 1980.

Going, R.E., Haugh, L.D., Grainger, D.A., and Conti, A.J.: Four-year Clinical Evaluation of a Pit and Fissure Sealant, *J. Am. Dent. Assoc.*, 95, 972, November, 1977.

Gourley, J.M.: A Two-year Study of a Fissure Sealant in Two Nova Scotia Communities, *J. Public Health Dent.*, 35, 132, Spring, 1975.

Jeronimus, D.J., Till, M.J., and Sveen, O.B.: Reduced Viability of Microorganisms Under Dental Sealants, *J. Dent. Child.*, 42, 275, July–August, 1975.

McCune, R.J., Bojanini, J., and Abodeely, R.A.: Effectiveness of a Pit and Fissure Sealant in the Prevention of Caries: Three-year Clinical Results, *J. Am. Dent. Assoc.*, 99, 619, October, 1979.

Meurman, J.H., Helminen, S.K.J., and Luoma, H.: Caries Reduction Over 5 Years From a Single Application of a Fissure Sealant, *Scand. J. Dent. Res.*, 86, 153, May, 1978.

Poulsen, S., Thylstrup, A., Christensen, P.F., and Ishøy, U.: Evaluation of a Pit- and Fissure-sealing Program in a Public Dental Health Service After 2 Years, *Community Dent. Oral Epidemiol.*, 7, 154, June, 1979.

Raadal, M.: Follow-up Study of Sealing and Filling With Composite Resins in the Prevention of Occlusal Caries, *Community Dent. Oral Epidemiol.*, 6, 176, July, 1978.

Rantala, E.V.: Caries Incidence in 7–9-year-old Children After Fissure Sealing and Topical Fluoride Therapy in Finland, *Community Dent. Oral Epidemiol.*, 7, 213, August, 1979.

Richardson, A.S., Gibson, G.B., and Waldman, R.: Chemically Polymerized Sealant in Preventing Occlusal Caries, *Can. Dent. Assoc. J.*, 46, 259, April, 1980.

Rock, W.P.: Fissure Sealants. Results of a 3-year Clinical Trial Using an Ultra-violet Sensitive Resin, *Br. Dent. J.*, 142, 16, January 4, 1977.

Rock, W.P., Gordon, P.H., and Bradnock, G.: The Effect of Operator Variability and Patient Age on the Retention of Fissure Sealant Resin, *Br. Dent. J.*, 145, 72, August 1, 1978.

Roder, D.M.: The Treatment of First Permanent Molars in a School Dental Programme: Implications for Fissure Sealants, *Aust. Dent. J.*, 20, 94, April, 1975.

Sheykholeslam, Z. and Houpt, M.: Clinical Effectiveness of an Autopolymerized Fissure Sealant After 2 Years, *Community Dent. Oral Epidemiol.*, 6, 181, July, 1978.

Simonsen, R.J.: Fissure Sealants: Deciduous Molar Retention of Colored Sealant With Variable Etch Time, *Quintessence Int.*, 9, 71, May, 1978.

Simonsen, R.J.: Fissure Sealants in Primary Molars: Retention of Colored Sealants with Variable Etch Times, at Twelve Months, *J. Dent. Child.*, 46, 382, September–October, 1979.

Simonsen, R.J.: Preventive Resin Restorations: Three-year Results, *J. Am. Dent. Assoc.*, 100, 535, April, 1980.

Simonsen, R.J. and Stallard, R.E.: Fissure Sealants: Colored Sealant Retention 3 Months Post Application, *Quintessence Int.*, 8, 81, February, 1977.

Speiser, A.M. and Segat, T.E.: The Influence of Technique Modifications on Sealant Leakage, *J. Dent. Child.*, 47, 93, March–April, 1980.

Stephen, K.W., Kirkwood, M., Young, K.C., Gillespie, F.C., MacFadyen, E.E., and Campbell, D.: Fissure Sealing of First Permanent Molars. An Improved Technique Applied by a Dental Auxiliary, *Br. Dent. J.*, 144, 7, January 3, 1978.

Thylstrup, A. and Poulsen, S.: Retention and Effectiveness of a Chemically Polymerized Pit and Fissure Sealant After 2 Years, *Scand. J. Dent. Res.*, 86, 21, January, 1978.

Rubber Dam Application

Bell, B.H. and Grainger, D.A.: *Basic Operative Dentistry Procedures*, 2nd ed. Philadelphia, Lea & Febiger, 1971, pp. 18–21.

Bell, R., Solomon, E., and Randell, S.: Application of Rubber Dam by the Dental Assistant, *Dent. Assist.*, 43, 20, November, 1974.

Castano, F.A. and Alden, B.A., eds.: *Handbook of Expanded Dental Auxiliary Practice*, 2nd ed. Philadelphia, J.B. Lippincott Co., 1980, pp. 103–107.

Cosgrove, D.J.: Rubber Dam in Routine Dentistry, *Dent. Assist.*, 39, 12, January, 1970.

Cunningham, P.R., Osborne, J.W., and Kaye, L.A.: *Controlling the Operative Field by Use of the Rubber Dam.* Buffalo, State University of New York, 1969.

Park, V.R., Ashman, J.R., and Shelly, G.J.: *A Textbook for Dental Assistants*, 2nd ed. Philadelphia, W.B. Saunders Co., 1975, pp. 355–357, 403–404.

Simon, W.J.: *Clinical Dental Assisting.* Hagerstown, Md., Medical Department, Harper & Row, 1973, pp. 170–175.

V

Instrumentation

INTRODUCTION

Instrumentation for scaling, root planing, gingival curettage, polishing of the teeth and restorations, and postoperative care is included in Part V. Postoperative procedures for dressing placement and removal, suture removal, and treatment of hypersensitive teeth are outlined. Immediate evaluation of techniques and their effects, short-term follow-up, and recall and maintenance evaluation are described.

The first objective of treatment is to create an environment in which the tissues can return to health. In the sequence of patient treatment, introduction to preventive measures is first, before professional instrumentation. After health has been attained, the patient's self-care on a daily basis is essential to keep the teeth and gingival tissues free from disease caused by the microorganisms of bacterial plaque. Professional instrumentation makes a limited contribution to arresting the progression of disease without daily plaque control measures by the patient.

I. Oral Prophylaxis: Definition Dilemma

The term *oral prophylaxis* means those specific treatment procedures aimed at removing local irritants to the gingiva and at smoothing the tooth surfaces. A smooth tooth surface resists the retention of dental deposits. The oral prophylaxis performed with these objectives is truly a *preventive periodontal treatment procedure.*[1]

There is a definite need for clarification and new terminology for the various services performed under the title "oral prophylaxis." Through common usage, an oral prophylaxis has taken on a variety of meanings.

Since *prophylaxis* means *prevention of disease,* then *oral prophylaxis,* as the *prevention of oral disease,* would include such preventive procedures as restoring individual teeth, replacing missing teeth, adjusting the occlusion, correcting faulty proximal contacts, and many other procedures, the basic purposes of which are preventive.[2] Unfortunately the term oral prophylaxis also is sometimes used to mean a superficial 5- to 10-minute application of a rubber polishing cup with an abrasive paste to the enamel surfaces that appear above the gingival margin. It is apparent that the term "oral prophylaxis" must be carefully and specifically defined if it is to be applied to the comprehensive treatment services of a dental hygienist.

II. Preventive Periodontal Treatment Procedure

In the development of a meaningful concept of the oral prophylaxis upon which the techniques and anticipated outcomes described in this book could be based, the acceptable definition could only be one based on the preventive aspects of periodontal diseases. Treatment procedures include the *complete* removal of all calculus and careful root planing to remove altered cementum. Instrumentation performed in this manner can be expected to contribute to the accomplishment of the objectives listed below.

III. Objectives of Instrumentation

Specific objectives for each type of instrumentation are included in the chapter which describes the details of technique. General objectives are that dental hygiene instrumentation will

475

A. Create an environment in which the tissues can return to health and then be maintained in health.

B. Aid in the prevention and control of gingival and periodontal diseases by removal of factors that predispose to the retention of bacterial plaque. Factors particularly implicated are dental calculus, irregular and overhanging restorations, and rough, altered cemental tooth surfaces.

C. Comprise the total treatment needed for certain patients with uncomplicated disease, and the initial preparatory phase of treatment for others with more advanced disease.

D. Assist in the maintenance phase of care.

E. Provide the patient with smooth tooth surfaces which are easier to clean and to keep plaque-free by self-care daily procedures.

F. Assist in instructing the patient in the appearance and feeling of a thoroughly clean mouth as a motivation toward the development of adequate habits of personal oral care.

G. Prepare the teeth for application of certain caries preventive agents.

H. Prepare the teeth and gingiva for dental operations, including those performed by the restorative dentist, prosthodontist, orthodontist, pedodontist, and oral surgeon.

I. Improve oral esthetics and sanitation.

IV. Appointment Sequence

In preparation for instrumentation, the patient history should be carefully reviewed and preappointment preparation such as premedication checked. The oral tissues are reexamined for orientation in a first appointment and evaluated for the effects of previous treatment when at a succeeding appointment.

Instruction is provided as needed and as designated by the treatment plan. Instrumentation, with explanation to the patient for complete patient understanding and cooperation, can then be carried out.

References

1. *World Workshop in Periodontics.* Ann Arbor, University of Michigan, 1966, p. 450.
2. Bunting, R.W.: *Oral Hygiene,* 3rd ed. Philadelphia, Lea & Febiger, 1957, p. 233.

Suggested Readings

Agerbaek, N., Poulsen, S., Melsen, B., and Glavind, L.: Effect of Professional Toothcleansing Every Third Week on Gingivitis and Dental Caries in Children, *Community Dent. Oral Epidemiol.,* 6, 40, Number 1, 1978.

American Dental Association, Council on Dental Care Programs: Reporting Periodontal Treatment Under Dental Prepayment Plans, *J. Am. Dent. Assoc.,* 102, 345, March, 1981.

Axelsson, P.: Concept and Practice of Plaque-control, *Pediatric Dent.,* 3, 101, Special Issue, May, 1981.

Axelsson, P. and Lindhe, J.: The Effect of a Preventive Programme on Dental Plaque, Gingivitis and Caries in Schoolchildren. Results After One and Two Years, *J. Clin. Periodontol.,* 1, 126, Number 2, 1974.

Badersten, A., Nilvéus, R., and Egelberg, J.: Effect of Nonsurgical Periodontal Therapy. 1. Moderately Advanced Periodontitis, *J. Clin. Periodontol.,* 8, 57, February, 1981.

Glavind, L.: Effect of Monthly Professional Mechanical Tooth Cleaning on Periodontal Health in Adults, *J. Clin. Periodontol.,* 4, 100, May, 1977.

Helldén, L.B., Listgarten, M.A., and Lindhe, J.: The Effect of Tetracycline and/or Scaling on Human Periodontal Disease, *J. Clin. Periodontol.,* 6, 222, August, 1979.

Hughes, T.P. and Caffesse, R.G.: Gingival Changes Following Scaling, Root Planing and Oral Hygiene, *J. Periodontol.,* 49, 245, May, 1978.

Nyman, S., Rosling, B., and Lindhe, J.: Effect of Professional Tooth Cleaning on Healing After Periodontal Surgery, *J. Clin. Periodontol.,* 2, 80, April, 1975.

Poulsen, S., Agerbaek, N., Melsen, B., Korts, D.C., Glavind, L., and Rölla, G.: The Effect of Professional Toothcleansing on Gingivitis and Dental Caries in Children After 1 Year, *Community Dent. Oral Epidemiol.,* 4, 195, Number 5, 1976.

Preventive Dental Services, Practices, Guidelines and Recommendations. Report of the Working Group on Preventive Dental Services, Health and Welfare, Canada, September, 1979, pp. 85–102.

Ripa, L.W., Barenie, J.T., and Leske, G.S.: The Effect of Professionally Administered Biannual Prophylaxes on the Oral Hygiene, Gingival Health, and Caries Scores of School Children, Two Year Study, *J. Prev. Dent.,* 3, 22, January–February, 1976.

Shaw, O., Shaw, B., Smith, D.M., and Swallow, J.N.: The Value of an Introductory Prophylaxis in the Alleviation of Children's Anxiety, *J. Int. Dent. Child.,* 6, 39, December, 1975.

Suomi, J.D., Smith, L.W., Chang, J.J., and Barbano, J.P.: Study of the Effect of Different Prophylaxis Frequencies on the Periodontium of Young Adult Males, *J. Periodontol.,* 44, 406, July, 1973.

Tagge, D.L., O'Leary, T.J., and El-Kafrawy, A.H.: The Clinical and Histological Response of Periodontal Pockets to Root Planing and Oral Hygiene, *J. Periodontol.,* 46, 527, September, 1975.

Talbot, K., Mandel, I.D., and Chilton, N.W.: Reduction of Baseline Gingivitis Scores with Repeated Prophylaxes, *J. Prev. Dent.,* 4, 28, November–December, 1977.

Torfason, T., Kiger, R., Selvig, K.A., and Egelberg, J.: Clinical Improvement of Gingival Conditions Following Ultrasonic Versus Hand Instrumentation of Periodontal Pockets, *J. Clin. Periodontol.,* 6, 165, June, 1979.

Vestergaard, V., Moss, A., Pedersen, H.O., and Poulsen, S.: The Effect of Supervised Tooth Cleansing Every Second Week on Dental Caries in Danish School Children, *Acta Odontol. Scand.,* 36, 249, Number 4, 1978.

Zander, H.A., Polson, A.M., and Heijl, L.C.: Goals of Periodontal Therapy, *J. Periodontol.,* 47, 261, May, 1976.

31

Principles for Instrumentation

Instrumentation begins with the identification of the various types of instruments for specific services to be performed and knowledge of the parts of those instruments. Then, to put the instruments into action to accomplish a particular task, requirements are stabilization by means of a correct grasp and finger rest, adaptation, angulation, and stroke.

A study of oral and dental anatomy and histology necessarily accompanies techniques. Development of a thorough, efficient, and safe procedure depends on an understanding of the characteristics of the dental and periodontal tissues being influenced.

Knowledge of the specific morphology and topography of each tooth and the relationship to the other teeth in the permanent, mixed, and primary dentitions is essential to the understanding and use of the instruments. Recognition of the characteristic signs of health and disease of the periodontal tissues provides the basis for application of instruments for treatment.

A high degree of skill in the care and use of the fine instruments is required. Skill is dependent on knowledge and understanding of the goals of therapy and of how the goals can be reached through application of the fundamental principles of instrumentation.

INSTRUMENT IDENTIFICATION

I. Recognition of Instruments

The instruments needed for examination and evaluation were described in Chapter 13, page 209, and instruments for scaling, planing, and gingival curettage are described in Chapter 32, page 487. Other instruments needed for various services may be found in other chapters.

Each instrument must be recognized by sight and distinguished at a glance by the profile of the instrument on the sterile tray. It is important to be able to designate the names and numbers, and to associate each instrument promptly with the various phases of instrumentation. Such spot identification contributes to neatness of tray arrangement and efficiency of operation through prompt selection of the proper instrument for the service to be performed.

II. Instrument Parts

There are three major parts: the working end, the shank, and the handle or shaft. The relationship of these parts is illustrated by the scaler in figure 31–1.

A. Working End

The working end refers to that part used to carry out the purpose and function of the instrument. Each working end is unique to the particular instrument.
  1. *Sharp Instruments.* The working end of a sharp instrument is called a *blade*. The parts of a sharp blade are the
     a. Cutting edge: a line where two surfaces meet. For example the face and

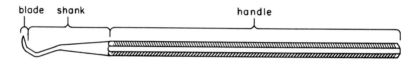

Figure 31–1. Scaler to illustrate the parts of an instrument. The working end of the scaler is the blade.

the lateral surfaces meet to form the sharp cutting edge of a sickle scaler (figures 32–1 and 32–2, page 488) or a curet (figure 32–6, page 491).

b. Lateral surfaces: the lateral surfaces meet or are continuous (as in the curved curet) to form the back of the instrument.

2. *Non-sharp Instruments.* The working end of a non-sharp instrument is a dull blade, or a *nib.* Although the term nib is most frequently applied to instruments for restorative dentistry, such as a condenser or burnisher, it may also apply to non-sharp ends such as the wood point at the end of the porte polisher (page 572) and the rubber cup of the prophylaxis angle (page 576).

B. Shank

1. Connects the working end with the handle.

2. May be angled, curved, or straight; the more restricted the access to an area, the greater number of shank angles are usually required. Anterior teeth are more accessible; therefore, straight-shanked instruments can be used. Posterior teeth need angled-shank instruments, particularly for proximal surfaces.

C. Handle

1. Double-ended instruments have paired (mirror image) or complementary working ends attached to one handle. Single-ended instruments have one working end.

2. Cone socket handles are separable from the shank and working end and permit instrument exchanges and replacements.

INSTRUMENT GRASP

Stability is essential for effective, controlled action of an instrument. The correct use de-

pends on maintaining *control* of the movement of the instrument through use of an effective *grasp* and the establishment and maintenance of an appropriate, firm, fulcrum *finger rest.*

I. Functions of the Instrument Grasp

The manner in which the instrument is held influences the entire procedure. A rigid grasp in which the instrument is gripped tightly, lessens the tactile sensitivity and hence the effectiveness of instrumentation. The appropriate grasp is firm, displays the confidence of the operator in the work being done, and provides the following effects:

A. Increased fingertip tactile sensitivity.

B. Positive control of the instrument with flexibility of motion.

C. Decreased hazard of trauma to the dental and periodontal tissues, which results in less postoperative discomfort for the patient.

D. Prevention of fatigue to operator's fingers, hand, and arm.

II. Types

A. Modified Pen Grasp

1. *Description.* The modified pen grasp is a three-finger grasp with the tips of the thumb, index finger, and middle (second) finger all in contact with the instrument. The ring finger is the finger rest. The instrument is held by the thumb and index finger at the junction of the shank and handle, with the middle (second) finger placed on the shank to hold and guide the movement (figure 31–2).

2. *Role of Middle Finger.* The shank of the instrument is held against the pad of the middle finger. The instrument is not held across the nail or the side of the middle finger as in a pen grasp usually used for writing (figure 31–3). The specific position of the middle finger is extremely important to instrument control in pre-

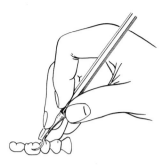

Figure 31–2. Instrument grasp and finger rest. In the *modified pen grasp* as shown, the instrument is held by the thumb and index finger near the junction of the handle and shank, with the middle finger placed on the shank to control and guide the movement. The finger rest is maintained by the ring and little fingers on a firm tooth surface near the area of operation.

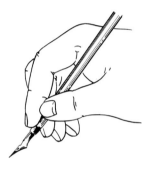

Figure 31–3. Pen grasp. For writing, a pen is frequently held with the side of the pen handle against the side of the middle finger. Compare this with figure 31–2 which shows a modified pen grasp as used during instrumentation.

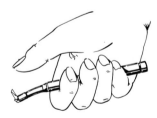

Figure 31–4. Palm grasp. Instrument handle is held in the palm by cupped index, middle, ring, and little fingers. Thumb is free and serves as the finger rest.

venting the instrument from slipping during manipulation.

B. Palm Grasp

1. *Description.* The handle of the instrument is held in the palm by cupped index, middle, ring, and little fingers. Thumb is free to serve as fulcrum (figure 31–4).

2. *Limitations of Use.* Instruments for scaling, planing, and gingival curettage are not used with a palm grasp. The possible exception is a chisel scaler when it is used to remove gross calculus by a push stroke (page 490). The palm grasp limits operation in that there is less tactile sensitivity and less flexibility of movement.

3. *Examples of Uses*
   a. Air syringe
   b. Rubber dam clamp holder
   c. Handpiece grasp for instrument sharpening (figure 32–15, page 501)
   d. Porte polisher for facial surfaces

FULCRUM: FINGER REST

A fulcrum must always be used when instruments are applied to the teeth and gingiva.

I. Definition

A. Fulcrum

The support, or point of rest, on which a lever turns in moving a body.

B. Finger Rest

The support, or point of finger rest on the tooth surface, on which the hand turns in moving an instrument.

II. Objectives

An effective, well-established finger rest is essential to the following:

A. Stability: for controlled action of the instrument.

B. Prevention of Injury: to the patient's oral tissues, which can result from irregular pressure and uncontrolled movement.

C. Comfort for the Patient: confidence in operator's ability, which results from the feeling of securely applied instruments.

D. Control of Length of Stroke: with instrument grasp, the finger rest limits the instrumentation to where it is needed.

III. Digits Used for Finger Rest

A. Modified Pen Grasp

1. *Ring Finger.* Little finger is held close beside ring finger (figure 31–2).

2. *Supplementary.* Pad of middle finger rests lightly on incisal or occlusal surface of tooth to which instrument is applied; ring finger maintains regular fulcrum position and middle finger maintains its grasp on instrument.

B. Palm Grasp: thumb.

IV. Location of Finger Rest

A. Purposes

The location of a finger rest is selected for the following reasons:
1. Convenience to area of operation.
2. Ease in instrument adaptation.
3. Maintenance of an effective grasp.
4. Application of the appropriate angulation.
5. Stability and control of instrument during the activation (strokes).
6. Safety of the operator: a finger rest placed in line of the stroke direction could result in a rubber glove puncture and/or a finger stab if the patient moved suddenly or the instrument slipped for any reason.

B. Principles

1. The first choice for a rest is usually the tooth adjacent to the one where the instruments are to be applied.
2. Maintain rest on firm solid tooth or teeth. The patient's chin, lips, and cheeks are mobile and flexible and therefore less reliable for stability.
3. Where possible, the rest should be on the same arch, maxillary or mandibular, as the instrumentation; also where possible, in the same quadrant.

V. Variations of Finger Rest

A. Need for Variation

A basic fulcrum location cannot always be used or may require supplementation. Variations may be used only after conventional fulcrum positioning has been tried and shown ineffective. Repeated attempts to vary fulcrum rests are inefficient and time-consuming.
1. A patient's facial musculature, oral anatomic features, dental anatomy, or a physical handicap affecting the oral cavity indirectly may interfere with customary positioning for instrumentation.
2. Tenacious calculus in difficult-access areas may not be displaced and root surfaces planed by the usual procedures. Greater support and pressure to the instrument are required.

B. General Categories of Variations[1,2]

When the problem in instrumentation seems to be related to space and accessibility, the height and position of the patient's oral cavity should be checked as well as a possible change in operator's working position.

When a variation in finger rest is used, apply basic rules for stability and control and avoid rests on movable tissues. Three types of variations are suggested here: *a substitute, supplementary,* or a *reinforced* finger rest.
1. *Substitute*
   a. Missing teeth where finger rest is usually applied. For an edentulous area, a cotton roll or gauze sponge may be packed into the area to provide a solid dry finger rest. Otherwise, a rest across the dental arch or in the opposite arch may be required to provide stability.
   b. Mobile teeth, or teeth with inadequate bony support. Avoid mobile teeth for finger rests or use only with minimal pressure for brief periods. Not only would the rest on a mobile tooth be unstable, but pressure, movement, and undue stress on the tooth could traumatize and tear the periodontal ligament fibers.
   c. Index finger of nondominant hand may be placed in the vestibule over a cotton roll. The usual finger rest can be placed on that. This aids retraction and visibility, particularly in the mouth of a small child.
2. *Supplemental.* Place the index finger of the nondominant hand on the occlusal surfaces of teeth adjacent to the working area. The finger rest can then be applied to the index finger. Such supplements

are not useful for distal surfaces where the mouth mirror is essential for vision.

3. *Reinforced*

   a. In this type, a support is placed between the instrument handle and the working end to provide additional strength and force, particularly for hard, tenacious calculus in pockets. Greater control of the instrument can result and, when applied correctly, reduce the danger of instrument breakage. A definite rest for both hands is needed.

   b. Index finger of nondominant hand can be rested on the tooth adjacent to the one being scaled while the thumb is placed on the instrument shank (or handle) for a reinforcement.

VI. Touch or Pressure Applied to Finger Rest

A. Balance

The fulcrum finger maintains a firm hold with moderate pressure to balance the action of the instrument being applied.

B. Effects of Excess Pressure

1. Decreased stability.
2. Diminished control.
3. Grasp overtightened to accommodate.
4. Mandibular fulcrums: heavy pressure on the movable mandible can cause fatigue in the temporomandibular joint and related muscles, and thus discomfort for the patient.
5. Fatigue in operator's fingers and hand.

ADAPTATION

With an appropriate grasp and finger rest, the instrument is next ready for application. The working end of the instrument is adapted to the surface of the tooth or tissue where instrumentation is to take place. *Adaptation* refers to the relationship between the instrument and the surface of the tooth or soft tissue.

I. Relation to Tooth Morphology

Adaptation of instruments is closely related to tooth and soft tissue morphology. Adaptation depends on a knowledge of oral anatomy and morphology. The adaptation of the instrument is of significance because of the need for completeness of service, as well as of the potential damage to the teeth and gingival tissue. Improperly adapted instruments can damage the tooth surface or remove excess tooth substance.

Areas in which instrument adaptation is most difficult and which require more attention, time, and careful application of skill, include the following:[3]

A. Line Angles

All line angles require that the instrument be rolled between the fingers to turn the working end as the instrument is activated. At each change of direction around a line angle, the instrument must be turned to keep it adapted to the surface.

B. Convex and Rounded Surfaces, particularly of narrow roots.

C. Cervical Area where the root is constricted.

D. Proximal Root Surfaces

Root surfaces may be concave, may have longitudinal grooves, and open furcations.

II. Characteristics of a Well-adapted Instrument

A. Working End

1. The working end of the instrument is correctly positioned for the task to be accomplished. For example, when scaling, the angle formed by the face of the instrument and the tooth surface is crucial for effective calculus removal. Angulation is described below.

2. As much as possible of the working end of the instrument is used. The instrument is adapted for maximum usefulness of the working end. For example, this may be 2 to 3 mm. of the end of a curet when on a "flat" surface, whereas at a convex surface of a narrow root, less than 2 mm. may be adaptable.

3. The working end is applied so that it fits closely to the surface; it is applied to conform to the contour of the surface.

4. As the instrument is activated, it can be adjusted to changes required by variations in the surface topography.

B. Tissue

It will not harm the tissue being treated nor the surrounding or adjacent tissues.

ANGULATION

A factor closely related to and directly influencing instrument adaptation is angulation. Angulation refers to the angle formed by a working end of an instrument with the surface to which the instrument is applied. Each instrument is applied to a surface in a specific manner for optimum operation.

I. Probe

The usual adaptation of a probe is to maintain the side of the working tip on the tooth, with the long axis of the working end nearly parallel with the tooth surface (pages 214–215).

As used for a bleeding index, the tip is placed inside the pocket wall and pressed slightly on the wall as the probe is moved horizontally around the tooth (figure 19–5, page 300).

II. Explorer

An explorer is held with the tip at a right angle to the occlusal surface when detecting occlusal pit or fissure caries; but on other surfaces, the side of the tip is kept on the tooth at all times. The angle is 5 degrees or less.

III. Scalers and Curets

Angulation for a scaler or a curet means the angle formed by the face of the instrument with the surface to which the instrument is applied. This is further described on page 531 with figure 34–1.

A. Scaling and Root Planing

An angle less than 90 degrees but not less than 45 degrees permits effective calculus removal and root planing with removal of altered cementum. The preferred angulation is between 60 and 80 degrees. Using a markedly closed angulation under 45 degrees may result in burnishing the calculus to produce a smooth veneer.

B. Gingival Curettage

The face is turned toward the soft-tissue wall of the pocket. It is angulated at less than 90 degrees but more than 45 degrees (figure 34–1, page 531).

ACTIVATION: STROKE

I. Definition

A stroke is a single unbroken movement made by an instrument. It is the action of an instrument in the performance of the task for which it was designed.

II. Characteristics of Strokes

A. Types

1. *Pull*. Example: scaler removing calculus.
2. *Push*. Example: exploratory stroke when a curet is being positioned.
3. *Combined Push and Pull*. Example: explorer in a walking stroke, which is moving the instrument up and down with equal pressure on the surface.
4. *Walking Stroke*. Example: probe is moved up and down, touching the bottom of the sulcus with each down stroke (figure 13–6, page 216).

B. Directions

1. *Vertical:* strokes parallel with the long axis of a tooth.
2. *Horizontal:* strokes perpendicular with the long axis of a tooth. They are sometimes called circumferential, which should not be interpreted to mean that a stroke can be made to go around a tooth or large segment of a tooth. A horizontal stroke necessarily must be a short stroke because of the constant changes in the topography.
3. *Diagonal or Oblique:* stroke that is diagonal to the long axis of the tooth.
4. *Circular:* stroke used with a porte polisher. A small 1- to 2-mm. diameter circular stroke is used with pressure, for example, to apply desensitizing paste (page 557).

III. Factors That Influence Selection of Stroke

A. Size, contour, and position of gingiva.
B. Surface and section of surface where the instrument is used.
C. Depth of sulcus or pocket.
D. Size and shape of instrument used.

IV. Nature of Stroke

A. Motion

The motion for a stroke is generated by a unified action of the shoulder, arm, wrist, and hand.

B. Grasp

The grasp of a scaler or curet is light while the working end is positioned for the stroke, and then the instrument is held more firmly during movement. An explorer and a probe should be held lightly for tactile sensitivity at all times.

C. Hand Stability

During a stroke the whole hand pivots or rotates around the fulcrum.

D. Length

1. The length of the stroke is limited by the action of the entire arm.
2. The stroke is short, controlled, decisive, and directed to protect the tissues from trauma.
3. The length of a stroke varies with each instrument and purpose. A description of strokes for each instrument is included in the respective chapters. The probe is described on pages 213–216; the explorer, page 224; scalers and curets, pages 513 and 517; curettage, page 531; handpiece, page 577.

V. Touch and Pressure

A. Explorers and Probe

A light touch is required for maximum degree of tactile sensitivity.

B. Scalers and Curets

A light but secure touch without pressure for the exploratory stroke is used in preparation for calculus removal or root planing (page 515), then a definite controlled pressure for deposit removal is required during the working stroke.

C. Porte Polisher

A firm, secure, even pressure during the polishing stroke is needed. A circular stroke may be used, and when the instrument is applied near the gingival margin, the stroke is lightened during that part of the circle that is directed toward the gingiva.

D. Prophylaxis Angle

A rubber cup is applied with light pressure in short but firm strokes.

VISIBILITY AND ACCESSIBILITY

I. Effects of Adequate Vision and Accessibility

A. Instrumentation will be more thorough with minimum trauma to the oral tissues.
B. Length of time required will be lessened, accompanied by less fatigue for patient and dental hygienist.
C. Patient cooperation will be increased because of shortened operating time and less discomfort.

II. Components

A. Patient and operator positions (pages 70–75).
B. Efficient use of direct or reflected (by mouth mirror) illumination for each tooth surface.
C. Adequate, yet gentle, retraction of lips, cheeks, and tongue with consideration for the patient's comfort and operator's convenience.

THOROUGHNESS OF PROCEDURE

During treatment, each particle of calculus and altered cementum must be removed from the tooth surfaces. A firm technique with a painstaking approach will achieve both the complete removal of deposits and comfort for the patient. Since time is involved, a happy medium is possible with time minimized, yet the patient's tissues treated with maximum respect.

Roughness is generally associated with carelessness, and neither has any place in dental hygiene procedures. Possible effects of roughness are:

1. Infliction of unnecessary pain during operation.
2. Prolonged postoperative discomfort.
3. Production of excessive bleeding and debris which hinder the efficiency of the operator.
4. Production of tissue lacerations which retard healing.

5. Gouging of tooth surfaces, which may produce a rough tooth surface subject to plaque retention and postoperative sensitivity.

6. Forcing of infected material into the deeper periodontal tissues, which can lead to increased incidence of bacteremia and postoperative infection.

DEXTERITY DEVELOPMENT FOR THE USE OF INSTRUMENTS

This section is included particularly for the beginning dental hygiene student and for the graduate dental hygienist who plans to return to practice after a period of retirement. A primary objective when learning or reviewing techniques for instrumentation is to develop the ability to hold instruments correctly while employing them for use.

However generally dexterous a person may be, the use of new or unusual instruments requires different procedures for coordination. Control is essential, and guided strength contributes to control.

Proficiency during techniques comes from repeated correct use of the instruments. Exercise for the fingers, hands, and arms supplement experience. Directed exercises are needed for both hands, separately and together. To facilitate the development of dexterity, certain exercises have been selected to supplement other types of practice such as the use of instruments on a manikin. A regular period of time each day during the training period should be set aside for exercises.

I. Squeezing a Ball

A. Purposes

1. To develop general muscles of hand and arm.
2. To develop strength and control for use of palm grasp.

B. Tennis Ball

1. Hold ball in palm of hand, grip with thumb and all fingers.
2. Tighten and release grip at regular intervals.
3. One hand rests while other is holding the ball.

C. Chip Blower

1. Hold bulb in palm of hand, grip with middle, ring, and little finger.
2. Use thumb and index finger to maintain nozzle in stationary position, such as that required when directing air on the teeth.
3. Rest one hand while other is exercising the chip blower.

II. Stretching a Rubber Band

A. Purposes

1. To strengthen finger and hand muscles.
2. To develop control of finger movements.
3. To develop ability to separate ring and middle fingers, while keeping ring and little fingers together and index and middle fingers together to simulate application of a finger rest.

B. Rubber Band on Finger Joints

1. Place rubber band at joint between first phalanx and second phalanx.
2. Stretch band by separating middle and ring fingers.
3. Place rubber band at joint between second phalanx and third phalanx and proceed as before.
4. Place rubber bands on both hands and do exercises together.
5. Use rubber bands of smaller diameter as strength and control increase.

C. Rubber Band on Finger Joints with Use of Fulcrum

1. Place rubber band on joint between first phalanx and second phalanx.
2. Establish fulcrum finger (ring finger) on tabletop with little finger closely adjacent to it; elbow and forearm free as they are during instrumentation. Stretch band by separating middle and ring fingers.
3. Touch thumb and index and middle fingers to simulate a modified pen grasp for instrument. Stretch band by separating middle and ring fingers.
4. Variations
   a. Hold instrument in modified pen grasp while doing the exercise.
   b. Do writing exercise with rubber band in place.
5. Rest one hand while other is being exercised.

III. Writing

A. Purposes

1. To develop correct instrument modified pen grasp.
2. To propel instrument by activation from wrist and arm, without moving fingers.
3. To practice use of instruments when mouth mirror is required.
4. To develop control and precision.

B. Circles and Vertical Lines

1. Hold long, well-sharpened, wooden lead pencil with modified pen grasp.
2. Establish fulcrum finger (ring finger) on tabletop; forearm and elbow free.
3. Inscribe counterclockwise small circles and vertical lines on paper, rapidly and lightly at first, slowly and with more pressure later.
4. Accomplish writing by activation of the hand by the upper arm, without flexing or extending the thumb and fingers holding the pencil.
5. Practice each hand separately at first; then use pencil in each hand at the same time, alternating writing action to simulate adaptation of, first, the mirror, and then the explorer or scaler.

C. Using Mouth Mirror

1. Hold mouth mirror with modified pen grasp in nondominant hand close to pencil while practicing writing exercises (III B) through the mirror. Reverse hands.
2. Using engineer's graph paper and modified pen grasp with fulcrum as described earlier, follow the lines of the small squares while looking in mirror held with opposite hand.

D. Everyday Penmanship

1. Use modified pen grasp whenever possible for writing.
2. Practice word writing with the left hand (with the right hand for left-handed person) to increase dexterity for handling mouth mirror.

IV. Mouth Mirror, Cotton Pliers, and Explorer

A. Purposes

1. To develop ability to turn mouth mirror at various angles.
2. To develop dexterity in holding objects with cotton pliers while operating.
3. To establish desired grasp of explorer to assure maximum touch sensitivity.

B. Mouth Mirror

1. Hold mouth mirror with modified pen grasp, ring finger on tabletop as fulcrum finger with little finger closely adjacent to it, elbow and forearm free.
2. Practice turning mirror with fingers, adjusting as to the several surfaces of the tooth.
3. Hold a small object in opposite hand for viewing in mirror.
4. Practice crossing the mirror over fulcrum finger as in position for retracting lower lip with fulcrum finger while viewing lingual surfaces of mandibular anterior teeth in mouth mirror.

C. Cotton Pliers

1. Make small, tight cotton pellets with thumb and index and middle fingers of each hand; then make one in each hand simultaneously.
2. Hold cotton pliers with modified pen grasp and establish fulcrum finger on tabletop; elbow and forearm free.
3. Practice picking up cotton pellets.
   a. Use in wiping motion on tabletop or other object.
   b. Move to different area to release pellet.

D. Explorer

1. Hold explorer with modified pen grasp and establish fulcrum finger on tabletop with upper arm and forearm free.
2. Use extracted teeth to feel with explorer tip until a light grasp permits maximum security of grasp and maximum sense of touch. Extracted teeth can provide a contrast between exploring enamel, cementum, calculus, or other rough area of tooth surface (page 205).

TECHNICAL HINTS

I. Time spent on exercises should be sufficient in any one period to cause moderate (but never severe) strain and fatigue of hand muscles.

II. To relax the muscles of the hands during a practice session, wash hands in warm water.

References

1. Pattison, G.L. and Pattison, A.M.: *Periodontal Instrumentation*. Reston, Virginia, Reston Publishing Co., 1979, pp. 185–190.
2. Cooper, N.P.: *Variations in Fulcrum* (mimeographed). Albuquerque, University of New Mexico, Dental Hygiene Program, 1974.
3. Terwilliger, D. and Schwindt, S.: *Instrument Adaptation as Related to Tooth Root Morphology*. Ann Arbor, School of Dentistry, University of Michigan, 1975, 80 pp.

Suggested Readings

Hard, D.: Oral Prophylaxis, in Bunting, R.W.: *Oral Hygiene*, 3rd ed. Philadelphia, Lea & Febiger, 1957, pp. 249–258.

Carranza, F.A.: *Glickman's Clinical Periodontology*, 5th ed. Philadelphia, W.B. Saunders Co., 1979, pp. 641–663.

Hirschfeld, L.: Subgingival Curettage in Periodontal Treatment, *J. Am. Dent. Assoc., 44*, 301, March, 1952.

Lieberman, N.W.: Your Best Dental Instrument, Your Hands: Exercises to Reduce Muscle Fatigue, *Dent. Surv., 49*, 56, April, 1973.

Taylor, M.: A Comparison of Three Methods of Initial Presentation of Instrument Adaptation, *J. Dent. Educ., 39*, 163, March, 1975.

Tondrowski, V.E.: Preclinical Procedures for the Dental Hygiene Student, *J. Dent. Educ., 20*, 321, November, 1956.

32

Instruments and Sharpening

Knowledge and understanding of the purpose and use of each instrument and the development of dexterity in the effective manipulation of the instruments are basic to clinical dental hygiene practice. The clinical results obtained for the patient depend in part on the proficiency and thoroughness with which the instrumentation is accomplished. *The main purpose of instrumentation is to create an environment about the teeth in which the tissues can heal and be maintained in health.*

I. Types of Instruments

Each instrument is designed for a specific type of application during treatment procedures. An instrument first can be categorized by whether it is designed primarily for supragingival treatment procedures (scalers) or for subgingival treatment (curets). Scalers and curets are then subdivided by their blade anatomy into the following types:

A. Scalers

1. Sickle scaler
   a. Curved sickle scaler
   b. Straight sickle scaler
2. Hoe scaler
3. Chisel scaler
4. File scaler

B. Curets

1. Universal
2. Area specific

II. Instrument Blade Anatomy

The parts of the blade of a scaler or a curet are the *face* (inner surface), *lateral surfaces, back, tip* or *toe*, and the *cutting edges*. The cutting edges are formed by the junction of the face and the lateral surfaces.

Each type of instrument is described in the next sections. The parts of each blade are labeled in figures 32–1, 32–2, and 32–6.

SCALERS

I. Sickle Scaler

By usual definition a sickle is considered curved. However, there are variations in the shapes of sickle scalers and in some forms the blade and cutting edges are straight. When reference is made to the instrument with a curved or straight blade, the types have frequently been called "curved sickle" or "straight sickle."

A. Curved Sickle Scaler

1. Two cutting edges on a curved blade (figure 32–1).
2. Face (inner surface between the cutting edges) is flat in cross section and curved lengthwise.
3. The face converges with the two lateral surfaces to form the tip of the scaler which is a sharp point.

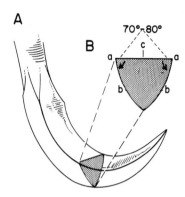

Figure 32–1. Curved sickle scaler. **A.** The curved blade terminates in a point. **B.** Cross section shows the two lateral surfaces (b and b) and the face (c). The two cutting edges (a and a) are formed where the lateral surfaces meet the face at a 70- to 80-degree angle.

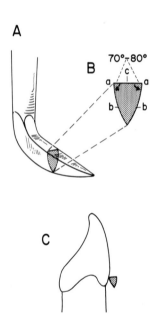

Figure 32–2. Straight sickle scaler. **A.** The two cutting edges meet at the pointed end. **B.** Cross section shows lateral surfaces (b and b) and face (c). Cutting edges (a and a) are formed where the lateral surfaces meet the face. **C.** The blade is applied to the tooth for scaling so that the face is at an angle of less than 90 degrees with the tooth surface but not less than 45 degrees.

4. Cross section of the blade: some are triangular (figure 32–1B); others are trapezoidal.
5. Internal angles of 70 to 80 degrees are formed where the lateral surfaces (b and b in figure 32–1B) meet the face (c) at the cutting edges (a and a).

B. Straight Sickle Scaler

1. Two cutting edges on a straight blade (figure 32–2).
2. Face (between the cutting edges) is flat.
3. The face converges with the two lateral surfaces to form the tip of the scaler which is a sharp point.
4. Cross section of the blade: triangular (figure 32–2B).
5. Internal angles of 70 to 80 degrees are formed where the lateral surfaces (b and b in figure 32–2B) meet the face (c) at the cutting edges (a and a).

C. Angulation of the Shank

Both curved and straight bladed sickles are available with angulated or straight shanks.

1. *Straight.* Single instrument in which the relationships of the shank, blade, and handle are in a flat plane; adaptable primarily for anterior teeth, although may be used for scaling premolars when the lips and cheeks permit retraction for correct angulation.
2. *Modified or Contra-Angle.* Paired instruments which are mirror images of each other to provide access to the proximal surfaces of posterior teeth; one adapts from the buccal and the other from the lingual.

D. Purposes and Use of Sickle Scalers

1. Principally for the *removal of supragingival calculus.*
2. May be useful for removal of gross calculus which is slightly below the gingival margin when the calculus is continuous with the supragingival calculus and when the gingival tissue is spongy and flexible to permit easy insertion of the instrument.
3. Contraindications for use of sickle scalers subgingivally:
   a. Cause undue trauma to the gingival tissue because of the large size, thickness, and length of the blade.
   b. Pointed tip and straight cutting edges cannot be adapted to the curved tooth surfaces: there is greater possibility for grooving or scratching the cemental surface.

c. Tactile sensitivity decreased with larger, heavier blades.

4. Small sickle scalers can be useful for fine supragingival deposits directly under contact areas and between overlapping teeth.

E. Application

1. Angulation: blade is applied to the tooth so that the inner surface or face of the scaler is at an angle of less than 90 degrees with the tooth surface but not less than 45 degrees (figure 32–2C). The preferred angulation is between 60 and 80 degrees.
2. Stroke: pull stroke only for this type of blade.

II. Hoe Scaler

A. Characteristics

1. Single, straight cutting edge (figure 32–3).
2. Blade turned at a 99- to 100-degree angle to the shank.
3. Cutting edge beveled at a 45-degree angle to the end of the blade (figure 32–3B).
4. Shank variously angulated for adaptation of cutting edges to accessible tooth surfaces; some are paired.

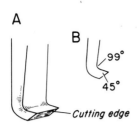

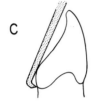

Figure 32–3. Hoe scaler. **A.** The hoe has a single cutting edge. **B.** The blade is turned at an angle of 99 degrees to the shank, and the cutting edge is beveled at a 45-degree angle. **C.** Adaptation to the tooth for removal of calculus is with a two-point contact when possible.

B. Purposes and Uses

1. Removes supragingival calculus, particularly large, accessible tenacious pieces.
2. May be useful to remove gross calculus 2 to 3 mm. below the gingival margin provided the tissue is spongy and flexible and is easily displaced.
3. Contraindications for use subgingivally
   a. Insertion of the thick-bladed instrument into the sulcus causes distention of the pocket wall.
   b. Lack of adaptability of the wide straight cutting edge to the curved root surface.
   c. Difficulty of use without gouging the cemental surface.
   d. Lack of sensitivity because of the bulk of the instrument and the marked angulation of the shanks of some hoes.
   e. Impossibility of reaching the bottom of the pocket without stretching and possibly tearing the gingival pocket wall unnecessarily because of the size and shape of the blade.

C. Application

1. With full width of the cutting edge in contact with the tooth surface and, when possible, a two-point contact with the tooth during the positioning and activation to stabilize the instrument. Two-point contact means contact of the cutting edge and the side of the shank with the tooth (figure 32–3C).
2. Positioning of the section of the shank adjacent to the blade: parallel or nearly parallel to the long axis of the tooth.
3. Hoes are not generally applied to proximal surfaces except the surface adjacent to an edentulous area.
4. Stroke: pull stroke toward occlusal or incisal.

III. Chisel Scaler

A. Characteristics

1. Single straight cutting edge (figure 32–4).
2. Blade is continuous with a slightly curved shank.
3. End of blade is flat and beveled at 45 degrees (figure 32–4B).

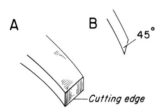

Figure 32–4. Chisel scaler. **A.** The chisel has a single cutting edge, and the blade is continuous with the slightly curved shank. **B.** There is a 45-degree bevel at the cutting edge.

B. Purposes and Uses

1. Useful for removal of supragingival calculus from exposed proximal surfaces of anterior teeth where interdental gingiva is missing.
2. Well suited for quick dislodgement of heavy calculus from the proximal areas of mandibular anterior teeth. When the calculus on the lingual forms a continuous bridge across several teeth, the chisel can be pushed horizontally from the labial to break up the large masses of calculus.
3. Useful for proximal surfaces of premolars when flexibility of the lips and cheeks permits retraction for proper positioning of the cutting edge.

C. Application

1. Full width of cutting edge should be applied, as the sharp corners can nick and groove the tooth surface.
2. Stroke: horizontal only, from labial to lingual on proximal surfaces of anterior, particularly mandibular teeth.

IV. File Scaler

A. Characteristics

1. Multiple cutting edges lined up as a series of miniature hoes on a round, oval, or rectangular base (figure 32–5A).
2. The multiple blades are at a 90- or 105-degree angle with the shank (figure 32–5B).
3. Shanks are variously angulated, similar to the hoes; some are paired instruments, others single.

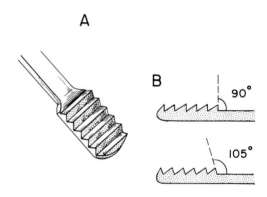

Figure 32–5. Periodontal file. **A.** A file has multiple cutting edges. **B.** Files are designed with each multiple blade at a 90- or 105-degree angle with the shank.

4. Reduced tactile sensitivity because of the size and shape; files are wide, flat, and bulky.

B. Purposes and Uses

In general, the file can be considered a supplementary instrument rather than the definitive instrument for routine use during scaling and root planing.

While never used by some dentists, the file is used by others for one or more of the following purposes:

1. Removal of calculus (accomplished by crushing or fragmentation).
2. Smoothing tooth surfaces: smoothing the tooth at the cementoenamel junction.
3. Root planing, primarily the exposed root surface following periodontal surgery.
4. Smoothing down overextended or rough amalgam restorations, particularly on proximal surfaces or in the cervical area.

C. Application

1. The entire working surface is placed flat against the area to be treated.
2. Adaptation to the curved tooth surfaces is difficult. In certain relationships the file has only a tangential contact.
3. Pressure applied permits the cutting edges to grasp the surface.
4. Stroke: pull only.
5. When the file is used to assist in root planing, it is advisable to follow the file with a curet, since research has shown that a greater degree of smoothness can be attained.[1,2]

CURETS

Characteristics

Blade

1. Two cutting edges on a curved, spoon-shaped blade (figure 32–6A); one cutting edge has a greater curvature than the other. The two cutting edges curve around to meet at the toe. In reality, a curet has one continuous cutting edge because the two sides are united without interruption by the rounded toe.
2. Face (inner surface between the cutting edges) is flat in cross section (figure 32–6B) and curved lengthwise.
3. Back or undersurface is rounded.
4. Cross section of the blade is shaped like a half circle (figure 32–6B).
5. Internal angles of 70 to 80 degrees are formed where the lateral surfaces meet the face (c) at the cutting edges (a and a in figure 32–6B).

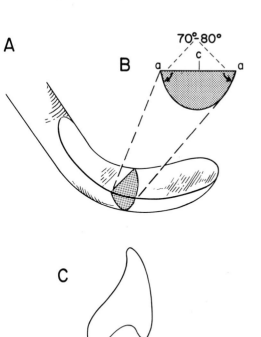

Figure 32–6. Curet. **A.** The two cutting edges are on the curved, spoon-shaped blade. **B.** Cross section is a half circle shape, with the face (c) between the two cutting edges (a and a). **C.** The blade is applied to the tooth so that the face is at less than a 90-degree but not less than a 45-degree angle with the tooth surface.

B. Shank

1. Shank, blade, and handle may be in a relatively flat plane for curets primarily adaptable to anterior teeth. For posterior teeth the shank is contra-angled for access to proximal surfaces.
2. Relationship of face and lower shank (the part of the shank next to the blade)
   a. Universal curet: a universal curet is one that can be adapted for instrumentation on any tooth surface. A truly universal instrument can be adapted so that the cutting edges on both sides of the face can be utilized when correctly angulated. The face of the blade is nearly perpendicular to the lower shank.
   b. Area specific curet: the Gracey curets are area specific. Only one cutting edge, on one side of the face, is used for instrumentation. The face of a Gracey curet is not perpendicular to the lower shank but is offset at an angle of approximately 60 degrees.[3]
3. Instruments are paired.

II. Purposes and Uses

A. Standard instrument for subgingival scaling and root planing (see also page 515).
B. Removal of fine supragingival calculus close to the gingival margin: the rounded instrument is best adapted to the cervical area.
C. Curettage of the lining of the gingival wall of the sulcus or pocket.

III. Application

A. Angulation: blade is applied to the tooth so that the face is at an angle less than 90 degrees but not less than 45 degrees with the tooth surface (figure 32–6C). The preferred angulation is between 60 and 80 degrees.
B. Curets are paired, mirror images of each other, with various angles of the shanks for access to all surfaces of all teeth. Curets for posterior use have greater curvatures of the shank.
C. Larger universal curets are used for subgingival scaling for removal of as much of the calculus as possible; smaller curets and area specific curets are for fine scaling and root planing.

D. The design of the curet allows easy entrance into the sulcus and the curved blade with rounded end permits access to the base of the sulcus or pocket. The slender shank permits entrance to the sulcus with a minimum of tissue distention.
E. Stroke: pull stroke only; applied in vertical, horizontal, or oblique directions.

SPECIFICATIONS FOR INSTRUMENTS FOR SCALING AND ROOT PLANING

I. Basic Qualities

Each instrument is designed for a specific purpose and is intended to be used for the purpose for which it was designed. Characteristics of instruments which influence their usefulness are listed below. An instrument should
A. Be effective and efficient for calculus removal and smoothing tooth surfaces with the least possible trauma to the gingival tissue or the tooth surface.
B. Provide comfort to the operator without causing fatigue or muscle cramp. Hollow handles have a comfortably wide diameter, and are light weight.
C. Permit maximum use of tactile sensitivity. Large, bulky instruments do not assist in transferring surface irregularities to the fingertips.
D. Have balance.
   1. The blade should be centered in line with the long axis of the handle (figure 32–7).
   2. The distance from the cutting edge (working end) of the blade to the junction of the shank and handle (where the instrument is held) should not be greater than 35 to 40 mm. ($1\frac{1}{2}$ inches). Too short a distance may limit the action; too long, may make the instrument unbalanced.
E. Have a blade of a size in keeping with
   1. Tooth anatomy; root curvatures.
   2. Location and extent of calculus deposits.
   3. Anatomy of the sulcus or pocket.
F. Be easy to care for when cleaning, sterilizing, sharpening.

II. Sharp Cutting Edges

Instruments must be sharp if scaling and root planing are to be completed efficiently with min-

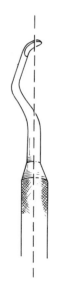

Figure 32–7. Instrument balance. The blade or working end should be centered over the long axis of the handle.

imal trauma to the tissues. With the instrument blade maintained with its original contour and cutting edges sharp, the following may be expected in contrast with the use of dull instruments:
A. Greater precision of operation, improved quality of results, with less operating time involved.
B. Increased tactile sensitivity during instrumentation: a sharp instrument does not have to be gripped as firmly as a dull one.
C. Greater control of the instrument possible with lighter grasp, less pressure required on the tooth being scaled or planed, and decreased pressure on the finger rest.
D. Fewer strokes required.
E. Less possibility of burnishing the calculus rather than removing it.
F. Prevention of unnecessary trauma to gingival tissues, and therefore, less discomfort experienced by the patient.
G. Decreased possibility of nicking, grooving, or scratching the tooth surfaces.
H. Less fatigue for the operator.

INSTRUMENT SHARPENING

Objectives for techniques of sharpening emphasize the *conservation of instrument blades* and the *preservation of their original shape.* Instruments designed for a particular purpose should continue to be used in the manner for which they were designed and not be distorted by inaccurate sharpening techniques.

Sharpening procedures are not easy to learn and require skill and patience to accomplish. It is no doubt true that more instruments are worn out from sharpening than from use.

This chapter includes sharpening procedures for the sickle, hoe, chisel, curet, and explorer, using various sharpening stones and devices. The principles of sharpening that are outlined and illustrated here may be applied to various types of sharpening stones and instruments that may be encountered.

I. Sharpening Stones

A. Materials and Their Sources

1. *Natural Abrasive Stones.* Quarried from mineral deposits, the hard Arkansas oilstone is used for dental instruments because of its fine abrasive particle size.
2. *Artificial Materials*
   a. Hard, nonmetallic substances impregnated with aluminum oxide, silicon carbide, or diamond particles; these are larger and coarser than particles of the Arkansas stone. Examples: ruby stone, carborundum stones, and the diamond hone.
   b. Solid aluminum oxide. Example: moonstone.[4]
   c. Steel alloys: metals that are harder than most dental instrument steel and therefore capable of sharpening the instrument. Example: tungsten carbide steel used in the Neivert Whittler.

B. Categories

Sharpening stones as they are manufactured for use may be classified into two general groups: the ones for manual (unmounted) sharpening and those for power-driven (mandrel mounted) sharpening. Examples of procedures using both unmounted and mounted stones are supplied in this chapter.

1. *Unmounted*
   a. Stationary flat stones: rectangular stones with square or rounded edges, or with one side grooved for the special adaptation of curved blades.
   b. Hand stones: cylindrical (tapered or straight) or rectangular with rounded edges.
   c. Other types: sharpening devices such as the Neivert Whittler.
2. *Mandrel Mounted.* Cylindrical (straight or tapered) small stones of various diameters designed to fit the various sizes of instrument blades.

C. Sterilization

A sterile sharpening stone should be a part of the basic clinic set-up for a scaling and root planing appointment. In that way, instruments may be sharpened throughout the procedure as they show signs of dullness. Efficiency will increase and the patient will benefit from receiving a more thorough treatment in less time.

Sterilization of stones may be accomplished by any of the four acceptable sterilization methods described in Chapter 3 (pages 33–37). Limitations of steam autoclave are that oil on the stone interferes with steam penetration and repeated autoclaving dries out a stone and may lead to chipping or breakage.

II. Facilities for Sharpening

The work area where instrument sharpening is accomplished should be arranged for convenience and comfort. Because sharpening is an everyday event, it needs to be planned so that available time can be utilized effectively without inconveniences.

A. Place

A definite place should be arranged where materials for sharpening can be kept together and work can be done from a seated position.

B. Lighting

A permanently fixed light which can be concentrated over the work area is needed; light must be shaded to protect the eyes.

C. Working Surface

The working surface should be firm and stationary. The bracket table or cervical tray is undesirable because of lack of stability.

D. Equipment

An adequate assortment of stones and the materials for their maintenance and cleanliness, magnifying glass, and other incidental materials related to specific procedures should be available.

III. Dynamics of Sharpening

A. Sharpening Stone Surface

A sharpening stone acts as an abrasive to reshape a dulled blade by grinding the surface until the cutting edge is restored. The surface of the stone is made up of masses of minute crystals which are the abrasive particles that accomplish the grinding of the instrument. A smaller particle size or a finer grain, as it is generally called, abrades or reduces more slowly and produces a finer cutting edge.

B. Cutting Edge

The cutting edge is a fine *line* formed where the face and lateral surface meet at an angle. The edge is a line and therefore has length but no thickness. The edge becomes dull by pressing it against a hard surface (the tooth), or it may be nicked when it is drawn over a rough surface. When the edge is dull, it is rounded and therefore has thickness. The object in sharpening is to reshape the cutting edge to a line.

C. Sharpening

Sharpening is accomplished by grinding the surface or surfaces that form the cutting edge.

IV. Tests for Instrument Sharpness

A. Visual or Glare Test

1. Examine the cutting edge under adequate light, preferably with a magnifying glass.
2. Since the sharp cutting edge is a fine *line*, it will not reflect light.
3. The dull cutting edge presents a rounded, shiny *surface*, which reflects light.

B. Plastic Testing Stick[5]

1. Use a plastic or acrylic ¼ inch rod, 3 inches long: the hardness and texture approximate a fingernail. A plastic disposable suction tip is also useful for this purpose.
2. Apply the instrument blade to the plastic stick at the correct angle for scaling; press lightly but firmly.
3. The sharp cutting edge will engage or grip the plastic and move with resistance if an attempt is made to draw the cutting edge over the surface.
4. The dull cutting edge will not catch without undue pressure, and will slide easily over the surface of the stick.
5. Test each area along an entire cutting edge since, during use, the edge is not uniformly dulled.

C. Fingernail Test

1. This test works similarly to the plastic testing stick: when the sharp cutting edge is applied to the nail at the appropriate angle, it will engage or grip the nail. The dulled instrument will not catch without undue pressure.
2. Although the fingernail test has been used widely over the years, it is not recommended for sanitary and esthetic reasons. The nail cannot be used when protective rubber gloves are worn.

V. Some Basic Principles

A. Sterilization

1. *Sharpening Before Sterilization.* When sharpening before sterilization, the instruments must first be cleaned and disinfected. An ultrasonic cleaner is recommended for sanitization. As an alternate, the instruments may be scrubbed thoroughly with soap and water, provided heavy-duty household gloves are worn and other procedures followed as described on pages 29–30. Steps for maximum precautions were outlined on page 64.

   After sharpening, the instruments are prepared for sterilization. When a dry stone is used, or when plain water is used on the stone, instruments and the stone are scrubbed thoroughly before packaging for sterilization.

   When oil is used during sharpening,

the instruments should be placed again in the ultrasonic cleaner or scrubbed thoroughly with soap and hot water to remove all of the oil. Oil on the instruments or stone can protect microorganisms and prevent complete sterilization. Rather than an oil which is penetrating and difficult to remove, petroleum jelly may be preferred because it is water soluble and therefore readily removed before sterilizing.

2. *Sterilization of the Sharpening Stone.* A sterile sharpening stone is a specific part of a clinic instrument tray, so that instruments can be sharpened as needed throughout the treatment.

B. Instrument Handling

All instruments must be handled with care to preserve sharpness and prevent accidental damage to the cutting edges.

C. Preparation of Stone for Sharpening

1. *Lubricated Stone.* Spread a thin layer of lubricant over the stone's surface. A clear, fine sterile oil or petroleum jelly may be used. An excess amount of oil or petroleum jelly can obscure the view of the cutting edge being sharpened.

   When sharpening during an appointment, a sterile swab is used to apply the lubricant to the sterile stone. The lubricant should be kept in a clinically clean covered jar or tube and set aside expressly for that purpose.

   The lubricant can provide the following effects:
   a. Facilitate the movement of the instrument blade over the stone and prevent scratching of the stone.
   b. Suspend the metallic particles removed during sharpening and so help prevent clogging of the pores of the stone (glazing).

2. *Dry Stone.* Because of the problems related to maintaining a sterile stone and preventing contamination when oil, tap water, or petroleum jelly is applied, the use of a dry stone provides a particular advantage.

   A dry stone contributes to the following effects:

   a. Sharpen the cutting edge without nicks in the blade which can be created from particles of metal suspended in a lubricant.[6]
   b. Allow the stone to be completely sterilized without the problem of interference by the oil left in and on the stone.

D. Sharpening

1. *Objectives.* The objectives during sharpening are to produce a sharp cutting edge and to preserve the original shape of the blade.
2. *When to Sharpen.* Sharpen at the first sign of dullness during an appointment. When instruments become grossly dulled, recontouring wastes the instrument, and it is difficult to restore the original contour and still have a strong blade.
3. *Choice of Method.* Select the sharpening method and sharpening stone or device consistent with the size and shape of the instrument being treated.
4. *Angulation.* Before starting to sharpen, analyze the cutting edge and establish the proper angle between the stone and the blade surface; maintain the angle through the firm grasp, secure finger rest, moderate pressure, short stroke, and other features of the technique appropriate to the individual instrument.
5. *Maintain Control.* Maintain control so that the entire surface is reduced evenly: care must be taken not to create a new bevel at the cutting edge.
6. *Prevent Grooving.* Prevent grooving of the sharpening stone by varying the areas for instrument placement. Resurfacing and stain removal procedures are described on page 504.

E. After Sharpening

Gently hone or burnish the nonbeveled surface adjacent to the cutting edge.
1. Honing: By definition, a *hone* is a sharpening stone and *honing* means sharpening. In common usage, honing has been applied to the process whereby the "bur" or "wire edge" is removed from

the side of the cutting edge that was not reduced.

2. During sharpening, some of the metal particles removed during grinding remain attached to the edge of the instrument and create the wire edge. If left, it is possible for the tiny particles to be removed when the instrument is applied to the tooth surface during treatment.

3. By sharpening into, toward, or against the cutting edge, the production of a wire edge will be minimized.

4. Method for removal: Using an even and light pressure, pass a flat Arkansas stone along the nonbeveled side of the cutting edge. One or two strokes is usually sufficient. If heavy pressure is applied, the bevel of the cutting edge can be altered.

SHARPENING CURETS AND SICKLES

Sharpening both the lateral surfaces and the face will preserve the original contour of the blade. For both curets and sickles, the internal angle at the cutting edge is 70 to 80 degrees (figures 32–1 and 32–6). To preserve this angle, sharpening stones must be placed and activated carefully.

Manual sharpening procedures are the methods of choice in order that the blade not be reduced unnecessarily by the rapid-cutting mounted stone. Techniques in this section show the use of a flat stone for manual sharpening of lateral surfaces. When sharpening lateral surfaces, the flat stone may be used in one of two ways: the stone may be moved while the instrument is stationary, or the stone may be stationary and the instrument moved over it.

MOVING FLAT STONE: STATIONARY INSTRUMENT

The side of the cutting edge formed by the lateral surface is reduced by this method. The technique described applies to both curets and sickles. Because the sickle is pointed and the curet is round on the toe end, there is a variation in the adaptation of the sharpening stone to that portion of the blade.

I. Prepare the Stone

Preparation of stones is described on page 495.

II. Examine the Cutting Edge to Be Sharpened

Test for sharpness to determine specific areas that are dull.

III. Stabilize the Instrument

A. Grasp the instrument in a palm grasp and hold the hand against the edge of a solid workbench or table under adequate light (figure 32–8A). The instrument should be low enough so that the operator will have no difficulty in seeing the cutting edges and the angle formed by the instrument and the sharpening stone.

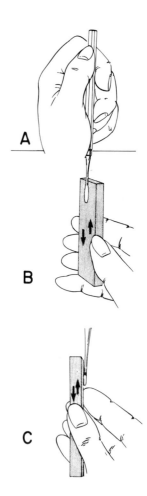

Figure 32–8. Sharpening a curet or scaler using a moving flat stone. **A.** Hold instrument with a firm grasp while stabilizing the hand on the edge of a stationary table or bench. **B.** Stone is angled with the face of the instrument at 100 to 110 degrees (figure 32–9) to maintain the internal angle of the blade at 70 to 80 degrees. **C.** Stone reversed to sharpen opposite cutting edge.

B. Turn the face of the instrument up and parallel with the floor.

IV. Apply Sharpening Stone

A. Apply the stone in a vertical position to the lateral surface at the heel of the cutting edge. Figure 32–8B shows the position for one side of the blade, and figure 32–8C shows the position for the other side.

B. Adjust the angle at which the stone is held to maintain the internal 70 to 80 degrees of the blade. The angle on the outside, between the instrument and the stone, will be 100 to 110 degrees (figure 32–9A and B).

V. Activate the Sharpening Stone

A. Keep the stone in contact with the blade and at the proper angle throughout the procedure.

B. Move the stone up and down with short rhythmical strokes about one-half to one-quarter inch high. Put more pressure on the down stroke.

C. Follow the cutting edge from heel to toe, applying several strokes to each millimeter.

D. Do not change the angle of the stone with the face of the instrument: when the angle is varied, an irregularity will be ground into the cutting edge.

E. Keep the wrist straight and use the whole arm to standardize the stroke and the adaptation of the stone to the instrument.

F. Variation at the toe-end
   1. Sickle: the stone is held straight as it nears the pointed tip.

2. Curet: adapt the stone's position so that sharpening continues around the round toe. The same angle between the stone and the face is maintained.

G. Finish with a down stroke.

VI. Test for Sharpness

Determine whether to repeat the first side before starting the second.

STATIONARY FLAT STONE: MOVING INSTRUMENT

I. Sickle Scaler

A. Prepare the stone (page 495) and place the stone flat on a firm table or bench top under adequate light. Do not tilt the stone while sharpening.

B. Examine cutting edges to be sharpened: test for sharpness.

C. Hold the instrument with a firm pen grasp, using thumb, index, and middle (second) fingers to prevent the instrument from rotating or changing angles during sharpening (figure 32–10B).

D. Establish finger rest on side of stone using ring and little fingers.

E. Stabilize stone with fingers of opposite hand.

F. Apply cutting edge to be sharpened to the stone: maintain 70 to 80 degree internal angle of the instrument (figure 32–9B). The portion of the cutting edge nearest the shank is applied first. Some sickles have flat lateral

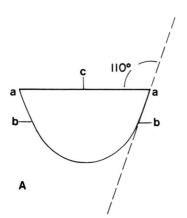

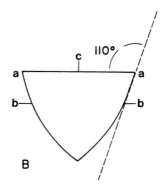

Figure 32–9. Angulation for sharpening. Cross sections of curet (A) and sickle scaler (B) to show correct angulation of the blade with the flat sharpening stone (broken line) when reducing the lateral surface (b). Angle shown on diagram between face (c) and the stone at the cutting edge (a) will be 100 to 110 degrees to maintain an internal angle of 70 to 80 degrees.

surfaces, and an entire side may be positioned at one time.

G. Apply moderate to light but firm pressure while instrument is in motion: heavy pressure can reduce control of instrument, cause scratching of the stone, and produce an unfavorable bevel at the cutting edge.

H. Use a short, slow stroke to maintain the exact relation of the cutting edge to the stone.
   1. Direction: pull blade forward, toward the cutting edge.
   2. All fingers move with the arm as a unit.
   3. Use a slow, steady stroke to maintain control and to assure that each portion of the cutting edge receives equal treatment.
   4. Turn the instrument continually to follow the arc-like shape of the blade to the pointed tip. A sickle with a flat lateral surface is not turned.

I. Test for sharpness after one or two strokes: repeat as needed for ideal sharpness.

J. Turn instrument and proceed to sharpen other lateral surface: when instrument placement is awkward for the modified contra-angled sickle, use a narrow side of the Arkansas stone.

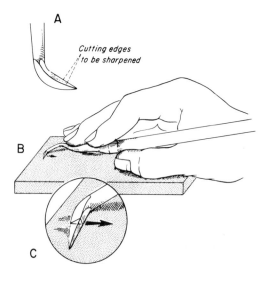

Figure 32–10. Sharpening the straight sickle scaler. **A.** The cutting edges to be sharpened. **B.** With a modified pen grasp and a finger rest firmly established on the side of the stone, the scaler is positioned for sharpening. **C.** The portion of the cutting edge nearest the shank is applied first with an angle of 100 to 110 degrees between the face and the stone. The instrument is turned continuously to follow the arc-like shape of the blade to the pointed tip.

K. Sharpening the face of a straight blade*
   1. Position the surface over a side of the flat stone with the tip pointed down.
   2. Apply entire face flat against the stone.
   3. With firmly established finger rest, apply moderate to light but firm pressure for a short slow stroke while the exact relation of the flat face is maintained on the stone.

II. Curet

A. Prepare the stone (page 495) and place it flat on a steady work bench or table.

B. Examine the cutting edges to be sharpened: test for sharpness.

C. Hold the instrument in a modifed pen grasp and establish a secure finger rest (figure 32–11B).

D. Apply the cutting edge to the stone. An angle of 110 degrees is formed by the stone and face.
   1. Since the curet is curved, only a small section of the cutting edge can be applied at one time.
   2. Sharpening is performed in a *series* of applications of the cutting edge to the stone, each overlapping the previous, as the instrument is turned and drawn steadily along the stone.
   3. The portion of the cutting edge nearest the shank is applied first (figure 32–11C, a).

E. Apply moderate to light but firm pressure while the instrument is activated.

F. Use a slow steady stroke to maintain control and to assure that each portion of the cutting edge receives equal treatment.

G. Move the blade forward into the cutting edge; turn the instrument continuously until the center of the round end of the blade is reached (figure 32–11C, b).

H. Test for sharpness along the entire cutting edge; reapply to stone as necessary for ideal sharpness.

I. Turn the instrument to sharpen the second cutting edge. Overlap at the center of the round tip.

J. Methods for sharpening the facial aspect: Use the hand sharpening cone (below) or the Neivert Whittler (page 500).

---

*Face of a curved sickle is sharpened with a hand sharpening cone (page 499) or the Neivert Whittler (page 500).

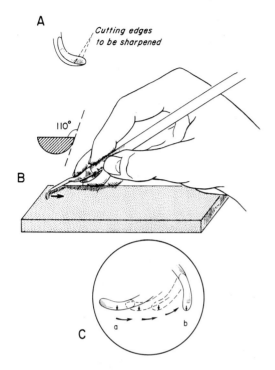

Figure 32–11. Sharpening a curet on a flat stone. **A.** Cutting edges to be sharpened. **B.** Position of the blade on the stone at the beginning of the stroke. With the finger rest stabilized on the edge of the stone, the cutting edge is maintained at the proper angulation (110 degrees) as the instrument is drawn along the stone with an even moderate pressure. **C.** To show the movement of the blade, the arrows indicate each portion of the cutting edge being sharpened as the blade is turned on the stone from the beginning (a) to the completion of the stroke (b) at the center of the rounded end of the curet. The instrument is turned over and the opposite cutting edge is sharpened.

HAND SHARPENING CONE

I. Description

A. Types

Hand stones are cylindrical (tapered or straight) Arkansas cones; or rectangular with rounded edges and tapered carborundum stones.

B. Uses

1. *Arkansas:* tapered cone is recommended for curved cutting edges of sickles and curets.
2. *Carborundum:* coarser grain is useful for preliminary shaping or sharpening of excessively dulled instruments; it is followed by use of a finer stone to refine the cutting edge.

II. Sharpening Procedure

A. Preparation of Stone (page 495).

B. Position

1. Hand-held instrument: hold in nondominant hand across palm with fingers and thumb grasping firmly; direct blade toward self with face of the blade up.
2. For additional support: place instrument over the edge of a firm hard block and maintain rigidly (figure 32–12).
3. Stabilize arms between the wrists and elbows on the edge of a solid table or bench top.
4. Tapered cone: with a firm grasp of the sharpening cone, position the appropriate diameter of the cone to fit the curvature of the surface to be sharpened; apply the stone straight across the face so that an even pressure can be applied to both cutting edges simultaneously to produce an evenly sharpened instrument (figure 32–12).

C. Motion

1. Rotate stone counterclockwise over the instrument with even, firm pressure.

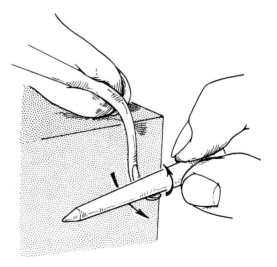

Figure 32–12. Hand sharpening cone. A cylindrical stone is applied to a curet. The instrument is stabilized over a firm block and the stone is positioned at the appropriate diameter to fit the curvature of the surface to be sharpened. An even pressure is applied across the face of the instrument so that both cutting edges will be sharpened evenly.

2. Continue rotation of stone upward (as in a circle) when approaching the end of the curet to prevent tapering off and reshaping the curvature of the tip. (Figure 32–15B illustrates this for the mounted stone. The same principle applies to the manually-operated instrument.)

3. A horizontal stroke may be used. The instrument is maintained stationary as described above, and the stone is moved back and forth across the face. Care must be taken to maintain the stone straight across so that an even pressure is applied simultaneously to both cutting edges.

D. Test for Sharpness

Test for sharpness after a few applications; repeat as necessary to obtain ideal sharpness.

THE NEIVERT WHITTLER

I. Description

A. Working End

The working end consists of five sharpening edges and a rounded burnishing edge of tungsten carbide.

B. Handle

The handle is made of stainless steel; it is bulky and hexagonal for comfortable grasping (figure 32–13).

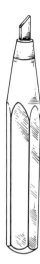

Figure 32–13. The Neivert Whittler. The drawing is approximately one third the instrument's size.

II. Uses

A. Manufacturer's instructions describe sharpening straight and curved blades: dental instruments, scissors, knives.

B. Particularly useful for the face of a curved scaler or curet.

C. Honing: the outer rounded edge is designed for honing (burnishing).

III. Sharpening Procedure

A. Position

Stability and control are most important.

1. Hold instrument to be sharpened firmly in the nondominant hand, across palm, grasping with all fingers and the thumb, with the surface to be sharpened turned toward self. The instrument can also be stabilized over the edge of a firm, hard surface as shown for the cone in figure 32–12.

2. Stabilize arms between the wrists and the elbows on the edge of a solid table or bench top.

3. Whittler is held in a palm grasp with thumb under handle adjacent to the working end and at the same time the thumb rest is applied beneath the instrument blade on the nondominant hand (figure 32–14A).

4. Working end: apply to the curvature of the surface to be sharpened straight across so that even pressure can be applied to both cutting edges and an evenly sharpened instrument will result (figure 32–14B).

B. Motion

1. Draw the Whittler edge across the length of the face with a moderate, even pressure.

2. As the end is approached, continue in an upward motion to prevent tapering off and reshaping curvature of the tip.

C. Test for Sharpness

Test for sharpness after a few applications.

D. Hone

Hone the lateral surfaces of blade next to cutting edges.

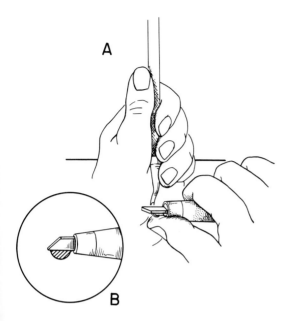

Figure 32–14. Sharpening a curet with a Neivert Whittler. **A.** The instrument to be sharpened is stabilized in the nondominant hand, while the sharpener is grasped in a palm grasp with the thumb rest close to the instrument to be sharpened. **B.** The blade of the sharpener is placed and maintained straight across the face of the curet to produce evenly sharpened cutting edges.

MANDREL MOUNTED STONES

I. Description

A. Types

1. *Arkansas:* fine grain.
2. *Ruby Stone:* coarser grain especially useful for recontouring excessively dull instrument; when used for routine sharpening, it should be applied conservatively.

B. Shapes

The stones are cylindrical with flat end or cone-shape.

C. Use

1. Applicable to most cutting edges: various sizes and grains of stones are selectively utilized.
2. Reshaping: coarse-grained ruby stone may be useful for this.
3. Stones may be sterilized and are used with water; therefore, they are useful for sharpening sterile instruments and for use during the patient's appointment.

II. Sharpening Procedure

A. Select Stone

Select a sharpening stone with a diameter appropriate to fit the blade of the instrument to be sharpened.

B. Prepare Stone

Apply oil to Arkansas stone; dip ruby stone in water and repeat at intervals during sharpening to aid in reducing heat production.

C. Position

1. Hold instrument to be sharpened in a palm grasp with blade face up.
2. Hold handpiece in other hand using a palm grasp with the thumb securely placed against the thumb of the hand holding the instrument (figure 32–15).
3. Stabilize arms between wrists and elbows on the edge of a solid table or bench top.
4. Apply stone to surface to be sharpened straight across so that light, even pressure can be applied to both cutting edges simultaneously and an evenly sharpened instrument will result.

D. Motion

1. *Use Low Speed*

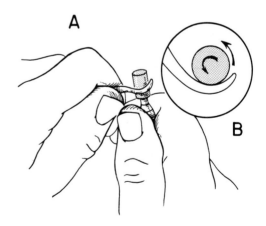

Figure 32–15. Sharpening with a mandrel mounted stone. **A.** A stone with a diameter appropriate for the curved blade to be sharpened is positioned across the face for even sharpening of the cutting edges. Hands and arms are stabilized for precision and control. **B.** With low speed to minimize heat production, the rotating stone is passed along the instrument surface. Near the end of the blade the stone is moved upward to prevent flattening off the instrument end.

a. To minimize heat production (alteration of the temper of the steel can result with repeated use).

b. To allow complete control of position of sharpening stone on blade.

2. *Apply Light Pressure.* To prevent undue reduction of instrument; yet heavy enough so that surface will be smooth.

3. *Maintain Blade Shape.* Pass the rotating stone upward when approaching the end of the blade to prevent tapering off and reshaping the tip.

E. Test for Sharpness

Test for sharpness after one or two applications; repeat when necessary.

F. Hone

Hone the lateral borders of the cutting edges.

III. Disadvantages of Power-Driven Sharpening

A. Inconsistent results because of variations in speed and difficulty of stabilization of instrument and sharpening stone.

B. Excess reduction of instrument during shorter period of use; less conservation of instruments than by manual methods.

C. Frictional heat may affect the temper of the steel.

SHARPENING THE HOE SCALER

Characteristics of the hoe scaler are described on page 489. The hoe has only one surface to be ground. Since placement of the small surface on the Arkansas stone is difficult to visualize, use of a magnifying glass can be particularly helpful.

I. Surface To Be Ground

Examine surface to be ground (figure 32–16A); test for sharpness.

II. Sharpening Procedure

A. Hold instrument in modified pen grasp; establish finger rest on the stone.

B. Apply the surface to be ground to the stone in correct relationship to maintain the 45-degree bevel (figure 32–16B).

C. With moderate, steady pressure, pull the instrument toward the cutting edge a short

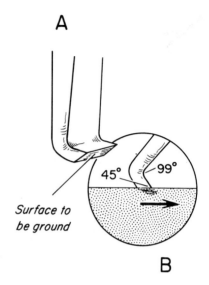

Figure 32–16.   Sharpening the hoe scaler. **A.** Surface to be ground. **B.** Hoe adapted to the surface of a flat stone at the proper angle to maintain the original bevel of 45 degrees. Arrow indicates direction of the sharpening stroke, which is toward the cutting edge.

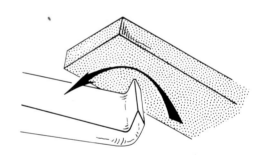

Figure 32–17.   Round the sharp corners of the hoe scaler. A flat stone is rubbed over the instrument with a gentle rolling motion.

distance, letting the whole hand move with the arm as a unit.

D. Release pressure and slide the instrument back; repeat.

E. Test for sharpness and reapply as needed for ideal sharpness.

F. Hone the undersurface of the blade adjacent to the cutting edge.

III. Round Corners

Corners should be rounded at each end of the cutting edge.

A. Purpose: to help prevent laceration of soft tissue or grooving of tooth surface.

B. Hold instrument in nondominant hand with corners of cutting edge directed inward.

C. Rub the surface of the sharpening stone across each corner with a gentle rolling motion (figure 32–17); two or three applications are usually sufficient.

SHARPENING THE CHISEL SCALER

Sharpening procedures for the chisel are similar to those for the hoe. Again, the surface is small, the angulation difficult to visualize, and the use of a magnifying glass recommended. Review the characteristics of the chisel scaler on pages 489–490.

I. Surface To Be Ground

Examine surface to be ground (figure 32–18A); test for sharpness.

II. Sharpening Procedure

A. Hold instrument with a modified pen grasp, establish finger rest, and apply the surface to be ground to the stone in the correct relationship to maintain the 45-degree bevel (figure 32–18B).
B. With moderate, steady pressure, push the instrument forward, toward the cutting edge, without changing the relationship with the stone.
C. After two or three applications, test for sharpness and reapply as necessary for an ideal cutting edge.
D. Hone the nonbeveled surface.

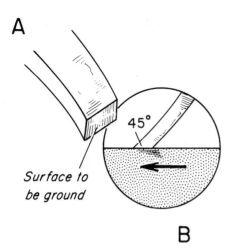

A

45°

Surface to be ground

B

Figure 32–18. Sharpening the chisel scaler. **A.** Surface to be ground. **B.** The chisel is adapted to the surface of a flat stone at the appropriate angle to maintain the original bevel of 45 degrees. Arrow indicates direction of the sharpening stroke, which is toward the cutting edge.

III. Round Corners

Round the corners at each end of the cutting edge. In a manner similar to that shown in figure 32–17 for the hoe scaler, rub the surface of the flat stone across each corner of the chisel with a gentle, even, rolling motion. Two or three applications are usually sufficient.

SHARPENING EXPLORERS

I. Tests for Sharpness

A. **Visual**

When examined under concentrated light, a dull explorer tip will appear rounded; the tip may reflect light.

B. **Plastic Testing Stick**

A sharp explorer will grip the plastic on light pressure and move with resistance when pulled over the surface; a dull explorer will not catch and will slide.

II. Recontour

Small-nosed pliers can be used to straighten a bent tip.

III. Sharpening Procedure

A. Prepare unmounted flat stone.
B. Instrument is held with a modified pen grasp; finger rest established on side of stone.
C. Placement and movement of the tip over the stone resembles somewhat the procedure for the curet on the unmounted stone (figure 32–11, page 499):
  1. Place side of tip on stone at approximately 15- to 20-degree angle of stone with shank of explorer.
  2. As tip is moved over the surface, the handle is rotated so that even pressure can be applied to each part of the tip.

CARE OF SHARPENING STONES

I. Flat Arkansas Stone

A. **Prepare for Sterilization**

Submerge in ultrasonic cleaner or scrub with soap and hot water to remove oil, petroleum jelly, and/or metal particles left from sharpening. Wrap and seal for sterilization.

B. Stain Removal

Periodically clean with ammonia, gasoline, or kerosene when stone becomes discolored. If the stone becomes "glazed" by metal particles ground into the surface, rub the stone over emery paper placed on a flat, solid surface.

C. Storage

Keep in sealed, sterilized package until needed for sharpening.

II. Mounted Stones

A. Arkansas Mounted Stones

Same basic procedures as for the flat stone.

B. Ruby Stone

1. Clean by scrubbing with soap and water.
2. Maintain an ungrooved surface: frequently apply the stone to a Joe Dandy disc (figure 32–19). A sandpaper disc is too flexible for this purpose.
3. Sterilize and store in a sealed bag.

III. Manufacturer's Directions

Follow manufacturer's directions for all artificial stones.

TECHNICAL HINTS

I. Prevent unnecessary dulling of instruments by applying the following suggestions.

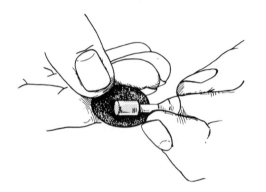

Figure 32–19. Care of the mounted ruby stone. A Joe Dandy disc is used to maintain a smooth surface without grooves.

A. When handling instruments for cleaning, sterilizing, or other reason, keep blades from hooking, bumping, or pressing against each other, as cutting edges become dull from contact with hard surfaces. Thinner instruments such as explorers and probes are subject to bending and breaking.
B. During instrumentation, utilize instruments at the appropriate angulation to the teeth; avoid pressing instrument against hard surface of metallic restorations.
C. Use of a tray system for sterilization and management of instruments can aid greatly in maintaining instruments separately.

II. Discard instruments that have been reduced so much from frequent sharpening that even moderate to slight pressure will flex the blade. There is danger of a tip breaking off in a pocket or between the teeth during instrumentation.

III. Sharpening of files has not been included in this chapter for several reasons. Since sharpening files is a difficult procedure because of the several parallel cutting edges, the amount of time consumed in sharpening with limited promise of effective results may not be justified. When sharpening a file is required, a jeweler's tang file may be obtained for the purpose. Use of a professional sharpening service or return of the files to the manufacturer for sharpening is highly recommended.

References

1. Barnes, J.E. and Schaffer, E.M.: Subgingival Root Planing: A Comparison Using Files, Hoes, and Curettes, *J. Periodontol.*, *31*, 300, September, 1960.
2. Green, E. and Ramfjord, S.P.: Tooth Roughness After Subgingival Root Planing, *J. Periodontol.*, *37*, 396, September–October, 1966.
3. Pattison, G.L. and Pattison, A.M.: *Periodontal Instrumentation.* Reston, Virginia, Reston Publishing Co., 1979, p. 150.
4. W.R. Case & Sons Cutlery Company, Bradford, Pennsylvania 16701.
5. Hu-Friedy Manufacturing Company, 3232 N. Rockwell Street, Chicago, Illinois 60618.
6. Juranitch, J.A.: Sharpening Secrets of a Pro, *Popular Science*, *210*, 118, February, 1977.

Suggested Readings

Antonini, C.J., Brady, J.M., Levin, M.P., and Garcia, W.L.:

Scanning Electron Microscope Study of Scalers, *J. Periodontol.*, *48*, 45, January, 1977.

Biller, I.R. and Karlsson, U.L.: SEM of Curet Edges, *Dent. Hyg.*, *53*, 549, December, 1979.

Carranza, F.A.: *Glickman's Clinical Periodontology*, 5th ed. Philadelphia, W.B. Saunders Co., 1979, pp. 674–686.

Green, E. and Seyer, P.C.: *Sharpening Curets and Sickle Scalers*, 2nd ed. Berkeley, California, Praxis Publishing Co., 1972, 40 pp.

Holmes, C.H. and Hoag, P.M.: The Sharpening of Scalers and Curets, in Boundy, S.S. and Reynolds, N.J., eds.: *Current Concepts in Dental Hygiene*, Volume 2. St. Louis, The C.V. Mosby Co., 1979, pp. 101–114.

Newell, K.J., Furry, C.A., Haider, M.L., and Lange, A.L.: Evaluating Sharpness of Gracey Curets, *Educ. Directions*, *5*, 25, August, 1980.

Paquette, O.E. and Levin, M.P.: The Sharpening of Scaling Instruments: I. An Examination of Principles, *J. Periodontol.*, *48*, 163, March, 1977.

Paquette, O.E. and Levin, M.P.: The Sharpening of Scaling Instruments: II. A Preferred Technique, *J. Periodontol.*, *48*, 169, March, 1977.

Pattison, G.L. and Pattison, A.M.: *Periodontal Instrumentation*. Reston, Virginia, Reston Publishing Co., 1979, pp. 308–333.

Schwindt, S.E.: A Review of Hand Instruments, *Dent. Hyg.*, *50*, 355, August, 1976.

Turley, L. and Janssen, J.: Instrument Sharpening, *Quintessence Journal*, *2*, 15, June, 1980.

United States Department of Health, Education, and Welfare, Project Acorde: *Instrument Sharpening*. Castro Valley, California, Quercus Corp., August, 1976, 107 pp.

Zimmer, S.E.: Instrument Sharpening—Sickle Scalers and Curettes, *Dent. Hyg.*, *52*, 21, January, 1978.

33

Scaling and Root Planing

Complete subgingival scaling, root planing, and gingival curettage are specific procedures in the treatment of inflammatory gingival and periodontal diseases. *Scaling* to remove calculus, *root planing* to remove residual calculus and altered cementum and produce a smooth tooth surface, and *curettage* to remove the diseased sulcular epithelial lining and underlying inflamed connective tissue are all directed toward an ultimate goal of pocket elimination and tissue health.

The success of treatment is dependent on the control of dental plaque by the patient. Therefore, instruction and supervision in plaque control procedures precedes, continues simultaneously with, and follows instrumentation for treatment.

To be effective, scaling and planing must be thorough. When calculus is left on the teeth, surfaces are not smooth, and areas of the root surface contain endotoxin and other bacterial products, gingival irritation and inflammation can persist.

Development of ability, skill, and efficiency in the successful removal of calculus through positive scaling procedures requires more than the development of dexterity for applying instruments to the tooth surfaces. In these refined and exacting techniques the dental hygienist must apply knowledge of the anatomic, histologic, and physiologic characteristics of the teeth and gingival tissues to the fullest advantage of the patient.

I. Definitions

A. Scaling

Scaling is the basic procedure by which calculus is removed from the surfaces of the teeth. Scaling is divided into supragingival and subgingival scaling, depending on the location of the calculus in relation to the gingival margin (figure 33–2, page 512).

B. Root Planing

Root planing is the process by which residual calculus and altered cementum are removed and the surfaces of the roots are made smooth. When the root surface is exposed following gingival recession or surgery, root planing is performed supragingivally; otherwise it is a subgingival procedure.*

II. Purposes

A few longitudinal studies have shown the important relationship between combined professional and supervised patient care. These studies demonstrated that, with periodic thorough scaling and root planing and controlled self-care by the patient, with instruction and review, various benefits resulted. The effects produced included

---

*Root planing is sometimes called root curettage. In this book the term curettage is reserved for curettage of the soft tissues. Gingival curettage is the process by which the diseased tissue lining the gingival sulcus or pocket wall is removed (Chapter 34).

reduced incidence of gingivitis, control of the quantity of calculus deposition, slower migration of the junctional epithelium, and generally cleaner mouths than observed in subjects of control groups who did not have such care.[1-7]

Scaling and planing will have limited short-term effects without self-care by the patient on a daily basis, without removal of other plaque retention factors such as overhanging margins, and without follow-up for other required dental and periodontal treatment. Plaque forms promptly, and calculus recurs within a few days in certain mouths.

The complete removal of calculus followed by root planing to remove altered cementum will contribute to the following:

A. Creation of an environment in which the gingival tissues can heal and inflammation can be resolved.
   1. Shrinkage of previously enlarged, spongy tissue.
   2. Reduction of pocket depth.
   3. Cessation of bleeding on provocation.
B. Regeneration of gingival tissues.
   1. Restoration of normal color, size, contour, consistency, and surface texture (table 11–1, page 196).
   2. Adaptation of the gingival tissue to the tooth surface.
C. Initial preparation prior to complicated and advanced periodontal therapy.
   1. Reduce etiologic and predisposing factors.
   2. Permit reevaluation: surgery may be lessened or confined to specific areas.
D. Removal of diseased altered cementum.
E. Increased effectiveness of plaque control measures. A smooth surface is easier for the patient to keep clean.
F. Removal of subsequent calculus deposits is easier because calculus will be less firmly attached to a smooth surface than to a rough one in which the calculus could become embedded in undercuts and other tooth surface irregularities.

PREPARATION FOR INSTRUMENTATION

I. Bacteremia Following Instrumentation

Bacteremia means the presence of bacteria in the blood. A transient bacteremia may occur after any type of oral surgery, periodontal treatment, scaling, and oral prophylaxis.[8-10]

A. **Factors Affecting Incidence**

The incidence of bacteremia has been directly related to the degree of trauma inflicted during surgery or instrumentation,[11] and especially related to the severity of the periodontal condition that was present at the time of instrumentation.[12,13] In one study,[13] patients with clinically healthy gingiva had a 21.6 percent incidence of bacteremia, those with gingivitis 29.0 percent, and those with periodontitis 51.2 percent following scaling and root planing. No difference in incidence of bacteremia was found associated with ultrasonic or manual instrumentation.[14]

B. **Precautions**

1. *Premedication.* Certain patients who require premedication for prevention of bacteremia are listed on pages 99–100. Although bacteremia is transient and of no known clinical significance in most instances, prophylactic antibiotic premedication must be planned in advance of an appointment for certain risk patients. The importance of obtaining a patient history and applying information from the history before instrumentation cannot be overemphasized.
2. *Antiseptic Mouthrinse.* The routine use of an antiseptic mouthrinse such as one containing povidone-iodine (Betadine) is recommended. Significant reductions in bacteria on oral surfaces have been shown.[15,16]

II. Use of Patient Records

The preliminary observations made during the preparation of the diagnostic workup provide basic information for planning procedures and indicating the number of appointments needed. A specific examination is required to conduct the treatment:

1. To determine exact location of calculus deposits.
2. To select instruments to be used.
3. To recognize irregularities of tooth sur-

faces, restorations, or other problem areas.

4. During instrumentation: to avoid unnecessary repetition and make each phase of the operation meaningful.

5. At expected completion of procedures: to assure complete removal of deposits.

III. Use of Radiographs

The radiographic survey can be a useful adjunct during scaling procedures and should always be available on a viewbox during appointments. Radiographic findings were outlined on pages 227–230. Limitations relative to the appearance of calculus in the radiograph were described. From the radiographs, factors related to plaque retention and treatment procedures, such as overhanging restorations and carious lesions, may interfere with scaling and planing.

IV. Supragingival Examination

A. Visual

Gross and moderate deposits and surface irregularities can be seen directly. Fine, unstained, white or yellowish calculus is frequently invisible when wet with saliva. Dry calculus is seen more readily than wet calculus. Procedures for calculus detection were described on pages 276 and 278.

B. Tactile Method

Without deposits the enamel surface is smooth; when an explorer is passed over, it slides freely, smoothly, and quietly. Calculus deposits are rough; the explorer does not slide freely but meets with resistance, and produces a scratchy sound.

V. Subgingival Examination

A. Anatomy of Subgingival Area

A pocket is a diseased sulcus. A pocket has an inner wall which is the tooth surface and an outer wall which is covered on the inside by the sulcular epithelium. The types of pockets were described on page 202. Total treatment is dependent on the type of pocket and the characteristics of the gingival tissue of the pocket wall.

B. Direct Visual Examination

1. Clinical appearance of the gingival tissues that reveals or is highly suggestive of the presence of subgingival calculus:

   a. Gingival tissue that is soft, spongy, nonresilient, bluish-red, with enlargement of the marginal gingiva, a rolled edge which tends to be separated from the tooth surface, and with a smooth shiny surface on which stippling is indistinct or missing.

   b. Dark-colored subgingival calculus may sometimes be seen as a dark area beneath relatively translucent marginal gingiva.

   c. Follow-up evaluation 1 to 2 weeks after scaling. The tissue appearance can be helpful in detecting remaining particles of calculus. Healing with tissue shrinkage will have occurred generally throughout, and only those areas of gingiva that cover remaining calculus will maintain the bluish-red color, enlargement, and other characteristics mentioned above.

2. Direct examination for subgingival calculus:

   a. When there are subgingival deposits under soft, spongy tissue, the lining of the pocket wall may be loose and resilient and can be separated or stretched away from the tooth surface.

   b. Procedure: apply compressed air gently to the gingival margin, deflect the tissue and look into the pocket. Subgingival calculus deposits which may be seen are generally dark brown or other dark color.

C. Tactile Examination: Periodontal Probe

The pocket depths recorded for the periodontal charting prepared during the initial patient examination can be used as a guide for subgingival scaling. Additional circumferential probing may be necessary for a complete definition of the working area. Probing techniques are described on pages 213–216.

1. *Irregularities of the Tooth Surface.* Various irregularities are listed on page 205. For example, as the probe passes over the tooth surface, it may be intercepted

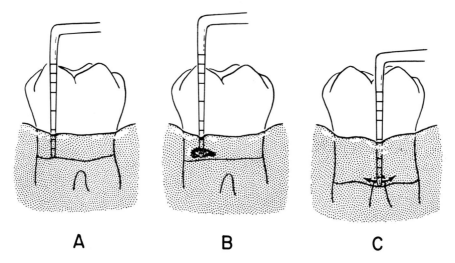

Figure 33–1. Subgingival examination with a periodontal probe. **A.** Probe is inserted to the bottom of the pocket until the resistance of the soft tissue attachment is felt. **B.** As the probe passes over the root surface, it may be intercepted by a hard mass of calculus. **C.** The probe is used to examine root topography: here the probe is in a furcation area.

by a hard mass of calculus (figure 33–1B). The calculus may be localized or may extend as a band around the entire tooth.

2. *Topography of the Tooth Surface.* Many grooves, curves, and furrow-like variations are found which can complicate instrumentation. When there is increased pocket depth, the anatomic features of the roots become evident. For example, the groove and the furcation between the roots of a mandibular molar can be probed (figure 33–1C).

Application of a curet into the furcation area for calculus removal and root planing is difficult and challenging. Such areas must also be examined with the explorer.

D. Tactile Examination: Explorer

1. *Purposes.* A subgingival explorer is used to determine the texture and character of the tooth surface and to distinguish by tactile means the cause and nature of surface roughness.

2. *Use.* The explorer is the instrument of evaluation. Before scaling and root planing, the extent and nature of the calculus deposits are evaluated and treatment procedures are planned. Progress and completion of techniques are also eval-

uated until the tooth surface is smooth to the critical touch of the explorer.

PROCEDURE FOR SCALING

I. Clinical Approach

Criteria for the determination of treatment sequence were described on page 327 in connection with treatment planning. Application of the concept of tissue conditioning by the patient in preparation for scaling and root planing contributes to more efficient treatment and more predictable and rapid postoperative healing.

Prerequisite to any selected procedure is the use of an efficient routine to minimize time. With respect to the use of individual instruments, one time-saver is to apply one instrument to all tooth surfaces where it is applicable within a quadrant or area being treated, followed by the next instrument; this minimizes transfer to and from the tray.

The advantages of a systematic procedure are that it

1. Ensures thoroughness in the completion of treatment.
2. Demonstrates ease and smoothness of operation.
3. Increases efficiency through repeated routine.
4. Decreases operating time.
5. Increases patient comfort.

6. Increases patient's confidence in the operator.

II. Overall System

A. Complete a Selected Area

Scale one quadrant (or selected group of teeth) thoroughly before moving on to the next, rather than move from area to area.

B. Single Appointment

When it is expected that scaling can be completed in a single appointment, it may be advisable to remove gross supragingival deposits throughout the entire dentition by manual or ultrasonic techniques and then return to concentrate on the finer scaling for each area. At the follow-up appointment 1 to 2 weeks later, when the response to treatment is observed, some additional localized scaling may be indicated.

C. Planned Multiple Appointments

When there is generalized supra- and subgingival calculus and extensive scaling and root planing to be done, a series of appointments must be planned as outlined on pages 328–331.
1. *Quadrant Scaling and Root Planing Appointments.*
   a. Scheduled at one week intervals to permit progressive healing.
   b. Local anesthesia for each quadrant is frequently indicated.
   c. Plaque control procedures can be reviewed and supplemented before scaling at each appointment.
2. *Initial Appointment.* A generalized scaling may be performed by manual, ultrasonic, or combined techniques after the patient has received basic plaque control instruction.
   a. Initial scaling should be as thorough as possible for the appointed time: generalized, random removal of gross deposits, without a directed effort to remove as much calculus as possible, may do more harm than good.
   b. Incomplete scaling in deep pockets and areas of furcation involvement is inadvisable, particularly for a patient who may be susceptible to infection or abscess formation (page 541).
      c. Calculus roughened by partial removal may be a source of greater irritation to the gingiva because of its ability to hold new plaque.
      d. During personal oral care, the gingival pocket wall may be pressed by the toothbrush against the roughened calculus. The continuing source of irritation prevents healing in the tissue and may even cause an acute inflammation.

III. Calculus Removal

Calculus is removed by systematic scaling from tooth to tooth and section by section of the calculus deposit on each tooth surface. Each scaling stroke overlaps the previous one as the scaler is positioned progressively along the area of the deposit.

A. Location of Instrumentation

Removal of calculus relates to the mode of attachment (page 280). Calculus removal from enamel is different from the calculus removal and root planing required for cementum. The nature of the strokes required varies for different parts of a tooth surface.

Figure 33–2 illustrates the location of instrumentation on the tooth surface. The type of pocket, the position of the margin of the free gingiva, and the level of periodontal tissue attachment, all determine the location of instrumentation and instrument selection for that instrumentation.

B. Steps

Scaling is not a shaving process in which layers are removed. Such a procedure tends to make the surface of the calculus smooth and burnished and sometimes indistinguishable from the tooth surface. The oldest calculus, that next to the tooth surface, is the hardest calculus.

There are five fundamental steps in the application of an instrument for calculus removal and root planing. In the sections following, the steps are described in detail for supragingival instrumentation and then followed by additional adaptations required for

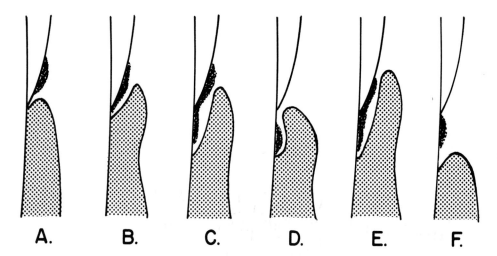

A.   B.   C.   D.   E.   F.

Figure 33–2.   Factors influencing instrumentation. Shown are varying conditions encountered which require different approaches. **A.** Supragingival calculus on enamel, **B.** Gingival pocket with both supra- and subgingival calculus, **C.** Periodontal pocket with both supra- and subgingival calculus, **D.** Periodontal pocket with subgingival calculus on cementum only, **E.** Periodontal pocket with subgingival calculus on both enamel and cementum, and **F.** Calculus on cementum over gingival recession.

subgingival instrumentation. The five steps, described on pages 478–483, are:

1. Grasp of instrument.
2. Establishment of finger rest.
3. Adaptation.
4. Angulation.
5. Activation
   a. Working stroke: activate the instrument.
   b. Completion of stroke: prepare for the next.

SUPRAGINGIVAL SCALING

I. Instruments

A. Scalers: Sickle, Hoe, Chisel

These instruments are designed for supragingival instrumentation. Sickles are sometimes used to remove gross calculus which is a millimeter or two below the gingival margin, provided the tissue of the gingival pocket wall is loose and the instrument can be inserted without force.

B. Curet

A curet is used primarily for subgingival instrumentation, but is recommended for supragingival scaling and planing in instances such as the following:

1. When a curved, rounded instrument is particularly adaptable for removing fine, hard deposits near the gingival margin.
2. When gingival recession has caused exposure of cementum and root planing techniques are required.

II. Steps for Calculus Removal

A. Grasp the Instrument

1. Apply modified pen grasp (figure 31–2, page 479).
2. Use a light grasp while instrument is positioned and at the completion of the stroke; tighten grasp during the working stroke.

B. Establish the Finger Rest

1. Use ring and little fingers on firm tooth or teeth for the major rest; apply supplementary rests for increased stability when indicated (page 480).
2. The fulcrum where the finger rest is applied must be dry for stability. Plaque and saliva make tooth surfaces slippery. Use a folded gauze sponge in the vestibular area with a corner over the fulcrum rest tooth; dry with compressed air or wipe with cotton, maintain retraction, and repeat the drying as needed for continued instrument control.

3. Finger rests are applied on the tooth adjacent to the one being scaled, or as close as possible and convenient. Long stretches between the rest and the point of instrument application can decrease control.
4. Use light but firm pressure on the finger rest while the instrument is being positioned and at the end of the stroke.
5. During the working stroke, the pressure on the fulcrum increases slightly to balance the pressure of the instrument on the tooth being scaled.

C. Adapt the Cutting Edge of the Blade

1. *Exploratory Stroke.* The exploratory stroke is a preliminary stroke in which the blade is applied lightly over the calculus until the base of the deposit is located, and then the blade is positioned for the working stroke. Use of the exploratory stroke has greatest application in the subgingival area when preparation for scaling is difficult because of invisibility. It also has particular use during supragingival instrumentation of the proximal surfaces.
2. *Angulation*
   a. Sickle scaler. Blade is applied beneath the calculus deposit so that the angle formed by the face and the tooth surface is between 60 and 80 degrees (less than 90 degrees but not less than 45 degrees) (figure 32–2, page 488).
   b. Hoe scaler. With the full width of the cutting edge in contact with the tooth, and with the shank adapted closely to the side of the tooth or with the shank in contact with the crown of the tooth (figure 32–3, page 489).
   c. Chisel scaler. With the full width of the cutting edge in contact with the tooth, and with the shank adapted closely to the tooth, in position for scaling from labial to lingual.
   d. Curet. At an angle formed by the face of the blade and the tooth surface between 60 and 80 degrees (less than 90 degrees but not less than 45 degrees) (figure 32–6, page 491).

3. *Preparation.* Hold the cutting edge firmly against the tooth surface in preparation for activating the instrument.

D. Activate the Instrument: Working Stroke

1. *Tighten the Grasp;* move the instrument firmly and deliberately.
2. *Maintain the Cutting Edge* evenly on the tooth surface during the stroke. The side of the tip or toe should always be adapted in contact with the tooth surface. Depending on the curvature of the tooth surface, only a few millimeters next to the tip or toe will be in contact.
3. *Direction of Strokes*
   a. Vertical pull strokes are used for scalers and hoes; horizontal and oblique strokes may be used when away from the cervical region near the gingival margin.
   b. Vertical, horizontal, and oblique strokes may be used for the curet.
   c. Horizontal push strokes only are used for the chisel from labial to lingual at right angles with the long axis of anterior teeth.
4. *Pressure of the Instrument* (on tooth surface). When the instrument is sharp, the minimum pressure applied will allow the cutting edge to grip the tooth surface; a balance of pressure is maintained between the pressure of the instrument, the grasp of the instrument, and the pressure on the finger rest.
5. *Control of Motion.* Without independent finger movement, the hand, wrist, and arm act as a continuum to activate the instrument.
6. *Length of Stroke:* short
   a. Short strokes permit accommodation of the cutting edge to changes in the topography of the tooth surface.
   b. Short strokes assist in maintaining *control* and *precision.*
   c. Strokes are confined to the area of the deposit on the tooth surface. The area in the vicinity of the cementoenamel junction where the majority of the deposits are located is called the *instrumentation zone.*[17] Extending the instrument up the side of the tooth in unnecessarily long strokes is

time-consuming, dulls the instrument, and decreases control by and
concentration of the operator.

E. Completion of Stroke

1. Hold instrument in place momentarily,
   maintain the finger rest, lighten the grasp
   on the instrument, and then return the
   instrument to position for a repeat stroke.
2. Repeat strokes until surface is smooth.

F. Continuation of Procedure

1. Move instrument laterally on the tooth
   surface to adjacent undisturbed deposit;
   maintain the same finger rest.
2. Overlap strokes to ensure complete removal of deposit. Roll the handle between the fingers of the grasp to maintain adaptation at line angles and other
   variations of tooth anatomy.
3. Repeat strokes until the tooth surface
   has been completely scaled.
4. Inspect surface with explorer assisted by
   compressed air and repeat as needed to
   produce a smooth surface that is free of
   calculus.

SUBGINGIVAL INSTRUMENTATION

Dexterity, deliberateness, and diligence are
key words in techniques for subgingival areas.
The principal objective is to remove the calculus
and to plane the root surface with a minimum
of trauma to the gingival tissue. Procedures are
guided by the recognized need for removal of
all calculus and altered cementum to assure maximum tissue response for oral health.

Root planing follows calculus removal. It is a
continuation of subgingival scaling and an integral part of it. Not all root planing is subgingival,
because when root surfaces are exposed as a result of recession or periodontal surgery for pocket
elimination, the cemental surface is supragingival (figure 33–2F).

**I. Comparison with Supragingival
Instrumentation**

Although the basic techniques described previously for removal of supragingival calculus are
applied in the subgingival area, techniques are
complicated by several factors, notably the following:

A. Accessibility

Instrumentation is necessary in areas
where access is difficult.

B. Invisible Working Area

Techniques are almost entirely dependent on tactile sensitivity. To locate and remove minute roughnesses of the tooth surface requires a keenly developed tactile
sensitivity.

C. Calculus Attachment

Attachment of calculus to the cementum
is more tenacious than to the enamel. On
the cementum, calculus attaches to minute
irregularities and in areas of cemental resorption, or by direct attachment of the calculus matrix to the root surface, which makes
removal difficult. Attachment to the enamel
is primarily by means of the acquired pellicle, which makes calculus removal much
easier (page 280).

D. Morphology of Calculus

Subgingival calculus is irregularly deposited, and occurs in nodular, ledge or ring-
like, smooth veneer, and other forms (table
17–1, page 277).

E. Variations in Root Surface Topography

Although many variations can be expected as part of the normal tooth anatomy,
others are unusual variations which complicate scaling primarily because of their invisibility (page 205).

F. Variations in Depth of Pockets

Pockets must be measured about each
tooth as variations in depth can occur on a
single surface; instruments must be adapted
to reach the bottom of the pocket around
the entire periphery of each tooth.

G. Gingival Wall

The gingival wall is close to the tooth surface with only a narrow area for manipulation of instruments. The width of the pocket
varies; it narrows down at the base next to
the attachment area.

II. Instrument Selection: Curets

As mentioned previously, gross calculus just

below the gingival margin may be removed during supragingival scaling, provided the tissue is loose and resilient enough to permit easy access by the instruments without having to force them into the sulcus. The ultrasonic scaler may also be used to remove gross subgingival deposits (pages 519–520).

Deeper in the pocket and close to the root surface, the curets are the instruments of choice for a number of reasons, including:

A. Fine, thin instruments permit increased tactile sensitivity which bulkier instruments cannot. Increased sensitivity is essential to thoroughness in areas with limited accessibility and visibility.

B. Root planing with curets produces smoother surfaces than planing with other instruments.[18–21]

C. The curved, narrow, fine curets with rounded ends can be adapted to the anatomic features of the subgingival area with less trauma to the tooth surface and the gingival tissue. Supragingival sickles, hoes, and chisels have sharp points or corners and are thick, bulky, and straight.

D. The sulcus or pocket narrows in the deeper area close to the attachment. The smallest, smoothest instruments are best applied to this narrow area to prevent the need for excess stretching of the gingival wall which can cause a splitting of the attachment from the tooth.

E. Because of the rounded end, a horizontal stroke can be used conservatively. The length of the horizontal stroke would depend on variations in pocket depth. When used in position for a vertical stroke, the round back of the curet can be placed against the bottom of the pocket.

III. Subgingival Procedures

The surface to be scaled must first be examined with probe and explorer to define the area and the calculus, as described on page 509. Then, the same basic five steps for calculus removal are followed as for supragingival scaling with variations listed below.

To remove heavier subgingival calculus, first, a larger, stronger curet is used for convenience and efficiency. The smaller, delicate curets should be reserved and kept sharp for fine scaling and root planing, particularly in the narrow depths of the pocket.

A. Grasp the Instrument

A modified pen grasp is used. The grasp is lightened as increased tactile sense is needed for refinement of the root surface with continued root planing.

B. Establish the Finger Rest

1. A definite finger rest on dry, firm tooth structure as close to the tooth being treated as possible and convenient is indicated.
2. Complete control is essential.

C. Position the Cutting Edge of the Blade

1. *Blade Position.* Position the blade on the tooth surface near the gingival margin where the instrument will be inserted for subgingival scaling.
   a. Hold at the appropriate angulation for scaling; that is, with the face at an angle between 60 and 80 degrees with the tooth surface (less than a 90-degree angle but not less than 45 degrees).
   b. The face of the blade will be directed toward the incisal or occlusal for a vertical stroke and tipped slightly for an oblique stroke; for a horizontal stroke, the curved tip of the blade is directed toward the apex of the tooth.
   c. Note the relationship of the handle, finger rest, grasp, blade, and tooth so that after insertion the blade may be promptly reangulated for calculus removal.
2. *Exploratory Stroke**
   a. Direct the tip of the curet gingivally; maintain contact with the tooth surface.
   b. With light grasp, insert the curet gently under the gingival margin (figure 33–3A).
   c. Keep the instrument tip in light contact with the tooth or calculus sur-

---

*The exploratory stroke is sometimes referred to as the preliminary or preparatory stroke. When the term "exploratory" is used, it should be distinguished from the meaning of the word as it applies to the use of an explorer. The curet is not used as an explorer, and the calculus has been identified previously by using an explorer.

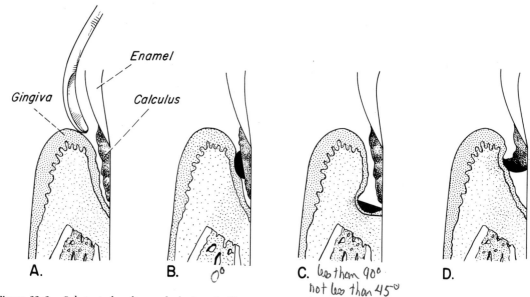

Annotations on figure: **C.** less than 90° not less than 45° **B.** 0°

Figure 33–3. Subgingival scaling and planing. **A.** The curet is gently inserted under the gingival margin. **B.** With an exploratory stroke, the blade is passed over the surface of the tooth or calculus. Note zero-degree angle of the face of the curet with the calculus. **C.** The curet is lowered to the base of the pocket until the tension of the soft tissue is felt, and then it is positioned at less than 90 degrees for scaling. **D.** The blade is moved along the root surface in a scaling stroke to remove calculus or a planing stroke to smooth the surface.

face. The blade is closed toward the tooth surface and held at or near an angle of zero degrees during the exploratory stroke (figure 33–3B).

d. Pass the instrument over the surface of the deposit to the base of the pocket until tension of the soft tissue attachment is felt.

e. Adjust the blade to the correct angulation with the tooth surface (as determined before insertion) just below the calculus deposit (figure 33–3C).

f. Utilize as much of the cutting edge of the blade as possible in accord with the anatomic contour of the tooth. The side of the toe or tip should be in contact with the tooth surface at all times.

D. Activate the Instrument: Working Stroke

1. *Tighten the Grasp* and move the instrument firmly and deliberately (figure 33–3D).
2. *Maintain the Cutting Edge* evenly on the tooth surface during the stroke and at the completion of the stroke.
3. *Direction of Strokes*

a. Vertical, oblique, or horizontal strokes may be applied.

b. All strokes are limited in length by the constant adjustment needed to conform with the curved tooth surfaces and the varying depths of the sulcus or pocket around the tooth.

c. Horizontal strokes cannot be applied to the bottom of the sulcus or pocket except where the probe measurements show the depth is uniform; otherwise the curet would be dragged into the attachment at the higher areas.

d. Not recommended: push-pull type strokes are not used subgingivally as these would tend to push particles and bacteria deep into the sulcus and into the soft tissue.

4. *Pressure of Instrument.* A balance of pressure between the pressure of the instrument, the grasp of the instrument, and the finger rest must be maintained. Undue pressure decreases control and lessens tactile sensitivity.

5. *Control of Motion.* Without independent finger movement, the hand, wrist,

and arm act as a continuum to activate the instrument.

6. *Length of Stroke*
   a. Short smooth decisive strokes, the length dependent on the height of the deposit (instrumentation zone, page 513).
   b. Within the confines of the pocket to prevent the need for repeated removal and reinsertion of the instrument, which is not only time-consuming but means that the instrument must pass over the more sensitive areas for the patient (the necks of the teeth and the gingival margin).

7. *Calculus Removal.* Calculus should not be shaved off in layers, but when possible, the whole thickness should be moved in one piece. By shaving, a thin veneer of calculus may be left which may be smooth and indiscernible from the tooth surface, yet contain endotoxin and other substances which can keep the gingiva from healing.

8. *Completion of Stroke.* Maintain finger rest, lighten grasp, repeat exploratory stroke within the pocket. Reposition for a repeat or adjacent stroke. Several strokes are generally required for each area.

E. Plane the Root Surface

The technique for planing is basically the same as for scaling. Instrument control, adaptation and angulation at the cutting edge, directions for strokes, and other principles are not essentially different. What is different is the ultimate perfection of resulting smoothness attained because of the high degree of tactile sensitivity involved and the precise instrumentation.

Specific differences in technique are related to touch and pressure. A lighter grasp must be used to increase tactile sensitivity. Since increased pressure is not needed, a lighter shaving-like stroke can be used for smoothing or finishing the root surface.

1. *Check the Sharpness of the Curets.* Generally, curets dulled during scaling should be resharpened or laid aside and a freshly sharpened set used for root planing.

2. *Strokes*
   a. Apply light pressure for maximum sensitivity to minute irregularities of the surface.
   b. Use smooth, even strokes that systematically overlap and cross over each other. As the surface becomes smoother, longer strokes with reduced pressure will help to remove small lines, scratches, or grooves.
   c. Directions: Vertical, then oblique, then, when applicable at levels away from the attachment epithelium, horizontal strokes should be used.
   d. Number of strokes: Many strokes frequently are needed, before a section of the root surface feels glassy smooth and hard.
   e. Adaptation of instrument: Careful application is necessary to adapt the curet to the morphologic features of the roots. The convex rounded surfaces, the constricted cervical area, the concavities and grooves of proximal surfaces, and furcations all require precise adaptation.
   f. As planing nears completion, there is a gradual change in the sound of the instrument on the root surface. At the completion, the instrument can be nearly as quiet as it would be on polished enamel.

3. *Examine* with a subgingival explorer to establish completion of instrumentation.

F. Irrigate All Sulci or Pockets

This should be done thoroughly with warm water under mild to moderate pressure to remove particles of cementum or calculus. Research has shown that bits of calculus, debris, or microorganisms can become implanted into the underlying tissue.[22-24]

EFFECTS OF SCALING AND PLANING

An evaluation by exploring immediately after completion of instrumentation is made to ascertain that the tooth surfaces are smooth and hard and that all detectable calculus has been removed. The real evaluation, the true test of successful treatment, cannot be made until 1 to 2 weeks after the initial scaling and root planing when the response of the gingival tissue will be apparent.

I. Effect on Gingiva

A. Coincidental Curettage

Without intentional curettage during scaling and root planing, there is some debridement (coincidental curettage) of the lining of the sulcus or pocket.[22–24] In the research, this effect was noted particularly in the deeper aspects, where the pocket narrows toward the attachment area. The partial curettage that occurs is due to the outer or unused side of the curet blade, even though a less than 90-degree angulation of the face of the blade to the tooth surface is maintained.

The soft tissue attachment may be partially removed, depending on the severity of the inflammation, the size of the instrument, and the amount of trauma inflicted by the operator. Partial curettage may be considered beneficial. The objectives of curettage are described on page 529.

B. Healing

With scaling, root planing, and plaque control, the adjacent gingival tissue heals by resolution of the inflammation. Edema recedes, necrotic cells are cleared away, and the tissue regenerates.

Healing has been shown to start with beginning epithelial regeneration within 2 days of scaling; new attachment to the tooth surface has been demonstrated as early as 5 days, and complete regeneration by approximately 2 weeks.[25,26] Healing time is generally related to the severity of the periodontal inflammation at the start of treatment.

C. Effect of Partial Scaling

When altered cementum or even a small amount of subgingival calculus is left on a tooth surface, an area of inflammation can persist. At examination on the subsequent appointment, some tissue shrinkage may have occurred, but the remaining deposit must be removed for complete resolution.

When large or small deposits are left after incomplete scaling, particularly in a deep pocket, an acute periodontal abscess may form (page 541). A periodontal abscess will result in pain, swelling, tooth sensitivity, and various symptoms.[27] Such abscesses can be prevented by completing calculus removal and planing.

Only as many teeth as can be completed in a given appointment should be undertaken. Other teeth should be left untouched except for plaque control instruction.

II. Effect on Tooth Surface

Research has shown that following careful subgingival scaling and root planing, some calculus frequently remains. During root planing, the altered cementum and residual calculus are removed. To obtain a smooth and hard root surface, the cementum is partly or wholly removed, the amount varying from surface to surface.[28,29] It is necessary to remove cementum because the surface, exposed after recession of the junctional epithelium during pocket formation, is rough, soft, and altered by bacterial and inflammatory substances from the contents of the pocket. Altered cementum contains endotoxin and other toxic substances which can prevent healing of the adjacent gingival tissue and can aggravate continuing inflammation.

The removal of endotoxin from diseased altered cementum has been measured.[30] When tooth surfaces were scaled but not root planed, the endotoxin content of the surface was much greater than values for healthy, unexposed tooth surfaces. However, after root planing, the tooth surfaces were found to be nearly as free of endotoxin as the healthy, unexposed surfaces.

Teeth that had been scaled were studied by electron microscopy.[29] The tooth surfaces that were under calculus were less mineralized than exposed root surfaces. An exchange of minerals occurs between the saliva and the tooth. Following exposure for 3 to 4 weeks after scaling, some surfaces became hypermineralized while others became decalcified and carious.

Knowledge of the processes involved in the surface changes can aid in the prevention of cemental caries, hypersensitivity, and calculus. Fluoride-containing dentifrice and mouthrinse should be routinely recommended following root planing when there is apparent recession and exposed cementum.

III. Effect on Pocket Microorganisms[31-34]

The subgingival bacterial flora is changed after scaling and root planing. Prior to instrumentation for treatment of periodontitis, the subgingival microorganisms are primarily anaerobic, gram-negative, motile forms, with bacterioides and spirochetes predominating.

After scaling and root planing, the total number of subgingival organisms decreases substantially. There is a shift to aerobic, gram-positive, nonmotile forms. Spirochetes and bacterioides are reduced and coccoid cells become more prominent.

USE OF ULTRASONICS

Ultrasonic instrumentation is an adjunct to manual scaling but not a substitute for it. Ultrasonic instruments are indicated primarily for adult patients with gross calculus.

Root planing is not accomplished by ultrasonic instruments and must be completed by curets. The ultrasonic method, therefore, is principally for treatment when deposits are gross, but is not applicable for preventive scaling measures when small deposits are removed at frequent recall appointments.

Histologic studies have shown postoperative healing following ultrasonic instrumentation to be at least as satisfactory and in some instances more satisfactory than hand scaling.[35,36,37]

When the energy output is low, the hand pressure light, and the tip of the instrument broad and polished where it touches the tooth, presumably no adverse effects on the tooth surfaces would be expected, at least not within a reasonable number of applications.[38]

While the instrument tip is on calculus, the tooth surface is unaffected, which brings out several operational factors. Tactile sensitivity is diminished appreciably. Therefore, the tooth surface should be examined with an explorer frequently during operation so that excessive application of the instrument to the tooth structure can be avoided. It is also important that minimal instrument application be made when there are small discrete calculus deposits or thin stains to be removed.

In addition to the removal of heavy calculus deposits, an ultrasonic instrument may be used in a variety of ways, including the removal of overhanging restorations and in periodontal curettage and surgery. In orthodontics, ultrasonic instrumentation has been found effective for scaling prior to fitting and cementing appliances, and for the removal of excess cement after initial cementation and when appliances are removed.

I. Mode of Action[38,39]

The ultrasonic unit consists of an electric generator, a handpiece assembly, a set of interchangeable prophylaxis inserts, and a foot control. The ultrasonic principle is based on the use of very high frequency sound waves.

A. The ultrasonic machine converts high frequency electrical energy into mechanical energy in the form of rapid vibrations.

B. The instrument tip vibrations vary for different models, but may be, for example, 25,000 cycles per second with an amplitude of 1/1000 cm. The vibratory action fractures the deposit and causes it to be removed from the tooth.

C. Ultrasonic waves are dissipated in the form of heat. The heat is reduced by keeping the handpiece cooled internally and the working end cooled by a constant flow of water which is expelled through a metal tube or by means of an internal flow through the working end.

D. Effects of water: the atomized water forms minute vacuum bubbles which collapse with release of tremendous local pressure; the effect is cleansing to the area. Since it is necessary to have the instrument in contact with the deposit on the tooth surface if the deposit is to be removed, the bubbling cavitational action of the water has little if any actual influence on deposit removal.

II. Procedure for Use[38,40,41]

A. Minimize Water Contamination

Run water through the tubing to the ultrasonic unit for a full 2 minutes prior to use. Cultures of samples from water lines showed very high microbial counts, particularly in water left in the tubing overnight. The use of contaminated water provides a potential source for disease transmission. If such contaminated water was forced into a pocket, bacteremia could be produced.[42]

B. Unit Adjustment

1. Tune according to the manufacturer's

specifications. Use the lowest effective power setting.

2. Adjust water to a maximum mist about the working tip. It is very important to prevent overheating.

C. Prophylaxis Tips

1. Sterilized tip is adapted to the handpiece after the unit water has cleared.
2. Instrument tips must be dull; if sharp or with small irregularities, the tooth surface could be nicked or gouged.

D. Patient Preparation

1. Review patient history
   a. Ultrasonic treatment is contraindicated for a patient with a cardiac pacemaker.[43]*
   b. Prophylactic antibiotic premedication is indicated for risk patients. Bacteremia is produced in a high percentage of patients treated by an ultrasonic as well as by manual instrumentation.[44]
2. Have the patient use an antiseptic mouth rinse for 30 seconds prior to ultrasonic scaling to lower the oral bacterial count and hence lower the bacterial count of the aerosols produced (pages 16–17).
3. Use coverall and towel.
4. Topical anesthetic may be applied to allay gingival sensitivity.

E. Instrumentation

1. Use an evacuator or effective saliva ejector.
2. Use modified pen grasp for handpiece and apply finger rest to appropriate, convenient tooth surfaces to stabilize the instrument and permit systematic coverage of tooth surfaces being scaled.
3. Application of working end: *keep tip parallel with long axis of the tooth or at no more than a 15-degree angle with tooth surface.* Adaptation to variations in tooth topography and morphology is difficult but necessary. To maintain a less than 15-degree angle in all positions takes practice and concentration.

4. Stroke
   a. *Keep the tip in motion at all times.*
   b. Check to be sure that the water reaches the operating area.
   c. Brush lightly over the deposit, moving in a vertical or diagonal direction: six strokes usually suffice. Pressure removes tooth structure.
   d. Move instrument with smooth, light, constant, and overlapping strokes.
   e. Increased number of strokes will not damage the tooth surface provided the instrument is blunt, the tip is not held perpendicular to the long axis of the tooth, and no positive pressure is used.
   f. Instrument tends to bind when inserted interproximally, and the excess pressure stops the vibration. Remove and reactivate the instrument.
5. Apply instrument with care when near porcelain jacket crowns or inlays. The vibration could fracture the porcelain.[45]
6. Release foot pedal switch at regular intervals to aid in water control; stop to evaluate the tooth surfaces with an explorer periodically.
7. Complete the procedure with manual instruments.
   a. Check subgingival areas with a subgingival explorer.
   b. Remove remaining subgingival irregularities and plane the surface smooth with curets.

F. Care of Prophylaxis Inserts

1. Sterilize.
2. Handle with care to avoid damage to working ends or internal mechanisms.

III. Advantages and Limitations

A. Advantages

1. Gross calculus removal may be accomplished with less effort than by manual instrumentation. More time can be devoted to thorough, careful root planing.
2. Requires minimum tissue manipulation for hypersensitive tissues.

---

*Attention must be paid to the proximity of any person in the dental office or clinic who may be wearing a pacemaker, whether a member of the dental team or a patient.

3. Operating time is reduced for removal of heavy stains and calculus.

B. Limitations

1. Contraindicated for use on young, growing tissues; therefore, it should not be used on children.
2. Lack of tactile perception during instrumentation.
3. Impeded visibility during operation; indirect vision with water-sprayed mouth mirror presents problems.
4. Will not complete the entire procedure: access to all areas is not possible, and fine subgingival calculus is not removed.
5. Patient and operator have discomfort and inconvenience of spraying or dripping of water.
6. Patient may experience pain and discomfort when the instrument is used on thin deposits or stains, or when it is used frequently.
7. Heat production. Potential damage to the pulp tissue has not been documented specifically, but the amount of heat produced by an uncooled ultrasonic compares with that produced by an uncooled conventional high-speed handpiece.[46] Constant motion of the instrument, correct angulation, and ample water for cooling are essential to operation.
8. Platelet aggregation. Human platelets are susceptible to damage by forces associated with ultrasonic cavitation at the level used clinically. If such damage were to occur in the pulp chamber of a tooth, thrombosis could result. The effect would be unlikely in large arteries but it could happen in a tooth because of the close area of enclosure. Pulpal thrombosis could lead to pulp death.[47]
9. Aerosols produced by an ultrasonic scaler may contain high bacterial counts.[48–51] The ultrasonic scaler should not be used for a patient with a communicable disease. A mask should be worn by the operator, and protective glasses are needed by both operator and patient.
10. Hearing shifts. Extended exposure to noises above a certain level such as the noise of a high-speed handpiece or an ultrasonic scaler is potentially damaging. Temporary hearing shifts have been demonstrated for a group of patients.[52]

USE OF A TOPICAL ANESTHETIC

A topical or surface anesthetic is a drug applied to the mucous membrane to produce a loss of sensation. A topical anesthetic can be used with a degree of success for short-duration desensitization of the gingiva. As a soft tissue anesthetic, a topical agent does not influence sensations in the teeth and, therefore, is not a substitute for local anesthetic administered by injection.

Pain reaction varies from person to person and even in the same person, depending on emotional state and degree of fatigue. A person with a low reaction to pain, who is hyporeactive, is said to have a *high pain threshold*. When there is a high reaction, the person is hyperreactive and has a *low pain threshold*.

In addition to emotional state and fatigue, other factors that influence pain threshold are age, sex, fear, and apprehension. Older individuals have a tendency to have a higher pain threshold than younger, males higher than females, but in fear or apprehension there will be a lowered pain threshold for either sex at any age.

I. Indications for Use

A local anesthetic should be used when indicated by the extent of the procedure, by the patient's pain threshold, or by evidence of fear and apprehension. Although a local anesthetic would be indicated primarily for deep subgingival scaling, root planing, and curettage, it may be indicated for any degree of scaling requirement.

Pain threshold can usually be detected during initial examination. A patient who hyperreacts to gentle, careful probing, may indeed have a low pain threshold, and a note should be made on the record to indicate possible need for anesthesia.

A topical anesthetic can be used for many dental hygiene and dental services, including the following:

A. Prior to injection for local anesthesia.
B. Prevention of gagging in radiographic techniques and impression making.

C. Relief of pain from localized diseased areas such as oral ulcers, wounds, or injuries.
D. During instrumentation for probing, exploring, scaling, and sometimes, root planing and gingival curettage. When root planing and curettage are deep and generalized, a local anesthetic is usually indicated.
E. Suture removal.
F. Dressing replacement after removal of a dressing. When pressure is needed for adaptation of the dressing, a topical application can provide relief.

II. Action of a Topical Anesthetic

The purpose is to desensitize the mucous membrane by anesthetizing the terminal nerve endings. A superficial anesthesia is produced that is related to the amount of absorption of the drug by the tissue.

The absorption varies with the thickness of the stratified squamous epithelial covering and the degree of keratinization. The skin and lips are highly resistant; the attached gingiva and cheek and palatal mucosa absorb drugs slowly; whereas the tissues without keratinization absorb more readily.

III. Requirements for an Adequate Topical Anesthetic

A. Produces effective lasting anesthesia.
B. Is miscible and stable in vehicle used.
C. Anesthetizing agent readily released from the preparation when applied.
D. Is nonirritating to the tissues.
E. Does not induce hypersensitivity reaction or other toxic effect at the concentration required for anesthesia.
F. Does not delay healing.
G. Can be readily washed off with water.

IV. Preparations Used: Characteristics

A number of preparations have been used in the form of gels, ointments, solutions, troches, or powders. The American Dental Association, Council on Dental Therapeutics evaluates and classifies topical anesthetics.[53]

General properties and characteristics of anesthetics for surface use are listed below.
A. Oils, alcohols, or glycols are used as the vehicle since most of the anesthetizing substances are only slightly soluble in water.
B. Most topical anesthetics are prepared in fairly concentrated form to allow for the resistance of the thick epithelial covering and viscid coating of saliva on the tissues. They are generally more concentrated than their counterparts used for local anesthesia.
C. The drugs are absorbed slowly due to their slight solubility and the resistance of the mucous membrane.
D. Alcohols or glycols in concentrated solutions may be irritating to the sensitive mucous membranes and therefore are inferior vehicles (percent of alcohol or glycol should not be greater than 10 percent).
E. Carbowaxes used as vehicles for topical anesthetics are somewhat hygroscopic, so that the jar in which the ointment is kept should be closed tightly.
F. Pressurized spray preparations need to be used with caution since it is difficult to control the amount of material expelled and to limit the area of application. Inhalation of the fine spray into the lungs can produce a toxic reaction. When the liquid flows into the throat (as may be possible with application of any type of preparation), coughing may be initiated.

V. Agents Used in Surface Anesthetic Preparations

The six drugs most commonly contained in surface anesthetics for dental use are listed here with brief notes about their characteristics.[53-56]

A. Benzocaine (ester type)

1. Slow absorption; may be applied to abrasions or open lesions.
2. May produce localized allergic reactions after prolonged or repeated use.

B. Tetracaine (ester type)

1. Rapid absorption and high toxicity; not for use on open abraded tissue.
2. Use in small quantities; avoid spray media where quantity used cannot be controlled.

C. Butacaine (ester type)

1. Good action through mucous membrane.

2. Toxic and should be used cautiously.

D. Lidocaine (amide type)

1. Allergy is rare; aqueous form is more toxic than nonaqueous lidocaine base.
2. May be applied to lacerated or incompletely healed tissue.

E. Chlorbutanol (aliphatic compound)

1. Has both antiseptic and anesthetic properties.
2. Has been used in preparations for alleviation of pain from pulpitis in a near pulp exposure and in dressings for postsurgical discomfort.

F. Dyclonine (ketone)

1. May be applied to lacerated or incompletely healed tissue because it is absorbed slowly.
2. Has low systemic toxicity; useful when other agents can not be used.

VI. Technique for Application of a Topical Anesthetic

A. Consult history and other records for pertinent information concerning a patient's previous experiences with anesthetics. When a patient reveals an allergy to a local anesthetic, there may also be an allergy to a surface anesthetic.
B. Explain purpose and anticipated effect to the patient.
C. Dry area with gauze sponge or cotton roll. Compressed air may be used with consideration for sensitive tissues.
D. Application
   1. Ointment
      a. A syringe with a bent needle may be used to introduce an ointment into a sulcus or pocket.
      b. Apply with a cotton pellet and rub into the proximal area. This method is less exact than the use of the syringe.
   2. Liquid: apply directly over the dry tissues with a cotton swab or pellet.
E. Wait briefly for anesthetic to take effect before proceeding.

VII. Precautions

A. Operator

Use agents on a swab and avoid contact. The repeated contacts with certain materials may lead to sensitization, which in turn may develop into an allergy.

B. Patient

1. Prevent absorption of agents into the system by the following:
   a. Limit the concentration and total amount of the agent applied.
   b. Limit the area of application.
   c. Avoid areas of sepsis and open traumatized tissue unless it is specified for the particular agent that it can be safely applied directly on an open wound.
2. Prevent respiratory reactions: avoid spray preparations.

C. Adverse Reactions[57]

1. Allergic-type reactions may occur; primarily, they are related to a topical anesthetic preparation that contains an ester-type agent.
2. Agents that are rapidly absorbed may cause an overdose reaction.

TECHNICAL HINTS

I. Summary: Methods to Minimize Patient Discomfort

A. Tissue Sensitivity

1. Gingival tissue: use topical anesthetic and/or local anesthetic as needed.
2. Exposed cementum or dentin: apply desensitizing agent (Chapter 37).
3. Protect lips and corners of mouth from irritation during instrumentation by application of petrolatum, cocoa butter, or other appropriate lubricant.
4. Use only *warm* water for rinsing.

B. Preventive Instrumentation

1. Use appropriate instrument, applied at the correct angulation, for each tooth surface.
2. Curets applied to base of sulcus or pocket must be small to prevent undue stretch-

ing of gingival wall and hence unnecessary detachment of the soft tissue attachment.

3. Instruments must be sharp, but the cementum can be scratched if sharp curets are not applied correctly and discriminately.

4. Maintain control of instrument at all times through effective grasp, appropriate finger rest, and correctly applied strokes to prevent accidental trauma to gingival tissue.

5. Apply minimum effective pressure on finger rest and of instrument on tooth to prevent patient from developing tired muscles and a stressed temporomandibular joint.

6. Finger rests on soft tissue give the patient a feeling of more pressure than finger rests on the teeth, and consequently, may give the impression that the dental hygienist is heavy-handed.

C. **Postoperative Care** (pages 598–599)

1. Massage of gingival tissue at completion of instrumentation can be soothing and restful for the patient.

2. An antiseptic may be applied or the patient requested to use mouthrinse to decrease discomfort.

3. Provide instruction for personal care, such as rinsing with warm salt water and other appropriate measures for postappointment follow-up.

II. Maintenance of a Clear Field

A. Use of saliva ejector and evacuator as needed.

B. Use of rolled gauze sponge or cotton rolls.

1. A gauze sponge rolled in the long dimension and placed in the mucobuccal fold beneath the teeth being treated can assist by
   a. Retracting the cheek or lip.
   b. Keeping teeth dry for secure finger rest.
   c. Drying the individual area for better vision.

2. Aid in retraction of tongue and keeping field free from saliva by placing cotton roll under tongue.

C. Maintenance of clear field and/or control of bleeding.

1. Application of pressure with cotton roll or pellet.

2. Application of 3% hydrogen peroxide with cotton pellet, followed by patient rinsing and/or dry pellet applied with pressure.

3. Use of compressed air to deflect tissue and remove debris.

III. Broken Instrument

The procedure to follow when an instrument blade tip breaks in the patient's mouth during operation should be in accord with the dentist's own policy. Therefore, it is recommended that this be discussed before an accident happens so that the procedure can be clarified.

The principal objective in the location of a broken instrument tip is to *know positively that the tip has been removed*. With this in mind, rinsing, use of suction or compressed air, or other procedures that could cause the removal of the tip unknowingly would be out of order. A general procedure is suggested here.

A. Cease operation, retain retraction without moving the patient's head unnecessarily, and isolate with gauze or cotton roll.

B. Do not alarm patient by describing the accident.

C. Examine the immediate field of operation, the floor of the mouth, and the mucobuccal fold. Blot the gingival tissue dry with a cotton roll and examine around the tooth.

D. Apply transilluminator or mouth light when available.

E. The gingival sulcus can be gently examined using a curet in a spooning-like stroke, but with care not to push the tip into the base of the sulcus (should the tip be there).

F. Consult the dentist for assistance in accord with previously discussed policy.

G. When tip is not removed by any means mentioned thus far, make a periapical radiograph of the area.

IV. Applications for Scaling Principles

A. Removal of excess cement following cementation of orthodontic bands.

B. Removal of pieces of periodontal dressings that adhere to the teeth when a dressing is removed (page 549).

V. Protection of the Dental Hygienist

Wear rimmed glasses for protection from bits of calculus or debris that could accidentally get into the eyes (figure 4–2, page 52). Calculus and debris are highly contaminated. Aerosols from the ultrasonic water spray contain large numbers of organisms and can be collected from the air of the room for long periods of time after scaling has ceased.[48]

FACTORS TO TEACH THE PATIENT

I. The nature, occurrence, and etiology of calculus.

II. The importance of the complete removal of calculus to the health of the oral tissues in the prevention of periodontal diseases.

III. Relationship of the accumulation of plaque to the patient's personal oral hygiene procedures.

IV. Basic reasons for need and advantages of more than one appointment to complete the scaling and root planing.

V. Needed frequency of recall appointments in relation to oral health.

References

1. Lovdal, A., Arno, A., Schei, O., and Waerhaug, J.: Combined Effect of Subgingival Scaling and Controlled Oral Hygiene on the Incidence of Gingivitis, *Acta Odontol. Scand.*, *19*, 537, December, 1961.
2. Ramfjord, S.P., Nissle, R.R., Shick, R.A., and Cooper, H.: Subgingival Curettage Versus Surgical Elimination of Periodontal Pockets, *J. Periodontol.*, *39*, 167, May, 1968.
3. Suomi, J.D., Green, J.C., Vermillion, J.R., Chang, J.J., and Leatherwood, E.C.: The Effect of Controlled Oral Hygiene Procedures on the Progression of Periodontal Disease in Adults: Results After Two Years, *J. Periodontol.*, *40*, 416, July, 1969.
4. Suomi, J.D., Greene, J.C., Vermillion, J.R., Doyle, J., Chang, J.J., and Leatherwood, E.C.: The Effect of Controlled Oral Hygiene Procedures on the Progression of Periodontal Disease in Adults: Results After Third and Final Year, *J. Periodontol.*, *42*, 152, March, 1971.
5. Lightner, L.M., O'Leary, T.J., Drake, R.B., Crump, P.P., and Allen, M.F.: Preventive Periodontic Treatment Procedures: Results Over 46 Months, *J. Periodontol.*, *42*, 555, September, 1971.
6. Glavind, L.: Effect of Monthly Professional Mechanical Tooth Cleaning on Periodontal Health in Adults, *J. Clin. Periodontol.*, *4*, 100, May, 1977.
7. Axelsson, P. and Lindhe, J.: Effect of Controlled Oral Hygiene Procedures on Caries and Periodontal Disease in Adults, *J. Clin. Periodontol.*, *5*, 133, May, 1978.
8. De Leo, A.A., Schoenknecht, M.D., Anderson, M.W., and Peterson, J.C.: The Incidence of Bacteremia Following Oral Prophylaxis on Pediatric Patients, *Oral Surg.*, *37*, 36, January, 1974.
9. Korn, N.A. and Schaffer, E.M.: Comparison of the Post-operative Bacteremias Induced Following Different Periodontal Procedures, *J. Periodontol.*, *33*, 226, July, 1962.
10. Royer, R., Gaines, R., and Kruger, G.: Bacteremia Following Exodontia, Prophylaxis, and Gingivectomy, *J. Dent. Res.*, *43*, 877, September–October, 1964, (Supplement).
11. Bender, I.B., Seltzer, S., Tashman, S., and Meloff, G.: Dental Procedures in Patients With Rheumatic Heart Disease, *Oral Surg.*, *16*, 466, April, 1963.
12. Winslow, M.B. and Kobernick, S.D.: Bacteremia After Prophylaxis, *J. Am. Dent. Assoc.*, *61*, 69, July, 1960.
13. Connor, H.D., Haberman, S., Collings, C.K., and Winford, T.E.: Bacteremias Following Periodontal Scaling in Patients with Healthy Appearing Gingiva, *J. Periodontol.*, *38*, 466, November–December, 1967.
14. Bandt, C.L., Korn, N.A., and Schaffer, E.M.: Bacteremias From Ultrasonic and Hand Instrumentation, *J. Periodontol.*, *35*, 214, May–June, 1964.
15. Randall, E. and Brenman, H.S.: Local Degerming With Povidone-iodine. I. Prior to Dental Prophylaxis, *J. Periodontol.*, *45*, 866, December, 1974.
16. Brenman, H.S. and Randall, E.: Local Degerming with Povidone-iodine. II. Prior to Gingivectomy, *J. Periodontol.*, *45*, 870, December, 1974.
17. Carranza, F.A.: *Glickman's Clinical Periodontology*, 5th ed. Philadelphia, W.B. Saunders Co., 1979, p. 656.
18. Barnes, J.E. and Schaffer, E.M.: Subgingival Root Planing: A Comparison Using Files, Hoes and Curettes, *J. Periodontol.*, *31*, 300, September, 1960.
19. Green, E. and Ramfjord, S.P.: Tooth Roughness After Subgingival Root Planing, *J. Periodontol.*, *37*, 396, September–October, 1966.
20. Kerry, G.J.: Roughness of Root Surfaces After Use of Ultrasonic Instruments and Hand Curettes, *J. Periodontol.*, *38*, 340, July–August, 1967.
21. Walker, S.L. and Ash, M.M.: A Study of Root Planing by Scanning Electron Microscopy, *Dent. Hyg.*, *50*, 109, March, 1976.
22. Ramfjord, S. and Kiester, G.: The Gingival Sulcus and the Periodontal Pocket Immediately Following Scaling of Teeth, *J. Periodontol.*, *25*, 167, July, 1954.
23. Moskow, B.S.: Response of the Gingival Sulcus to Instrumentation: A Histological Investigation. I. The Scaling Procedure, *J. Periodontol.*, *33*, 282, July, 1962.
24. Schaffer, E.M., Stende, G., and King, D.: Healing of Periodontal Pocket Tissues Following Ultrasonic Scaling and Hand Planing, *J. Periodontol.*, *35*, 140, March–April, 1964.
25. Stahl, S.S., Weiner, J.M., Benjamin, S., and Yamada, L.: Soft Tissue Healing Following Curettage and Root Planing, *J. Periodontol.*, *42*, 678, November, 1971.
26. Tagge, D.L., O'Leary, T.J., and El-Kafrawy, A.H.: The Clinical and Histologic Response of Periodontal Pockets to Root Planing and Oral Hygiene, *J. Periodontol.*, *46*, 527, September, 1975.
27. Carranza: op. cit., p. 269–270.
28. Schaffer, E.M.: Histological Results of Root Curettage of Human Teeth, *J. Periodontol.*, *27*, 296, October, 1956.
29. Selvig, K.A.: Biological Changes at the Tooth-saliva Interface in Periodontal Disease, *J. Dent. Res.*, *48*, 846, September–October, 1969, (Supplement).
30. Jones, W.A. and O'Leary, T.J.: The Effectiveness of *in vivo* Root Planing in Removing Bacterial Endotoxin from the Roots of Periodontally Involved Teeth, *J. Periodontol.*, *49*, 337, July, 1978.
31. Listgarten, M.A. and Hellden, L.: Relative Distribution of Bacteria at Clinically Healthy and Periodontally Dis-

eased Sites in Humans, *J. Clin. Periodontol.*, 5, 115, May, 1978.

32. Listgarten, M.A., Lindhe, J., and Hellden, L.: Effect of Tetracycline and/or Scaling on Human Periodontal Disease. Clinical, Microbiological, and Histological Observations, *J. Clin. Periodontol.*, 5, 246, November, 1978.

33. Mousquès, T., Listgarten, M.A., and Phillips, R.W.: Effect of Scaling and Root Planing on the Composition of the Human Subgingival Microbial Flora, *J. Periodont. Res.*, 15, 144, March, 1980.

34. Slots, J., Mashimo, P., Levine, M.J., and Genco, R.J.: Periodontal Therapy in Humans. I. Microbiologic and Clinical Effects of a Single Course of Periodontal Scaling and Root Planing, and of Adjunctive Tetracycline Therapy, *J. Periodontol.*, 50, 495, October, 1979.

35. Walsh, T.F. and Waite, I.M.: A Comparison of Postsurgical Healing Following Debridement by Ultrasonic or Hand Instruments, *J. Periodontol.*, 49, 201, April, 1978.

36. Bhaskar, S.N., Grower, M.F., and Cutright, D.E.: Gingival Healing After Hand and Ultrasonic Scaling—Biochemical and Histologic Analysis, *J. Periodontol.*, 43, 31, January, 1972.

37. Donzé, Y., Krüger, J., Ketterl, W., and Rateitschak, K.H.: Treatment of Gingivitis With Cavitron or Hand Instruments: A Comparative Study, *Helv. Odontol. Acta.*, 17, 31, April, 1973.

38. Clark, S.M.: The Ultrasonic Dental Unit: A Guide for the Clinical Application of Ultrasonics in Dentistry and in Dental Hygiene, *J. Periodontol.*, 40, 621, November, 1969.

39. Ewen, S. and Glickstein, C.: *Ultrasonic Therapy in Periodontics*. Springfield, Illinois, Charles C Thomas, 1968, pp. 12–45.

40. Schaffer, E.M.: Objective Evaluation of Ultrasonic Versus Hand Instrumentation in Periodontics, *Dent. Clin. North Am.*, p. 165, March, 1964.

41. Jacobson, L.: Ultrasonic Scaling, *Aust. Dent. J.*, 19, 379, December, 1974.

42. Gross, A., Devine, M.J., and Cutright, D.E.: Microbial Contamination of Dental Units and Ultrasonic Scalers, *J. Periodontol.*, 47, 670, November, 1978.

43. Ore, D.E. and Shriner, W.A.: Doctor: Don't Shut Off That Pacemaker, *Chicago Dent. Soc. Rev.*, pp. 22–23, August, 1974.

44. Bandt, C.L., Korn, N.A., and Schaffer, E.M.: Bacteremias from Ultrasonic and Hand Instrumentation, *J. Periodontol.*, 35, 214, May–June, 1964.

45. American Dental Association, Council on Dental Materials, Instruments and Equipment: *Dentist's Desk Reference: Materials, Instruments and Equipment*, 1st ed. Chicago, American Dental Association, 1981, pp. 288–291.

46. Frost, H.M.: Heating Under Ultrasonic Dental Scaling Conditions, HEW Publication (FDA) 78–8048, Rockville, Maryland, Public Health Service, Bureau of Radiological Health, pp. 64–76, December, 1977.

47. Williams, A.R. and Chater, B.V.: Mammalian Platelet Damage *in vitro* by an Ultrasonic Therapeutic Device, *Arch. Oral Biol.*, 25, 175, Number 3, 1980.

48. Larato, D.C., Ruskin, P.F., and Martin, A.: Effect of an Ultrasonic Scaler on Bacterial Counts in Air, *J. Periodontol.*, 38, 550, November–December, 1967.

49. Holbrook, W.P., Muir, K.F., MacPhee, I.T., and Ross, P.W.: Bacteriological Investigation of the Aerosol from Ultrasonic Scalers, *Br. Dent. J.*, 144, 245, April 18, 1978.

50. Muir, K.F., Ross, P.W., MacPhee, I.T., Holbrook,

W.P., and Kowolik, M.J.: Reduction of Microbial Contamination from Ultrasonic Scalers, *Br. Dent. J.*, 145, 76, August 1, 1978.

51. Williams, G.H., Pollok, N.L., Shay, D.E., and Barr, C.E.: Laminar Air Purge of Microorganisms in Dental Aerosols: Prophylactic Procedures With an Ultrasonic Scaler, *J. Dent. Res.*, 49, 1498, November–December, 1970.

52. Möller, P., Grevstad, A.O., and Kristoffersen, T.: Ultrasonic Scaling of Maxillary Teeth Causing Tinnitus and Temporary Hearing Shifts, *J. Clin. Periodontol.*, 3, 123, May, 1976.

53. American Dental Association, Council on Dental Therapeutics: *Accepted Dental Therapeutics*, 39th ed. Chicago, American Dental Association, 1982, pp. 158–163.

54. Cianco, S.G. and Bourgault, P.C.: *Clinical Pharmacology for Dental Professionals*. New York, McGraw-Hill, 1980, pp. 91, 221–222.

55. Cowan, F.F.: *Pharmacology for the Dental Hygienist*. Philadelphia, Lea & Febiger, 1978, pp. 121–127.

56. Holroyd, S.V., ed.: *Clinical Pharmacology in Dental Practice*, 2nd ed. St. Louis, The C.V. Mosby Co., 1978, pp. 147–148.

57. Malamed, S.F.: *Handbook of Medical Emergencies in the Dental Office*. St. Louis, The C.V. Mosby Co., 1978, pp. 214, 228.

Suggested Readings

Armitage, G.C.: *Biologic Basis of Periodontal Maintenance Therapy*. Berkeley, California, Praxis Publishing Co., 1980, pp. 79–115.

Bellini, H.T. and Johansen, J.R.: Average Time Required for Scaling and Surgery in Periodontal Therapy, *Acta Odontol. Scand.*, 31, 283, Number 5, 1973.

Carranza, F.A.: *Glickman's Clinical Periodontology*, 5th ed. Philadelphia, W.B. Saunders Co., 1979, pp. 606–615, 641–664, 711–724.

Goldman, H.M. and Cohen, D.W.: *Periodontal Therapy*, 6th ed. St. Louis, The C.V. Mosby Co., 1980, pp. 441–443, 454–494.

Grant, D.A., Stern, I.B., and Everett, F.G.: *Periodontics*, 5th ed. St. Louis, The C.V. Mosby Co., 1979, pp. 571–599.

Handleman, S.L. and Hess, C.: Effect of Dental Prophylaxis on Tooth-surface Flora, *J. Dent. Res.*, 49, 340, March–April, 1970.

Hirschfeld, L.: Subgingival Curettage in Periodontal Treatment, *J. Am. Dent. Assoc.*, 44, 301, March, 1952.

Parr, R.W., Green, E., Madsen, L., and Miller, S.: *Subgingival Scaling and Root Planing*. Berkeley, California, Praxis Publishing Co., 1976, 90 pp.

Parr, R.W., John, R., and Ratcliff, P.A.: *Tooth Preparation*. Berkeley, California, Praxis Publishing Co., 1974, 52 pp.

Pattison, G.L. and Pattison, A.M.: *Periodontal Instrumentation*. Reston, Virginia, Reston Publishing Co., 1979, pp. 143–306.

Ramfjord, S.P. and Ash, M.M.: *Periodontology and Periodontics*. Philadelphia, W.B. Saunders Co., 1979, pp. 362–396.

Anatomic Features

Bower, R.C.: Furcation Morphology Relative to Periodontal Treatment. Furcation Entrance Architecture, *J. Periodontol.*, 50, 23, January, 1979.

Bower, R.C.: Furcation Morphology Relative to Periodontal Treatment. Furcation Root Surface Anatomy, *J. Periodontol.*, 50, 366, July, 1979.

Gher, M.E. and Vernino, A.R.: Root Morphology—Clinical

Significance in Pathogenesis and Treatment of Periodontal Disease, *J. Am. Dent. Assoc.*, *101*, 627, October, 1980.

Harris, J.H. and Overton, E.E.: Cementoenamel Defects in an Unusual Location, *J. Am. Dent. Assoc.*, *97*, 221, August, 1978.

Effects of Scaling: Soft Tissue

Caton, J.G. and Zander, H.A.: The Attachment Between Tooth and Gingival Tissues After Periodic Root Planing and Soft Tissue Curettage, *J. Periodontol.*, *50*, 462, September, 1979.

Hughes, T.P. and Caffesse, R.G.: Gingival Changes Following Scaling, Root Planing and Oral Hygiene, *J. Periodontol.*, *49*, 245, May, 1978.

Lopez, N.J. and Belvederessi, M.: Subgingival Scaling With Root Planing and Curettage: Effects Upon Gingival Inflammation: A Comparative Study, *J. Periodontol.*, *48*, 354, June, 1977.

Morrison, E.C., Lang, N.P., Löe, H., and Ramfjord, S.P.: Effects of Repeated Scaling and Root Planing and/or Controlled Oral Hygiene on the Periodontal Attachment Level and Pocket Depth in Beagle Dogs. I. Clinical Findings, *J. Periodont. Res.*, *14*, 428, September, 1979.

Pihlstrom, B.L., Ortiz-Campos, C., and McHugh, R.B.: A Randomized Four-year Study of Periodontal Therapy, *J. Periodontol.*, *52*, 227, May, 1981.

Ribbons, J.W.: A Clinical Investigation into the Changes in the Periodontal Tissues of Man, Following the Removal of Subgingival Calculus, *Br. Dent. J.*, *139*, 350, November 4, 1975.

Stahl, S.S.: Repair Potential of the Soft Tissue-root Interface, *J. Periodontol.*, *48*, 545, September, 1977.

Waerhaug, J.: Healing of the Dento-epithelial Junction Following Subgingival Plaque Control. I. As Observed in Human Biopsy Material, *J. Periodontol.*, *49*, 1, January, 1978.

Waerhaug, J.: Healing of the Dento-epithelial Junction Following Subgingival Plaque Control. II. As Observed on Extracted Teeth, *J. Periodontol.*, *49*, 119, March, 1978.

Effects of Scaling: Tooth Surface

Frisch, J., Levin, M.P., and Bhaskar, S.N.: Calculus Removal. Effectiveness of Scaling, *J. South. Calif. Dent. Assoc.*, *38*, 36, January, 1970.

Garrett, J.S.: Root Planing: A Perspective, *J. Periodontol.*, *48*, 553, September, 1977.

Green, E.: Root Planing With Dull and Sharp Curettes, *J. Periodontol.*, *39*, 348, November, 1968.

Rabbani, G.M., Ash, M.M., and Caffesse, R.G.: The Effectiveness of Subgingival Scaling and Root Planing in Calculus Removal, *J. Periodontol.*, *52*, 119, March, 1981.

Retief, D.H. and Denys, F.R.: Finishing of Enamel Surfaces After Debonding of Orthodontic Attachments, *Angle Orthod.*, *49*, 1, January, 1979.

Rosenberg, R.M. and Ash, M.M.: The Effect of Root Roughness on Plaque Accumulation and Gingival Inflammation, *J. Periodontol.*, *45*, 146, March, 1974.

Ruben, M.P.: Significance of Root Surface Preparation in Periodontal Therapy, *Quintessence Int.*, *9*, 57, January, 1978.

Ultrasonic Scaling

Belting, C.M. and Spjut, P.J.: Effects of High-speed Periodontal Instruments on the Root Surface During Subgingival Calculus Removal, *J. Am. Dent. Assoc.*, *69*, 578, November, 1964.

Clark, S.M., Grupe, H.E., and Mahler, D.B.: The Effect of Ultrasonic Instrumentation on Root Surfaces, *J. Periodontol.*, *39*, 135, May, 1968.

D'Silva, I.V., Nayak, R.P., Cherian, K.M., and Mulky, M.J.: An Evaluation of the Root Topography Following Periodontal Instrumentation—A Scanning Electron Microscopic Study, *J. Periodontol.*, *50*, 283, June, 1979.

Glick, D.H. and Freeman, E.: Postsurgical Bone Loss Following Root Planing by Ultrasonic and Hand Instruments, *J. Periodontol.*, *51*, 510, September, 1980.

Green, G.H. and Sanderson, A.D.: Ultrasonics and Periodontal Therapy—A Review of Clinical and Biologic Effects, *J. Periodontol.*, *36*, 232, May–June, 1965.

Jones, S.J., Lozdan, J., and Boyde, A.: Tooth Surfaces Treated *in situ* with Periodontal Instruments, *Br. Dent. J.*, *132*, 57, January 18, 1972.

Lie, T. and Meyer, K.: Calculus Removal and Loss of Tooth Substance in Response to Different Periodontal Instruments, *J. Clin. Periodontol.*, *4*, 250, November, 1977.

McQuade, M.J., Huget, E.F., de Simon, L.B., and Levin, M.P.: Effect of Ultrasonic Instrumentation on the Retention of Simulated Cast Crowns, *J. Prosthet. Dent.*, *39*, 640, June, 1978.

Meyer, K. and Lie, T.: Root Surface Roughness in Response to Periodontal Instrumentation Studied by Combined Use of Microroughness Measurements and Scanning Electron Microscopy, *J. Clin. Periodontol.*, *4*, 77, May, 1977.

Moore, L.: Ultrasonic Devices vs. Hand Instruments: The Scientific Rationale, *Dent. Hyg.*, *49*, 356, August, 1975.

Moskow, B.S. and Bressman, E.: Cemental Response to Ultrasonic and Hand Instrumentation, *J. Am. Dent. Assoc.*, *68*, 698, May, 1964.

Nishimine, D. and O'Leary, T.J.: Hand Instrumentation Versus Ultrasonics in the Removal of Endotoxins from Root Surfaces, *J. Periodontol.*, *50*, 345, July, 1979.

Pameijer, C.H., Stallard, R.E., and Hiep, N.: Surface Characteristics of Teeth Following Periodontal Instrumentation: A Scanning Electron Microscope Study, *J. Periodontol.*, *43*, 628, October, 1972.

Stewart, J.L., Briggs, R.L., Drisko, R.R., and Jamison, H.C.: Relative Calculus and Tooth Structure Loss with Use of Power-driven Scaling Instruments, *J. Am. Dent. Assoc.*, *83*, 840, October, 1971.

Suppipat, N.: Ultrasonics in Periodontics, *J. Clin. Periodontol.*, *1*, 206, Number 4, 1974.

Torfason, T., Kiger, R., Selvig, K.A., and Egelberg, J.: Clinical Improvement of Gingival Conditions Following Ultrasonic Versus Hand Instrumentation of Periodontal Pockets, *J. Clin. Periodontol.*, *6*, 165, June, 1979.

Van Volkinburg, J.W., Green, E., and Armitage, G.C.: The Nature of Root Surfaces After Curette, Cavitron and Alpha-sonic Instrumentation, *J. Periodont. Res.*, *11*, 374, November, 1976.

Wilkinson, R.F. and Maybury, J.E.: Scanning Electron Microscopy of the Root Surface Following Instrumentation, *J. Periodontol.*, *44*, 559, September, 1973.

Woodruff, H.C., Levin, M.P., and Brady, J.M.: The Effects of Two Ultrasonic Instruments on Root Surfaces, *J. Periodontol.*, *46*, 119, February, 1975.

34

Gingival Curettage

Gingival or soft tissue curettage is a planned systematic procedure to remove the diseased sulcular epithelial lining and underlying inflamed connective tissue of a gingival or periodontal pocket. It contributes to the control of disease and may be the definitive treatment by which a pocket can be reduced in depth or eliminated. It also may be part of the preparatory or initial phase of treatment. Reevaluation can then be made to determine whether more complex periodontal therapy will be required.

Coincidental curettage occurs as a result of the movement of the inactive side of a curet blade along the pocket wall during scaling and root planing. It was described in Chapter 33, page 518.

Although terminology varies, *gingival curettage* generally means treatment of a pocket wall and *subgingival curettage* includes removal of the attachment area and connective tissue apical to the attachment. The term *surgical curettage* refers to preparation of a flap in an open curettage procedure.

I. The Pocket Wall

In health, the lining of the sulcus is nonkeratinized stratified squamous epithelium. In disease, the pocket wall is characterized by degenerative changes in the sulcular epithelium with partial destruction, ulceration with exposure of the underlying connective tissue, and suppuration (cells and fluid) from the inflamed connective tissue.

Soft, spongy enlargement is related to edema and local circulatory stasis. On the other hand, hard, firm enlargement is due to long-standing chronic inflammation with fibrosis in the connective tissue.

II. Purposes of Gingival Curettage

A. Overall Objectives

As a part of the treatment for the restoration of gingival health, with effective plaque control, curettage can contribute to
1. Reduction or elimination of inflammation.
2. Reduction or eradication of gingival or periodontal pockets.

B. Specific Objectives

Removal of the inflamed, ulcerated soft tissue of the pocket wall can
1. Allow inflammation to subside by establishing drainage for edema and hyperemia.
2. Cause shrinkage of the free gingiva, and hence reduce pocket depth.
3. Promote fibrosis and healing.
4. Permit replacement of the diseased pocket lining with newly formed connective tissue and sulcular epithelium which can be maintained in health.

5. Contribute to a return of the gingiva to a normal contour.

III. Indications for Gingival Curettage

A. Gingival tissue with a soft, spongy consistency and other signs of inflammation (table 11–1, page 196).
B. Pockets that are relatively shallow (4 to 5 mm.) and are suprabony.
C. Persistence of hyperemia, edema, and pocket depth after complete scaling and root planing.
D. Deep pockets that cannot be expected to shrink enough for elimination; but curettage may be used to reduce inflammation and pocket depth for maintenance in a patient who cannot have surgery for other health reasons or may be required to postpone surgery.
E. Presurgical tissue preparation to lessen inflammation and make the tissue more fibrotic for surgical management.

IV. Contraindications for Gingival Curettage

A. Gingival tissue with a firm, fibrous consistency contains fibrotic, collagenous elements that do not permit shrinkage of a pocket wall. Pocket elimination, therefore, cannot be an objective.
B. Except for presurgical tissue preparation, curettage is not indicated for mucogingival involvement, frenal attachments, intrabony pockets, or other complications that require specific surgical procedures.

TREATMENT

I. Relation to Scaling and Root Planing

Curettage is performed after scaling and planing. For certain patients, it is done immediately after, in the same appointment; whereas for others, it is postponed a few weeks to observe the tissue changes following scaling and root planing. At that time, if healing is adequate and the tissues have responded favorably, curettage would not be indicated. Other patients may have only localized, isolated areas that need curettage and those may be done at the time of the root planing or later.

II. Appointment Plan

At an appointment, treatment is confined to one or possibly two quadrants. However, the plan for treatment depends on the severity of the condition, depth of pockets, and whether treatment is localized or generalized. The extent of treatment is also influenced by the use of anesthesia, whether topical application is adequate, or local anesthetic is to be administered.

The treatment plan outlined on page 330 is illustrative of the steps needed. With local anesthetic and the use of periodontal dressings, several appointments are needed in a series over several weeks for continuing evaluation.

III. Preparation of the Patient

A. Instruction in Personal Care

When plaque is not yet under control, additional help must be provided, because after curettage, healing is dependent on plaque removal on a daily basis.

B. Complete Scaling and Planing

When part or all is performed on the same day as curettage, the pockets must be carefully irrigated, using suction to remove particles of calculus, cementum, and other debris so they cannot be forced into the tissue during curettage.

C. Anesthesia for Pain Control

Topical anesthetic may be sufficient for some patients and some areas, particularly when the pockets are shallow. The anesthetic may be applied to a group of teeth, and then curets dipped in the agent and carried into the sulcus for additional benefit.

D. Assessment

Careful probing and examination of each pocket is needed to define the depth and working area.

IV. Instrumentation

A. Instruments

Only precisely sharp, fine curets are used. Instruments used for curettage are best kept separate from others used for scaling and planing, to preserve their sharpness and have them ready for use. When scaling and planing immediately precede curettage, the same instruments should not be used without re-sharpening.

B. Grasp

Use modified pen grasp and lead with the fulcrum finger to the rest near the area of operation.

C. Adaptation and Angulation

1. *Position the Blade* on the tooth surface over the pocket to be treated.
   a. Hold blade in correct position with cutting edge on tooth. Angulation will be greater than 90 degrees with the tooth surface in order that a less than 90-degree angle will be applied to the sulcular epithelium.
   b. The blade is open, that is, both cutting edges can be seen. When the curet is in correct position for scaling or planing, only the rounded back of the blade can be seen. A comparison of angulation during scaling and curettage is shown in figure 34–1.
2. *Prepare for Insertion.* With the curet in position at the gingival margin, note the relation of the handle, fulcrum, grasp, and angulation of the face of the curet with the tooth, so that, after insertion, the blade can be properly repositioned at the bottom of the pocket.

D. Insertion of Curet Into Sulcus

1. Direct the toe of the blade toward the

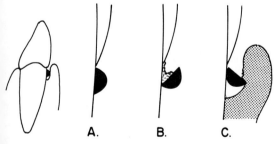

Figure 34–1. Angulation of a curet during instrumentation. **A.** Enlargement of pocket area diagrammed on left showing a cross section of the blade of a curet in black, angulated at zero degrees with the tooth surface as used for an exploratory or insertion stroke. **B.** Blade angulated for scaling and root planing at less than 90 degrees but greater than 45 degrees. **C.** Blade angulated with the gingival wall of the pocket for gingival curettage at the correct angle which is greater than 45 degrees but less than 90 degrees.

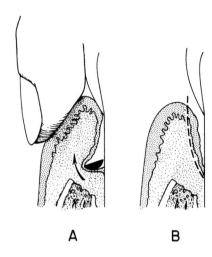

A   B

Figure 34–2. Gingival curettage. **A.** Curet positioned at the bottom of the pocket with the cutting edge toward the gingival wall. Pressure can be applied with a thumb or finger to the outside of the pocket for support while the curet is activated. **B.** The objective of curettage is to remove the lining of the pocket so that new healthy tissue can replace the old.

gingival margin, and open the blade more so that it can be slipped under the margin without trauma.

2. Slide the curet to the bottom of the sulcus; use toe-end to determine bottom of the pocket. Tension of the soft tissue will be felt.
3. Reposition the blade to the correct angulation for curettage (figure 34–2).

E. Strokes

Vertical and oblique strokes are used near the bottom of the pocket; horizontal strokes may be used nearer the top.

1. *Support the Pocket Wall.* Apply finger of non-working hand to outside of the pocket wall to offset pressure applied by the instrument on the inner surface. For treatment of an interdental papilla, apply pressure against the adjacent tooth.
2. *Number of Strokes.* Only a few are needed when the curet is sharp. The number of strokes may vary from as few as 2 or 3 to 12 or 15. An experienced sense of touch can be developed to distinguish the soft mushy granulation tissue from the underlying firm connective tissue.

3. *Removal of Diseased Tissue.* The debris and soft particles of pocket lining are brought out of the sulcus to be removed by evacuation.

F. Proceed Systematically Around Each Tooth

Strokes should overlap from the lingual and facial at the proximal.

V. Irrigation

Debris removal by irrigation is important to aid healing.

VI. Tissue Adaptation and Hemostasis

Press the area with gauze to adapt the gingival margins to the tooth. All bleeding should be stopped by pressure applied on the tissues for a short while. Although a blood clot is essential to healing, excess pressure from a large clot can permit the gingival tissue to heal away from the tooth. Physiologic form is an objective of healing.

VII. Apply Periodontal Dressing

The objectives of the dressing are described on page 545. A dressing is needed particularly when there is tissue separation from the teeth and when pressure of the dressing can aid in molding the tissue to heal in a physiologic form. The dressing usually is left in place for one week before removal.

POSTOPERATIVE CARE

I. Postoperative Instructions

A. Dressing Placed

Printed instructions are advisable. Suggestions for care following dressing placement are found on page 548 (table 36–1).

B. Without Dressing

1. Plaque removal is very important. Use soft (.006 inch filament diameter) toothbrush with rounded ends. Definite plaque removal, but care not to traumatize the healing tissue, is necessary.
2. Rinse with warm weak saline solution (pages 373–374).

II. Follow-up

A. Dressing Removal

Dressing should be removed in approximately one week. Specific plaque removal instructions given.

B. Tooth Sensitivity

Advise the patient that most sensitivity is transient. Toothbrushing with a fluoride dentifrice and use of a fluoride mouthrinse daily can be most effective. Desensitizing agents can be applied to persistent spots (page 557).

C. Polishing

Polishing is not advised immediately following dressing removal because curettage leaves a wide healing area. An abrasive would be an irritant. Instruction for daily complete plaque removal by the patient is necessary to prevent re-infection.

HEALING

I. Effects of Instrumentation

Removal of the chronically inflamed ulcerated pocket lining and underlying inflamed connective tissue creates a surgical wound. Healing follows a pattern of epithelialization and collagenation and resolution of inflammation in the connective tissue. The effects are as follows:
A. Shrinkage of the gingival walls with fluid drainage.
B. Reepithelialization with coverage of the exposed connective tissue.
C. Formation of new connective tissue beneath the new epithelial lining of the sulcus and attachment.
D. Return to normal circulation.

II. Steps in Healing[1]

A. Formation of a blood clot immediately after curettage. The clot fills the pocket area, which is adapted against the tooth by pressure and a dressing.
B. Initial tissue reaction of inflammation as with any wound.
C. Proliferation of fibroblasts and new vessels to form granulation tissue.
D. Epithelial cells arise from the epithelium at the margin of the gingiva. The epithelium

migrates in and over the granulation tissue. This begins by approximately 24 hours following the curettage.

E. New epithelium covers the sulcus lining within 5 to 6 days, and the new junctional epithelium is formed by 5 days.

F. Connective tissue healing proceeds and is well organized by 2 weeks.

G. Keratinization of oral (outer) epithelium may be observed by 2 weeks. It reaches normal thickness by 28 to 40 days.

III. Interferences with Healing

A. Residual and newly formed calculus. Repeated root planing is frequently necessary.

B. Plaque and other local irritants. Meticulous self-care must be supervised over several weeks following curettage.

C. Systemic factors may be involved when healing delay cannot be otherwise accounted for, but local factors must be rechecked first.

IV. Clinical Appearance of the Healed Tissue

When healing is complete, the usual signs of healthy gingiva as outlined in table 11–1 on page 196 should be evident. There should be minimal probe measurement in the sulcus, the sulcus should be free from bleeding on probing, stippling should be apparent, and the color, size, shape, and other characteristics, normal.

FACTORS TO TEACH THE PATIENT

I. Why pockets need to be treated; how curettage contributes to pocket reduction or elimination.

II. Reasons for periodontal dressing placement.

III. Postoperative care with and without a dressing. Care of teeth and gingiva not involved in the curettage.

IV. Relationship of plaque and plaque control to healing.

V. Desensitization, using proper toothbrushing technique applied to cervical areas, and a fluoride dentifrice and mouthrinse.

Reference

1. Goldman, H.M. and Cohen, D.W.: *Periodontal Therapy*, 6th ed. St. Louis, The C.V. Mosby Co., 1980, pp. 677–682.

Suggested Readings

Ainslie, P.T. and Caffesse, R.G.: A Biometric Evaluation of Gingival Curettage (I), *Quintessence Int.*, *12*, 519, May, 1981.

Chace, R.: Subgingival Curettage in Periodontal Therapy, *J. Periodontol.*, *45*, 107, February, 1974.

Grant, D.A., Stern, I.B., and Everett, F.G.: *Periodontics*, 5th ed. St. Louis, The C.V. Mosby Co., 1979, pp. 621–643.

Green, M.L. and Green, B.L.: Aggressive Curettage, *Dent. Hyg.*, *53*, 409, September, 1979.

Houston, M.: Gingival Curettage, in Boundy, S.S. and Reynolds, N.J., eds.: *Current Concepts in Dental Hygiene*. St. Louis, The C.V. Mosby Co., 1977, pp. 183–194.

Knowles, J., Burgett, F., Morrison, E., Nissle, R., and Ramfjord, S.: Comparison of Results Following Three Modalities of Periodontal Therapy Related to Tooth Type and Initial Pocket Depth, *J. Clin. Periodontol.*, *7*, 32, February, 1980.

Oshrain, H.I., Salkind, A., and Mandel, I.D.: Bacteriologic Studies of Periodontal Pockets Ten Minutes After Curettage, *J. Periodontol.*, *43*, 685, November, 1972.

Pattison, G.L. and Pattison, A.M.: *Periodontal Instrumentation*. Reston, Virginia, Reston Publishing Co., 1979, pp. 351–363.

Ramfjord, S.P.: Root Planing and Curettage, *Int. Dent. J.*, *30*, 93, June, 1980.

Ramfjord, S.P. and Ash, M.M.: *Periodontology and Periodontics*. Philadelphia, W.B. Saunders Co., 1979, pp. 521–541.

Ramfjord, S.P., Knowles, J.W., Nissle, R.R., Burgett, F.G., and Shick, R.A.: Results Following Three Modalities of Periodontal Therapy, *J. Periodontol.*, *46*, 522, September, 1975.

Schluger, S., Yuodelis, R.A., and Page, R.C.: *Periodontal Disease*. Philadelphia, Lea & Febiger, 1977, pp. 380–384.

Stahl, S.S., Weiner, J.M., Benjamin, S., and Yamada, L.: Soft Tissue Healing Following Curettage and Root Planing, *J. Periodontol.*, *42*, 678, November, 1971.

Stone, S. and Kalis, P.J.: Periodontics, in Dunn, M.J., ed.: *Dental Auxiliary Practice*, Module 6. Baltimore, Williams & Wilkins, 1975, pp. 187–194.

Tandy, R.B.: Gingival Curettage, Literature Review, *Periodont. Abstr.*, *18*, 100, June, 1970.

35
Treatment of Acute Gingival Conditions

The dental hygienist frequently participates in clinical treatment procedures for acute gingival lesions. The dentist determines the diagnosis and treatment plan and supervises and directs the instruction and clinical techniques to be carried out.

NECROTIZING ULCERATIVE GINGIVITIS

Necrotizing ulcerative gingivitis (NUG), as the name suggests, is an acute inflammatory, destructive disease of the periodontium. It is commonly referred to as "ANUG," which means acute necrotizing ulcerative gingivitis.

When the condition is superimposed over existing periodontitis, or when with recurrent attacks of the disease, there is bone loss and other symptoms of periodontitis, it should then be called necrotizing ulcerative periodontitis (NUP).[1] Other names that have been used include trench mouth, Vincent's Infection, Vincent's Disease, and ulceromembranous gingivitis.

Although NUG may occur at any age, the majority of cases are seen among young people between ages 15 and 30. It is rare in children under 10 years in the United States, but is not uncommon in young children from low socioeconomic groups studied in South America.[2] Malnutrition and lowered resistance to infection are significant predisposing factors. Individuals with Down's Syndrome have been shown to have an increased incidence of NUG, as described on page 736.

I. Clinical Recognition

A. Initial Signs and Symptoms

The patient reports
1. Sudden onset.
2. Pain and soreness caused by slight pressure such as during chewing and toothbrushing; may be intensified by hot or highly seasoned foods. Gentle probing may produce an exaggerated pain response.
3. Bleeding: spontaneous or on slight pressure.
4. Poor appetite.
5. Metallic or other unpleasant taste.

B. Characteristic Clinical Findings

1. Interdental necrosis with ulceration of the papillae. Crater-like defects in the col area result. In early disease, only the tips of papillae are involved, followed by progressive destruction of the entire papillae and extension to the marginal gingiva facially and lingually.
2. Pseudomembrane. A gray, loose, necrotic slough forms over the necrotic area. When it is wiped off, red and shiny hemorrhagic gingiva is exposed.
3. The membranous ulceration may be seen locally, that is, between two or three

teeth, or it may be generalized throughout both maxillary and mandibular arches.

C. Other Clinical Findings

The following usually accompany the characteristic signs and symptoms:
1. Debris, materia alba, and plaque collect profusely because the patient avoids brushing the sensitive teeth and gingiva.
2. Fetor oris (bad breath) is often severe. It is caused by necrotic tissue, stagnant saliva, and breakdown products of blood and debris.
3. Increased salivation.

D. Systemic Signs

An occasional patient will have apparent systemic involvement. Examination should always be made to detect the presence of the following:
1. Malaise.
2. Adenopathy of submaxillary and cervical nodes.
3. Possible slight elevation of body temperature.[3]

II. Predisposing Factors

A specific cause has not been determined, but certain predisposing factors are usually associated. When the condition occurs, local factors, stress factors, and factors related to general health and resistance to disease are involved.

A. Local Factors

NUG is rarely, if ever, seen in a clean, healthy, cared-for, and professionally supervised mouth. Many of the factors that can be considered predisposing are the same as those that predispose to chronic marginal gingivitis.

Predisposing factors include
1. Preexisting gingivitis and/or periodontitis.
2. Inadequate personal oral care with general neglect.
3. Tobacco smoking.
4. Factors related to retention of microorganisms and deposits.
   a. Calculus as a retainer for plaque and debris.
   b. Open contacts encourage food impaction and stagnation.
   c. Oral habits, for example, mouth breathing.
   d. Periodontal pockets retain microorganisms and debris.
   e. Malposition of teeth; overcrowding.
   f. Iatrogenic causes: overhanging fillings.
   g. Tissue flap, for example, over a partially erupted third mandibular molar.
   h. Open carious lesions.

B. Stress Factors

1. Acute anxiety related to life situations is a common characteristic of patients with NUG. In susceptible people, the condition has been found to occur or recur during periods of stress. Examples include students during examination periods, military men in combat, and people at times of important decision-making.
2. Emotional stress is frequently accompanied by poor oral care, improper diet, excessive smoking, overexertion with interrupted sleep, and other deviations in health habits.

C. Systemic: Disease-resistance Factors

1. Dietary and nutritional inadequacies; vitamin deficiencies.
2. Recent illnesses; frequent upper respiratory infections; debilitating diseases such as infectious mononucleosis, pernicious anemia, or hepatitis.
3. Fatigue; insufficient sleep.

III. Etiology

Bacteriologic and immunologic factors are implicated. For many years, bacteriologic smears were made from the NUG lesion and examined by microscope for the presence of fusiform bacilli and spirochetes. It is now realized that the smear test is not significant when making a diagnosis.

NUG has not been identified as a communicable disease. Research has shown that a transfer of organisms from an infected patient does not produce the typical disease.

IV. Course of Development

A. Description of the Lesion

1. NUG is superimposed over gingivitis or periodontitis.
2. Ulceration and necrosis begin in the col area.
3. Both epithelial tissue and connective tissue are involved.
4. The disease process progresses to involve the entire papilla, and eventually, to the marginal gingiva on the facial and lingual.
5. The pseudomembrane covering the lesion is a necrotic slough of the surface epithelium. It contains leukocytes, bacteria, epithelial cells, and fibrin.
6. Connective tissue shows the signs of acute inflammation. It is hyperemic and filled with leukocytes, and its capillaries are engorged. When the pseudomembrane is lifted, the red inflamed connective tissue can be seen.

B. Microscopic Examination

There are four layers in the lesion which have been described from observations made by electron microscopy.[4] All layers contain spirochetes.

1. *Bacterial Zone.* The most superficial zone consists primarily of a mass of varied bacteria, including a few spirochetes.
2. *Neutrophil-rich Zone.* Under the bacterial zone is a layer of leukocytes, predominantly neutrophils. Microorganisms, including many spirochetes, are found among the leukocytes.
3. *Necrotic Zone.* This zone contains disintegrating tissue cells, many spirochetes, and other bacteria.
4. *Spirochetal Infiltration Zone.* In this non-necrotized layer where tissue components are still preserved, spirochetes have invaded, but other microorganisms have not. In other forms of gingival diseases it is unusual for bacteria to be found within tissues. The action of toxins and other bacterial products was described with pocket formation on pages 202–204.

TREATMENT

Patient instruction and motivation for self-care are needed along with skillful subgingival instrumentation. After the initial symptoms have subsided, complete therapy must be carried out. The tissue destruction usually has left the gingiva deformed, with interdental flattening or cratering. Surgical treatment may be needed to restore a physiologic form that can be maintained by the patient in the plan to prevent recurrence of the disease.

I. Preparation for Diagnosis

Initially, certain data must be collected for use by the dentist in making the diagnosis and treatment plan. To prepare a complete diagnostic work-up may be impractical, considering the emergency nature of the patient's condition. Basic information needed is suggested by the steps described here.

A. History

1. Describe the chief complaint. The history of the current disease is recorded by date of onset, duration, symptoms as described, and what self-treatment the patient had already performed.
2. Record whether this is a recurrence and, if so, note details of previous episodes with the treatment given.
3. Obtain information needed for preliminary treatment.
   a. Conditions needing medical consultation.
   b. Need for premedication for prevention of bacteremia (see the list on pages 99–100).
   c. Allergies.
4. Use knowledge of predisposing factors in NUG to gather pertinent information.
   a. Tobacco smoking habits.
   b. Recent illnesses or types of therapy may explain a lowered resistance.
   c. Dietary habits: record immediately previous 24-hour food intake. When the mouth has been sore and it has been painful to eat, a diet recording may not be typical of the patient's usual intake. Later a 5-day or weeklong diet diary will be requested as part of the continuing preventive program.
   d. Sleeping hours: variations of normal routine.

B. Examination

1. Record the patient's temperature.
2. Extraoral examination.
   a. Palpate submaxillary and cervical nodes (figure 8–6, page 120).
   b. Observe face and skin: flushed, damp.
   c. Observe signs of malaise.
3. Oral examination. Without instrumentation, the dental hygienist can make a preliminary examination and record the overall appearance of the gingival tissue. The dentist may prefer to see the gingiva as it appeared initially, before instrumentation or rinsing, in order to make the diagnosis and prepare the treatment plan. Instrumentation may be temporarily delayed for patients requiring premedication.

II. Treatment Plan

The dental hygiene treatment plan is formulated within the total treatment plan. Only a partial treatment plan is made until after the acute phase of the disease has passed. After the initial treatment, the diagnostic work-up can be completed and full evaluation made.

A. Systemic Treatment

1. Directions concerning diet, rest, and other systemic influences.
2. Multivitamin supplements are sometimes prescribed.
3. Antibiotics. After the diagnosis is made, the dentist will indicate whether systemic therapy is required. Except for those requiring antibiotic coverage for instrumentation to prevent bacteremia, antibiotics are prescribed conservatively.

B. Relief of Acute Symptoms

1. Personal care instruction for rinsing, brushing, smoking limitation.
2. Debridement of teeth and gingiva.
3. Subgingival scaling and root planing.

C. Basic Therapy

1. Complete diagnostic work-up.
2. Reevaluation and preparation of total treatment plan.

3. Preventive program.
   a. Instruction for prevention of recurrence of NUG.
   b. Dietary analysis and counseling.
   c. Self-care fluoride; professional application when indicated.
4. Complete scaling and root planing.
5. Reduction or elimination of predisposing factors to NUG.
   a. Removal of overhanging margins and other retention factors.
   b. Restoration of teeth and contact areas.
6. Evaluation for periodontal surgery: need for restoration of tissue contour and elimination of craters.
7. Restoration of occlusion; prosthetic replacements and all other dental needs.

DENTAL HYGIENE CARE

A series of appointments for a typical NUG patient is outlined here. The number of appointments and the exact procedure at each appointment will depend on the severity of the disease and the response of the gingiva as treatment progresses.

Usually four or five appointments will be needed during the acute stage, and at least the first three should be at 24-hour intervals. After that, when the acute stage has subsided, a regular appointment is established for continued supervision and for proceeding with basic therapy.

I. Acute Phase: First Appointment

The first part of this appointment has been described under *History* on page 537. After the dentist has examined the patient and made the diagnosis, the dental hygienist will be directed to follow a procedure such as the following:

A. History Review

Check the history for a patient requiring prophylactic premedication for prevention of bacteremia, and arrange accordingly. Parenteral administration may be indicated which should be discussed with the patient's physician.

B. Patient Instruction

1. Explain local causes and control measures.

2. Demonstrate plaque with a disclosing agent.
3. Show plaque removal procedures using a soft brush moistened with warm water.

C. General Debridement

1. Apply hydrogen peroxide (3% solution with equal parts of water) with cotton pellets at proximal areas; spray with water, and request patient to rinse.
2. Apply topical anesthetic and when painful, treat by quadrants, using block anesthesia.
3. Supragingival instrumentation. Use ultrasonic or manual scaling instruments or a combination for scaling. Use warm water for frequent irrigation while scaling. When time is limited, more time should be spent on calculus at the gingival margin and in the subgingival areas. Supragingival calculus, which does not contact the gingival margin, can be left for future appointments since it does not immediately influence gingival healing.

D. Subgingival Instrumentation

The gingiva will respond sooner if subgingival scaling and curettage can be started at the first visit.

1. Perform instrumentation carefully to prevent tissue damage.
2. Irrigate and evacuate frequently to clear all debris and diseased tissue removed by curettage.

E. Patient Instruction

1. Instructions for home procedures must be carefully explained. Written directions are needed.
2. Inform the patient that treatment will not be complete when the pain is eliminated. Explain the underlying gingival or periodontal disease and how NUG recurs if the periodontal condition is not treated.
3. Rinsing directions. Vigorous rinsing with hot weak salt water (page 374) (hydrogen peroxide 3% with equal parts water is preferred by some dentists) is necessary every hour for 5 minutes during the period of acute symptoms.

4. Toothbrushing. Use a soft nylon brush (.006 inch filament) gently, but thoroughly. Clean the teeth as much as possible after each meal and before going to bed. When a brush is not given the patient at the clinic or office, write down the names of specific brushes for the patient to purchase.
5. Avoid smoking tobacco. The heavy smoker can be asked to limit the amount.
6. Diet[5]
   a. Recommend frequent small nutritious meals that incorporate daily requirements from the Basic 4 (table 28–1, page 424).
   b. A liquid diet is advised for the first day, particularly for the patient with systemic symptoms or pronounced sensitivity when chewing. A semi-liquid or soft solids diet can be used on the second day. Examples of foods to include in a liquid and a soft solid diet are listed on pages 668–669.
   c. Increased nutrients should be used from the milk and meat food groups, and fruits and juices containing vitamin C.
   d. Avoid highly seasoned foods and alcoholic beverages.

II. Acute Phase: Second Appointment

A. Patient Examination

In 24 hours it is usual to see a remarkable improvement. It would be expected that the pain and discomfort would have subsided, the pseudomembrane would have disappeared, and the tissue swelling would have been reduced.

B. Scaling and Root Planing

Continue from previous appointment after checking areas previously treated. The objective is to be as thorough as possible, since plaque retained over residual calculus and altered cementum can keep the tissues from complete healing.

C. Instruction: Second Day

1. *Rinsing.* When healing is progressing favorably, change rinsing schedule to every 2 hours.

2. *Toothbrushing.* Emphasize thorough coverage of the entire dentition, using sulcular brushing.
3. *Proximal Surfaces.* The use of floss is advised and demonstrated at this or the third appointment, depending on the readiness of the patient and the tissues. Other proximal cleaning devices may be useful. When the interdental embrasures are open as a result of papillary necrosis, an interdental brush or other device is usually indicated. The importance of complete plaque removal must be explained.
4. *Diet.* A liquid diet is not usually indicated after the first day and the patient can use the soft solids diet or a regular diet adapted with bland foods that will not irritate the healing tissues.
5. *Instructions.* Provide specific written instructions.

III. Acute Phase: Third Appointment

A. Observe and Evaluate the Gingival Tissues

Continued improvement should be expected each day. Areas where healing has not progressed will need additional personal plaque control, scaling, and root planing.

B. Instruction in Self-care Procedures

Instructions are continued. Follow Lesson I or Lesson II (pages 413–414), depending on the extent of previous instruction.

C. Scaling and Root Planing

Treatment is continued, with particular attention to areas where healing has not been complete.

D. Home Care Instruction

1. *Rinsing.* Discontinue peroxide if that was the selected rinse. Request the patient to use warm mild saline solution vigorously after brushing and flossing.
2. *Review Instructions.* Review and emphasize previous instruction.

IV. Successive Appointments

After daily supervision during the acute stage, regular appointments for basic treatment are planned. The gingiva is evaluated, and repeated scaling and root planing, performed as needed to complete that part of the treatment.

A. Preparation of a Diagnostic Work-up

The complete diagnostic work-up is prepared as directed by the dentist, and the patient instructed for continued treatment.

B. Recurrence of NUG

When the gingival and bony craters that remain after the initial healing phase are not treated, they are vulnerable to continuing disease and recurrence of NUG. Plaque and debris can collect readily in the misshapen proximal areas, and the areas are difficult to clean with plaque control techniques. Gingival craters invite further tissue breakdown, leading to periodontal pocket formation.

Surgical treatment may involve gingivoplasty when the bone is not involved. When bony craters exist, treatment may involve flap surgery with osseous reshaping.

PERIODONTAL ABSCESS

An abscess is a collection of pus in a circumscribed or walled-off area. Gingival and periodontal abscesses occur within the peridontal tissues. An abscess is called *gingival* when it is located in the marginal area, and *periodontal* when it is in the deeper periodontal tissues. They may also be known as *lateral abscesses* because they occur along the lateral surfaces of a tooth, which is in contrast to a periapical abscess which is usually associated with the apex.

I. Development of a Periodontal Abscess

Pus collects in the tissue as a result of bacterial infection. The infection may be a complication of an already existing periodontal disease or it may be an immediate result of purulent microorganisms forced into the tissue by some form of trauma. The body's reaction is to send large numbers of defense cells to the area, particularly polymorphonuclear leukocytes (PMNs), which are the major constituents of the purulent exudate (pus) that collects.

Pus is a thick fluid product of inflammation. It contains many living and dead PMNs mixed with debris from cells and tissues that have been destroyed by the enzymes released by the PMNs. Unless there is a means for drainage, the pus collects and forms an abscess.

A sinus or fistula may form. A fistula is a pathologic sinus or abnormal passage that leads from an abscess to the surface of the gingiva or mucosa. Drainage may occur through the sinus and release the pressure within the abscess, which in turn, can relieve the pain the patient may be experiencing.

II. Etiologic Factors

A. Periodontal Pockets

Deep pockets of chronic inflammatory periodontal disease provide an environment for abscess formation. Special anatomic variations predispose to abscess formation. Instrumentation applied within the pocket and the effects of the instrumentation may be the precipitating factors that initiate abscess formation.

1. *Anatomic Features.* Intrabony pockets, pockets that extend into bi- or trifurcation areas, and complex pockets that develop in winding or irregular shapes, are particularly susceptible to becoming closed and therefore susceptible to abscess formation.
2. *Instrumentation.*[6] Incomplete scaling and root planing in the depth of a pocket may allow the tissue at the opening of the pocket to heal, tighten, and prevent drainage from the infectious material deep in the pocket. Plaque and calculus remaining in the sealed off part of the pocket attract the collection of more PMNs, and an abscess develops.

B. Trauma

Foreign objects may enter by way of the sulcus or pocket and become embedded along with microorganisms. The infection leads to abscess formation.

1. *Implanted or Impacted Material*[7]
   a. Popcorn husk, small fish bone or shellfish fragment, seeds, seed coverings, or other material from food.
   b. Oral hygiene devices include toothbrush bristle or filament, or a sliver from a toothpick.

2. *Instrumentation.* Trauma during subgingival instrumentation may force infectious material into the pocket wall.

C. Patient Susceptibility to Infection

The possibility for abscess formation within the gingival tissue is increased from any of the etiologic factors mentioned above when the patient's resistance to infection is lowered. A patient with uncontrolled diabetes or one who is receiving immunosuppressive medication are examples.

III. Clinical Signs and Symptoms

Although variable, classic signs and symptoms are listed here.

A. Clinical Appearance

The area of the abscess is enlarged, with a red, shiny, smooth surface. It may appear dome-like or pointed, and on slight digital pressure, pus may appear.

B. The Tooth

1. *Sensitivity.* The tooth may be sensitive to percussion. When it is extruded, it may be sensitive to touching the tooth in the opposing jaw. It may have slight mobility.
2. *Pulp Vitality Test.* Pulp testing will usually reveal a vital tooth, responding at normal levels.
3. *Radiographs.* Radiographically, there may be a radiolucency along the lateral wall of the tooth, but such a finding is variable. The early lesion will show no bone loss. The amount of bone destruction and the location of the abscess will influence the possible radiographic finding.

C. General Physical Condition

Occasionally, a patient will have evidence of systemic involvement. There may be a slight elevation in body temperature, malaise, and adenopathy.

D. Chronic Abscess

In the chronic state, there is usually a sinus tract that opens on the gingival surface and drains periodically. Before drainage, there may be a dull pain from pressure of the fluid within the abscess area. Acute symptoms may be expected from time to time unless definitive periodontal therapy is completed.

IV. Comparison of Periapical and Periodontal Abscesses

Differentiation between a periapical and a periodontal abscess must frequently be made by the dentist during diagnosis. Certain signs and symptoms are nearly the same for both. A few of the potentially distinguishing findings are noted here.

A. Pulp Test

The tooth with a periapical lesion will not respond normally to a pulp tester.

B. Sinus Tract Formation

The opening from a sinus tract from a periapical abscess will usually be positioned more apically, whereas the opening from a periodontal abscess will be more coronal.

C. Pain

Sharp steady pain is typical of a periapical lesion, whereas the pain from a periodontal abscess varies.

D. Periodontal Examination

A tooth with a periapical lesion is not necessarily periodontally involved. Probing may reveal no pocket depth of note, and there may be no bone loss in the radiograph.

Occasionally, there may be a combined periodontic and endodontic lesion. Communication between a deep periodontal pocket and an apical lesion is not unusual. There also may be communication from a periodontal pocket into the pulp by way of a lateral or accessory canal through the dentin.

E. Dental Caries

A diseased pulp leading to a periapical abscess is caused by either trauma to the tooth or dental caries extending inward until the pulp becomes infected. A carious lesion may also be present when there is a periodontal abscess, which may complicate the differential diagnosis.

F. Radiographic Examination

Early stages of either a periapical or a periodontal abscess will not be evident in a radiograph. A thickening of the periodontal ligament space may appear.

V. Treatment

There are two phases of treatment for the patient with a periodontal abscess. The first is for immediate relief of acute symptoms, and the second is the definitive treatment followed by preventive maintenance. The entire plan should be explained to the patient at the outset.

A. Objectives of Emergency Treatment

1. Relieve pain.
2. Establish drainage.
3. Determine need for systemic antibiotic therapy.

B. Review Medical History

Determine necessary preappointment precautions such as the need for antibiotic premedication (pages 99–100).

C. Examination for Systemic Involvement

Antibiotic medication is frequently prescribed by the dentist when there is definite systemic involvement.
1. Determine and record the patient's body temperature (pages 103–104).
2. Examine submaxillary and neck lymph nodes for adenopathy.

D. Provide Anesthesia

When the abscess is confined to the gingival area, and the drainage may be expected to cause little if any discomfort, a topical anesthetic may suffice.[8] Usually, block anesthesia is indicated.

E. Methods for Drainage

1. *Via Pocket or Sulcus Opening.* Isolate the area, swab with a topical antiseptic, and use a probe to gain admission into the sulcus or pocket. Gently probe circumferentially until an opening into the abscess is found. Drainage usually begins promptly.

   Use a curet to open the area and locate and remove a foreign body irritant when known to be present from the history obtained from the patient. Scaling, root planing, and gingival curettage are performed as needed.

2. *Direct Incision.* The type of incision varies. A horizontal or semilunar incision may be made directly over the abscess.[9,10] A vertical incision from the abscess straight to the gingival margin has also been used.[8,11] A drain may be needed to keep the incision open long enough for complete drainage. Either a piece of rubber dam or iodophor gauze may be used.

All incisions should be avoided, if possible, to prevent gingival recession from a vertical incision, unsightly scars from any type of incision, or complications during healing.

F. Postoperative Instructions

Rinsing with hot saline solution every 2 hours is advised. The patient should return for observation in 24 to 48 hours. Relief from pain and discomfort can be expected and appointments for definitive treatment planned. Plaque control instruction is initiated or continued, and scaling and root planing completed.

G. Anticipated Results

1. Acute symptoms resolved.
2. Pain relief within a short time following the initiation of drainage, because the pressure is released from within the abscessed area.
3. Extruded tooth returns to its normal position.
4. Swelling is reduced.
5. Temporary comfort for the patient: the lesion is reduced to a standard chronic lesion that requires additional treatment.
6. Incomplete treatment. If drainage is not complete, an acute lesion may develop into a lesion with a chronic sinus.

VI. Definitive Therapy

Whatever pocket elimination procedures are indicated should be completed within a reasonable time to prevent further complications. Careful and regular plaque control with scaling,

root planing, and gingival curettage are usually needed.

TECHNICAL HINTS

I. Provide explicit directions concerning rinsing with hydrogen peroxide. Extended use of oxygenating drugs can cause tissue changes such as chemical trauma, surface necrosis or "burn," and black hairy tongue.[12]

II. Instructions for patients can be printed or written. Since each day during the acute phase the instructions change, individual slips should be prepared using paper of different colors. Printed instructions can be personalized with added written notations.

FACTORS TO TEACH THE PATIENT

I. Premature discontinuation of treatment for NUG because acute signs have subsided can lead to recurrence of the disease.

II. The role of diet, rest, and plaque control in the prevention of NUG.

III. Avoid use of an oral irrigating device in the presence of acute inflammatory conditions.[13] Microorganisms may be forced into the tissues beneath a pocket, and bacteremia can be produced.

References

1. Grant, D.A., Stern, I.B., and Everett, F.G.: *Periodontics*, 5th ed. St. Louis, The C.V. Mosby Co., 1979, pp. 340–358.
2. Jimenez L., M. and Baer, P.N.: Necrotizing Ulcerative Gingivitis in Children: A 9 Year Clinical Study, *J. Periodontol.*, 46, 715, December, 1975.
3. Schluger, S., Yuodelis, R.A., and Page, R.C.: *Periodontal Disease.* Philadelphia, Lea & Febiger, 1977, pp. 243–250.
4. Listgarten, M.A.: Electron Microscopic Observations on the Bacterial Flora of Acute Necrotizing Ulcerative Gingivitis, *J. Periodontol.*, 36, 328, July–August, 1965.
5. Nizel, A.E.: *Nutrition in Preventive Dentistry: Science and Practice*, 2nd ed. Philadelphia, W.B. Saunders Co., 1981, pp. 485–488.
6. Armitage, G.C.: *Biologic Basis of Periodontal Maintenance Therapy.* Berkeley, California, Praxis Publishing Co., 1980, pp. 154–159.
7. Gillette, W.B. and Van House, R.L.: Ill Effects of Improper Oral Hygiene Procedures, *J. Am. Dent. Assoc.*, 101, 476, September, 1980.
8. United States Navy Dental Corps: *Periodontics Syllabus.* Washington, D.C., Superintendent of Documents, United States Government Printing Office, NAVMED P-5110, 1975, p. 156.
9. Grant, Stern, and Everett: op cit., pp. 363–372.

10. Schluger, Yuodelis, and Page: op. cit., pp. 240–242.

11. Carranza, F.A.: *Glickman's Clinical Periodontology*, 5th ed. Philadelphia, W.B. Saunders Co., 1979, pp. 268–274, 688–695.

12. McCarthy, P.L. and Shklar, G.: *Diseases of the Oral Mucosa*, 2nd ed. Philadelphia, Lea & Febiger, 1980, p. 343.

13. American Dental Association, Council on Dental Materials, Instruments and Equipment: *Dentist's Desk Reference: Materials, Instruments and Equipment*, 1st ed. Chicago, American Dental Association, 1981, pp. 342–343.

Suggested Readings

Necrotizing Ulcerative Gingivitis

American Dental Association, Council on Dental Therapeutics: *Accepted Dental Therapeutics*, 39th ed. Chicago, American Dental Association, 1982, p. 50.

Armitage, G.C.: *Biologic Basis of Periodontal Maintenance Therapy*. Berkeley, California, Praxis Publishing Co., 1980, pp. 146–154.

Barnes, G.P., Bowles, W.F., and Carter, H.G.: Acute Necrotizing Ulcerative Gingivitis: A Survey of 218 Cases, *J. Periodontol.*, 44, 35, January, 1973.

Becker, S.L.: Treating ANUG Patients, *Quintessence Int.*, 11, 75, February, 1980.

Brown, R.H.: Necrotizing Ulcerative Gingivitis in Mongoloid and Non-Mongoloid Retarded Individuals, *J. Periodont. Res.*, 8, 290, Number 5, 1973.

Burket, L.W. and Greenberg, M.S.: Diseases Primarily Affecting the Gingivae, in Lynch, M.A., ed.: *Burket's Oral Medicine*, 7th ed., Philadelphia, J.B. Lippincott Co., 1977, pp. 176–182.

Carranza, F.A.: *Glickman's Clinical Periodontology*, 5th ed. Philadelphia, W.B. Saunders Co., 1979, pp. 135–147, 696–706.

Cianco, S.G. and Bourgault, P.C.: *Clinical Pharmacology for Dental Professionals*. New York, McGraw-Hill, 1980, pp. 51–52.

Coslet, R.B.: The Psychogenic Factor in the Etiology of Acute Necrotizing Gingivitis, *Dent. Hyg.*, 53, 257, June, 1979.

Davis, R.K. and Baer, P.N.: Necrotizing Ulcerative Gingivitis in Drug Addict Patients Being Withdrawn from Drugs, *Oral Surg.*, 31, 200, February, 1971.

Dolby, A.E.: Acute Ulcerative Gingivitis: Immune Complex, *J. Dent. Res.*, 51, 1639, November–December, 1972.

Enwonwu, C.O.: Epidemiological and Biochemical Studies of Necrotizing Ulcerative Gingivitis and Noma (Cancrum Oris) in Nigerian Children, *Arch. Oral Biol.*, 17, 1357, September, 1972.

Formicola, A.J., Witte, E.T., and Curran, P.M.: A Study of Personality Traits and Acute Necrotizing Ulcerative Gingivitis, *J. Periodontol.*, 41, 36, January, 1970.

Goldman, H.M. and Cohen, D.W.: *Periodontal Therapy*, 6th ed. St. Louis, The C.V. Mosby Co., 1980, pp. 185–186, 226–238, 774.

Harding, J., Berry, W.C., Marsh, C., and Jolliff, C.R.: Salivary Antibodies in Acute Gingivitis, *J. Periodontol.*, 51, 63, February, 1980.

Hawkins, B.F.: Stress Factor in Necrotizing Ulcerative Gingivitis, *Q. Natl. Dent. Assoc.*, 32, 63, April, 1974.

Hooper, P.A. and Seymour, G.J.: The Histopathogenesis of Acute Ulcerative Gingivitis, *J. Periodontol.*, 50, 419, August, 1979.

Kardachi, B.J.R. and Clarke, N.G.: Aetiology of Acute Necrotising Ulcerative Gingivitis: A Hypothetical Explanation, *J. Periodontol.*, 45, 830, November, 1974.

Lehner, T.: Immunoglobulin Abnormalities in Ulcerative Gingivitis, *Br. Dent. J.*, 127, 165, August 19, 1969.

Listgarten, M.A. and Lewis, D.W.: The Distribution of Spirochetes in the Lesion of Acute Necrotizing Ulcerative Gingivitis: An Electron Microscopic and Statistical Survey, *J. Periodontol.*, 38, 379, September–October, 1967.

Loesche, W.J., Syed, S.A., Laughon, B.E., and Stoll, J.: The Bacteriology of Acute Necrotizing Ulcerative Gingivitis, *J. Periodontol.*, 53, 223, April, 1982.

Meister, F., Rank, D.F.P., and Davies, E.E.: Importance of Patient Motivation in the Treatment of Acute Necrotizing Ulcerative Gingivitis, *Quintessence Int.*, 12, 199, February, 1981.

Page, L.R., Bosman, C.W., Drummond, J.F., and Ciancio, S.G.: Acute Recurrent Gingivitis, *Oral Surg.*, 49, 337, April, 1980.

Ranney, R.R.: Pathogenesis of Periodontal Disease, in *International Conference on Research in the Biology of Periodontal Disease*. Chicago, University of Illinois, June, 1977, pp. 227, 247–250, 306, 402.

Shannon, I.L., Kilgore, W.G., and O'Leary, T.J.: Stress as a Predisposing Factor in Necrotizing Ulcerative Gingivitis, *J. Periodontol.*, 40, 240, April, 1969.

Shields, W.D.: Acute Necrotizing Ulcerative Gingivitis. A Study of Some of the Contributing Factors and Their Validity in an Army Population, *J. Periodontol.*, 48, 346, June, 1977.

Silver, J.G., Southcott, R.J., and Wade, A.B.: Acute Necrotizing Ulcerative Gingivitis—An Evaluation of the Ulcer Improvement Index, *J. Periodontol.*, 45, 308, May, 1974.

Wilton, J.M., Ivanyi, L., and Lehner, T.: Cell-mediated Immunity and Humoral Antibodies in Acute Ulcerative Gingivitis, *J. Periodont. Res.*, 6, 9, Number 1, 1971.

Wirthlin, M.R. and Devine, L.: Venery and Vincent's? 15 Case Reports and Discussion, *J. Periodontol.*, 49, 449, September, 1978.

Periodontal Abscess

Collins, W.J.N., Forrest, J.O., and Walsh, T.F.: *A Handbook for Dental Hygienists*. Bristol, England, John Wright, 1978, pp. 180–181.

Epstein, S. and Scopp, I.W.: Antibiotics and the Intraoral Abscess, *J. Periodontol.*, 48, 236, April, 1977.

Goldman, H.M. and Cohen, D.W.: *Periodontal Therapy*, 6th ed. St. Louis, The C.V. Mosby Co., 1980, pp. 307–308, 744–745, 1018–1019.

Miyasato, M.C.: The Periodontal Abscess, *Periodont. Abstr.*, 23, 53, Summer, 1975.

Ranney, R.R.: Pathogenesis of Periodontal Disease, in *International Conference on Research in the Biology of Periodontal Disease*. Chicago, University of Illinois, June, 1977, pp. 227, 247.

36

Periodontal Dressings and Sutures

A periodontal dressing may be placed over the surgical wound following periodontal surgery. A dressing is frequently indicated after gingival curettage.

I. Purposes and Uses

A. Provide mechanical protection for the surgical wound and therefore facilitate healing.
B. Prevent postoperative bleeding by maintaining the initial clot in place.
C. Support mobile teeth during healing.
D. Aid in shaping or molding the newly formed tissues; aid in holding a flap in place or immobilizing a graft.
E. Provide patient comfort during the healing period by isolating the wound from external irritations and injuries.

II. Characteristics of an Acceptable Dressing

An acceptable periodontal dressing should have the following characteristics:
A. Have no risk for dental team member or patient.
B. Be nontoxic and nonirritating to oral tissues.
C. Not contain asbestos or other ingredient that may be injurious to the health of the person who prepares the dressing.
D. Is conveniently prepared, placed, and removed with minimal discomfort for the patient.
E. Be able to maintain adhesion to itself and to the teeth and tissue where it is placed.
F. Should not damage or stain restorative materials with which it may have oral contact.

III. Types of Dressings

Dressings are usually classified into two groups: eugenol-containing and those without eugenol. Healing has been shown to progress at about the same rate under either dressing, so selection by the dentist can be based on such factors as firmness of the material, durability, consistency, ease of manipulation, or personal preference.

A. Eugenol-containing

1. *Basic Ingredients*
   a. Powder: zinc oxide, powdered rosin, and tannic acid. Formerly, asbestos fiber was used as a binder in some formulae. Since airborne asbestos is a recognized pulmonary health hazard, dental team members responsible for mixing periodontal dressings frequently and in quantity may become over-exposed. Asbestos fiber is no longer an acceptable ingredient of dressings.[1,2]
   b. Liquid: eugenol, with an oil such as peanut or cottonseed, and thymol.

545

2. *Examples.* Well-known dressings are Ward's (Wonderpack), Periodontal Dressing Powder and Liquid ("PPC"), and Kirkland. Formulae for the last two are given below as examples of the ingredients and their proportions.[1]

    a. Kirkland Periodontal Pack
       Powder: each 100 grams contains

Zinc oxide	40.00 g.
Rosin	40.00 g.
Tannic acid	20.00 g.

       Liquid: each 100 milliliters contains

Eugenol	46.5 ml.
Peanut oil	46.5 ml.
Rosin	7.7 g.

    b. Periodontal Dressing Powder and Liquid ("PPC")
       Powder: each 100 grams contains

Zinc oxide	42.9 g.
Powdered rosin	38.1 g.
Tannic acid	9.5 g.
Kaolin	2.4 g.
Mica	7.1 g.

       Liquid: each 100 milliliters contains

Eugenol	98.0 ml.
Thymol	2.0 g.
Color	

B. Non-Eugenol-containing

Eugenol has an unpleasant, sharp taste, and can be irritating to the mucous membrane. Over the years, in search for a substitute for eugenol, other formulae have been developed. Other ingredients such as antibiotics that would provide bacteriostatic effects have been tried.

1. *Hydrogenated Fat Dressing.*[3] The powder contains zinc oxide and rosin powder to which may be added bacitracin. The powder is mixed with an ointment containing zinc oxide with hydrogenated fat. It is mixed to a putty-like consistency and may be stored by wrapping in foil and refrigerating.

2. *Coe-Pak.* Prepared by mixing pastes from two tubes: one containing metallic oxides with a fungicide and the other non-ionizing carboxylic acids with a germicide-fungicide. It sets within a few minutes and cannot be prepared in advance.

When it is desirable to have a firmer dressing, some powder from a eugenol-containing dressing can be added to the Coe-Pak during mixing.

CLINICAL APPLICATION

I. Eugenol-containing Dressing

A. Mixing

1. Mix powder and liquid on a paper mixing pad, incorporating the powder gradually to form a thick paste. Use a metal spatula or wooden tongue depressor.

2. Knead additional powder into the paste with the fingers until the consistency is firm and thick, but not sticky. (Orange solvent will aid in cleaning the hands afterwards, but wearing rubber gloves is recommended.)

3. Divide the mass into quantities appropriate for application to a quadrant or other specific area. Wrap pieces in foil or waxed paper for storage in freezer.

B. Application

1. Roll the mixed dressing into a round strip.

2. Examine area to be sure bleeding has stopped.

3. Quadrant application: apply continuous (one strip) from lingual to facial; or two strips may be used to cover a quadrant, the first to extend from the distal of the most posterior tooth over the facial surfaces, and the second to overlap the first on the distal and extend along the lingual.

4. Moisten the fingers with water or dip the fingers in dressing powder to prevent sticking during application.

5. Press at the interproximal areas to gain retention and provide complete coverage for the treatment area. Adapt with a plastic instrument.

6. Edentulous areas can usually be filled to make the dressing continuous between the teeth unless too great a gap exists.

7. Muscle trim (border mold) the cheeks, lips, and tongue to prevent movement or dislodgment of the dressing.

8. Check frena for freedom of movement.
    a. Lingual: request patient to touch palate with tip of tongue.

b. Buccal: retract cheek up and out over maxillary premolars and out from mandibular premolars.

c. Anterior: retract upper lip up and out over maxillary central incisors and retract lower lip out and up for mandibular midline frenum.

d. Adjust dressing by rolling and folding back the border, unless there is gross excess, which should be removed.

9. Check the occlusion: the dressing should extend only to the height of the contour of the teeth and should not be in occlusal contact during closure.

10. Variation for open interproximal embrasures with missing papillae and recession: use small sections of dressing to mold into wedge shapes to press interproximally from facial and from lingual. It is very important that the proximal gingiva be completely and firmly covered. A strip of dressing can then be added facially and lingually for complete coverage.

II. Non-Eugenol Dressing (Coe-Pak)

A. Mixing

1. Place equal lengths of material from each tube beside each other (but not touching) on the mixing pad. Prepare only the amount needed, which can be readily estimated after a few experiences.

2. Since working time is relatively brief, prepare the patient by stabilizing the head and placing a gauze sponge over the area that will receive the dressing. Request the patient to close.

3. Mix the two pastes together quickly until the colors are blended and neither color is perceptible separately. Mix over a small area, not across width of pad.

4. When mixing is complete, gather the material together with the spatula and place on the edge of a tongue depressor. If using a metal spatula, wipe it clean promptly, before dressing hardens.

B. Application

1. After one minute, touch the mixture with a finger coated with petroleum jelly. As soon as the mixture feels warm, it usually can be managed and should be placed promptly. Coat the fingers with a thin layer of petroleum jelly or use water.

2. Roll the dressing into a strip the approximate length and thickness needed for the specific area. Application of excess material should be avoided since removal of the excess is unnecessarily time-consuming and awkward.

3. Apply in a continuous piece: for a quadrant, place center of the roll at the posterior surface of the most posterior tooth and bring around to facial and lingual. Press the dressing at the interproximal areas (lingual and facial can be done simultaneously).

4. Mold the dressing into place to the height of contour, and border mold to prevent displacement by the tongue, cheeks, lips. Check frena (I.,B.,8. above).

5. Check the occlusion: patient may feel the excess, or teeth prints will show the location. When excess dressing is removed, use a cutting motion with a plastic instrument or scaler. Do not pull on a section of the dressing as the whole dressing is very cohesive and can be dislodged in one piece.

III. Characteristics of a Well-Placed Dressing

Dressings must be placed in keeping with biologic principles, which will contribute to healing and yet be tolerated by the patient. A satisfactory dressing has the following characteristics:

A. Is secure and rigid. A movable dressing is an irritant and can promote hemorrhage.

B. Has as little bulk as possible, yet is bulky enough to give strength.

C. Is locked mechanically interdentally and cannot be displaced by action of tongue, cheek, or lips.

D. Covers all of the surgical wound without unnecessary overextension.

E. Fills interdental area to cover the surgerized area and discourage food retention.

IV. Patient Dismissal and Instructions

A. Patient must not be dismissed until bleeding or oozing from under dressing has ceased.

B. Written instructions are more effective than verbal. Table 36–1 lists items for which instructions should be given to a patient who has a periodontal dressing. Printed instructions can be prepared from these items. Other instructions for the patient after general oral surgery or tooth removal may be found on page 661.

Table 36–1.   Instructions for Postoperative Care

Factor	Instructions to Patient	Purpose of Instruction
Information about the Dressing	Dressing to protect the surgery and to help it heal Do not disturb it; keep it on until the next appointment	Understanding and cooperation by the patient
Care During the First Few Hours	Dressing will not be hard for a few hours. Do not eat anything that requires chewing Use only cool liquids Keep quiet; get rest	Dressing must harden and be undisturbed
Anesthesia	Be careful not to bite the lip or cheek Avoid foods that require chewing until the anesthesia has worn off	Prevent trauma to lip or cheek
Discomfort After the Anesthesia Wears Off	When a prescription is given, have the prescription filled and follow the directions for taking the medication; do not take more than directed	Pain control
Ice Pack or Cold Compress	Use as directed only Apply every 30 minutes for 15 minutes; or 30 minutes on and 30 minutes off	Prevent swelling from edema
Bleeding	Slight temporary bleeding within the first few hours is not unusual Do not suck on the area or use straws. The blood clot should be left undisturbed Persistent or excessive bleeding should be reported to the dentist for treatment as indicated	Alleviate patient alarm over small amount of bleeding, but assure patient of help as needed
Dressing Care and Retention	Avoid pressing the dressing with the tongue or trying to clean under it Small particles may chip off during the week: no problem, unless the sharp edge bothers the tongue or the dressing seems to have loosened Call the dentist if the whole dressing or a large portion of it falls off before the fifth day: it should be replaced. If after the fifth day, call for an early replacement appointment when area is unusually sensitive: otherwise rinse with saline solution and cover the area with white petrolatum	Dressing needed for wound protection Epithelium covers wound by fifth day in normal healing
Smoking	Do not smoke A heavy smoker should make every effort to decrease quantity of tobacco used	Heat and smoke irritate the gingiva and delay healing

Table 36–1. *continued*

Factor	Instructions to Patient	Purpose of Instruction
Rinsing	Do not rinse on the day of the surgery Second day: use saline solution made with one-half teaspoon (measured) in one-half glass of warm water every 2 to 3 hours Third and subsequent days: use the saline solution or a pleasant tasting mouthrinse diluted one-third mouthrinse to two-thirds water	Might disturb clot Saline may aid healing Pleasant flavored mouthrinse may reduce mouth odors from debris on the dressing
Toothbrushing and Flossing	Use better-than-usual brushing and flossing on unoperated areas Brush occlusal surface over dressing Use soft brush with water carefully on surface of dressing to clean off debris and film Brush the tongue	Plaque control Oral sanitation Odor and taste control Reduce number of oral microorganisms
Eating	Highly nutritious food is needed during healing. Check the Basic 4 Use soft-textured diet Omit foods that are highly seasoned, spicy, hot Avoid sticky, crunchy or coarse foods that could break the dressing	Healing Protect the dressing from breakage or displacement
Mastication	Avoid foods that require excessive chewing. Use ground meat, or cut meat into small pieces Chew only on unoperated side Take small bite-sized pieces at a time	Dressing protection

V. Dressing Removal

During healing, epithelium will cover a wound in 6 days and complete restoration of epithelium and connective tissue can be expected by 21 days. The dressing may be left in place from 7 to 10 days as predetermined by the dentist.

When the dressing breaks or falls off before the appointed time for removal, it usually should be replaced rather than patched because the remaining segment is generally loose.

A. Patient Examination

1. Question patient and record postoperative effects or discomfort. When part or all of the dressing was broken off, record its duration.
2. Examine mucosa about the dressing and record appearance.

B. Procedure for Removal

1. Insert a large scaler, hoe, or plastic instrument under the border of the dressing (coronal or apical border or both); apply lateral pressure.
2. Watch for sutures that may be caught in the dressing. They may need to be cut for release. Use principles for suture removal as on pages 551–553.
3. Remove pieces of dressing gently with cotton pliers to avoid scratching the thin epithelial covering of the healing tissue with the rough edges of dressing.
4. Observe tissue condition and record appearance. Note any deviations from the normal healing expected in the length of time since the treatment.
5. Use a scaler for removal of pieces attached to tooth surfaces; use curet for particles near the gingival margin. Some root planing may be indicated, and all calculus and roughness should be eliminated to prevent plaque retention.
6. Syringe with a gentle stream of *warm* water, and provide *warm* diluted mouthrinse for the patient's comfort.

C. Plaque Control Follow-up

Plaque control follow-up is essential after dressing removal.

1. Use a soft brush (.006 inch filaments) on treated area with careful attention to plaque removal at the gingival margin. Use usual methods for all other areas of the mouth.
2. Increase intensity of care on the treated area each day, with a return to complete procedures by 3 or 4 days.
3. Rinse with warm mild saline solution, forcing the liquid between the teeth, to encourage healing.
4. When teeth are sensitive, a fluoride dentifrice containing monofluorophosphate may be advisable. Other suggestions for coping with sensitivity may be found on pages 556–557.

D. Follow-up

Return for observation of complete healing in one week to one month depending on the individual patient's progress and total treatment plan.

VI. Dressing Replacement

A. Indications

1. Dressing broken or displaced before time for removal.
2. A second dressing for an extended period of time may be indicated and depends on the
   a. Extent of the surgery and degree of periodontal disease involvement.
   b. Need for additional healing period for certain types of surgery.

B. Procedural Suggestions

1. Use a topical anesthetic to prevent patient discomfort.
2. Use a soft dressing with minimal pressure during application over a partly healed area.

SUTURE REMOVAL

A suture is a strand or fiber used to unite parts of the body. Sutures are necessary in many oral operations wherever a surgical wound must be closed, a flap positioned, or tissue grafted.

I. Purposes of Sutures

A. Maintain the sutured tissues until healing is great enough to provide the tissues with sufficient strength to undergo normal physiologic activity.
B. By holding and stabilizing the replaced and readapted tissue, sutures contribute to the following:
   1. Maintaining the clot during the initial healing period.
   2. Reducing the size of the wound, therefore lessening the time required for healing.
   3. Protecting the area from foreign debris and trauma.

II. Types of Sutures and Needles

Sutures are classified as absorbable and nonabsorbable. Absorbable sutures are digested by body tissue fluids and enzymes, carried away by phagocytic action, and with the normal healing process, are replaced by scar tissue. In medical surgery, absorbable sutures can be used internally. Nonabsorbable sutures are made of inert materials and, when used on the surface, must be removed after 5 to 10 days as indicated by the type of surgery.

A. Absorbable Sutures

1. *Surgical Gut.* Prepared from the submucosa of sheep intestines, and prepared for use as plain or chrome.
   a. Plain. Processed, sterilized, and tested.
   b. Chrome. Special treatment of the suture material with chromic acid to control and lengthen the absorption time.
2. *Polyglycolic Acid (PGA).* Synthetic material that tends to produce a milder tissue reaction than surgical gut or nonabsorbable materials, it inhibits bacterial growth.

B. Nonabsorbable Sutures

1. *Surgical Silk:* black twisted or braided. Most widely used, particularly in oral surgery.
2. *Surgical Cotton and Linen*
3. *Wire:* tantalum, silver, stainless steel, vitallium.

4. *Synthetic Fibers:* polyester (example: Dupont Mersilene), nylon, Dermalon, orlon.

C. **Characteristics**

1. Braided, twisted, plain. Braiding provides more retention, but the suture is more permeable to bacteria.
2. Monofilament or multifilament. Monofilament gives less tissue reaction, but multifilament gives better retention.
3. Sizes described from 0 to 8–0. For example, 4–0 silk is frequently used in periodontal surgery.

D. **Needles**

Many types of suturing needles are available, and their use and selection are based on the patient's needs and the dentist's preference. The three basic characteristics of suture needles are as follows:

1. *Shape of Needle:* straight, half circle, 3/8 circle, half-curved.
2. *Cross-sectional Shape:* round or triangular (has cutting edge). The tip may be a taper point or a trocar (triangular) point.
3. *Eye*
   a. Regular eye: eye may be round or square, or a French spring eye which grips suture material.
   b. Atraumatic: No eye. The needle and an end of the suture material are swaged. The suture and needle are a continuous unit.

III. Suturing Techniques

Many different patterns of suturing are used. A dental hygienist who will be removing sutures as part of postoperative patient care needs to become familiar with the methods preferred by the dentist-surgeon. Assisting and observing at the time of the operation can be especially educational. When the patient is one for whom the hygienist participated in the initial preparation, knowledge of the surgical procedures used adds to the continuity of treatment.

At the time of the operation, the number and type or description of the sutures placed should be recorded in the patient's record. At the time of removal, the information is necessary, since, during healing, sutures may become loosened, misplaced, or sometimes covered with tissue.

All sutures should be accounted for at the time of removal.

General types frequently used in the oral cavity are described here briefly to introduce terminology and to help orient the dental hygienist to the various sutures that may be encountered during removal.

A. **Interrupted**

Each stitch is taken and tied separately (figure 36–1B).

B. **Continuous Uninterrupted**

A series of stitches tied at one or both ends. Examples of sutures that may be applied in a series are the sling or suspension and the blanket.

C. **Circumferential**

A term applied to a suture that encircles a tooth for suspension and retention of a flap.

D. **Blanket**

Each stitch is brought over a loop of the preceding one, thus forming a series of loops on one side of the incision and a series of stitches on the incision (figure 36–1A). It is also called a continuous lock. It is used, for example, for approximation of the gingival margins after alveolectomy.

E. **Sling or Suspension**

When a flap is only on one side, facial or lingual, the sutures are passed through the interdental papilla, through the proximal, around the tooth, and then into the adjacent papilla (figure 36–1D). The suture is adjusted so that the flap can be positioned for correct healing.

F. **Interdental**

Where there are lingual and facial flaps, interdental ligation joins the two by passing the suture through each interdental area (figure 31–1C). Coverage for the interdental area can be accomplished by coapting the edges of the papillae.

IV. Procedure for Removal

When a dressing has been placed over sutures, the steps will overlap with V.B.2., Dressing Removal, page 549. A suture can become

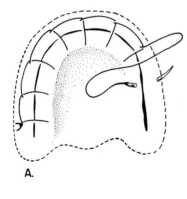

A.

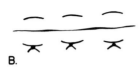

B.

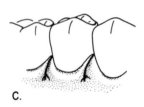

C.

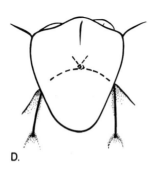

D.

Figure 36–1. Types of sutures. **A.** blanket stitch, **B.** interrupted, individual sutures, **C.** interdental individual sutures, and **D,** sling or suspension suture tied on the lingual (dotted line).

caught in dressing material, and may need to be cut and removed while the dressing is being removed. The same principles for removal are to be observed.

A. Supplies for Suture Removal

> Mouth mirror
> Cotton pliers
> Curved sharp scissors with pointed tip (suture scissors)
> Gauze sponge
> Topical anesthetic: Use type that can be applied safely on an abraded or incompletely healed area (pages 522–523).
> Topical antiseptic
> Cotton pellets
> Saliva ejector tip

B. Patient Examination

1. Observe healing tissue about the suture(s).
2. Record any deviations of color, size, shape of the tissue, adaptation of a flap, or coaptation of an incision healing by first intention.

C. Preparation of the Patient

1. Debridement of area: rinse the area and remove debris particles, using a cotton tipped applicator or a cotton pellet dipped in 3% peroxide. Follow with another rinse, or wipe gently with a gauze sponge.
2. Place and adjust saliva ejector.
3. Retract and pat area with gauze sponge to remove surface moisture.
4. Swab area with topical antiseptic. Maintain retraction to prevent dilution.
5. Apply topical anesthetic.

D. Retraction

Three hands are really needed: one for retraction, one for cotton pliers to hold and remove the suture, and one for cutting the suture. When an assistant is not available, a cotton roll placed in the vestibule may provide enough retraction along with the finger rest and little finger of the nondominant hand holding the cotton pliers.

E. Steps for Removal

As described here and illustrated in figure 36–2, removal is for a single interrupted suture. The same principles apply for the ends and each segment of a continuous suture, wherever septic suture material could pass through the soft tissue.

1. Grasp the suture knot with the cotton plier held in the nondominant hand. Draw the suture gently up about 2 mm. and hold with slight tension. A finger rest is needed for control.
2. Insert tip of sharp scissors under the suture, slightly depress the tissue with the back of the scissor blade, and cut the suture in the part that was previously buried in the tissue.
3. Hold knot end up with the cotton plier and pull gently to allow suture to come out through the side opposite where it was cut. This prevents any part of the external segment of the suture from passing through the tissue and introducing infectious material.

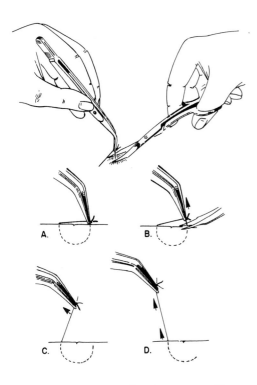

Figure 36–2. Suture removal. **A.** Suture grasped by cotton pliers near entrance into tissue. **B.** Suture pulled up gently while scissor is inserted close to tissue. Suture is cut in the part previously buried in the tissue. **C.** Suture held up for vertical removal. **D.** Suture pulled gently to pass the suture out on the side opposite from the cut. The object is to prevent the external part of the suture from passing through the tissue and introducing infection.

4. Withdraw gently and steadily.
5. Place each suture on a sponge for final counting and proceed to remove the next suture.
6. Count total sutures and confirm with the patient's record of the surgical procedures of the previous appointment.
7. Apply gauze sponge with slight pressure on bleeding spots.
8. Request dentist to observe the area.
9. Request patient to close on the sponge while dressing is readied (when a dressing replacement is indicated).

F. Precautions

In summary of the points brought out in the above description, precautions are as follows:

1. Count sutures; record number placed and number removed.
2. Record all observations of the tissues by dentist and hygienist and note any adverse reactions or bleeding problems. Record comments made by the patient.
3. Sutures should not be left longer than 5 to 10 days. Special arrangements for removal need to be made for the patient who cannot return for a scheduled appointment.
4. Take care when removing a periodontal dressing to prevent ripping out a suture that may have become imbedded in the dressing.
5. Provide proper postappointment instructions for the patient.

TECHNICAL HINTS

I. Sutures placed without a dressing may have a crust over them at the time of removal. Apply mineral oil by cotton swab or pellet, and in a short time, the crust will soften and can be wiped away. Removing the suture with the crust can cause unnecessary discomfort for the patient.

II. Adaptation and retention of a dressing can be improved when the dressing is covered with a well-adapted adhesive periodontal foil when this is in accord with the dentist's philosophy. Place the foil over the lingual, occlusal, and facial, but do not cover the margins of the dressing in order to prevent irritating the mucosa.

FACTORS TO TEACH THE PATIENT

I. Care of the mouth during the period of treatment while wearing dressings. See table 36–1.

II. Maintenance and follow-up care after treatment is formally over.

References

1. American Dental Association, Council on Dental Therapeutics: *Accepted Dental Therapeutics*, 39th ed. Chicago, American Dental Association, 1982, pp. 303–305.
2. American Dental Association, Council on Dental Materials, Instruments and Equipment: *Dentist's Desk Reference: Materials, Instruments and Equipment*, 1st ed. Chicago, American Dental Association, 1981, p. 18.
3. Baer, P.N., Sumner, C.F., and Miller, G.: Periodontal Dressings, *Dent. Clin. North Am.*, *13*, 181, January, 1969.

Suggested Readings

Bradley, R.E. and Malena, D.E.: Postoperative Care, in Clark, J.W., ed.: *Clinical Dentistry, Volume 3*, Chapter 15. Hagerstown, Maryland, Harper & Row, 1981, pp. 1–10.

Carranza, F.A.: *Glickman's Clinical Periodontology*, 5th ed. Philadelphia, W.B. Saunders Co., 1979, pp. 791–802, 832–842.

Castano, F.A. and Alden, B.A., eds.: *Handbook of Expanded Dental Auxiliary Practice*, 2nd ed. Philadelphia, J.B. Lippincott Co., 1980, pp. 186–189.

Grant, D.A., Stern, I.B., and Everett, F.G.: *Periodontics*, 5th ed. St. Louis, The C.V. Mosby Co., 1979, pp. 613–616, 683–696.

Levin, M.P.: Periodontal Suture Materials and Surgical Dressings, *Dent. Clin. North Am.*, *24*, 767, October, 1980.

Pattison, G. and Pattison, A.M.: *Periodontal Instrumentation.* Reston, Virginia, Reston Publishing Co., 1979, pp. 369–392.

Ramfjord, S.P. and Ash, M.M.: *Periodontology and Periodontics.* Philadelphia, W.B. Saunders Co., 1979, pp. 504–519, 699–703.

Periodontal Dressings

Addy, M. and Dolby, A.E.: The Use of Chlorhexidine Mouthwash Compared With a Periodontal Dressing Following the Gingivectomy Procedure, *J. Clin. Periodontol.*, *3*, 59, February, 1976.

Addy, M. and Douglas, W.H.: A Chlorhexidine-containing Methacrylic Gel as a Periodontal Dressing, *J. Periodontol.*, *46*, 465, August, 1975.

American Dental Association, Council on Dental Therapeutics and Council on Dental Materials and Devices: Hazards of Asbestos in Dentistry, *J. Am. Dent. Assoc.*, *92*, 777, April, 1976.

Bakdash, M.B. and Frydman, A.: Asbestos in Periodontal Dressings: A Possible Health Hazard, *Quintessence Int.*, *7*, 61, October, 1976.

Haugen, E., Espevik, S., and Mjör, I.A.: Adhesive Properties of Periodontal Dressings—An *in vitro* Study, *J. Periodont. Res.*, *14*, 487, November, 1979.

Haugen, E. and Gjermo, P.: Clinical Assessment of Periodontal Dressings, *J. Clin. Periodontol.*, *5*, 50, February, 1978.

Haugen, E., Gjermo, P., and Ørstavik, D.: Some Antibacterial Properties of Periodontal Dressings, *J. Clin. Periodontol.*, *4*, 62, February, 1977.

Heany, T.G. and Appleton, J.: The Effect of Periodontal Dressings on the Healthy Periodontium, *J. Clin. Periodontol.*, *3*, 66, February, 1976.

Jones, T.M. and Cassingham, R.J.: Comparison of Healing Following Periodontal Surgery With and Without Dressings in Humans, *J. Periodontol.*, *50*, 387, August, 1979.

Kozam, G. and Mantell, G.M.: The Effect of Eugenol on Oral Mucous Membranes, *J. Dent. Res.*, *57*, 954, November–December, 1978.

Levin, M.P., Cutright, D.E., and Bhaskar, S.N.: Cyanoacrylate as a Periodontal Dressing, *J. Oral Med.*, *30*, 40, April–June, 1975.

McGraw, V.A. and Caffesse, R.G.: Cyanoacrylates in Periodontics, *Periodont. Abstr.*, *26*, 4, Number 1, 1978.

Newman, P.S. and Addy, M.: A Comparison of a Periodontal Dressing and Chlorhexidine Gluconate Mouthwash After the Internal Bevelled Flap Procedure, *J. Periodontol.*, *49*, 576, November, 1978.

Nezwek, R.A., Caffesse, R.G., Bergenholtz, A., and Nasjleti, C.E.: Connective Tissue Response to Periodontal Dressings, *J. Periodontol.*, *51*, 521, September, 1980.

O'Neil, T.C.A.: Antibacterial Properties of Periodontal Dressings, *J. Periodontol.*, *46*, 469, August, 1975.

Pihlstrom, B.L., Thorn, H.L., and Folke, L.E.A.: The Effect of Periodontal Dressing on Supragingival Microorganisms, *J. Periodontol.*, *48*, 440, August, 1977.

Poulsom, R.C.: An Anaphylactoid Reaction to Periodontal Surgical Dressing: Report of Case, *J. Am. Dent. Assoc.*, *89*, 895, October, 1974.

Smith, D.C.: A Materialistic Look at Periodontal Packs, *Dent. Pract. (London)*, *20*, 263, April, 1970.

Watts, T.L.P. and Combe, E.C.: Adhesion of Periodontal Dressings to Enamel *in vitro*, *J. Clin. Periodontol.*, *7*, 62, February, 1980.

Watts, T.L.P. and Combe, E.C.: Periodontal Dressing Materials, *J. Clin. Periodontol.*, *6*, 3, February, 1979.

Sutures

Boundy, S.S.: Suture Removal, in Boundy, S.S. and Reynolds, N.J., eds.: *Current Concepts in Dental Hygiene*, Volume 2. St. Louis, The C.V. Mosby Co., 1979, pp. 130–133.

Castelli, W.A., Nasjleti, C.E., Caffesse, R.E., and Diaz-Perez, R.: Gingival Response to Silk, Cotton, and Nylon Suture Materials, *Oral Surg.*, *45*, 179, February, 1978.

Ebert, J.R.: Method for Scanning Electron Microscopic Study of Plaque on Periodontal Suture Material, *J. Dent. Res.*, *53*, 1298, September–October, 1974.

Macht, S.D. and Krizek, T.J.: Sutures and Suturing—Current Concepts, *J. Oral Surg.*, *36*, 710, September, 1978.

Nelson, E.H., Funakoshi, E., and O'Leary, T.J.: A Comparison of the Continuous and Interrupted Suturing Techniques, *J. Periodontol.*, *48*, 273, May, 1977.

Project Acorde, United States Department of Health, Education, and Welfare: *Assisting With Suture Placement and Sutures: Placing and Removing Medication for Dry Sockets.* Castro Valley, California, Quercus, 1979, pp. 7–61.

Racey, G.L., Wallace, W.R., Cavalaris, C.J., and Marquard, J.V.: Comparison of a Polyglycolic-polylactic Acid Suture to Black Silk and Plain Catgut in Human Oral Tissues, *J. Oral Surg.*, *36*, 766, October, 1978.

37

Care of Hypersensitive Teeth

Sensitivity in the cervical area of a tooth can produce considerable discomfort. Care must be taken during instrumentation and application of air to prevent a hypersensitive reaction. Since tooth sensitivity is frequently related to the accumulation of plaque in the exposed cervical area, instruction in exacting plaque removal techniques is indicated.

Patients are appreciative of clinical procedures directed at desensitizing the area involved. A number of chemical and mechanical means have been used successfully to reduce or eliminate pain. No known method is universally effective for desensitization.

I. Factors Contributing to Hypersensitivity

A. Exposure of Cementum and Dentin

1. *Gingival Recession*[1,2]
   a. Pathologic (localized or generalized): inflammation that may stimulate proliferation of the junctional epithelium along the root surface.
   b. Traumatic: toothbrush with abrasive dentifrice.
2. *Periodontal Surgery:* for pocket elimination.

B. Anatomy of the Cementoenamel Junction

Zone of dentin occurs between the enamel and the cementum in approximately 10 percent of teeth[3,4] (figure 12–2, page 205).

C. Loss of Cementum Denudes the Dentin

Cementum is lost through abrasion, erosion, dental caries, scaling, or root planing.

D. Sensitivity of Dentin

In most teeth, the dentin is more sensitive on its outer surface.[5] The sensitivity could be related to the branching of the odontoblastic processes. By branching, a wider area of cytoplasm is exposed.

II. Types of Pain Stimuli[6]

A. Mechanical

Toothbrush filaments or bristles, eating utensils, periodontal and dental hygiene instruments, friction from denture clasps or other appliances.

B. Chemical

Acids formed from fermentable carbohydrates in debris and plaque, citrus fruit acids, or condiments.

C. Thermal

Hot or cold foods or beverages; air entering the oral cavity.

III. Mode of Action of Densensitizing Agents[6]

A. Mechanism

The exact mechanism of pain transmission

is not known. It is probable that sensitivity is due to irritation of the organic matter or "nerve elements" in the dentinal tubules, which is transmitted to the nerves of the pulp.

B. Types of Agents

Agents used for desensitization may be classified as those acting in one of the following ways:
1. Precipitation or denaturing of the organic peripheral ends of the odontoblastic processes (Tome's fibers).
2. Stimulation of the formation of secondary dentin.
3. Deposition of inorganic insoluble salts at the ends of the tubules to plug them and seal them off.
4. Adhesion of substances over the ends of the tubules to cover and seal off.

IV. Useful Characteristics of a Desensitizing Agent

When selecting a method for desensitization, practical aspects are important. When possible, the patient's daily personal care can be used to incorporate treatment on a self-care basis. When an agent is applied professionally, the following considerations are suggested. An agent needs
A. Rapidity of action.
B. Ease of application.
C. Biologic acceptance by the body tissues.
D. Long-lasting or permanent effects.
E. No side effects such as discoloration of the teeth.

METHODS FOR DESENSITIZATION

Few patients respond to a single form of treatment. For all, keeping the teeth as free of plaque, particularly at the gingival third where sensitivity areas occur, and the use of a form of self-applied topical fluoride are basic procedures. When that program is established, specific agents can be selected for professional application to persistent areas of sensitivity.

I. Self-care by the Patient

A. Plaque Control

Root surfaces subjected to vigorous plaque control measures by brushing, flossing, and using other aids such as a Perio-aid, develop a smooth hard surface with increased luster and less hypersensitivity. The dentinal tubules are blocked off by increased mineralization.

When plaque is retained at the cervical third, the root surfaces may develop root caries, and usually are hypersensitive. A concentrated program of instruction and supervision would be indicated. A sulcular technique (page 346) with a soft nylon brush, flossing, use of the Perio-aid, and other appropriate measures must be instituted.

B. Dentifrice

Dentifrices containing strontium chloride 10%* and sodium monofluorophosphate 0.76%† have been shown to reduce sensitivity when used routinely. Research has compared the two dentifrices.[7,8] Potassium nitrate 5%** has also been shown to be effective in lessening hypersensitivity.[9]

An advantage of the dentifrice with sodium monofluorophosphate over the others is its caries preventive action. In the prevention of cemental caries, the use of a fluoride dentifrice is an important part of the total program.

C. Self-applied Fluoride

In addition to fluoride dentifrice, the patient's treatment plan should include daily applications of fluoride by mouth rinsing, custom tray with gel, chewable tablet, brushing with a gel, or other mode for regular use. The various procedures were described on pages 456–458. With an increase in surface fluoride, hypersensitivity usually will decrease.

D. Diet

A food diary kept for 5 to 7 days, from which a dietary analysis is made with the patient, can be valuable. Foods that aggravate the hypersensitivity can be identified, and substitutes can be selected with the patient. Excessive fermentable carbohydrates, citrus fruits, or condiments of pronounced flavors may initiate a reaction.

---

*Sensodyne
†Colgate, Aim, Maclean's, Aquafresh.
**Denquel

II. Professional Applications

Without effective personal plaque removal measures, professional applications have limited, and frequently temporary, effects. Dentists have used albumin precipitants such as 40% formalin, 40% zinc chloride, or 40% silver nitrate to seal the dentinal tubules and hence reduce sensitivity. Cavity varnishes, thin mixes of crown and bridge cement, zinc oxide and eugenol packs, or Gottlieb's solution have been used to protect the tooth surface against thermal shock.

A. Preparation for Densensitization

1. Complete scaling and planing.
2. Anesthesia. When teeth are too sensitive for scaling and planing, a local anesthetic is indicated. Note areas where a desensitizing agent is to be applied before the anesthetic is given.

B. Fluoride Preparations

1. *Sodium Fluoride Aqueous Solution* (2 to 4%). Apply as in the topical application for the prevention of dental caries (pages 452–454).
2. *Sodium Fluoride Desensitizing Paste.* 33% sodium fluoride, 33% kaolin, and 33% glycerin.[10]
   a. Clean and isolate the sensitive tooth, using cotton rolls, cotton roll holder for mandibular, and saliva ejector.
   b. Wipe exposed area with cotton pellet moistened in 2% sodium fluoride solution.
   c. Dry area thoroughly, using cotton pellets or cotton roll.
   d. Place small amount of desensitizing paste on area with tip of wood point in porte polisher. A narrow wood point may fit the cervical area more effectively than a wide one.
   e. Massage paste on area gently but firmly with wood point, using small circular strokes. If patient suffers acute pain response at beginning of application, wipe off paste, have patient rinse with warm water, and begin again immediately.
   f. Continue massage for 3 minutes: use timer.
   g. Wipe off excess paste with cotton pellet.
   h. Remove cotton rolls and saliva ejector and request patient to rinse with warm water.
   i. Repeat at future appointment if desensitization has not been accomplished.
3. *Sodium Silicofluoride Solution* (0.7 to 0.9%)[11]
   a. Clean and isolate the sensitive tooth using cotton rolls, cotton roll holder for mandibular, and saliva ejector.
   b. Dry the area thoroughly, using cotton pellets or cotton roll.
   c. Apply solution with cotton pellet or applicator.
   d. Keep area glistening (but not dripping) wet for 5 minutes.
   e. Remove excess solution with cotton pellets.
   f. Repeat weekly for maximum of three applications as needed: if desensitization is to occur, it will have occurred after three applications.

C. Iontophoresis[12,13]

Iontophoresis is the impregnation of tissue with ions from dissolved salts with the aid of an electric current. Iontophoresis utilizes a direct current to promote ionic transport of fluoride, a negatively charged ion, onto a tooth surface.

The actual mechanism of action may be deposition of fluoride ions deeper into the dentin to obtain more extensive protoplasmic precipitation or formation of secondary dentin. A short-lived paresthesia of the odontoblastic processes may be produced. Manufacturer's instructions should be followed for use of the equipment.

1. Isolate with rubber dam or cotton rolls.
2. Low-voltage batteries ($1\frac{1}{2}$ to 9 volts) supply positive current to patient's tooth. A special direct-current source has been developed.[13]
3. Circuit completed by contact of brush applicator for negatively charged aqueous fluoride solution (2% sodium fluoride).
4. Check patient's medical history before use of a current. A patient wearing a pacemaker should not receive treatment by such means as pulp tester, ultrasonic,

or other current-producing instrument (page 789).

TECHNICAL HINTS

I. Do not use compressed air on sensitive teeth. Dry only with cotton pellets or cotton roll.

II. Sodium silicofluoride solution and sodium fluoride desensitizing paste contain enough fluoride to cause nausea if swallowed in excess. Prevent by using only small amounts, wiping excess off with cotton pellets before removing cotton rolls, requesting the patient to rinse thoroughly, and using the saliva ejector to prevent the need for swallowing before the mouth can be rinsed.

III. Prepare solution of sodium silicofluoride weekly and store in polyethylene container. A chemical reaction results when a plain glass bottle is used.[11]

IV. Keep jar containing sodium fluoride desensitizing paste tightly closed. Its shelf-life can be indefinite because of its glycerin base.

FACTORS TO TEACH THE PATIENT

I. General causes of gingival recession.

II. Causes of hypersensitivity of teeth.

III. Importance of toothbrushing for plaque removal in the cervical area as a method of desensitization.

IV. Probability that the hypersensitivity will subside in time with daily plaque removal whether a desensitizer is applied or not.

V. Specific foods that should and should not be used in the diet if relief from sensitivity is to be obtained.

References

1. Grant, D.A., Stern, I.B., and Everett, F.G.: *Periodontics*, 5th ed. St. Louis, The C.V. Mosby Co., 1979, pp. 373–382.
2. Carranza, F.A.: *Glickman's Clinical Periodontology*, 5th ed. Philadelphia, W.B. Saunders Co., 1979, pp. 100–104.
3. Melfi, R.C.: *Permar's Oral Embryology and Microscopic Anatomy*, 7th ed. Philadelphia, Lea & Febiger, 1982, p. 85.
4. Bhaskar, S.N., ed.: *Orban's Oral Histology and Embryology*, 9th ed. St. Louis, The C.V. Mosby Co., 1980, p. 193.
5. *Ibid.*, p. 138.
6. Grant, Stern, and Everett: op. cit., pp. 559–563.
7. Shapiro, W.B., Kaslick, R.S., Chasens, A.I., and Weinstein, D.: Controlled Clinical Comparison Between a Strontium Chloride and a Sodium Monofluorophosphate Toothpaste in Diminishing Root Hypersensitivity, *J. Periodontol.*, *41*, 523, September, 1970.
8. Hernandez, F., Mohammed, C., Shannon, I., Volpe, A., and King, W.: Clinical Study Evaluating the Desensitizing Effect and Duration of Two Commercially Available Dentifrices, *J. Periodontol.*, *43*, 367, June, 1972.
9. Tarbet, W.J., Silverman, G., Stolman, J.M., and Fratarcangelo, P.A.: Clinical Evaluation of a New Treatment for Dentinal Hypersensitivity, *J. Periodontol.*, *51*, 535, September, 1980.
10. Hoyt, W.H. and Bibby, B.G.: Use of Sodium Fluoride for Desensitizing Dentin, *J. Am. Dent. Assoc.*, *30*, 1372, September 1, 1943.
11. Stout, W.C.: Sodium Silicofluoride as a Desensitizing Agent, *J. Periodontol.*, *26*, 208, July, 1955.
12. Murthy, K.S., Talim, S.T., and Singh, I.: A Comparative Evaluation of Topical Application and Iontophoresis of Sodium Fluoride for Desensitization of Hypersensitive Dentin, *Oral Surg.*, *36*, 448, September, 1973.
13. Gangarosa, L.P. and Park, N.H.: Practical Considerations in Iontophoresis of Fluoride for Desensitizing Dentin, *J. Prosthet. Dent.*, *39*, 173, February, 1978.

Suggested Readings

Anderson, D.J.: Human and Animal Studies on Sensory Mechanisms in Teeth, *Int. Dent. J.*, *22*, 33, March, 1972.

Brännström, M., Johnson, G., and Nordenvall, K.-J.: Transmission and Control of Dentinal Pain: Resin Impregnation for the Desensitization of Dentin, *J. Am. Dent. Assoc.*, *99*, 612, October, 1979.

Dayton, R.E., DeMarco, T.J., and Swedlow, D.: Treatment of Hypersensitive Root Surfaces With Dental Adhesive Materials, *J. Periodontol.*, *45*, 873, December, 1974.

Gangarosa, L.P.: Iontophoretic Application of Fluoride by Tray Techniques for Desensitization of Multiple Teeth, *J. Am. Dent. Assoc.*, *102*, 50, January, 1981.

Gedalia, I., Brayer, L., Kalter, N., Richter, M., and Stabholz, A.: The Effect of Fluoride and Strontium Application on Dentin: *in vivo* and *in vitro* Studies, *J. Periodontol.*, *49*, 269, May, 1978.

Green, B.L., Green, M.L., and McFall, W.T.: Calcium Hydroxide and Potassium Nitrate as Desensitizing Agents for Hypersensitive Root Surfaces, *J. Periodontol.*, *48*, 667, October, 1977.

Hiatt, W.H. and Johansen, E.: Root Preparation I. Obturation of Dentinal Tubules in Treatment of Root Hypersensitivity, *J. Periodontol.*, *43*, 373, June, 1972.

Hodosh, M.: A Superior Desensitizer–Potassium Nitrate, *J. Am. Dent. Assoc.*, *88*, 831, April, 1974.

Minkov, B., Marmari, I., Gedalia, I., and Garfunkel, A.: The Effectiveness of Sodium Fluoride Treatment With and Without Iontophoresis on the Reduction of Hypersensitive Dentin, *J. Periodontol.*, *46*, 246, April, 1975.

Peden, J.W.: Dental Hypersensitivity, *Periodont. Abstr.*, *25*, 75, Number 2, 1977.

Seltzer, S.: Hypothetic Mechanisms for Dentine Sensitivity, *Oral Surg.*, *31*, 388, March, 1971.

Shapiro, W.B., Kaslick, R.S., and Chasens, A.I.: The Effect of a Strontium Chloride Toothpaste on Root Hypersensitivity in a Controlled Clinical Study, *J. Periodontol.*, *41*, 702, December, 1970.

Simon, W.J. and Hilborn, L.B.: Hypersensitive Dentin, *Dent. Assist.*, *46*, 16, September, 1977.

Tarbet, W.J., Silverman, G., Stolman, J.M., and Fratarc-angelo, P.A.: An Evaluation of Two Methods for the Quantitation of Dentinal Hypersensitivity, *J. Am. Dent. Assoc.*, *98*, 914, June, 1979.

Uchida, A., Wakano, Y., Fukuyama, O., Miki, T., Iwayama, Y., and Okada, H.: Controlled Clinical Evaluation of a 10% Strontium Chloride Dentifrice in Treatment of Dentin Hypersensitivity Following Periodontal Surgery, *J. Periodontol.*, *51*, 578, October, 1980.

Wei, S.H.Y., Lainson, P.A., Henderson, W., and Wolfson, S.H.: Evaluation of Dentifrices for the Relief of Hypersensitive Tooth Surfaces, *Quintessence Int.*, *11*, 67, January, 1980.

Zinner, D.D., Duany, L.F., and Lutz, H.J.: A New Desensitizing Dentifrice: Preliminary Report, *J. Am. Dent. Assoc.*, *95*, 982, November, 1977.

38

Introduction to Polishing

After treatment by scaling, root planing, and other periodontal therapy, the teeth are evaluated for polishing. Polishing is a selective procedure and not every patient needs to have the teeth polished, especially on a routine basis.

When the evaluation is made, several factors must be taken into consideration. These will be described in this chapter.

I. Indications for Polishing

The objectives for polishing may need clarification, since polishing has been a routine procedure in many offices and clinics. The indications may be summarized as follows:

A. Remove Extrinsic Stains not Otherwise Removed During Toothbrushing and Scaling

Stains on the teeth have never been considered etiologic factors for any disease or destructive process. Therefore, the removal of stains is for esthetics, not for a health service. The need for removal by polishing should be evaluated after the plaque is under control, since some stains are incorporated in plaque and can be removed during brushing and flossing by the patient.

When the stain is to be removed by the professional person, as much stain as possible must first be removed with the calculus during scaling. Certain stains can be scaled away readily even without being incorpo-

rated within calculus. Black line stain, for example, has been called a type of calculus. It resembles calculus in that it is composed of microorganisms, has a similar mode of attachment to enamel, and similar signs of calcification under a microscope.[1] Another reason why black line stain should be scaled rather than polished is that it is most commonly found on the teeth of children. Newly erupted teeth are more porous and less mineralized, and should not be damaged by polishing. The effect of heat created by power-driven instruments is not completely known, except that excess heat can produce pulp damage.

For stains on adult teeth that are not removed with calculus, a polishing paste that is the least abrasive should be selected. The toothpaste manufactured for daily home use may be amply abrasive for professional use when very little stain removal is needed.

The source of an extrinsic stain should be discussed with the patient and a preventive plan initiated. When the recurrence of a stain is preventable, or when the etiologic factor is controllable, the patient should be encouraged to make the necessary habit changes to prevent the stain from collecting again. Improved techniques of personal plaque removal and more frequent attention to oral hygiene can result in a significant improvement.

B. Polish Restorative Materials

Polished amalgam resists tarnish and corrosion. Polishing increases the life of the restoration. With recontouring of overhanging margins, finishing and polishing contributes to the prevention of bacterial plaque accumulation, which in turn, may lead to dental caries. Polishing of restorations is described in Chapter 41, page 592.

C. Prepare the Teeth for Caries Preventive Agents

1. *Pit and Fissure Sealant.* The manufacturer's directions should be followed relative to preparation of the teeth for sealant application. Since commercial prophylaxis pastes contain oils, fluoride, flavoring substances, or other agents that may interfere with the integrity of the sealant, a plain, fine pumice with water is indicated (page 468).
2. *Professional Application of Fluoride Solutions or Gels.* Traditionally, tooth polishing after scaling has preceded a topical application because of the original history-making research of Knutson.[2] Current research shows that plaque and debris removal can be accomplished adequately by the patient using a toothbrush and dental floss, rather than requiring the more drastic means of polishing with a rubber cup and abrasive cleaning agent. New evidence has shown that the pellicle on the tooth surface does not act as a barrier to fluoride.[3] Tinanoff[4] showed that fluoride uptake in the enamel was similar from a fluoride application whether the teeth had been brushed by the patient or polished with pumice.

   Having a patient brush and floss prior to a topical application provides an excellent opportunity to combine patient instruction with treatment and utilize the educational principle of participation of the learner. Such an objective has unquestionable value.

   Excellent benefits, many similar or better in caries prevention than those accomplished by professional topical applications, have been obtained from home and school fluoride rinsing programs.[5,6] When considering whether the use of a rubber cup with prophylaxis paste is necessary prior to topical application, the effects of rinsing on a weekly or daily basis without prior polishing should be recognized.

   A polishing procedure may be deemed necessary prior to professional fluoride application when stains were not removed during scaling. In that case, it is advised that a fluoride-containing prophylaxis paste with minimal abrasiveness be used. The fluoride from the paste may replace in part that removed by the abrasive action.[7]

D. Contribute to Patient Motivation

Polishing should never be a substitute for complete calculus removal and root planing as a means for making the tooth surfaces smooth. Smoothing of tooth surfaces is a part of the basic instrumentation and is performed during the final series of strokes for scaling and planing.

Smooth polished tooth surfaces may contribute in part to the following effects:
1. Help the instructed patient to obtain more satisfactory results from self-care procedures. A smooth surface should be easier to clean.
2. Show the patient the appearance and feeling of a clean mouth for motivational purposes. However, the greatest change in behavior, the true learning, can usually be obtained through patient participation in the use of a disclosing agent and personal removal of plaque with floss and toothbrush.

E. Relationship Between Polishing and Plaque Removal

Removal of plaque must be a *daily* procedure carried out *by the patient*. It must be accomplished thoroughly at least once or twice daily, and for some patients, three times daily if disease is to be controlled and the sanitation of the mouth maintained.

One removal of soft deposits from the teeth at a dental hygiene appointment does not accomplish any purpose since deposits return promptly. It is known that pellicle returns to cover the teeth within minutes after complete polishing, and that plaque bacteria begin to collect on the pellicle within an hour or two, increasing in thickness until by 12 to 24 hours plaque is thick enough to show clearly when a disclosing agent is applied. Undisturbed, calculus forms from the plaque in a few days.

Except for a minority of patients who practice superior plaque control, the deposits return promptly. Effects of polishing as a preventive measure for gingival disease or dental caries have not been proven.

II. Effects of Polishing

Because of the detrimental effects, the needs of an individual patient must be reviewed prior to polishing. Professional judgment based on patient need decides when a service is to be included in a treatment plan.

A. Bacteremia

Since bacteremia can be created during the use of a rubber cup with a polishing agent, the *medical history* must be taken initially and then reviewed and updated at succeeding recall appointments. All patient histories should be carefully updated at least annually.

Bacteremias result from manipulation of the gingival tissues. In one research study, 11 of 39 children (mean age, 9 years) had a bacteremia following application of a rubber cup with a prophylaxis paste.[8] It is recommended that use of a rubber cup be withheld until the plaque is under control and the gingiva do not bleed when the patient brushes.

For risk patients, particularly those with damaged or abnormal heart valves, prosthetic valves, joint replacements, rheumatic heart disease, and others listed on pages 99–100, antibiotic prophylaxis as outlined by the American Heart Association is needed.

B. Environmental Factors

1. *Aerosol Production.* Aerosols are created during use of all rotary instruments including a prophylaxis handpiece with a polishing paste and the air and water sprays used during rinsing.[9] The biologic contaminants of aerosols stay suspended for long periods and provide a means for disease transmission to dental personnel as well as for succeeding patients (page 17).

   Rotary instruments should be avoided when a patient is known to have a communicable disease. Precautions for hepatitis B and other diseases were described on pages 63–65.

2. *Splatter.* Protective eyeglasses are needed for all dental team members and for the patient. Serious eye damage has occurred as a result of splatter in the eye from a polishing paste, or from instruments. Constituents of commercial prophylaxis pastes may include various chemicals such as oils that can aggravate a severe inflammatory response.[10]

C. Effect on Teeth

1. *Removal of Tooth Structure.* It has been shown that polishing for 30 seconds with a pumice paste may remove as much as 4 μm of the outer enamel.[7] Performed repeatedly over the years, the tooth loss could be substantial. The effect has particular significance for children because the surface of young, newly erupted teeth is incompletely mineralized.

   Cementum and dentin are softer and more porous, so greater amounts can be removed than during polishing of the enamel.[11,12] When cementum is exposed because of gingival recession, polishing of the exposed surfaces should be avoided. Also to be avoided are areas of decalcification. It has been shown that nearly three times more surface enamel is lost from abrasive polishing over white spots than over intact enamel.[13]

   A coarse abrasive may create a rougher tooth surface than existed before polishing. Grooves and scratches created by an abrasive applied with a rubber cup have been studied microscopically.[14,15]

   Removal of tooth structure in the cervical portion of the tooth, where enamel is thin and cementum is exposed, can create unnecessary sensitivity. Special treatment problems may follow. These areas should not be polished.

2. *Removal of Fluoride-rich Surface.* More important than the amount of enamel lost during polishing is the fact that the outermost layer of tooth structure has been shown to contain the greatest amounts of fluoride.[16] The surface fluoride protects against dental caries. The concentration of fluoride drops quickly inward toward the dentin, so that if the surface layer is polished away the protection is greatly diminished.

The fluoride-rich surface is important and should not be removed. Certain conditions increase caries susceptibility and therefore preclude removal through polishing. Patients with xerostomia from any cause, for example drug or radiation therapy, cannot afford to have the enamel surface weakened by polishing. In contrast, their therapy must include daily addition of concentrated fluoride, usually through self-applied methods such as rinsing or gel tray.

When upon evaluation it appears that polishing is required and therefore loss of the fluoride-rich surface is unavoidable, topical fluoride (gel or solution) must be applied in the attempt to replace the lost protection.[17] Fluoride uptake is minimal from prophylaxis pastes as compared to topical solutions or gels; therefore, a paste is not a substitute. In addition to topical application, daily self-applied fluoride should be recommended and prescribed. All patients need a fluoride-containing dentifrice, and in addition, a rinse, chewable tablet, or gel tray can be used, depending on age and caries susceptibility.

3. *Heat Production.* Steady pressure with a rapidly revolving rubber cup or bristle brush and a minimum of wet abrasive agent can create sufficient heat to cause pain and discomfort for the patient. The damage to the pulp by the heat has not been documented, but the pulps of young people are large and may be more susceptible to heat.

D. Effect on Gingiva

Trauma to the gingival tissue can result, especially when the prophylaxis angle is run at a high speed and the rubber cup is applied for an extended period. In one study a rubber cup with pumice rotated for 2 minutes caused a total removal of the epithelium inside the crest of the free gingiva.[18] Complete healing from such a wound would take from 8 to 14 days. The patient's sore and sensitive tissues could prevent adequate plaque removal during that time and a severe inflammation could result along with calculus reformation.

With the fast rotation of a rubber cup, particles of a polishing agent can be forced into the subepithelial tissues and create a source of irritation. Polishing after gingival and periodontal treatments, including scaling, root planing, and curettage, is not recommended on the same day. The diseased lining of the pocket usually has been removed and the pocket wall is wide open to receive particles that may become imbedded, out of reach of the most careful irrigation and rinsing.

By rotation of the rubber cup, microorganisms can be forced into the tissues. An inflammatory response can be expected, and bacteria may gain access to the blood stream to create a bacteremia.

Foreign body reactions to abrasives have been tested. A number of agents have been shown to have potential for creating reactions. Some explanation for delayed healing following tissue trauma may be found in this concept.[19]

III. Clinical Application of Selective Polishing

Because of the number of health and safety factors involved, as described above, decision to polish should be based on consideration for the individual patient. Instruction for stain prevention is important along with minimizing for all or omitting for selected patients the use of the abrasive paste with the rubber cup.

A. Summary of Contraindications for Polishing

The following list suggests some of the specific cases when polishing is either contraindicated indefinitely or should be postponed.

1. When there is no unsightly stain: The principle of selective polishing is not to polish unless it is needed. Appearance is important to patients, but it is also important to maintain the integrity of the enamel surface for disease prevention. When stain is noted on specific tooth surfaces, polishing can be applied to selected areas without having to cover all the teeth in a generalized procedure.[20]
2. Newly erupted teeth.
3. Decalcified areas.
4. Exposed root surfaces.
5. When instruction for personal plaque removal (daily care) has not yet been given or when the patient has not demonstrated adequate plaque control.
6. Soft spongy tissue that bleeds on brushing or gentle instrumentation.
7. Immediately following deep subgingival scaling, root planing, and gingival curettage.
8. Gold and other restorations that may be scratched by an abrasive.

B. Suggestions for Clinic Procedure

1. *Remove Stain by Scaling.* Whenever possible, stains can be removed during scaling. Unsightly stains will need removal for the new patient initially. At that time, an explanation of the selective polishing principle can be presented and assistance on a preventive plan for stain control given.
2. *Remove Stain During Root Planing.* The end product of root planing is a smooth, glassy surface that does not need further polishing.
3. *Minimize Polishing.* Correct application using a light intermittent stroke with the rubber cup should be always observed. Factors affecting the rate of abrasion are described in the next section.

CLEANING AND POLISHING AGENTS

Abrasive agents are applied with polishing instruments to remove extrinsic dental stains. Abrasives selected should produce smooth tooth surfaces but not remove tooth structure unnecessarily, abrade gingival epithelium, or produce excessive frictional heat.

I. Definitions

A. Abrasive

A material composed of particles of sufficient hardness and sharpness to cut or scratch a softer material when drawn across its surface.

B. Abrasion

The wearing away of surface material by friction. Marked or severe abrasion would be destructive to a tooth surface.[21]

C. Polishing

The production, especially by friction, of a smooth, glossy, mirror-like surface that reflects light.[21] A very fine agent is used for polishing after a coarser agent is used for cleaning.

II. Factors Affecting Abrasive Action

During polishing, sharp edges of abrasive particles are moved along the surface of a material, abrading it by producing microscopic scratches or grooves. The rate of abrasion, or speed with which structural material is removed from the surface being polished, is governed by characteristics of the abrasive particles as well as by the manner in which they are applied.

A. Characteristics of Abrasive Particles[21]

1. *Shape.* Irregularly shaped particles with sharp edges produce deeper grooves and thus abrade faster than rounded particles with dull edges.
2. *Hardness.* Particles must be harder than the surface to be abraded; harder particles abrade faster.
3. *Body Strength.* Particles that fracture into smaller sharp-edged particles during use are more abrasive than those that wear down with use and become dull and rounded.
4. *Attrition Resistance.* Effective abrasive particles do not dull or become impregnated in the surface being abraded; particles with greater attrition resistance abrade faster.

5. *Particle Size (Grit)*
   a. The larger the particles, the more abrasive they are with less polishing ability. Finer abrasive particles achieve a glossier finish.
   b. Grades: Abrasive and polishing agents are graded from coarse to fine based on the size of the holes in a standard sieve through which they will pass. The finer abrasives are called powders or flours and are graded in order of increasing fineness as F, FF, FFF, etc. Particles imbedded in papers are graded 0, 00, 000, etc.

B. **Method of Application of Abrasives**
   1. *Quantity Applied.* The more particles applied per unit time, the faster the rate of abrasion.
      a. Particles suspended in water or other vehicles are present in quantities proportional to the thickness of the paste. These vehicles act as lubricants to reduce the amount of frictional heat produced.
      b. Dry powders or flours represent the greatest quantity that can be applied per unit time. Frictional heat produced is proportional to the rate of abrasion; therefore, the use of *dry agents* is *contraindicated* for polishing natural teeth because of the potential danger of thermal injury to the dental pulp.
   2. *Speed of Application.* The greater the speed of application, the faster the rate of abrasion.
      a. With increased speed of application, pressure must be reduced.
      b. *Rapid abrasion* is *contraindicated* because it increases frictional heat.
   3. *Pressure of Application.* The heavier the pressure applied, the faster the rate of abrasion.
      a. Particles to which pressure is applied produce deep grooves at first, but fracture according to their impact strength. With sufficient pressure, the particles may disintegrate.
      b. *Heavy pressure* is *contraindicated* because it increases frictional heat.

4. *Summary.* When cleaning and polishing are indicated after patient evaluation, the following should be observed:
   a. Use wet agents.
   b. Apply a rubber polishing cup using low speed (page 577).
   c. Use a light, intermittent touch.

III. **Abrasive Agents**[21,22]

The abrasives listed below are examples of commonly used agents. Some are available in several grades, and the specific use varies with the grade. For example, while a superfine grade might be used for polishing enamel surfaces and metallic restorations, a coarser grade would be used for laboratory purposes only.

Abrasives for use daily in a dentifrice must necessarily be of a finer grade than those used for professional polishing accomplished a few times each year. Dentifrice abrasives are described on page 371.

A. **Silex** (silicon dioxide)
   1. *XXX Silex:* fairly abrasive.
   2. *Super-fine Silex:* can be used for stain removal from enamel.

B. **Pumice**

   Powdered pumice is of volcanic origin and consists chiefly of complex silicates of aluminum, potassium, and sodium. The specifications for particle size are listed in the *National Formulary*[23] as follows:
   1. *Pumice Flour or Superfine Pumice:* least abrasive, and may be used to remove stains from enamel.
   2. *Fine Pumice:* mildly abrasive.
   3. *Coarse Pumice:* not for use on natural teeth.

C. **Calcium Carbonate** (whiting, calcite, chalk)

   Various grades are used for different polishing techniques.

D. **Tin Oxide** (putty powder, stannic oxide)

   Polishing agent for teeth and metallic restorations.

E. **Emery** (corundum)

   Not used directly on the enamel.

1. *Aluminum Oxide* (alumina): the pure form of emery.
2. *Levigated Alumina:* extremely fine particles of aluminum oxide, which may be used for polishing metals but are destructive to tooth surfaces.

F. Rouge (jeweler's rouge)

Iron oxide, a fine red powder sometimes impregnated on paper discs. It is useful for polishing gold and precious metal alloys in the laboratory.

IV. Preparation of Abrasives

Agents used for polishing the natural teeth and restorations are mixed with water or other lubricant to facilitate particle movement across the tooth surface and to reduce frictional heat. A quantity of polishing paste can be prepared in advance and kept in a closed jar. Glycerin is added to help as a spreading factor and to prevent splashing during application of the polishing cup.

A. Preparation of Single Quantity

1. Place water or flavored mouthrinse in a dappen dish. Some agents require a specific amount of water.
2. Add the dry agent to saturation and stir.

B. Consistency: moist as possible, but transportable between dappen dish and the teeth.

C. Two Separate Containers and Rubber Cups
are used when a cleaning abrasive is used first and followed by a polishing agent.

V. Commercial Preparations

Numerous dental prophylactic cleaning and polishing preparations are available. Some of these have been studied for their relative abrasive effect on enamel and dentin, and their cleaning properties.[11]

A. Constituents

. Most commercially prepared polishing pastes contain an abrasive, water, a humectant, a binder, and agents for sweetening, flavoring, and color. Approximate proportions and purposes of each constituent with examples are as follows:
1. *Abrasive* 50 to 60 percent, main ingredient.

Examples: pumice, silicon dioxide.
2. *Water* 10 to 20 percent, solvent, and to provide desired consistency.
3. *Humectant* 20 to 25 percent, moisture-retainer, stabilize the ingredients. Examples: glycerin, sorbitol.
4. *Binder* 1.5 to 2.0 percent, prevent separation, non-splatter. Examples: agar-agar, sodium silicate powder.
5. *Sweetener,* artificial, noncariogenic.
6. *Flavoring,* coloring agents.

B. Packaging

Commercial preparations are in the forms of pastes, powders, or tablets. Some are available in measured amounts, contained in small plastic or other individual packets which contribute to the cleanliness and sterility of the procedure.

C. Selection

1. *General.* Selection of a preparation has been based on its qualities of abrasiveness, consistency for convenient use, or flavor for patient pleasure.
2. *Surface Fluoride Replacement.* The use of an abrasive on the tooth surface removes the outer layer of enamel that contains the highest concentration of fluoride (figure 29–2, page 443). Fluoride in a polishing paste is intended to provide fluoride to replace at least a part of that lost while polishing.

    A number of laboratory and clinical studies have been conducted to determine the effectiveness of incorporating fluoride into prophylactic pastes. Stannous fluoride and acidulated phosphate fluoride have been used primarily. Abrasives have included silex (silicon dioxide), lava pumice, and flour of pumice.

    Problems in the development of an effective paste are incompatibilities between the fluoride and the abrasive or other components of polishing pastes.

FACTORS TO TEACH THE PATIENT

I. Stains and deposits removed by polishing will return promptly if plaque control is not carried out faithfully.

II. Polishing agents employed in the dental office are too abrasive for routine daily home use.

III. The meaning of selective polishing, and why it is not necessary to polish all teeth at every recall appointment.

References

1. Theilade, J., Slots, J., and Fejerskov, O.: The Ultra-structure of Black Stain on Human Primary Teeth, *Scand. J. Dent. Res., 81*, 528, Number 7, 1973.
2. Knutson, J.W.: Sodium Fluoride Solutions: Technique for Application to the Teeth, *J. Am. Dent. Assoc., 36*, 37, January, 1948.
3. Tinanoff, N.: The Significance of the Acquired Pellicle in the Practice of Dentistry, *J. Dent. Child., 43*, 20, January–February, 1976.
4. Tinanoff, N., Wei, S.H.Y., and Parkins, F.M.: Effect of a Pumice Prophylaxis on Fluoride Uptake in Tooth Enamel, *J. Am. Dent. Assoc., 88*, 384, February, 1974.
5. Birkeland, J.M. and Torell, P.: Caries-preventive Fluoride Mouthrinses, *Caries Res., 12*, 38, Supplement 1, 1978.
6. Jones, J.C., Murphy, R.F., and Edd, P.A.: Using Health Education in a Fluoride Mouthrinse Program: The Public Health Hygienist's Role, *Dent. Hyg., 53*, 469, October, 1979.
7. Vrbic, V., Brudevold, F., and McCann, H.G.: Acquisition of Fluoride by Enamel From Fluoride Pumice Pastes, *Helv. Odontol. Acta, 11*, 21, April, 1967.
8. DeLeo, A.A.: The Incidence of Bacteremia Following Oral Prophylaxis on Pediatric Patients, *Oral Surg., 37*, 36, January, 1974.
9. Micik, R.E., Miller, R.L., Mazzarella, M.A., and Ryge, G.: Studies on Dental Aerobiology: I. Bacterial Aerosols Generated During Dental Procedures, *J. Dent. Res., 48*, 49, January–February, 1969.
10. Hartley, J.L.: Eye and Facial Injuries Resulting From Dental Procedures, *Dent. Clin. North Am., 22*, 505, July, 1978.
11. Whitehurst, V.E., Stookey, G.K., and Muhler, J.C.: Studies Concerning the Cleaning, Polishing, and Therapeutic Properties of Commercial Prophylactic Pastes, *J. Oral Thera. and Pharm., 4*, 181, November, 1967.
12. Stookey, G.K.: *In vitro* Estimates of Enamel and Dentin Abrasion Associated With a Prophylaxis, *J. Dent. Res., 57*, 36, January, 1978.
13. Zuniga, M.A. and Caldwell, R.C.: The Effect of Fluor-ide-containing Prophylaxis Pastes on Normal and "White-spot" Enamel, *J. Dent. Child., 36*, 345, September–October, 1969.
14. Brasch, S.V., Lazarou, J., Van Abbé, N.J., and Forrest, J.O.: The Assessment of Dentifrice Abrasivity *in vivo*, *Br. Dent. J., 127*, 119, August 5, 1969.
15. Jefferies, R.W.: Polishing Dental Enamel, *New Zeal. Dent. J., 69*, 167, July, 1973.
16. Brudevold, F., Gardner, D.E., and Smith, F.A.: The Distribution of Fluoride in Human Enamel, *J. Dent. Res., 35*, 420, June, 1956.
17. Vrbic, V. and Brudevold, F.: Fluoride Uptake From Treatment With Different Fluoride Prophylaxis Pastes and From the Use of Pastes Containing a Soluble Aluminum Salt Followed by Topical Application, *Caries Res., 4*, 158, Number 2, 1970.
18. Löe, H.: Reactions of Marginal Periodontal Tissues to Restorative Procedures, *Int. Dent. J., 18*, 759, December, 1968.
19. Miller, W.A.: Experimental Foreign Body Reactions to Toothpaste Abrasives, *J. Periodontol., 47*, 101, February, 1976.
20. Sheiham, A.: Prevention and Control of Periodontal Disease, in *International Conference on Research in the Biology of Periodontal Disease*. Chicago, University of Illinois, June, 1977, p. 332.
21. Phillips, R.W.: *Skinner's Science of Dental Materials*, 7th ed. Philadelphia, W.B. Saunders Co., 1973, pp. 623–630.
22. Craig, R.G., O'Brien, W.J., and Powers, J.M.: *Dental Materials. Properties and Manipulation*, 2nd ed. St. Louis, The C.V. Mosby Co., 1979, pp. 88–97.
23. American Pharmaceutical Association: *National Formulary XIII*. Washington, D.C., American Pharmaceutical Association, 1970, p. 611.

Suggested Readings

Brooks, E.B. and Voigt, J.P.: Particle Configuration of Prophylaxis Pastes as Observed by Scanning Electron Microscopy, *J. Periodontol., 45*, 23, January, 1974.

Bruun, C. and Stoltze, K.: *In vivo* Uptake of Fluoride by Surface Enamel of Cleaned and Plaque-covered Teeth, *Scand. J. Dent. Res., 84*, 268, September, 1976.

Clarke, P. and Seabrook, I.: Effectiveness of Self Prophylaxis and Rubber Cup Prophylaxis for Improving Paedodontic Home Care, *Can. Dent. Assoc. J., 41*, 511, September, 1975.

Davis, W.B.: Cervical Enamel: A Danger Zone, *J. Oral Rehabil., 6*, 385, October, 1979.

Handleman, S.L. and Hess, C.: Effect of Dental Prophylaxis on Tooth-surface Flora, *J. Dent. Res., 49*, 340, March–April, 1970.

Hunter, E.L., Biller-Karlsson, I.R., Featherstone, M.J., and Silverstone, L.M.: The Prophylaxis Polish—A Review of the Literature, *Dent. Hyg., 55*, 36, September, 1981.

Kidd, E.A.M., Thylstrup, A., Fejerskov, O., and Bruun, C.: Influence of Fluoride in Surface Enamel and Degree of Dental Fluorosis on Caries Development *in vitro*, *Caries Res., 14*, 196, Number 4, 1980.

Mellberg, J.R.: The Relative Abrasivity of Dental Prophylactic Pastes and Abrasives on Enamel and Dentin, *Clin. Prev. Dent., 1*, 13, January–February, 1979.

Nagle, S.: Prophylaxis Prior to Topical Fluoride Application: A Questionable Procedure? *Can. Dent. Hyg., 15*, 19, Spring, 1981.

Phillips, R.W.: *Elements of Dental Materials*, 3rd ed. Philadelphia, W.B. Saunders Co., 1977, pp. 343–354.

Primosch, R.E.: Rubber Cup Prophylaxis: A Reevaluation of Its Use in Pediatric Dental Patients, *Dent. Hyg., 54*, 525, November, 1980.

Putt, M.S., Kleber, C.J., and Muhler, J.C.: Studies of Prophylaxis Pastes Containing Sodium-potassium Aluminum Silicate and Fluoride, *J. Dent. Res., 58*, 1659, July, 1979.

Putt, M.S., Kleber, C.J., Davis, J.A., Schimmele, R.G., and Muhler, J.C.: Physical Characteristics of a New Cleaning and Polishing Agent for Use in a Prophylactic Paste, *J. Dent. Res., 54*, 527, May–June, 1975.

Richmond, G.: Applying Fluoridated Prophylaxis Paste to Interproximal Surfaces, *Quintessence Journal, 3*, 135, March, 1981.

Rootare, H.M., Powers, J.M., and Craig, R.G.: Wear of Composites by Abrasives of Varying Hardness, *J. Dent. Res., 58*, 1097, March, 1979.

Roulet, J.F. and Roulet-Mehrens, T.K.: The Surface Roughness of Restorative Materials and Dental Tissues After Polishing with Prophylaxis and Polishing Pastes, *J. Periodontol.*, *53*, 257, April, 1982.

Schifter, C.C., Hangorsky, C.A., and Emling, R.C.: A Philosophy of Selective Polishing, *R.D.H.*, *1*, 34, March, 1981.

Stookey, G.K. and Schemehorn, B.R.: Studies Evaluating a Fluoride-containing Prophylactic Cup, *Dent. Hyg.*, *50*, 253, June, 1976.

Stookey, G.K. and Schemehorn, B.R.: A Method for Assessing the Relative Abrasion of Prophylaxis Materials, *J. Dent. Res.*, *58*, 588, February, 1979.

Swan, R.W.: Dimensional Changes in a Tooth Root Incident to Various Polishing and Root Planing Procedures, *Dent. Hyg.*, *53*, 17, January, 1979.

Zampa, S.T. and Green, E.: Effect of Polishing Agents on Root Roughness, *J. Periodontol.*, *43*, 125, February, 1972.

39

The Porte Polisher with Wood Point

The porte polisher is a prophylactic hand instrument constructed to hold a wood polishing point at a contra-angle. A comparison of the porte polisher and the prophylaxis angle is made in table 39–1.

Manual polishing is accomplished by pressure of the wood point on the tooth surfaces as a moist abrasive is applied. The firm, carefully directed, rhythmic strokes impart a vigorous massage to the periodontal tissues. This is considered beneficial to the periodontal ligament because the periodontal fibers serve as a cushion for the slight movement of the tooth that occurs as the pressure of the instrument is applied. Fones described the beneficial effects to the gingival margin.[1] He suggested that the slight bumping of the wood point on the tissue causes a light pressure and release which has a massaging effect in producing a stimulation of the peripheral circulation.

I. Purposes and Uses

The entire polishing procedure may be accomplished with the porte polisher, although this is unusual in routine practice because of the time factor. Patients can be highly appreciative of smooth, quiet, hand polishing. With certain patients, under particular circumstances and for selected procedures, porte polishing is specifically indicated. Functions, purposes, and uses are suggested here.

A. Removes stains from the natural and restored surfaces of the teeth.
B. Provides a high, smooth polish which may help the tooth surfaces to resist deposit accumulation.
C. Effectively polishes cervical areas and exposed cementum or dentin of teeth that are hypersensitive to the heat produced by even a slowly revolving rubber polishing cup. A superfine, unflavored abrasive mixed with water only is appreciated by the patient and causes less abrasion of tooth structure.
D. Adapts to tooth surfaces that are inaccessible to a prophylaxis angle, such as the following:
   1. Exposed proximal surfaces of the teeth of patients who have undergone periodontal surgery.
   2. Lingual surfaces of lingually inclined mandibular molars, or distal surfaces of maxillary third permanent molars.
E. Method of choice for application of certain desensitizing agents for exposed cementum and dentin (page 557).
F. Useful for the homebound or bedridden patient when portable power-driven equipment is not available.
G. Helpful for orientation of small children, handicapped, or other patients apprehensive of power-driven equipment.

II. Characteristics of a Porte Polisher

Several types of porte polishers are available

571

Table 39–1.   Comparison of the Porte Polisher and the Prophylaxis Angle

Characteristic	Porte Polisher	Prophylaxis Angle
Massaging effect	Provided for gingival margin and periodontal ligament	No effect
Protection of gingiva from trauma	Easy by use of slow, even strokes	Difficult because of speed at which rubber cup is moving
Danger of abrading enamel and cementum	Minimized	Greater because of faster speed and decreased sense of touch
Stain removal	Removes all stains	Time saved in the removal of gross stains, but steady application of rubber cup could produce more heat than the patient could tolerate
Polish	High	Superficial cleaning
Heat	None	Much heat produced
Accessibility to tooth surface	Readily adapted to all surfaces	Limited because of size and weight of handpiece
Operator's sense of touch	Greater control of instrument is possible because sense of touch is present	Sense of touch is decreased because of weight and size of handpiece
Comfort to patient	Increased because of quietness and lack of discomfort from heat	Decreased because of noise, vibration, and heat produced
Comfort to operator	Light instrument, less tiring to trained hands	Heavy instrument is tiring to hold
Polishing agent	Less damage because of fewer strokes; agent must be applied wet	Only very fine grain powder should be used; must be applied very wet
Portability	Is portable, therefore useful at any time (for example, for bedridden patient)	Useful only in dental office, or with portable motor, with electricity
Care of instrument	Simple to sterilize	More time required for cleaning, oiling, sterilizing

for use. Practical features that influence selection are suggested below.

A. Can be taken apart conveniently for cleaning and sterilization.
B. Will not rust or discolor when given ordinary care.
C. Has convenient adjustment for attachment of wood points of various widths.
D. Is light weight for comfort of operator during use.
E. Has handle of diameter convenient to type of instrument grasp required.
F. Has handle with a finish that resists slipping in the hand during operation.

III. Selection and Preparation of Wood Points

Although several kinds of wood, including cedar, maple, and hard pine, have been used for polishing points, orangewood is preferred because it is hard enough to withstand pressure without fraying readily, yet porous enough to hold polishing agents. Ready-made wood points are available commercially in standard sizes and shapes.

A supply of wood points of routinely used sizes and shapes should be cut, sterilized, and stored in small sealed packages. Wood points can be included on a preprepared tray (page 32).

A. Length

1. Short
   a. To maintain rigidity of wood.
   b. To prevent unnecessary retraction of cheek and tongue.

2. Long enough to gain access to tooth surfaces without interference of shank of the porte polisher.

B. Width

1. Narrow
   a. For adaptation to the variety of tooth surfaces and contours.
   b. To prevent damage to the gingival margins as the point is adapted to the curved tooth surfaces.
2. Wide enough for efficiency in polishing.
3. Recommended average width: equal to the diameter of the circular wood point holder of the porte polisher.

C. Shape

1. *Wedge:* for facial, lingual, and proximal surfaces, and inclined planes of cusps.
2. *Cone (pointed):* for occlusal pits and grooves.

IV. Techniques for Use of Porte Polisher

The principles of technique described in Chapter 31 are applied during hand polishing. A systematic order of procedure from one tooth surface to the next surface is prerequisite to thoroughness. Applications of the general principles are included here.

A. Instrument Grasps (pages 478–479)

1. *Modified Pen*
   a. Recommended for all surfaces except maxillary anterior facial.
   b. Hold middle finger as near working end of instrument as possible as a guide and support.
2. *Palm*
   a. Recommended for maxillary anterior labial surfaces.
   b. Adapt to posterior maxillary facial surfaces when indicated by existing stains.

B. Finger Rest

Securely maintained on firm tooth.

C. Strokes

1. *Circular:* $1/16$ to $1/8$ inch diameter; apply at cervical third and when adjacent to gingival margin.

2. *Linear*
   a. Horizontal: back and forth on buccal and lingual of posterior teeth and to proximal surfaces as applicable.
   b. Vertical: up and down over labial and lingual surfaces of anterior teeth.
3. *Selection of Type and Size*
   a. Provide greatest protection for gingiva.
   b. Provide greatest efficiency in technique in accord with the anatomy of the tooth and the nature and location of the stains.

D. Manner of Operation

1. Apply appropriate grasp and finger rest, then position wood point on the tooth surface.
2. Hand, wrist, and arm rotate to propel the porte polisher.
   a. Fulcrum remains positioned as hand pivots around it.
   b. Fingers remain immobile, except for turning the instrument for adaptation.

E. Pressure Applied

1. Apply a directed, firm, moderate pressure with the use of slow deliberate strokes.
2. Apply increased pressure when circular stroke is directed away from free gingiva; decrease pressure when directed toward free gingiva.
3. Vary pressure with the tenacity of the deposit or stain to be removed.
4. Balance pressure applied to wood point with finger rest pressure.
5. Effect of excess pressure
   a. Increases hazard of injury to the margin of the free gingiva.
   b. Decreases stability and control during stroke.

TECHNICAL HINTS

I. Edges of wood points should be trimmed and the wood grain smoothed to minimize splinters that may harm the gingival tissues.

II. Place wood point flush with porte polisher attachment to prevent possible irritation to cheek, lip, or tongue.

III. Change wood point frequently during polishing procedure as it becomes saturated with moisture and splintered.
   A. To prevent wood slivers from damaging free gingiva.
   B. To increase efficiency by having well-shaped wedge for polishing.
IV. When more than one polishing agent is to be applied, use fresh wood points to prevent mixing the abrasives.
V. Avoid undue pressure on pontics and mobile teeth.
VI. Thorough flossing and irrigation of sulci following polishing is important because retained particles of polishing agent can be a source of irritation to the gingiva and increase postoperative discomfort.
VII. An iodine disclosing solution applied to green stain prior to polishing tends to facilitate its removal.

FACTORS TO TEACH THE PATIENT

I. The nature, occurrence, and etiology of stains.
II. Reasons for polishing the teeth.
III. Benefits of hand polishing.
IV. Relationship of plaque and stain accumulation to the frequency and thoroughness of patient's personal oral care habits.

Reference

1. Fones, A.C.: *Mouth Hygiene*, 4th ed. Philadelphia, Lea & Febiger, 1934, p. 277.

Suggested Readings

Alper, M.N.: An Evaluation of Tooth Polishing Techniques, *J. Am. Dent. Hyg. Assoc.*, *43*, 137, 3rd Quarter, 1969.

Carranza, F.A.: *Glickman's Clinical Periodontology*, 5th ed. Philadelphia, W.B. Saunders Co., 1979, p. 632.

Fones, A.C.: *Mouth Hygiene*, 4th ed. Philadelphia, Lea & Febiger, 1934, pp. 277–289.

Hall, W.B.: Oral Prophylaxis, in Steele, P.F., ed.: *Dimensions of Dental Hygiene*, 2nd ed. Philadelphia, Lea & Febiger, 1975, pp. 177–179.

Hard, D.: Oral Prophylaxis, in Bunting, R.W.: *Oral Hygiene*, 3rd ed. Philadelphia, Lea & Febiger, 1957, pp. 255–258.

Miller, S.C.: *Textbook of Periodontia*, 3rd ed. Philadelphia, Blakiston, 1950, pp. 278–280.

Sorrin, S., ed.: *The Practice of Periodontia*. New York, Blakiston Division, McGraw-Hill, 1960, pp. 182–183.

Woodall, I.R., Dafoe, B.R., Young, N.S., Weed-Fonner, L., and Yankell, S.L.: *Comprehensive Dental Hygiene Care*. St. Louis, The C.V. Mosby Co., 1980, pp. 303–304.

40

Polishing Procedures

As described on page 561, cleaning and polishing for stain removal is a selective procedure. After scaling and other periodontal treatment, an evaluation is made to determine the need for polishing of teeth, restorations, and dental prostheses. In preparation for polishing, a review should be made of pertinent information on stains (page 286), pellicle and plaque (page 261), fluoride in the surface enamel (page 443), and abrasives (page 566).

I. Patient Preparation for Polishing

Preparation of the patient includes instruction in plaque control procedures, complete scaling and planing, and overhang removal. The patient should be informed of the limited value of polishing and why it is a selective procedure performed as needed.

A. Plaque Control

Polishing should be withheld until the patient's plaque removal on a daily basis is adequate, in order that the deposition of stains can be controlled. When a patient is informed of the relationship between self-care and the recurrence of stains, cooperation may be obtained. When a stain such as tobacco stain returns, polishing frequency should be limited and, with each polishing, topical fluoride applied.

B. Scaling

As much stain as possible should be re-moved during scaling for calculus removal from the enamel. All stain should be removed during root planing, since the stain is located within the diseased, altered cementum.

II. Environmental Preparation

Environmental factors were described in Chapter 3, including handpiece and prophylaxis angle sterilization and care. Special needs for patients who require maximum precautions were identified on page 64. A topical summary is provided here.

A. Procedures to Lessen the Extent of Contaminated Aerosols

1. Avoid use of power-driven instruments for a maximum precautions patient with a communicable disease that could be disseminated by way of aerosols.
2. Clear the water that will be used for rinsing. Flush water through the tubing for 5 to 6 minutes at the beginning of each work period, and for 30 seconds after each appointment.
3. Request patient to rinse with a povidone-iodine mouthrinse to reduce the numbers of oral microorganisms before starting instrumentation.
4. Use high velocity evacuation.

B. Protective Eyeglasses and Mask

Both patient and operator must wear protective eyeglasses, and the operator needs a face mask (pages 50–53).

III. Instruments

Both power-driven and manual instruments may be useful when polishing. All polishing instruments should be used with discretion and in a manner requiring minimal abrasion of the tooth surface. Since tooth structure is removed when an abrasive is used on the enamel, and still more when used on dentin or cementum, only a mild abrasive agent is appropriate.

Power-driven implements, floss, and finishing strips will be outlined first, followed by procedures for cleaning a removable prosthesis. In the next chapter, finishing of amalgam restorations will be described.

THE INSTRUMENTS

I. Handpiece

A handpiece is an instrument used to hold rotary instruments in the dental unit. It is connected by an arm, cable, belt, or tube to the source of power. Rotary instruments have been classified according to their rotational speeds designated by revolutions per minute (r.p.m.) as high speed, mid speed, and low speed.[1]

A. Ultra or High Speed (Type I)

Class A: Greater than 160,000 r.p.m.
Class B: 100,000 to 160,000 r.p.m.

B. Mid Speed (Type II)

Between 20,000 and 100,000 r.p.m. Some high speed handpieces can be adjusted to speeds from zero to their capacity, which makes it possible to use them with the proper attachments for tooth polishing.

C. Low Speed (Type III)

Typical range under 20,000 r.p.m. Lowest speeds are used for polishing and finishing procedures.

II. Prophylaxis Angle

Contra or right-angle attachment for the handpiece to which polishing devices (rubber cup, bristle brush) are attached.

A. Characteristics

Many types of prophylaxis angles are available. They are generally made of stainless steel and may have hard chrome, carbon steel, or brass bearings. A few types are reversible in their action.

B. Service Life

The length of time a prophylaxis angle is serviceable is related in part to the quality of materials used and the manner of construction. Primarily, however, *the length of life is directly proportional to the care provided in cleaning and lubricating after each use.*

III. Prophylaxis Angle Attachments

A. Rubber Polishing Cups

1. *Types*
   a. Slip-on: with ribbed cup to aid in holding polishing agent.
   b. Slip-on: with bristles inside cup.
   c. Threaded (screw type): with plain ribbed cup or flange (webbed) type.
2. *Materials*
   a. Natural rubber: more resilient and will not stain the teeth.
   b. Synthetic: stiffer than natural rubber; white cups must be used since synthetic black may stain the teeth.

B. Bristle Brushes

1. *Types*
   a. For prophylaxis angle: slip-on or screw type.
   b. For handpiece: mandrel mounted.
2. *Materials:* nylon or natural bristles.

IV. Uses for Attachments

A. Handpiece With Straight Mandrel

1. Dixon bristle brush (Type C, soft) for polishing removable dentures (page 581).
2. Mounted stone for sharpening instruments (page 501).
3. Rubber cup on mandrel for polishing labial surfaces of anterior teeth.

B. Prophylaxis Angle With Rubber Cup or Brush

1. Rubber cup for removal of stains from the tooth surfaces and polishing restorations.

2. Brush
   a. For removing stains from deep pits and fissures and enamel surfaces away from gingival margin. A brush is not recommended for use on exposed cementum or dentin. They are easily grooved by such an instrument.
   b. For preliminary polishing of amalgam restorations.

USE OF THE PROPHYLAXIS ANGLE

I. Effects on Tissues: Precautions

The use of power-driven instruments can cause discomfort for the patient if care and consideration for the oral tissues are not exercised to prevent unnecessary trauma.

Awareness of the potential tissue damage that may result is important. Tactile sensitivity of the operator while using a thick, bulky handpiece is diminished, and unnecessary pressure may be applied inadvertently. Frictional heat may cause pain or discomfort.

Some loss of tooth structure occurs during polishing when an abrasive agent is used. Research on the effects on tooth structure was reviewed on page 563.

The greater the speed of application of a polishing agent, the faster the rate of abrasion (page 566). Therefore, the speed at which the handpiece is operated should be a low r.p.m.

Trauma to the gingival tissue can result from too high a speed, extended application of the rubber cup, and use of an abrasive polishing agent. Tissue damage and the need for antibiotic premedication for risk patients was described on pages 99–100.

II. Prophylaxis Angle Technique

The first technique principle is to apply the polishing agent only where it is needed, that is, where there is unsightly stain.[2] Contraindications were listed on pages 564–565.

As with all oral procedures, a systematic order of polishing should be followed. A variety of skills must be learned in using and caring for the equipment.

A. Instrument Grasp: Modified pen (page 478)

B. Finger Rest (page 479)

1. Establish firmly on tooth structure.

2. Use a wide fulcrum area when practical to aid in the balance of the large instrument. Example: place cushion of fulcrum finger across occlusal surfaces of premolars while polishing the molars.
3. Avoid use of mobile teeth as finger rests.

C. Speed of Handpiece

1. Use slowest available speed to minimize frictional heat.
2. Adjust r.p.m. by changing the position of the rheostat foot pedal.

D. Use of Rheostat Pedal

1. Apply steady pressure with foot to produce an even, slow speed.
2. Keep sole of the foot that activates rheostat pedal flat on the floor. Use toe to activate rheostat pedal.

E. Preparation of Polishing Agent

1. Agent is mixed as wet as possible, but not so wet that it cannot be carried conveniently in the rubber cup from the dappen dish to the teeth.
2. Wetness aids in alleviating the frictional heat produced.

F. Stroke and Procedure

1. *Rubber Cup*
   a. Observe where polishing is needed to prevent unnecessary rubber cup application.
   b. Distribute polishing agent over group of tooth surfaces to be polished.
   c. Fill rubber cup with polishing agent, establish finger rest, and bring rubber cup almost in contact with tooth surface before starting motor.
   d. Using slowest r.p.m., apply revolving cup lightly to tooth surface for 1 or 2 seconds.
   e. Move cup to adjacent area on tooth surface, using a patting motion.
   f. Move cup from tooth to tooth, frequently replenishing supply of polishing agent.
   g. Turn handpiece to adapt rubber cup to fit each surface of the tooth, including proximal surfaces and gin-

gival surfaces of fixed partial dentures.

h. When two polishing agents of different abrasiveness are to be applied, use a separate rubber cup for each.

i. Discard a rubber cup as it becomes less firm and before it wears on the edges. Cups that cannot be sterilized are used only once.

2. *Bristle Brush.* Bristle brushes should be used selectively. Lacerations of the gingiva and grooves and scratches in the tooth surface, particularly roots, may result.

a. Soak stiff brush in hot water to soften bristles.

b. Distribute mild abrasive polishing agent over occlusal surfaces of teeth to be polished.

c. Place fingers of nondominant hand in a position that will both retract and protect cheek and tongue from the revolving brush.

d. Establish a firm finger rest and bring brush almost in contact with the tooth before starting motor.

e. Using slowest r.p.m., apply revolving brush lightly to the occlusal surface only, avoiding contact of bristles with soft tissues.

f. Use a short stroke in a brushing motion, following the inclined planes of the cusps.

g. Move from tooth to tooth to prevent generation of excessive frictional heat. Replenish supply of polishing agent frequently.

G. Irrigation

Teeth and interdental areas should be irrigated thoroughly several times with water from the syringe to remove abrasive particles. The rotary movement of the rubber cup or bristle brush tends to force the abrasive into the gingival sulci, which may be a source of irritation to the soft tissues.

POLISHING PROXIMAL SURFACES

Considerable care must be exercised in the use of floss, tape, and finishing strips. Understanding the anatomy of the interdental papillae and their relationship to the contact areas and proximal surfaces of the teeth is prerequisite to the prevention of tissue damage. Inadequate contacts between teeth provide potential areas of food impaction and plaque retention. These contacts should be charted for consideration by the dentist during treatment planning.

As much polishing as possible of accessible proximal surfaces is accomplished during the use of the rubber cup in the prophylaxis angle. This is followed by the use of dental tape with polishing agent when necessary. Finishing strips are used only in selected instances when all other techniques fail to remove a stain.

The use of dental floss or tape for dental plaque control on proximal tooth surfaces is an essential part of self-care by the patient. This is described on pages 360–363.

I. Dental Tape and Floss

A. Description

Floss and tape are made of spun silk or nylon thread and are available unwaxed or coated with wax. The wax covering affords some protection for the tissues, facilitates the movement of the floss or tape, prevents excessive absorption of moisture, and assists in the prevention of shredding.

Tape is flat and has relatively sharp edges, whereas floss is round. Either floss or tape may injure the tissue when used incorrectly or carelessly.

B. Uses

1. *Tape for Polishing*
   a. Proximal tooth surfaces.
   b. Gingival surface of fixed partial denture.

2. *Floss for Removing*
   a. Debris and food particles. Patient instruction and review at beginning of appointment prepares the teeth for scaling.
   b. Particles of polishing agents at completion of polishing procedures.
      (1) From interproximal areas and gingival sulci.
      (2) From gingival surface of fixed partial dentures.
   c. Retained abrasive particles after use of finishing strips.

C. Technique for Dental Floss and Tape

Techniques for tape and floss application are described on pages 360–363 and illustrated in figures 23–1, 23–2, and 23–3. The same principles apply whether the patient or the operator is using the floss. Finger rests must be used to prevent snapping through contact areas.

1. *Polishing with Dental Tape.* Polishing agent is applied to the tooth, and the tape is moved gently back and forth over the area where stain was observed.
2. *Polishing Gingival Surface of a Fixed Partial Denture.* A floss threader is used to position the floss or tape over the gingival surface. Floss threaders are described and illustrated on page 381. Polishing agent is applied under the pontic, and the floss or tape moved back and forth.
3. *Floss after Polishing.* Particles of abrasive agent should be removed by irrigation and by using a clean length of floss applied in the usual manner.
4. *Rinse and Irrigate.* Irrigate with water spray syringe to clean out all abrasive agent.

II. Finishing Strips

A. Description

Finishing strips are also known as linen abrasive strips. They are thin, flexible, tape-shaped, and are available in four widths—extra narrow, narrow, medium, and wide.

Finishing strips are made of linen or plastic with one smooth side and the other that serves as a carrier for abrasive agents bonded to the side. "Gapped" strips are available with an abrasive-free portion to permit sliding the strip through the contact area without abrading the enamel.[3]

They are available in extra fine, fine, medium, or coarse grit. *Only extra narrow or narrow strips with fine grit are suggested for stain removal and then only with discretion.*

B. Use

1. *For Stain Removal on Proximal Surfaces of Anterior Teeth.* When other polishing techniques are unsuccessful.

2. *Precautions for Use*
   a. Edge of strip is sharp and may cut gingival tissue or lip.
   b. Rough working side of strip is capable of removing tooth structure and may make nicks or grooves, particularly in the cementum.
   c. Use of a finishing strip should be limited to enamel surfaces.

C. Technique for Finishing Strip

1. *Grasp and Finger Rest.* A strip no longer than 6 inches is most conveniently applied. The grasp and fulcrum must be well controlled. Protection of the lip by retraction with the thumb and index finger holding the strip is mandatory.

2. *Positioning*
   a. Direct the abrasive side of strip toward the proximal surface to be treated, as the strip is worked slowly and gently between the teeth with a slightly sawing motion. Bring strip just through the contact area. If the strip breaks, immediately use floss to remove particles of abrasive.
   b. When a space is clearly visible through an interproximal area and the interdental papilla is missing, a narrow finishing strip may be threaded through. Prepare strip by cutting the end on the diagonal to facilitate threading.

3. *Stain Removal*
   a. Press abrasive side of strip against tooth. Draw back and forth in a $\frac{1}{8}$ inch arc two or three times, rocking on the established fulcrum.
   b. Remove strip and insert for adjacent proximal surface. Do not attempt to turn the strip while it is in the interdental area.

4. *Use Dental Floss.* Follow each application of finishing strips with dental floss to remove abrasive particles.

CLEANING THE REMOVABLE DENTURE

A complete patient service includes the scaling and polishing of all natural teeth and their replacements. Complete and partial dentures may accumulate calculus, soft deposits, and stains which may affect the adaptation of the dentures in the mouth as well as afford a source of irritation to adjacent mucous membranes. The parts of a complete denture are illustrated in figure 24–9, page 385, and the parts of a partial in figure 24–12, page 391.

A learning experience in the proper care of the dentures can be provided for the patient while the dentures are cleaned professionally. Specific instruction for the patient is described on pages 385–393.

I. Objectives

With professional cleaning of a removable denture, the following benefits can be expected:
A. Aid in preserving the natural teeth associated with a removable partial denture.
B. Removal of calculus and stains, thereby smoothing the surfaces of the denture to lessen plaque and debris retention.
C. Improvement of the appearance and sanitation of the denture.
D. Provide the patient with a feeling of complete oral cleanliness.
E. Understanding by the patient of the importance of routine personal and professional care of the denture.

II. Removal of Denture

Generally, the patient removes the denture. The dental hygienist will have occasion to remove dentures for certain patients, particularly those who may be handicapped or helpless, or as an emergency measure.

Although denture removal may be complicated by anatomic features of an individual mouth, a general procedure is outlined here. The procedure should be reviewed with the dentist in order to follow a preferred technique.

A. Wear Rubber Gloves

When the patient is known to have, or is suspected of having, a communicable disease or when a generally septic condition exists in the oral cavity, rubber gloves should be worn.

B. Complete Maxillary Denture

1. Grasp the denture firmly with the thumb on the facial surface at the height of the border of the denture under the lip and the index finger on the palatal surface.

2. With the other hand, elevate the lip to expose the border of the denture to break the seal.
3. Remove the denture gently in a downward and forward direction.
4. If the retention of the denture cannot be overcome by elevation of the lip, request the able patient to blow into the mouth with the lips closed. This generally will break the seal.

C. Complete Mandibular Denture

1. Grasp the denture firmly on the facial surface with the thumb and the lingual with the index finger.
2. With the other hand, retract the lower lip forward and remove the denture gently.

D. Partial Denture with Clasps

Exert an even pressure on both sides of the denture simultaneously as the clasps are lifted over their abutment teeth. Usually, the line of insertion and removal of a partial denture is designed and constructed for an even, vertical removal.

III. Care of Dentures During Intra-oral Procedures

A. Provide a cleansing tissue for the patient's use when requesting the patient to remove or insert the denture.
B. Receive removable denture in a paper cup or container with a fitted cover.
C. Wear rubber gloves and scrub the denture with surgical soap.
D. Immerse in antiseptic solution (page 64).
E. Place container in a safe place away from working area to minimize hazard of breakage.

IV. Procedure for Cleaning

Ultrasonic cleaning is the procedure of choice for the safety of the denture, for the preservation of the surface finish, to eliminate the possibility of scratching the denture surface through the use of scalers, polishing agents, or other devices, and for the time saved. When ultrasonic equipment is not available, manual and power-driven instruments must be used.

A. **Ultrasonic**

1. Principles and procedures were described on pages 30–31.
2. Use the solution designated for stain and calculus removal and follow the manufacturer's directions specifically.
3. Rinse thoroughly and scrub free of solution and loosened debris with a moderately stiff brush before returning the denture to the patient. Brushes reserved for this purpose should be sterilized.

B. **Manual and Power-driven**

1. *Removal of Calculus.* Remove calculus by careful scaling. Care must be taken not to scratch the denture.
2. *Method for Holding Denture.* Grasp firmly and securely in the palm of the nondominant hand (figure 24–10, page 388); avoid excessive pressure on a partial denture bar or clasps to prevent bending.
3. *Polishing the Denture.* Polish only the external polished surface of a denture; abrasive applied to the internal impression surface could alter the fit of the denture.
4. *Polishing at the Dental Chair*
   a. With a conventional dental chair, polishing over the cuspidor (lined with a towel) is sometimes convenient. Focus the dental light over the work area.
   b. Polish nonmetal parts with a mounted brush (Dixon C softened in warm water), using very wet superfine pumice or other appropriate abrasive. The finger rest is maintained on the denture.
   c. Polish metal parts lightly with a rubber polishing cup. A fine polishing agent should be used to prevent scratching of the metal.
5. *Polishing on the Dental Lathe in the Laboratory*
   a. Prevention of cross contamination in the laboratory.[4]
      (1) Wear a mask and safety glasses while working over a lathe.
      (2) Use sterile rag wheel and pumice.
      (3) Soak the prosthesis in an antiseptic solution for 2 to 3 minutes

before returning it to the patient. The solution should be fresh for each patient.
      b. Use a wet rag wheel with fine wet abrasive for nonmetal parts, and whiting or tin oxide on a separate rag wheel for the metal parts other than clasps. Keep denture and polishing agent wet at all times.
      c. Hold the denture in a two-handed grip. Cover the clasps and denture teeth with fingers to prevent abrasive from scratching the teeth and the clasps from hooking into the rag wheel. The clasps are cleaned later with a wood point in the porte polisher.
      d. Run the lathe at low speed and apply denture carefully. Constantly change the surface applied to the rag wheel to prevent excess frictional heat.
6. *Rinsing the Denture.* Rinse the denture thoroughly under warm (never hot) running water.
   a. Line the sink with a towel, or fill half-full with water to avoid breakage in case the denture is dropped.
   b. Brush the internal impression surface of the denture using a mild soap or a detergent; rinse thoroughly.
7. *Evaluation.* Evaluate the cleanliness of the denture: examine under bright light and apply compressed air stream to detect calculus or dental plaque.
8. *Disinfection.* Disinfect, rinse and return the denture to the patient on a paper towel. The denture should be wet for comfortable insertion.

TECHNICAL HINTS

I. Maintain several prophylaxis angles in practice to facilitate use during successive appointments. When this is done, care of the prophylaxis angles should be accomplished as soon as possible after use: within a few hours at the most.
II. Test staining potential of a black synthetic rubber cup by using it as an eraser on white paper. If black appears, the teeth can be stained.

III. Prevent rheostat from sliding on highly polished floor by placing one or two drops of carbon tetrachloride under the rheostat.
IV. Wear eyeglasses and mask for protection from flying material and aerosols when using handpiece, prophylaxis angle, and dental lathe.
V. Protect patient's lips and intraoral soft tissues during the use of floss, tape, finishing strips, and discs.

FACTORS TO TEACH THE PATIENT

I. How plaques and stains form on the natural teeth and their replacements and why too frequent polishing in the dental office is not advisable. When adequate self-care is carried out, polishing is not necessary.
II. The need for adapting toothbrushing and flossing techniques to cleanse abutment teeth.
III. The importance of regular cleansing of dentures with special attention to clasps.
IV. How to handle and cleanse a denture.

References

1. American Dental Association, Council on Dental Materials, Instruments and Equipment: *Dentist's Desk Reference: Materials, Instruments and Equipment*, 1st ed. Chicago, American Dental Association, 1981, pp. 14–15, 223–227, 230.
2. Sheiham, A.: Prevention and Control of Periodontal Disease, in *International Conference on Research in the Biology of Periodontal Disease.* Chicago, University of Illinois, June, 1977, p. 332.
3. Project Acorde, United States Department of Health, Education, and Welfare: *Recontouring, Finishing, and Polishing.* Castro Valley, California, Quercus, 1976, pp. 27–28.
4. Katberg, J.W.: Cross-contamination via the Prosthodontic Laboratory, *J. Prosthet. Dent., 32,* 412, October, 1974.

Suggested Readings

Eames, W.B., Reder, B.S., Smith, G.A., Satrom, K.D., and Dwyer, B.M.: Ten High-speed Handpieces: Evaluation of Performance, *Gen. Dent., 28,* 22, March–April, 1980.
Galil, K.A.: An *in vitro* Assessment of Oral Prophylaxis Procedures. A Scanning Electron Microscopy Study, *Can. Dent. Assoc. J., 43,* 370, August, 1977.
Hartley, J.L.: Eye and Facial Injuries Resulting from Dental Procedures, *Dent. Clin. North Am., 22,* 505, July, 1978.
Kilpatrick, H.C.: High Speed Handpieces–Update (I), *Quintessence Int., 10,* 93, February, 1979.
Kilpatrick, H.C.: High Speed Handpieces–Update (II), *Quintessence Int., 10,* 63, March, 1979.
Larato, D.C.: Disinfection of Pumice, *J. Prosthet. Dent., 18,* 534, December, 1967.
Morant, G.A.: Burs and Rotary Instruments. Introduction of a New Standard Numbering System, *Br. Dent. J., 147,* 97, August 21, 1979.
Nicholson, R.J., Stark, M.M., and Scott, H.E.: Calculus and Stain Removal from Acrylic Resin Dentures, *J. Prosthet. Dent., 20,* 326, October, 1968.
Park, P.R.: Effects of Sound on Dentists, *Dent. Clin. North Am., 22,* 415, July, 1978.
Peyton, F.A.: Status Report on Dental Operating Handpieces, *J. Am. Dent. Assoc., 89,* 1162, November, 1974.
Sockwell, C.L.: Dental Handpieces and Rotary Cutting Instruments, *Dent. Clin. North Am., 15,* 219, January, 1971.
Walsh, R.F. and Ames, M.I.: Reinforcing the Aseptic Chain in Hospital Dental Practice, *J. Hosp. Dent. Pract., 6,* 57, April, 1972.
Willmann, D.E., Norling, B.K., and Johnson, W.N.: A New Prophylaxis Instrument: Effect on Enamel Alterations, *J. Am. Dent. Assoc., 101,* 923, December, 1980.
Woodall, I.R., Dafoe, B.R., Young, N.S., Weed-Fonner, L., and Yankell, S.L.: *Comprehensive Dental Hygiene Care.* St. Louis, The C.V. Mosby Co., 1980, pp. 297–307.

41

Finishing and Polishing Amalgam Restorations

The finishing of an amalgam restoration includes the procedures that collectively produce a restoration with normal tooth contours, refined margins, smooth corrosion-resistant surfaces, functional effectiveness, and an acceptable appearance. With such characteristics, the restoration can be expected to contribute to the patient's oral health for a long period of time. The economic benefit is especially notable when preventive measures are emphasized.

There are two applications for finishing procedures; namely, for the newly placed restoration, and for the previously placed restoration, which for various reasons, has irregular margins and surfaces. Basic procedures to follow when treating both the old and the new restorations are similar.

The extent of necessary finishing for a new restoration depends on the carving and burnishing performed at the time the restoration was placed. The neatly and carefully carved restoration which fulfills ideal, normal anatomic and functional requirements will require little smoothing of margins and surfaces before polishing. On the other hand, an "old" filling may have many irregularities of the margins and surfaces which have resulted either from inadequate finishing when the restoration was placed originally or from changes over the years.

Principles and procedures are presented in this chapter. A study of amalgam and its properties should precede learning to finish and polish.[1,2,3]

RATIONALE FOR FINISHING AND POLISHING

Finishing and polishing of amalgam restorations contribute to the following effects:

A. Increased length of service of the restoration by eliminating factors that lead to surface changes and recurrent dental caries.
B. Decreased amalgam tarnish and corrosion.
C. Increased integrity of the junction of tooth surface and amalgam.
D. Improved gingival health because of less plaque retention by amalgam irregularities.
E. Improved maintenance by the patient: plaque is more easily removed by brush and floss from smooth surfaces.
F. Improved compatibility of the restorative material with the oral soft tissues.
G. Increased comfort for the patient because the restorations are smooth to the tongue.
H. Improved appearance of the restorations.

THE AMALGAM RESTORATION

A large majority of restorations for both primary and permanent teeth are made of dental amalgam. Amalgam is an important restorative material, and when scientific principles are used while a restoration is placed and the restored tooth is cared for daily by the patient, the restoration can be expected to last many years, some, even a lifetime.

The initial factors that influence the longevity of an amalgam restoration include the design of the cavity preparation, the mix and manipulation of the dental material, the condensation, prevention of contamination and moisture, and the finishing and polishing.[1] After the restoration has been completed, factors that contribute to the continued serviceability relate to the patient's daily preventive program through plaque control, low-cariogenic diet, and fluoride application, combined with maintenance supervision at professional recall appointments.

A review of selected amalgam properties and changes with age that are pertinent to finishing and polishing will be considered first. That will be followed by descriptive definitions of types of marginal irregularities of an amalgam restoration encountered during examination.

I. Amalgam Properties and Age Changes

A. Surface Changes

1. *Tarnish.* Tarnish is a surface discoloration, principally a sulfide. It is usually caused by lack of oral cleanliness, with resultant plaque collection, and certain foods, especially foods containing sulfur. Tarnish is less frequently found on properly finished and polished restorations.

2. *Corrosion.* Corrosion is an actual chemical deterioration of the metal, which usually begins as a tarnish and is caused by environmental factors such as air, moisture, acid or alkaline solutions, and other chemicals.[4] Smoothly polished amalgam resists corrosion.

   Corrosion at the margin of a restoration can cause deterioration and fracture of the margin. An open gap where plaque can collect is the usual result. The products of corrosion may be carried into the dentinal tubules, and the entire area around the restoration may appear bluish-black.

B. Dimensional Changes[1,2]

Expansion can occur as a result of incom-

plete trituration and condensation or contamination from moisture entering the amalgam during the mixing and placing of the restoration. When expansion occurs in excess, the filling appears extruded above the cavosurface margin. Expansion can also produce postoperative pain or tooth sensitivity because of pressure on the pulp.

When contraction occurs, the amalgam may pull away from the cavosurface margin. Contraction is one of the causes of "ditching," a term used to describe a space between the filling material and the tooth structure, as defined on page 586.

C. Amalgam Strength

Fractures are a result of insufficient strength. A fracture may be seen as a gross irregularity, a crack-line across an entire restoration, or a marginal chip. Several factors can be involved in amalgam fractures, including the following:

1. *Manipulation of the Filling Material.* Undertrituration of amalgam results in low strength.

2. *Overload of Pressure on a Restoration Before Setting is Complete.* Strength of the amalgam is low during the first few hours after placement. After carving, the occlusal relationship should be checked for high contact spots, which if subjected to masticatory stress, could lead to fracture.

3. *Inadequate Strength of Surrounding Tooth Structure.* Strength and support for an amalgam restoration depend in part on the strength of the surrounding tooth structure. When dental caries requires wide extension of the cavity preparation, the tooth walls may be subject to fracture. Both the amalgam and the tooth may fracture together.

4. *Improper Carving of the Restoration.* Marginal strength can be compromised when a thin excess of amalgam is left extending over the cavosurface margin. If the small overhang (flash) breaks off, a part of the margin of the restoration may also break off with the flash (figure 41–1). The fracture may be caused by occlusal pressures or finishing procedures.

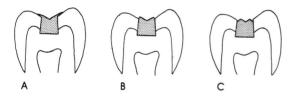

Figure 41–1. Occlusal surface irregularities of amalgam restorations. **A.** Flash; **B.** Irregular margin when flash breaks off; **C.** Ditching resulting from broken off flash.

II. Types of Marginal Irregularities: Definitions

When an amalgam restoration is to be finished and polished, it is first examined by moving an explorer over the surfaces and margins. A variety of irregularities or defects may be found. The defects represent excesses or deficiencies of amalgam.

The finished functional restoration will follow the normal contours of the tooth. All cavosurface junctions will be smooth to an explorer.

It is necessary to recognize and differentiate excesses and deficiencies, so that finishing and polishing procedures can be carried out effectively. When deficiencies of amalgam occur, correction by finishing techniques could require removal of excess tooth structure. Usually, deficiencies must be corrected by replacement of the restoration.

The common irregularities and defects of amalgam restorations are defined and described below.

A. Overhanging Margin

An amalgam overhang is an area of excess amalgam that extends beyond the cavosurface margin of a cavity preparation (figure 41–2A). Proximal overhangs result primarily from improper placement of the matrix band and wedge. Overhangs may occur on any tooth surface, supra- or subgingivally, in any class of cavity. They may be caused by errors of manipulation, carving, and/or finishing.

B. Flash

A flash is a type of overhang in which a thin layer of amalgam extends beyond the cavosurface margin. It is sometimes referred to as a feather ledge.

1. *Occlusal.* Figure 41–1A illustrates a feather ledge or flash that was left during carving. Carving, correctly performed, brings the cavosurface margin into view and makes the filling material flush with the enamel.

2. *Proximal–Gingival.* A flash-type overhang can result when an amalgam is packed between a matrix band and the tooth surface below the cavity preparation (figure 41–2B). The irregularity can occur when a proximal wedge is not used or not positioned to adapt the matrix tightly against the tooth surface. A tooth with a concave proximal surface is most vulnerable to flash.

C. Open Margin

An open margin is found when there is a distinct space between the amalgam and the wall of the cavity preparation (figure 41–2C). The causes include the following:

1. Too much time elapses after trituration before condensation. The amalgam material begins to set and becomes difficult to condense properly.

2. Too large an amount of the amalgam mix is inserted into the cavity preparation at one time.

D. Undercontoured

The opposite of an overhang is a deficiency of amalgam between the margin of the amalgam and the cavity wall as shown in figure 41–2D. Causes could be related on the proximal to improper placement of the matrix or wedge or both or misdirected carving with poorly selected instruments.

Undercontouring is exemplified also by missing contact areas, flattened cervical

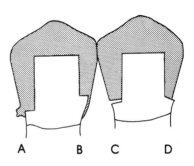

Figure 41–2. Marginal irregularities of amalgam restorations. **A.** Overhang; **B.** Flash on proximal surface; **C.** Open margin; **D.** Undercontoured.

ridges, incomplete marginal ridges, and incomplete filling of the cavity preparation.

E. Overcontoured

An overcontoured restoration has an excess of amalgam in such a position as to change the normal anatomic form of the restoration. Interproximally overcontoured surfaces may widen the contact area or narrow the embrasure. When the crown is overcontoured, the effect can be plaque retention and pressure on the gingival margin.

In figure 25–1C, on page 398, overcontoured crowns of a double abutment have narrowed the embrasure. Problems of plaque control for the overcontoured crowns are illustrated in figure 25–4 on page 402.

F. Ditch or Groove

The formation of a gap between the cavity preparation margin and the amalgam, as shown in figure 41–1C, is usually referred to as ditching. Plaque retention can lead to recurrent caries in such an area.

OVERHANGING RESTORATIONS

The recontouring of overhanging restorations is an essential part of the dental and periodontal treatment of patients. Treatment planning for initial therapy, or Phase I periodontal therapy, must include the correction of overhangs if inflammation is to be controlled.[5,6]

I. Description

An overhang is identified by its relation to the gingival margin, location on a specific tooth surface, shape, and size or extent. From those data, the required finishing procedures can be selected for a specific treatment plan.

A. Relation to Gingival Margin

1. Supragingival.
2. Subgingival.

B. Tooth Surfaces: Location

1. Occlusal, mesial, distal, buccal, lingual, or combination.
2. Tooth surface margin.
   a. Enamel only.
   b. Enamel and cementum.
   c. Cementum only.

C. Size Determined by Visual and Tactile Examination[7]

Overhangs are found by running a sharp explorer back and forth over the junction between the tooth and the amalgam.
1. *Type I:* small overhang; slight catch with explorer in at least one section.
2. *Type II:* moderately large overhang with definite catch with explorer, usually involving more than one side of the restoration.
3. *Type III:* large, gross overhang clearly apparent by exploration and often visually apparent on direct observation.

D. Radiographic Examination

Overhangs on surfaces other than proximal are rarely visible on radiographic examination. Visibility of proximal surface overhangs depends on angulation of the x-ray. In other words, radiographic examination for overhangs should be a supplementary procedure to examination using an explorer. The entire outline of each restoration can be explored.

A magnifying glass is recommended for examining radiographs for small type I overhangs. Adjacent and undermining carious lesions are more definitively seen when magnification is used.

II. Effects of Overhangs

A. Relation to Periodontal Disease

Because overhanging restorations harbor plaque and hinder plaque removal by the patient, they are considered significant iatrogenic contributing factors in periodontal disease development. In the presence of overhangs, plaque collects in greater amounts and inflammation is more severe than in relation to teeth that do not have overhangs.[8,9,10] Increased bone loss adjacent to overhangs has been demonstrated.[8,11]

Removal of overhangs is beneficial to the periodontal tissues. Combined with scaling and plaque control, a marked improvement in the periodontal condition has been shown after overhang removal.[9,12]

B. Problems of Plaque Control

1. Irregular margins of overhangs catch and tear dental floss.
2. Inaccessible areas
   a. Area under the ledge of the overhang, particularly a proximal overhang, is inaccessible for direct application of a toothbrush and other plaque removal aids.
   b. Gingival enlargement resulting from inflammation caused by plaque that is held by the overhang may cover a portion of the overhang, and thus make the subgingival part inaccessible for plaque removal. After overhang removal and shrinkage of the soft tissue pocket wall, the restoration may be wholly supragingival, and therefore, accessible for maintenance.
3. Debris retention contributes to a general lack of oral sanitation and to halitosis from breakdown products in dental plaque and food debris held by the overhang.

C. Dental Caries

Marginal irregularities harbor microorganisms and sucrose in an environment conducive to the formation of secondary caries. The process is described on pages 269–271.

III. Indications and Contraindications for Removal of Overhangs

All overhanging restorations should be corrected or removed and replaced for the health of the periodontium. Large overhangs cannot usually be treated by finishing procedures and are therefore indicated for total removal of the restoration. If replacement will be delayed, the gross overhang should be reshaped and smoothed so that plaque control will be possible. The periodontal tissues can recover, inflammation be reduced, and continuing treatment be more satisfactory.

Whether a certain overhang can be removed by finishing techniques or whether it must be removed and replaced with a new properly prepared, contoured, and finished restoration, is the professional decision that must be made. Guidelines for selection of the correct procedure are suggested here. Contraindications for finishing procedures apply to restorations of any size or location.

A. Indications for Finishing

1. Tooth anatomy can be maintained or improved to conform with normal morphology.
2. The overhang is small or moderate in size.
3. Proximal contact is intact.
4. No adjacent secondary dental caries can be detected.
5. There are no fractures of the cavity margin either of the tooth or the filling, and no large fractures of the bulk of the restoration.
6. The overhang is accessible for the instrumentation necessary for finishing and polishing without damaging the adjacent tooth structure or unduly traumatizing the gingival tissues.

B. Indications for Removal and Restoration

1. The overhang is extensive and would require an excess of time for complete recontouring.
2. Secondary marginal or undermining dental caries is present.
3. The contact area must be restored.
4. Fractures, chips, cracks, or broken margins are apparent that could not be corrected by finishing and polishing procedures.

FINISHING PROCEDURES

I. Definitions

A. Carving

Carving is the removal of excess filling material, using specially designed instruments, immediately after condensation of the amalgam into the cavity preparation. The goal of carving is to produce accurate anatomic contours which approximate the normal for the particular tooth.

B. Contouring

Contouring includes procedures to reproduce the size, shape, grooves, and other details of tooth form in the restoration. The term *contouring* is usually used when a new restoration is being prepared, whereas the term *recontouring* is used when an old or previously placed restoration is being corrected and reshaped.

C. Burnishing

Burnishing is the production of a smooth, lustrous surface of a restoration by rubbing lightly (to prevent heat production) with a metal, specially designed instrument for amalgam burnishing or rubbing with a cotton pellet. The effects are improved marginal adaptation, increased hardness, and increased resistance to corrosion.[1]

D. Margination

Margination procedures are carried out to remove excess restorative material and apply finishing techniques to establish a smooth, well-adapted junction between the enamel surface (or cementum in a restoration of root surface) and the restoration. The resultant enamel-amalgam junction should conform in shape to the normal anatomic characteristics of the particular tooth.

E. Polishing

Polishing procedures are applied after other finishing techniques to produce a visually smooth, unscratched, lustrous, homogenous amalgam surface. Abrasive agents are used during polishing to remove final surface roughness, make the surface resistant to corrosion, and eliminate grooves or pits left after carving.

II. Technique Objectives

At the completion of finishing procedures, the restoration and the tooth will have the following characteristics:
A. Normal anatomic tooth form has been restored or preserved and there are no signs of gouges or other damage.
B. Margins between tooth structure and restoration are smooth, so that no irregularity is detectable when a fine explorer is passed back and forth over the entire outline of the restoration. There is neither an area of deficient margin nor overhanging margin.
C. Contact is maintained with the adjacent tooth.
D. Embrasures provide normal spacing and appear functional.

E. The surface of the restoration is smooth, lustrous, glossy, free from visible and tactile irregularities, and functionally adequate.

APPOINTMENT PLANNING

I. Patient Preparation

A. Patient History Review

A review of the patient's medical and dental history and the entire current appointment record will reveal essential appointment features that will be required. For a risk patient, prophylactic antibiotic premedication may be indicated.

B. Protective Glasses

Both patient and operator must wear protective eyeglasses. The use of rotary instruments and polishing agents creates a potential hazard of splatter and aerosols (pages 16–18).

II. Sterile Procedures

Prevention of disease transmission procedures are followed as described in Chapters 3 and 4. A specific tray arrangement is planned. The specific instruments, burs, and stones can be kept in sealed sterilized packages, or a preset tray system can be used.

III. Patient Instruction

A. Explain the purposes and need for finishing restorations.
B. Explain possible detrimental effects of rough restorations, particularly in relation to plaque retention, gingival disease, and dental caries.
C. For new restorations, describe why finishing procedures are to be performed 24 to 48 hours after the restoration was placed.

IV. Examination

A. Review charting and treatment plan for restoration to be treated.
B. Make certain that a new restoration has been placed for a minimum of 24 hours and preferably for 48 hours.[1,2]
C. Study the radiographs for available information to supplement the clinical visual examination.
D. Evaluate an unpolished restoration visually by noting small shiny spots which may in-

dicate specific occlusal contacts. Call the spots to the attention of the dentist for checking the occlusal relationship before the spots are obliterated during finishing procedures.

E. Examine with an explorer to determine the nature of any irregularities such as the following:
1. Margins with excess amalgam.
2. Roughness of amalgam surfaces.
3. Entire outline of the restoration.

V. Technique Selection

A. Assessment

During careful examination by direct observation, radiographs, and exploring, the need for finishing is determined and the technique treatment plan outlined. As mentioned previously, a newly placed, neatly carved restoration may require only polishing, whereas much more instrumentation is required to recontour overhanging margins.

The extent of instrumentation is limited to that required. Unnecessary overinstrumentation must be avoided.

B. Procedural Plan

There are many technique routines used in practice.[7,13,14,15,16] Procedures may be carried out using manual instruments primarily, power-driven instruments primarily, or a combination of manual and power-driven. It is important to work out a practical routine for efficiency and time conservation.

General suggestions are provided below, describing procedures for finishing in which the excess amalgam and overhanging margins are removed, margins and surfaces are smoothed, and a careful check with an explorer is made before the polishing procedures are carried out.

VI. Rubber Dam Placement

A. Purposes

Whenever possible, a rubber dam should be placed. It would be indicated particularly when there are several restorations to polish in a given quadrant. The rubber dam serves to
1. Protect the patient's soft tissues.

2. Aid in control of debris, moisture, and aerosols created during the finishing procedures to prevent inhalation of particles of amalgam and polishing agents.
3. Improve vision and accessibility.
4. Decrease time of operation by eliminating difficulties in maintaining a clear field.

B. Problems of Isolation

1. *Anesthesia.* Although the use of anesthesia can be helpful while finishing restorations, patients are not routinely anesthetized. Placing the rubber dam clamp without anesthesia may cause discomfort for the patient.
2. *Tooth Temperature.* With the rubber dam in place, keeping the tooth cool during finishing may be more difficult. The use of air spray for cooling may lead to scattering of amalgam particles. Central suction evacuation is required. Mercury hygiene practices are listed in the Technical Hints at the end of this chapter.
3. *Use of Cotton Rolls*
   a. Rotating instruments catch the cotton rolls.
   b. Repeated need for cooling and rinsing away debris from finishing and polishing procedures requires considerable time in changing cotton rolls.

VII. Selection of Instruments

Development of a workable set of instruments is accomplished with experience. As knowledge of normal tooth morphology is applied during finishing and polishing, instruments will be used with increased skill and efficiency. Not all of the instruments listed below are needed for each restoration.

A. Factors Affecting Selection of Instruments

1. *Location of the Restoration:* accessibility and visibility.
2. *Instrument Size, Shape, and Form:* to fit the tooth surface and area without traumatizing adjacent tooth structure and gingival tissues.
3. *Abrasiveness of Discs and Polishing Agents.* The character of the surface of

the restoration defines the degree of abrasiveness. As mild an abrasive as possible should be used to prevent unnecessary removal of amalgam and tooth structure adjacent to the cavosurface margin. Replenishment of tooth surface fluoride will be described later in this chapter.

B. Manual Instruments

Amalgam or gold knives
Files (heavy, medium, fine)
Cleoid–discoid carver
Scaler, curet
Finishing strips (fine grit, single surface, narrow)
Waxed dental tape

C. Power-driven Instruments

1. *Bladed Instruments*
   Finishing burs (12-bladed)
2. *Abrasive*
   Stones: green or white
   Discs: waterproof, fine grit, in garnet or cuttle
3. *Polishing*
   Rubber cup
   Mandrel-mounted brushes

VIII. Principles and Precautions

A. Anatomic Considerations

1. *Cementum.* When a restoration extends near or into cementum, care must be taken to prevent ditching or grooving the cementum. Cementum is softer than enamel and therefore more easily damaged.
2. *Tooth Morphology and Position.* Concave surfaces such as the mesial of the maxillary first premolars and the mesials of the mandibular first molars require special adaptations of instruments. Other problem areas are created by tooth rotations, inclinations, and other malpositions.
3. *Gingival Tissues.* Restorations may be partially or wholly covered by enlarged gingival tissue related to plaque accumulation as described previously.

   When the papillae are bulbous, enlarged, and bleed easily on manipulation, it is usually advisable to provide plaque control instruction and supervision and to wait until the health of the tissue has improved before undertaking margination procedures. Waxed floss can be used by the patient so there will be less tearing and shredding when the floss is passed under the overhang.

B. Instrumentation

1. *Finger Rests.* Use secure finger rests to allow precision techniques. Prevention of damage to surrounding tooth structure as well as preservation of tooth anatomy is essential.
2. *Contact Area.* Avoid the contact area. It was created for a new restoration by a smooth, polished matrix band and usually requires no additional smoothing. Polishing agents can remove amalgam and alter the contour and contact.

MARGINATION

I. Margination Procedures Summarized

A. Remove excess amalgam and overhangs.
B. Finish all cavosurface margins to assure continuous, uninterrupted smooth relationships.
C. Smooth all surfaces of the restoration.

II. Manual Instruments

A. General Suggestions for Use of Manual Instruments

1. Maintain sharp instruments. The object is to cut, not burnish, excess amalgam in small increments and prevent amalgam fracture.
2. Work deliberately and carefully to prevent damage to gingival tissue and uninvolved tooth surfaces, especially cementum.
3. Use the tooth surface as a guide to the contour of the restoration. The instrument is moved parallel with or diagonal to, the margin.

B. Amalgam Knife

1. Hold knife blade across tooth structure and amalgam, and activate the knife diagonally across the junction.
2. Use short, overlapping, shaving strokes to remove amalgam in small increments. Prevent risk of fracture of the margins.

3. For proximal adaptation, move knife away from gingiva to prevent amalgam bits from being pushed into the pocket. Continuous evacuation is recommended.

C. File

1. Determine from the design of each file whether it is designed for a pull or a push stroke, and position the file accordingly.
2. Bulk of amalgam is removed by coarser files; margin smoothness can be refined with finer files.
3. Overlap tooth and amalgam together during a stroke to prevent ditching, gouging, or leaving a deficiency (undercontour).

D. Cleoid–Discoid Carver

1. Refine fossae and fissures with a small sharp cleoid (the pointed tip). The discoid is not used in occlusal fossae because the effect would be one of scooping out and making a round channel.
2. Use discoid as aid for refining cavosurface margins.

E. Finishing Strips

1. Use narrow, fine or medium strips after gross amalgam has been removed by amalgam knife or file.
2. Avoid contact area with abrasive finishing strip
   a. Cut end of strip on diagonal to thread the strip through the embrasure. The slanted tip may be dipped in cavity varnish to facilitate sliding the strip through.[17]
   b. Strips with a gap or middle area without abrasive are available to make it possible to position the strip from the occlusal or incisal.
3. Position strip over the amalgam at the cavosurface margin. Avoid pressure of the abrasive strip on the adjacent tooth structure, especially cementum, as grooves can be made.
4. Curve the strip and move gently and carefully to prevent damage to the interdental gingival tissue (page 579).

F. Scaler

Only a strong scaler should be used. A scaler tip could be easily broken if applied with much force. It should also be remembered that using a metal cutting edge on metal (the amalgam) will dull the instrument rapidly.

III. Power-driven Instruments

A. General Suggestions for Power-driven Instruments

Power-driven instruments can create heat, which is detrimental. With careful techniques, ill effects can be prevented.

1. Effects of overheating
   a. Irreversible pulp damage.
   b. Alteration of the chemical structure of the amalgam. Properties of the amalgam can be changed and the longevity of the restoration can be decreased.
   c. Patient discomfort from tooth sensitivity.
2. Use only low speed handpiece (maximum 6,000 r.p.m.) with intermittent, light strokes.
3. Use water and/or air for cooling.

B. Finishing Burs and Stones

1. Select the shape appropriate for accessibility and visibility.
2. Position the bur or stone to permit the remaining enamel to guide the contour produced. The instrument is held across the cavosurface margin and then moved diagonally to prevent fracture or ditching.
3. Keep the bur or stone in constant motion, with a light, sweeping movement to reduce the possibility of leaving marks and grooves.

C. Discs[14]

1. Select abrasivity of disc in accord with objective. Coarse discs will remove bulk more readily, but also may be more damaging to surrounding tissues and tooth structure. Follow each grit with a disc of the next finer grit.
2. Do not reduce tooth structure.

3. Activate the disc for proximal surface contouring and smoothing to prevent flattening of the restoration and removing amalgam near the contact area.

4. Use short, overlapping strokes with a sweeping motion diagonally across the cavosurface margin. Rotate the disc from the tooth structure to the amalgam to reduce chance of ditching.

D. Ultrasonic

Certain models of ultrasonic machines have special tips designed for removal of overhanging amalgam. The device can be helpful for removal of gross amalgam prior to use of finer instruments. The precautions for use of ultrasonics are listed on page 521.

POLISHING

After margination and surface smoothing, the amalgam is polished.

I. General Suggestions for Polishing Amalgam

A. Use Very Wet Polishing Agents

1. Heat factors described previously for power-driven instruments apply alike to polishing instruments.
2. Avoid dry polishing powders and discs.
3. Avoid rubber devices such as rubber polishing or finishing points because of heat production. Rubber polishing cups should always be separated from the tooth and restoration by a wet abrasive agent.

B. Do Not Overpolish

Overpolishing, even with a fine abrasive agent, can alter the morphology of the restoration, destroy the contact area, and remove excess surrounding tooth structure, especially when cementum is involved.

C. Use Slow Speed: with light, intermittent strokes.

D. Do Not Extend Polishing Brushes or Cups Over the Cementum

The abrasive polishing agent can groove and scratch the cementum.

II. Instruments

A. Bristle brushes: pointed, cup-shaped, disc-shaped.
B. Rubber cups.
C. Waxed dental tape.

III. Procedures

A. Initial Polish

1. Agent: fine silex or fine pumice in a very wet slurry with water.
2. Bristle brushes
   a. Prepare by soaking in warm water.
   b. Apply with copious amounts of the slurry.
3. Application
   a. Apply the agent over the tooth and restoration before starting the power-driven instrument.
   b. Use the pointed brush in the pits and fissures and cup-shaped brush or rubber cup for convex surfaces.
   c. Keep the brush or cup in constant motion with light, intermittent strokes to prevent heat generation. Replenish slurry often.
   d. Apply polishing agent to proximal surfaces with waxed dental tape. Avoid the contact area. Curve the tape around the tooth to prevent damage to the interdental gingival tissue.
4. Rinse and inspect frequently to prevent overpolishing.

B. Fine Finish

1. Agent: tin oxide in a thin, wet slurry with water.
2. Use a new rubber cup or brush to prevent mixing the agents.
3. Apply with light, intermittent strokes.
4. Rinse and inspect to prevent overpolishing.

IV. Final Evaluation

The finished and polished restoration has the characteristics described in Technique Objectives, page 588.

FLUORIDE APPLICATION

The use of abrasive stones and polishing agents at the margin of a restoration removes a layer of the surface enamel and, with it, the concentration of fluoride that is protective against dental caries. Commercially prepared paste containing fluoride may restore in part the lost fluoride (page 458), and can be used during the polishing procedure.

After polishing, a topical application of fluoride should be made, followed by periodic applications at succeeding recall appointments, depending on individual needs. Self-application on a daily basis, using a mouthrinse, custom tray, or chewable tablet, may also be recommended to supplement fluoride derived from the use of a dentifrice.

TECHNICAL HINTS

I. Mercury Pollution of Environment

The mercury vapor level in a dental operatory is higher than in the normal atmosphere.[1] Although a dentist or an auxiliary rarely exhibits symptoms of toxicity, the potential danger is there, and certain precautions are necessary. The American Dental Association lists sources of mercury that include the following:[18]

A. Direct contact or handling of mercury.

B. Inhalation of vapors from mercury.

C. Exposure to accidental spills and leaky or contaminated amalgamator capsules and amalgamators.

D. Wringing excess mercury from amalgam.

E. Vaporization of mercury from contaminated instruments in sterilizers.

F. Amalgam condensation, especially with ultrasonic compactors.

G. Scrap amalgam improperly stored.

H. Milling old amalgam restorations.

II. Mercury Hygiene Practices[18]

Recommendations from the American Dental Association include the following:

A. Work in well ventilated areas.

B. Monitor the office or clinic periodically for atmospheric mercury.

C. Require yearly urinalysis for mercury for all personnel.

D. Store mercury in unbreakable, tightly sealed containers away from heat sources.

E. Keep amalgam scrap in a tightly sealed container.

F. Handle amalgam with caution and without direct contact; clean up spilled mercury immediately.

G. Use water stream and high volume evacuation when removing or finishing amalgam restorations.

H. Avoid heating mercury or amalgam, mercury-containing solutions, and carpeting for treatment rooms.

I. Do not eat, drink, or smoke in dental and dental hygiene treatment rooms.

FACTORS TO TEACH THE PATIENT

I. Advantages of having restorations smooth and well finished.

II. Reasons for having to wait 24 to 48 hours to have finishing procedures completed.

III. The importance of having inadequate contact areas restored rather than using floss repeatedly to alleviate the discomforts of food impaction.

IV. The need for daily and professional applications of fluoride to preserve the tooth structure around each restoration. Daily mouthrinse, brush-on gel, gel in a tray, chewable tablet, or other form of fluoride is advised.

V. Advantages of maintaining amalgam restorations by daily plaque control measures, limiting cariogenic foods, and all possible preventive procedures.

References

1. Phillips, R.W.: *Elements of Dental Materials for Dental Hygienists and Assistants*, 3rd ed. Philadelphia, W.B. Saunders Co., 1977, pp. 193–227.
2. Craig, R.G., O'Brien, W.J., and Powers, J.M.: *Dental Materials. Properties and Manipulation*, 2nd ed. St. Louis, The C.V. Mosby Co., 1979, pp. 73–87.
3. American Dental Association, Council on Dental Materials, Instruments and Equipment: *Dentist's Desk Reference: Materials, Instruments and Equipment*, 1st ed. Chicago, American Dental Association, 1981, pp. 33–43.
4. Phillips: op. cit., pp. 185–190.
5. Carranza, F.A.: *Glickman's Clinical Periodontology*, 5th ed. Philadelphia, W.B. Saunders Co., 1979, pp. 717–720.
6. Schluger, S., Yuodelis, R.A., and Page, R.C.: *Periodontal Disease*. Philadelphia, Lea & Febiger, 1977, pp. 322–323.
7. Langslet, J.: *Margination—Rationale and Technique*, Seattle, Washington, Department of Dental Hygiene, University of Washington, 1976, 28 pp.
8. Gilmore, N. and Sheiham, A.: Overhanging Dental Restorations and Periodontal Disease, *J. Periodontol.*, 42, 8, January, 1971.
9. Highfield, J.E. and Powell, R.N.: Effects of Removal of Posterior Overhanging Metallic Margins of Restorations Upon the Periodontal Tissues, *J. Clin. Periodontol.*, 5, 169, August, 1978.
10. Gorzo, I., Newman, H.N., and Strahan, J.D.: Amalgam

Restorations, Plaque Removal and Periodontal Health, *J. Clin. Periodontol.*, 6, 98, April, 1979.

11. Jeffcoat, M.K. and Howell, T.H.: Alveolar Bone Destruction Due to Overhanging Amalgam in Periodontal Disease, *J. Periodontol.*, 51, 599, October, 1980.

12. Rodriguez-Ferrer, H.J., Strahan, J.D., and Newman, H.N.: Effect on Gingival Health of Removing Overhanging Margins of Interproximal Subgingival Amalgam Restorations, *J. Clin. Periodontol.*, 7, 457, December, 1980.

13. Goldfogel, M.H., Smith, G.E., and Bomberg, T.J.: Amalgam Polishing, *Operative Dent.*, 1, 146, Autumn, 1976.

14. Project Acorde, United States Department of Health, Education, and Welfare: *Recontouring, Finishing, and Polishing.* Castro Valley, California, Quercus, 1976, 85 pp.

15. Murphy, M.P.: *Finishing and Polishing Dental Amalgam.* Halifax, Nova Scotia, School of Dental Hygiene, Dalhousie University, 1978, 16 pp.

16. Muhler, S.A.: *Amalgam Polish.* Pennsylvania EFDA Faculty Institute, Philadelphia, University of Pennsylvania, 1979.

17. Chapman, M.K.: Role of the Auxiliary in Restorative Dentistry, in Castano, F.A. and Alden, B.A., eds.: *Handbook of Clinical Dental Auxiliary Practice*, 2nd ed. Philadelphia, J.B. Lippincott Co., 1980, pp. 96–102.

18. American Dental Association, Council on Dental Materials, Instruments and Equipment: op. cit., pp. 21–23.

Suggested Readings

Bushee, E.J.: Polishing and Scaling Restorations, in Boundy, S.S. and Reynolds, N.J., eds.: *Current Concepts in Dental Hygiene, Volume 2.* St. Louis, The C.V. Mosby Co., 1979, pp. 93–100.

Chan, K.C., Edie, J.W., and Svare, C.W.: Scanning Electron Microscope Study of Marginal Adaptation of Amalgam in Restoration Finishing Techniques, *J. Prosthet. Dent.*, 38, 165, August, 1977.

Charbeneau, G.T.: A Suggested Technic for Polishing Amalgam Restorations, *J. Mich. Dent. Assoc.*, 47, 320, November, 1965.

Cooley, R.L., Barkmeier, W.W., and White, J.H.: Heat Generation During Polishing of Restorations, *Quintessence Int.*, 9, 77, December, 1978.

Creaven, P.J., Dennison, J.B., and Charbeneau, G.T.: Surface Roughness of Two Dental Amalgams after Various Polishing Techniques, *J. Prosthet. Dent.*, 43, 289, March, 1980.

Cunningham, J.: Finishing Amalgam Restorations, *Br. Dent. J.*, 142, 9, January 4, 1977.

Dahi, F., Dorfman, R.L., Asgar, K., and Corpron, R.E.: Microscopic Observations of Amalgams Carved by Different Methods and Subsequently Polished, *J. Am. Dent. Assoc.*, 97, 197, August, 1978.

Dahl, J.E. and Eriksen, H.M.: Reasons for Replacement of Amalgam Dental Restorations, *Scand. J. Dent. Res.*, 86, 404, September, 1978.

Full, C.A., Svare, C.W., and Kerber, P.E.: A Scanning Electron Microscope Study of One Year *in Vivo* Amalgam-enamel Interfaces, *Pediatric Dentistry*, 1, 235, December, 1979.

Fusayama, T., Nagata, N., Iwaku, M., Sakai, Y., and Hisamitsu, H.: Development of New Polishing Agents for Dental Amalgam, *J. Prosthet. Dent.*, 36, 409, October, 1976.

Going, R.E.: Reducing Marginal Leakage: A Review of Materials and Techniques, *J. Am. Dent. Assoc.*, 99, 646, October, 1979.

Goldberg, J., Tanzer, J., Munster, E., Amara, J., Thal, F., and Birkhed, D.: Cross-sectional Clinical Evaluation of Recurrent Enamel Caries, Restoration of Marginal Integrity, and Oral Hygiene Status, *J. Am. Dent. Assoc.*, 102, 635, May, 1981.

Goldschmidt, P.R., Cogen, R.B., and Taubman, S.B.: Effects of Amalgam Corrosion Products on Human Cells, *J. Periodont. Res.*, 11, 108, April, 1976.

Gough, J.E.: Amalgam Material as an Occupational Hazard, *Dent. Assist.*, 50, 28, March/April, 1981.

Grajower, R., Kaufman, E., and Rajstein, J.: Temperature in the Pulp Chamber During Polishing of Amalgam Restorations, *J. Dent. Res.*, 53, 1189, September–October, 1974.

Leidal, T.I. and Dahl, J.E.: Marginal Integrity of Amalgam Restorations, *Acta Odontol. Scand.*, 38, 81, Number 2, 1980.

Nitkin, D.A. and Goldberg, A.J.: Placing and Polishing Amalgam in One Visit, *Quintessence Int.*, 10, 23, June 1979.

O'Brien, W.J., Johnston, W.M., and Heinkel, D.E.: Surface Properties of Dental Amalgam: Roughness Produced by Setting Reaction, *J. Am. Dent. Assoc.*, 94, 891, May, 1977.

Saltzberg, D.S., Ceravolo, F.J., Holstein, F., Groom, G., and Gottsegen, R.: Scanning Electron Microscope Study of the Junction Between Restorations and Gingival Cavosurface Margins, *J. Prosthet. Dent.*, 36, 517, November, 1976.

Smales, R.J. and Creaven, P.J.: Evaluation of Clinical Methods for Assessing the Surface Roughness of Restorations, *J. Prosthet. Dent.*, 42, 45, July, 1979.

Swedlow, D.B., Kopel, H.M., Grenoble, D.E., and Katz, J.L.: Dental Amalgam Polishing with Discs as Observed by Scanning Electron Microscopy, *J. Prosthet. Dent.*, 27, 536, May, 1972.

Tidmarsh, B.G. and Gavin, J.B.: Finishing Amalgam Restorations—A Scanning Electron Microscope Study, *N.Z. Dent. J.*, 69, 175, July, 1973.

Vale, J.D.F. and Caffesse, R.G.: Removal of Amalgam Overhangs. A Profilometric and Scanning Electron Microscopic Evaluation, *J. Periodontol.*, 50, 245, May, 1979.

Vernetti, J.P. and Baynton, D.B.: Placement, Carving, and Polishing of Amalgam Restorations, in Boundy, S.S. and Reynolds, N.J., eds.: *Current Concepts in Dental Hygiene, Volume 2*, St. Louis, The C.V. Mosby Co., 1979, pp. 9–19.

Restorations and Gingival Health

Blank, L.W., Caffesse, R.G., and Charbeneau, G.T.: The Gingival Response to Well-finished Composite Resin Restorations, *J. Prosthet. Dent.*, 42, 626, December, 1979.

Carranza, F.A. and Romanelli, J.H.: The Effects of Fillings and Prosthetic Appliances on the Marginal Gingiva, *Int. Dent. J.*, 23, 64, March, 1973.

Coxhead, L.J., Robertson, J.B., and Simpson, E.F.: Amalgam Overhangs—A Radiographic Study, *N.Z. Dent. J.*, 74, 145, July, 1978.

Gullo, C.A.O. and Powell, R.N.: The Effect of Placement of Cervical Margins of Class II Amalgam Restorations on Plaque Accumulation and Gingival Health, *J. Oral Rehabil.*, 6, 317, October, 1979.

Leon, A.R.: Amalgam Restorations and Periodontal Disease, *Br. Dent. J.*, 140, 377, June 1, 1976.

Leon, A.R.: The Periodontium and Restorative Procedures, *J. Oral Rehabil.*, 4, 105, April, 1977.

Sotres, L.S., Huysen, G.V., and Gilmore, H.W.: A Histologic Study of Gingival Tissue Response to Amalgam,

Silicate and Resin Restorations, *J. Periodontol.*, *40*, 543, September, 1969.

Trivedi, S.C. and Talim, S.T.: The Response of Human Gingiva to Restorative Materials, *J. Prosthet. Dent.*, *29*, 73, January, 1973.

Turgeon, J., LeMay, L.-P., and Cléroux, R.: Periodontal Effects of Restoring Proximal Tooth Surfaces with Amalgam: A Clinical Evaluation in Children, *Can. Dent. Assoc. J.*, *38*, 255, July, 1972.

Volchansky, A., Cleaton-Jones, P., and Retief, D.H.: Study of Surface Characteristics of Natural Teeth and Restorations Adjacent to Gingivae, *J. Prosthet. Dent.*, *31*, 411, April, 1974.

Waerhaug, J.: Effect of Rough Surfaces Upon Gingival Tissue, *J. Dent. Res.*, *35*, 323, April, 1956.

Waerhaug, J.: Presence or Absence of Plaque on Subgingival Restorations, *Scand. J. Dent. Res.*, *83*, 193, July, 1975.

Wagman, S.S.: The Role of Coronal Contour in Gingival Health, *J. Prosthet. Dent.*, *37*, 280, March, 1977.

Weitman, R.T. and Eames, W.B.: Plaque Accumulation on Composite Surfaces after Various Finishing Procedures, *J. Am. Dent. Assoc.*, *91*, 101, July, 1975.

Wise, M.D. and Dykema, R.W.: The Plaque-retaining Capacity of Four Dental Materials, *J. Prosthet. Dent.*, *33*, 178, February, 1975.

Yuodelis, R.A., Weaver, J.D., and Sapkos, S.: Facial and Lingual Contours of Artificial Complete Crown Restorations and Their Effects on the Periodontium, *J. Prosthet. Dent.*, *29*, 61, January, 1973.

42

Evaluation, Maintenance, and Recall

The objective of treatment is oral health for the patient, and individually performed services are steps toward total health. To evaluate the health of the gingival tissues, a period of time must be allowed for healing to take place and for the benefits of the professional treatment and the patient's self-care on a daily basis to become apparent. After health has been attained, it must be maintained. Dental hygiene care is an integral part of total care and cannot be thought of as isolated appointment procedures.

There are three basic phases for evaluation. The *first* is the immediate observation at the completion of each appointment; the *second* is short-term follow-up one week to 10 days after completion of a treatment or series of treatments; and the *third* is long-term recall to evaluate maintenance.

IMMEDIATE EVALUATION

I. Objectives

A. Teeth

Observation and exploration will reveal the immediate effects of instrumentation on the teeth. An objective has been to produce a smooth glassy tooth surface, free from deposits and stains. The effect of specific instrumentation is to facilitate the patient's self-care by removing signs of disease and local factors, particularly calculus and over-hanging fillings which encourage plaque retention.

B. Gingiva

The gingival changes are not apparent immediately after instrumentation. Tissue regeneration and healing takes approximately one week to 10 days for initial healing, and even longer for maturation of connective tissue and keratinization of epithelium.

The objective at the treatment appointment is to *create an environment in which the gingival tissue can heal and be maintained in health by the patient.*

II. Examination

When scaling is accomplished over a series of appointments, each previously scaled quadrant or area is examined and rescaled as needed at each appointment. For the final evaluation, visual and tactile methods are applied carefully to each tooth surface. Instruments, methods, and procedures were described on pages 509–510.

A. Visual

1. Use compressed air with mouth mirror and adequate lighting for supragingival examination and just below the gingival margin.
2. Transillumination methods are applied.
3. A disclosing agent can reveal small areas of remaining deposits.

B. Tactile

Use subgingival explorer to assure smoothness of tooth surfaces to the bottom of each pocket (pages 224–225).

III. Appearance of the Teeth after Instrumentation

The experienced eye will recognize the bright luster of thoroughly clean teeth. All deposits have been removed and the surfaces are smooth to tactile examination.

To evaluate completion of instrumentation, the following observations are made:

A. Supragingival Nondecalcified Tooth Surfaces

1. Surfaces are visually clean and lustrous.
2. No calculus or extrinsic stains are evident after drying the surfaces with compressed air.
3. Metallic restorations are free from tarnish.
4. Enamel surfaces are smooth to tactile examination; root surfaces in areas of gingival recession feel smooth and hard.
5. Gingival surfaces of pontics are free of deposits.

B. Subgingival Nondecalcified Tooth Surfaces

1. Surfaces feel free of calculus and diseased altered cementum.
2. Surfaces are smooth and hard to tactile examination with a subgingival explorer.

C. Overhanging Fillings

1. Excess amalgam has been removed.
2. Junctions between restorations and tooth surfaces are smooth and uninterrupted when an explorer tip is passed over.
3. Normal tooth contour has been restored.

D. Removable Appliance

1. Outer polished surfaces have no visible calculus, soft deposits, or stains, and are smooth and unscratched.
2. Impression surfaces are free of deposits and unmarred.
3. Attachments or metal parts are smooth and shiny.

POSTOPERATIVE PROCEDURES

Postoperative care immediately following instrumentation includes flossing, careful irrigation, and postoperative instructions for the patient to carry out after leaving the office or clinic. Depending on the service performed, postoperative care may also include the placing of a periodontal dressing, application of a topical antiseptic, and gingival massage. Postoperative care may also include a postappointment telephone contact concerning patient comfort and adherence to instructions.

Long-range postoperative care may include suture and dressing removal and dressing replacement. These have been described on pages 549–553.

Postoperative care and instruction can have a direct bearing on the progress of healing and hence the follow-up evaluation which is planned for a week or 10 days after treatment is completed. Healing may be influenced by rinsing, brushing, and other self-care by the patient.

I. Gingival Massage

A firm but gentle massage of the gingival tissue may be performed after completion of scaling and planing. It would not be wise to massage the tissue over partially completed scaling because of mechanical injury to the pocket lining by the rough calculus.

Massage can be soothing to the patient and temporarily stimulating to the circulation of the gingiva. It is performed prior to application of an antiseptic solution.

A. Effects of Massage

Massage is the systematic mechanical application and removal of pressure. The application of pressure forces stagnant blood from the tissues and produces a temporary ischemia; the removal of pressure allows arterial blood to enter the capillaries and produce a temporary hyperemia.

B. Technique for Massage

A toothpaste may be applied to the gingiva as a lubricating agent, or the massage may be performed with the fingers moistened with water.
1. Follow the routine order of technique used for other procedures or start from the midline to massage each quadrant.

2. Place the thumb and index finger over the teeth onto the attached gingiva.

3. Apply moderate, firm pressure, moving the fingers in the direction of the gingival papilla, toward the incisal or occlusal surfaces.

4. Release pressure at the tip of the papilla and return fingers to the attached gingiva above the adjacent tooth. Repeat rhythmically around the mouth.

II. Application of an Antiseptic

When an antiseptic is applied, the limitations should be realized. Although some temporary reduction in bacterial count may be expected, sterilization would be impossible.

The antiseptics usually employed for postoperative applications are iodine or mercury preparations in the proper dilutions for application to the oral mucous membrane. Merthiolate (1:1000), Metaphen (1:200), or Merbromin (2%) (Mercurochrome) are commonly used for this purpose.

A. Purposes

1. Reduces the possibility of infection.
2. Reduces postoperative discomfort.

B. Technique for Application

1. Hold small cotton pellet with cotton pliers and saturate it in the antiseptic to be used. Express excess solution.

2. Provide adequate retraction of lip, cheek, and tongue, and apply solution to the crest of each interdental papilla on both facial and lingual surfaces. Solution will flow into sulcus/pocket.

3. Do not allow the patient to rinse.

III. Postoperative Instruction

Instruction pertaining to periodontal dressings is outlined in table 36–1 on page 548. Many of the same principles can be applied for postoperative instruction when a dressing has not been applied.

Postoperative instruction is essential following scaling, particularly when the patient's gingiva has been hypersensitive or has hemorrhaged excessively, or when there has been extensive subgingival instrumentation. Directions for postoperative care include suggestions for rinsing and toothbrushing. An explanation of

what discomfort may be expected should also be given.

Dietary and nutritional factors may be discussed. The temporary use of bland foods lacking in strong, spicy seasonings, as well as continuing use of nutritional foods to promote healing can be helpful.

It is best to prepare directions for postoperative care in printed or mimeographed form. This can prevent incomplete or inaccurate interpretation of orally delivered directions.

A. Rinsing

A warm solution will be soothing to the tissue and improve the circulation for healing. A suggested solution would be one that provides the appropriate concentration for osmotic balance of the salts of the solution with the salts of the oral tissue fluids.

1. *Solutions Suggested for Use*
   a. Hypertonic salt solution: level $1/2$ teaspoonful of table salt in 4-ounce glass of warm water.
   b. Sodium bicarbonate solution: level $1/2$ teaspoonful baking soda in $3/4$ glass (8-ounce) warm water.

2. *Directions for Rinsing*
   a. Every 2 hours; after eating; after toothbrushing; before retiring.
   b. Use the rinse mouthful by mouthful, forcing the solution between the teeth.

B. Toothbrushing

The use of a soft brush is advisable after scaling and root planing, but the patient must clearly understand the need for complete plaque removal.

FOLLOW-UP EVALUATION

In order that the response of the gingival tissues to treatment and the patient's personal daily care can be observed, an appointment is planned for approximately 10 days after instrumentation has been completed. Such reevaluation after an interval in which the tissues can heal provides the opportunity to locate areas where additional treatment and instruction may be indicated.

It should not be assumed that, because the teeth were apparently free from deposits and were smooth and glassy at the immediate evaluation following instrumentation, gingival healing, pocket wall shrinkage, resolution of inflammation, and other favorable treatment effects will inevitably result. Follow-up examination may reveal a variety of complications that may point to a need for additional root planing, curettage, self-care instruction, or referral for periodontal therapy.

A six-step evaluation plan is described here.

I. Evaluate the Gingival Tissue

A. Examine with the patient to observe
   1. Color, size, shape, consistency, surface texture. By 10 days, the tissues should assume normal characteristics. Use table 11–1 on page 196 for guidelines.
   2. Areas of damage to the gingiva, resulting from incorrect brushing or flossing.
B. Compare findings and indices with previous examination and notes from treatment appointments when these characteristics were observed before.

II. Evaluate Pocket Depths

A. Use probe, and measure around each tooth.
B. Record and compare with initial measurements.
C. Shrinkage of pockets when tissue is spongy and soft can be expected as healing progresses.

III. Evaluate Gingival Bleeding

A. Run the probe along the inside of the pocket wall. The technique is illustrated in figure 19–5 on page 300. If bleeding was apparent during probing for pocket depth in Step II (above), evaluation can be made without additional probing for bleeding.
B. Ask the patient whether bleeding occurred during toothbrushing.
C. Healthy tissue does not bleed. As healing progresses, bleeding should be eliminated.

IV. Evaluate Plaque

A. Apply disclosing agent and examine with the patient for areas where plaque has not been removed by the patient's personal care.
B. Relate areas of plaque on the teeth to the areas of gingival redness, enlargement, and other signs of disease.

V. Evaluate Plaque Control Methods and Techniques

A. Request patient to demonstrate techniques with emphasis on areas where the disclosing agent revealed plaque and where the gingiva has not responded.
B. Help the patient to evaluate and make corrections.
C. Introduce or substitute new methods when applicable.
D. Learning is a slow process and repeated review and encouragement is usually needed.

VI. Examine for Residual Calculus

A. Use a subgingival explorer to examine areas where gingival redness and enlargement have persisted, whether marginal plaque was observed or not.
B. Remaining particles of calculus or areas of root surface roughness, however small, may be sufficient to encourage plaque collection and prevent complete healing.
C. Because the detection and removal of calculus in a pocket requires intricate and exacting instrumentation, even the most skilled operator must expect to recheck and complete the scaling and planing as indicated. The most frequent areas for residual calculus are proximal surfaces of molars, premolars, and crowded anteriors.

VII. Continuation of Evaluation

In practice, a patient should not be placed in the recall category until there is complete healing and the dentist and dental hygienist are satisfied that optimum tissue health has been obtained. Sometimes a series of short appointments can be arranged in conjunction with dental appointments for restorative procedures by the dentist. At each appointment, the patient may meet with the dental hygienist for continuing supervision of self-care procedures and observation of tissue response.

Notes concerning the status of gingival health and the instruction for the patient should be made in the patient's permanent record at each appointment. The observations are important to long-range planning for patient care and can provide a basis for determining the frequency of recall.

RECALL: THE MAINTENANCE PHASE

Through common usage, the term "recall" is

applied to the system of appointments for the long-term maintenance phase of patient care which has as its primary objective the *prevention of the recurrence of disease* through supervised control. This program requires the cooperative efforts of the patient and all members of the dental team.

Initially, the success of the program depends on the understanding of the patient relative to the recall procedure. The patient must realize that oral diseases do recur, but control is possible by combined personal and professional care.

I. Recall Interval

There can be no fixed schedule by which all patients are recalled, because the frequency depends on the needs of each patient. Appointments may vary from 2 to 6 months, and an occasional patient needs only an annual recall. The time interval needs to be reevaluated periodically and changed in accord with changing needs.

A. The First Recall

The gingival or periodontal treatment may be completed or nearly completed by the time appointments for restorative phases of treatment are under way. The first recall appointment should be dated from the completion of the gingival and periodontal treatment. When extensive restorative, prosthetic, or other treatment is to follow, tissue maintenance during long-term therapy is essential.

B. Frequent Recall Requirements

2- and 3-month intervals are required by many patients. Examples of patients in this category are those with the following conditions:

1. *Rampant Dental Caries.* Recall for continuation of a caries control effort which includes topical fluoride applications, dietary supervision, and personal care factors for dental plaque control.
2. *Periodontal Disease.* Following periodontal surgery or deep scaling and curettage, many patients need a long period of supervision before it is certain that the etiologic factors are under control.

3. *Orthodontic Therapy.* Appliances make cleaning and plaque control difficult; frequent topical fluoride applications may be indicated; response of gingival tissue to irritants can be marked.
4. *Mentally or Physically Handicapped.* There may be difficulty in managing the toothbrush; when the handicap involves the mouth area, there may be problems of opening the mouth.
5. *Diabetes* or other disease that predisposes to a lowered resistance to infection; tissues must not be allowed to develop advanced disease.
6. *Cardiovascular Diseases or Other Conditions.* Brushing is a difficult procedure to carry out and only short appointments at the dental office can be tolerated because of the fatigue factor.

II. Recall Procedures

Preparation of data for the recall follows the same plan as for a new patient. A diagnostic work-up is prepared. At least annually, every patient needs a medical history review, an intraoral and extraoral examination for soft tissue lesions, particularly for cancer, and a blood pressure determination.

At every appointment for recall, whether 3, 6, or other number of months, a patient of any age who has had periodontal therapy needs a complete pocket probing and special evaluations for the particular problems of previous treatments. The patient with complete oral rehabilitation needs a detailed examination every few months (page 402).

Basic to all recall examinations are the periodontal examination (page 320) and the dental examination (page 321) with charting.

Steps in preparation of a recall diagnostic work-up include the following:

A. Review Patient History

Supplementary questions are asked to determine the present state of health, recent illnesses, present medications, and other pertinent data (page 99).

B. Blood Pressure Determination (pages 107–111).

C. Extraoral and Intraoral Examination for oral pathology, particularly cancer (pages 114–116 and table 8–1, pages 117–119).

602

Instrumentation

D. **Radiographs,** frequency in accord with dentist's determination of an indvidual patient's need.

E. **Periodontal Examination**

Details are outlined on pages 211–220. Minimum examination includes clinical tissue examination of color, size, shape, consistency, surface texture, pocket charting, determination of tooth mobility, examination of mucogingival line, furcations, occlusion, and tooth deposits. Bleeding on probing should be correlated with a bleeding index.

F. **Examination of the Teeth** (page 234)

A new charting with restorations and caries, examination for pulp vitality when indicated, and a record of tooth sensitivity, if reported by the patient or detected during examination, should be made.

G. **Evaluation of Oral Cleanliness and Adequacy of Self-care Measures**

Relate plaque on teeth as observed after applying a disclosing agent, with areas of gingival redness, enlargement, and other signs of disease.

H. **Examination of Specific Areas by the Dentist**

Areas of special problems include endodontically treated teeth, postsurgery, occlusal factors, prosthetic appliances.

III. Recall Treatment Plan

The dentist reviews the data collected and a treatment plan is outlined, based on the new diagnosis and evaluation of the patient's oral condition. For the dental hygienist's treatment plan, scaling, planing, topical fluoride or other preventive application, and patient instruction provide the basis for the continuing preventive program.

TECHNICAL HINTS

Methods for maintenance of a recall plan vary. Two systems in current use are described here.

I. Make each patient's appointment before the patient leaves the office. An appointment card is given the patient who is asked to enter it on the calendar ahead of time, and an envelope is prepared for mailing a duplicate card a week before the appointment is to be held.

II. Individual file cards (3 × 5 or 4 × 6 inches) are maintained for each patient to show name, address, telephone number, and instructions concerning the recall frequency as well as the available appointment time. Cards are filed by the month in which the patient is due for recall. Each month the cards are pulled, and appointments are mailed or telephoned well in advance.

FACTORS TO TEACH THE PATIENT

I. Appearance and feeling of a clean mouth.
II. Relationship of personal oral care habits to maintenance of cleanliness provided through professional scaling and planing.
III. Purposes of postoperative care by the dental hygienist and the patient.
IV. How to prepare solutions for postoperative rinsing.
V. Directions for postoperative care.
VI. Purposes of follow-up and recall appointments.

Suggested Readings

Boggs, D.G. and Schork, M.A.: Determination of Optimal Time Lapse for Recall of Patients in an Incremental Dental Care Program, *J. Am. Dent. Assoc.*, 90, 644, March, 1975.

Carranza, F.A.: *Glickman's Clinical Periodontology*, 5th ed. Philadelphia, W.B. Saunders Co., 1979, pp. 663, 1042–1054.

Chace, R.: Retreatment in Periodontal Practice, *J. Periodontol.*, 48, 410, July, 1977.

Goldman, H.M. and Cohen, D.W.: *Periodontal Therapy*, 6th ed. St. Louis, The C.V. Mosby Co., 1980, pp. 1155–1178.

Gottlieb, M.A.: Recall and Maintenance Procedures in Pedodontics—An Overview, *Alpha Omegan*, 72, 52, September, 1979.

Grant, D.A., Stern, I.B., and Everett, F.G.: *Periodontics*, 5th ed. St. Louis, The C.V. Mosby Co., 1979, pp. 917–939.

Hirschfeld, L. and Wasserman, B.: A Long-term Survey of Tooth Loss in 600 Treated Periodontal Patients, *J. Periodontol.*, 49, 225, May, 1978.

Lerner, M.H.: The Three-month Recall for Children—The "Self-prophy." Good Learning Low Overhead Profit Center, *J. Am. Soc. Prev. Dent.*, 6, 14, October, 1976.

Ogilvie, A.L.: Maintenance of the Periodontal Patient, in Schluger, S., Yuodelis, R.A., and Page, R.C.: *Periodontal Disease*. Philadelphia, Lea & Febiger, 1977, pp. 704–721.

Parr, R.W.: *Periodontal Maintenance Therapy*. Berkeley, California, Praxis Publishing Co., 1974, 86 pp.

Parr, R.W., Green, E., and Miller, S.R.: *Hygienists in Per-*

iodontal Maintenance Therapy. Berkeley, California, Praxis Publishing Co., 1978, 67 pp.

Roberts, B.W.: The Recall System. A Necessary Part of a Partial Denture Service, *Br. Dent. J.*, *149*, 46, July 15, 1980.

Ross, I.F. and Thompson, R.H.: A Long Term Study of Root Retention in the Treatment of Maxillary Molars With Furcation Involvement, *J. Periodontol.*, *49*, 238, May, 1978.

Schmid, M.O.: The Maintenance Phase of Dental Therapy, *Dent. Clin. North Am.*, *24*, 379, April, 1980.

VI

Applied Techniques for Patients with Special Needs

INTRODUCTION

To understand each patient's general and/or oral health problems requires particular study. Actually, each patient is a "special" patient and must be considered according to individual needs. However, certain patients have problems peculiar to their age group and/or unusual health factors which may complicate the routine of care generally provided. These special patients require more skillful application of dental hygiene knowledge and ability to accomplish a comparably favorable result than does what might be called the "normal" patient.

Optimum oral health is frequently an important contributing factor in maintaining or restoring the patient's physical, emotional, vocational, economic, and social usefulness to the extent of individual capabilities. *The dental hygienist's obligation is to see that no patient needs special rehabilitative dental services because of any condition that could have been prevented by dental hygiene care.*

To consider the patient as a whole requires attention to general physical and emotional problems as well as oral problems. Basic psychologic needs for affection, belonging, independence, achievement, recognition, and self-esteem frequently influence the outcome of treatment as well as the patient's whole attitude toward dental and dental hygiene care.

With certain disabilities, oral health has assumed less importance in the mind of the patient because other health problems have demanded so much attention. For some of these patients, neglect has intensified the need for oral care.

The patients with special needs who will be considered in the chapters following include patients with oral and general systemic conditions. Variations with respect to age and degree of disability are considered.

SPECIAL ORAL PROBLEMS

In each specialty of dentistry, patients present problems that can be helped by the services performed by the dental hygienist. For example, patients with fixed or removable dentures require particular attention. Patients with dentofacial handicaps who have missing teeth or congenital malformations, patients requiring surgery, and patients afflicted with habits conducive to the initiation of dental caries need special adaptations of the preventive care and instruction the dental hygienist can provide.

SYSTEMIC DISEASES

Oral manifestations may be evident in association with certain acute and chronic systemic diseases, particularly nutritional deficiencies, endocrine disturbances, blood diseases, and many chronic degenerative diseases. The presence of oral diseases may complicate and delay the rehabilitation of a patient with systemic illness. When an oral manifestation suggests the possibility of an undiagnosed systemic disease, dental personnel have a responsibility to refer the patient for medical examination.

Patients with chronic conditions may or may not be able to go to a dental office or clinic for appointments. Certain conditions, particularly during the advanced stages of a disease, require the patient to remain confined and, in some instances, bedridden. Dental hygienists need to understand the special procedures for care in these instances.

The basic approach to oral problems of the patient with a chronic disease or a physical or mental disability is through prevention. Individual initiative is vital if the impact of preventive measures is to be understood and necessary action taken. The public, including dental personnel, must incorporate into daily living fundamental health practices that contribute to optimum health and hence to the prevention of chronic disease. Dental hygiene care can improve the general health and influence the resistance to infection of the oral cavity.

INTEGRATION OF APPLICATIONS TO SPECIAL NEEDS

It should be realized that a patient may have more than one special need. For example, the patient who requires dental hygiene care prior to oral surgery may have a blood disorder. The pregnant patient may be diabetic. The use of the patient's medical history plays an important role when the total needs of the patient are outlined.

In Part VI, there is an attempt to integrate learning from other areas of medical and social sciences into the dental and dental hygiene aspects. The dental hygienist is encouraged to supplement knowledge and appreciation of the special needs of patients through the use of additional readings such as those suggested at the end of each chapter. By application of understanding of the patient's needs, clinical techniques and patient instruction may be directed more skillfully to provide *complete dental hygiene care.*

43

The Pregnant Patient

During pregnancy, attention is focused on good health practices for the mother. She is anxious and concerned for the health of her baby and for herself. This alertness to total health, of which oral health is an important part, provides an unusual opportunity to help the patient learn principles that may be applied to the future care of the child.

The term *prenatal care* refers to the supervised preparation for childbirth that helps the mother enjoy optimum health during and after her pregnancy and the reward of a healthy baby. Such a program involves the combined efforts of the obstetrician, nurse, dentist, dental hygienist, and the expectant parents. Pregnancy is arbitrarily divided into three periods of three months each, referred to as the first, second, and third trimesters, respectively.

Unfortunately, there are still many women who do not seek care until delivery. Oral health is neglected along with general health. Some of these patients will appear for emergency dental service, and may be receptive to a program of care and instruction to prevent further emergencies. The dental hygienist in public health will participate in community educational programs with public health nurses, whereby some of the less informed or less motivated women may learn of the need for professional dental care and advice during pregnancy.

Obstetricians routinely recommend dental care early in pregnancy. This brings to the dental office or clinic many women who previously would not have had a regular plan for obtaining professional service. Many of these women have not known the advantages of personal habits of daily care and diet related to the health of the oral tissues. There are numerous misconceptions or "old wives' tales" to counteract when providing up-to-date information about the relationship of pregnancy and oral health.

I. Gingival Conditions During Pregnancy[1-3]

The condition of the gingiva is the result of an exaggerated response of the tissues to bacterial plaque. When the mouth is in good health and the patient uses adequate personal oral care measures for plaque control, no adverse gingival changes may be expected.

Pregnancy will tend to aggravate an existing gingival condition, and is, therefore, a secondary or conditioning factor. Since the principal gingival reaction in pregnancy is an inflammatory one, the pregnancy itself cannot be the cause.

From 36 to 100 percent of pregnant patients have been shown in surveys to have gingival inflammation.[4,5] The severity tends to increase during pregnancy, when untreated, but with controlled periodontal care and plaque control, as few as 0.03 percent of pregnant patients may have gingivitis.[4]

Gingivitis may be particularly noticed during the second trimester or late in the first trimester.[6] During that period, the patient may become more aware of her mouth than she was during the earlier period.

Exaggerated symptoms abate after the birth of the child, but it should not be expected that a completely healthy condition will result. Patients with a gingival disturbance during pregnancy will continue to have the disturbance, even if somewhat lessened in degree.

A. Generalized Gingival Enlargement

1. *Clinical Appearance.* Symptoms are generally limited to the free gingiva. The appearance varies, as suggested by the possible characteristics of inflamed tissues listed below.
    a. Enlargement: hyperplasia, edema.
    b. Shiny, smooth surface.
    c. Bleeds readily with probing and slight trauma.
    d. Color: may be bluish-purple or raspberry red.
    e. Loss of normal resiliency.
2. *Predisposing Factors*
    a. Local irritation due to an unhygienic oral condition and bacterial plaque on the teeth and gingiva related to laxity in personal care procedures.
    b. Hormonal changes during pregnancy may alter the tissue reaction.

B. Isolated Gingival Enlargement

An isolated or discrete gingival enlargement may occur, which has been called a "pregnancy tumor." The use of the word tumor is misleading since the lesion is not a tumor but a hyperplasia, and may correctly be called an epulis gravidarum[6] or pyogenic granuloma.[7]

1. *Clinical Appearance*
    a. Location: superficially on the free gingiva, usually associated with an interdental papilla.
    b. Mushroom-like flattened mass.
    c. Smooth, glistening surface.
    d. Color: purplish-red, magenta, or deep blue, sometimes dotted with red; color depends on vascularity.
2. *Symptoms*
    a. Bleeds readily with slight trauma.
    b. Painless unless it becomes large

enough to interfere with occlusion and mastication.

II. Personal Factors

Mental hygiene of the expectant mother is influenced by her attitude toward herself, her husband, her other children, and her unborn child. Normally, in a large majority of cases, when the husband is pleased and there is security in the marriage, there will be genuine happiness and anticipation or at least tranquil acceptance. When there is emotional instability, the mother may exhibit degrees of apprehension or even open rebellion in her rejection of the baby.

The first few months are usually the most difficult, and anxiety may be observed, since pregnancy provides an emotional experience with many adjustments to be made. Generally, these early problems resolve themselves, and if they continue throughout the pregnancy, may disappear when the baby is born. A few of the possible characteristic emotional manifestations of pregnancy are listed below with suggestions for the dental hygiene appointment.

A. Changes in Mood from Happiness to Depression

At times the change may be abrupt. Adapt conversation and instruction to receptiveness of patient.

B. Hypersensitivity

Be cautious about joking over personal matters and avoid calling attention to size or appearance.

C. Irritability

Minimize disturbances, interruptions, or noises; make operations smooth; adjust room temperature; avoid topics of discussion that might bring patient reaction.

D. Increased Introversion, Passivity, Dependence on Others

Help patient to feel the concern for her oral health being taken by the dentist and dental hygienist, yet interest her in the need for her own personal care.

E. Physical and Mental Indifference

May explain lack of conscientiousness in the patient's personal oral care habits.

1. Plan sufficient appointments for dental hygiene care to counteract patient's own limited care.
2. Plan for telephoning to remind a patient who is indifferent to keeping appointments.
3. Be firm with patient instruction in plaque control; take advantage of teachable moments.

F. Impaired Judgment

Be specific in outlining the plan for oral care, both professional and personal. Help the patient visualize realistically the possible effects of neglect.

G. Hidden Fears Not Recognized or Admitted

Fear of the pregnancy, the child's health, her own health, or of adjustments that must be made after the birth of the child. Offer reassurance. Conversation should dwell on positive factors, not morbid.

H. Changes in Appetite; Craving for Unusual Foods

Provide specific information concerning the use of foods other than fermentable carbohydrates, particularly as snacks.

III. Aspects of Patient Care

The dental hygienist needs to be well informed concerning aspects of dental care in order to motivate the patient and dispel fears related to certain services. The patient may consult the dental hygienist for reassurance and interpretation concerning the dentist's recommendations and procedures.

A. Oral Examination and Treatment Planning

The patient should be seen as early in pregnancy as possible. Consultation with the patient's physician is of particular importance in order that the total prenatal care may be integrated.

B. Radiography

Cover the patient with a lead apron, and use a second apron for the back to prevent secondary radiation from reaching the abdomen. Apply all current methods for radiation safety and protection including optimum filtration, collimation, use of speed group D or E film, and extended target film distance.

Determine the minimum number of film exposures that will produce the required diagnostic information. The use of a paralleling technique should not require angulation directed toward the patient's abdomen, as compared with steep angulation needed for bisection technique applied to maxillary teeth. Careful and skillful film placement, angulation, processing, and all phases of technique will prevent the need for remaking any radiographs.

C. Periodontal Treatment

Areas of food impaction should be corrected and all overhanging restorations reshaped or replaced. All scaling and root planing procedures should be carefully and thoroughly completed.

The patient's general health, the severity of the periodontal disease, and particularly, the advice of the obstetrician will determine the plan of action when a surgical procedure is indicated. In general, the second trimester is considered most favorable for any type of required surgical procedure. Elective procedures, particularly those requiring general anesthesia, should be deferred until after the baby is born.[8]

D. Restorative Dentistry

All required work should be completed with permanent restorations. One important contraindication for the use of temporary restorations lies in the fact that after the baby is born, the mother may be much too busy to attend to appointments, and may postpone them.

DENTAL HYGIENE CARE

Gingival disease need not be expected when the patient is motivated to practice conscientious self-care procedures for oral cleanliness and plaque control. This calls for a specific recall appointment plan for scaling and instruction.

A concentrated plan for dental caries control is indicated. A multiple fluoride program and limitation of cariogenic foods are basic to the preventive efforts.

I. Appointment Planning

A. Recall Intervals

Monthly appointments or appointments three times during the 9-month period may be required, depending on the individual mouth and the patient's motivation in personal care.

B. Length of Individual Appointments

Short, for patient comfort. A series of appointments is needed when there is heavy calculus.

C. Recall Postpartum

For the patient who has not been on a regular recall plan prior to pregnancy, emphasis must be placed on motivating the patient to continue regular appointments for dental hygiene and dental care after the baby is born.

II. Appointment Procedures

A. Patient History

The history must be reviewed carefully, since the prenatal patient may require applied techniques for conditions other than pregnancy. For example, diabetes or cardiovascular diseases can involve serious complications. Special procedures for these and other systemic conditions have been described in other chapters.

When the expectant mother is an adolescent, consideration for her own health takes on a different perspective than for the mature woman. Aspects of adolescent development and psychology will be described in Chapter 44.

B. Consultation with Physician

The dentist and the physician benefit mutually through discussion of patient treatment. The need for particular precautions before, during, or after treatment becomes known to the dentist and dental hygienist.

When a patient seeks dental and dental hygiene care and is not under the care of a physician, she should be strongly urged to obtain medical supervision, have examinations, and thereby improve her health as well as that of the baby. She must under-stand the relationship of general health to oral health.

III. Clinical Aspects

It is not within the scope of this book to review all of the physiologic changes that occur during pregnancy. There are common disturbances that should be identified since they can affect appointment procedures. Nearly every pregnant woman is bothered by one or more minor complaints.

Attention to small details will provide the patient with comfort and motivate her to continuing oral care. Table 43–1 lists the more common minor physical disturbances of pregnancy and suggests a few appointment considerations.

A. Instrumentation

When the patient is seen with gingival enlargement and inflammation, it is usually advisable to spend the first appointment on instruction in plaque control and other preventive measures. At the second appointment, evaluation is made and instruction continued.

Careful instrumentation for scaling and planing is indicated. Bleeding may be excessive. If polishing is needed, it is advisable to postpone it until the tissue has responded to the plaque control measures.

B. Fluoride Program

1. *Professional Topical Application.* As described in the chapter on fluoride treatment (pages 451, 455), applications are not advised on inflamed, enlarged gingival tissue immediately following scaling. At a second appointment, after the patient has practiced the recommended plaque control procedures and the tissue has healed, the fluoride application can be made.
2. *Self-application.* A fluoride dentifrice is recommended for all patients. A daily mouthrinse, gel tray, or other mode of application is essential, depending on the individual evaluation. A concentrated fluoride effort can be particularly important to the teeth of the adolescent mother-to-be.

Table 43–1. Appointment Adaptations for the Prenatal Patient

Characteristic	*Dental Hygiene Implication*
Fatigues easily, may even fall asleep	Short appointments; several in series, as needed
Discomfort of remaining in one position too long	Interrupt in middle of appointment to change chair position Assistance with evacuation during intraoral instrumentation can lessen operating time
Backache	Adjust chair appropriately for comfort
Frequent urination	Allow long enough appointment time for interruptions. Suggest at beginning of appointment that patient mention need for interruption
General awkwardness because of size and shape	Attend to details such as gently lowering chair and straightening it for patient to get out Make sure rinsing facilities are convenient; or preferably, an assistant attends to evacuation
Faintness and dizziness	Be prepared for emergency (table 58–1, pages 845–852). Place the patient on her *side* and not in supine or Trendelenburg position because pressure from the enlarged uterus and the abdominal organs on the inferior vena cava can interfere with venous return; placental separation could result

Nausea and vomiting
  a. Unpleasant taste in mouth
  b. Gagging
  c. Reactions to odors and flavors of medicaments and other office materials
 	
  d. Physician's recommendations for alleviation of symptoms: frequent eating of small amounts of foods
	Suggest toothbrushing or rinsing at frequent intervals
	Care in instrument and radiographic film placement
	Attention to cleanliness of cuspidor
	Determine particularly obnoxious odors for an individual patient and remove them
	Encourage use of foods that are noncariogenic

Unusual food cravings	If cravings are for sweets, clearly define relationship of frequent nibbling of cariogenic foods to dental caries

PATIENT INSTRUCTION

During pregnancy, the emphasis on general health provides the ideal situation for the dental hygienist to instruct relative to many aspects of oral health for the mother, her expected new child, as well as for other members of the family. New developments in disease prevention and control should be explained.

Printed materials concerning the prevention of periodontal diseases and dental caries and the development and care of children's teeth are available from the American Dental Association.* Reading material to supplement personal

discussions can contribute to patient understanding and appreciation.

I. Plaque Control

A rigid schedule for self-care must be demonstrated and supervised. A series of instructional periods is usually needed.

Emphasis should not be placed on the hormonal changes of pregnancy as influential in producing gingival changes. The patient may be all too willing to use the systemic factor as an excuse for her lack of attention to adequate self-care.

II. Diet

A majority of expectant mothers will base their diets on the recommendations of their physicians. However, instruction must be provided

---

* An American Dental Association catalog for the current year may be obtained by writing the Order Section, 211 East Chicago Avenue, Chicago, Ill. 60611.

in dental caries prevention and the health of the supporting structures of the teeth. The use of a varied diet containing the essential protective basic four food groups, with a minimum of cariogenic foods, is necessary.

A. Purposes of Adequate Diet During Pregnancy

1. To maintain daily strength.
2. To prepare for labor by building up the muscle tone of the body to meet the crisis of labor and delivery.
3. To shorten the period of convalescence after delivery.
4. To prepare the patient to be better able to nurse the baby.
5. To provide the essential building materials for the developing fetus.
6. To protect and promote the health of the oral tissues of the mother.

B. Dietary Needs of Pregnancy

In the *Recommended Daily Dietary Allowances* from the Food and Nutrition Board of the National Research Council[9] the increased allowances during pregnancy and lactation are specified. Since the embryo or fetus is a parasite and thrives at the mother's expense, the mother's diet must be adequate to maintain her own nutritional status as well as to meet the needs of the fetus.

The particular needs of the fetus are
1. Proteins, for general tissue construction.
2. Minerals, especially calcium and phosphorus, for bone and tooth calcification; and iron for blood corpuscles.
3. Vitamins.

C. Dietary Adjustments[10,11]

Foods from the four food groups (table 28–1, page 424) are selected. To meet the needs for calcium, phosphorus, and riboflavin, a quart of milk or its equivalent in milk products is sufficient, except for the teen-age mother who needs a quart and one-half if her own maturing body requirements are to be met.

An added citrus fruit or other good source of vitamin C, a dark green or deep yellow vegetable daily for vitamin A, along with sources for iron, thiamine, and vitamin D are indicated. Proteins of high physiologic value are important, that is, proteins from meat, eggs, fish, and fowl rather than of vegetable origin only. Calories may be increased in accord with exercise and tendency for weight gain. A decreased use of cariogenic foods is important for general nutrition and weight problems, as well as in the prevention of dental caries.

III. Dental Caries Control

A. Incidence During Pregnancy

Certain patients believe that they have more dental caries during and because of pregnancy. Research has shown that this is not true, and that any relationship is an indirect one. Factors that result in dental caries formation are the same during pregnancy as at other times.

B. Factors That May Contribute to Apparent Increase in Dental Caries Rate

1. *Previous Neglect:* a patient may not have kept a regular appointment plan, so that the existing dental caries during pregnancy represents an accumulation, possibly even of years.
2. *Diet During Pregnancy:* possible increase in intake of fermentable carbohydrates
   a. Unusual cravings may be for sweet foods.
   b. Frequency of eating: patient may be eating every few hours for prevention of nausea and these foods may be cariogenic.
3. *Neglect of Personal Oral Care Procedures:* lack of interest or laxity in toothbrushing or rinsing immediately following intake of fermentable carbohydrates.

C. Calcium and the Mother's Teeth[12]

There has been widespread misconception concerning the withdrawal of calcium from the mother's teeth and its relationship to dental caries. It is important to review the known facts and provide references for further reading on the subject, since the patient's beliefs may need clarification. In discussing the problem with the patient, a summary of the process of dental caries initiation can be helpful (pages 269–271).

1. Minerals contained in the erupted tooth enamel and dentin are not available and no removal of minerals can occur by way of the pulp.

2. Minerals contained within the alveolar bone are available as they are from other bones of the body. When the mother's diet does not contain sufficient calcium and phosphorus, her own reserve is utilized.

3. Majority of calcium and phosphorus of bones and teeth is added to the fetus during the third trimester. Incidence of dental caries in the mother is not different during that period although the carious lesions may be larger if the teeth have been neglected throughout the pregnancy.

4. There is a definite tendency for the teeth of the fetus to develop and calcify normally in spite of the diet of the mother since the reserve in her bones is used.

D. Relationship of Fluoride

There is no direct evidence to show that prenatal fluoride intake will influence the dental caries rate in the child.[13,14] When the community water supply is not fluoridated, dietary fluoride by prescription is advised for the baby after birth (pages 447–448).

References

1. Ramfjord, S.P. and Ash, M.M.: *Periodontology and Periodontics*. Philadelphia, W.B. Saunders Co., 1979, pp. 196, 438–441.
2. Carranza, F.A.: *Glickman's Clinical Periodontology*, 5th ed. Philadelphia, W.B. Saunders Co., 1979, pp. 119–120, 516–519, 945.
3. Goldman, H.M. and Cohen, D.W.: *Periodontal Therapy*, 6th ed. St. Louis, The C.V. Mosby Co., 1980, pp. 161–164.
4. Chaiken, B.S.: Incidence of Gingivitis in Pregnancy, *Quintessence Int.*, 8, 81, October, 1977.
5. Löe, H.: Periodontal Changes in Pregnancy, *J. Periodontol.*, 36, 209, May–June, 1965.
6. McCarthy, P.L. and Shklar, G.: *Diseases of the Oral Mucosa*, 2nd ed. Philadelphia, Lea & Febiger, 1980, pp. 354–355, 391–392, 430.
7. Shafer, W.G., Hine, M.K., and Levy, B.M.: *A Textbook of Oral Pathology*, 3rd ed. Philadelphia, W.B. Saunders Co., 1974, p. 324.
8. Sexton, J., Edelin, K., Booth, D.F., and Kilgore, T.: Surgery in a Gravid Patient, *J. Oral Surg.*, 36, 878, November, 1978.
9. National Research Council, Committee on Dietary Allowances, Food and Nutrition Board: *Recommended Dietary Allowances*, 9th ed. Washington, D.C., National Academy of Sciences, Office of Publications, 1980.
10. Nizel, A.E.: *Nutrition in Preventive Dentistry*, 2nd ed., Philadelphia, W.B. Saunders Co., 1981, pp. 364–368.
11. Gibbs, C.E. and Seitchik, J.: Nutrition in Pregnancy, in Goodhart, R.S. and Shils, M.E., eds.: *Modern Nutrition in Health and Disease*, 6th ed. Philadelphia, Lea & Febiger, 1980, pp. 743–752.
12. Miller, M.F.: Diseases of the Endocrine Organs, in Lynch, M.A., ed.: *Burket's Oral Medicine*, 7th ed. Philadelphia, J.B. Lippincott Co., 1977, pp. 446–447.
13. Driscoll, W.S.: A Review of Clinical Research on the Use of Prenatal Fluoride Administration for Prevention of Dental Caries, *J. Dent. Child.*, 48, 109, March–April, 1981.
14. Thylstrup, A.: Is There a Biological Rationale for Prenatal Fluoride Administration? *J. Dent. Child.*, 48, 103, March–April, 1981.

Suggested Readings

Adams, D., Carney, J.S., and Dicks, D.A.: Pregnancy Gingivitis: A Survey of 100 Antenatal Patients, *J. Dent.*, 2, 106, February, 1974.

American Dental Association, Council on Dental Therapeutics: *Accepted Dental Therapeutics*, 39th ed. Chicago, American Dental Association, 1982, pp. 30–36, 134–135, 246–247.

Arafat, A.H.: Periodontal Status During Pregnancy, *J. Periodontol.*, 45, 641, August, 1974.

Blinkhorn, A.S.: Dental Preventive Advice for Pregnant and Nursing Mothers—Sociological Implications, *Int. Dent. J.*, 31, 14, March, 1981.

Cheney, H.G. and Cheney, V.C.: The Dental Hygienist as a Health Educator in Prenatal Care, *Dent. Hyg.*, 48, 150, May–June, 1974.

Cheney, V.C. and Cheney, H.G.: Prescription for the Pregnant Patient, in DePaola, D.P. and Cheney, H.G., eds.: *Preventive Dentistry*. Preventive Dental Handbook Series, Volume 2, Littleton, Massachusetts, PSG Publishing, 1979, pp. 177–192.

Cohen, D.W., Friedman, L., Shapiro, J., and Kyle, G.C.: A Longitudinal Investigation of the Periodontal Changes During Pregnancy, *J. Periodontol.*, 40, 563, October, 1969.

Goins, S.R.: A Dental Health Education Program in a Hospital Prenatal Clinic, *Dent. Hyg.*, 51, 115, March, 1977.

Kornman, K.S. and Loesche, W.J.: The Subgingival Microbial Flora During Pregnancy, *J. Periodont. Res.*, 15, 111, March, 1980.

Lloyd, P.F.: Pregnancy and Dentistry, *J. Dent. Assoc. So. Africa*, 34, 763, November, 1979.

Nowak, A.J., Casamassimo, P.S., and McTigue, D.J.: Prevention of Dental Disease From Nine Months in Utero to Eruption of the First Tooth, *J. Am. Soc. Prev. Dent.*, 6, 6, October, 1976.

O'Neil, T.C.A.: Maternal T-lymphocyte Response and Gingivitis in Pregnancy, *J. Periodontol.*, 50, 178, April, 1979.

O'Neil, T.C.A.: Plasma Female Sex-hormone Levels and Gingivitis in Pregnancy, *J. Periodontol.*, 50, 279, June, 1979.

Rosenlicht, J., Murphy, J.B., and Maloney, P.L.: Fetal Alcohol Syndrome, *Oral Surg.*, 47, 8, January, 1979.

Sanger, R.G.: Preventive Dental Health Program for the Infant, *Dent. Hyg.*, 51, 408, September, 1977.

Samant, A., Malik, C.P., Chabra, S.K., and Devi, P.K.: Gingivitis and Periodontal Disease in Pregnancy, *J. Periodontol.*, 47, 415, July, 1976.

Utian, W.H.: Dental Obstetrics, *J. Dent. Assoc. So. Africa*, 30, 405, April, 1975.

Weir, J.C., Silberman, S.L., and Cohen, L.A.: Recurring Oral Pregnancy Tumors, *Obstet. Gynecol.*, *54*, 358, September, 1979.

Williamson, T.L.: The Pregnant Patient—Problems, Management, and Treatment, *Dent. Assist, 48*, 24, January–February, 1979.

Wood, N. and Turner, J.W.: Fetal Alcohol Syndrome: A Review, *J. Dent. Child.*, *48*, 198, May–June, 1981.

Diet and Nutrition

Anderson, G.J.: Nutrition and Dental Health During Pregnancy, *Educ. Directions, 1*, 26, November, 1976.

Hook, E.B.: Dietary Cravings and Aversions During Pregnancy, *Am. J. Clin. Nutr.*, *31*, 1355, August, 1978.

Karolus, J.A.: A Dental Hygienist's Approach to Pregnancy and Nutrition, *Dent. Hyg.*, *54*, 267, June, 1980.

Krause, M.V. and Mahan, L.K.: *Food, Nutrition and Diet Therapy*, 6th ed. Philadelphia, W.B. Saunders Co., 1979, pp. 275–295.

Pack, A.R.C. and Thomson, M.E.: Effects of Topical and Systemic Folic Acid Supplementation on Gingivitis in Pregnancy, *J. Clin. Periodontol.*, *7*, 402, October, 1980.

Randolph, P.M.: The Role of Diet and Nutrition in Pregnancy and Lactation, in Boundy, S.S. and Reynolds, N.J., eds.: *Current Concepts in Dental Hygiene*, Volume 2, St. Louis, The C.V. Mosby Co., 1979, pp. 179–191.

Adolescent Pregnancy

Alton, I.R.: Nutrition Services for Pregnant Adolescents Within a Public High School, *J. Am. Dietet. Assoc.*, *74*, 667, June, 1979.

Berg, M., Taylor, B., Edwards, L.E., and Hakanson, E.Y.: Prenatal Care for Pregnant Adolescents in a Public High School, *J. School Health, 49*, 32, January, 1979.

Edwards, L., Steinman, M., and Hakanson, E.: An Experimental Comprehensive High School Clinic, *Am. J. Public Health, 67*, 765, August, 1977.

11 Million Teenagers: What Can Be Done About the Epidemic of Adolescent Pregnancies in the United States. New York, Alan Guttmacher Institute, 1976, 64 pp.

Steinman, M.E.: Reaching and Helping the Adolescent Who Becomes Pregnant, *Am. J. Maternal Child Nurs.*, *4*, 35, January/February, 1979.

44

Patients During Puberty, Adolescence, and Menopause

INTRODUCTION

The endocrine glands are glands of internal secretion. They secrete highly specialized substances—the hormones—which, with the nervous system, maintain body homeostasis.

A hormone is a chemical product of an organ or of certain cells within an organ, which has a specific regulatory effect upon cells remote from its origin. Hormones are transported by the blood or lymph. They may act directly on body cells or may act to control the hormones of other glands. Their complex and unified action augments and regulates many vital functions, including growth and development, energy production, food metabolism, reproductive processes, and the responses of the body to stress.

The major endocrine glands are the pituitary, thyroid, parathyroids, pancreas, adrenals, and gonads. The anterior pituitary is called the master gland, because it is the regulator of the output of hormones by other glands. In turn, the pituitary itself is regulated by the hormones of the other glands.

Both hyposecretion and hypersecretion of a hormone can cause physical and mental disturbances. Regulation of hormonal secretion is complex, and the mechanisms are not fully known. Normally, hormones are secreted when needed. The external temperature, for example, can in-

fluence the production of thyroxin of the thyroid gland. The calcium level of the blood affects parathyroid activity.

Treatment for endocrine disturbances is accomplished either by decreasing the output of an overactive gland or, when there is a hormone deficiency, by stimulating glandular activity or supplying the deficient hormone. An example is the use of insulin or a hypoglycemic agent in the treatment of diabetes.

Hormones of the reproductive system have a controlling influence on the development and function of the individual. Some of the relationships to oral health and patient care will be discussed in this chapter.

PUBERTY AND ADOLESCENCE

Puberty is the period during which the gonads mature and begin to function. *Adolescence* is the period extending from the time of puberty to the attainment of complete maturity.

I. Pubertal Changes

Chronologic age is an unreliable means for designation, because puberty may begin normally in either sex between 9 and 17 years of age. In a majority, the secondary sex characteristics begin to appear between 10 and 13 in girls, whereas in boys, changes are later, starting at about 13 or 14 years. The major changes are usually complete in 3 to 4 years.

A. Hormonal Influences

Pituitary hormones control the hormones produced by the ovaries and testes. The several hormones produced by the ovaries are known collectively as *estrogens,* and those produced by the testes are called *androgens.* They are responsible for the development of the sex organs, the accessory sex organs, and the secondary sex characteristics, and have strong influences throughout the body.

B. Female Development

1. Beginning of menstruation and ovulation. Menstruation precedes ovulation.
2. Development in accessory sex organs: Fallopian tubes, uterus, vagina, and breasts.
3. Appearance of secondary sex characteristics
   a. Growth of pubic and axillary hair.
   b. Skeletal development: especially enlargement of the pelvis.
   c. Fat deposition on the hips.
   d. Voice drops one or two tones.

C. Male Development

1. Increase in size of testes and beginning of spermatogenesis.
2. Development in accessory sex organs: vas deferens, seminal vesicles, prostate, and penis.
3. Appearance of secondary sex characteristics
   a. Growth of beard and pubic and axillary hair.
   b. Voice deepens.

II. Characteristics of Adolescence

A. Growth Spurt

1. Varies in age of occurrence, extent, and duration; with boys generally between 12 and 16, girls 11 to 14.
2. Marked by rapid, extensive growth in height, weight, and muscle mass.
3. Obesity: overeating with underexercise along with psychologic problems make obesity a difficult and serious problem,

particularly among those young adolescents where food is not limited by scarcity or cost.
4. Young adolescents: poor coordination and awkwardness may result from irregular, uneven stages of growth.

B. Nutritional Requirements

1. Highest of any time in life for boys; will be exceeded only during pregnancy for girls.
2. Undernutrition is common; in boys, because of overactivity and poor food selection; in girls, because of voluntary diet restrictions with poor food selection and fad diets in the attempt to keep slim.
3. Iron-deficiency anemia is not uncommon among teen-age girls, particularly after menstruation starts.

C. Skin Disorders

Acne vulgaris is common; improves with improved diet and skin care.

D. Fatigue

Many adolescents require an unusual amount of sleep.

III. Personal Factors

Adolescents are no longer children, and yet they have not reached adulthood. They may respond and wish to be treated as adults or as children at different times. They are learning to adapt to body changes, sexual impulses, and secondary sex characteristics. The most likely causes of anxiety in adolescents are sex, performance in school, family relationships, acceptance by their own age group, confusion over their beliefs, and concern about their futures.[1]

There is no fixed picture that can be described, but characteristics listed here are exhibited to one degree or another by many adolescents.

A. Increased Self-interest

1. Adolescents have a great deal of concern for themselves and respond best to those who show concern for them.
2. They want attention and tend to reject those who do not listen.

B. Growing Independence

1. Adolescence is a period of rapidly growing independence of thought and action.
2. Childhood dependence on parents is given up: idea of infallibility of parents is lost; teachers and others in authority are questioned.
3. Personal identity is sought: they are uncertain about their place and role in society.
4. Independence from parents frequently means increased confidence in and respect for other adults.

C. Concern over Physical Characteristics[1]

1. Girls mature earlier than boys, and young female adolescents are usually taller than males, which presents social problems.
2. Increased interest in personal appearance: want to dress and be like their peers.
3. Problems such as delayed growth and sexual development and obesity can be of extreme importance.

IV. Oral Conditions

A. Dental Caries

The incidence of dental caries is higher during adolescence than in any other age group. This can be directly related to the dietary and eating habits of most adolescents. Appetite becomes intensified by the demands of rapid growth as well as by the emotional problems confronted, which leads to frequent eating. Many cariogenic foods are utilized, particularly for between-meal use.

B. Gingivitis

A large majority of adolescents has gingivitis. An exaggerated response to local irritants sometimes occurs during puberty and has been thought to be related to hormonal influences which may be conditioning factors.[2,3]

The tissue presents with gingival enlargement, particularly of the papillary gingiva, relative pockets, bluish-red color, and pronounced inflammation. Local aggravating factors include dental plaque, other tooth deposits, mouth breathing, erupting teeth, and orthodontic appliances.

C. Necrotizing Ulcerative Gingivitis

Although found infrequently in children, necrotizing ulcerative gingivitis has its highest frequency in older adolescents and young adults. Stress, undernutrition, lack of plaque control, neglect of oral health, as well as psychosomatic factors are implicated as predisposing influences in its development (page 536).

D. Periodontal Disease

Bone destruction and other signs of periodontal involvement occur in adolescents.[4] Careful probing and study of radiographs are indicated for each patient in order that all precautions can be taken and early treatment initiated.

Localized juvenile periodontitis, a rare condition formerly called periodontosis, is characterized by early bone destruction during circumpubertal or mid-teen years.[5] Symmetrical bone loss associated with the incisors and first permanent molars occurs more severely than can usually be explained by bacterial plaque and local predisposing factors. As the disease progresses and when plaque and calculus accumulate, chronic inflammatory periodontitis becomes clearly apparent with tooth mobility and migration, deep pockets, and other typical signs of severe periodontal disease.

DENTAL HYGIENE CARE

Dental and dental hygiene care during adolescence can influence oral health throughout the patient's lifetime. Preventive measures are even more critical than in younger age groups because of the increased incidence of dental caries and gingival diseases.

Adolescents will be parents within a few years. Knowledge, attitudes, and practices acquired and developed during adolescence can influence the oral health of their families.

I. Patient Approach

Adolescence is a period of transition. Working with adolescents offers a real challenge, and each situation requires its own approach. Some of the physical and psychologic characteristics have been listed in this chapter to provide a framework for what may be expected. A few basic suggestions for approach include the following:

A. Treat adolescents as adults. Physically many of them are mature, although their emotional development may be at various levels.
B. Set the stage to let them know of your interest in them and their problems. Encourage them to talk, and then listen.
C. Suggest and advise, but do not become impatient or take offense when they try to make their own decisions.
D. They are usually interested in health matters and details about their physical condition, although they may act indifferent. Cleanliness and attractiveness are important to the teen-age patient.
E. Health, including oral health, may be a real concern. Adolescents need to be well informed about their oral conditions, and explanations on a scientific basis are generally appreciated.

II. Patient History

Adolescents should provide their own information for the medical and dental histories. It may also be necessary to consult the parents for information, but not in the same interview with the patient and not without the patient's knowledge.

Adolescents need to begin to take increasing responsibility for their own health. Although frequently, the initial dental visit may be at the insistence of the parents, every effort of the dentist and dental hygienist should be to focus the evaluation and treatment on the patient, not the parents.

The adolescent patient may present with other health problems. The patient with diabetes, heart disease, a mental, physical, or sensory handicap, or other systemic involvement will require special methods for approach as described in the various chapters of this book. Medical clearance will be necessary for conditions requiring antibiotic coverage or other medication.

III. Preventive Dental Hygiene Program

A clear explanation of the causes of dental caries and periodontal conditions, with the methods for prevention, is important. Adolescents need to understand the effects of accu-

mulation of bacterial plaque, the purposes of calculus removal, and the relation of the daily self-care plaque control program to the health status of the gingiva.

For dental caries prevention, they must appreciate the effects of fluoride and the need for restriction of cariogenic foods that cling to the teeth. The program is outlined and conducted on the basis of these clear-cut preventive measures.

IV. Plaque Control

A. Instruction in self-care procedures is given in sequential steps (pages 411–416).
B. Continuing review over a series of appointments is necessary to develop daily practices that can be carried on into adult life.
C. Gingival enlargement: when gingival response to local irritants appears unusually pronounced, the treatment plan outlined by the dentist may call for gingival curettage along with root planing or gingival surgery. The dental hygienist will be responsible for providing postsurgical instruction for a rigid plaque control program to prevent recurrence of the gingival enlargement.

V. Instrumentation

A. Schedule

A series of appointments is frequently required for the patient with gingivitis associated with puberty, depending on pocket depth and extent of calculus deposits. Careful and complete scaling and root planing and removal of all local irregularities and predisposing factors are the basic treatment procedures.

B. Relation to Gingival Surgery

When the gingival enlargement has developed over a long period of time and the tissue is firm (fibrotic) rather than spongy (edematous), which can be treated with gingival curettage, a surgical procedure may be necessary. Follow-up root planing with frequent recall is indicated for adequate supervision.

VI. Fluoride Treatment Program

A combined fluoride program is generally indicated for most adolescent patients. In addition to the topical applications made in conjunction with dental hygiene professional appointments, self-administered methods should include a fluoride dentifrice along with a mouthrinse following toothbrushing, or a daily application of a fluoride gel in a custom-made tray. The methods are described in Chapter 29.

VII. Diet Control

A. Dietary Analysis (pages 423–432)

A study of the patient's diet and counseling relative to general nutrition and dental caries control can provide important learning experiences for many adolescents. The parent or other person who is in charge of shopping and food preparation will have to be included, in order that appropriate foods will be available for selection. As much responsibility as possible should be placed on the patient.

B. Instruction Suggestions

1. *Advise Foods From the Four Food Groups (page 424):* for growth, energy, clear complexion, and prevention of illness.
2. *Emphasize a Good Breakfast:* teen-agers tend to slight or omit breakfast, particularly if they have to prepare it for themselves.
3. *Snack Selection:* from the nutritious foods, with recognition of cariogenic foods. Snacks suggested can include raw fruits and vegetables, nuts, milk, use of sugar-free foods when possible, and sugarless chewing gum if used.

MENSTRUATION

The menstrual cycle refers to the cyclic structural changes in the uterus, instigated by hormones, which represent periodic preparation of the lining of the uterus for fertilization of the ovum and pregnancy. When fertilization does not take place, changes in the mucous membrane lining the uterus (the endometrium) lead to the menstrual discharge. The fluid discharged is composed primarily of blood with fragments of the disintegrated endometrium.

I. Characteristics

A. Occurrence

The cyclic changes occur from puberty to menopause except during pregnancy. Although the average cycle is complete in about 28 days, the normal range is from 22 to 34 days.[6]

B. Menarche

Menstruation may begin any time from age 9 to 17. The mean age in the United States is between 12 and 13 years.

Menarche, the beginning of menstruation, frequently occurs before ovulation, that is, before the pituitary and ovarian hormones are synchronized and ovulation becomes a part of the menstrual cycle. There may be irregularity in timing and extent of flow for several months or even a few years after the start of menstruation.

II. Irregularities

Variations in menstruation and the cycle are common. The pattern of the cycle may be upset by such factors as changes in climate, changes in work schedule, emotional trauma, or acute or chronic illnesses.

Menstruation may have strong emotional impact, and associated disturbances may have psychologic bases. Some girls have intense conflicts with a major problem related to the inability to accept the feminine role and assume the responsibilities of womanhood. Some or all of the symptoms of premenstrual tension and dysmenorrhea described below may continue beyond adolescence and even to menopause.

A. Premenstrual Tension

This disorder is associated with fluid retention in the body and psychologic depression occurring within 10 days prior to menstruation. Symptoms include headache, fatigue, weight gain, heaviness in the lower abdomen, and fullness and tenseness of the breasts. Feelings of depression and irritability with mood variations are common. The symptoms disappear when menstrual flow begins.[6]

B. Dysmenorrhea

Difficult or painful menstruation may be

due to conditions such as tumors or inflammatory diseases in women past adolescence. In adolescents, causes are generally related to physiologic and psychologic factors. Dysmenorrhea is frequently an indication of the adolescent's emotional status, which may result from poor preparation for the arrival of puberty and menstruation, or from parental example.

Although a high percentage of girls may have some discomfort, a smaller percentage suffer severe pain with "cramps," sometimes accompanied by nausea and vomiting. They may be bedridden, seek sympathy, and behave in a dependent, childlike manner. A few girls may need psychiatric help, but others are relieved of the severity of their symptoms when a mature relationship with their parents has been acquired, when they obtain security about maturing into womanhood, or with childbirth.[6]

III. Dental Hygiene Care

A. Patient History

Menstruation is a normal process and should not be referred to as a "sick period" or a "monthly illness." When presenting questions for the patient history, use of terms such as the "period" or "monthly period" is preferable.

The menstrual history may provide indications of a woman's general health. Regular excessive menstrual flow may be related to an anemic state.

B. Oral Findings[2,7]

There are no specific gingival changes related to the menstrual cycle. An exaggerated response to local irritants or unusual gingival bleeding during or following scaling may be noted in an occasional patient. With control of local irritants by plaque control, self-care measures, and removal of calculus at regular recall appointments, bleeding can be controlled.

Recurrent aphthous ulcers have been associated with the menstrual cycle in the susceptible patient. A recurrence of more severe symptoms of necrotizing ulcerative gingivitis when treatment has not been completed has been observed.

MENOPAUSE AND CLIMACTERIC

Menopause is the cessation of menstruation. It occurs normally between the ages of 42 and 55, with the average between 47 and 49. It may be induced by surgical removal of the ovaries or by radiation therapy.

The female *climacteric* is that period of change during the gradual decline of ovarian efficiency when ovulation is less regular and finally ends, through the menopause, and including the period after menopause when the body is adjusting to endocrine and other changes. While adolescence is considered the transitional period from childhood into maturity, climacteric has been described as the transitional period from maturity into senescence. The male climacteric occurs at a later age, with few if any definite symptoms.

I. Characteristics

Prior to menopause, menstruation decreases in frequency, duration, and amount of flow over a period of about 12 to 24 months. Although many women may experience minor symptoms, only about 10 percent have any pronounced effects from menopause.

A. General Symptoms

With diminishing estrogen, as ovarian function declines, physiologic changes in body function take place. Vasomotor reactions in the form of hot flashes, in which there are sudden, periodic surges of heat involving the whole body and accompanied by drenching sweats may occur during the day or night. Although a strict distinction is not always made between flush and flash, the term hot flush may be used to mean a reaction of lesser degree in which there is a wave of warm feeling over the face, neck, and upper thorax. Headaches, heart palpitations, and sleeplessness may occur.

Emotional disturbances are not caused specifically by estrogen deficiencies but are frequently related to personal and family circumstances and a fear of growing old. Reactions generally are most severe in women who had premenopausal neurotic or prepsychotic tendencies. Anxiety, tension, irritability, with depression and feelings of uselessness may appear.

B. Postmenopausal Effects

1. Reproductive organs atrophy.
2. Bone: changes may lead to osteoporosis. This condition is less frequent among people who have used drinking water containing fluoride over the years.
3. Skin and mucous membranes: decreased thickness with decreased keratinization.
4. Predisposition to other conditions including atherosclerosis, diabetes, hypothyroidism, and cancer of the sex organs.

II. Oral Findings

Oral disturbances are relatively uncommon. Findings are nonspecific and may be noted only because they appear when the patient has reached menopause, a time when she may be more sensitive to minor changes.

A. Gingiva

Gingival changes associated with menopause usually represent an exaggerated response to local irritation, which reflects the conditioning influence of the hormonal changes taking place. When local factors are controlled through preventive dental hygiene recall and personal oral care, unusual gingival changes will rarely be noted.

Rarely, a condition that has been called menopausal gingivostomatitis may develop.[8] It may also occur after removal of or radiation therapy to the ovaries.

B. Mucous Membranes and Tongue

1. Dryness, with burning or unusual taste sensations may be present.
2. Epithelium may become thin and atrophic with decreased keratinization; tolerance for removable prostheses may be diminished.
3. Relation to diet and undernutrition: inadequate diet and eating habits may contribute to the adverse changes of the mucosal tissues. The appearance and symptoms frequently resemble those associated with vitamin deficiencies, particularly B vitamins.

III. Dental Hygiene Care

In the approach to the patient, a specific relationship of oral conditions to menopause should not be made, because the patient may tend to overemphasize such a relationship and deemphasize the need for self-care measures. Because of the importance of local factors, attention should be directed to the need for regular and frequent professional care as well as to increased efforts for daily plaque control.

A. Appointment Suggestions

The symptoms of physical and emotional changes should be kept in mind when planning and conducting the appointment. The patient's possible tenseness and irritability can be anticipated, and attention to details, such as not keeping the patient waiting unduly, handling materials and instruments with calm assurance, and maintaining conservativeness in conversation to prevent annoyances, may be significant.

B. Instruction of Patient

Preservation of oral health is of particular importance to the woman who has her natural teeth. Because of the possible difficulties and discomforts of wearing prostheses, every effort should be made to prevent the need for tooth removal. A saliva substitute may provide a degree of relief from xerostomia (page 680).

Measures for the prevention of periodontal diseases should be carefully explained, and emphasis placed on reasons for frequent calculus removal supplemented by meticulous daily care. Since good general health practices are very important to this age group, the relationship of general and oral health can be brought out.

C. Diet

A dietary survey may prove to be a helpful teaching–learning experience (page 425). Because of the tendency toward inadequately balanced food selection, the patient may be helped by seeing and analyzing her own inadequacies better when illustrated by a daily food diary. When a patient tends to indulge in between-meal eating, caries prevention through selection of nutritious and noncariogenic foods is emphasized.

References

1. Adams, W.: Adolescence, in Gabel, S. and Erickson,

M.T., eds.: *Child Development and Developmental Disabilities*. Boston, Little, Brown & Co., 1980, pp. 59–81.

2. Carranza, F.A.: *Glickman's Clinical Periodontology*, 5th ed. Philadelphia, W.B. Saunders Co., 1979, pp. 120–121, 515–516.

3. McCarthy, P.L. and Shklar, G.: *Diseases of the Oral Mucosa*, 2nd ed. Philadelphia, Lea & Febiger, 1980, pp. 354–355, 391.

4. Poulsen, S.: Epidemiology and Indices of Gingival and Periodontal Disease, *Pediatr. Dent.*, 3, 82, May, 1981.

5. Newman, M.G.: Localized Juvenile Periodontitis (Periodontosis), *Pediatr. Dent.*, 3, 121, May, 1981.

6. Gallagher, J.R.: *Medical Care of the Adolescent*, 2nd ed. New York, Appleton-Century-Crofts, 1966, pp. 266–299.

7. Miller, M.F.: Diseases of the Endocrine Organs, in Lynch, M.A., ed.: *Burket's Oral Medicine*, 7th ed. Philadelphia, J.B. Lippincott Co., 1977, pp. 445–446.

8. Carranza: op. cit., p. 519.

Suggested Readings

Basker, R.M., Sturdee, D.W., and Davenport, J.C.: Patients With Burning Mouths. A Clinical Investigation of Causative Factors, Including the Climacteric and Diabetes, *Br. Dent. J.*, 145, 9, July 4, 1978.

Cebi, S. and Stephen, K.W.: Caries Prevalence and Oral Contraception, *Community Dent. Oral Epidemiol.*, 7, 183, June, 1979.

Croley, T.E. and Miers, C.: Epithelial Changes in the Oral Mucosa Resulting From a Variation in Hormone Stimulus, *J. Oral Med.*, 33, 86, July–September, 1978.

Darzenta, N.C. and Giunta, J.L.: Radiographic Changes of Mandible Related to Oral Contraceptives, *Oral Surg.*, 43, 478, March, 1977.

Kerr, D.A., Ash, M.M., and Millard, H.D.: *Oral Diagnosis*, 5th ed. St. Louis, The C.V. Mosby Co., 1978, pp. 72–73 (menopause).

Pearlman, B.A.: An Oral Contraceptive Drug and Gingival Enlargement; The Relationship Between Local and Systemic Factors, *J. Clin. Periodontol.*, 1, 47, Number 1, 1974.

Segal, A.L., Katcher, A.H., Brightman, V.J., and Miller, M.F.: Recurrent Herpes Labialis, Recurrent Aphthous Ulcers, and the Menstrual Cycle, *J. Dent. Res.*, 53, 797, July–August, 1974.

Wingrove, F.A., Rubright, W.C., and Kerber, P.E.: Influence of Ovarian Hormone Situation on Atrophy, Hypertrophy, and/or Desquamation of Human Gingiva in Premenopausal and Postmenopausal Women, *J. Periodontol.*, 50, 445, September, 1979.

Puberty and Adolescence

Brunswick, A.F. and Nikias, M.: Dentist's Ratings and Adolescents' Perceptions of Oral Health, *J. Dent. Res.*, 54, 836, July–August, 1975.

Casamassimo, P.S., Pinkham, J.R., and Steinke, D.: Dental Health Needs of the Adolescent, *Pediatr. Dent.*, 1, 129, June, 1979.

Chertkow, S.: Tooth Mineralization as an Indicator of the Pubertal Growth Spurt, *Am. J. Orthod.*, 77, 79, January, 1980.

Currier, G.F.: The Child and the Adolescent: New Rights for an "Old" Minority, *Dent. Clin. North Am.*, 21, 605, July, 1977.

Hägg, U. and Taranger, J.: Menarche and Voice Change as Indicators of the Pubertal Growth Spurt, *Acta Odontol. Scand.*, 38, 179, Number 3, 1980.

Linn, E.L.: Teenagers' Attitudes, Knowledge, and Behaviors Related to Oral Health, *J. Am. Dent. Assoc.*, 92, 946, May, 1976.

Lourie, R.S.: Adolescence: Normal Psychological Development and Psychiatric Problems, *J. Periodontol.*, 42, 525, August, 1971.

Marino, D.D. and King, J.C.: Nutritional Concerns During Adolescence, *Pediatr. Clin. North Am.*, 27, 125, February, 1980.

Mickelsen, O.: Adolescent Nutrition, *J. Periodontol.*, 42, 460, August, 1971.

Shank, S.E. and Guthrie, H.A.: Nutritional Counseling for Prevention of Dental Caries in Adolescents, *J. Am. Dent. Assoc.*, 92, 378, February, 1976.

Taranger, J. and Hägg, U.: The Timing and Duration of Adolescent Growth, *Acta Odontol. Scand.*, 38, 57, Number 1, 1980.

Workshop on Periodontal Disease in the Circumpubertal and Adolescent Periods, *J. Periodontol.*, 42, 452–537, August, 1971.

Periodontal Disease During Adolescence

Biswas, S., Duperon, D.F., and Chebib, F.S.: Study of Periodontal Disease in Children and Young Adolescents. I. Effect of Age, Sex and Gingival Inflammation on Crevice Fluid Volume, Pocket Depth, pH of Supragingival Plaque and Crevice, Collagenase Activity and Urea, *J. Periodont. Res.*, 12, 250, July, 1977.

Blankenstein, R., Murray, J.J., and Lind, O.P.: Prevalence of Chronic Periodontitis in 13–15-year-old Children, *J. Clin. Periodontol.*, 5, 285, November, 1978.

Bowden, D.E.J., Davies, R.M., Holloway, P.J., Lennon, M.A., and Rugg-Gunn, A.J.: A Treatment Need Survey of a 15-year-old Population, *Br. Dent. J.*, 134, 375, May 1, 1973.

Davies, P.H.J., Downer, M.C., and Lennon, M.A.: Periodontal Bone Loss in English Secondary School Children. A Longitudinal Radiological Study, *J. Clin. Periodontol.*, 5, 278, November, 1978.

Hoover, J.N., Ellegaard, B., and Attström, R.: Periodontal Status of 14–16-year-old Danish Schoolchildren, *Scand. J. Dent. Res.*, 89, 175, April, 1981.

Lennon, M.A. and Davies, R.M.: Prevalence and Distribution of Alveolar Bone Loss in a Population of 15-year-old Schoolchildren, *J. Clin. Periodontol.*, 1, 175, Number 3, 1974.

Ranney, R.R., Debski, B.F., and Tew, J.G.: Pathogenesis of Gingivitis and Periodontal Disease in Children and Young Adults, *Pediatr. Dent.*, 3, 89, May, 1981.

Juvenile Periodontitis (Periodontosis)

Baer, P.N. and Kaslick, R.S.: Periodontosis: A Confusion of Terminology, *J. Periodontol.*, 49, 153, March, 1978.

Hangorsky, C.: Juvenile Periodontitis/Periodontosis: Historical Overview and Update, *Dent. Hyg.*, 56, 29, June, 1982.

Hørmand, J. and Frandsen, A.: Juvenile Periodontitis. Localization of Bone Loss in Relation to Age, Sex, and Teeth, *J. Clin. Periodontol.*, 6, 407, December, 1979.

Liljenberg, B. and Lindhe, J.: Juvenile Periodontitis. Some Microbiological, Histopathological and Clinical Characteristics, *J. Clin. Periodontol.*, 7, 48, February, 1980.

Rowat, J.S. and Rowe, D.J.: The Role of Impaired Host Defense Mechanisms in the Pathogenesis of Juvenile Periodontitis, *Dent. Hyg.*, 54, 529, November, 1980.

Saxén, L.: Juvenile Periodontitis, A Review, *J. Clin. Periodontol.*, 7, 1, February, 1980.

Saxén, L.: Heredity of Juvenile Periodontitis, *J. Clin. Periodontol.*, 7, 276, August, 1980.

Sonis, A.L.: Periodontosis of the Primary Dentition: A Case Report, *Pediatr. Dent.*, 2, 53, March, 1980.

45

The Gerodontic Patient

Preventive measures for the aged through care and instruction require greater emphasis as the number of people involved in this group increases steadily. Currently, the population over age 65 represents nearly 11 percent of the total population of the United States, and by the year 2000 it will have increased to nearly 12 percent.[1] The population of those aged 75 years and over will increase from 4.1 to 5.2 percent during the same period.

Only 5 percent of persons 65 or over are in institutions such as mental hospitals, chronic disease hospitals, nursing homes, and other long-term care institutions for the aged. In mental hospitals, nearly one third of the patients are from the older age group.

Dentists and dental hygienists are challenged by the need to help the aging population learn about personal care and seek professional care that will provide continuing oral comfort and function. As the percentage of people in the older group has increased, the total number of patients in a general or adult practice has grown. An increasing number of dental hygienists specialize in the care of the elderly and are employed in long-term care and resident facilities for the aged.

Tooth loss increases with age, but not because of age. Dental caries and periodontal diseases are the major causes of tooth loss. Terminal periodontal disease in the older population represents the cumulative effects of long-standing neglected disease, which may have had its origin in childhood. With application of current knowledge of preventive measures for all oral diseases in younger age groups, it is to be hoped that future generations of older people will not be subjected to the severe effects of uncontrolled and untreated oral diseases.

AGING

According to the World Health Organization, people between 65 and 80 years of age are "old" and people over 80 are "very old." The aging of an individual denotes a "physiological process that begins at conception and entails changes, characteristic for the species, throughout the whole life cycle."[2]

Biologic age is not synonymous with chronologic age, and hence, signs of aging appear at different chronologic ages in different individuals. In other words, some people are old at 45 years, while others are not old at 75 years.

Senescence, the process or condition of growing old, has sociocultural, as well as physiologic and chronologic implications. Normal aging should not be confused with the effects of pathologic influences that accelerate the aging process. Each age period brings changes in body metabolism, activity of the cells, endocrine balance, and mental processes.

An older person's health status is influenced by many factors. Both biologic and environmental factors influence longevity. Genetically, a person may belong to a family of healthy people who have exhibited great resistance to disease factors. Another person may have inherited a specific disease state. Even inherited diseases, for example diabetes or sickle cell anemia, may be controllable through treatment or genetic counseling.

Investigations have shown that significant variables that adversely affect longevity are lack of physical activity, diet, obesity, excess cigarette smoking, use of alcohol to excess, psychologic stress, work dissatisfaction, and unhappiness.[3]

CHARACTERISTICS OF AGING

Changes with aging vary among individuals and among organs and tissues of the same individual. It is difficult to separate physiologic manifestations of aging from those of disease or the after effects of disease.

I. General Physiologic Changes

During aging, an overall reduction in functional capacities occurs in most organs, with a decrease in cell metabolism and numbers of active cells. When cells age, they lose their capacity to proliferate. The tissues may show signs of dehydration, atrophy, fibrosis, reduced elasticity, and diminished reparative ability, although many of these characteristics cannot be separated from pathologic changes.

A. Skeletal System

Skeletal integrity is significantly influenced by an insufficient calcium, phosphorus,[4] and fluoride intake (page 445). Osteoporosis is common in individuals over age 60, and the incidence increases with age. It is most predominant in postmenopausal women.

B. Basal Metabolism

Lowered.

C. Skin

Thin, wrinkled, dry, loss of tone, pigmented spots, atrophy of sweat glands and slower healing of surface wounds.

D. Muscular System

Loss of muscle tone, development of unsteadiness and tremor, lack of muscular strength, decreased speed of response.

E. Digestive System

1. Gradual decrease in production of hydrochloric acid and other secretions necessary for digestion.
2. Peristalsis slowed; decreased absorptive functions.

F. Glandular Secretions

Diminished.

G. Cardiovascular System

1. Tendency toward increased blood pressure.
2. Arteriosclerosis, with decreased circulation to the tissues.
3. Reduced cardiac output; increased heart size.
4. Postural hypotension; with dizziness or weakness when sitting up from recumbent position.

H. Respiratory System

1. Vital capacity progressively diminished.
2. Loss of pulmonary efficiency.
3. Shortness of breath (apnea).

I. Special Senses

1. *Vision: reduced acuity.* The more common eye problems are cataracts, degeneration of central vision, glaucoma, and diabetic retinopathy.[5]
2. *Hearing:* reduced hearing ability, with a loss of sensitivity to high tones.
3. *Pain Sensitivity:* decreased.

II. Diseases in the Elderly

A. Response to Disease

1. *Course and Severity.* Although the diseases that affect the elderly also occur in younger persons, the course and effects of the diseases may differ. In the elderly, disease may occur with greater severity and have a longer course, with slower recovery.
2. *Pain Sensitivity:* may be lessened.
3. *Temperature Response:* may be altered so that a patient may be very ill without an expected temperature increase.
4. *Healing*
   a. Decreased healing capacity.
   b. More prone to secondary infection.

c. Postoperative bleeding may occur more frequently because of increased capillary fragility.

B. Causes of Disability

According to the World Health Organization,[2] the most prevalent long-term diseases that cause the greatest incapacity or disability in persons over 65 years of age include the cardiovascular and cerebrovascular diseases, cancer, diseases of the locomotor system, mental illness, accidents, and pathologic conditions affecting hearing and vision. Handicapping conditions, such as hemiplegia, Parkinsonism, osteoarthritis, fracture, or amputation, are not uncommon.

III. Oral Findings

As mentioned earlier in this chapter, it is difficult to separate changes related to aging from the long-term effects of chronic diseases.

A. Lips

1. *Tissue Changes.* Dry, purse-string opening results from dehydration and loss of elasticity within the tissues.
2. *Angular cheilosis or cheilitis.*[6] Angular cheilitis or cheilosis is not specifically an age-related lesion, but is frequently seen among the elderly. It appears as skin folds with fissuring at the angles of the mouth, and is related to reduced vertical dimension or inadequate support of the lips. Etiologic factors are summarized on page 642.

B. Oral Mucosa

Degenerative changes take several forms. The surface texture is affected by changes in lubrication of the tissue with decreased secretion of salivary and mucous glands.
1. *Atrophic Changes.* The tissue may become thinner and less vascular, with a loss of elasticity. Clinically, the smooth shiny appearance is related to thinning of the epithelium.
2. *Hyperkeratosis.* White, leukoplakic areas develop as a result of irritation from sharp edges of broken teeth, restorations, or dentures, and smoking.
3. *Capillary Fragility.* Facial bruises and petechiae of the mucosa are common.

C. Tongue

1. *Atrophic Glossitis (burning tongue).* The tongue appears smooth, shiny, and bald, with atrophied papillae. The condition is related to anemia, which results from a deficiency of folic acid, iron, or vitamin B_{12}, or combinations of deficiencies. Elderly people have deficiency anemias more frequently than other age groups because of nutritional factors, but not because of aging specifically.
2. *Taste Sensations.* Taste may be reduced or there may be abnormal taste reactions, primarily in people with a disease condition, but changes are not routinely observed in the healthy elderly.[7]
3. *Sublingual Varicosities*
   a. Clinical appearance: deep red or bluish nodular dilated vessels on either side of the midline on the ventral surface of the tongue.
   b. Significance: although frequently occurring, there is not necessarily a direct relation to systemic conditions.

D. Xerostomia

1. *Etiologies.* Dryness of the mouth is found frequently in older people in conjunction with pathologic states, drug-induced changes, or radiation-induced degeneration of the salivary glands.[8] Healthy people continue to have normal salivary flow.[9]
   a. Pathology of the salivary glands, such as neoplasm, may require surgical removal of the glands, which in turn, leads to xerostomia.
   b. Pharmacologically-induced. Older people take a variety of medications and some may require several prescriptions. At least 300 drugs have been listed that are common prescription items and that produce dry mouth as an adverse symptom.[10] The major tranquilizers and the tricyclic antidepressants are examples.
   c. Radiation. Treatment for cancer of the oral region near or over the salivary glands alters their function, so there may be partial or complete loss of salivary production. The problems

and treatment of these patients are described in Chapter 49.

2. *Effects of Xerostomia.* The functions of saliva relate to taste acuity, mechanical cleansing, buffering acid produced by bacteria in plaque and on soft tissue surfaces, anti-bacterial activities, lubrication, and preservation of teeth. When saliva is missing, the patient has problems of oral health and comfort.

   a. Predisposition to dental caries, particularly cemental caries.

   b. Problems of denture wearing (page 639).

   c. Discomfort, especially when eating. There may be dietary changes or use of large quantities of liquid to soften food for swallowing.

   d. Plaque retention on the oral mucosa, gingiva, and teeth.

E. Teeth

1. *Color.* The teeth may show color changes from long use of tobacco or foods with coloring agents such as tea or coffee. Dark intrinsic stains from dental restorations may be evident.

2. *Attrition.* The teeth of elderly people frequently show signs of wear, which may be the long-term effects of diet, occupational factors, or bruxism. Figure 14–3, page 238, illustrates incisal wear. Attrition may be accompanied by chipping; teeth may seem more brittle, particularly when compared with teeth of young people.

3. *Abrasion.* Abrasion at the neck of a tooth may be the result of extended use of a hard toothbrush in a horizontal direction with an abrasive dentifrice. With current preventive measures, use of soft-textured brushes, and attention to abrasiveness of dentifrices, future generations will be less likely to exhibit such tooth alterations.

4. *Dental Caries.* Although nearly 37 percent of people 60 years and older wear dentures at the present time (page 637), the percentage will decrease as more of the population is exposed to fluoridation and other preventive measures.

   a. Cemental caries. With roots exposed

by periodontal diseases, an increase in caries of the cementum can result. Cemental caries is described on page 239. Studies have shown an increase in cemental caries with age. In one report, the prevalence was 27 to 36 percent in those from 30 to 39 years of age, compared with 58 to 64 percent in the 50 to 59 age group.[11]

Periodontal therapy with continuing recall maintenance may influence the extent of cemental caries after age 60. In one group of patients with untreated moderate to severe periodontitis, root caries steadily increased with age, until in the over-60 age group, 86 percent were affected. In another group, comparable by age and disease severity but which had received periodontal treatment and regular maintenance, the dental caries incidence tapered off after 60 years, from 51 percent in the 50 to 59 age group to 42 percent in those over 60.[12]

   b. Rampant caries. Sometimes called "retirement caries,"[13] a noticeable increase in dental caries after age 65 may occur. The caries can be related to xerostomia, which deprives the mouth of the tooth-protection factors of the saliva. Other people may be victims of diet changes related to oral health problems or life style changes of aging and retirement.

5. *Dental Pulp.*[14,15] Whether pulpal changes can be considered results of aging is questionable. The pulpal changes develop as reactions to dental caries, restorations, bruxism, and other assaults during the elderly person's long life of usage. The changes noted here may be observed at younger ages, but are seen more frequently in older people.

   a. Narrowing of pulp chambers and root canals; increased deposition of secondary dentin.

   b. Progressive deposition of calcified masses (pulp stones or denticles).[16]

F. Periodontium

1. *Clinical Findings.* The appearance of the

periodontal tissues reflects the health and disease of the patient over the years. One of the following may apply to any patient.

a. The healthy periodontium. Healthy tissues that have been maintained over the years may have had a minimum of disease. The radiographs show little if any bone recession, the gingiva are firm, and the appearance is normal in every way. Probing reveals minimal sulcus depth with no bleeding.

b. The treated patient. Although the patient was subject to periodontal disease, treatment was completed, and the tissues were maintained in health through personal care and professional supervision. The tissues may show the effects of the treated disease such as scar tissue. Areas of recession with exposed cementum may also be evident.

c. The patient with periodontal disease. Neglect or omission of preventive measures and therapy over the years may have resulted in a slow developing condition of chronic periodontal disease, with extension of tissue destruction into the bone, periodontal ligament, and cementum. There may be loss of attachment, deep periodontal pockets, and radiographic signs of periodontitis. Of the 50 percent of the people over 65 who have remaining natural teeth, a high percentage have periodontal disease.

2. *Tissue Changes Related to Aging*

a. Bone. Osteoporosis is evident, which may be related to aging, but more specifically, to nutritional and hormonal factors. Depressed vascularity, a reduction in metabolism, and reduced healing power affect bone.

b. Cementum. Increased thickness has been demonstrated. In one series of measurements, the average overall thickness of the cementum at 20 years of age was 0.095 mm., while teeth from 60-year-olds measured 0.215 mm.[17]

c. Periodontal ligament. Arterioscle-rotic vascular changes with smaller lumen, calcifications, and increased fibrosis of the principal fibers have been shown.[18,19]

d. Gingiva. Most gingival changes can be traced to the effects of disease, or the effects of anatomic factors. For example, gingival recession, seen frequently in older individuals, may have been predisposed throughout the patient's lifetime by a lack of sufficient attached gingiva, malposition of the teeth, bony dehiscences, or a combination of the three. Precipitating factors may be vigorous inappropriate toothbrushing, laceration, inflammation, or a result of dental treatment such as the placement of a rubber dam on an area with minimum attached gingiva.[20]

IV. Personal Factors

The list below should not be considered typical of all elderly patients since many are well-adjusted. These characteristics are suggested to help the dental hygienist understand possible patient attitudes and actions.

A. Insecurity

1. Related to reduced economic status, self-respect, and feeling of being needed due to inability to work.
2. Reduced activity
   a. Physical limitations.
   b. Overprotection by family.
3. Rejection by family.
4. Anxiety over health.

B. Depression

1. Limited physical power; sensitivity about shortcomings of impaired vision, hearing, and lack of motor control.
2. Changes in physical appearance.
3. Loneliness: desire for attention.

C. Inability to Adjust to Changes in Mode of Life

Tendency to develop fixed habits and ideas.

D. Slowing of Voluntary Responses

Voluntary responses, association of thoughts, and speed of vocalization may all be slowed.

E. Tendency to Introspection

Narrowing of interests; living in the past.

DENTAL HYGIENE CARE

When planning and conducting appointments for a gerodontic patient, knowledge of the physical, oral, and personal problems of this group is applied. Any differences in procedure are not differences in the actual dental hygiene techniques or procedures, but rather differences related to the management of an individual patient.

Care for the older patient should be planned in terms of comprehensive, not palliative treatment. Long-term results with regular maintenance, directed to prevent additional complex problems or more severe disease, must be the basic objective.

Many elderly people do not seek dental and dental hygiene care except when an emergency or other self-perceived need arises. There are several reasons for the lack of attention to professional care. Primary reasons are limited personal finances and lack of financial aid sources. Other reasons relate to physical and mental disabilities, chronic disease, and physical barriers, such as transportation or accessibility of the dental office.[21] Recognition of possible fears and deterrents to care will help the dental hygienist to help an older patient.

I. Appointment Factors

A. Office or Clinic Facilities

Attention to dental office arrangement that may provide physical barriers is important. The aged person's impaired vision, feebleness, or lack of motor control must be considered.

There is need for elimination of hazards such as small rugs, which can slide on polished floors, corners of rugs, which can be tripped over, and irregularities in floor levels. Other considerations related to architectural barriers and how to assist an elderly person who may be disabled are described on pages 691–694.

B. Patient History

Preparation of a careful and detailed medical and dental history takes on particular significance. Basic procedures for preparation of the history are in Chapter 6.

1. *Suggestions for Patient Approach*[22]
   a. Eliminate distracting background music or sounds.
   b. Sit facing the patient, since hearing may be a problem.
   c. Be courteous at all times; show respect for age. Do not call the patient by his/her first name unless the patient suggests it.
   d. Present one idea at a time; be a good listener; older people do not like to be hurried.
   e. Develop trust; reduce anxiety.

2. *Areas of Emphasis*
   a. Chronic diseases. The incidence of chronic disease is high, and many people in the older age group have more than one condition. The prevalence of diabetes in persons over 65 years of age is 78.5 per 1000.[23] Principles of dental hygiene care for diabetics have special application for the gerodontic patient (pages 826–828).

      When a chronic disease is present, the patient's physician should be contacted. All details of the patient's condition may not have been revealed to the patient. The patient may not report health problems that appear unrelated to the mouth and teeth.
   b. Medications. Asking the patient to bring in either the bottles containing the various medications or a written copy of the labels can aid in obtaining a more accurate listing when the patient is not sure. The patient's physician is the best source for an accurate list of prescribed medications.

3. *Need for Antibiotic Premedication.* Many conditions that require prophylactic coverage are found fairly frequently in the elderly. Those with diabetes or those who receive chemotherapeutic or steroid treatments may have an increased susceptibility to infection. When the pa-

tient has a prosthetic joint replacement, heart valve or aortic prosthesis, or a history of other condition listed on pages 99–100, premedication is indicated.

C. Vital Signs

Blood pressure determination is recommended for each visit (pages 107–111).

D. Intraoral and Extraoral Examination

The need for careful, periodic examination of the oral mucosa from lips to throat cannot be overstressed at any age, but especially for the elderly, since oral cancer occurs with increasing frequency with advancing years. Many, in fact most, oral lesions exist without the patient being aware of them. In a survey of 785 healthy people, most of whom were between ages 60 and 90, 81 percent showed some form of notable, grossly visible, potential pathology in the soft tissues.[24] Two patients were found to have squamous cell carcinoma.

For some early surface lesions, biopsy is definitely indicated. For others, the dental hygienist may prepare the cytologic smear as directed by the dentist (pages 122–124).

II. Preventive Treatment Program

Older patients need to have frequent appointments to maintain their oral health at a high level through supervision on a regular basis. The contents of a treatment plan resemble that for other age groups, and emphasis on plaque control dominates. Appointment suggestions are summarized in table 45–1. The dental hygiene appointments may include the following:

A. Plaque Control: described in detail in III, below.

B. Periodontal Care

Treatment with complete scaling, root planing, and follow-up to assess need for additional therapy.[25]

C. Dental Caries Control

1. Diet survey covering several days (page 425).
2. Diet adjustment to eliminate cariogenic foods and make appropriate substitutions.

3. Emphasis on prevention of rampant cemental caries.[13]
4. Fluoride therapy: use of daily self-applied preparations by dentifrice, rinse, or gel tray as needed (pages 456–458).

D. Xerostomia: use of a saliva substitute (page 680).

III. Plaque Control

A. Objectives

Basic objectives do not differ from those for younger people: infection must be eliminated, the masticatory apparatus must be maintained for general health related to diet utilization, and esthetic factors are very important for the patient's sense of well-being and importance.

Older individuals need to be as interested in their health and appearance as people of any age. Esthetic deterioration may create emotional unhappiness, and when the aged feel insecure or unwanted they may lose their interest in personal oral care and diet. Motivation through expression of sincere interest on the part of dental personnel can be an influencing factor in helping the patient to better health.

In the younger age groups, many still believe it inevitable and normal to lose the teeth eventually. With older people who still have their teeth, there is a tendency to be very resistant about the loss of them. Certain people fear dentures because they associate them with "old" people. Patients with partial dentures may already have been impressed with the need for preservation of the remaining teeth. Here, in the desire to save the teeth, lies the appeal for preventive measures for both the teeth and their supporting structures, and good use should be made of this very real motivating force.

In patient instruction, it is important not to try to change all life-long habits since this may create frustration and unhappiness. Self-confidence, which has diminished because of lowering of physical capabilities and emotional satisfaction, must be built up. Major changes required because previous habits are detrimental must be brought about gradually if cooperation is to be ex-

Table 45–1. Adaptations in Treatment Procedures for the Gerodontic Patient

Appointment Factors	Characteristic of the Gerodontic Patient	Suggested Procedure Effect During an Appointment
Medical History Review	Many forms of chronic diseases Variety of medications used	Poor medical prognosis may limit extent of total treatment Need for premedication: antibiotic premedication for decreased immune response
Appointment Planning	Low stress tolerance Tires more easily than younger patient	Morning appointments Shorter appointments Need for frequent recall to provide high level preventive care Appreciation of the real effort patient has made to get there
	Slower voluntary responses Sensitivity about shortcomings of lack of motor control	Do not rush. Do not make the patient feel old by obvious physical assistance
	Lowered tolerance to extremes of heat and cold; less body cooling through perspiration Impaired hearing; difficulty in hearing when there are distractions	Adjust room temperature Cover with blanket Speak clearly and slowly; provide written memorandum of date and time of each appointment Eliminate background noises and music
Instrumentation	Loss of elasticity of lips and oral mucosa	Difficulty in retraction may provide patient discomfort
	Slowing of voluntary responses Cannot adjust to sudden muscular demands	Do not demand quick response to request for change of position of head, rinsing
	Pulp recession: variable pain threshold	Ask patient before administering anesthesia, as the patient may not need it
	Reduction in growth and repair processes Decreased resistance to infection Healing slowed	Provide as little trauma to gingiva as possible during instrumentation Suggest postoperative care procedures to promote healing
	Inability to recover readily from stresses and strains Unsteadiness; tendency to postural hypotension	At completion of appointment, straighten chair back slowly and let patient sit up for short time before dismissing; assist out of chair

pected. There is need for a more optimistic attitude about the degree of oral health the elderly patient can be expected to achieve.

B. Dental Plaque Formation

The incidence and severity of periodontal disease increase with age as an effect of disease accumulation. The amount of periodontal destruction reflects the length of time the tissues have been exposed to etiologic factors, primarily plaque.

Experimental gingivitis studies have compared plaque accumulation and gingivitis development over a 21-day period (page 271). In an experimental gingivitis study comparing young and aged individuals, it was shown that the older people developed plaque more rapidly and the inflammation was more severe than the younger.[26] After 21 days, when oral hygiene procedures were reinstated, the rate of healing and the reduction of inflammation clinically was not different between the age groups. It has also been shown that the microbial population of plaque is different in young and elderly persons.[27]

Several factors can contribute to a more rapid accumulation of plaque in the older patient. Some of these are listed here.

1. *Anatomic*
   a. Gingival recession with large embrasures that result from periodontal disease destruction. Characteristics of the periodontium after periodontal therapy were described on page 198.
   b. Exposed cementum with areas of abrasion or dental caries at the neck of a tooth can create undercut areas where special adaptations of plaque removal devices are needed.
2. *Plaque Retention and Removal*
   a. Exposed cementum may hold plaque more readily than does enamel. When the cementum is planed to a glassy smoothness it would be less likely to hold plaque, and plaque removal efforts would be more successful.
   b. Decreased saliva production reduces or eliminates the cleansing and lubricating effects of saliva.
   c. Restorations and prostheses provide a more complex dentition for personal care. Plaque removal requires more time, patience, and motivation.
   d. Deficient restorations, worn or broken from long years of use, may present with deficient margins which provide areas of plaque retention.
   e. Lack of dexterity related to handicapping conditions resulting from chronic diseases such as arthritis and Parkinsonism.

C. **Specific Recommendations**

Toothbrushing and other plaque control procedures as well as methods for the care of fixed and removable prostheses are selected as for other adult patients (page 333). A powered brush may help certain patients, particularly those with impaired motor function. Adaptations to alter the handle of a manual brush are described on pages 700–702.

Because of increased exposure of root surfaces, attention must be paid to dentifrice selection to prevent effects of abrasion and to prevent root caries. Certain patients may need instruction in desensitizing procedures (pages 556–558). The use of a fluoride dentifrice and a daily fluoride mouthrinse can contribute to both dental caries prevention and desensitization.

When a saliva substitute is recommended for patients with dry mouth, specific instruction must be given. Available preparations are described on pages 680–681.

Instruction and motivation techniques are best applied gradually and regularly, at frequent intervals. Suggestions for adaptations of instruction to the physical and personal characteristics are listed in table 45–2.

IV. **Diet and Nutrition**

A. **Dietary Habits**

1. *Nutritional Deficiencies.* Dietary and resulting nutritional deficiencies are common in older people. For example, characteristic changes such as burning tongue, angular cheilosis, and atrophic glossitis may be related to vitamin B deficiencies. Unfortunately, many people believe that a diet rich in nutritive elements is important only for children.
2. *Factors Contributing to Dietary and Nutritional Deficiencies*
   a. Limited budget.
   b. Lives alone or eats alone.
   c. Does not eat regular meals; frequently uses non-nutritious snacks and foods for entertaining.
   d. Lacks interest in shopping for food or preparing it.
   e. Acuteness of senses lowered; may seek highly seasoned or sweetened foods.
   f. Childish likes and dislikes; unusual cravings.
   g. Tendency to follow food habits of lifetime; ignores newer knowledge of food preparation methods and dietary needs.

Table 45—2. Characteristics Affecting Instruction for the Gerodontic Patient

Characteristic of the Gerodontic Patient	*Suggested Relation to Appointment Procedure*
Tendency for introspection; desire for attention	Patience needed in taking time to listen to complaints and accounts of past experiences
Feelings of insecurity Deprivation of physical capabilities	Sympathetic understanding needed
Touchy sensitiveness, exaggerated imaginary or real pains, or attitudes of suspicion	Build up self-confidence
Resistance to change; tendency to maintain fixed habits	Should not attempt to change all life-long habits, only detrimental ones
Vision impaired	For the patient who wears prescription eyeglasses: make sure the glasses are worn while instruction is being given. Recommend that eyeglasses be worn at home while performing plaque control procedures
Hearing impaired; loss of sensitivity to higher tones	Speak distinctly in normal voice. Look directly at patient while speaking; many are lip readers (page 770)
Slowing of voluntary responses Slowing of speed of thought associations Difficulty in timing sequential events; skills become separate movements, as by a child Least comfortable when must respond quickly to demanding sequential stimuli Rate of learning changed, ability to learn not changed Changes in speed of vocalization	Make suggestions gradually, over a series of appointments Do not demand learning a completely new procedure; adapt procedure already used Guide patient's demonstration of toothbrushing to prevent embarrassment Do not expect perfection; go slowly, anticipate difficulties, give cues, clues Distinguish between slowness of learning and inability
Memory shortened, due mainly to lack of attention, lack of interest, or more selection of what patient wants to remember	Use motivating factors carefully. Provide written instructions; spoken instructions may be forgotten or misunderstood
Need for personal achievement	Help patient gain sense of accomplishment; commend for any success, however minor Never compare the patient's condition with other patients

h. Inadequate masticatory efficiency through tooth loss or dentures that no longer fit properly.

i. Adverse food selection may result from social embarrassment over inability to chew.

j. Adaptations in eating habits, made to compensate for deficiency, may interfere with adequate digestion and absorption of nutrients.

k. May follow dietary fads which provide only a limited and unbalanced diet.

l. Loss of appetite: may have physiologic, social, or economic causes.

m. Lack of self-discipline; feeling that aging brings privilege to eat only preferred foods.

B. Dietary Needs of the Aged

The total nutritional needs are not different from those of younger persons, but there is a need to cut down the quantity, particularly calories. Caloric intake must be decreased to control weight and because of a lowered metabolic rate. Protein, vitamins, and minerals are particularly important for body function, repair, and resistance to disease. Exercise and activity are necessary for proper utilization.

A necessary objective in geriatric nutrition is to retard the progression of diet-induced chronic diseases.[28] Examples of these are arteriosclerosis related to disorders of glucose and lipid metabolism, anemias related to iron and folic acid deficiencies, and osteoporosis resulting from disorders of calcium, magnesium, and phosphorous metabolism with a negative calcium balance.[4]

In addition to a better intake of calcium in the diet, recent research has shown that fluoride intake over the years is beneficial in the prevention of osteoporosis and fractures of the bones.[29] The relationship between fluoride in the drinking water and the decreased prevalence of osteoporosis was described on page 445.

C. Instruction in Diet and Oral Health

1. *Dietary Analysis.* A 4- or 5-day record of the patient's diet can provide information to guide recommendations to be made. Difficulties in showing the procedure to the patient and obtaining accurate results may seem insurmountable. Inaccuracy of recent memory is a problem with some elderly people, so that even the 24-hour dietary record prepared during the appointment, may not be complete.

   The first consideration in making recommendations for aging patients is that a well-balanced diet be used with limited fermentable carbohydrate for dental caries prevention. Food for an adequate diet is listed in table 28–1 on page 424.

2. *Motivation.* Appeal to the patient is made through personal concerns for the relationships of dietary deficiencies to appearance, lowered resistance to disease, and premature aging, which may inspire the patient to improve daily habits. Educational materials are available to study with, and to give to, the patient.

TECHNICAL HINTS

Sources of Materials

A Guide for Food and Nutrition in Later Years
   Society for Nutrition Education
   2140 Shattuck Ave., Suite 1110
   Berkeley, California 94704

Oral Health for Long-term Care Patients
   American Society for Geriatric Dentistry
   1121 West Michigan Street
   Indianapolis, Indiana 46202

Caring for Natural Teeth

Caring for Dentures
   Asuman Kiyak
   Department of Community Dentistry
   University of Washington
   Seattle, Washington 98195

The Why, When, and How, Preventive Oral Hygiene Care for the Elderly, Homebound or Nursing Home Residents
   Barbara L. Wilson
   Department of Dental Hygiene
   University of Rhode Island
   Kingston, Rhode Island 02881

References

1. United States Bureau of the Census: *Current Population Reports Special Studies*, Series P–23, Number 59, May, 1976, p. 9.
2. World Health Organization: *Planning and Organization of Geriatric Services*. World Health Organization, Technical Report Series, Number 548, 1974, p. 11.
3. Eisdorfer, C.: Some Variables Relating to Longevity in Humans, in Ostfeld, A.M. and Gibson, D.C., eds.: *Epidemiology of Aging*. Bethesda, United States Department of Health, Education, and Welfare, Public Health Service, DHEW Publication Number (NIH) 77–711, 1972, pp. 100–105.
4. Massler, M.: Geriatric Nutrition. I. Osteoporosis, *J. Prosthet. Dent.*, 42, 252, September, 1979.
5. Kornzweig, A.I.: Visual Loss in the Elderly, *Hosp. Pract.*, 12, 51, July, 1977.
6. Shafer, W.G., Hine, M.K., and Levy, B.M.: *A Textbook of Oral Pathology*, 3rd ed. Philadelphia, W.B. Saunders Co., 1974, pp. 360–361.
7. Baum, B.J.: Current Research on Aging and Oral Health, *Special Care*, 1, 105, May–June, 1981.
8. Shafer, Hine, and Levy: op. cit., p. 31.
9. Baum, B.J.: Evaluation of Stimulated Parotid Saliva Flow Rate in Different Age Groups, *J. Dent. Res.*, 60, 1292, July, 1981.
10. Lyons, D.C.: The Dry Mouth Adverse Reaction Syndrome in the Geriatric Patient, *J. Oral Med.*, 27, 110, October–December, 1972.
11. Sumney, D.L., Jordan, H.V., and Englander, H.R.: The Prevalence of Root Surface Caries in Selected Populations, *J. Periodontol.*, 44, 500, August, 1973.
12. Hix, J.O. and O'Leary, T.J.: The Relationship between Cemental Caries, Oral Hygiene Status and Fermentable Carbohydrate Intake, *J. Periodontol.*, 47, 398, July, 1976.
13. Chase, R.H.: The Management of "Retirement Caries," *J. Mich. Dent. Assoc.*, 57, 178, April, 1975.
14. Bernick, S. and Nedelman, C.: Effect of Aging on the Human Pulp, *J. Endod.*, 1, 88, March, 1975.
15. Seltzer, S. and Bender, I.B.: *The Dental Pulp. Biologic Considerations in Dental Procedures*, 2nd ed. Philadelphia, J.B. Lippincott Co., 1975, pp. 291–314.
16. Shafer, Hine, and Levy: op. cit., pp. 292–293.

17. Zander, H.A. and Hurzeler, B.: Continuous Cementum Apposition, *J. Dent. Res.*, 37, 1035, November–December, 1958.
18. Grant, D. and Bernick, S.: Arteriosclerosis in Periodontal Vessels of Ageing Humans, *J. Periodontol.*, 41, 170, March, 1970.
19. Grant, D. and Bernick, S.: The Periodontium of Ageing Humans, *J. Periodontol.*, 43, 660, November, 1972.
20. Hall, W.B.: Present Status of Soft Tissue Grafting, *J. Periodontol.*, 48, 587, September, 1977.
21. Gift, H.C.: The Seventh Age of Man: Oral Health and the Elderly, *J. Am. Coll. Dent.*, 46, 204, October, 1979.
22. Ettinger, R.L., Beck, J.D., and Glenn, R.E.: Eliminating Office Architectural Barriers to Dental Care of the Elderly and Handicapped, *J. Am. Dent. Assoc.*, 98, 398, March, 1979.
23. United States Department of Health, Education, and Welfare: *Diabetes Data. Compiled 1977.* Washington, D.C., Public Health Service, National Institutes of Health, DHEW Publication Number (NIH) 78–1468, p. 9.
24. Bhaskar, S.N.: Oral Lesions in the Aged Population, a Survey of 785 Cases, *Geriatrics*, 23, 137, October, 1968.
25. Robinson, P.J.: Periodontal Therapy for the Ageing Mouth, *Int. Dent. J.*, 29, 220, September, 1979.
26. Holm-Pedersen, P., Agerbaek, N., and Theilade, E.: Experimental Gingivitis in Young and Elderly Individuals, *J. Clin. Periodontol.*, 2, 14, February, 1975.
27. Holm-Pedersen, P., Folke, L.E.A., and Gawronski, T.H.: Composition and Metabolic Activity of Dental Plaque from Healthy Young and Elderly Individuals, *J. Dent. Res.*, 59, 771, May, 1980.
28. Schroeder, H.A.: Nutrition, in Steinberg, F.U., ed.: *Cowdry's The Care of the Geriatric Patient*, 5th ed. St. Louis, The C.V. Mosby Co., 1976, pp. 191–214.
29. Jowsey, J., Riggs, B.L., and Kelly, P.J.: Fluoride in the Treatment of Osteoporosis, in Johansen, E., Taves, D.R., and Olsen, T.O.: *Continuing Evaluation of the Use of Fluorides.* AAAS Selected Symposium Number 11, Boulder, Colorado, Westview Press, 1979, pp. 111–123.

Suggested Readings

Adler, S.S.: Anemia in the Aged: Causes and Considerations, *Geriatrics*, 35, 49, April, 1980.
American Dental Association: Council on Dental Health and Health Planning: *Oral Health Care for the Geriatric Patient in a Long-term Care Facility; an Educational Program.* Chicago, American Dental Association, 1979, 40 pp.
Banting, D.W., Ellen, R.P., and Fillery, E.D.: Prevalence of Root Surface Caries Among Institutionalized Older Persons, *Community Dent. Oral Epidemiol.*, 8, 84, April, 1980.
Baum, B.J.: Research on Aging and Oral Health: An Assessment of Current Status and Future Needs, *Special Care*, 1, 156, July–August, 1981.
Bishop, J.L.: A Study of Dental Hygienists' Attitudes Towards Working with Elderly Patients, *Dent. Hyg.*, 53, 125, March, 1979.
Chauncey, H. and House, J.E.: Dental Problems in the Elderly, *Hospital Practice*, 12, 81, December, 1977.
Chauncey, H.H. and Wayler, A.H.: The Modifying Influence of Age on Taste Perception, *Special Care*, 1, 68, March–April, 1981.
Dummett, C.O.: Dental Health Problems of the Geriatric Population, *J. Natl. Med. Assoc.*, 71, 182, February, 1979.

Eichner, K.: Conservative and Prosthetic Rehabilitation Procedures in the Dentition of Old People, *Int. Dent. J.*, 29, 285, December, 1979.
Ford, M.A.: Care of the Elderly Patient, *Dent. Assist.*, 45, 14, December, 1976.
Franks, A.S.T. and Winter, G.B.: Management of the Handicapped and Chronic Sick Patient in the Dental Practice, 4. Dental Care of the Elderly, *Br. Dent. J.*, 136, 145, February 19, 1974.
Freedman, K.A.: Geriatric Oral Health Care, in DePaola, D.P. and Cheney, H.G., eds.: *Preventive Dentistry.* Postgraduate Dental Handbook Series, Volume 2. Littleton, Massachusetts, PSG Publishing, 1979, pp. 193–204.
Freedman, K.A.: *Management of the Geriatric Dental Patient.* Chicago, Quintessence, 1979, 148 pp.
Garverick, C.M. and Ortman, L.F.: The Geriatric Patient, *Dent. Clin. North Am.*, 21, 637, July, 1977.
Giddon, D.B. and Hittelman, E.: Psychologic Aspects of Prosthodontic Treatment for Geriatric Patients, *J. Prosthet. Dent.*, 43, 374, April, 1980.
Gunn, W.G.: Radiation Therapy for the Aging Patient, *Ca— A Cancer Journal for Clinicians*, 30, 337, November/December, 1980.
Harris, C.S.: *Fact Book on Aging: A Profile of America's Older Population.* Washington, D.C., National Council on the Aging, February, 1978.
Johnson, D.L. and Stratton, R.J.: Special Considerations in the Elderly Prosthodontic Patient, *Quintessence Int.*, 11, 47, February, 1980.
Kiyak, H.A.: Psychosocial Factors in Dental Needs of the Elderly, *Special Care*, 1, 22, January–February, 1981.
Langer, A.: Oral Signs of Aging and Their Clinical Significance, *Geriatrics*, 31, 63, December, 1976.
Massler, M.: Geriatric Dentistry: Root Caries in the Elderly, *J. Prosthet. Dent.*, 44, 147, August, 1980.
Massler, M.: Geriatric Dentistry: The Problem, *J. Prosthet. Dent.*, 40, 324, September, 1978.
Massler, M.: Oral Aspects of Aging, *Postgrad. Med.*, 49, 179, January, 1971.
Nedelman, C.I. and Bernick, S.: The Significance of Age Changes in Human Alveolar Mucosa and Bone, *J. Prosthet. Dent.*, 39, 495, May, 1978.
Peterson, B.A. and Kennedy, B.J.: Aging and Cancer Management. Part I. Clinical Observations, *Ca—A Cancer Journal for Clinicians*, 29, 322, November–December, 1979.
Silverman, S.I.: Geriatric Dentistry, in Boundy, S.S. and Reynolds, N.J., eds.: *Current Concepts in Dental Hygiene, Volume 2.* St. Louis, The C.V. Mosby Co., 1979, pp. 47–68.
Siskind-Houle, B.: The Dental Hygienist's Role in Care of the Elderly, *Dent. Hyg.*, 53, 507, November, 1979.
Swoope, C.C., Smith, D.E., and Lukens, E.M.: Geriatric Dentistry, in Clark, J.W., ed.: *Clinical Dentistry, Volume 1*, Chapter 34. Hagerstown, Maryland, Harper & Row, 1981, pp. 1–15.

Periodontal Conditions

Borden, S.M., Golub, L.M., and Kleinberg, I.: The Effect of Age and Sex on the Relationship between Crevicular Fluid Flow and Gingival Inflammation in Humans, *J. Periodont. Res.*, 12, 160, May, 1977.
Carranza, F.A.: *Glickman's Clinical Periodontology*, 5th ed. Philadelphia, W.B. Saunders Co., 1979, pp. 72–77.
Grant, D.A., Stern, I.B., and Everett, F.G.: *Periodontics*, 5th ed. St. Louis, The C.V. Mosby Co., 1979, pp. 90–104.
Hansen, G.C.: An Epidemiologic Investigation of the Effect

of Biologic Aging on the Breakdown of Periodontal Tissue, *J. Periodontol.*, *44*, 269, May, 1973.

Holthuis, A.F., Holm-Pedersen, P., and Folke, L.E.A.: Interepithelial Lymphocytes in Experimental Gingivitis in Young and Elderly Individuals, *J. Periodont. Res.*, *12*, 166, May, 1977.

Newman, M.G., Grinenco, V., Weiner, M., Angel, I., Karge, H., and Nisengard, R.: Predominant Microbiota Associated with Periodontal Health in the Aged, *J. Periodontol.*, *49*, 553, November, 1978.

Roper, R.E., Knerr, G.W., Gocka, E.F., and Stahl, S.S.: Periodontal Disease in Aged Individuals, *J. Periodontol.*, *43*, 304, May, 1972.

Severson, J.A., Moffett, B.C., Kokich, V., and Selipsky, H.: A Histologic Study of Age Changes in the Adult Human Periodontal Joint (Ligament), *J. Periodontol.*, *49*, 189, April, 1978.

Socransky, S.S. and Manganiello, S.D.: The Oral Microbiota of Man from Birth to Senility, *J. Periodontol.*, *42*, 485, August, 1971.

Tonna, E.A.: Factors (Aging) Affecting Bone and Cementum, *J. Periodontol.*, *47*, 267, May, 1976.

Nutrition

Berger, R.: Nutritional Needs of the Aged, *J. Calif. Dent. Assoc.*, 7, 45, November, 1979.

Dreizen, S., ed.: Symposium on Nutrition, *Geriatrics*, *29*, 55–178, May, 1974.

Feldman, R.S., Kapur, K.K., Alman, J.E., and Chauncey, H.H.: Aging and Mastication: Changes in Performance and in the Swallowing Threshold with Natural Dentition, *J. Am. Geriatr. Soc.*, *28*, 97, March, 1980.

Franks, A.S.T. and Hedegard, B.: *Geriatric Dentistry.* Oxford, Blackwell Scientific Publications, 1973, pp. 103–118.

Jowsey, J.: Why Is Mineral Nutrition Important in Osteoporosis? *Geriatrics*, *33*, 39, August, 1978.

Krause, M.V. and Mahan, L.K.: *Food, Nutrition and Diet Therapy*, 6th ed. Philadelphia, W.B. Saunders Co., 1979, pp. 343–354.

Massler, M.: Geriatric Nutrition: The Role of Taste and Smell in Appetite, *J. Prosthet. Dent.*, *43*, 247, March, 1980.

Massler, M.: Geriatric Nutrition II. Dehydration in the Elderly, *J. Prosthet. Dent.*, *42*, 489, November, 1979.

Nizel, A.E.: *Nutrition in Preventive Dentistry. Science and Practice*, 2nd ed. Philadelphia, W.B. Saunders Co., 1981, pp. 373–374, 524–546.

Nizel, A.E.: Role of Nutrition in the Oral Health of the Aging Patient, *Dent. Clin. North Am.*, *20*, 569, July, 1976.

O'Hanlon, P. and Kohrs, M.B.: Dietary Studies of Older Americans, *Am. J. Clin. Nutr.*, *31*, 1257, July, 1978.

Schafer, S.: Malnutrition in the Aged, *Dent. Hyg.*, *54*, 233, May, 1980.

Shank, R.E.: Nutrition and Aging, in Ostfeld, A.M. and Gibson, D.C., eds.; *Epidemiology of Aging.* Bethesda, United States Department of Health, Education, and Welfare, National Institutes of Health, 1972, DHEW Publication Number (NIH) 77–711, pp. 199–213.

Slavkin, H.C.: The Aging Process and Nutrition: Conception to Senescence, *Special Care*, *1*, 31, January–February, 1981.

Watkin, D.M.: Nutrition for the Aging and Aged, in Goodhart, R.S. and Shils, M.E., eds.: *Modern Nutrition in Health and Disease*, 6th ed. Philadelphia, Lea & Febiger, 1980, pp. 781–813.

46

The Edentulous Patient

The completely edentulous patient needs at least annual recall for careful observation of the oral tissues, as well as for supervision of plaque control for the dentures and care of the mucosa. Instruction for the patient who receives new dentures is also a concern, since preventive procedures are necessary for the patient's general and oral health.

Approximately 11 percent of the population in the United States is completely edentulous. A survey of complete-denture wearers has shown that the percentage increases with age from 0.6 percent of persons under 30 years of age to 36.8 percent of those 60 years and over.[1]

Of the completely edentulous, particularly in the older age groups, some individuals have dentures they do not wear, others have dentures but wear only one, while others have no dentures. When there is a single denture, more frequently it is the maxillary denture that is worn. It is not unusual to find that the same dentures have been worn for many years without having the dentures or the supporting oral tissues examined.

Dentures to replace primary teeth must occasionally be constructed. The teeth may be congenitally missing (anodontia) or may have required extraction because of rampant caries or trauma. Nursing caries syndrome, which can result in severe breakdown soon after eruption, was described on page 241.

To provide esthetics and function, dentures can be constructed for the accepting child who will be able to cooperate. As the permanent teeth begin to erupt, parts of the denture will be cut away (figure 46–1). A supervised caries prevention program is initiated for protection of the permanent dentition.

I. Types of Complete Dentures[2]

A. Complete Denture

A dental prosthesis that replaces the entire dentition and associated structures of the maxilla or mandible. The components of a complete denture are described on page 385.

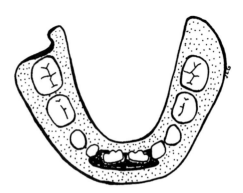

Figure 46–1. Denture for a young child. As the permanent teeth erupt, parts of the denture are cut away. Shown are denture alterations for the mandibular right first permanent molar and the mandibular central incisors.

B. Immediate Denture

A denture constructed for insertion immediately following the removal of natural teeth.

C. Overdenture

A denture supported by both retained natural teeth and the mucosa. The overdenture is described on pages 389–391.

D. Implant Denture

A denture that receives its stability and retention from a substructure that is partially or wholly implanted under the soft tissues of the denture basal seat.

E. Obturator

A prosthesis used to close a congenital or acquired opening in the palate. When the teeth are missing, the obturator is connected to the complete denture.

II. The Edentulous Mouth

A. Bone

1. *Residual Ridges.* After the teeth are removed, the residual ridges enter into a continuing process of remodelling. The alveolar bone which had supported the teeth undergoes resorption. The rate and amount of bony resorption varies with each individual. The major bony changes occur during the first year after the teeth are removed, but changes continue throughout life. Mandibular bone loss is generally as much as four times greater than maxillary.[3] Because of the oral changes, it is usually necessary to have dentures rebased or remade at intervals.
2. *Torus Palatinus.*[4] A torus palatinus may be present in the midline of the palate. Tori are benign bony outgrowths of varying shapes. Occasionally, because of size or shape, it may be necessary to remove a torus surgically before a denture is constructed.

B. Mucous Membrane

As described on page 186, the oral mucosa is composed of masticatory, lining, and specialized mucosa. The edentulous ridges and the hard palate are covered with masticatory mucosa, which is continuous with the lining mucosa that covers the floor of the mouth, vestibules, and cheeks.

The mucous membrane covering the bony ridges is made up of two layers, the lamina propria and the surface stratified squamous epithelium which is keratinized in the healthy mouth. Underneath the mucous membrane is the submucosa which is attached to the underlying bone.

The submucosa is composed of connective tissue with vessels, nerves, adipose tissue, and glands. The support or cushioning effect for the denture is dependent on the make-up of the submucosa, which varies in different parts of a mouth.

When an edentulous mouth is examined clinically, and the lips and cheeks are retracted using a tension test technique (page 217), a line of demarcation similar to the mucogingival junction is apparent, separating the attached tissue over the bony ridge and the loose lining mucosa of the vestibule. Frenal attachments can be observed readily.

III. The Patient With New Dentures

A. Patient Counseling

The preparation for denture insertion has to begin well in advance of the day the dentures are delivered. The patient needs a clear idea of what to expect and what procedures will be followed. Successful after-care and denture satisfaction depend to a large extent on the conditioning of the patient toward the adjustments to be made and the period of practice and learning with the new dentures that can be expected.[5]

Many dentists prepare their own printed educational materials, while others use those available from outside sources. Titles of selected printed materials and their sources are listed in the Technical Hints at the end of this chapter.

Dental auxiliaries are frequently responsible for presenting phases of the instruction to the edentulous patient. The preliminary counseling is followed through the initial postinsertion appointments, particularly to teach denture hygiene and to arrange for continuing maintenance appointments during the following years.

B. Postinsertion Care

1. *Immediate Denture.* The patient receiving an immediate denture will be instructed to leave the denture in place for 24 to 48 hours to aid in the control of bleeding and swelling. When the patient returns and the denture is removed, the mouth is rinsed and appropriate instructions given. After initial healing, the denture care and other instructions are similar to those presented in table 46–1.

2. *New Dentures over Healed Ridges*

   a. Appointments. Following insertion, adjustment appointments are scheduled routinely because adjustments can be expected. The first appointment is made within 48 hours of the time of insertion, and additional appointments are made in accord with individual needs.

   b. Instructions.[6] Too many instructions given on the day of insertion may only confuse the patient. Basic denture care and other procedures of immediate concern can be reviewed. Slow repetition over several periods will help the patient to develop adequate denture management and hygiene habits.

   Basic information for the new denture wearer is provided in table 46–1. Denture cleaning methods are described with other plaque control procedures for the care of dental appliances on pages 385–391.

IV. Denture Related Oral Changes

The condition of the mucous membranes, salivary glands, and alveolar bone is influenced by dietary and nutritional deficiencies, age, and various chronic diseases. Tissue alterations for an older patient were described on pages 624–625. Some of the denture related changes are listed here.

A. Bone Changes

1. *Alveolar Ridge Remodeling.*[7] There is a continuing reduction in size of the residual ridge, which leads to loss of denture support, loss of facial height and lip support, increased prominence of the chin, possible temporomandibular joint manifestations, and occlusal disharmony.

2. *Compensations by the Patient.*

   a. Patients may adapt to the bone changes by making compensating adjustments in the way they wear and manage the dentures.

   b. Other patients may resort to drug store remedies such as pads, adhesives, or self-reline materials, which may be detrimental and cause further oral damage.[8]

3. *Treatment by the Dentist.* Dentures will need relining, rebasing, or remaking periodically.

B. Oral Mucosa

The tissue reaction under a denture varies a great deal between individuals. Whereas one mouth may have an absence of keratinization, thinning of the mucosa, submucosa, and particularly the epithelium, others may have normal keratinization or hyperkeratinization.

Factors that influence the mucosa are systemic conditions that alter host response, aging, denture and tissue hygiene, wearing constantly, and fit and occlusion of the denture itself.

C. Xerostomia

The causes of xerostomia were described on page 625. Diminished salivary flow can influence denture retention and tissue lubrication, as well as reduce the resistance of the oral mucosa to trauma and infection.

1. *Lubrication.* The oral mucosa needs saliva for protection against frictional irritation by the denture.

2. *Retention.* The film of saliva between the denture and the mucosa contributes to retention of the denture.

D. Sensory Changes

1. *Tactile Sense.* With the dentures in place, there may be a diminished sensitivity to small objects in the mouth such as small bones or bits of nut shells.

2. *Taste.* An occasional patient will indicate that there has been a change in food flavors since wearing dentures or that food

Table 46–1. Patient Instruction for Complete Dentures

Item	Factors to Teach

Food Selection	Use foods from the Basic 4 (page 424)
	 Check each day's diet to fulfill needs for a balanced diet
	 Older patients: use foods to prevent diet-induced chronic diseases (pages 631–633)
	
	 New denture wearer:
	    Avoid foods that need incising
	    Avoid raw vegetables, fibrous meats, and sticky foods until experience has been gained
	    Cut food into small pieces
	
	 Practiced denture wearer:
	    Select a variety of foods, but do not expect the same efficiency as with natural teeth

Incision or Biting	Use the canine and premolar area. Insert for biting at the angle of the mouth Push back as the food is incised; do not pull or tear the food in a forward direction
Chewing	Take small portions Try to chew with some food on each side at the same time to stabilize the denture Be patient and practice
Salivary Flow	Anticipate an increased flow of saliva when a new denture is worn
Speaking	Speak slowly and quietly Practice by reading aloud at home, preferably in front of a mirror Repeat and practice words that seem the most difficult
Sneezing, Coughing, Yawning	Anticipate loss of denture retention Cover mouth with hand and handkerchief
Denture Hygiene	Thoroughly clean dentures twice each day Immerse dentures in chemical solution and brush for plaque removal. Rinse thoroughly Complete denture care is described on pages 385–391 Devices to aid a handicapped person are shown on page 703
Mucosa	Tissues need to rest each day. Preferable to leave the dentures out while sleeping Brush and massage the mucosa to clean away plaque and debris and stimulate circulation
Storage of Dentures	Store the dentures in water (or cleaning solution) in a covered container Place in a safe place inaccessible to children or house pets
Over-the-Counter Products	Never attempt to alter the denture for relief of discomfort Do not buy and use self-reline materials, adhesives, or other additives without consulting the dentist. They may be harmful to the dentures and/or the oral tissues. Consult the dentist for advice about all denture problems
Recall and Maintenance	Understand the importance of the dentist's examination of the denture fit, occlusion, and wear, and the condition of the oral mucosa First year: expect reline, rebase, or remake of dentures as the bone remodeling will be greatest during the first year Subsequent recall period: an examination each year for most patients, provided the denture hygiene is ideal. Other patients in cancer-susceptible category need three months' examination (page 674)

does not taste the same as before wearing dentures. Although the taste buds that are located in the tongue papillae are not affected by the dentures, the taste buds of the palate are covered by the maxillary denture and therefore are ineffective for taste perception. Denture hygiene must be meticulous to assure that the denture does not develop thick odoriferous plaque, which may alter food flavors.

V. Denture-Induced Oral Lesions

When the extraoral and intraoral examinations are made, the dentures are removed and a careful, thorough review of the mucosa is completed. The patient may tell of an area that has been sensitive and thus helpfully call attention to a specific visible lesion. On the other hand, a patient may be unaware of chronic mucosal lesions, which are often asymptomatic. Because tissue changes may be important indicators of serious disease such as oral cancer, the intraoral examination must be conducted thoroughly with good illumination.

A. Principal Causes of Lesions Under Dentures

The three factors which singly or in combination cause most oral lesions under dentures are ill-fit of the dentures, inadequate oral hygiene, and wearing the dentures all the time, without relief for the tissues.

1. *Ill-fitting Dentures.* Because tissue changes under dentures occur gradually over a long period, the patient may not be aware of developing disease. The patient may not realize or may not have been informed of the importance of having regular professional examinations of the dentures and the oral mucosa.

2. *Lack of Oral Hygiene.* The dentures and the oral mucosa need daily care. Neglected dentures can accumulate heavy plaque and calculus which irritate the mucosa.

3. *Continuous Wearing of Dentures.* Dentures need to be removed for a part of every 24 hours so that the mucosa can have a rest from the pressure of the hard acrylic during occlusion, bruxism, and clenching. The rest period also allows

the tissue to recover in its natural environment, where the tongue and saliva provide a cleansing effect.

B. Inflammatory Lesions

1. *Localized Inflammation (sore spots)*
   a. Appearance: isolated red inflamed area, sometimes ulcerated.
   b. Etiologic factors: trauma from an ill-fitting denture, rough spot on a denture surface, tongue bite.

2. *Generalized Inflammation*
   a. Other names: "denture sore mouth;" "denture stomatitis"
   b. Appearance: generalized redness over the tissues that support the denture. The patient may have pain and a burning sensation. This occurs more frequently in the maxilla.
   c. Etiologic factors
      The following may occur singly or in combinations.
      (1) Denture trauma from the fit, occlusion, or parafunctional habits.
      (2) Inadequate denture hygiene and care of the mucosa.
      (3) Chemotoxic effect from residual cleaning paste or solution not thoroughly rinsed from the denture.
      (4) Allergy to the denture base: rare.
      (5) Continuous denture wearing without relief for the tissues.
      (6) Patient self-treatment with over-the-counter products for relining.
      (7) Systemic influence on the tolerance of the tissues to trauma and lowered resistance to infection; for examples, vitamin and other nutritional deficiencies and immunosuppressant therapy, such as chemotherapy.
      (8) Candida albicans, parasitism or infection.[9,10] C. albicans is a customary member of the oral flora of people with or without teeth. In denture stomatitis, or in recognizable candidiasis or moniliasis, the numbers of the yeast-like fungus increase. Conditions that promote C. albicans over-

growth are depression of defense mechanisms by immunosuppressants, radiation therapy, or prolonged antibiotic therapy.

C. **Ulcerative Lesions**

Localized ulcer-shaped lesions usually are related to an overextended denture border. The ulcer may resemble a cancerous lesion and should be biopsied if it persists longer than expected of a healing traumatic ulcer.[11]

D. **Papillary Hyperplasia**

1. *Appearance*. Papillary hyperplasia is located on the palatal vault, rarely outside the confines of the bony ridges (figure 46–2). The overall lesion appears as a group of closely arranged pebble-shaped, red, edematous projections.
2. *Etiologic Factors*. The cause is unknown but it is associated with poor denture hygiene, ill-fitting dentures, and possible monilia infection.

E. **Denture Irritation Hyperplasia (Epulis fissuratum)**

Long-standing, chronic inflammatory tissue appears in single or multiple elongated folds related to the border of an ill-fitting denture.

F. **Leukoplakia**

Leukoplakia is a clinical white patch on the mucosa. It may be due to a variety of predisposing factors including local irritation and excess use of tobacco and alcohol. A few leukoplakias microscopically may be precancerous.

G. **Angular Cheilosis or Cheilitis**

1. *Appearance*. Angular cheilosis appears as fissuring at the angles of the mouth, with cracks, ulcerations, and erythema. Sometimes it is dry with a crust; otherwise, it is moist from saliva.
2. *Etiologic Factors*. It is usually initiated by lack of support of the commissure because of overclosure or incorrect position of denture teeth, and moistness from salivation. Secondarily, a riboflavin deficiency or an infection by Candida albicans or other organisms may be involved.[12]

PREVENTION AND MAINTENANCE

I. Development of Patient Attitude and Understanding

For continuing oral health and appropriate denture service, the patient needs to understand the following:

A. Purposes of regular maintenance appointments for finding early signs of disease, particularly chronic irritations and oral cancer.
B. Reasons why the dentist must supervise the function and fit of the dentures.
C. Damage that can result from wearing ill-fitting dentures for long periods of time (years) without tissue and denture examination.
D. Harmful effects to the oral tissue and damage to the dentures that can result from the unsupervised use of commercial products for denture retention or relief, or home repair kits.[13]

II. Daily Preventive Measures

A. **Denture Hygiene**

Dentures must be cleaned at least once daily (page 387).

B. **Oral Mucosa**

1. Brush to clean and massage.
2. Digital massage.

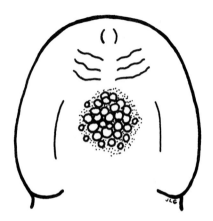

Figure 46–2. Papillary hyperplasia. Outline of an edentulous palate to show characteristic location of papillary hyperplasia within the bony ridges.

C. Rest for the Tissues

For most patients, having the dentures out while sleeping is the best procedure to provide rest for the oral tissues. When this is impossible, the patient should remove the denture for as long a daytime period as possible, such as while bathing. While the dentures are out of the mouth, they can be placed in a container with cleaning solution, and the mucosa can be cleaned and massaged.

D. Diet and Nutrition

The teaching of food selection cannot be overemphasized. For denture wearers, an emphasis on using foods from the Basic Four food groups is necessary. Control of weight and avoidance of foods that are related to specific chronic conditions are important. A dietary analysis can provide a foundation for making specific recommendations.

The diet problems of the elderly patient have been described on pages 631–633. Factors that contribute to dietary deficiencies in patients of any age are magnified when dentures are ill-fitting and masticatory efficiency is decreased. The patient will tend to overlook food value and select foods that are within the limits of chewing ability or that can be swallowed without chewing.

E. Relief from Xerostomia

The use of a saliva substitute may be recommended (page 680).

III. Professional Supervision

A. Frequency of Recall

1. *First year.* After the initial adjustments, the patient can expect the dentures to need reline, rebase, or remake in 6 months to 1 year.
2. *Subsequent Recall Period*
   a. For most patients, one appointment each year will be adequate.
   b. For patients who are careless with denture and tissue care, at least two appointments each year are advised.
   c. For patients who are at high cancer risk because of age, smoking and alcohol-drinking habits, tendency to have leukoplakia, or a previous history of cancer, examination three to four times per year should be scheduled.

B. Recall Appointment

Recall procedures as described on pages 601–602 are followed with necessary adaptations for the edentulous patient.

1. *Procedures for the Dental Hygienist*
   a. Review patient history; make necessary additions to the record.
   b. Determine blood pressure.
   c. Perform an extraoral and intraoral examination and record suspicious lesions for the dentist's review.
   d. Examine dentures for cleanliness and evidences of patient care
      (1) Ask patient to describe the home care procedures used routinely.
      (2) Supplement with additional demonstration and instruction when the care is less than adequate.
   e. Clean the dentures to remove calculus and stain. Procedures are described on pages 387–389.
2. *Procedures for the Dentist*
   a. Review all findings recorded by the dental hygienist.
   b. Examine the oral tissues and the fit and occlusion of the dentures.
   c. Treatment as needed.
3. *Subsequent Appointment*
   Make necessary appointments for continuing current treatment or for next official recall.

DENTURE MARKING FOR IDENTIFICATION

The need for denture marking is apparent in a variety of situations. A universal system for marking would be ideal. Marking is required by law in some countries and in certain states of the United States. In forensic dentistry, or for identification of victims of war, disasters such as flood or fire, or transportation catastrophe, the dentition has been used increasingly as a means for identification.

Dentures provide a method for immediate identification. Prompt identification could be urgent when an individual is found unconscious from illness or injury or suffering from amnesia due to psychiatric or traumatic causes as well as senility.

The dentures of people in long-term residence or care facilities should be marked. Mislaid dentures can be returned, and mix-ups by the direct care staff can be prevented. Dental hygienists are able to make an important contribution to an oral health program by introducing a plan for denture marking.

I. Criteria for an Adequate Marking System

Information on the denture must be specific so that rapid identification is possible.

A. Relative to the Denture

1. Must have no adverse effects on denture material.
2. Must not change the strength, surface texture, or fit of the denture.
3. Must be cosmetically acceptable: the label placed in an inobtrusive position.

B. Relative to the Procedure

1. Readily learned and simple to carry out.
2. Inexpensive.
3. Durable result. When the information is incorporated during denture processing, indefinite durability can be expected. A surface marker for a denture already in use should be able to withstand denture cleaning methods for a reasonable period of time.

C. Characteristics of the Material Used

1. *Fire and Humidity Resistant.* When the label is placed inside the posterior section of a denture, the surrounding tongue and maxillofacial parts offer protection except in the most severe conflagration.
2. *Radiopaque.* A metal marker can be of use as a means of identification by radiographic examination in the event the radiolucent acrylic denture is accidentally swallowed.[14]

II. Methods of Marking

The types used fall into two general categories, inclusion and surface markers.

A. Inclusion

1. *New Dentures.* A typewritten or printed

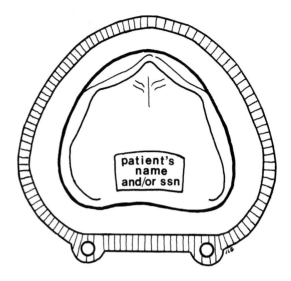

Figure 46–3. Inclusion markers for new dentures. The label is inserted on the impression surface as the denture is being processed. On the flasked maxillary denture shown, the marker is positioned near the posterior border. The patient's name and social security number (ssn) or other identification may be included as described in the text.

enclosure is inserted as a denture is being processed. Labels are positioned on the impression surfaces of the maxillary and mandibular dentures (figure 46–3). They are covered just before the final closure of the flask, with a clear acrylic material.

A label may be typewritten on onionskin paper or the tissue paper that separates sheets of packaged baseplate wax.[15,16,17] Another system uses a thin metal strip for the insert. Stainless steel matrix bands, orthodontic bands, and thin metal strips (shim stock) have been used.[14,18,19]

2. *Old Dentures.*[20]
   a. Clean the dentures thoroughly.
   b. Use a Number 6 or 8 round bur and an inverted cone to cut small, shallow, box-like preparations in the posterior buccal flange of the maxillary denture and the lingual posterior flange of the mandibular denture (figure 46–4). Do not go through to the impression surface.
   c. Typewrite two copies of the patient's initials (or other choice of identification) on onionskin paper, and trim

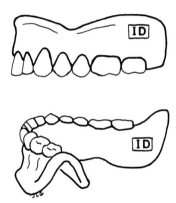

Figure 46–4. Location of markers for dentures. The labels are placed on polished external denture surfaces. As shown, the markers are on the maxillary buccal flange and the mandibular lingual flange.

the papers to fit the box-like preparations.

    d. Cover the paper with cold cure clear acrylic and fill to a slight excess; after the acrylic has cured, polish to a smooth finish.

B. Surface Markers

Surface markers are not as durable, but instruction can be provided for persons not trained in dental laboratory methods. In a skilled nursing facility or other long-term institution where there is no resident dentist or dental hygienist, it may be important to teach a nurse or other staff member to mark dentures of residents as they are admitted. The two methods described below have been used for this purpose.

1. *Indelible Pen.* After cleaning and drying the denture, a small area near the posterior of the outer or polished denture surface is rubbed with an emery board until it is rough (figure 46–4). The name, initials, or other identification is printed on the roughened area with an indelible pen and dried. Two or three coats of a finger nail acrylic (heavy nail protector) are painted over the area; each layer is dried before applying the next. Surface markings have been found to last at least 6 months.[21,22]

2. *Engraving Tool.* An engraving tool is used to enter the name on the denture, and the grooves created are darkened with a special pencil before the appli-

cation of a sealing liquid. Materials are available in a commercial kit.[23,24,25]

III. Information to Include on a Marker

For residents of a home or institution, using only the person's name and initials should suffice for temporary surface marking.

In a community, country, or international situation, the name alone would not provide enough identification, and the social security number, armed services serial number, or the equivalent in other countries, should be included.

Other identification such as blood type and vital drug or disease condition have been suggested. In certain countries, the dentist's registration or hospital number has been used. In Sweden, the patient's date of birth and national registration number have been marked on the dentures.[18]

TECHNICAL HINTS

Sources of Materials
G-26 *Don't Do It Yourself*
G-35 *Dentures: What You Don't Know Can Hurt You*
G-4 *Your New Dentures*
G-18 *Immediate Dentures*
    American Dental Association
      Order Department
    211 East Chicago Ave.
    Chicago, Illinois 60611
Here Are Some Helpful Tips for the New Denture Patient
    American Prosthodontic Society
    919 North Michigan Ave. (Suite 2108)
    Chicago, Illinois 60611

FACTORS TO TEACH THE PATIENT

    I. Dentures are not permanent appliances.
   II. Dentures and tissues must be examined at least once a year. Teach frequency of recall for the individual, depending in part on that individual's ability to clean the dentures and maintain them free from plaque, stain, and calculus.
  III. Dentures may need replacement periodically. Tissues under the denture change.
  IV. Avoid use of drug store remedies, reliners, and other home-applied materials unless

the dentist has provided specific instruction.

V. Specific methods of care for dentures.

VI. Leaving the dentures out of the mouth overnight in accord with dentist's directions.

VII. Where to obtain and how to use a saliva substitute.

References

1. American Dental Association, Bureau of Economic Research and Statistics: *Prosthodontic Care: Number and Types of Denture Wearers*, 1975. Chicago, American Dental Association, October, 1976, Table 1.
2. American Academy of Denture Prosthetics, Nomenclature Committee: *Glossary of Prosthodontic Terms*, 4th ed. *J. Prosthet. Dent.*, 38, 70, July, 1977.
3. Tallgren, A.: The Continuing Reduction of the Residual Alveolar Ridges in Complete Denture Wearers: A Mixed-Longitudinal Study Covering 25 Years, *J. Prosthet. Dent.*, 27, 120, February, 1972.
4. Shafer, W.G., Hine, M.K., and Levy, B.M.: *A Textbook of Oral Pathology*, 3rd ed. Philadelphia, W.B. Saunders Co., 1974, pp. 154–156.
5. American Dental Association, Council on Dental Health: Guidelines on After Care for Denture Patients, *J. Am. Dent. Assoc.*, 94, 1187, June, 1977.
6. Gallagher, J.B.: Insertion and Postinsertion Care, in Clark, J.W., ed.: *Clinical Dentistry, Volume 5*, Chapter 14. Hagerstown, Maryland, Harper & Row, 1981, pp. 1–27.
7. Atwood, D.A.: Bone Loss of Edentulous Alveolar Ridges, *J. Periodontol.*, 50, 11, Special Issue, 1979.
8. Welker, W.A.: Prosthodontic Treatment of Abused Oral Tissues, *J. Prosthet. Dent.*, 37, 259, March, 1977.
9. Renner, R.P., Lee, M., Andors, L., and McNamara, T.F.: The Role of C. albicans in Denture Stomatitis, *Oral Surg.*, 47, 323, April, 1979.
10. Shafer, Hine, and Levy: op. cit., pp. 355–358.
11. Ibid., p. 501.
12. Ibid., p. 360.
13. Ortman, L.F.: Patient Education and Complete Denture Maintenance, in Winkler, S.: *Essentials of Complete Denture Prosthodontics*. Philadelphia, W.B. Saunders Co., 1979, pp. 473–476.
14. Jerman, A.C.: Denture Identification, *J. Am. Dent. Assoc.*, 80, 1358, June, 1970.
15. Dentsply International Inc.: *Method for Placing Permanent Record Data in Denture Base, Without Affecting Tissue Adaptation*, Technical Bulletin. Dentsply International, Inc., York, Pennsylvania, 17404.
16. Lose, F.M.: Denture Identification, *J. Prosthet. Dent.*, 8, 940, November–December, 1958.
17. Woodward, J.D.: Denture Marking for Identification, *J. Am. Dent. Assoc.*, 99, 59, July, 1979.
18. Harvey, W.: Identity by Teeth and the Marking of Dentures, *Br. Dent. J.*, 121, 334, October 4, 1966.
19. Turner, C.H., Fletcher, A.M., and Ritchie, G.M.: Denture Marking and Human Identification, *Br. Dent. J.*, 141, 114, August, 17, 1976.
20. Bauer, T.L.: Technique for Denture Identification, *J. Indiana Dent. Assoc.*, 58, 28, Number 6, 1979.
21. Pugnier, V.A. and Jordan, W.A.: Denture Identification in Nursing Homes, *Northwest Dent.*, 48, 312, November–December, 1969.
22. Deb, A.K. and Heath, M.R.: Marking Dentures in Ger-

iatric Institutions. The Relevance and Appropriate Methods, *Br. Dent. J.*, 146, 282, May 1, 1979.
23. Identure, Geri, Inc., P.O. Box 2086, St. Paul, Minnesota, 55109.
24. Johns, L.D., Boone, M.E., and House, J.E.: Use of *in Vitro* Test Methods as Applied to Denture Surface Identification, *J. Prosthet. Dent.*, 33, 454, April, 1975.
25. Avery, K.T.: Marking Dentures for Nursing Home Residents, *Dent. Hyg.*, 51, 358, August, 1977.

Suggested Readings

Bastiaan, R.J.: Denture Sore Mouth, Aetiological Aspects and Treatment, *Aust. Dent. J.*, 21, 375, October, 1976.

Budtz-Jörgensen, E.: Clinical Aspects of Candida Infection in Denture Wearers, *J. Am. Dent. Assoc.*, 96, 474, March, 1978.

Burket, L.W.: Oral Medicine in the Edentulous Patient, in Lynch, M.A., ed.: *Burket's Oral Medicine, Diagnosis and Treatment*, 7th ed. Philadelphia, J.B. Lippincott Co., 1977, pp. 568–581.

Langer, A.: Prosthodontic Failures in Patients with Systemic Disorders, *J. Oral Rehabil.*, 6, 13, January, 1979.

Miller, E.L.: Clinical Management of Denture-induced Inflammations, *J. Prosthet. Dent.*, 38, 362, October, 1977.

Nater, J.P., Groenman, N.H., Wakkers-Garritsen, B.G., and Timmer, L.H.: Etiologic Factors in Denture Sore Mouth Syndrome, *J. Prosthet. Dent.*, 40, 367, October, 1978.

Ritchie, G.M. and Fletcher, A.M.: A Radiographic Investigation of Edentulous Jaws, *Oral Surg.*, 47, 563, June, 1979.

Russotto, S.B.: The Role of *Candida albicans* in the Pathogenesis of Angular Cheilosis, *J. Prosthet. Dent.*, 44, 243, September, 1980.

Winkler, S.: The Geriatric Complete Denture Patient, *Dent. Clin. North Am.*, 21, 403, April, 1977.

Zakhari, K.N. and McMurry, W.S.: Denture Stomatitis and Methods Influencing Its Cure, *J. Prosthet. Dent.*, 37, 133, February, 1977.

Personal Factors

Breustedt, A.: Physiological and Social Factors of Importance for the Older Edentulous Patient, *Int. Dent. J.*, 29, 276, December, 1979.

Chierici, G., Parker, M.L., and Hemphill, C.D.: Influence of Immediate Dentures on Oral Motor Skill and Speech, *J. Prosthet. Dent.*, 39, 21, January, 1978.

Engels, M. and Tijmstra, T.: Characteristics and Experiences of Women with and without Full Dentures in a City of the Netherlands, *Community Dent. Oral Epidemiol.*, 7, 227, August, 1979.

Guckes, A.D., Smith, D.E., and Swoope, C.C.: Counseling and Related Factors Influencing Satisfaction with Dentures, *J. Prosthet. Dent.*, 39, 259, March, 1978.

Nassif, J.: A Self-administered Questionnaire—An Aid in Managing Complete Denture Patients, *J. Prosthet. Dent.*, 40, 363, October, 1978.

Smith, J.M. and Sheiham, A.: How Dental Conditions Handicap the Elderly, *Community Dent. Oral Epidemiol.*, 7, 305, December, 1979.

Straus, R., Sandifer, J.C., Hall, D.S., and Haley, J.V.: Behavioral Factors and Denture Status, *J. Prosthet. Dent.*, 37, 264, March, 1977.

Patient Instruction

Abere, D.J.: Post-placement Care of Complete and Removable Partial Dentures, *Dent. Clin. North Am.*, 23, 143, January, 1979.

Bauman, R.: Survey of Dentists' Attitudes Regarding Instructions for Home Care for Patients Who Wear Dentures, *J. Am. Dent. Assoc.*, *100*, 206, February, 1980.

Bauman, R.: Inflammatory Papillary Hyperplasia and Homecare Instructions to Denture Patients, *J. Prosthet. Dent.*, *37*, 608, June, 1977.

Ortman, L.F.: Patient Education and Complete Denture Maintenance, *Dent. Clin. North Am.*, *21*, 359, April, 1977.

Nutrition

Barone, J.V.: Nutrition—Phase One of the Edentulous Patient, *J. Prosthet. Dent.*, *40*, 122, August, 1978.

Ettinger, R.L.: Diet, Nutrition, and Masticatory Ability in a Group of Elderly Edentulous Patients, *Aust. Dent. J.*, *18*, 12, February, 1973.

Hartsook, E.I.: Food Selection, Dietary Adequacy, and Related Dental Problems of Patients with Dental Prostheses, *J. Prosthet. Dent.*, *32*, 32, July, 1974.

Miller, E.L. and Ringsdorf, W.M.: Diet and Residual Ridge Resorption, *Quintessence Int.*, *10*, 135, October, 1979.

Nizel, A.E.: Role of Nutrition in the Oral Health of the Aging Patient, in Winkler, S.: *Essentials of Complete Denture Prosthodontics*. Philadelphia, W.B. Saunders Co., 1979, pp. 480–492.

Nizel, A.E.: *Nutrition In Preventive Dentistry. Science and Practice*, 2nd ed. Philadelphia, W.B. Saunders Co., 1981, pp. 546–550.

Denture Identification

Cavalier, M.: Early Neoplastic Change Related to a Denture Identification Mark, *Br. Dent. J.*, *140*, 23, January 6, 1976.

Key, M.C. and Forcucci, C.: A Simplified Identification Technique for Removable Prostheses, *Gen. Dent.*, *28*, 59, November–December, 1980.

MacEntee, M.I. and Campbell, T.: Personal Identification Using Dental Prostheses, *J. Prosthet. Dent.*, *41*, 377, April, 1979.

Todo, J. and Lukens, E.M.: A Technique for Placing Names in Dentures, *J. Prosthet. Dent.*, *37*, 469, April, 1977.

Denture Repairs and Self Repair

Koudelka, B.M., Nelson, J.F., and Webb, J.G.: Denture Self-repair: Experimental Soft Tissue Response to Selected Commercial Adhesives, *J. Prosthet. Dent.*, *43*, 143, February, 1980.

Lamb, D.J.: Denture Adhesives: A Side Effect, *J. Dent.*, *8*, 35, March, 1980.

Means, C.R.: The Home Reliner Materials: The Significance of the Problem, *J. Prosthet. Dent.*, *14*, 1086, November–December, 1964.

Means, C.R.: A Study of the Use of Home Reliners in Dentures, *J. Prosthet. Dent.*, *14*, 623, July–August, 1964.

Tarbet, W.J. and Grossman, E.: Observations of Denture-supporting Tissue During Six Months of Denture Adhesive Wearing, *J. Am. Dent. Assoc.*, *101*, 789, November, 1980.

Terry, J.M., Lutes, M., and Ellinger, C.: Do-it-yourself Denture Reline Materials: A Contourator Study, *J. Prosthet. Dent.*, *18*, 31, July, 1967.

Woelfel, J.B., Kreider, J.A., and Berg, T., Jr.: Deformed Lower Ridge Caused by the Relining of a Denture by a Patient, *J. Am. Dent. Assoc.*, *64*, 763, June, 1962.

Woelfel, J.B., Berg, T., Mann, A.W., and Kreider, J.A.: Documented Reports of Bone Loss Caused by Use of a Denture Reliner, *J. Am. Dent. Assoc.*, *71*, 23, July, 1965.

Woelfel, J.B., Winter, C.M., and Curry, R.L.: Additives Sold Over the Counter Dangerously Prolong Wearing Period of Ill-fitting Dentures, *J. Am. Dent. Assoc.*, *71*, 603, September, 1965.

47

The Patient with a Cleft Lip or Palate

The patient with a cleft lip or palate or both may be a dental cripple unless there is extensive rehabilitative supervision. Treatment and care require the united efforts of nearly all of the dental specialists as well as the family physician, plastic surgeon, speech therapist, psychiatrist, otolaryngologist, audiologist, social worker, and vocational counselor. The dental hygienist is an important member of the team responsible for oral care.

Cleft lip, cleft palate, or both are found in one of approximately 750 live births. Speaking ability and appearance are necessarily the first factors considered when the long-range treatment program is planned since the objective is to help the patient lead a normal life. Dental personnel need to maintain a current list of the health agencies, clinics, and other community resources where the patient and family may obtain assistance for the various phases of treatment and habilitation.

DESCRIPTION

I. Classification of Cleft Lip and Palate

The classification is based on the disturbances in embryologic formation of the palate as it develops from the premaxillary region toward the uvula in a definite pattern. There may be an interference with normal development of the palate at one age level of the embryo and the normal pattern may be reestablished at a later age. Such interferences would modify the classification suggested below.

All degrees are found from an insignificant notch in the mucous membrane of the lip or uvula, which produces no functional disability, to the complete cleft defined by Class 6 of this classification. The first six classes are illustrated in figure 47–1.

Class 1. Cleft of the tip of the uvula.

Class 2. Cleft of the uvula (bifid uvula).

Class 3. Cleft of the soft palate.

Class 4. Cleft of the soft and hard palates.

Class 5. Cleft of the soft and hard palates that continues through the alveolar ridge on one side of the premaxilla; usually associated with cleft lip of the same side.

Class 6. Cleft of the soft and hard palates that continues through the alveolar ridge on both sides, leaving a free premaxilla; usually associated with bilateral cleft lip.

Class 7. Submucous cleft in which there is imperfect muscle union across the soft palate. The palate is short, the uvula often bifid, a groove is situated at the midline of the soft palate, and the closure to the pharynx is incompetent.

II. Etiology

A. Embryology[1,2]

Cleft lip and palate represent a failure of

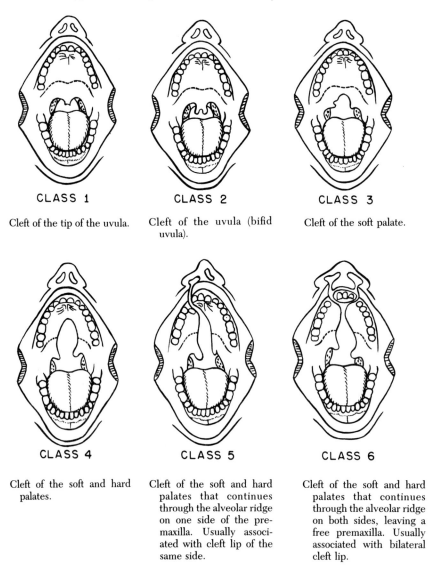

CLASS 1

Cleft of the tip of the uvula.

CLASS 2

Cleft of the uvula (bifid uvula).

CLASS 3

Cleft of the soft palate.

CLASS 4

Cleft of the soft and hard palates.

CLASS 5

Cleft of the soft and hard palates that continues through the alveolar ridge on one side of the pre-maxilla. Usually associated with cleft lip of the same side.

CLASS 6

Cleft of the soft and hard palates that continues through the alveolar ridge on both sides, leaving a free premaxilla. Usually associated with bilateral cleft lip.

Figure 47–1.   Classification of cleft lip and palate. (Courtesy of O.E. Beder.)

normal fusion of embryonic processes during development in the first trimester of pregnancy. Formation of the lip occurs between the fourth and seventh weeks in utero. The development of the palate takes place during the eighth to twelfth weeks. Fusion begins in the premaxillary region and continues backward toward the uvula.

B. Predisposing Factors

Heredity (genetic predisposition) is believed to exert a major influence. A number of other factors have been considered and some of these have been shown effective in animal experimentation. Examples are in-fectious diseases in the mother, nutritional deficiencies, or mechanical interferences in the fetus. It is generally believed that both genetic and environmental forces are involved.

III. Oral Characteristics

A. Tooth Development

Disturbances in the normal development of the tooth buds occur more frequently in patients with clefts than in the general population. There is a higher incidence of missing and supernumerary teeth, as well as other abnormalities of tooth form.

B. Malocclusion

A high percentage of cleft lip and palate patients require orthodontic care.

C. Open Palate

Provides direct communication with the nasal cavity.

D. Muscle Coordination

A lack of coordinate movements of lips, tongue, cheeks, floor of mouth, and throat may exist and lead to compensatory habits formed in the attempt to produce normal sounds while speaking.

E. Gingival Disturbances

These are created by effects of bacterial plaque accumulation influenced by malocclusion, displaced teeth, possible inability to keep lips closed, as well as difficulties in accomplishing adequate personal oral care.

F. Dental Caries

The incidence of dental caries should be no different from noncleft patients, except that predisposing factors such as malocclusion, problems of mastication, and dietary selection factors may be intensified.

G. Treated Case

1. Suture lines from surgery may be evident.
2. Removable prosthodontic appliance. Types of appliances are defined on page 652.

IV. General Physical Characteristics

A. Other Congenital Anomalies

Incidence is higher than in noncleft people.

B. Facial Deformity

Depression of nostril on the side with the cleft lip; deficiency of upper lip in which it may be short or retroposed, lower lip may be overprominent.

C. Infections

Predisposition to upper respiratory and middle ear infections.

D. Hearing Loss

The incidence of hearing loss is significantly higher in individuals with cleft palate than in the non-cleft population.

E. Speech

Difficulty in making certain sounds; nasal tones produced. Anatomic structure is not considered the only contributing factor to the speech problem. It may be related to the hearing loss or psychologic factors related to inferior feelings or parental attitude.

F. Undernourishment

Undernourishment may result when feeding problems continue for a long period.

V. Personal Factors

Most cleft lip and palate patients do not have personality problems, but realization of the social effects of speech and appearance makes it easy to understand why some of them exhibit evidences of maladjustment. The ridicule of contemporaries soon leads even small children to think they are "different." Parental acceptance or rejection no doubt can be a strong influence in adjustment. A few possible characteristics are suggested here.

A. Self-consciousness

Hypersensitivity to taunts or obvious pity.

B. Feelings of Inferiority

The result may be a person who is quiet, unresponsive, and withdrawn or one who is openly brash or rebellious until rapport is established.

VI. Treatment

Treatment is coordinated by a team of specialists and based on the child's progress at each age period. Several reviews provide overviews of the types of treatment and the objectives of each.[3,4,5]

A. Cleft Lip

Surgical union of the cleft lip is made early, usually when the child weighs 10 pounds and is 10 weeks old. The infant's general health is a determining factor, and some surgeons wait until the birth weight is regained or the weight has reached 12 pounds.

The closure aids in feeding, development of the premaxilla and growth of the lip, and may also help to partially close the palatal cleft. The operation has a favorable effect on parents and family members in that it helps to lessen their apprehension and concern.

At the time of lip surgery, an obturator may be made for the palate to make feeding easier and provide support for the lip and premaxilla. It is remade periodically to accommodate for the growth and development of the child. For each step in treatment, the parents, or other person responsible, need instruction for the daily care of the patient's oral cavity and frequent, meticulous cleaning and care of the appliance.

B. Cleft Palate

It is generally agreed that repair of the palate should be undertaken between ages 1 and 2 years. Occlusion has a strong influence on the development of palatal dimensions and growth is rapid during this period. Surgical intervention too early could interfere with normal growth. The combined efforts of many specialists are required.

1. *Purposes for Early Treatment*
    a. Improve child's appearance.
    b. Aid child's mental development.
    c. Prevent malnourishment by improving the feeding apparatus.
    d. Aid in development of the speech pattern.
    e. Reduce possibilities of repeated infections of the nasopharyngeal region.
2. *Maxillofacial Surgery.* Closure of the palate is accomplished by surgery or prosthodontics or both. Surgery provides direct union of the existing tissue that has been moved to a more desirable position for function.

C. Prosthodontics

A removable appliance is designed to provide closure of the palatal opening and/or to complete the palatopharyngeal valving required for speech.

1. *Types of Appliances*

a. Prosthesis. Artificial replacement for a missing part.
b. Obturator. Removable appliance designed to close an opening such as a cleft of the hard palate.
c. Speech aid. A removable appliance related to the soft palate which provides a means for palatopharyngeal valving for speech.

2. *Purposes of the Appliance* (it may be designed to accomplish one or all of the following factors)
    a. Closure of the palate.
    b. Replacement of missing teeth.
    c. Scaffolding to fill out the upper lip.
    d. Masticatory function.
    e. Restoration of vertical dimension.
    f. Postorthodontic retainer.

D. Orthodontics

Treatment may be initiated as early as 3 years of age, depending on the problems of dentofacial development.

E. Speech Therapy

Training may be started with very young children, and is particularly emphasized after the surgical or prosthodontic treatment has been accomplished.

F. Operative Dentistry (Pedodontist or General Dental Practitioner)

A major problem can be dental caries leading to tooth loss. With missing teeth, major difficulties arise related to all phases of treatment, particularly the retention of the prosthesis. Preservation of the primary teeth is very important.

DENTAL HYGIENE CARE

Preventive measures for preservation of the teeth and their supporting structures are essential to the success of the special care needed for the habilitation of the cleft palate patient. Each phase of dental hygiene care and instruction, important for all patients, takes on even greater significance in the light of the magnified problems of the dental cripple.

Every attempt should be made to avoid the need for removal of teeth since the patient has enough oral problems without also being edentulous. Primary and permanent teeth are needed for the stabilization of a speech aid or obturator and success of all treatment procedures. Understanding by the patient and the parents of the value of preventive procedures is accomplished through explanation and instruction.

When the patient has not had specialized care, the dental hygienist has a responsibility in working with the dentist to arrange referral to an available agency, clinic, or private practice specialist.

I. Objectives for Appointment Planning

Frequent recall appointments, scheduled every 3 or 4 months, are usually needed during the maintenance phase of the patient's care.
A. To review plaque control measures and provide encouragement for the patient in maintaining the health of the supporting structures and the cleanliness of the obturator or speech aid.
B. To remove all calculus and smooth the surfaces as a supplement to the patient's personal daily care procedures.
C. To make topical fluoride applications at proper intervals for both primary and permanent dentitions, and supervise self-applied daily fluoride.

II. Appointment Psychology

A. A patient who has often been in a hospital for oral surgery may be very apprehensive about dental and dental hygiene care.
B. Speech may be almost indiscernible although with repeated contact, understanding is developed.
   1. Avoid embarrassment produced by constantly asking the patient to repeat what has been said.
   2. Provide pencil and paper for the older child to write requests or comments.
   3. Let parent or other person accompanying small child interpret.
C. Hearing loss: depending on severity, approach is similar to that for speech difficulties listed above. Suggestions for care of patients with hearing problems are described on page 770.
D. Avoid solicitousness or obvious pity. Approach as a normal patient.
E. Provide motivations for quiet unresponsive or bold rebellious types which will help them

gain an objective approach to the care of their mouths.

III. Sterile Techniques

Although procedures for asepsis should be the same for all patients, it should be remembered that the open fissure lines make the cleft palate patient particularly susceptible to infections.

IV. Instrumentation

Techniques are adapted to the oral characteristics. All objectives of scaling and other instrumentation have particular implications for the patient with a cleft palate.

A. **Malaligned Teeth:** adjust scaling and root planing procedures.

B. **Free Premaxilla (unoperated older patient):** related to bilateral cleft of alveolar ridge; avoid undue pressure with finger rests or instrument to prevent movement of the part.

C. **Area of Recent Surgery:** avoid pressure.

D. **Sensitive, Enlarged Gingival Tissue that Bleeds Readily**
   1. Begin plaque control instruction first before any instrumentation.
   2. Continue plaque control instruction as small sections of scaling are done over several appointments.
   3. Arrange follow-up appointments to check response of tissue.

E. **Open Fissures:** prevent debris or pieces of calculus from passing into or being retained in the clefts. Whenever possible, use rubber dam for indicated procedures.

F. **Lack of Coordinated Movements:** small children especially may need instruction in how to rinse when this is a new procedure for them.

G. **Prosthesis or Speech Aid:** use same procedures and precautions as for cleaning a removable denture (pages 391–393, 579–581).

V. Topical Application of Fluoride Agent

Free premaxilla or short upper lip may complicate cotton roll or tray placement.

VI. Patient Instruction

A. Personal Oral Care Procedures

The self-conscious patient with an inferiority complex may actually fear or exhibit rejection toward the oral cavity. With a small child, the parents may be afraid of damaging the deformed areas or hurting the child if cleansing methods are employed. The dental hygienist must have an empathetic and sympathetic approach and plan for continued instruction over a long period of time.

1. *Teeth and Gingiva*
   a. Select toothbrush, brushing method, and auxiliary aids according to the individual needs.
   b. Adapt techniques for patient with free premaxilla to prevent its movement. A soft nylon brush with end-rounded filaments is indicated.
   c. Instigate daily self-applied fluoride: mouth rinse, fluoride dentifrice, and diet supplements for a young child in a nonfluoridated community (pages 447–448, 456–457).
2. *Prosthesis or Speech Aid.* Halitosis may be a real problem when the prosthesis forms the soft palate and the floor of the nasal cavity because of the accumulation of mucus secreted by the nasal cavity surfaces.
   a. Instruct patient in the need for frequent removal of appliance for cleansing, particularly following eating.
   b. Method for cleaning prosthesis: same as for removable partial denture (pages 391–393).

B. Diet

1. *Need for a Varied Diet:* should include adequate proportions of all essential food groups (table 28–1, page 424).
2. *Need for Prevention of Dental Caries:* limitation of cariogenic foods, particularly for between-meal snacks. Procedures of a dental caries control study are recommended (pages 432–435).

VII. Dental Hygiene Care Related to Oral Surgery

A. Presurgery (pages 658–661, 670)

Objectives have particular significance because the cleft palate patient is unusually susceptible to infections of the upper respiratory area and middle ear. Every precaution should be taken to prevent complications.

B. Postsurgery Personal Oral Care

In certain of the palate operations, arm restraints are applied to prevent accidental damage to the repaired region. After each feeding (liquid diet for several days, soft diet for the next week), the mouth must be rinsed carefully. Brushing must be accomplished with great care, usually by the parent or hospital attendant, to avoid damage to the healing suture lines. In some cases, the toothbrush with suction attachment may be useful (pages 718–719).

References

1. Bhaskar, S.N., ed.: *Orban's Oral Histology and Embryology,* 9th ed. St. Louis, The C.V. Mosby Co., 1980, pp. 19–21.
2. Melfi, R.C.: Permar's *Oral Embryology and Microscopic Anatomy,* 7th ed. Philadelphia, Lea & Febiger, 1982, pp. 22–36.
3. Berkowitz S.: State of the Art in Cleft Palate Orofacial Growth and Dentistry. A Historical Perspective, *Am. J. Orthod.,* 74, 564, November, 1978.
4. Krogman, W.M.: The Cleft Palate Team in Action, in Cooper, H.K., Harding, R.L., Krogman, W.M., Mazaheri, M., and Millard, R.T., eds.: *Cleft Palate and Cleft Lip: A Team Approach to Clinical Management and Rehabilitation of the Patient.* Philadelphia, W.B. Saunders Co., 1979, pp. 145–161.
5. Harris, R.: Summary of a Conference on Cleft Lip and Cleft Palate, *J. Am. Dent. Assoc.,* 100, 396, March, 1980.

Suggested Readings

Ames, J.R. and Maki, K.A.: The Autogenous Particulate Cancellous Bone Marrow Graft in Alveolar Clefts, A Report of Forty-one Cases, *Oral Surg.,* 51, 588, June, 1981.

Bennington, I.C., Watson, I.B., Jenkins, W.M.M., and Allan, G.R.J.: Restorative Treatment of the Cleft Palate Patient, 1–Introduction, *Br. Dent. J.,* 146, 14, January 2, 1979; 2–Examination and Treatment Planning, *Br. Dent. J.,* 146, 47, January 16, 1979; 3–Preventive and Periodontal Aspects, *Br. Dent. J.,* 146, 79, February 6, 1979; 4–Fixed Prostheses, *Br. Dent. J.,* 146, 115, February 20, 1979; 5–Removable Prostheses, *Br. Dent. J.,* 146, 144, March 6, 1979; 6–Complete Dentures, *Br. Dent. J.,* 146, 183, March 20, 1979.

Carl, W.: Preoperative and Immediate Postoperative Obturators, *J. Prosthet. Dent.,* 36, 298, September, 1976.

Crosthwaite, G.H.: Dental Consideration for the Child With Cleft Palate, *J. Am. Dent. Assoc.,* 91, 1042, November, 1975.

Desjardins, R.P.: Prosthodontic Management of the Cleft-palate Patient, *J. Prosthet. Dent.,* 33, 655, June, 1975.

Droschl, H.: Orthodontic Therapy of Clefts of the Lips, Jaw, and Palate, *Quintessence Int.,* 12, 27, January, 1981.

Dungy, A.F.: General Dental Care of the Cleft Palate Patient, *Can. Dent. Assoc. J.*, *42*, 356, July, 1976.

Ettinger, R.L.: Use of Teeth With a Poor Prognosis in Cleft Palate Prosthodontics, *J. Am. Dent. Assoc.*, *94*, 910, May, 1977.

Fletcher, S.G., Berkowitz, S., Bradley, D.P., Burdi, A.R., Koch, L., and Maue-Dickson, W.: Cleft Lip and Palate Research: An Updated State of the Art (Six Parts), *Cleft Palate J.*, *14*, 261–328, October, 1977.

Joffe, L., Judes, G., and McCollum, A.G.: The Role of the Dentist in the Management of the Cleft Palate Patient, *J. Dent. Assoc. So. Africa*, *31*, 375, July, 1976.

Jones, J.E.: Early Management of Severe Bilateral Cleft Lip and Palate in an Infant, *J. Dent. Child.*, *48*, 50, January–February, 1981.

Kennedy, T.J., Miller, S.H., Tooze, F.M., Harding, R.L., Davis, T.S., and Graham, W.P.: The Team Approach to Treatment of the Cleft Lip and Palate, *Am. Family Physician*, *18*, 74, July, 1978.

Kwon, H.J., Waite, D.E., Stickel, F.R., Chisholm, T., and McParland, F.: The Management of Alveolar Cleft Defects, *J. Am. Dent. Assoc.*, *102*, 848, June, 1981.

Lang, N.P., Braegger, U., and Schuerch, E.: Periodontal Conditions in Adolescents With Cleft Lip and Palate, *J. Dent. Res.*, *60*, 388, Abstract 310, Special Issue A, March, 1981.

Moore, D.J.: The Continuing Role of the Prosthodontist in the Treatment of Patients With Cleft Lip and Palate, *J. Prosthet. Dent.*, *36*, 186, August, 1976.

Nizel, A.E.: *Nutrition in Preventive Dentistry: Science and Practice*, 2nd ed. Philadelphia, W.B. Saunders Co., 1981, pp. 521–523.

Pannbacker, M.: Survey of Publications for Parents of Cleft Palate Children: A Preliminary Report, *Cleft Palate J.*, *13*, 57, January, 1976.

Pashayan, H.M. and McNab, M.: Simplified Method of Feeding Infants Born With Cleft Palate With or Without Cleft Lip, *Am. J. Dis. Child.*, *133*, 145, February, 1979.

Razek, M.K.A.: Prosthetic Feeding Aids for Infants With Cleft Lip and Palate, *J. Prosthet. Dent.*, *44*, 556, November, 1980.

Schneiderman, C.R. and Mann, M.B.: Air Flow and Intelligibility of Speech of Normal Speakers and Speakers With a Prosthodontically Repaired Cleft Palate, *J. Prosthet. Dent.*, *39*, 193, February, 1978.

Shah, C.P. and Wong, D.: Management of Children With Cleft Lip and Palate, *Can. Med. Assoc. J.*, *122*, 19, January 12, 1980.

Shaw, W.C.: Orthodontic Treatment of Malocclusion Associated with Repaired Complete Clefts of the Lip and Palate, *Br. J. Orthod.*, *6*, 73, April, 1979.

Stephen, K.W. and MacFadyen, E.E.: Three Years of Clinical Caries Prevention for Cleft Palate Children, *Br. Dent. J.*, *143*, 111, August 16, 1977.

Strohaver, R.A.: Button Obturator for a Soft Palate Defect, *J. Prosthet. Dent.*, *43*, 229, February, 1980.

Thayer, R.: Cleft Palate Speech Defects Associated With Dental Malocclusions, *Dent. Assist.*, *47*, 19, May/June, 1978.

Wolford, L.M. and Epker, B.N.: Sequencing and Timing of Treatment in the Correction of Dentofacial Deformities in Adult Patients With Clefts, *J. Am. Dent. Assoc.*, *96*, 835, May, 1978.

Etiology and Development

Bixler, D.: Heritability of Clefts of the Lip and Palate, *J. Prosthet. Dent.*, *33*, 100, January, 1975.

Cohen, M.M., Jr.: Syndromes With Cleft Lip and Cleft Palate, *Cleft Palate J.*, *15*, 306, October, 1978.

Ericson, A., Kallen, B., and Westerholm, P.: Cigarette Smoking as an Etiologic Factor in Cleft Lip and Palate, *Am. J. Obstet. Gynecol.*, *135*, 348, October 1, 1979.

Haring, F.N.: Dental Development in Cleft and Noncleft Subjects, *Angle Orthod.*, *46*, 47, January, 1976.

Poole, A.E.: Genetics of Cleft Lip and Cleft Palate, *Dent. Clin. North Am.*, *19*, 171, January, 1975.

Schroeder, D.C. and Green, L.J.: Frequency of Dental Trait Anomalies in Cleft, Sibling, and Noncleft Groups, *J. Dent. Res.*, *54*, 802, July–August, 1975.

Psychosocial Aspects

Beder, O.E. and Weinstein, P.: Explorations of the Coping of Adolescents With Orofacial Anomalies Using the Cornell Medical Index, *J. Prosthet. Dent.*, *43*, 565, May, 1980.

Glass, L. and Starr, C.D.: A Study of Relationships Between Judgments of Speech and Appearance of Patients with Orofacial Clefts, *Cleft Palate J.*, *16*, 436, October, 1979.

Kommers, M.S. and Sullivan, M.D.: Written Language Skills of Children With Cleft Palate, *Cleft Palate J.*, *16*, 81, January, 1979.

MacDonald, S.K.: Parental Needs and Professional Responses: A Parental Perspective, *Cleft Palate J.*, *16*, 188, April, 1979.

McWilliams, B.J. and Matthews, H.P.: A Comparison of Intelligence and Social Maturity in Children With Unilateral Complete Clefts and Those With Isolated Cleft Palates, *Cleft Palate J.*, *16*, 363, October, 1979.

Renalli, D.N.: Psychosocial Considerations in the Dental Treatment of Individuals With Congenital Orofacial Clefting: A Summary for Clinicians, *Special Care*, *1*, 65, March–April, 1981.

Richman, L.C.: Parents and Teachers: Differing Views of Behavior of Cleft Palate Children, *Cleft Palate J.*, *15*, 360, October, 1978.

Richman, L.C.: Behavior and Achievement of Cleft Palate Children, *Cleft Palate J.*, *13*, 4, January, 1976.

Richman, L.C. and Harper, D.C.: Personality Profiles of Physically Impaired Young Adults, *J. Clin. Psychol.*, *36*, 668, July, 1980.

Richman, L.C. and Harper, D.C.: Observable Stigmata and Perceived Maternal Behavior, *Cleft Palate J.*, *15*, 215, July, 1978.

Simonds, J.F. and Heimburger, R.E.: Psychiatric Evaluation of Youth With Cleft Lip-palate Matched With a Control Group, *Cleft Palate J.*, *15*, 193, July, 1978.

Starr, P.: Cleft Type, Age, and Sex Differences in Teenagers' Ratings of Their Own Behavior, Self-esteem, and Attitude Toward Clefting, *Rehabil. Lit.*, *4*, 177, July–August, 1980.

Starr, P.: Facial Attractiveness and Behavior of Patients With Cleft Lip and/or Palate, *Psychol. Rep.*, *46*, 579, April, 1980.

Starr, P.: Self-esteem and Behavioral Functioning of Teenagers With Oral-facial Clefts, *Rehabil. Lit.*, *39*, 233, August, 1978.

Starr, P., Chinsky, R., Canter, H., and Meier, J.: Mental, Motor, and Social Behavior of Infants With Cleft Lip and/or Cleft Palate, *Cleft Palate J.*, *14*, 140, April, 1977.

Starr, P. and Heiserman, K.J.: Factors Associated With Missed Appointments of Patients in a Cleft Lip and Palate Clinic, *Cleft Palate J.*, *12*, 461, October, 1975.

Starr, P. and Zirpoli, E.: Cleft Palate Patients—The Social Work Approach, *Health Soc. Work*, *1*, 104, May, 1976.

Walesky-Rainbow, P.A. and Morris, H.L.: An Assessment of Informative-counseling Procedures for Cleft Palate Children, *Cleft Palate J.*, *15*, 20, January, 1978.

48

The Oral Surgery Patient and the Patient with a Fractured Jaw

A mouth is not considered a good surgical risk when the teeth are covered with debris and calculus and the gingiva show signs of inflammation and possible nutritional deficiency. It is recommended that unless emergency surgery is required, the appointment be postponed until the mouth is in a better state of cleanliness and health.

I. Overview of Oral and Maxillofacial Surgery

The term *oral and maxillofacial surgery* has been defined professionally as the diagnosis and treatment, surgical and adjunctive, of the diseases, injuries, and defects of the human jaws and associated structures.

Included among the many types of operations performed are (1) the removal of hopelessly diseased or impacted teeth; (2) the removal of cysts, tumors, and obstructions of the salivary glands; (3) correction of congenital or developmental defects such as cleft lip and palate; (4) reduction and fixation of fractured jaws and other facial bones; and (5) procedures to prepare the mouth for orthodontic or prosthodontic treatments.

Surgery for treatment of diseases and correction of defects of the periodontal tissues is categorized specifically as *periodontal surgery*. Within the scope of periodontal surgery are procedures for pocket elimination, gingivoplasty,

treatment of furcation involvements, correction of mucogingival defects, and treatment for bony defects about the teeth. Preparation for periodontal surgery is not specifically described in this chapter.

II. Objectives

Dental hygiene care and instruction prior to oral and maxillofacial surgery may contribute to the patient's health and well-being by one or more of the following:

A. Remove Debris and Reduce Oral Bacterial Count[1]

1. Aid in the preparation of an aseptic field of operation.
2. Make postoperative infection less likely or less severe.

B. Reduce Inflammation of the Gingiva and Improve Tissue Tone

1. Lessen local hemorrhage at the time of the operation.
2. Promote postoperative healing.

C. Remove Calculus Deposits

1. Remove a source of plaque retention and thus improve gingival tissue tone.
2. Prevent interference with placement of surgical instruments.

3. Prevent pieces of calculus from breaking away during tooth removal.
   a. Danger of inhalation, particularly when a general anesthetic is used.
   b. Possibility of calculus falling into socket or other surgical area and acting as a foreign body to inhibit healing.

D. Instruct in Preoperative Personal Oral Care Procedures

This will contribute to reducing inflammation and thus improve tissue tone.

E. Instruct in the Use of Foods

The patient should be instructed about those foods that provide the elements essential to tissue building and repair during pre- and postoperative periods.

F. Interpret the Dentist's Directions

This should be done for the immediate preoperative preparation with respect to rest and dietary limitations, particularly when a general anesthetic is to be administered.

G. Motivate the Patient Who Will Have Teeth Remaining

The patient who will have teeth remaining after surgery should be motivated to prevent further tooth loss through routine dental and dental hygiene professional care and personal oral care procedures.

H. Emphasize the Importance of Diet

For the patient who will have all teeth removed and dentures inserted, the importance of a diet containing all essential food groups should be emphasized.

III. Personal Factors

The extent of the operation to be performed and previous experiences will affect the patient's attitude. A majority of the patients who are in greatest need for preoperative dental hygiene care and instruction may be people who have neglected their mouths for many years. They have been indifferent toward or unaware of the importance of obtaining adequate care. Their only visits to a dentist may have been to have a toothache relieved by extraction. Their knowledge of preventive measures may be limited. A few of the characteristics that may confront the dental hygienist are suggested below.

A. Apprehensive and Fearful

1. Apprehensive and indifferent toward need for personal care of teeth that are to be removed.
2. Fearful of all dental procedures, particularly oral surgery and anesthesia.
3. Fearful of personal appearance after surgery.

B. Impatient

When teeth have caused discomfort and pain it may be difficult to understand need for delay while dental hygiene procedures are accomplished.

C. Ashamed

Of appearance or of having neglected teeth.

D. Resigned

Feeling of inevitableness of the situation; lack of appreciation for natural teeth.

E. Discouraged

Over tooth loss or development of soft tissue lesions.

F. Resentful

1. Toward time lost from work.
2. Toward the financial aspects of dental care.
3. Toward inconvenience and discomfort.

DENTAL HYGIENE CARE

A review of the patient's record will show preliminary procedures that need to be completed. For example, a thorough intraoral and extraoral examination, a recording of vital signs, photographs, and additional radiographs may be required. The patient's medical and dental history will reveal essential information relative to the need for prophylactic antibiotics or other precautions.

I. Presurgery Treatment Planning

At least two appointments frequently are needed, but the pending date for the operation and the patient's attitude may limit the time to be spent.

A. First Appointment

Develop patient rapport; explain and demonstrate initial plaque control principles; present a dietary record form for completion before the next appointment; and remove calculus deposits. Scaling may be limited to one quadrant or one side, depending on the severity of the periodontal condition and the nature of the deposits.

B. Second Appointment

1. Observe gingival tissue response; apply disclosing agent; and review disease control procedures. Introduce the use of dental floss or other interdental aids when applicable.
2. Receive the dietary record and review it with the patient (page 425). Present diet recommendations.
3. Complete or continue the scaling. More than two appointments will be needed for patients who will have surgery for oral cancer, cardiovascular or other condition in which it is necessary to complete all periodontal and dental treatment. When radiation or chemotherapy will be used following surgery for oral cancer, or when a prosthetic heart valve or total joint replacement will be involved, complete oral care is necessary as described on pages 677, 791.

C. Preoperative Instructions[2]

At the appointment just prior to the oral surgery appointment, instructions relative to the surgery should be discussed with the patient. The objective is to let the patient know what to expect so that full cooperation is possible. The patient may have concerns about the anesthesia, the surgical procedure, and the outcome.

1. Explain the general procedures for anesthesia and surgery.
2. Provide printed preoperative instructions. Information in the printed instructions would include the following:
   a. Food and liquid intake. Specify the number of hours prior to the time of the operation when there should be no further intake of food or fluids.
   b. Alcohol and medications restrictions. Certain proprietary self-medications are not compatible with the anesthetic and drugs to be used during and following the surgical procedure.
   c. Transport to and from the appointment. When a general anesthetic is used, the patient should not drive. Plans for someone to accompany and assist the patient should be made.
   d. The night before the appointment. In addition to food and alcohol restrictions, a good night's rest is advocated.
   e. Personal items
      (1) Clothing: the clothing worn should be loose and comfortable. The sleeves should be easily drawn up over the elbows.
      (2) Care of contact lens and prostheses: the patient will be asked to remove contact lens and prostheses, and should bring containers for their safe keeping.

II. Patient Instruction: Plaque Control

A. Toothbrushing

1. *Brush:* soft, nylon type.
2. *Technique:* For a patient who may not have practiced careful brushing on a regular plan, a simple technique is preferred. Time for establishing habits may be limited until postoperative healing is complete. Use of disclosing agent for the patient's own evaluation is important.

B. Auxiliary Procedures

Interdental plaque removal and care of fixed and removable appliances are included in instruction (Chapters 23 and 24). The patient who will have multiple extractions for an immediate denture or other appliance, such as an obturator or other prosthesis following cleft palate, tumor, or other surgery, will need postoperative instruction for the specific care of the appliance.

III. Instrumentation

Scaling techniques are of primary importance. Frequently, polishing procedures are contraindicated because of the condition of the gingival tissues.

A. Scaling

1. *Problems*
   a. Teeth with large carious lesions.
   b. Mobile teeth.
   c. Edentulous areas.
   d. Sensitive, enlarged gingival tissue that bleeds readily.

2. *Suggestions for Technique*
   a. Use topical or local anesthetic.
   b. Maintain a clear field, using evacuation techniques.
   c. Use alternate finger rests to adapt to mobile teeth or edentulous areas; stabilize mobile teeth during scaling strokes.
   d. Ultrasonic scaling techniques may be particularly appropriate when there are gross deposits, provided an iodophore mouthrinse is used first to lessen the bacterial count of the aerosols produced.

B. Polishing

1. *Contraindications*
   a. Enlarged, inflamed, sensitive gingiva.
   b. Deep pockets.
   c. Profuse hemorrhage.

2. *Effects* (page 564)
   a. Irritation to tissue by polishing abrasive and action of rubber polishing cup.
   b. Movement of rubber cup forces abrasive particles into the gingival tissues.

C. Rinsing Instruction

1. *Objectives:* to promote tissue healing following scaling and to remove debris; to initiate the habit of rinsing for postoperative care later.

2. *Rinsing Solution:* warm mild hypertonic salt solution (page 599).

3. *Frequency:* recommended for several times each day; after surgery as instructed by oral surgeon.

D. Follow-up Evaluation

Scaling and planing should be planned for a few weeks after oral surgery. Such an appointment should not be scheduled until healing has progressed favorably.

IV. Patient Instruction: Diet Selection[3]

The nutritional state can influence the resistance to infection and wound healing, as well as the general recovery powers. Specific recommendations of what to include and not to include in the diet should be given to the patient.

Postoperative suggestions may differ from preoperative; for example, when difficulty in chewing is a postoperative problem, a liquid or soft diet may be required. When major oral surgery requires hospitalization, tube feeding may be necessary during the initial healing period. Tube feeding is described on page 668.

A. Nutritional and Dietary Needs

Diets outlined are designed to include the essential foods from the Four Food Groups (table 28–1, page 424).

1. *Essential for Promotion of Healing:* protein and vitamins, particularly vitamin A, vitamin C, and riboflavin.

2. *Essential for Building Gingival Tissue Resistance:* a varied diet that includes adequate portions of all essential food groups.

3. *Essential for Providing Gingival Stimulation:* firm, fibrous foods that require mastication, especially fresh fruits and vegetables. Possibilities for making recommendations in this area are limited by the patient's masticatory deficiencies.

4. *Essential For Dental Caries Prevention:* foods without fermentable carbohydrate. When a patient has not been able to masticate properly, the diet employed frequently may have included many soft cariogenic foods.

B. Suggestions for Instruction

1. Provide instruction sheets that show specific meal plans for pre- and postsurgery. Foods for liquid and soft diets are listed on pages 668–669.

2. Express nutritional needs in terms of quantity or servings of foods so that the patient clearly understands.

3. For the patient who will receive dentures, careful instruction must be provided over a period of time. At the preoperative appointment only an introduction can be given, particularly

because the patient is probably more concerned about the operation than about the after effects.

When the patient will lose the teeth because of dental caries, the diet has likely been high in fermentable carbohydrates. Emphasis should be placed on helping the patient include nutritious foods for the general health of the body and more specifically the health of the alveolar processes that will support the dentures.

V. Postoperative Care

A. Immediate Instructions

Basic instructions following tooth extraction and other dental operations: printed or mimeographed postoperative instructions should be given to each patient after the prepared material is reviewed with the patient after surgery. Specific details will vary, but basic information for postoperative instruction sheets includes the following:

1. *Control Bleeding.* Keep the sponge in the mouth over the surgical area for one-half hour, then discard it. When bleeding persists at home, place a gauze pad or cold wet teabag over the area and bite firmly for 30 minutes.
2. *Rinsing.* Do not rinse for 24 hours after the surgery. Then use warm salt water (about one-half teaspoonful salt in an 8-ounce glass of warm water), after toothbrushing and every 2 hours.
3. *Plaque Control.* Brush the teeth as usual; use dental floss.
4. *Rest.* Get plenty of rest: at least 8 to 10 hours sleep each night. Avoid strenuous exercise during the first 24 hours, and keep the mouth from excessive movement.
5. *Diet.* Use a liquid or soft solid diet high in protein. Drink water and fruit juices freely. Avoid foods that require excessive chewing.
6. *Pain.* If needed, use pain-relieving preparation prescribed by the dentist.
7. *Icepack.* Following a flap operation or when there is swelling, apply icepack (ice cubes in a plastic bag) for 30 minutes followed by 30 minutes off, or apply for

15 minutes after 30 minutes off, as directed by the dentist. Heat is not used for swelling.
8. *Complications.* Instructions should include the telephone number to call after office hours, should complications arise; complications may include uncontrollable pain, marked bleeding, temperature rise, difficulty in opening the mouth, or unusual swelling a few days after the surgery.

B. Follow-up Care

The dental hygienist may participate in suture removal, irrigation of sockets, and other postoperative procedures when the patient returns. Appropriately, instruction concerning plaque control, rinsing, oral irrigation, and other personal care as well as diet supervision can be continued.

PATIENT WITH A FRACTURED JAW

The limited access for personal oral care procedures and the effect of the liquid diet required for most cases define the need for special dental hygiene care for the patient with a fractured jaw. Attention to rehabilitation of the oral tissues during the period following the removal of appliances takes on particular significance lest permanent tissue damage result or inadequate oral care habits be continued indefinitely.

The patient with a fractured jaw may be hospitalized. A dental hygienist employed in a hospital would be called upon to assume a part of the responsibility for patient care or to give oral hygiene instruction to direct care personnel. After dismissal from the hospital, the patient may require special attention in the private dental office for a long period of time.

Treatment of a fractured jaw may be very complex, and the patient may suffer considerably, both physically and mentally. Some basic knowledge of the nature of fractures and their treatment is helpful in understanding the patient's needs.

I. Causes

A. Traumatic

From automobile, bicycle, and sports injuries, industrial accidents, and physical violence (blows, fistfights).

B. Predisposing

Pathologic conditions such as tumors, cysts, osteoporosis, or osteomyelitis weaken the bone, thus slight trauma or even tooth removal can cause fracture.

II. Emergency Care

Immediate attention must be paid to measures for care of the patient's general condition. Emergency care is given for airway, breathing, and circulation ("A B C," page 838). Hemorrhage, shock, and skull or internal head injuries are next in the sequence of concern.

Almost any category of emergency care may be required (table 58–1, page 845). Although treatment for the fractured jaw must not be postponed for any great length of time, its immediate care takes second place in the light of the vital aspects of patient care.

Tetanus prophylaxis may be indicated as soon as medical treatment is available.

III. Recognition

A. History

Except for a pathologic fracture, a history of trauma would be available.

B. Clinical Signs

The patient has pain, especially on movement, and tenderness on slight pressure over the area of the fracture. Teeth may be displaced, fractured, or show mobility. Because of muscle pull or contraction, segments of the bones may be displaced, and the occlusion of the teeth irregular.

Muscle spasm is a common finding, particularly when the fracture is at the angle or ramus of the mandible. Crepitation can be heard if the parts of bone are moved.

The soft tissue in the area of the fracture may show laceration and bleeding, discoloration (ecchymosis), and enlargement.

IV. Types

A fracture is classified by using a combination of descriptive words for its location, direction, nature, and severity. Fractures may be single or multiple, bilateral or unilateral, complete or incomplete.

A. Classification by Nature of the Fracture (figure 48–1)

1. *Simple:* has no communication with outside.
2. *Compound:* has communication with outside.
3. *Comminuted:* shattered.
4. *Incomplete:* "greenstick" fracture has one side of a bone broken and the other side bent. It occurs in incompletely calcified bones (young children, usually). The fibers tend to bend rather than break.

B. Mandibular (described by location)

1. Alveolar process
2. Condyle
3. Angle
4. Body
5. Symphysis

C. Maxillary

1. *Alveolar Process.* The alveolar process fracture does not extend to the midline of the palate.
2. *Le Fort I.*[4] The Le Fort classification is used widely to identify the three general levels of maxillary fractures as shown in figure 48–2.

   Le Fort I is a horizontal fracture line above the roots of the teeth, above the palate, across the maxillary sinus, below the zygomatic process, and across the pterygoid plates.
3. *Le Fort II.* The midface fracture extends over the middle of the nose, down the medial wall of the orbits, across the infraorbital rims, and posteriorly, across the pterygoid plates.
4. *Le Fort III.* The high level craniofacial fracture extends transversely across the bridge of the nose, across the orbits and the zygomatic arches, and across the pterygoid plates.

TREATMENT OF FRACTURES[5,6,7]

Each fracture differs from the next, and the methods used in treatment vary with the individual case. Many factors are involved when the

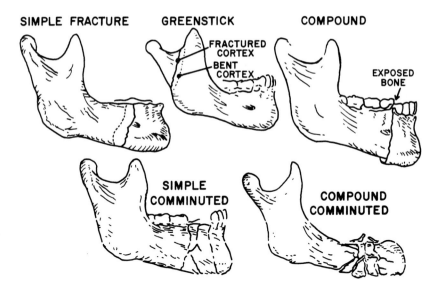

Figure 48–1. Types of fractures. (From Kruger, G.O.: Textbook of Oral and Maxillofacial Surgery, 5th ed. St. Louis, The C.V. Mosby Co., 1979.)

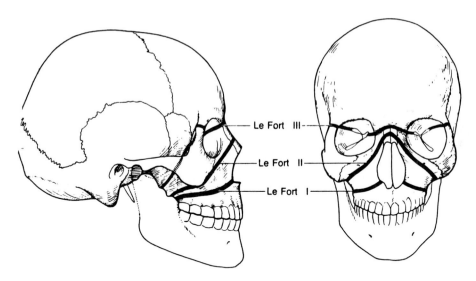

Figure 48–2. Le Fort classification of fractures of the maxilla. Le Fort I, horizontal fracture above the roots of the teeth, below the zygomatic process, and across the pterygoid plates; Le Fort II, midface fracture over the middle of the nose and across infraorbital rims; Le Fort III, transversely across bridge of nose, across the orbits and the zygomatic bone. (From Archer, W.H.: Oral and Maxillofacial Surgery, 5th ed. Philadelphia, W.B. Saunders Co., 1975: From Committee on Trauma, Amer. Coll. of Surgeons: Early Care of the Injured Patient. Philadelphia, W.B. Saunders Co., 1972.)

oral surgeon selects the methods to be used, particularly the location of the fracture or fractures, the presence or absence of teeth, existing injuries to the teeth, other head injuries, and the general health and condition of the patient.

Treatment of a fracture consists of *reduction* of the fracture, *fixation* of the fragments, and *immobilization* of the jaw. A temporary remov-able splint may be necessary when a patient must be transported to another location for specialized treatment. An accident or war casualty may occur many miles from a professional treatment facility.

I. Reduction

Reduction means the positioning of the parts

on either side of the fracture so they are in apposition for healing and restoration of function. The closure of the teeth is the guide for position in the dentulous patient.

A. Closed Reduction

1. Manual manipulation of the parts.
2. Elastic traction. The most common traction is applied with elastic bands hooked to arch bars which are also part of the method for fixation. The method is described below under the topic intermaxillary fixation.

B. Open Reduction

The bone fracture ends are exposed surgically by a flap procedure and the two ends are brought together. They are then fixed as described below under transosseous wires or bone plate.

II. Fixation

The fracture is first reduced or positioned, and then fixed or stabilized in that position. Fractures take several weeks to heal, and fixation apparatus is left in place long enough to assure union of the bony parts.

A. Transosseous Wires or Metal Plate

When the bony parts are reduced by open reduction, they are fastened together by either a wire suture threaded through holes drilled on either side of the fracture line (figure 48–3), or by a metal plate. The metal plate is designed to cross over the fracture

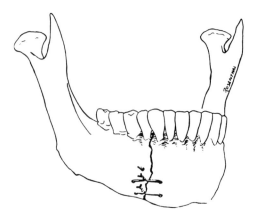

Figure 48–3. Open reduction for a mandibular fracture. Transosseous wiring is shown to hold bony parts in position for healing at the fracture line. (From Waite, D.E.: Practical Oral Surgery, 2nd ed. Philadelphia, Lea & Febiger, 1978.)

line and is held in place by screws on either side.

B. Intermaxillary Fixation

Intermaxillary fixation is fixation obtained by applying wires or elastic bands between the maxillary and mandibular arches. This is sufficient treatment for many fractures. More complicated types of fractures may require additional or supplemental types of therapy.

Ready-made, contoured, metal arch bars are available, or wires may be custom made with loops on which to hook wires or elastics to connect the mandible and maxilla in occlusion. The arch bars are adapted carefully to fit accurately to each tooth, and then wired into place so that the hooks project up in the maxilla and down in the mandible.

Elastics are positioned to provide a steady, gradual pull to aid in reducing the fracture (figure 48–4). A small horizontal elastic may be positioned across the fracture line to reduce the lateral displacement (figure 48–4D).

C. External Skeletal Fixation

1. *Indications.* Management of a fracture cannot always be accomplished satisfactorily by intermaxillary wiring alone. The following are situations in which external skeletal fixation is usually indicated.
   a. Insufficient number of teeth in good condition for intermaxillary fixation.
   b. Supplementary to intermaxillary fixation when there are no teeth in the fractured portion of the mandible.
   c. Loss of bone substance. When bone substance is lost because of an accident, a gunshot wound, or a pathologic condition, a bone graft may be indicated. The extraoral fixation is used first to hold the fractured parts in a normal relationship, and then to immobilize the area during healing following the bone graft surgery.
   d. Patients unable to have the jaws closed for a long period
      (1) Patient with a vomiting problem, such as during pregnancy.

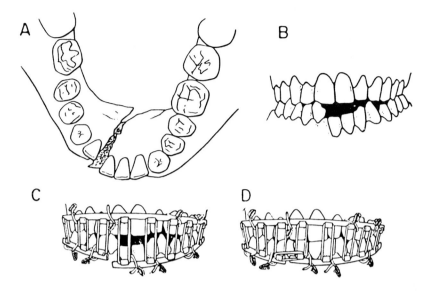

Figure 48–4. Intermaxillary fixation. **A.** Location of fracture of the mandible, **B.** Segments of bone on either side of the fracture are displaced, usually related to muscle pull or contraction, **C.** Metal arch bars wired in place with elastics positioned to provide a steady pull for fracture reduction, **D.** Note small horizontal elastic extending from the hook at the mandibular right central incisor to the mandibular right canine to reduce the lateral displacement. (From Archer, W.H.: Oral and Maxillofacial Surgery, 5th ed. Philadelphia, W.B. Saunders Co., 1975.)

     (2) Patient with a mental or physical disability such as cerebral palsy, epilepsy, or mental retardation.

  e. Edentulous mandible when the fracture fragments are greatly displaced, when the fracture is at the angle of the mandible, or when the mandible is atrophic or thinned.

  2. *Description.* Two special bone screws are placed via skin incisions on either side

of the fracture. An acrylic bar is molded, and while still pliable, is pressed over the threads of the bone screws and locked into position with the screw nuts (figure 48–5).

III. Edentulous Patient

    The use of external skeletal fixation for an edentulous mandible was described above. Other procedures are included here.

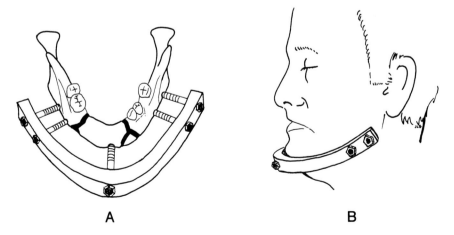

Figure 48–5. External skeletal fixation. **A.** Precision bone screws placed on either side of the fractures shown in heavy black lines, **B.** Acrylic bar molded, positioned over the bone screws, and locked into position with nuts.

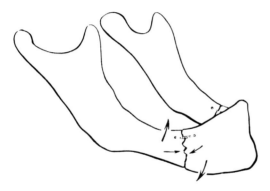

Figure 48–6. Edentulous mandible to show use of open reduction with transosseous wiring. (From Archer, W.H.: Oral and Maxillofacial Surgery, 5th ed. Philadelphia, W.B. Saunders Co., 1975: From Dingman, R.A. and Natvig, P.: Surgery of Facial Fractures, Philadelphia, W.B. Saunders Co., 1964.)

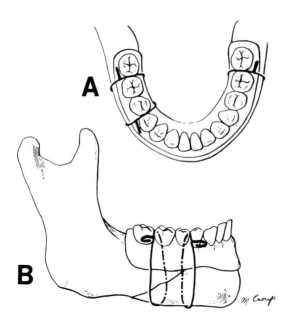

Figure 48–7. Use of patient's denture to splint a mandibular fracture. **A.** Wires are placed around the denture and the dental arch and twisted together to stabilize the reduction, **B.** Note line of fracture with the denture positioned to cover it. (From Archer, W.H.: Oral and Maxillofacial Surgery, 5th ed. Philadelphia, W.B. Saunders Co., 1975.)

A. Open Reduction Using Transosseous Wiring

Transosseous wiring for an edentulous mandible is similar to that described for the dentulous mandible in II.A. above. The bony parts are brought together and held in place by wire sutures (figure 48–6).

B. Circumferential Wiring

The patient's denture is used for a splint. If the denture was broken when the mandible was fractured, it may be repaired immediately or a temporary edentulous splint may be fabricated. Wires are placed around the denture and the arch together by threading the wire, using surgical procedures (figure 48–7). The line of fracture must be under the denture-covered area, or additional procedures are needed for the uncovered portion.

Since considerable trauma may be associated with the fracture, there may be swelling which prevents denture placement. In addition, the insertion of circumferential wires may cause more trauma to the soft tissues. An external skeletal fixation may be a preferred treatment.

C. Intermaxillary Fixation

The mandibular denture may be wired to the maxillary complete denture for additional mobilization. Mandibular anterior teeth may be cut away in order that the patient may feed by straw or glass feeding tube.

IV. Maxillary Fracture

Maxillary fractures are more difficult to handle because of the number of bones, the associated anatomy, and the complications of basal skull fractures.

A. Intermaxillary Fixation

Whether the fracture is Le Fort I, II, or III (figure 48–2), intermaxillary fixation is completed first to establish the occlusal relationship (figure 48–4). The next step is to accomplish craniomaxillary immobilization.

B. Craniomaxillary Immobilization

A rigid craniomaxillary fixation is necessary. A variety of methods has been used, some internal and others external.
1. *Cranial Suspension to the Nearest Superior Unfractured Bone.* Pins are used to provide a connection for the attachment of wires from a stable bone, such as the supraorbital area, to the mandibular arch bar.

2. *Head Cap.* A plaster headcap can provide a means for extraoral traction. This method is no longer frequently used.

3. *Internal Suspension Wires.* A maxilla with a Le Fort I fracture may be suspended by internal wires over the zygoma. In the oral cavity, the wires are connected to the mandibular arch bar. When the zygoma is also fractured, another method must be selected.

V. Alveolar Process Fracture

The most common fracture of all is of the alveolar process, maxillary or mandibular.

A. Clinical Appearance

Lacerations of lips and gingiva, mobility, fracture or displacement of teeth, swelling, bruising, and hemorrhage are usual signs.

B. Treatment[8]

1. Reimplantation of displaced teeth.
2. Immobilization with interdental wiring. A temporary fixed splint of acrylic may be placed over the wires. The teeth must be tested periodically for vitality.
3. Endodontic therapy may be required later.

VI. Healing

Union is affected by the location and character of the fracture. Much depends on the patient's general health and resistance and cooperation. Six weeks is considered the average for the uncomplicated mandibular case and 4 to 6 weeks for the maxillary. The major cause of complication is infection.

DENTAL HYGIENE CARE

I. Problems

Fixation apparatus, however carefully placed to prevent tissue irritation, interferes with normal function. The length of time the appliances must be in place is sufficient for considerable disturbance of tissue metabolism. Identification of possible effects of treatment provides the basis for planning dental hygiene care.

A. Development of Gingivitis or Periodontal Complications

1. Thick plaque formation and food debris

accumulation provide sources of irritation to the gingiva.

2. Lack of normal stimulation to the circulation of the periodontium and cleansing effects usually provided by the action of the tongue, lips, and facial muscles, contribute to stagnation of saliva and bacterial plaque accumulation.

3. Tender, sensitive gingiva makes plaque control more difficult even on available surfaces.

B. Dental Caries Initiation

It is difficult to plan an interesting soft or liquid diet using limited cariogenic foods for dental caries prevention.

C. Loss of Appetite

Loss of appetite related to monotonous liquid or soft diet leads to weight loss and lowered physical resistance. Secondary infections, including those of the oral tissues, may result.

D. Difficulty in Opening the Mouth

1. When there has been injury to the temporomandibular joint, the patient wearing fixation appliances that involve only the mandible has difficulty in applying a toothbrush to the lingual surfaces of teeth.

2. After removal of appliances, all patients have a degree of muscular trismus which hinders toothbrushing and mastication.

II. Instrumentation

A. Preoperative

Gross calculus is removed insofar as possible before wiring or the placement of metal or acrylic splints. Trauma to surrounding soft tissues of lip, tongue, and cheeks, limits accessibility.

B. During Treatment

Periodic scaling in conjunction with plaque control contributes to oral health. Although access is only from the facial for a patient with intermaxillary wiring, some benefit can be obtained. It is essential to have an assistant to provide continual suction during treatment.

C. After Removal of Appliances

A few weeks after removal of appliances, when the patient can open the mouth normally and plaque control procedures have been initiated, complete scaling and planing can be performed.

III. Diet

Many patients with fractured jaws tend to lose weight, which is generally related to an inadequate nutrient and caloric intake. Objectives in planning the diet are to help the patient maintain an adequate nutritional state, to promote healing, and to increase resistance to infection.

Attention must be given to the patient's willingness and ability to follow the recommendations made. The patient may be in the hospital for a few days to a few weeks depending on the severity of other injuries. A greater length of time is spent as an outpatient, when the diet is much more difficult to supervise. It has been suggested that the patient's understanding of dietary instructions and what is expected appears to be much more significant than the actual type of diet recommended.

A. Nutritional Needs

After any surgery, the diet must be planned to promote tissue building and repair.[3]

1. All essential food elements.
2. Emphasis on protein, vitamins, particularly A and C, and minerals, particularly calcium and phosphorus.
3. Usual caloric requirements for patient's age, taking into consideration lack of physical exercise and loss of appetite while ill.

B. Methods of Feeding

1. *Plastic Straw.* Liquid is sucked through the teeth or through an edentulous area. Straw can be bent to acccommodate a patient who can not sit up.
2. *Spoon Feeding.* When a patient's arms are not functional, direct assistance will be needed. The mouth may have injuries that prevent sucking food through a straw.

3. *Tube Feeding.*[9] Tube feeding may be indicated following various types of extensive oral surgery, facial trauma, burns, immobilized fractured jaw, and other conditions that prevent taking sufficient caloric and nutritional ingestion of food by way of the mouth.

A nasogastric tube is used (figure 48–8). Blenderized food can be prepared or special tube formulas are available commercially. When commercial preparations are used, contents may be selected to meet specific nutritional and caloric requirements of an individual patient.

C. Liquid Diet

1. *Indications*
   a. All patients with jaws wired together.
   b. All patients with no appliance or single jaw appliance who have difficulty in opening mouth due to condition such as temporomandibular joint involvement, or tongue or lip injury that will hinder insertion of food or manipulation of food in the mouth.
2. *Examples of Foods:* fruit juices; milk; eggnog; meat juices and soups; cooked thin cereals; canned baby foods. Strained

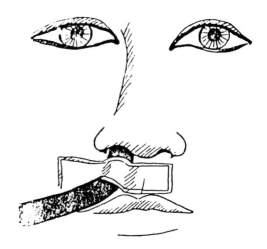

Figure 48–8. Nasogastric tube in position for feeding. To prevent injury to the nasopharyngeal passages, the tube is taped securely between the upper lip and the nares. (From Lewis, C.M.: Nursing Considerations in Tube-Fed Patients. Philadelphia, F.A. Davis Co., 1976.)

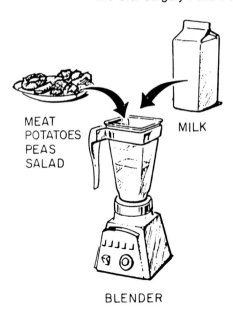

MEAT
POTATOES
PEAS
SALAD

MILK

BLENDER

Figure 48–9. Food blender for preparation of liquid diet. Regular table foods can be blenderized with milk or other nutritious liquid. (From Schultz, R.C.: Facial Injuries, 2nd ed. Copyright © 1977 by Yearbook Medical Publishers, Inc., Chicago.)

vegetables and meats (baby foods) may be added to meat juices and soups.

3. *Use of a Blender.* Regular table foods can be mixed in a food blender. With liquid such as clear soup or milk added, a fluid consistency can be obtained that will pass through a straw (figure 48–9).

D. Soft Solids Diet

1. *Indications*
   a. Patient with no appliance or with single jaw appliance without complications in opening the mouth or in movement of the lips and tongue.
   b. Patient who has been maintained on liquid diet throughout treatment period: after appliances are removed, the soft diet is recommended for several days to a week to provide the stomach with foods that are readily digestible rather than making drastic change to regular diet. A soft solids diet can also aid by protecting tender oral tissues from rough textures of regular diet until tissues have a chance to respond to softer foods and regular plaque control routine.

2. *Examples of Foods:* soft poached, scrambled, or boiled eggs; cooked cereals; mashed soft cooked vegetables, including potato; mashed fresh or canned fruits; soft, finely divided meats; custards; plain ice cream.

E. Hints for Diet Planning With the Nonhospitalized Patient

1. Provide instruction sheets that show specific meal plans.
2. Express nutritional needs in quantities or servings of foods.
3. Show methods of varying the diet. A liquid or soft diet is at best monotonous because of sameness of texture.
4. Suggest limitation of cariogenic foods as an aid to prevention of dental caries.

IV. Personal Oral Care Procedures

Every attempt to keep the patient's mouth as clean as possible for comfort and sanitation, and as plaque-free as possible for disease prevention should be made. The extent of possible care depends on the appliances, the condition of the lips, tongue, and other oral tissues, and the cooperation of the patient.

Encouragement must be given to the patient to begin toothbrushing as soon as possible after the surgery, but until the patient is able, a plan for care is outlined for an attendant.

A. Irrigation

1. *Indications:* during first few days after surgery while mouth may be too tender for brushing, frequent irrigations are required; irrigation also serves as an adjunct to toothbrushing.
2. *Method:* spray bottle and suction tube. Power spray at least once each day aids in removing microorganisms and debris that have accumulated interproximally.
3. *Mouthrinse Selection.* The oral surgeon should be consulted for specific instructions.
   a. Physiologic saline
   b. Sodium bicarbonate
   c. Fluoride rinse after toothbrushing to aid caries prevention.

B. Early Mouth Cleansing

Before a toothbrush can be used effectively, it may be necessary to use a pre-moistened swab or toothette to clean and lubricate the lips, mucosa, and gingiva. Because plaque removal should be attempted as soon as possible, a very soft toothbrush with suction can be applied. The toothbrush with suction is described on pages 718–719.

C. Personal Care by the Patient

As soon as possible, the patient is instructed in personal care. A toothbrushing method and other aids such as are used for orthodontic appliances are recommended and demonstrated (pages 382–384).

The patient must be shown why care must be taken not to entangle the toothbrush filaments with the wires. When the tongue is not injured, the patient can be instructed to use the tongue as an aid in cleaning the lingual surfaces of the teeth and massaging the gingiva.

The ambulatory patient can use a water irrigator. Specific instructions must be provided, showing the patient how to lower the head over a sink. A low pressure setting is used and the spray carefully directed to prevent tissue injury (pages 369–370).

D. After Appliances Are Removed

A step-by-step series of lessons is usually necessary before the patient can carry out adequate plaque control.

A method for daily self-applied fluoride, such as a mouthrinse or gel tray, should be introduced along with the use of a fluoride dentifrice. Decalcification and dental caries can result from plaque retention about the appliances.

DENTAL HYGIENE CARE PRIOR TO GENERAL SURGERY

Completing dental and dental hygiene treatment and bringing the oral cavity to a state of health has special significance for certain patients who will have surgery other than oral. When emergency surgery is performed, preparation of the mouth is not possible, and postoperative examination and care may be complicated by various limitations.

When surgery is elective, or planned well in advance, the patient can be encouraged to have complete dental and periodontal treatment.[10]

Protection against complications related to broken appliances or restorations, which may have been prevented, can be very meaningful to the hospitalized patient. Types of patients will be discussed briefly here. Other examples are to be found in the various special patient chapters throughout this book section.

I. Patient Whose Surgery Changes the Risk Status

Susceptibility to infection is greatly increased in certain patients, for example, those with prosthetic heart valves, prostheses for joint replacement, and transplanted organs.[11,12] Patients who receive chemotherapeutic agents as partial treatment after surgery for various types of cancer, and others who use immunosuppressant drugs, require special management to prevent complications during dental and dental hygiene appointments. Antibiotic premedication to prevent infective endocarditis and other infections is mandatory for certain patients (pages 99–100).

Prior to general surgery for prostheses, transplants, cancer, and other serious conditions, patients can be informed of the need for completing oral care treatments. A mouth in health, with preventive personal care, is much less a problem in the risk patient.

II. Preparation of the Mouth Prior to General Inhalation Anesthesia

Plaque control and professional instrumentation aid in reducing the oral bacterial count.[1] Since the mouth is the entrance to the respiratory chamber, there is always the possibility of the inhalation of debris and fluids from the mouth. This could occur during the administration of an anesthetic, or when the patient coughs.

III. Patient With Long Convalescence

Patients whose surgery will require a long convalescence will be unable to keep a regular recall appointment. When the patient has a healthy mouth before the hospitalization and convalescence, the problems of postoperative oral care are lessened, but not eliminated.

Instruction for the person who will provide direct care may be needed. A home visit by the dentist and dental hygienist may be required.

TECHNICAL HINTS

I. Written Consent

Surgery is not provided to minors without consent of parent or guardian. Written consent is mandatory.

II. Accident Prevention

Encourage patients to use the seat belts in their cars. Professional people should set the example by using their own seat belts.

III. Sources of Materials

What to Do After Extraction of a Tooth (G20)
American Dental Association,
Order Department
211 East Chicago Avenue
Chicago, Illinois 60611

Facial Trauma (P5)
Impacted Teeth (P3)
Nutrition Following Oral and Maxillofacial Surgery (P9)
American Association of Oral and
Maxillofacial Surgeons
211 East Chicago Avenue
Chicago, Illinois 60611

References

1. Whitacre, R.J., Robins, S.K., Williams, B.L., and Crawford, J.J.: *Dental Asepsis.* Seattle, Stoma Press, 1979, p. 50.
2. Atterbury, R.A.: Preoperative Guidelines for Oral Surgery Patients, *Dent. Surv.*, 52, 35, October, 1976.
3. Nizel, A.E.: *Nutrition in Preventive Dentistry: Science and Practice, 2nd ed.* Philadelphia, W.B. Saunders Co., 1980, pp. 507–521.
4. Hargis, H.W.: Early and Emergent Care of Maxillofacial Injuries, in Clark, J.W., ed.: *Clinical Dentistry, Volume 3*, Chapter 33. Hagerstown, Maryland, Harper & Row, 1981, pp. 6–8.
5. Archer, W.H.: *Oral and Maxillofacial Surgery,* 5th ed. Philadelphia, W.B. Saunders Co., 1975, pp. 1031–1363.
6. Cawson, R.A. and Rowe, N.L.: Fracture of the Jaws and Facial Skeleton, in Cawson, R.A.: *Essentials of Dental Surgery and Pathology,* 3rd ed. Edinburgh, Churchill Livingstone, 1978, pp. 252–273.
7. Kruger, G.O., ed.: *Textbook of Oral and Maxillofacial Surgery,* 5th ed. St. Louis, The C.V. Mosby Co., 1979, pp. 341–412.
8. Quinn, T.: Department of Oral Surgery, Tufts University School of Dental Medicine, Boston, Massachusetts, personal communication, July, 1980.
9. Shils, M.E. and Randall, H.T.: Diet and Nutrition in the Care of the Surgical Patient, in Goodhart, R.S. and Shils, M.E., eds.: *Modern Nutrition in Health and Dis-*

ease, 6th ed. Philadelphia, Lea & Febiger, 1980, pp. 1115–1118, 1312, 1327–1330.
10. Robinson, H.B.G.: Some Very Special Patients, *Dent. Surv.*, 54, 4, March, 1978.
11. Westbrook, S.D.: Dental Management of Patients Receiving Hemodialysis and Kidney Transplants, *J. Am. Dent. Assoc.*, 96, 464, March, 1978.
12. Mulligan, R.: Late Infections in Patients with Prostheses for Total Replacement of Joints: Implications for the Dental Practitioner, *J. Am. Dent. Assoc.*, 101, 44, July, 1980.

Suggested Readings

Bresner, M.: Nutrition for the Surgical Patient, *J. Oral Surg.*, 35, 200, March, 1977.
Byrne, J.E. and Byrne, L.R.: The Dietary Management of the Patient with a Fractured Jaw, *Oral Surg.*, 29, 666, May, 1970.
Jones, N.B.: Dietary Needs of the Oral Surgery Patient with Comparison of Dietary Supplements, *J. Oral Surg.*, 28, 892, December, 1970.
Krause, M.V. and Mahan, L.K.: *Food, Nutrition and Diet Therapy,* 6th ed. Philadelphia, W.B. Saunders Co., 1979, pp. 680–693.
Olson, R.E., Mincey, D.L., and Graber, T.M.: Orthosurgical Teamwork, *J. Am. Dent. Assoc.*, 90, 998, May, 1975.
Schultz, R.C.: *Facial Injuries.* Chicago, Year Book, 1970, pp. 202–206.
Simon, W.J.: Rationale for the Use of Cold Packs, *Quintessence Journal*, 1, 15, October, 1979.
Snyder, B.S.: Oral Surgery, in Steele, P.F., ed.: *Dental Specialties for the Dental Hygienist,* 2nd ed. Philadelphia, Lea & Febiger, 1978, pp. 173–198.

Fractured Jaw

Banks, P.: Fixation of Facial Fractures. Current Concepts, *Br. Dent. J.*, 138, 129, February 18, 1975.
Barclay, J.K.: Intermaxillary Fixation—A Safety Measure, *Br. J. Oral Surg.*, 17, 77, July, 1979.
Ciola, B.: Pathologic Fractures of the Mandible Following Invasive Oral Carcinomas, *Oral Surg.*, 46, 725, November, 1978.
Goracy, E. and Stratigos, G.T.: Successive Mandibular Fractures in the Alcoholic–Epileptic Patient, *Oral Surg.*, 32, 701, November, 1971.
Hale, M.L.: Fractures of the Jaws, in Waite, D.E.: *Textbook of Practical Oral Surgery,* 2nd ed. Philadelphia, Lea & Febiger, 1978, pp. 297–316.
Lanigan, D.T. and Stoelinga, P.J.W.: Fractures of the Supraorbital Rim, *J. Oral Surg.*, 38, 764, October, 1980.
Marciani, R.D. and Hill, O.J.: Treatment of the Fractured Edentulous Mandible, *J. Oral Surg.*, 37, 569, August, 1979.
Maw, R.B.: A New Look at Maxillomandibular Fixation of Mandibular Fractures, *J. Oral Surg.*, 39, 187, March, 1981.
Nash, E.S. and Addy, M.: The Use of Chlorhexidine Gluconate Mouthrinses in Patients with Inter-Maxillary Fixation, *Br. J. Oral Surg.*, 17, 251, March, 1980.
Souyris, F., Lamarche, J.P., and Mirfakhrai, A.M.: Treatment of Mandibular Fractures by Intraoral Placement of Bone Plates, *J. Oral Surg.*, 38, 33, January, 1980.
Vogl, W., Baker, G., and Chapnick, P.: Compound Mandibular Fracture Treatment (without Intermaxillary Fixation), *Can. Dent. Assoc. J.*, 46, 772, December, 1980.
Wagner, W.F., Neal, D.C., and Alpert, B.: Morbidity Associated with Extraoral Open Reduction of Mandibular Fractures, *J. Oral Surg.*, 37, 97, February, 1979.

49

The Patient With Oral Cancer

Care of the cancer patient before, during, and after therapy has as its main purposes attaining and maintaining oral health at the highest possible level and contributing to the patient's general and mental health. The patient may be under the care of a team of medical and dental specialists including the dentist, oral surgeon, dental hygienist, physician, radiation oncologist, registered nurse, and other paramedical auxiliaries. Special rehabilitation personnel, such as a plastic surgeon, speech therapist, psychiatrist, and maxillofacial prosthodontist, are frequently involved after the treatment phase.

DESCRIPTION

A *neoplasm* is an abnormal, uncontrolled new growth generally classified as benign or malignant. A *benign neoplasm* is slow-growing, does not invade, does not metastasize to other organs, and is not a threat to life. A *malignant neoplasm,* in contrast, is faster-growing, invades surrounding tissues, may metastasize to other parts of the body, and is life-threatening. The principal locations of oral neoplasms are shown in the diagram in figure 8–7 on page 121.

I. Incidence

Early recognition of suspicious lesions was described on pages 121–122. Since the patient suffers no pain or other symptoms from early cancer, detection is dependent on oral examination by a dentist and a dental hygienist during routine examinations. When discovered early, removal or other treatment can increase the cure rate at the local site, before invasion to adjacent tissues and lymph nodes of the neck. By the detection of early lesions, serious post-treatment sequelae can be prevented or minimized.

A. Number of Oral Cancers

Including the lips and salivary glands, there are approximately 19,100 new cancers of the oral cavity proper, and another 7700 of the oropharynx annually in the United States. Of those in the oral cavity, about 50 percent occur on the lip and tongue.[1] Males between ages 40 and 65 have the highest numbers of lip and tongue cancers.

B. Deaths

Cancer is the second ranking cause of death in the United States. Only diseases of the heart rank higher in adults, and accidents in children under 15 years of age. Approximately 9150 deaths result from cancers of the oral cavity proper and the oropharynx. Of the 4950 in the oral cavity, 2000 are from cancers of the tongue. Estimated annual deaths from lip cancer total 175, of which 150 are males and 25 females.[1] The fewer deaths from lip cancer can be attributed to the accessibility and visibility for early treatment.

673

II. Etiology and Predisposing Factors

Although the specific etiology of cancer is not known, extensive research is being conducted. There are a number of contributing factors to oral cancers. These are very important in the prevention, control, and particularly in early recognition by dentists and dental hygienists. Factors that are believed to contribute to the initiation and development of oral cancer in susceptible people are listed here.[2]

A. Long-term Exposure to the Sun's Rays

1. Squamous cell carcinoma of the lower lip has been related to overexposure. Occupations that require outdoor activity and work have been found in a high percentage of those with lip cancer.
2. Pigmentation appears to intervene, so that carcinoma of the lower lip is relatively rare in black people.

B. Heavy Smoking

1. Smoking increases the chances of developing oral cancer. Long term exposure to the chemical carcinogens of tobacco as well as trauma from the heat on the tissues are significant factors.
2. Holding chewing tobacco or snuff on an area of the oral mucosa will lead to tissue changes and premalignant lesions.
3. The risk of developing a second primary oral cancer is greatly increased by continued smoking.[3]

C. Chronic Alcoholism

Chronic alcoholism increases the tendency to develop cancer. Chronic alcoholics have more lesions of the tongue and floor of the mouth than of other locations in the oral cavity.

TYPES OF TREATMENT AND ORAL EFFECTS

I. Surgical Procedures

Small lesions may be removed by simple excision. Some are totally removed when a biopsy is used for diagnosis.

Radical neck dissection is a procedure that includes wide removal of tissues around a tumor. This is necessary when the oropharynx and neck are involved, in order to prevent the spread of the cancer to the lymph nodes.

II. Radiation[4,5]

Therapeutic radiation may be given as the only treatment or it may be used in conjunction with surgery.

A. Objectives

1. *Given as a Total Treatment.* Exposures are usually made in fractions, as daily doses.
2. *Given in Conjunction with Surgery*
   a. Preoperative: to reduce the size of the neoplasm as an aid to surgery by limiting the surgical area.
   b. Postoperatively: to control residual disease.

B. Types

1. *External*
   a. Orthovoltage. Low-yield radiation may be used for superficial lesions. It has high skin and bone absorption factors, and is not used currently as much as it was before megavoltage radiation was developed.
   b. Mega- or supervoltage. High-yield radiation includes cobalt-60. It has a sparing effect on skin and bone and less scatter radiation to surrounding tissues than orthovoltage.
2. *Internal.* The source of radiation is placed within the body. There is less radiation to surrounding tissues than when an external source is utilized. Radium needles and radon and gold seeds which are radioactive are used.

C. Effects of Radiation Therapy

Irradiation is the exposure of tissues to x-rays or other forms of radiation. The purpose is to destroy cancerous cells. Damage to surrounding normal tissue cannot be avoided, but the severity of damage can be minimized.

Ionizing radiation induces tissue changes, some of which are apparent during the treatment period and may continue for a few weeks or months after cessation of irradiation. Other changes may not be evident until after treatment and may have long-term significance.

Principal effects are on the mucosa, salivary glands, bones, teeth, and taste sensations. Early changes result from damage to the epithelium and include dermatitis, mucositis, alopecia, and at first, an increased salivary flow. Later changes include atrophy of the salivary glands with diminished salivary flow and diminished bone vascularity.

1. *Mucosa*
   a. Mucositis. Inflammation of the mucosa may appear as early as one week after radiation therapy is started. An unpleasant odor usually is present.
      (1) Cellular changes. Initially, there is an inflammatory response with edema. The tissues may become ulcerated and necrotic with sloughing. Later fibrosis develops.
      (2) Clinical signs. Sensitivity to temperature extremes and pressure, an unpleasant odor from the necrotic tissue and plaque collection are commonly found. The patient with dentures may not be able to tolerate wearing them.
      (3) Recovery. The severe signs will heal and disappear within a few weeks after radiation is stopped, but the epithelium never completely recovers and tends to be thin and more fragile than normal.
   b. Effects on patient. Toothbrushing and other personal care may be neglected because of the sensitivity of the tissues. A flavored dentifrice may not be tolerated. A soft diet may be required.
2. *Salivary Glands.* Radiation to the salivary glands may be unavoidable, depending on the location of the cancerous lesion. The radiation primarily affects the serous gland cells with a lessening of secretion.
   a. Xerostomia. A reduced quantity of saliva may be noticed as early as the third or fourth day after the beginning of radiation.

   b. Saliva is thickened and sticky, which makes swallowing difficult.
   c. Dry mucosa may be prone to cracks and bleeding.
   d. Effects on patient
      (1) Difficulty in speaking and swallowing.
      (2) Difficulty in wearing prostheses.
      (3) Increased dental caries.
3. *Bone.* Radiation damages bone cells and blood vessels within the bone. Changes in the endothelial cells lead to sclerosis of the vessels. The result is change in the growth potential of the bone and lowered resistance to infection.
   a. The lowered resistance to infection predisposes the bone to infection that may reach the bone through an ulcer in the mucosa, deep periodontal pocket, periapical lesion, open socket from tooth extraction, or other potential channel for microorganisms. Such infection may develop many years after radiation because the bone changes are not reversible. Osteoradionecrosis occurs more frequently in the mandible because of the limitation of the blood supply.
   b. Symptoms. Osteoradionecrosis is characterized by pain, trismus, exposed bone, sequestration, and pathologic fracture. The infection can be suppurative, and halitosis is usually present. Treatment is difficult and may involve extended antibiotic therapy and surgery for the removal of the sequestra, or even part of the mandible.
   c. Prevention. Correct pre- and postradiation procedures have had a definite effect on lowering the incidence of osteoradionecrosis. Maintenance of oral cleanliness and health are contributing preventive factors.
4. *Teeth*
   a. "Radiation caries"
      (1) Description. Teeth with exposed root surfaces are especially susceptible. The lesions develop in the cervical thirds and gradually encircle the necks of the teeth.

They appear black or dark brown.

(2) Predisposing factors. Xerostomia, neglect of plaque control measures, soft cariogenic diet, sore mouth, and changes in oral flora are responsible, not radiation directly.

(3) Prevention. Intensified preventive measures for fluoride application and plaque control are needed. The use of a saliva substitute containing fluoride is also indicated (page 680).

b. Tooth development. Radiation in children can affect the odontogenic cells. A tooth bud may be completely destroyed if irradiated before calcification has started.

c. Sensitivity of teeth. The teeth with marked dental caries are particularly sensitive, but all teeth may react to temperature extremes.

5. *Taste.* Taste can be altered by degeneration of taste buds or by changes in the saliva quantity.

6. *Loss of Appetite.* Because of sore mouth, loss of taste sensation, diminished saliva, and related symptoms, interest in eating fades, and there is a loss of appetite followed by weight loss. Denture wearers who cannot wear their dentures have an added eating problem.

7. *Trismus.* Trismus is spasm of the muscles of mastication. It can result from fibrosis in the muscle fibers that were irradiated. It may occur 3 to 6 months after therapy has stopped, and it makes opening of the mouth very difficult. Exercises and stretching appliances have been used for treatment.

III. Chemotherapy[6,7]

A. Objectives

Chemotherapeutic drugs are used in the control of widely scattered neoplasms and to supplement treatment by surgery and/or radiation. The objective is to destroy or deactivate the cancer cells with as little destruction of normal cells as possible. Side effects from the drugs are significant, and frequently involve the oral tissues.

B. Types of Chemotherapeutic Agents[6]

There are four major groups of chemotherapeutic drugs and others that are occasionally used or are in an experimental category. The drugs may be used singly, but more commonly are used in combinations. The types of drugs are alkylating agents, antimetabolites, antibiotics, and plant alkaloids. Others include hormones, steroids, and enzymes.

C. Side Effects of Chemotherapy

Rapidly proliferating normal cells are susceptible to the suppressive action of chemotherapeutic agents. These include hair, bone marrow, and oral and intestinal mucosal epithelial cells. The drugs are *immunosuppressive* by inhibiting antibody responses and inducing leukopenia. They are *myelosuppressive* by depressing bone marrow activity, which results in leukopenia and thrombocytopenia.

D. Oral Complications

Whether or not chemotherapeutic drugs are administered for malignancies of the head and neck or elsewhere in the body, oral effects are common. Nearly 40 percent of adult and 90 percent of child patients with malignancies not of the head and neck were shown to have oral problems.[8] In that study, ulceration was the most common complication.

Loss of appetite, nausea, vomiting, and diarrhea are frequent side effects of chemotherapy. When there are oral lesions, and the mouth is sore, eating can be difficult. Oral lesions may become so severe that the patient's health and nutritional state are affected. Chemotherapy may have to be stopped, which changes the degree of success that can be expected from the treatment as well as the patient's chances of survival.[7]

Principal oral effects may be grouped as cytotoxic, hemorrhagic, and infectious, in addition to the nutritional problems mentioned above.[6,7,9] Different effects are produced by the various drugs used.

1. *Cytotoxic.* Toxic effects to the oral mucosal cells result in ulcerations and loss of surface characteristics. There is a greater incidence in younger patients. Loss of nutritional elements may complicate the problem. Fewer oral lesions develop when plaque is under control and the tissues present with signs of health.[10]

2. *Hemorrhagic.* Bone marrow suppression leads to thrombocytopenia, and clinically, there may be petechiae and spontaneous gingival bleeding. The frequency and severity of bleeding are directly related to whether the patient already has mucositis and/or periodontitis, and also has received radiation therapy. The state of health of the gingiva is highly significant.

3. *Infectious.* As a result of immunosuppression and myelosuppression, chronic infections may increase in severity and become acute. Changes occur in the oral microflora, with a shift to predominantly gram negative microorganisms and fungi. Candidiasis is the most frequent fungal infection. Viral infections are relatively infrequent except for herpes simplex. Necrotizing ulcerative gingivitis may occur in the neglected mouth.[9]

PERSONAL FACTORS[11,12,13]

Patient attitudes and feelings are similar to those of any patient with a major chronic disease or disability. As with other diseases with limited hope for cure, strong feelings of hopelessness and despair predominate.

The course of the illness of cancer patients and their survival rates are well known. The very word *cancer* brings fear and anxiety to the patient who knows the diagnosis and of what the treatment will consist. The concerns of a patient may differ at different stages of treatment.

I. Patient Problems

A. Early Fears and Anxieties

1. Imminent surgery, radiation, or other treatment.
2. Disfigurement, changes in appearance, and pain.
3. Extended hospitalization.
4. Financial stress.
5. Outcome of the treatment.

B. During and Following Therapy

1. Preoccupation with details of examinations, treatments, symptoms, or medications.
2. Depression and grief, which may lead to withdrawal and isolation.
3. Major concerns include obvious facial deformity, speech difficulty, swallowing difficulty, drooling, and odors from debris collection and tissue changes.

II. Suggestions for Approach to Patient

A. Provide explanations before and after therapy to prevent misconceptions and apprehensions, and attempt to allay fears.

B. Provide paper and pencil for patient with a speech difficulty to write questions and requests.

C. Show acceptance. Acknowledge the appropriateness of the patient's concerns.

D. Express empathy, but avoid oversolicitousness.

E. Help to direct thoughts and efforts toward restoration of function activity.

F. Instill trust and security by demonstrating genuine interest.

G. Assist the patient who was an alcoholic, smoked heavily, or had other habits that have to be eliminated. The patient may need the help of psychiatry, Alcoholics Anonymous, or other type of organization.

PREPARATION FOR TREATMENT

Time may be a factor for the patient with advanced malignancy. The aim in preparation of a patient for treatment for cancer is to restore the mouth to optimal health before the surgery, radiation, or chemotherapy. The extent and severity of the after effects of cancer therapy are related to the condition of the teeth and soft tissues before therapy.

Basic preparation follows the same general outline as described on page 658 for a patient with oral surgery. Objectives and treatment include steps to reduce the oral microbial count and provide a better environment for surgical procedures, as well as to improve the conditions for healing.

I. Oral Findings

Many patients with an oral cancer may not have sought dental treatment for many years. They may have neglected personal care that could have maintained oral cleanliness. Therefore, it is not unusual to find some or all of the following:

A. Broken-down teeth, some with exposed pulps.
B. Severe periodontal involvement.
C. Ill-fitting dentures.
D. Extremely poor oral hygiene.

II. Dental Treatment Plan

When the patient is to have therapy by radiation, particular attention must be paid to eliminating sources of infection in the oral cavity. It has been shown that when consideration is given to proper preparation for treatment and supervision of preventive measures during and after treatment, the incidence of harmful effects can be reduced.

Because of the effect of radiation on the bone and other tissues, dental procedures, such as tooth removal, periodontal surgery, and endodontic treatment, which could open a channel for infection to reach the bone, are contraindicated after therapy. Therefore, the objectives in dental and dental hygiene care prior to radiation are to reduce the incidence of complications of radiation, particularly osteoradionecrosis and postirradiation caries.

The patient's total treatment plan should include at least the following:

A. Removal of nonrestorable teeth. Extensively involved teeth may need extraction due to severity of bone loss, mobility, and other signs of advanced periodontal disease, large carious lesions with pulpal exposures not conducive to endodontic therapy, or periapical radiographic findings.

In the past, treatment frequently called for complete extraction of all teeth that would be in the pathway of radiation whether or not they were broken down or diseased. Now, only teeth that are definitely beyond salvaging are removed. There are patients with such badly broken-down teeth that all will have to be removed. When extractions are needed, trimming of the bone and careful surgical removal of all spicules is necessary. As long a healing period as possible should be allowed before starting radiation because, when bone is irradiated, healing and remodeling will stop.

B. Removal of residual root tips and other subsurface pathologic areas which are found in radiographs of edentulous areas.
C. Endodontic therapy for essential abutment teeth. Treatment planning for prosthetic replacements must be made in advance so that abutment teeth can receive proper treatment before radiation.
D. Periodontal therapy
    1. Complete scaling and planing with curettage as indicated.
    2. Surgical procedures when time permits follow-up for healing.
    3. Occlusal adjustment.
E. Restoration of carious lesions.
F. Complete preventive program for plaque control and fluoride therapy started at the first appointment.

DENTAL HYGIENE CARE

In the not too distant past, the patient with an oral cancer was doomed to complete tooth removal or at least removal of all teeth in the line of radiation. When the teeth were left in the mouth, inevitable severe radiation caries developed. A high percentage of patients had osteoradionecrosis. Now, many teeth are saved, restored, and preserved by an intensive daily preventive program of plaque control and self-applied fluoride by gel trays or brush-on.

The dental hygienist's contribution to the preparation of the patient for cancer therapy, and the continued supervision of oral health and preventive techniques, during treatment and regularly thereafter, has special significance. Plaque control, irrigation, rinsing, fluoride application, dietary factors for general health and dental caries prevention, along with specific instrumentation for the health of the periodontal tissues, are major areas of attention for the dental hygienist.

I. Patient Instruction

A. Plaque Control

A complete instruction series (pages

410–416) should be started prior to cancer treatment with careful supervision. The patient must understand the reasons for intensive oral health care. Scaling and planing can be accomplished within the same series of appointments as those for the series of lessons for plaque control. Time is usually an important factor when a malignant tumor is involved.

1. *Toothbrushing.* Sulcular brushing with a soft nylon brush is recommended for the following reasons:
   a. Radiation caries occurs primarily at the cervical third, about the necks of the teeth. Emphasis must be placed on keeping the cervical areas plaque-free.
   b. Control of gingival health with prevention of gingivitis is necessary. Fewer side effects develop from chemotherapy when optimum oral health is maintained.[10]
   c. Sensitivity of teeth is most frequently associated with the cervical third. Brushing with monofluorophosphate dentifrice can help alleviate sensitivity and prevent dental caries (page 556).
2. *Tongue Brushing.* Bacteria and debris collect on the dry tongue.
3. *Dental Floss.* Proximal surface plaque must be removed. Other interdental devices may be helpful.

B. Nutrition and Diet

Every possible attempt to improve the general health must be made. If the patient is malnourished and debilitated, a high protein diet is needed. Reduction of cariogenic foods is essential to the dental caries prevention program.

A hospitalized patient will be under the supervision of a physician who gives diet prescription orders to the hospital dietitian. The private or clinic physician may make specific recommendations to the patient. Within the framework of the physician's orders, the dental hygienist may also help the patient and the person who will prepare the patient's food at home. Instructions in the preparation of food in a blender may be needed.

Because the mouth may be sore and tender, a topical anesthetic in the form of a troche may be needed before eating. During the treatment phase and immediately following radiation therapy, there may be difficulty in swallowing, and because of xerostomia, liquids will be needed with a meal to moisten the food for swallowing. Since the patient suffers from a loss of appetite and difficulty in eating, weight loss is common. Diet selection can be very important so that proper nutrients will be included within the limited diet.

C. Other Instruction

1. *Reduction of Sources of Irritation to the Mucosa.* There must be no smoking or use of alcohol.
2. *Care of Dental Prostheses.* Frequently, prostheses are not worn during the period of cancer therapy. When new dentures are to be made, there may be a waiting period of at least 6 months and sometimes up to 2 years before the tissues can tolerate dentures.[14] The use of a saliva substitute can provide relief and make it possible to wear dentures with comfort.

   Meticulous denture hygiene must be maintained when the dentures are worn. Instruction and frequent supervision of cleaning procedures can be very important to most patients.

II. Instrumentation

A. Mouth Preparation for Radiation and Surgery

Although complete periodontal treatment prior to treatment of oral cancer would be ideal, time frequently contraindicates prolonged procedures. Minimum preparation, therefore, would include complete calculus removal with root planing. Excessive manipulation of tissues and instrumentation within the few days preceding oral surgery should be avoided.

Whenever possible, the following should be completed:

1. Complete scaling, planing, and curettage. These may be accomplished in con-

junction with plaque control instruction in a series of quadrant treatments.

2. Removal of all rough and overhanging margins and finishing and polishing of all restorations.

B. Continuing Treatment

Repeated scaling and planing is needed at each appointment to supplement plaque control efforts by the patient.

III. Fluoride

A. Dentifrice

Basic to fluoride therapy is the use of a fluoride dentifrice. When the dentifrice is highly flavored, the tissues may not tolerate it during the period when the mucosa is inflamed. A bland dentifrice with fluoride may be recommended.[15]

B. Gel Tray Applications

The patient must receive daily fluoride applications while receiving radiation therapy. The incidence of postirradiation caries can be reduced by use of a custom tray with a fluoride gel or by brushing with the gel after regular brushing.[16,17]

1. *Application by Patient.* The patient can be trained to make the application. During radiation therapy, the patient may be preoccupied or too uncomfortable to have interest in carrying out the procedure since it may appear to have no immediate benefit.

   When it seems apparent that the patient may neglect the fluoride, the dental hygienist or other dental or medical auxiliary must plan to make the daily application. If that is not feasible, a family member can be trained in the procedure.

2. *Procedure.* Prepare custom trays before the radiation therapy starts, one for each dental arch. Fluoride gel is placed in the tray and fitted over the teeth for five minutes. The patient does not rinse after removal.

3. *Effect on Sensitivity of the Teeth.* Topical fluoride on a daily basis benefits the patient by lessening tooth sensitivity.

IV. Saliva Substitute

A patient undergoing radiation therapy for cancer of the head and neck may have a drop in saliva flow up to 60 percent during the first week and 95 percent by the sixth week.[18] Severe discomfort with drying, cracking, and bleeding of the mucosa, difficulty during mastication and swallowing which can affect nutritional factors, food particles clinging to the teeth and gingiva with increased bacterial plaque, inability to wear prostheses, and increased susceptibility to dental caries are major effects from xerostomia. The increase in dental caries following irradiation is due to a lack of saliva and not to the direct radiation to the tooth.

A. Objectives of Use of Saliva Substitute

1. Prevent dental caries.
2. Induce remineralization of exposed tooth surfaces.
3. Lubricate the mucosa to relieve discomfort and pain, facilitate mastication and swallowing, and permit wearing of prostheses.

B. Composition

Various rinses, troches, and mixtures containing glycerin have been tried in the attempt to provide comfort and function for the patient with a dry mouth. A saliva substitute has been developed that contains electrolytes and other components and that provides a viscosity and consistency similar to natural saliva.[19] Sodium fluoride (2 ppm) has been added to promote remineralization of exposed tooth surfaces. It has been shown that calcium, phosphorus, and fluoride are necessary for maximal mineralization.[19]

C. Use

Instructions to a patient are simple, and there are no limitations on the frequency of use. The patient is instructed to place a drop or two in the mouth and spread the gel around with the tongue. Although prepared originally for patients receiving radiation therapy, the saliva substitute can be recommended to any patient with xerostomia from any cause (pages 625, 639).

V. Recall and Maintenance

A. Preventive Self-care

The importance of prevention and control throughout the patient's life cannot be over-emphasized. All the steps for care of the gingiva and teeth should be continued daily.

B. Frequency of Recall

Examination of the oral mucosa and supervision of gingival and dental health are carried out daily during therapy, weekly following the completion of therapy, and then monthly as indicated by the condition of the oral tissues.

The dental hygiene recall will include at least the following:
1. Extraoral and intraoral soft tissue examination.
2. Gingival examination with pocket measurements and evaluation of bleeding, tooth mobility, and other checks of periodontal disease.
3. Evaluation of plaque and plaque removal procedures. Review of techniques to motivate and encourage the patient.
4. Instrumentation. Scaling and planing as needed must be completed at each recall. Patients receiving immunosuppressive drugs need antibiotic premedication prior to instrumentation (page 100).
5. Review of fluoride procedures with a check to be certain the patient has refilled the fluoride prescription.

TECHNICAL HINTS

I. Preparation of History

Preparation of a medical and dental history should include questions relative to radiation therapy received by all patients. Radiation during childhood should be recorded as well as that during adulthood.

II. Patient Referral

When a patient is referred to a specialist or specialty clinic, a check must be made to ascertain that the patient arrives for the appointment. Frightened patients may become confused or may postpone the visit if they do not realize the urgency of the condition.

III. Source of Material

American Cancer Society
777 Third Avenue
New York, New York 10017.

State cancer society addresses can be obtained from the New York office.

IV. Sources of Saliva Substitute

Orex
Young Dental Manufacturing Company
2418 Northline Industrial Boulevard
Maryland Heights, Missouri 63043

Xero-lube
Scherer Laboratory Inc.
P.O. Box 400009
14335 Gillis Road
Dallas, Texas 75240

FACTORS TO TEACH THE PATIENT

I. Plaque control methods, gel-tray application, use of saliva substitute, and all other details of personal care.
II. Why smoking and use of alcohol must be stopped.
III. Instruction for family members in oral health care for the sick and helpless patient.

References

1. Cancer Statistics, 1982. *Ca—A Cancer Journal for Clinicians*, 32, 22, January/February, 1982.
2. Osterkamp, R.W. and Whitten, J.B.: The Etiology and Pathogenesis of Oral Cancer, in *Oral Cancer, Diagnosis, Treatment and Rehabilitation*. American Cancer Society, Professional Education Publication, 1972, 1973, pp. 48–52.
3. Silverman, S. and Griffith, M.: Smoking Characteristics of Patients With Oral Carcinoma and the Risk for Second Oral Primary Carcinoma, *J. Am. Dent. Assoc.*, 85, 637, September, 1972.
4. Beumer, J. and Curtis, T.A.: Radiation Therapy of Head and Neck Tumors, Oral Effects and Dental Manifestations, in Beumer, J., Curtis, T.A., and Firtell, D.N.: *Maxillofacial Rehabilitation, Prosthodontic and Surgical Considerations*. St. Louis, The C.V. Mosby Co., 1979, pp. 23–89.
5. Rubin, R.L. and Doku, H.C.: Therapeutic Radiation—The Modalities and Their Effects on Oral Tissues, *J. Am. Dent. Assoc.*, 92, 731, April, 1976.
6. Matvias, F.M.: Chemotherapy and Its Dental Manifestations, in Beumer, J., Curtis, T.A., and Firtell, D.N.: *Maxillofacial Rehabilitation, Prosthodontic and Surgical Considerations*. St. Louis, The C.V. Mosby Co., 1979, pp. 11–22.
7. Dreizen, S.: Stomatotoxic Manifestations of Cancer Chemotherapy, *J. Prosthet. Dent.*, 40, 650, December, 1978.

8. Sonis, S.T., Sonis, A.L., and Lieberman, A.: Oral Complications in Patients Receiving Treatment for Malignancies Other Than of the Head and Neck, *J. Am. Dent. Assoc.*, 97, 468, September, 1978.

9. Lockhart, P.B. and Sonis, S.T.: Relationship of Oral Complications to Peripheral Blood Leukocyte and Platelet Counts in Patients Receiving Cancer Chemotherapy, *Oral Surg.*, 48, 21, July, 1979.

10. Lindquist, S.F., Hickey, A.J., and Drane, J.B.: Effect of Oral Hygiene on Stomatitis in Patients Receiving Cancer Chemotherapy, *J. Prosthet. Dent.*, 40, 312, September, 1978.

11. Rosillo, R.H., Welty, M.J., and Graham, W.P.: The Patient With Maxillofacial Cancer. II. Psychologic Aspects, *Nurs. Clin. North Am.*, 8, 153, March, 1973.

12. Turns, D. and Sands, R.G.: Psychological Problems of Patients With Head and Neck Cancer, *J. Prosthet. Dent.*, 39, 68, January, 1978.

13. Ross, B.R.: The Clinician and the Head and Neck Cancer Patient, Psychodynamic Interactions, in Beumer, J., Curtis, T.A., and Firtell, D.N.: *Maxillofacial Rehabilitation, Prosthodontic and Surgical Considerations.* St. Louis, The C.V. Mosby Co., 1979, pp. 1–10.

14. Osbon, D.B., Marshall, K.J., and Lavelle, W.E.: Management of the Irradiated Patient, in Clark, J.W., ed.: *Clinical Dentistry, Volume 3*, Chapter 38. Hagerstown, Maryland, Harper & Row, 1981, pp. 1–11.

15. Greenspan, D. and Silverman, S.: Study of a Bland Dentifrice for Persons With Radiation-induced Mucositis and Vesiculo-erosive Disease, *J. Am. Dent. Assoc.*, 99, 203, August, 1979.

16. Miller, J.T. and Shannon, I.L.: A Clinical Report. Water-free Stannous Fluoride Gel and Post-irradiation Caries, *J. Public Health Dent.*, 32, 127, Spring, 1972.

17. Dreizen, S., Brown, L.R., Daly, T.E., and Drane, J.B.: Prevention of Xerostomia-related Dental Caries in Irradiated Cancer Patients, *J. Dent. Res.*, 56, 99, February, 1977.

18. Shannon, I.L., Starcke, E.N., and Wescott, W.B.: Effect of Radiotherapy on Whole Saliva Flow, *J. Dent. Res.*, 56, 693, June, 1977.

19. Shannon, I.L., Trodahl, J.N., and Starcke, E.N.: Remineralization of Enamel by a Saliva Substitute Designed for Use by Irradiated Patients, *Cancer*, 41, 1746, May, 1978.

Suggested Readings

Braham, R.L.: The Role of Dentistry in the Treatment of Malignant Disease, *J. Prev. Dent.*, 4, 28, January–February, 1977.

Buckingham, R.W.: Dental Care Policies for Treating the Terminal Cancer Patient, *Dent. Hyg.*, 55, 23, April, 1981.

Cawson, R.A.: *Essentials of Dental Surgery and Pathology.* Edinburgh, Churchill Livingstone, 1978, pp. 420–429.

Greene, S.L.: Treating the Head and Neck Cancer Patient, *Dent. Hyg.*, 54, 23, January, 1980.

Hall, G.L., Melrose, R.J., and Abrams, A.M.: Education in Early Detection of Oral Squamous Cell Carcinoma: A Community Outreach Program, *J. Am. Dent. Assoc.*, 100, 362, March, 1980.

Lavelle, C.L.B.: Prevention of Oral Infections in Patients Receiving Cancer Therapy, *Can. Dent. Assoc., J.*, 42, 551, November, 1976.

Lindquist, C., Pukkala, E., and Teppo, L.: Second Primary Cancers in Patients With Carcinoma of the Lip, *Community Dent. Oral Epidemiol.*, 7, 233, August, 1979.

Lunin, M.: Oral Pathology of the Child, in Forrester, D.J.,

Wagner, M.L., and Fleming, J., eds.: *Pediatric Dental Medicine.* Philadelphia, Lea & Febiger, 1981, pp. 192–196.

Sanner, J.R., Ramin, J.E., and Yang, C.-H.: Carcinoma of the Lung Metastatic to the Gingiva: Review of the Literature and Report of Case, *J. Oral Surg.*, 37, 103, February, 1979.

Saunders, T.R.: Development, Utilization, and Evaluation of Educational Programs for Patients With Maxillary and Mandibular Defects, *J. Prosthet. Dent.*, 42, 665, December, 1979.

Wheeler, R.L., Logemann, J.A., and Rosen, M.S.: Maxillary Reshaping Prostheses: Effectiveness in Improving Speech and Swallowing of Postsurgical Oral Cancer Patients, *J. Prosthet. Dent.*, 43, 313, March, 1980.

WHO Collaborating Centre for Oral Precancerous Lesions: Definition of Leukoplakia and Related Lesions: An Aid to Studies on Oral Precancer, *Oral Surg.*, 46, 518, October, 1978.

Radiation

Bennett, J.: Oral Care of Cancer Patients Undergoing Head and Neck Irradiation, *Dent. Hyg.*, 53, 209, May, 1979.

Beumer, J. and Brady, F.A.: Dental Management of the Irradiated Patient, *Int. J. Oral Surg.*, 7, 208, June, 1978.

Beumer, J., Curtis, T.A., and Morrish, R.B.: Radiation Complications in Edentulous Patients, *J. Prosthet. Dent.*, 36, 193, August, 1976.

Beumer, J. and Seto, B.: Dental Extractions in the Irradiated Patient, *Special Care*, 1, 166, July–August, 1981.

Beumer, J., Silverman, S., and Benak, S.B.: Hard and Soft Tissue Necroses Following Radiation Therapy for Oral Cancer, *J. Prosthet. Dent.*, 27, 640, June, 1972.

Brown, L.R., Dreizen, S., Daly, T.E., Drane, J.B., Handler, S., Riggan, L.J., and Johnston, D.A.: Interrelations of Oral Microorganisms, Immunoglobulins, and Dental Caries Following Radiotherapy, *J. Dent. Res.*, 57, 882, September–October, 1978.

Carl, W. and Wood, R.: Effects of Radiation on the Developing Dentition and Supporting Bone, *J. Am. Dent. Assoc.*, 101, 646, October, 1980.

Carpenter, J.S.: Dental Care for Children Who Have Received Head and Neck Therapeutic Radiation, *J. Pedod.*, 3, 36, Fall, 1978.

Donaldson, S.S.: Nutritional Consequences of Radiotherapy, *Cancer Res.*, 37, 2407, July, 1977.

Dreizen, S., Brown, L.R., Daly, T.E., and Drane, J.B.: Prevention of Xerostomia-related Dental Caries in Irradiated Cancer Patients, *J. Dent. Res.*, 56, 99, February, 1977.

Dreizen, S., Daly, T.E., Drane, J.B., and Brown, L.R.: Oral Complications of Cancer Radiotherapy, *Postgrad. Med.*, 61, 85, February, 1977.

Floyd, B.R.: Oral Care of the Oral Radiation Therapy Patient, *Dent. Hyg.*, 52, 577, December, 1978.

Gunn, W.G.: Radiation Therapy for the Aging Patient, *Ca—A Cancer Journal for Clinicians*, 30, 337, November–December, 1980.

Karmiol, M. and Walsh, R.F.: Dental Caries After Radiotherapy of the Oral Regions, *J. Am. Dent. Assoc.*, 91, 838, October, 1975.

Murray, C.G., Daly, T.E., and Zimmerman, S.O.: The Relationship Between Dental Disease and Radiation Necrosis of the Mandible, *Oral Surg.*, 49, 99, February, 1980.

Reynolds, W.R., Hickey, A.J., and Feldman, M.I.: Dental Management of the Cancer Patient Receiving Radiation Therapy, *Clin. Prev. Dent.*, 2, 5, September–October, 1980.

Robinson, J.E.: Characteristics of Irradiated Soft and Hard Tissues, *J. Prosthet. Dent.*, 35, 549, May, 1976.

Schofield, I.D.F., Abbott, W., and Popowich, L.: Osteo-radionecrosis of Maxillae, *Oral Surg.*, 45, 692, May, 1978.

Starcke, E.N. and Shannon, I.L.: How Critical Is the Interval Between Extractions and Irradiation in Patients With Head and Neck Malignancy? *Oral Surg.*, 43, 333, March, 1977.

Wescott, W.B., Starcke, E.N., and Shannon, I.L.: Chemical Protection Against Postirradiation Dental Caries, *Oral Surg.*, 40, 709, December, 1975.

Chemotherapy

Bottomley, W.K., Perlin, E., and Ross, G.R.: Antineoplastic Agents and Their Oral Manifestations, *Oral Surg.*, 44, 527, October, 1977.

Carl, W.: Cancer Chemotherapy and Dentistry, *Quintessence Int.*, 8, 9, December, 1977.

Dreizen, S., Bodey, G.P., and Rodriguez, V.: Oral Complications of Cancer Chemotherapy, *Postgrad. Med.*, 58, 75, August, 1975.

Greenberg, M.S.: Ulcerative, Vesicular and Bullous Lesions, in Lynch, M.A., ed.: *Burket's Oral Medicine, Diagnosis and Treatment*, 7th ed. Philadelphia, J.B. Lippincott Co., 1977, pp. 33–65.

Hickey, A.J., Vergo, T.J., Nathanson, L., and Parkinson, D.R.: Survey of Oral/Dental Needs of Patients Receiving Chemotherapy for Malignant Disease, *Compendium Cont. Ed.*, 2, 92, March/April, 1981.

Shipman, B.: Clinical Evaluation of Oral *Candida* in Cancer Chemotherapy Patients, *J. Prosthet. Dent.*, 41, 63, January, 1979.

Saliva Substitute

Klestov, A.C., Webb, J., Latt, D., Schiller, G., McNamara, K., Young, D.Y., Hobbes, J., and Fetherston, J.: Treatment of Xerostomia: A Double-blind Trial in 108 Patients With Sjogren's Syndrome, *Oral Surg.*, 51, 594, June, 1981.

Nakamoto, R.Y.: Use of a Saliva Substitute in Postradiation Xerostomia, *J. Prosthet. Dent.*, 42, 539, November, 1979.

Shannon, I.L. and Edmonds, E.J.: Effects of Fluoride Concentration on Rehardening of Enamel by Saliva Substitute, *Int. Dent. J.*, 28, 420, December, 1978.

Shannon, I.L., McCrary, B.R., and Starcke, E.N.: A Saliva Substitute for Use by Xerostomic Patients Undergoing Radiotherapy to the Head and Neck, *Oral Surg.*, 44, 656, November, 1977.

Vergo, T.J. and Kadish, S.P.: Dentures as Artificial Saliva Reservoirs in the Irradiated Edentulous Cancer Patient with Xerostomia: A Pilot Study, *Oral Surg.*, 51, 229, March, 1981.

Types and Pathology of Neoplasms

Bhaskar, S.N.: *Synopsis of Oral Pathology*, 6th ed. St. Louis, The C.V. Mosby Co., 1981, pp. 539–573.

Bolden, T.E.: The Prevention and Detection of Oral Cancer, in Caldwell, R.C. and Stallard, R.E., eds.: *A Textbook of Preventive Dentistry*. Philadelphia, W.B. Saunders Co., 1977, pp. 265–324.

Donlan, C.P.: Radiation Therapy of Lesions of the Oral Cavity, in Archer, W.H.: *Oral and Maxillofacial Surgery*, 5th ed. Philadelphia, W.B. Saunders Co., 1975, pp. 1732–1830.

Giunta, J.: Oral Pathology, in Dunn, M.J., ed.: *Dental Auxiliary Practice*, Module 3. Baltimore, Williams & Wilkins, 1975, pp. 98–115.

Hamner, J.E.: Oral Cancer, in Lynch, M.A., ed.: *Burket's Oral Medicine, Diagnosis and Treatment*, 7th ed. Philadelphia, J.B. Lippincott Co., 1977, pp. 607–650.

Scopp, I.W.: *Oral Medicine*, 2nd ed. St. Louis, The C.V. Mosby Co., 1973, pp. 325–368.

Shafer, W.G., Hine, M.K., and Levy, B.M.: *A Textbook of Oral Pathology*, 3rd ed. Philadelphia, W.B. Saunders Co., 1974, pp. 81–211.

Wright, J.C., Mersheimer, W.L., Miller, D.G., and Rotman, M.: Cancer, in Steinberg, F.U., ed.: *Cowdry's The Care of the Geriatric Patient*, 5th ed. St. Louis, The C.V. Mosby Co., 1976, pp. 35–65.

50

Care and Management of Patients with Disabilities

Many types of disabilities or handicaps require special attention and adaptations during dental and dental hygiene appointments. The general term disability refers to any reduction of a person's activity that has resulted from an acute or chronic health condition and affects motor, sensory, or mental functions.

A disability may be permanent or temporary. A temporary disability may be physical such as a fracture of a leg, or physiologic with physical limitations such as during pregnancy. Chronic systemic diseases may result in crippling disabilities. The causes of disabilities may be factors of heredity, systemic disease, trauma, or combinations of these.

The Developmental Disabilities Assistance and Bill of Rights Act of 1978 defined the term *developmental disability* as a severe, chronic disability of a person which

A. is attributable to a mental or physical impairment or combination of mental or physical impairments;
B. is manifested before the person attains age twenty-two;
C. is likely to continue indefinitely;
D. results in substantial functional limitations in three or more of the following areas of major life activity:
   (i) self-care,
   (ii) receptive and expressive language,
   (iii) learning,
   (iv) mobility,
   (v) self-direction,
   (vi) capacity for independent living, and
   (vii) economic self-sufficiency; and
E. reflects the person's need for a combination and sequence of special, interdisciplinary, or generic care, treatment, or other services which are of lifelong or extended duration and are individually planned and coordinated.[1]

According to the 1970 United States census, 1 in every 11 Americans, or over 9 percent in the 16 to 64 working age group of the noninstitutionalized population was disabled.[2] Of the total population, including those 65 years and over and children under 16, 12 to 15 percent are disabled.

Current trends toward deinstitutionalization have brought alternative living, educational, and work arrangements to many individuals with physical and mental disabilities. Specially staffed community housing for group living has been made available. Children taken out of institutional life and trained for community living in transitional homes are being integrated into regular school and health programs.

The term *normalization* is used to mean the attempt to provide a normal pattern of daily living. *Mainstreaming* is the integration of people with handicaps into their communities. Through a program of rehabilitation, persons with disabilities receive vocational, educational, placement, medical, and dental services as needed.

DENTAL AND DENTAL HYGIENE CARE

Oral health for the individual with a handicap takes on more than usual significance and presents a challenge to dental personnel. For the patient, the handicap provides enough of a burden without additional oral problems which can reduce an already lowered potential for normal living. Preventive measures, particularly fluoridation and other means for protecting the teeth with fluoride, must be encouraged and promoted through community effort and personal instruction to minimize oral problems in this group of special patients.

Imagination, ingenuity, and flexibility are necessary for those involved in treating people with handicaps. Individualization and modification of usual procedures will be necessary in addition to the material described in this chapter. Patience, calmness, and kindness are keys to approaching the special patient.

I. Objectives

The dental hygienist is able to make a significant contribution to the well-being, independent mobility, and sense of personal value of a patient with a handicap. Whether employed in private practice, an institutional or community clinical and educational setting, or contributing on a volunteer basis, the objectives are to
A. Make dental hygiene appointments pleasant and comfortable experiences.
B. Motivate the patient and those who provide daily care for the patient. Personal oral care practices conducive to maintaining healthy oral tissue with freedom from infection must be developed.
C. Contribute to the patient's general health, of which oral health is an integral part. Prevention of tooth loss increases the ability to masticate food, which in turn, is essential to prevent malnutrition and to increase resistance to infection.
D. Prevent the need for extensive dental and periodontal treatment which the patient may not be able to undergo because of lowered physical stamina or ability to cooperate.

Dentures or other removable appliances can be hazardous for certain patients or impossible for others.
E. Aid in the improvement of appearance which contributes to social acceptance. An untidy person with unclean teeth and halitosis (from local causes) is much less acceptable socially than one with a clean mouth.

II. Types of Conditions

A variety of disabling conditions are found among persons with handicaps. An individual may have more than one type of crippling or limiting problem. The list below is not intended to include all possibilities, but it is representative.[3] Many of the diseases and syndromes in which these symptoms occur or from which they result are described in the various chapters throughout Section VI of this book.
A. Mental retardation.
B. Seizure disorders; convulsive states.
C. Sensory impairments
   1. Visual.
   2. Speech.
   3. Hearing.
D. Learning disabilities
   1. Perceptual handicaps.
   2. Hyperkinesis.
   3. Dyslexia.
E. Surgical disfigurement, such as amputation of limbs or maxillofacial defects after oral cancer surgery.
F. Congenital defects: cleft lip and/or palate.
G. Paralysis
   1. Spastic and athetoid paralysis (cerebral palsy).
   2. Paraplegia, hemiplegia, quadriplegia (tetraplegia).
H. Respiratory problems
I. Neuromotor/locomotor
   1. Muscle dystrophy, weakness.
   2. Joint symptoms (including temporomandibular).
   3. Bone deformity.
J. Chronic disease limitations
   1. Cardiovascular.
   2. Blood diseases.
   3. Diabetes.
   4. Malignancies.
K. Aging.

III. Pretreatment Planning

A large majority of patients with disabilities

can be treated in the private dental office setting. Only a relatively few will need hospitalization because of marked difficulties in management or because of a systemic condition that would require special medical supervision.

A. Preliminary Information

Information about the younger, dependent, mentally retarded, or elderly senile patient will be obtained from a parent, relative, advocate, or other person responsible. To facilitate planning and expedite the initial appointment, as much information as possible should be obtained in advance, by telephone if a personal interview cannot be arranged.

Medical and other record forms can be mailed to the home for completion. Advance information permits the dental team to be prepared for the patient so that valuable appointment time is not wasted, and complete attention can be devoted to the patient's needs.

B. Records and Forms

1. *Medical History.* In addition to the usual topics covered by questions (pages 90–91), information relative to the handicapping condition is needed. At least the following should be included:
   a. Specific handicapping condition: when diagnosed, history of treatments, hospitalizations, current medications and other therapy, names and addresses of specialists involved.
   b. Record of institutionalization.
   c. History of hepatitis; most recent blood tests.
   d. Seizures: history, frequency, treatment.
   e. Muscular coordination: mobility, dexterity.
   f. Communication: speech, vision, hearing.
   g. Mental capacities: schooling, special classes.
   h. Degree of independence: self-care, ability to dress and feed self, perform own oral care with brush, floss, other aids.
   i. Dietary restrictions.

2. *Dental History*
   a. Previous dental experiences: patient's attitude, ability to cooperate.
   b. Difficulties in obtaining appointments in other locations.
   c. Most recent care: scaling, restorations, extractions, other.
   d. Oral infections; oral habits.
   e. Fluoride history: fluoridation, dietary supplements, self- or professionally-applied topical methods; with years, ages, and frequency.
   f. Current home care methods (aids and special devices, frequency, degree of self-care).
   g. Patient/parent concepts of perceived needs; attitudes and apparent emphasis on dental care.

3. *Consent Forms.* Consent forms for minors, mentally retarded, or brain damaged patients must be signed by parent or legal guardian.

C. Consultations with Physicians and Other Specialists

Medical aspects of the patient's care are integrated into treatment planning for oral care. The physician can supply information the dentist can apply in the selection of antibiotic, sedative, or other necessary pharmaceutical agents. Additional pertinent information may be obtained from other medical specialists and the social worker.

D. Discussion with Parent or Other Direct-care Person

1. Determine familial interrelationships. Many parents devote their lives to the care of their child who is handicapped. Dental personnel need to make every effort to learn from the parents the capabilities of the patient and the methods most effective for gaining cooperation. The names, ages, and interrelationships of other family members can prove helpful.

   Families may overindulge the special child: sweets may be used as rewards or bribes to pacify. Poor behavior may be condoned.

2. Describe to the parent the cooperation and assistance needed. Special help may

be needed during the appointment and for supervision of oral care on a daily basis in the total preventive care program.

3. Solicit parental help in preparing the patient for the appointments. Ask that procedures and facilities be described in advance in a pleasant and positive manner to reassure the patient.
4. Request that if possible the patient be brought to the office or clinic before the appointment to see the facility and become familiar with the surroundings and staff.
5. List special aids the patient needs to bring to the appointment, such as a transfer board for transfer into the dental chair, hearing aid, dental prostheses, and any special plaque control devices currently in use.

E. Appointment Scheduling

1. *Determine Special Requirements.* Determine whether special requirements of the patient's daily schedule influence time selection.[4] The cooperation of the patient may be decreased if basic routines are disturbed. Some examples are as follows:
   a. Diabetic patient's appointment must not interfere with medication, meal, or between-meal eating schedules.
   b. Elderly person who rises early may feel better for a morning appointment.
   c. Arthritic patient may have greater mobility late in the morning or in the afternoon.
   d. Child's nap schedule should be respected.
   e. Early morning appointment may be very difficult for a patient who requires a long time for morning preparation, such as a patient with a spinal cord injury or colostomy.
2. *Effect of Transportation Requirements*
   a. Availability of family member who accompanies patient; the person should not be expected to lose a day's work if the dental appointment can be accommodated otherwise. Fami-

lies may have limited financial resources because of expenses related to treatment of the person with the handicap.
   b. Wheelchair patient may need to reserve a public wheelchair transport vehicle and be limited by the schedule.
3. *Time of Appointment*
   a. Arrange at a time when the patient will not have to wait a long time after arrival. If daily appointments tend to be increasingly off schedule by late morning or afternoon, the patient with a disability needs the appointment at the start of the day or first in the afternoon.
   b. Dentist and dental hygienist should try to schedule a patient who taxes their resources of energy or patience at a time when their own condition is at a maximum potential.
   c. Allow sufficient time so that the patient does not feel rushed; many people with handicaps cannot hurry.
4. *Recall*

   The recall frequency needs to be individualized. The time depends on the patient's oral problems and general disabilities. A frequent recall is encouraged for the following reasons:
   a. To decrease length of single appointment by keeping the oral tissues at an optimum level of health.
   b. To assist the patient whose handicap limits the ability to perform personal oral hygiene techniques.
   c. To provide motivation through plaque monitoring and review of procedures for the patient and the parent or other direct care person involved.

BARRIER-FREE ENVIRONMENT

A variety of factors can explain the general lack of dental and dental hygiene care of the elderly or individuals of any age who are handicapped. One of the more significant reasons is the existence of physical barriers confronting patients who may attempt to keep appointments.[5] Fear of not being able to cope with architectural barriers, fear of falling, or fear of attracting attention in an embarrassing way, can all be hindrances to seeking oral care.

The elimination of barriers such as steps and stairs, narrow passageways and doorways, heavy doors, rest room inaccessibility, and other features that prohibit free and safe movement by all, can be difficult when a building is not previously accessible. When a new office or clinic is being planned, provision can be made to accommodate all patients.

In general, when a facility is barrier-free for a patient in a wheelchair, all other individuals will have adequate access. The patient in a wheelchair requires more space for turning and positioning than a patient with crutches, a walker, or a patient with another person walking at the side to guide or provide support. In addition to space requirements, special features are needed for other specific disabilities. An example is having braille floor indicators beside the numbers on elevators.

Basic uniform specifications for a barrier-free environment have been prepared in explicit detail. A list of the various sources with the addresses is provided under *Suggested Readings* at the end of this chapter. The descriptions below represent general features based on architectural standards, along with suggested applications for a dental clinic or office.

I. External Features

A. Parking

A reserved area, clearly marked, should be close to the building entrance and 13 feet wide to permit a person with a handicap to open car doors for exiting and reboarding.

B. Walkways

A 4-foot wide walkway is needed for wheelchair accommodation. The surface must be solid and nonslip without irregularities. Curb ramps (cuts) from the street and from the parking area are necessary.

C. Entrance

At least one entrance to the building should be on ground level or reached by a gently sloping ramp (rise of 1 inch for every 12 inches). An easily grasped handrail (height 32 inches) is needed on at least one side, and preferably both sides, to accommodate

left- and right-handed cane and one-crutch users.

D. Door

The light weight door with a lever type handle must open at least 32 inches for a wheelchair and tall crutch user (figure 50–1).

II. Internal Features

Official regulations specify dimensions for accessibility of all aspects, including passageways, floors, drinking fountains, and restrooms. A few will be described.

A. Passageways

The passageways should be at least 4 feet wide with handrails along the sides, and free from obstructions such as hanging signs with which a tall blind person could collide.

B. Floors

Level floors with nonslip surfaces are important. Thick or small unattached movable rugs or carpets present obstacles for wheelchairs or walkers and hazards for a patient with crutches, cane, or leg brace.

C. Reception Area

At least part of the furniture should permit easy access during seating and rising. Preferred are chairs with 18-inch high flat,

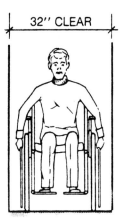

Figure 50–1. Wheelchair accessibility. To accommodate adult wheelchairs, which vary in width from 2 feet 3 inches to 2 feet 8 inches, a clear door width of 32 inches has been accepted as the official regulation. (From Coons, M. and Milner, M. eds.: Creating an Accessible Campus. Washington, D.C., Association of Physical Plant Administrators, 1978.)

firm seats, arms for support when pushing oneself up by the arms, and which cannot slide or tip as the person rises.

III. The Dental/Dental Hygiene Treatment Room

In a group of several operatories, where a limited number of patients in wheelchairs are served, only one room needs to be able to accommodate the wheelchair. Dental personnel should be versatile in exchanging rooms to serve special patients.

A. Dimensions

The operatory should have space for both the dental chair and related dental equipment and the wheelchair. The doorway will be a standard 32 inches wide. The wheelchair is placed beside and parallel to the dental chair for patient transfer. In a small operatory, the dental chair can be rotated to give room for turning the wheelchair.[6]

When planning or redesigning an operatory for wheelchair accessibility, the dental chair selected should be able to be lowered to 19 inches from the floor, and be accessible from both sides for wheelchair transfer. Having an x-ray machine in the same operatory can simplify the problems of moving the patient into a separate radiography room.

B. Wheelchair Used During Treatment

For a patient confined to a wheelchair and unable to transfer easily, if at all, the wheelchair is positioned for direct utilization.
1. *Portable Headrest.*[7] A portable headrest may be attached to the wheelchair handles.
2. *Position of Dental Chair.* The dental chair can be swiveled to permit the wheelchair to be backed up to place the patient's head in a usual operating position. The dental lamp can then be directed into the patient's oral cavity and adjusted for access to the equipment.
3. *Wheelchair Lift.* An automatic wheelchair lift that tilts the chair back to a usual working position can be obtained for a clinical situation where wheelchair patients are treated frequently.[7]

IV. Plaque Control Facility

When a teaching area is planned for patient instruction, attention must be given to assure accessibility for a patient in a wheelchair. The same facility can be used by a seated nondisabled patient.

A. Dimensions

The usual 32-inch doorway and turnabout space for a wheelchair would be indicated. The tabletop and washbasin built at a height of 32 to 34 inches permit clearance underneath for knees and wheelchair arms (figure 50–2). The same regulations are used for a lavatory sink.

B. Wash Basin

Lever- or blade-type handles on faucets are usable by patients who cannot grip round handles or who have no hands. Under the sink, hot pipes must be covered or insulated, since patients who have no sensation in their legs could be burned.[8] The hot water temperature may be able to be regulated.

C. Mirror

Mirrors and dispensers are positioned low. A tilt mirror could provide better viewing

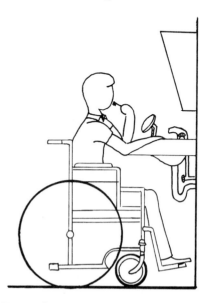

Figure 50–2. Plaque control facility and lavatory. With the tabletop and washbasin built at a height of 32 to 34 inches, clearance is available underneath for knees and arms of a wheelchair. Hot pipes under the sink must be covered or insulated since patients with no sensation in their legs could be burned.

of the teeth during instruction. A tilt mirror with a hinge has more adaptability for tall and short patients and patients with bifocal eyeglasses.

An unattached hand mirror, preferably one on a pedestal that tilts, will be necessary to supplement the wall mirror. A close-up magnifying mirror can provide an excellent aid for viewing the disclosed plaque and devices for plaque removal.

PATIENT RECEPTION

I. The Initial Appointment

The orientation of a patient with a handicapping condition paves the way for long-term dental and dental hygiene supervision and care even as it does for a patient with no disability. When a patient is passive, follows instructions, and may have received sedative medication, the situation is quite different from that of a patient who is apprehensive and fearful, perhaps because of past medical and dental experiences. Other patients have difficulties of communication, or limitations of body movement and control. The problems of management and care become greatly intensified for such patients.

A. Orientation

The first appointment includes, and when necessary is devoted entirely to, a basic orientation to the facilities, the dental chair, and the personnel. The examination of the oral cavity is started if possible, and, depending on the degree of patient cooperation, various steps in the examination may be completed. Preventive personal care procedures to alleviate gingival inflammation are initiated, and participation of the direct care person is solicited.

A number of orientation visits may be necessary since hurrying or forcing a patient may cause more severe problems. For the dental hygienist in a dental clinic of a long-term care facility where patients live on the premises, daily short visits to the clinic may be possible to condition or desensitize a patient.

B. Communication

Each patient is different, and the dentist and auxiliaries must watch, listen, and learn procedures that will develop the patient's trust. Parents and others who work with and care for the patient can explain how best to communicate. The parent will help to interpret the changing moods of the patient.

Even for the patient who cannot or will not speak and may appear withdrawn, the ability to understand what is being said should not be underestimated.

Nonverbal communication using facial expression, pointing, body language, and demonstration will help certain patients to respond. Other patients will write messages on a pad of paper, use sign language, a language board, or other devices the dental personnel can learn. Suggested procedures for the deaf patient are described on page 770.

C. Preventive Care Introduction

Whether or not the examination and treatment plan are completed at the initial visit, the personal oral daily care program should be introduced. After finding out what the current daily care has been, instruction for the parent or other person who cares for the patient is provided along with that for the patient.

It must be made clear from the start that the first step in treatment is to eliminate infection of the gingiva, which is accomplished primarily by daily plaque removal. When dental caries is present, or routinely in keeping with practice policy, a food diary form is explained in preparation for daily recording at home. It can be requested that the completed form be brought in or mailed in so that it can be ready for review at the next appointment.

The complete instruction and prevention program is described on pages 698–707.

II. Wheelchair Transfers[9,10]

Three basic transfer techniques will be described here. The size, weight, and mobility of the patient along with any special physical conditions influence the choice. The patient may prefer to transfer from the left or the right side of the dental chair depending on which side of the body is stronger.

When the patient is in a total support wheelchair, transfer to the dental chair may not be advisable. However, dental and dental hygiene care may be hampered unless there is a portable headrest and possibly a wheelchair lift as described on page 690.

A. Preparation for Transfer

1. *Clear the Area.* Before starting a transfer, clear the area by moving the operating stool, bracket tray, portable unit, and dental light. After the transfer, release the wheelchair brake to move it aside. In a small operatory, the wheelchair may be folded and set aside.

2. *Special Needs of Patient*[10]
   a. Chair padding. Special padding is usually used in a wheelchair as a protection from pressure sores. Depending on the length of the appointment, the patient will decide whether the padding should be moved to the dental chair. Pressure sores are described on page 745.
   b. Bags and catheters. A patient, such as one with paraplegia or quadriplegia, who does not have control of urine discharge will have a bag with tubing for collection. The bag may be attached to the leg of the patient or to the wheelchair. To prevent dislodging the appliance, its location must be determined. After transfer, the tubing must be checked to be sure it is not bent or twisted.
   c. Spasms. Ask the patient about susceptibility to spasms, and what procedures to follow for prevention.
   d. Advice concerning transfer. Ask the patient, family member, or attendant how best the operator can help during the transfer. The patient must be allowed to do as much as possible.

B. Mobile Patient Transfer

When a patient can support his or her own weight, the "stand and pivot" technique can be used.

1. Position the wheelchair facing in the same direction as the dental chair at approximately an angle of 30 degrees; set brakes; remove footrests. The patient will adjust a power-driven chair and set the brakes before turning it off.

2. Adjust dental chair to same height as or lower than the wheelchair.

3. Clear path for transfer by moving the dental chair arm and removing the arm of the wheelchair.

4. Face the patient and place feet outside the patient's feet for pivoting. Operator's knees should be close to or against the patient's knees to prevent buckling.

5. Place hands under the patient's arms and grasp the waist belt in back. Patient places arms around operator's neck or places hands on wheelchair arms to push up. Operator lifts patient to standing position.

6. Pivot together slowly until the patient is backed up to the side of the dental chair with the backs of the legs touching. The patient is gently lowered to sitting position. Reposition the arm of dental chair.

7. Grasp patient's legs together between the ankles and knees, and lift them onto the dental chair.

8. After the appointment, the patient is returned to the wheelchair in the reverse order of procedure.

C. Immobile Patient Transfer

The patient is unable to support his or her own weight. Two operators are required. The parent, advocate, or other attendant may serve as the second person.

1. Position wheelchair in the same direction as the dental chair and parallel to it; set brakes; remove footrests.

2. Adjust the dental chair to the same height as or lower than the seat of the wheelchair.

3. Move arm of dental chair out of transfer area and remove arm of wheelchair.

4. Operator I from behind the wheelchair: place feet, one on either side of the rear wheel nearest the dental chair; place hands under the patient's folded arms, and clasp the patient's arms below the elbows, pressing forearms against the patient's lower thorax area.

5. Operator II may do either of the following, depending on the size and weight of the patient:
   a. Face patient and grasp hands under the patient's knees.

b. Face dental chair and place one arm under the thighs and the other under the calves of the lower legs.

6. On a prearranged signal, with a steady motion, the patient is lifted and gently transferred to the dental chair.

7. After the appointment, the patient is returned to the wheelchair in the reverse order of procedure.

D. Sliding Board Transfer

A patient may bring a sliding board or one may be kept in the office or clinic. Two persons will be needed when the patient is heavy or less mobile.[10]

1. Position the wheelchair in the same direction as the dental chair and parallel with it; set the brakes; remove the footrests if they will be in the way of the sliding board.

2. Adjust the seat of the dental chair to slightly lower than the wheelchair seat.

3. Move the arm of the dental chair out of transfer area and remove the arm of the wheelchair.

4. Patient or operator: place the sliding board well under the hip, and extending across to the dental chair.

5. Patient slides by shifting weight, balancing on hands, and walking the buttocks across the board. The operator who faces the patient can assist or even do the transfer by holding the patient under the axillae.

6. Board is removed and replaced after the appointment.

7. Dental chair is positioned slightly higher than the wheelchair seat for the transfer back.

III. Walking Frame, Crutches, Cane

The operator asks the patient for instructions in how to assist.

A. Walking Frame to the Dental Chair

1. Adjust dental chair upright with arm out of the way and seat to level of back of patient's knees.

2. Patient backs up to dental chair until back of legs touch, then lowers into the chair. Operator stabilizes the walking frame.

3. Operator takes patient by the ankles to lift legs and turn patient onto the dental chair.

4. Remove walker to a place out of the way of dental personnel.

B. Walking Frame from the Dental Chair

1. Raise dental chair to upright and ask patient to wait while the walker is positioned. Allow ample time for patient to adjust to upright position to prevent effects of postural hypotension.

2. Move arm of dental chair; position chair to approximate height of patient's knees.

3. Grasp ankles, gently turn patient and swing legs down.

4. Reposition walker.

5. Patient uses one hand to push up and other to grasp walker. When walker is used for balance, one hand must be in the middle to prevent tipping.

6. If patient wants assistance when rising, operator hooks an arm under the patient's arm on left side if patient is right-handed. The patient's right hand is used to grasp the walker.

C. Crutches

1. Dental chair is positioned upright at a level with patient's knees. Some patients need the chair higher so seating does not require knees to be bent.

2. Operator assists, as directed by patient, while patient lowers into the chair; the legs are lifted onto the dental chair.

3. After the appointment, with patient seated on the side of the dental chair, pass the crutches together to one hand. The patient usually will use the other hand to push up. If assistance in rising is requested, hook arm under the patient's arm as directed.

D. Cane

1. Dental chair is positioned at the level of the patient's knees or higher if the patient may have difficulty in bending the knees.

2. Patient may need assistance in lifting the legs onto the dental chair.

3. After the appointment, when the patient is seated on the side of the dental chair,

operator passes the cane to the patient and assists patient to rise only as directed.

IV. Patient Position and Stabilization

The objectives in patient positioning and stabilization are to let the patient feel comfortable and secure while the professional person performs in a position that provides adequate illumination, visibility, and accessibility. A hyperactive patient or one with involuntary muscle movements can wear a special stabilizing device to make it possible for the operator to work and to prevent damage to the oral tissues by accidental movement of instruments.

A. Chair Position

1. *Tip Chair Back Slowly.* Immediately after a patient with cerebral palsy or other condition that involves a lack of muscle control is in the dental chair, start to tip the chair back to provide balance so that the patient cannot fall. While tipping back the chair, place one hand on the patient's shoulder to offer assurance and support. Never place the chair back quickly. Advance in steps to allow the patient to adjust.

2. *Chair Up.* A patient with a respiratory complication will need to have the chair back up. A patient with a cardiac disease or one wearing a pacemaker should be asked a question such as "How many pillows do you use at night?" and the chair can be adjusted accordingly.

B. Body Adjustments

During the appointment, patients with a spinal cord injury need to do a "push up" and quadriplegics need to shift their weight every 20 minutes for 10 to 15 seconds. This enables the patient to maintain good circulation and healthy tissue of the buttocks where there is no sensation. The procedure is a preventive measure for decubitus ulcers and should be a consideration during long dental procedures.

C. Body Stabilization[11]

A restraint can be used to limit body movement and provide support for paralyzed limbs. When a restraint of any type is

to be used, it should be explained to the patient. It must be understood that the devices are used to help the dentist and make the patient more comfortable, and not in any way for punishment.

1. *Body Enclosure Restraints.* Although a small patient may be held by a parent, such positioning can be tiring and insecure. Better cooperation is usually obtained by the use of positive restraints such as commercial wraps, which are available, or an improvised wrap.
   a. Pediwrap.
      The *Pediwrap* is made of nylon mesh and encloses the patient from neck to ankles. It is available in three sizes to fit infants and children through 10 years of age.[12] It is frequently used with support straps about the patient's legs and arms.
   b. Papoose board.
      A *Papoose board* is a board with padded wraps to enclose a patient. It is available in three sizes from a small child size to an adult size.[13]
   c. Bedsheet or blanket.
      The parent can bring a blanket or sheet from home which is familiar to the patient. The sheet or blanket is folded firmly around the patient twice and held securely by a velcro strap around the body. Support straps about the legs and body provide the patient with additional control.

2. *Support Straps.* Adhesive tape (2 or 3 inches wide), canvas, or velcro straps may be used with or without a body enclosure restraint. A soft restraint may be made from a soft material such as flannel with a padded section to place over the wrists, ankles, or where needed. Ties 4 to 6 inches wide may be passed around the dental chair or be tied to the arms of the chair.

3. *Hand Restraint or Support Mitt.* A mitt without a thumb made from unbleached cotton can have long ties attached at the wrist line. The ties are first tied at the wrist and then looped around the arm of the dental chair and secured.[14]

4. *Head Stabilization*
   a. Arm of operator. From a working po-

sition at 12:00 (top of patient's head), the nondominant arm placed around the patient's head will hold it in position.

b. Automated head stabilizer. A fitted head support helmet has been designed for a patient with cerebral palsy to control movements and hold the head in position for dental hygiene treatment.[15]

c. Mouth prop (page 710).

CLINIC PROCEDURES FOR EVALUATION OF PATIENT

I. Precautions for Hepatitis

As described in Chapter 53 (page 736), a significant number of institutionalized or previously institutionalized individuals, particularly among those with Down's Syndrome, have been shown to be carriers of hepatitis B antigen. The medical history, consultation with physician, and/or the health records of the institution will provide necessary information to guide procedures.

A. Label the Record

"HEPATITIS PRECAUTIONS" can be printed in large, clear letters on and within the record as needed for the attention of all concerned.

B. Clinical Procedures

Precautions relative to sterilization and the use of disposable items were described on page 64, and must be followed explicitly. A mask, gloves, and eyeglasses must be worn. Aerosol-producing handpieces, sprays, and ultrasonic scaling instruments should be avoided. The use of a rubber dam is indicated for appropriate procedures.

II. Patient Evaluation Procedures

As many as possible of the procedures for evaluation are accomplished at the first appointment. The goals should be the same for all patients; namely, to prepare the evaluation material to be reviewed and analyzed by the dentist for treatment planning.

The patient may not be able to complete all of the steps in evaluation, and extra time must be spent on orientation. Each clinic procedure is prefaced by an explanation and demonstration. Several trials may be needed.

A. Patient Histories (pages 99–100)

Certain patients will need prophylactic antibiotics prior to instrumentation.

B. Vital Signs: Blood Pressure Determination

For the patient who will be examined in a body enclosure restraint, blood pressure determination must be accomplished early in the appointment, before application of the restraint.

C. Extraoral and Intraoral Examination

When a mouth prop is needed to perform intraoral procedures, the intraoral pathology examination can be made in conjunction with the gingival and dental examinations. The mouth prop would be placed first on one side and then the other.

D. Photographs

Depending on the treatment, photographs may be requested by the dentist. In some instances, photographs of the teeth and gingiva are made for patient instruction. A patient requiring orthodontic therapy, maxillofacial surgery, or other special treatment may need to be photographed.

E. Radiographic Survey[16,17]

1. *Periapical Survey.* Since the most diagnostic information can be gained from periapical and bitewing surveys, the attempt should be made to obtain as many of the essential exposures as possible.

   a. Use a mouth prop, film holder, and much patience. When help is needed, the parent or other attendant can assist.

   b. Patient and attendant wear lead aprons; person holding film in mouth can wear a lead glove. Dental personnel never hold film for a patient.

2. *Extraoral, Occlusal, Panoramic.* The overall views provided by occlusal or extraoral surveys can aid in locating anomalies, retained root tips, impactions, and other pathology, but such surveys are not substitutes for the detail pro-

vided by periapical radiographs. For example, a periapical film would be needed to identify root fracture and apical pathology which may be present in the patient with cerebral palsy who bruxes heavily and may traumatize anterior teeth.

F. Study Casts[18]

Study casts would be needed for orthodontic, prosthetic, and phases of restorative therapy or for documentation and record purposes. With adequate patient preparation and orientation, cooperation can be obtained. Suggestions for technique are listed here.
1. Use a comfortable tray and bead with a soft wax (pages 169–171). A flexible tray may prove easier to insert.
2. Practice the insertion and removal several times to prepare the patient. Practicing tray insertion may be started at one appointment and the actual impression made at another.
3. Apply a topical anesthetic to the intraoral tissues when the patient has a gag reflex.
4. Use fast-setting alginate and warm water.

G. Gingival Examination

Despite difficulties, a thorough evaluation must be made. Procedures for examination were described on pages 209–230. Clinical aspects including the degree of inflammation, pockets, mucogingival involvement, frenal attachments, and tooth mobility are detected and recorded. Information from the radiographs is used to confirm the presence and degree of periodontal destruction.

Evaluation of the amount, extent, and location of calculus is needed in order that an appropriate estimate of scaling requirements may be made for the dental hygiene treatment plan. Overall oral cleanliness and the presence of plaque and materia alba provide a prevue to plaque control instruction needs.

H. Dental Examination

1. Number, size, color, and occlusion of the teeth.

2. Malformations, supernumerary, and other irregularities that frequently are associated with certain developmental disabilities.

III. Oral Manifestations[19]

Oral diseases of disabled individuals are not different in kind than those of nondisabled persons. The two principal diseases found are dental caries and periodontal diseases. Other oral findings described below include congenital malformations, oral injuries, and malocclusions. In the chapters devoted to describing specific individuals with disabilities, oral characteristics of each are included.

For a majority of patients with disabilities, once the patient is in the dental chair, sedated if needed, and stabilized physically, dental and dental hygiene treatment is not different. For a few other patients, an oral manifestation can be caused by, or a result of, the patient's disabling condition. Examples are included here.

A. Congenital Malformations

1. Cleft lip or palate.
2. Other craniofacial anomalies.
3. Tooth defects.[20] An increased incidence of malformations has been observed with developmental disabilities; for example,
    a. Variations in number and morphology of teeth.
    b. Dentinogenesis imperfecta, amelogenesis imperfecta, enamel hyperplasia, and other abnormalities of tooth structure.

B. Oral Injuries

1. *Attrition.* Attrition due to bruxism is particularly common among individuals with cerebral palsy and mental retardation.[21]
2. *Trauma to Teeth and Soft Tissues.* Trauma to teeth and soft tissues may result from accidents (instability, falling), self-abuse, or seizures. The individual with epilepsy is particularly susceptible to accidents. Chipped and fractured teeth as well as residual scars in the tongue and lips may be seen frequently.

    Because of personal limitations and living a protected life, many patients with disabilities are not exposed to contact sports, traffic accidents, and other accident-prone situations. The incidence of facial trauma may be expected to be less.

C. Facial Weakness or Paralysis

When a patient has muscle weakness or paralysis of one side of the face, it is not possible to masticate bilaterally. Plaque usually collects more heavily and food debris is retained on the involved side. Certain patients may have bilateral weakness.

D. Malocclusion

An increased incidence of malocclusion has been reported among people with developmental disabilities.[19,21,22] Factors contributing to problems of occlusion include skeletal and muscular deformities, oral habits such as tongue thrust, macroglossia, mouth breathing, and/or congenitally missing teeth.

E. Dental Caries

Survey summaries vary, so generalizations cannot be made concerning the prevalence of dental caries. Studies have shown a high incidence of untreated dental caries as well as many missing teeth, which appears to be a reflection of the type of dental care the patient has or has not received. The dentist may have been unable to cope with the problems presented by the individual with a handicap and, therefore, more extractions than restorations were performed.[23]

The more fortunate patients with fewer carious lesions and extractions may have lived in a community with fluoridated water or had the benefit of supplements such as tablets, rinses, or topical fluoride applications professionally. They may also have had knowledgeable parents who were able to control the exposures to carbohydrates in the diet.

F. Gingival and Periodontal Diseases[24,25]

Gingival and periodontal diseases have been shown to be increased in incidence, especially among individuals with mental retardation and those with physical conditions that prevent daily self-care. Patients with Down's Syndrome have an increased incidence of severe periodontal disease with bone loss at an earlier age than other individuals with mental retardation (page 736).

Many patients with disabilities have poor oral hygiene and heavy calculus deposits. Factors related to plaque control are described on page 698 and calculus is discussed on page 711.

G. Therapy-related Oral Findings

1. *Phenytoin-induced Gingival Overgrowth.* Patients whose treatment for seizures requires phenytoin (Dilantin) are susceptible to a slight to severe gingival enlargement. The severity of the enlargement is usually dependent on the maintenance of healthy gingival tissue associated with adequate daily plaque control. A description of phenytoin-induced gingival overgrowth is included in Chapter 52, page 724.

2. *Chemotherapy.* Oral ulcerations, mucositis, and susceptibility to infection are frequent manifestations following cancer chemotherapy (pages 676–677). Patients with leukemia have a high incidence of oral manifestations, including lymphadenopathy, gingival changes with bleeding, and petechiae, more severe following chemotherapy. In Hodgkin's Disease, an increased incidence of necrotizing ulcerative gingivitis has been noted along with other oral problems.[26]

3. *Radiation Therapy.* When radiation therapy of the head and neck area involves the cells of the salivary glands, xerostomia can result and contribute to an increased incidence of dental caries. The symptoms and treatment aspects of radiation therapy are described on pages 674–676.

IV. Dental Hygiene Treatment Plan

Parts of the total treatment plan that are to be accomplished by the dental hygienist can be identified under educational, therapeutic, and preventive services. Choice of procedures depends on the findings of the clinical examination, and will include some or all of the items listed below.

A. Educational

1. Patient orientation to each dental hygiene and dental procedure.
2. Parental counseling starting as early as possible when an infant is known to have a disability.
3. Instruction in disease control
   a. Plaque control for natural teeth and appliances.
   b. Daily fluoride: systemic and/or topical.
   c. Dietary and nutritional effects.

B. Therapeutic

1. Patient's plaque control for therapeutic purposes until tissue health is attained.
2. Complete scaling and root planing.
3. Removal of overhanging fillings.
4. Gingival curettage.
5. Reevaluation for additional periodontal therapy.
6. Restorative phase; polishing restorations.

C. Preventive Therapy

1. Fluoride program
   a. Supervision of self-applied daily fluoride.
   b. Periodic professionally topically applied fluoride.
2. Pit and fissure sealants.
3. Use of artificial saliva for xerostomia.

DISEASE PREVENTION AND CONTROL

I. Preventive Program Components[27,28,29]

A. Plaque control.
B. Fluorides.
C. Pit and fissure sealants.
D. Diet counseling.
E. Regular professional examinations and treatment at intervals as recommended by the dentist and dental hygienist.

II. Functioning Levels

For a patient who does not have a mental or physical disability, personal oral hygiene neglect usually can be explained by either a lack of knowledge and understanding about the need for plaque removal and how it is accomplished, or a lack of motivation to carry out the necessary daily routines. For certain patients with disabilities, the problem of disease control becomes greatly magnified because of a lack of the necessary mental and/or physical coordination to carry out even the simplest of oral hygiene measures.

Depending on the severity of the disability, many patients need either complete or partial assistance. Assistance must be provided by parents and other family members when living at home, or by an aide or other person responsible for the patient's care in a residence or institutional setting. The dental hygienist has a twofold responsibility to teach and supervise the patient and those who care for the patient. Suggestions for in-service education are on page 707.

A *high, moderate* or *low* functioning level refers to what daily living skills (bathing, toothbrushing, dressing, for examples) an individual can do alone, what range or degree of assistance is needed, or whether the person is dependent on others for complete care. The functioning levels have also been called *self-care, partial-care,* or *total care.*[30] In another concept, the terms *supervised, supervised/assistance,* and *maintenance (by others)* have been used.[31]

A. High Functioning Level

The high functioning, self-care group are those capable of flossing and brushing their own teeth. Many, particularly children and patients of all ages who are mentally retarded, will need varying degrees of encouragement, motivation, and supervision.

B. Moderate Functioning Level

The moderate functioning, partial-care group are those capable of carrying out at least part of their oral hygiene needs, but who require considerable training, assistance, and direct supervision. The assistance may be verbal, gestural, or hand-over-hand.

C. Low Functioning Level

The low functioning, total care group are those unable to attend to their own care, and therefore are dependent. Patients in this group may be bedridden and nonambulatory, although others may be confined to wheelchairs. With training, some may be able to attempt a part of their own care.

III. Preparation for Instruction

A. Basic Planning Questions

1. What is the patient's functioning level?
2. Will the patient do all or part of the plaque removal personally or require partial or total care?
3. Is the patient involved in any community dental health programs (home, school, or day activity) and can the dentist and/or dental hygienist in such a program be contacted to coordinate the instruction given?
4. Will the parent or attendant do part or all of the oral care?
5. What disabilities have the greatest influence on the extent of self-care possible and the anticipated success of the overall preventive program? Mental? physical? sensory? learning? oral?
6. Which techniques and procedures will best fit the situation of the particular patient and the parent or attendant?
7. How can the patient be helped to be as independent as possible?

B. Introduction

From the answers to the questions above, an initial plan is made, with the realization that the system is on a trial and error basis. As the skills of the patient and parent improve and less plaque is observed and recorded on succeeding appointments, adaptations can be made. In the meantime, communication improves and the patient's trust develops as the sincere concern of the dental hygienist is realized.

For all patients, with or without a disability, the aim is complete daily plaque control. Such an ideal result may seem far from reality with a moderate- or low-functioning person, but with continuing reinforcement and inspiration, progress can be made. Patient and parental attitudes, willingness to participate, and acceptance of the recommended procedures must be taken into consideration.

PLAQUE CONTROL METHODS

I. Components

General procedures for instruction and methods for toothbrushing, interdental plaque removal, and care of fixed and removable prostheses were described in Chapters 22 through 27. Individualization for each patient's needs and abilities is necessary. Each step must be explained slowly and carefully.

A. Provide Basic Information

Plaque formation and disease development is described on a level at which the patient and parent can learn and be motivated.

B. Disclose and Show Plaque

An on-going record of the extent of plaque in graphic form by which the patient and parent can watch progress may help to motivate many patients.

C. Toothbrushing

1. Provide a soft toothbrush and ask patient to remove the disclosed plaque from the teeth. For the completely dependent patient, the parent will demonstrate. Alternative positions for the parent are described in Section IV, on page 704.
2. Brushing procedure: plaque removal is more important than the specific technique used, as long as damage is not done to the gingiva or teeth. A scrub-brush or circular Fones' method is usually appropriate and within the capability of most patients (pages 349–350).
3. Adaptations for brush handles and other devices to promote or make possible a patient's independent performance are described on pages 700–702.
4. Patients who are carriers of hepatitis or who have any known communicable disease should keep their toothbrushes and related materials apart and use a separate sink from other people in the same residence. The use of a powered brush would be contraindicated because of aerosol formation. Nonimmune direct care personnel should protect themselves with gloves and mask when helping with or performing plaque control for a patient with a communicable disease.

D. Dentifrice

When a dentifrice is used, one that contains fluoride can be recommended. An ingestible dentifrice may prove useful. The factors to consider when deciding whether a standard noningestible dentifrice should be used include the following:[27]

1. When a patient cannot rinse or expectorate, a dentifrice should not be used. The person who is institutionalized and severely handicapped may be treated with a suction brush as described on pages 718–719.
2. When a parent, aide, or other person is performing the brushing,
   a. The paste may limit visibility for thorough plaque removal.
   b. When a paste is used, the brushing has to be done near a sink where rinsing is possible, which may not be convenient for a patient in a seated or supine position.
3. Dentifrice may increase gag reflex for certain patients.
4. For the patient whose problem is brush manipulation, and for whom special adaptations of the brush are recommended, management of the dentifrice may be awkward and messy.
5. Dentifrice is not essential to plaque removal, and other means for daily fluoride application may prove easier for certain patients. A brush-on gel or tray with gel may be recommended.

E. Dental Floss

With time and continued instruction, many patients with disabilities can learn to use dental floss, and some will learn to use other interdental aids. The use of a floss holder can make flossing possible for certain patients, such as those with limited digital dexterity or the use of only one hand.

The holder may also be useful for the parent or other person who cares for the patient. Floss holders were described on page 362. Methods for increasing the size of a toothbrush handle may be adapted for the handle of a floss holder.

II. Evaluation

Many patients, parents, and direct care personnel can learn with demonstration and practice how to examine the teeth and gingiva. The signs of healthy gingiva can be noted; especially color and absence of bleeding on brushing.

For most patients, the brushing thoroughness can be improved if a disclosing agent is used at the start. The visible objective then is to remove all of the color. Another system is to apply a disclosing agent after brushing to determine completion of plaque removal, and then brush any additional plaque noted.

When a patient brushes first, followed by the parent or direct care person, the disclosing agent might be applied by the parent so the task of removal can be completed. Since the patient is encouraged to do as much as possible and praised for whatever successes are accomplished, the plaque disclosed for the parent to remove may be a factor of discouragement to the patient who really had done the very best to the extent of individual capability. A better plan could be for the patient to do all of the brushing and flossing once a day, and for the parent to do it all at a different time.

III. Self-care Aids

Although a parent or attendant may be willing to brush the patient's teeth, as much as possible should be carried out by the patient. Psychologic benefits to the patient result in feelings of self-esteem and accomplishment when able to manage the important and worthwhile task of brushing.

For patients of all ages whose main deterrent to personal self-care is related to grasp, manipulation, or control of a toothbrush, adaptations of the brush have been devised.[32,33,34,35] Modifications to accommodate specific needs include enlarged handles, hand attachments, and elongated handles.

A. General Prerequisites for a Self-care Aid
1. Cleanable.
2. Durable: can withstand exposure to water and saliva.
3. Resistant to absorption of oral fluids.

B. For Patient with Fingers Permanently Fixed in a Fist

Insert the brush handle into the grasp.

C. For Patient Who Cannot Grasp and Hold
1. *Objective:* to fasten the brush handle to the open hand

2. *Methods*

   a. Velcro strap around hand with a slit on the palm side to insert the brush handle. A vinyl pocket with an adjustable velcro strap is commercially available. The toothbrush handle fits into the pocket (figure 50–3A). The device is used to hold other utensils for the patient, such as eating utensils.[36]

   b. Handle of fingernail brush attached to toothbrush by adhesive water-resistant tape (figure 50–3B).

   c. Wide rubber strap or a length of small-diameter rubber tubing attached through the hole in the toothbrush handle and tied adjacent to the brush head so the patient's hand can be slipped under the rubber and be held firmly (figure 50–3C).

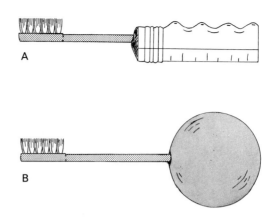

A

B

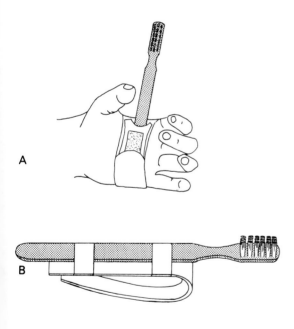

A

B

C

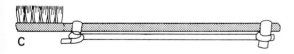

C

Figure 50–3. Aids for a patient who cannot grasp and hold. **A.** adjustable velcro strap around hand has pocket to hold the toothbrush handle. **B.** Handle of fingernail brush attached to toothbrush by adhesive tape. **C.** Rubber tubing attached firmly to toothbrush handle to hold brush across the palm of the patient's hand. A floss holder may be held by any of these methods.

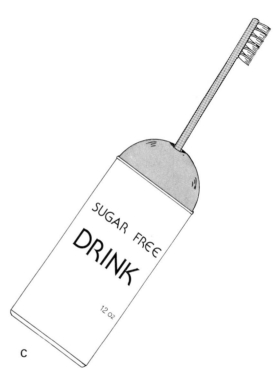

C

Figure 50–4. Aids for a patient with limited hand closure or grasp. **A.** Toothbrush inserted into a bicycle handle grip. **B.** Toothbrush inserted into a soft rubber ball. **C.** Toothbrush in soft rubber ball inserted into a juice or pop can.

D. For Patient with Limited Hand Closure (unable to manipulate usual toothbrush handle or floss holder)

1. *Objective:* enlarge the diameter of the handle

2. *Methods*

   a. Bicycle handle grip: insert toothbrush handle (figure 50–4A).

b. Soft rubber ball: push brush handle in (figure 50–4B).

c. Juice or pop can: place the rubber ball with toothbrush inside the can (figure 50–4C).

d. Foam rubber hair roller: insert brush handle.

e. Quick-cure acrylic: Obtain an impression of the patient's hand grasp by having him grasp a cylinder of base plate wax; then fill the wax cylinder with quick-cure acrylic. Insert the toothbrush handle before the acrylic sets. The angle may be adjusted to set the brush head for the patient's convenient use. Polish the acrylic.

E. For Patient Unable to Lift Hand or Arm (with limited shoulder or elbow movement)

1. *Objective:* lengthen the handle of the brush.

2. *Prerequisite:* the material must be strong or rigid enough to maintain the brush contact with sufficient lateral pressure to remove plaque from the tooth surfaces.

3. *Methods*

a. Cylinder of wood with brush handle cemented inside.[35]

b. Two brushes: cut the head from an old used brush and fasten the handle to the end of the new brush handle (glue, tape, heat).

c. Tongue depressors taped to the brush handle, then one or two other tongue depressors taped to overlap and provide an extension.

d. Commercially available stiff metal extender with bolt attachment and wing nut to attach through a hole in the toothbrush. Brush may be used full length or cut off.[36]

e. Bicycle spoke, coat hanger, or other means for elongation fixed with a handle of acrylic resin. The metal tip may be heated and pushed into the toothbrush handle.[32,33] Use double or triple thickness to avoid flexibility.

F. For Patient Who Can Hold and Position the Toothbrush But Cannot Manipulate To Make Strokes for Plaque Removal

Guide patient to learn to move the head

up and down or from side to side while brush is held against the teeth.[33]

G. Use of a Powered Toothbrush

A powered brush can serve as a motivational adjunct for selected patients (page 353). For an uncoordinated patient, a powered brush could be harmful. The various models present different characteristics.

1. *Advantages and Disadvantages*[38]

a. The extra weight of the handle may prove advantageous for some patients and not for others with limited arm strength.

b. The on/off mechanism may require more strength and finger coordination to operate than certain patients can manage.

c. The brush handle is thick, and therefore helpful for a patient with grasping problems.

d. The vibration created during use could not be tolerated by certain patients.

2. *Suggestions for Use*

a. For use without hands: attach the brush handle by means of a clamp in a stationary upright position lower than the patient's mouth when bending down. Patient can insert the brush and apply to the teeth, moving the head for application to all surfaces. The use of a dentifrice probably would be contraindicated, since splashing might be uncontrollable.

b. An elastic cuff around the hand and the brush can aid in brush control.

3. *Institutional Use.* Although not possible for many institutionalized patients to use for themselves, direct care staffs have found powered brushes effective in certain situations.[39,40,41] One handle for 10 or 12 clients has been used. Handles must be replaced promptly when out of order, which may present problems in some institutions.

Cross-contamination is a problem even when individual tips are labeled, washed, and kept apart. Handles have to be sanitized routinely between brushings. Special instruction for the direct care people is necessary, and repeated motivation for any toothbrushing program is important. Using a powered brush is not encouraged by many dental hygienists associated with long-term care institutions.

H. Cleaning Removable Dental Appliances[34,35,37]

The details for cleaning removable appliances were described on pages 391–393. The same materials and procedures are recommended for the patient with a handicap or other person who will care for the appliance. Management of both the appliance and the brush requires attention and skill, and instruction in methods that will prevent accidents is necessary. In all procedures, the sink must be partially filled with water and/or a face cloth or small towel be placed in the sink to serve as a cushion if the denture should be dropped.

1. For the patient with difficulty grasping or holding the brush, a denture brush handle may be adapted by any of the methods described for the regular toothbrush (figure 50–4). A fingernail brush may be used instead of a standard denture brush, provided all denture surfaces can be reached for plaque removal.
2. For the patient handicapped by hemiplegia or the patient with use of two hands but who needs to grasp the denture with two hands to prevent accidents, the following are recommended:
    a. Denture brush with suction cups to attach low inside the sink bowl (figure 50–5B).
    b. Fingernail brush with suction cups.
    c. Denture brush in mounting that has suction cups. These are available commercially (figure 50–5A).[36]

IV. Instruction For Direct-care Person

The individual who needs partial or total care will present with varying degrees of ability to cooperate, depending on the nature of the handicap. The size of the patient and whether the patient is ambulatory, bedridden, or in a wheelchair are among the factors that influence the technique for management.

The instruction for the parents or the other direct-care persons should be given where the

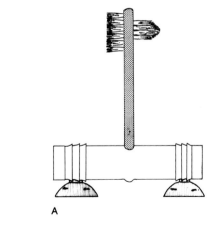

A

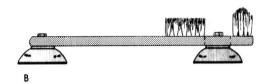

B

Figure 50–5.   Denture brushes with suction cups. **A.** Denture brush in commercially available mounting. **B.** Suction cups attached to the denture brush. The brush may be positioned in the sink to aid the person with one hand, or who needs to grasp the denture with two hands to prevent accidents.

specific techniques can actually be demonstrated as they will be done at home, rather than attempting to use a dental chair. When the patient will lie down with the head in the parent's lap, for example, a suitable couch should be used, or chairs can be placed together. Time and repeated practice sessions are needed for successful plaque removal for a difficult patient.

A. Self-care and Attitude

Whenever possible, instruction for the parents, other family members, or direct-care persons begins with their own personal oral care. The most success will come when those who care for the patient have knowledge and understanding of the purposes and techniques and can demonstrate their own plaque removal.

An appreciation for the need for preventive care, and why the health of the teeth and gingiva are of great importance to the well-being and overall health of the patient, can help those responsible to develop the patience and take the necessary time from their own busy schedules.

B. **General Suggestions**

1. *Place.* The plaque removal procedures need to be performed where both the patient and the parent can be comfortable and relaxed. A bathroom may be the least desirable place, since positioning the patient may be awkward except when a standing position can be used.

    Good light, easy visibility of the teeth, and control of the head of the person with the disability are prerequisites.

2. *Teaching Techniques for Plaque Removal*

    a. Use of finger and hand rests. The person performing the plaque removal needs to learn how to balance the toothbrush, dental floss, floss aid, or any other implement with a finger or hand rest on the side of the patient's face or chin. Such contact contributes to total patient control in addition to effective use of the plaque removal device.

    b. Use of a mouth prop. For certain patients, plaque removal will be impossible without a mouth prop, and demonstration for insertion on both sides will be needed. For home use, a washable, rubber prop will be practical.

C. **Positions**

    General positions are suggested below which involve one or two people.[27,30,32,42] When the patient is young, hyperactive, and unable to cooperate and assistance of a second person is not available, the use of a blanket or sheet wrap may be necessary (page 694).

    In the descriptions below, the term "parent" is used to mean whichever family member or other direct-care person may be performing the plaque removal.

1. *Parent Standing.* With the parent standing from behind, the arm is brought around the patient's head and the chin is cupped while using the thumb and index finger to retract the lips and cheeks. The other hand will apply the toothbrush, floss aid, or other device. This technique requires that the patient be able to bend the head back far enough for the parent to see the maxillary teeth. The procedure may be applicable for the following:

    a. Short patient standing in front of, backed up to, the parent.

    b. Tall patient seated in a chair with the head tipped back to lean against the parent, or seated in a large chair or sofa with the head stabilized against the top of chair back.

    c. Patient in a wheelchair leaning back against the parent. Wheelchair brakes are set.

2. *Parent Seated*

    a. Patient seated on pillow on floor in front of parent, with back close to the chair and head turned back into parent's lap (figure 50–6A). The parent may place his/her legs over the shoulders of the patient to restrain arms and body movements (figure 50–6B).

    b. Parent is seated at the end of a sofa or couch and patient is lying down with the head in parent's lap (figure 50–6C).

    c. For a bedridden patient, the parent may sit at the patient's head and place the head in the lap. When it is necessary to control body and arm movements, the parent can sit beside the patient, lean across the patient's chest, and hold the patient's arm against the body with the elbow. The hand of the restraining arm can hold the mouth prop, retract, or whatever is necessary. If the patient is particularly difficult, a sheet or blanket wrap would be indicated.

3. *Two People.* In any of the positions previously mentioned, the parent may need the assistance of a second person to hold the hands and arms or otherwise restrain the patient.

    A small child may be placed across the laps of two persons seated facing each other. One stabilizes the head and brushes and flosses while the other per-

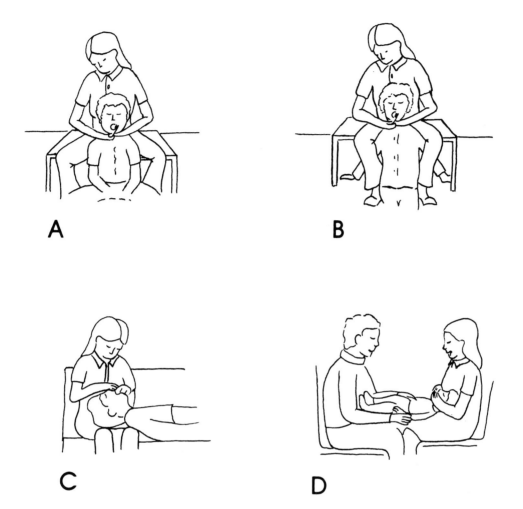

Figure 50–6. Positions for child or disabled patient for plaque control by parent or other direct-care person. **A.** Patient seated on floor with head turned back into parent's lap. **B.** Patient's arms restrained by legs of parent. **C.** Patient reclining with head in parent's lap. **D.** Two people participating with small child between. One holds the patient for stabilization, while the other holds the head and performs toothbrushing and flossing.

son holds hands, arms, legs, as needed (figure 50–6D).

FLUORIDES

Selection of a multiple fluoride program for an individual patient is dependent on the age, the caries status, and the concentration of fluoride in the water supply. In addition, for a patient with a handicap, the abilities to cooperate, to accept the vehicle and mode of application, and to master the technique required for a self-administered preparation, will dictate the final recommendation. Detailed reference tables have

been prepared by a special fluorides task force of the National Foundation of Dentistry for the Handicapped.[43]

I. Fluoridation

A. Community Water Fluoridation

As more communities begin to fluoridate the water supplies, more of the total population, including persons with handicaps, will benefit.

B. Institutional Water Fluoridation

Research has shown the benefits derived

from fluoridation of a school water supply when the community in which the school is located cannot or does not have fluoridation. These programs were summarized in Chapter 29, page 446.

Institutions where individuals with disabilities reside may have a water supply that could be fluoridated. Installation is a relatively inexpensive procedure when the health benefits and the decreased need for professional care are realized.

II. Dietary Supplements

When the community water supply is deficient in fluoride content, the fluoride level is below optimum, or the water intake by a child is low, a supplement is recommended as described on page 448. Depending on the masticatory function of the child, whether chewing or rinsing is possible, the fluoride can be prescribed in the form of a chewable tablet, lozenge, drops, or mouthwash to swallow after swishing.

III. Professionally Applied Topical Fluoride

When there is no water fluoridation, or to supplement the benefits of water fluoridation, at least two topical applications per year are indicated, and more frequently if the dental caries rate is high. The method for application and system for isolation of the teeth will depend on the patient's ability to cooperate.

IV. Self-applied Procedures

Whether the individual with a disability is a child or an adult, a home fluoride program is indicated.

After disease control techniques for flossing and toothbrushing have been completed before the patient retires, either a mouthrinse, for the patient who can rinse, a gel applied by tray or toothbrush, or a chewable tablet, for the patient who can chew and who needs a fluoride supplement may be advised. For a young, dependent, low-functioning person, brushing with a gel or swabbing with a fluoride rinse might be most applicable.

Parental supervision and cooperation are essential. Motivation of the parent or direct care person needs regular reinforcement by the dental team.

PIT AND FISSURE SEALANTS

Pit and fissure sealants have been used for children with developmental disabilities with satisfactory results.[44,45] The principles for application are the same as those described for all patients (page 468). The use of a rubber dam is especially important for patients with excess saliva, hyperactivity of the tongue, or other management difficulties.

When a severely disabled patient will be having general anesthesia for restorative procedures, the pit and fissure sealant should be placed in all noncarious occlusal surfaces while the patient is under control. For all young patients, the sealant can be placed as soon after eruption as the tooth will hold a rubber dam.[27]

DIET INSTRUCTION

Efforts to help adults who are disabled and the parents, family members, advocates, and others responsible to understand the general dietary requirements for oral health and how to put the principles into daily practice are a distinct part of the total preventive program. Information from Chapter 28 is applicable to patients with special needs as well as to all patients.

A careful analysis of current habits and knowledge, family customs, and economic factors as they relate to a patient's condition is necessary before specific recommendations can be made. In an institutional setting, efforts can be directed to contact and work with the administrative people, teachers, dietitians, and aides. Coordination of plaque control, snack selection, as well as snack availability, together with the fluoride program, opens the way to caries control.

A. Factors That Influence Diet Habits

For certain patients, diet selection and utilization centers around problems of mastication; while with others, the transport of food to the mouth is a major undertaking. The problems of the elderly were described on pages 631–633.

The following partial list of problems is suggested to help during dietary analysis and counseling. Many of the problems are directly related to increases in plaque accumulation and resultant dental caries and periodontal diseases.

1. Masticatory or feeding problems, which can result in the use of a soft diet, often composed mainly of carbohydrates.

2. Overindulgence in sucrose-containing foods, particularly as rewards or bribes by unsuspecting family members or teachers involved in behavior modification procedures in training programs.

3. Inability to accomplish personal plaque control measures on a daily basis because of physical disability or lack of assistance from a parent or aide, combined with a diet high in cariogenic foods, which has led to dental caries development.

4. Lack of professional care and instruction due to unavailability, inability to obtain care because of physical barriers, inadequate financial support, lack of knowledge of the importance of oral health, or preoccupation with other major health problems.

5. Nonambulatory or otherwise confined patient may have less access to between-meal foods, therefore may eat more regularly, as served. On the other hand, the confined person may have snacks and sweets readily available, which can lead to dental destruction.

6. Medications may influence diet
   a. Limitations because of chronic diseases, allergies, or inborn errors of metabolism.
   b. Medications with a side effect of xerostomia contribute to dental caries.
   c. Medications that diminish appetite as a side effect.
   d. Medications contained within a sucrose base designed to mask the flavor of the agent or to pacify the patient.

7. Obesity is a problem with certain patients who suffer from inactivity, overeating, boredom, or lack of knowledge of proper food selection.

8. Difficulty of food preparation can be a major limitation to diet selection for adults with neuromuscular disorders. Wheelchair confinement, lack of muscular coordination, hemiplegia or paraplegia, and dependence on others for grocery shopping are examples of problems encountered.

B. Diet Analysis and Counseling

1. *Food Diary.* A high-functioning patient, except the very young, may be able to keep the food diary, and participation should be encouraged. The parent, advocate, or other responsible person can assist, or in the case of a low or moderate functioning person, may complete the entire diary. With the diary and the information from the medical and dental histories, items for counseling can be selected.

2. *Recommendations.* General procedures for analysis and counseling were described on pages 428–432. Adaptations involve long-range planning for gradual modification of each patient's diet. The person who selects and prepares the food must be involved in the planning. Sugarless snacks and sugarless rewards during behavior modification training are especially important to control.

   Parents need instruction as early as possible after a newborn is known to be developmentally disabled, so that fluoride, diet, early personal hygiene, and the prevention of nursing caries syndrome can be coordinated into the daily program.

GROUP IN-SERVICE EDUCATION

Dental hygienists are called upon to carry out in-service education in a variety of situations. In-service programs may be provided for teachers, registered nurses, other health professionals, parents, and volunteers in school and community preventive programs. For example, all of those mentioned could be involved in the preparation for a program of classroom weekly rinsing with a fluoride mouthrinse. When a program is citywide and many dental hygienists are involved, in-service preparation for the dental hygienists themselves is necessary.

There is a special need for in-service instruction in oral health measures for the direct-care personnel in extended care institutions. Many patients in such facilities are unable to care for their own needs and may require total care, partial assistance, supervision, or regular reminders. The dental hygienist is able to work with the direct-care personnel to teach them appropriate techniques and to motivate them to incorporate oral care into the daily routine for each resident or patient.

The general suggestions outlined below pertain to preparation and content for in-service workshops for the oral care of long-term patients. To supplement this brief introduction, a section of the *Suggested Readings* at the end of this chapter contains references that describe programs where in-service education has been included.

I. Preparation for an In-Service Program

An in-service program needs careful planning. For many groups, time for in-service is taken from an already busy work schedule. Nonmotivated participants require special considerations. The most important factor contributing to the success of a program is the genuine concern and enthusiasm of the dental hygienist in motivating the participants.[46]

The material must be clear and to the point, interestingly presented with appropriate visual aids, and stimulating for learning. Objectives should be defined in writing and serve as a guide to preparation and evaluation. Problems of the staff must be recognized. Some members may have negative oral health attitudes, minimal educational background, and poor personal oral health.

Initially, basic preparation would include learning about the functioning levels of the clients and assessing the procedures used for their oral care. A survey of the plaque control materials and devices available and in current use, methods for labeling or storing individual brushes, and the frequency of use is important.

Clinic records for each patient should be examined for information relative to the dental status and to those who wear dentures. Medical histories must be reviewed so that special general or oral health problems can be considered and necessary precautions taken. For example, disposable gloves will be needed when dealing with certain groups because of the higher incidence of hepatitis carriers.

When a dental hygienist is employed regularly within an institution, a much more complete assessment can be made. The dental hygienist invited to the institution for the specific purpose of presenting the workshop might only have a telephone conversation with the supervisor to determine facts about the residents and their oral health.

The use of a gingival or plaque index (pages 299–309) can provide a baseline of information from which progress can be evaluated.[47] The direct-care personnel could carry out the daily plaque control program and see the changes that take place by comparing survey results at a later date. Such continuing participation could provide a real motivation to the group.

II. Program Content

A. The Participants' Own Plaque Control

Based on the premise that people who are motivated to care for their own mouths have a clearer understanding of the effects and importance of oral care and give a higher priority to the time spent daily, an in-service education group needs to participate in a personal plaque control program. A plaque-free score (page 305) or other evaluation device can be used. A group may be willing to work in pairs and learn to evaluate and score each other, thereby learning the techniques to be applied to their clients.

B. Facts About Etiology and Prevention

Basic information about plaque, its formation, and how gingivitis and dental caries develop will be important to most groups. The progress of disease from reversible gingivitis to severe periodontitis can be explained, as can the process of dental caries from a small cavity to a diseased pulp. Prevention through plaque control, fluoride, dietary controls, sealants, and early treatment for restorations must be carefully presented. Handout materials and colorful visual aids will promote learning.

C. Oral Examination

1. *Oral Mucosa.* Techniques demonstrated and practiced by the participants on each other should include the use of a tongue depressor to retract and a disposable mirror and a light source to see the oral mucosa. How to hold the tongue, using

a sponge to lift and inspect all parts can be shown. Patients with dentures need the supporting tissues examined periodically by the dentist, but the direct-care person will be able to notice changes that should be called to the dentist's attention on a day-to-day basis while cleaning and massaging the mucosa under the denture.

2. *Gingiva.* Color, size, and bleeding that occurs spontaneously or while brushing can be explained and demonstrated. When projection is possible, slides can be included for all aspects of the instructional material. When a camera is available for intraoral photography, "before" and "after" pictures of the patients can be shown. Changes effected by the plaque control supervised by the direct-care aides will be more meaningful than pictures of strangers.

3. *Dental Plaque.* Inspection for plaque can be demonstrated when the disclosing agent is used prior to plaque scoring and removal.

4. *Dentures.* Sample dentures may be used to help the participants learn to examine each denture for cracks or sharp edges. Examination for deposits can be made by the patient and the direct-care person and compared with the denture after it has been cleaned.

D. Techniques of Mouth Care and Disease Control

Staff members can be trained to work in pairs.[48] Working in pairs is more efficient, particularly in the care of difficult patients.

A plan for each client can be worked out with the aides so that individual problems relative to dental caries prevention, gingival disease control, or complete or partial denture care can be solved. Teaching some or all of the following may be included, depending on the needs of the clients.

1. *Plaque Control.* Instruction includes positioning of the patient (pages 704–705), application of disclosing agent, examination for plaque on the teeth, toothbrush selection and use, use of a mouth prop, and flossing with or without a floss aid. The use of a portable or bedside suction unit for removing debris from a patient's mouth, can be practiced by a paired team.[48]

2. *Fluoride Application.* The objectives and techniques for brushing with a gel, swabbing with a mouthrinse, assisting the patient with a chewable tablet, or applying a gel tray can be included.

3. *Denture Care.* Care of dentures and of the mucosa under the denture are shown.

4. *Saliva Substitute.* Use of saliva substitute for dry mouth is demonstrated.

E. Denture Marking Procedure

Not all members of the staff need to learn the technique for marking dentures for personal identification. Since dentures should be marked soon after arrival, personnel involved with admissions of new clients or patients are most in need of the instruction. In a large hospital or rehabilitation center, new dentures made in the dental clinic would be marked during processing. The techniques for denture marking are outlined in Chapter 46 pages 643–645.

III. Records

A record form to be completed for each client is essential to follow-up and evaluation. During the instruction periods, the staff can learn how to complete the record and where to file the copies.

The form can be designed with spaces to record information obtained during the oral examination, the functioning level and degree of cooperation, the procedures needed for dental caries control, periodontal health, and/or denture care. In addition, the instruction provided, the implements and materials used, the planned future instruction, the prognosis, and any other personal notes, can be included.

IV. Follow-up

After direct-care personnel have had an opportunity to try their newly learned procedures, an opportunity to have questions answered should be provided. Direct observation by the dental hygienist of techniques performed with and for the clients, advice concerning oral problems of particular patients, and corrections when necessary can motivate and encourage both client and aide.

Disclosing and recording the plaque for comparison of scores before and after the program can show the progress being made.

V. Continuing Education

A. Individual instruction should be provided for each new employee during the orientation period for that employee.
B. Periodic updating for all employees can be accomplished by presenting new and review information at regular intervals. Questions and problems can be discussed, and plans introduced for changing a certain procedure based on new research evidence.
C. A specific plan for scheduled oral health programs may be a requirement for licensure of a health care facility.[49]

INSTRUMENTATION

Customary techniques must be adapted. With basic knowledge of methods for maintaining patient stability, adequate visibility of working area, secure instrument grasps and finger rests, and well controlled strokes, instrumentation for calculus removal and root planing can be effectively accomplished.

Patients who are hyperactive, lack muscular control, or have a mental deficiency provide many challenges. With some patients, the tasks of keeping the head and mouth positioned, the profuse saliva and the oversized or hyperactive tongue controlled may seem insurmountable. Patience, a gentle but firm touch, and continuing experience are essential.

I. Preparation For Instrumentation

A. Premedication

1. Antibiotic coverage as indicated for susceptible patients (pages 99–100).
2. Sedative for control of selected patients.

B. Plaque Control Instruction Precedes Scaling

1. Disclose and present or review information on plaque.
2. Continue practice on plaque removal methods that were selected for the particular patient. The patient, parent, attendant demonstrate.

II. Stabilization

For certain patients, opening the mouth is difficult and maintaining the mouth in an open position is impossible. A mouth prop can be used to assist the patient. Verbal encouragement of the patient must continue throughout the appointment.

A. Ratchet Type (Molt's Mouth Gag)

The preferred, most stable mouth prop is a sterilizable prop that can be nearly closed for insertion between the teeth. It can gradually be opened to hold the jaws at the necessary position. The tips are covered with rubber tubing and are positioned over the maxillary and mandibular teeth on one side while the operator treats the opposite side.

B. Rubber Bite Block

A long piece of dental floss should be tied through the holes in a commercially available rubber mouth prop, so that, in case of a sudden respiratory change, the prop can be quickly pulled out and breathing normalized.

C. Tongue Depressors

A practical, disposable mouth prop can be made from three to six tongue depressors taped together. A folded sponge should be placed under the tape to provide a cushion.

D. Precautions for the Use of a Mouth Prop

1. Mobile teeth could be knocked out and aspirated
   a. Loose primary teeth in young patient.
   b. Mobile teeth in advanced periodontal disease.
2. Fatigue of the patient's facial and masticatory muscles and temporomandibular joint.
3. Patient must know that all stabilization devices are for comfort and to make the work easier and in no way meant to hurt or punish.

III. Treatment by Quadrants

For many patients, particularly those with generalized heavy supra- and subgingival calculus, treatment by quadrants under local anesthesia is the procedure of choice. Removal of calculus and overhanging fillings can be completed more efficiently by that system.

A. Scaling Requirements

At the initial appointment for dental hygiene care, many patients with handicaps are found to have generalized heavy calculus deposits. The reason is usually inadequate personal and professional care, intensified by factors related to the handicapping condition.

Certain groups have been studied, and it has been suggested that the heavy calculus deposits may be related to metabolic factors. For example, in a group of children ages 10 to 15 with cystic fibrosis, 90 percent had calculus, and in a group of the same age with asthma, 100 percent had calculus. Only 43 percent of the able-bodied children measured in the study had calculus deposits. The occurrence of calculus in the children with cystic fibrosis and asthma was believed to be related to their elevated salivary calcium and phosphorus.[50]

The objective of the technique is the complete removal of calculus and planing of root surfaces. To compromise or rationalize complete treatment is to neglect the patient's needs and to permit advanced periodontal disease to develop.

B. Anesthesia

1. *Local Anesthesia.* Profound local anesthesia is indicated to assure continued cooperation from the patient. The need for anesthesia varies with the type of disability and the age of the patient.
2. *Nitrous Oxide–Oxygen Analgesia or Psychosedation.*[51] Care must be taken to determine the patient's ability to tolerate the use of analgesia. Attention is directed especially to those with breathing, swallowing, or coughing problems. The physician's approval should be sought. A patient may be fearful of the nasal inhalor.

C. Evacuation

1. *Need for Assistance.* A dental assistant is needed while treating many types of patients with disabilities. Many patients will have excess saliva, while others will have uncontrollable tongue movements as well as general body movements, all of which can hinder instrumentation. With assistance for stabilization, visibility, and maintenance of a clear field, the procedure will be less traumatic for the patient and less timeconsuming for all.
2. *Precaution During Evacuation.* Patients such as those with chronic lung disorders, asthma, or cystic fibrosis and patients with cerebral palsy are considered "aspiration risks." For example, a sudden spasm in the facial, neck, or throat areas could cause a cerebral palsy patient to aspirate foreign matter from the mouth into the airway.

D. Instruments

1. Unbreakable mirrors are recommended for use with a patient subject to spasm or sudden closure.
2. Use of an ultrasonic scaler is contraindicated for an aspiration risk patient. It also should not be used for patients who over-react to sensory stimuli, such as a patient with autism (page 737).

E. Technique Suggestions

1. *Introduce Each Procedure and Sound to Prevent Startling a Patient.* Follow the basic instruction rule to "show, tell, then do." When a patient is blind or deaf, the rule has double significance.
2. *Finger Rests.* Firm, dependable finger rests are needed. Supplemental or reinforced rests can contribute to instrument stability. With certain patients, external finger and hand rests may be safer for the operator.[52]
3. *Periodontal Dressing.* Patients with severe or profound retardation, muscular problems, and other oral physical difficulties cannot tolerate the wearing of periodontal dressings. When treatment for phenytoin-induced gingival overgrowth is planned, a technique should be used that does not depend on a dressing for success during healing.[53]

TECHNICAL HINTS

Sources of Materials

Caring for Your Handicapped Child's Dental Health (S6)
> American Dental Association
> Order Department
> 211 East Chicago Avenue
> Chicago, Illinois 60611

Casamassimo, P.: *Toothbrushing and Flossing. A Manual of Home Dental Care for Persons Who Are Handicapped*
Nowak, A.J.: *Helping Handicapped Persons Clean Their Teeth*
> National Easter Seal Society for Crippled Children and Adults
> 2023 West Ogden Avenue
> Chicago, Illinois 60612

Schey, L.S.: *Home Dental Care for the Handicapped Child*
> New England Developmental Disabilities Communication Center
> 200 Trapelo Road
> Waltham, Massachusetts 02154

> National Foundation of Dentistry for the Handicapped and Academy of Dentistry for the Handicapped
> 1726 Champa (Suite 422)
> Denver, Colorado 80202
> Request list of available materials.

References

1. United States Developmental Disabilities Assistance and Bill of Rights Act of 1978, P.L. 95–602.
2. Hershkowitz, M.: *One in Eleven.* Handicapped Adults in America, A Survey Based on 1970 U.S. Census Data. Washington, D.C., President's Committee on Employment of the Handicapped, U.S. Government Printing Office: 1977, 0-241-016/32.
3. American Association of Dental Schools and the National Foundation of Dentistry for the Handicapped, Joint Committee: Curriculum Guidelines for Dentistry for the Handicapped, *J. Dent. Educ.*, 43, 37, September, Part 2 of 2, 1979.
4. Ettinger, R.L., Beck, J.D., and Glenn, R.E.: Eliminating Office Architectural Barriers to Dental Care of the Elderly and Handicapped, *J. Am. Dent. Assoc.*, 98, 398, March, 1979.
5. Bramer, M.L.: Barriers in Dental Practice-Architectural and Structural, *J. Am. Coll. Dent.*, 32, 315, October, 1965.
6. Hale, J., Snow, M., and Stiefel, D.J.: Providing Office Accessibility to the Disabled Patient, *J. Dent. Handicap.*, 3, 10, Summer, 1977.
7. Metal Dynamics Corporation, 9324 State Road, Philadelphia, Pennsylvania, 19114.
8. Mace, R.I.: *Accessibility Modifications.* Special Office for the Handicapped, North Carolina, Department of Insurance, pp. 43, 45.
9. Posnick, W.R. and Martin, H.H.: Wheel Chair Transfer Techniques for the Dental Office, *J. Am. Dent. Assoc.*, 94, 719, April, 1977.
10. Stiefel, D.J., Schubert, M.M., Hale, J.M., and Friedel, C.A.: *Wheelchair Transfers in the Dental Office.* Disability Dental Instruction, 4919 Northeast 86th Street, Seattle, Washington 98115, 42 pp.
11. Luke, D.J.: People with Physical and Mental Disabilities, in Boundy, S.S. and Reynolds, N.J., eds.: *Current Concepts in Dental Hygiene.* St. Louis, The C.V. Mosby Co., 1977, pp. 205–232.
12. Clark Associates, 370 Park Avenue, Worcester, Massachusetts, 01610.
13. Olympic Medical Corporation, 4400 7th Avenue South, Seattle, Washington, 98108.
14. Northup, H.L., State of Rhode Island, Department of Mental Health, Retardation, and Hospitals, Dr. Joseph H. Ladd Center, North Kingstowne, Rhode Island, personal communication, 1981.
15. Harris, F.A. and Nicholls, J.I.: An Automated Head Stabilizer to Facilitate Dental Care for Cerebral Palsied Patients, *J. Hosp. Dent. Pract.*, 12, 92, July–September, 1978.
16. Braff, M.E.: X-Raying the Handicapped Patient, *Dent. Hyg.*, 51, 449, October, 1977.
17. Posnick, W.R. and Posnick, I.H.: Dental Care in the Private Practice, in Nowak, A.J.: *Dentistry for the Handicapped Patient.* St. Louis, The C.V. Mosby Co., 1976, pp. 199–201.
18. Koster, S.: Orthodontic Treatment of Handicapped Persons, in Wei, S.H.Y. and Casko, J., eds.: *Orthodontic Care for Handicapped Persons*, Proceedings of a Workshop, University of Iowa, Iowa City, Iowa, 1977, p. 31.
19. Franks, A.S.T. and Winter, G.B.: Management of the Handicapped and Chronic Sick Patient in Dental Practice. 3—Common Dental Disorders in the Handicapped, *Br. Dent. J.*, 136, 107, February 5, 1974.
20. Jorgenson, R.J., Levin, L.S., and McKusick, V.A.: Heritable Oral Handicaps, *Dent. Clin. North Am.*, 18, 579, July, 1974.
21. Rosenbaum, C.H., McDonald, R.E., and Levitt, E.E.: Occlusion of Cerebral-Palsied Children, *J. Dent. Res.*, 45, 1696, November–December, 1966.
22. Gullikson, J.S.: Oral Findings of Mentally Retarded Children, *J. Dent. Child.*, 36, 133, March–April, 1969.
23. Nowak, A.J.: Dental Care for the Handicapped Patient—Past, Present, Future, in Nowak, A.J.: *Dentistry for the Handicapped Patient.* St. Louis, The C.V. Mosby Co., 1976, p. 11.
24. Steinberg, A.D.: Periodontal Evaluation and Treatment Considerations with the Handicapped Patient, in Nowak, A.J.: *Dentistry for the Handicapped Patient.* St. Louis, The C.V. Mosby Co., 1976, pp. 302–328.
25. Kramer, R.B.: Management of the Periodontium in Handicapped Children, *J. Dent. Handicap.*, 2, 12, Winter, 1976.
26. Sonis, S.T., Sonis, A.L., and Lieberman, A.: Oral Complications in Patients Receiving Treatment for Malignancies Other Than of the Head and Neck, *J. Am. Dent. Assoc.*, 97, 468, September, 1978.
27. Nowak, A.J.: *Dentistry for the Handicapped Patient.* St. Louis, The C.V. Mosby Co., 1976, pp. 167–192.

28. Franks, A.S.T. and Winter, G.B.: Management of the Handicapped and Chronic Sick Patient in the Dental Practice. 2—Dental Care of Handicapped Children, *Br. Dent. J.*, *136*, 62, January 15, 1974.

29. Sonnenberg, E.M. and Shey, Z.: A Review of Preventive Dentistry for the Handicapped Individual, *Clin. Prev. Dent.*, *1*, 16, July–August, 1979.

30. Troutman, K.C.: Prevention of Dental Disease for the Handicapped, in DePaola, D.P. and Cheney, H.G., eds.: *Preventive Dentistry.* Preventive Dental Handbook Series, vol. 2. Littleton, Massachusetts, PSG Publishing, 1979, pp. 205–224.

31. Meador, H.G.: Toothbrushing: A Sensible Approach for the Mentally Retarded, *Dent. Hyg.*, *53*, 462, October, 1979.

32. Albertson, D.: Prevention and the Handicapped Child, *Dent. Clin. North Am.*, *18*, 595, July, 1974.

33. Ettinger, R.L. and Pinkham, J.R.: Oral Hygiene and the Handicapped Child, *J. Int. Assoc. Dent. Child.* 9, 3, July, 1978.

34. Price, V.E.: Toothbrush Modifications for the Handicapped, *Dent. Hyg.*, *54*, 467, October, 1980.

35. Duncan, J.L.: Incorporating Oral Hygiene Procedures in Geriatric Nursing Homes, *Dent. Hyg.*, *53*, 519, November, 1979.

36. Fred Sammons Inc., Box 32, Brookfield, Illinois, 60513.

37. Ettinger, R.L. and Pinkham, J.R.: Dental Care for the Homebound—Assessment and Hygiene, *Aust. Dent. J.*, *22*, 77, April, 1977.

38. Mulligan, R.A.: Design Characteristics of Electric Toothbrushes Important to Physically Compromised Patients, *J. Dent. Res.*, *59*, 450, Abstract 731, Special Issue A, March, 1980.

39. Lucente, J.: Use of an Electric Toothbrush in Severely Retarded Children, *J. Dent. Child.*, *33*, 25, January, 1966.

40. Harrison, C.C.: Desirable Characteristics of an Electric Toothbrush for Institutional Use, *J. Periodontol.*, *39*, 270, September, 1968.

41. Miller, G.I.: Oral Health Care for the Retarded Institutional Patient: One Hospital's Experience, *J. Hosp. Dent. Pract.*, *13*, 147, Fourth Quarter, 1979.

42. McIver, F.T. and Machen, J.B.: Prevention of Dental Disease in Handicapped People, in Wessels, K.E., ed.: *Dentistry and the Handicapped Patient.* Postgraduate Dental Handbook Series, Volume 5. Littleton, Massachusetts, PSG Publishing, 1979, pp. 77–115.

43. National Foundation of Dentistry for the Handicapped, Fluorides Task Force: *A Guide To The Use of Fluorides With Alternative Recommendations for Patients With Handicaps.* 1726 Champa, Suite 422, Denver, Colorado 80202.

44. Ripa, L.W. and Cole, W.W.: Occlusal Sealing and Caries Prevention: Results 12 Months After a Single Application of Adhesive Resin, *J. Dent. Res.*, *49*, 171, January, 1970.

45. Richardson, B.A., Smith, D.C., and Hargreaves, J.A.: Study of a Fissure Sealant in Mentally Retarded Canadian Children, *Community Dent. Oral Epidemiol.*, *5*, 220, September, 1977.

46. Albertson, D. and Johnson, R.: Plaque Control for the Institutionalized Child, *J. Am. Dent. Assoc.*, *87*, 1389, December, 1973.

47. Full, C.A., Kerber, P.E., Boender, P., and Schneberger, N.: Oral Health Maintenance of the Institutionalized Handicapped Child, *J. Am. Dent. Assoc.*, *94*, 111, January, 1977.

48. Gertenrich, R.L. and Hart, R.W.: Utilization of the Oral Hygiene Team in a Mental Health Institution, *J. Dent. Child.*, *39*, 174, May–June, 1972.

49. Title 22, California Administrative Code, Section 72301 (e) and CFR 405.1129(a).

50. Wotman, S., Mercadante, J., Mandel, I.D., Goldman, R.S., and Denning, C.: The Occurrence of Calculus in Normal Children, Children with Cystic Fibrosis, and Children with Asthma, *J. Periodontol.*, *44*, 278, May, 1973.

51. Fox, L.A.: The Handicapped Child, A Prelude to Care, *Dent. Clin. North Am.*, *18*, 535, July, 1974.

52. Pattison, G. and Pattison, A.M.: *Periodontal Instrumentation. A Clinical Manual.* Reston, Virginia, Reston Publishing Co., 1979, pp. 187–189.

53. Murphy, J.B., Nersasian, R., and Clark, A.: The Management of Drug Induced Gingival Hyperplasia in Mentally Retarded Patients with Hemophilia: A Report of Two Cases, *J. Periodontol.*, *49*, 44, January, 1978.

Suggested Reading

Bender, P.A.: Behavior Management for the Special Child, in Snawder, K.D.: *Handbook of Clinical Pedodontics.* St. Louis, The C.V. Mosby Co., 1980, pp. 54–61.

Bramer, M.L.: Dental Treatment for the Severely Handicapped Child. The Handicap May be Mental, Physical, or Behavioral, *Dent. Radiogr. Photogr.*, *50*, 16, Number 1, 1977.

Brown, J.P. and Schodel, D.R.: A Review of Controlled Surveys of Dental Disease in Handicapped Persons, *J. Dent. Child.*, *43*, 313, September–October, 1976.

Cramer, J.J. and Wright, S.A.: The Bean Bag Chair and the Pedodontic Patient with Cerebral Palsy, *Dent. Hyg.*, *49*, 167, April, 1975.

Curson, I.: Dental Treatment for Handicapped Adults, *Int. Dent. J.*, *25*, 15, March, 1975.

Entwistle, B.A.: Dental Needs, in Siantz, M.L.: *The Nurse and the Developmentally Disabled Adolescent.* Baltimore, University Park Press, 1977, pp. 119–138.

Funakoshi, Y., Kushida, Y., Kanomi, R., and Hieda, T.: Dental Management of Handicapped Children, *J. Pedod.*, *4*, 249, Spring, 1980.

Giddon, D.B., Rude, C.M., and Belton, D.E.: Psychological Problems of the Physically Handicapped Patient, *Int. Dent. J.*, *25*, 199, September, 1975.

Gravois, S.L.: Inpatient Preventive Dentistry Within a Veterans Administration Medical Center, *Dent. Hyg.*, *53*, 513, November, 1979.

Hargreaves, J.A.: Preventive Dentistry for Handicapped Children, *Can. Dent. Assoc. J.*, *42*, 352, July, 1976.

Jedrychowski, J.R.: The Handicapped Patient in Dental Practice, *Dent. Hyg.*, *50*, 165, April, 1976.

Kanar, H.L.: Cerebral Palsy and Other Gross Motor or Skeletal Problems, in Wessels, K.E., ed.: *Dentistry for the Handicapped Patient.* Littleton, Massachusetts, PSG Publishing, 1979, pp. 33–62.

Kostiw, U.: Dental Hygiene Care for the Handicapped Patient, *Dent. Hyg.*, *55*, 14, January, 1981.

Leeds, J.J.: Clinical Modifications for Treatment of Handicapped Children, *J. Dent. Child.*, *43*, 42, January–February, 1976.

Libman, R.H., Coke, J.M., and Cohen, L.: Complications Related to the Administration of General Anesthesia in 600 Developmentally Disabled Dental Patients, *J. Am. Dent. Assoc.*, *99*, 190, August, 1979.

Miller, J.B. and Taylor, P.P.: A Survey of the Oral Health of a Group of Orthopedically Handicapped Children, *J. Dent. Child.*, *37*, 331, July–August, 1970.

Poland, C. and Davis, W.B.: Dental Problems of the Handicapped Child, in McDonald, R.E. and Avery, D.R.: *Dentistry for the Child and Adolescent*, 3rd ed. St. Louis, The C.V. Mosby Co., 1978, pp. 488–503.

Reiner, M.L.: Psychological Concomitants of Disability, *J. Oral Med.*, *30*, 47, April–June, 1975.

Richman, L.C. and Harper, D.C.: Observable Stigmata and Perceived Maternal Behavior, *Cleft Palate J.*, *15*, 215, July, 1978.

Smith, F.B.: Management of the Child Patient and the Handicapped Patient, in Clark, J.W., ed.: *Clinical Dentistry*, Volume 1, Chapter 33, Hagerstown, Maryland, Harper & Row, 1981, pp. 1–27.

Soble, R.K.: Sociologic and Psychologic Considerations in Special Patient Care: the Dentist, the Patient, and the Family, *Dent. Clin. North Am.*, *18*, 545, July, 1974.

Spock, B.: *Baby and Child Care*, 4th ed. New York, Hawthorn, 1976, pp. 612–627.

Willard, D.H. and Nowak, A.J.: Communicating With the Family of the Child With a Developmental Disability, *J. Am. Dent. Assoc.*, *102*, 647, May, 1981.

Plaque Control

Albertson, D. and Johnson, R.: Plaque Control for the Institutionalized Child, *J. Am. Dent. Assoc.*, *87*, 1389, December, 1973.

Clemens, C. and Taylor, S.: Toothbrushing to Music, *Dent. Hyg.*, *54*, 125, March, 1980.

Nowak, A.J.: The Effect of Dietary and Brushing Habits on Dental Caries in Noninstitutionalized Handicapped Children, *J. Dent. Handicap.*, *3*, 15, Summer, 1977.

Price, P.A.S.: An Aid for the Manipulation of Partial Dentures by Handicapped Patients, *Aust. Dent. J.*, *19*, 420, December, 1974.

Williams, B.J.: Practical Oral Hygiene for Handicapped Children, *J. Dent Child.*, *46*, 408, September–October, 1979.

Barrier-Free Environment

American Institute of Architects, 1735 New York Avenue, N.W., Washington, D.C. 20006.

American National Standard: *Specifications for Making Buildings and Facilities Accessible to and Usable by Physically Handicapped People*, ANSI A117.1-1980, American National Standards Institute, Inc., 1430 Broadway, New York, New York, 10018.

Hale, J.M., Snow, M., Stiefel, D.J., and Jones, W.C.: *The Accessible Dental Office*. Disability Dental Instruction, 4919 Northeast 86th Street, Seattle, Washington, 98115.

Kliment, S.A.: *Into the Mainstream, A Syllabus for a Barrier-Free Environment*. American Institute of Architects, and The Rehabilitation Services Administration, HEW, 1976. Superintendent of Documents, U.S. Government Printing Office, Washington, D.C. 20402.

National Center for a Barrier Free Environment, 1140 Connecticut Ave. N.W. (Suite 1006) Washington, D.C. 20036.

Selected Resources for Accessibility. Architectural and Transportation Barriers Compliance Board, Washington, D.C. 20201.

United States Department of Health, Education, and Welfare: *Technical Handbook for Facilities, Engineering and Construction Manual*. 4.00 Architectural, Section 4.12 Design of Barrier-free Facilities. Department Technical Handbook Series DHEW-TH 4.12 Barrier Free, Office of Facilities Engineering, 330 Independence Ave., S.W. Washington, D.C. 20201.

Equipment Modifications

Anderson, C.F.: Modified Dental Chair for Patients in Wheelchairs, *J. Am. Dent. Assoc.*, *74*, 1255, May, 1967.

Beach, P.: Wheelchair Transfer (Letter to the Editor), *J. Am. Dent. Assoc.*, *95*, 18, July, 1977.

Carsen, R.A.: Stable Head Support for the Wheelchair Patient, *J. Hosp. Dent. Pract.*, *4*, 112, October, 1970.

Kilfoil, J.O. and Popovitch, P.P.: Auxiliary Headrest Mounting Bracket for Handicapped Patients, *J. Prosthet. Dent.*, *38*, 347, September, 1977.

McGhay, R.M.: A Simple Headrest for Patients Confined to Wheelchairs, *J. Prosthet. Dent.*, *44*, 347, September, 1980.

McGowan, R.H.: Headrest for Patients in Wheelchairs, *Br. Dent. J.*, *136*, 203, March 5, 1974.

Smith, H.P. and King, D.L.: A Postural Support Device for Handicapped Children, *J. Dent. Handicap.*, *4*, 14, Fall/Winter, 1978.

Programs With In-Service Education

American Dental Association, Council on Dental Health and Health Planning: *Oral Health Care for the Geriatric Patient in a Long-term Care Facility: An Educational Program*. Chicago, American Dental Association, 1979, pp. 15–16, 24–32.

Block, P.L.: An Oral Care Program for Hospitalized Patients: A Project for the Dental Health Committee, *Milit. Med.*, *145*, 42, January, 1980.

Casamassimo, P.S. and Nowak, A.J.: Planning a Preventive Dentistry Program for the Handicapped Patient in an Intermediate Facility, *Rehabil. Lit.*, *38*, 251, August, 1977.

Craig, T.T. and Freedman, K.A., ed.: *Oral Health For Long-Term Care Patients*. American Society for Geriatric Dentistry, 1977.

Duncan, J.L.: Incorporating Oral Hygiene Procedures in Geriatric Nursing Homes, *Dent. Hyg.*, *53*, 519, November, 1979.

Kass, L.: Dental Health Program for the Institutionally Mentally Retarded, *Dent. Hyg.*, *53*, 76, February, 1979.

Kowitz, M.D., Ness, J.C., Campbell, J.G., Clapham, E., Moretti, G.M., Gallagher, T.M., and Spate, D.J.: Prosthetic Maintenance Research Program for the Geriatric Patient, *J. Calif. Dent. Assoc.*, *7*, 37, November, 1979.

Luke, D.J.: People with Physical and Mental Disabilities, in Boundy, S.S. and Reynolds, N.J., eds.: *Current Concepts in Dental Hygiene*. St. Louis, The C.V. Mosby Co., 1977, pp. 222–223.

Lukens, E.M., Saxton, R.N., and Bolender, C.L.: Development of a Nursing-home Dental Program, *J. Prosthet. Dent.*, *33*, 22, January, 1975.

Meador, H.G.: Toothbrushing: A Sensible Approach for the Mentally Retarded, *Dent. Hyg.*, *53*, 462, October, 1979.

Miller, G.I.: Oral Health Care for the Retarded Institutional Patient: One Hospital's Experience, *J. Hosp. Dent. Pract.*, *13*, 147, Fourth Quarter, 1979.

Moak, L.B.: Working with the Mentally Retarded, *Dent. Hyg.*, *52*, 392, August, 1978.

Nordbye, M.: Oral Prophylaxis in a Home for the Retarded Adult, *Quintessence Journal*, *2*, 33, May, 1980.

Schmidt, S.M., Leach, M., Nicolaci, A.B., Sutton, R.B., and O'Donnell, J.P.: The Dental Health Educator and Programs for Institutions with Persons Who are Mentally Retarded, *Special Care*, *1*, 174, July–August, 1981.

Thornton, M.A.: Preventive Dentistry in the Veterans Administration, *Dent. Hyg.*, *53*, 121, March, 1979.

Winchell, S.: Rancho Los Amigos Hospital—A Hygiene Program, *Dent. Hyg.*, *50*, 29, January, 1976.

51

The Patient Who is Homebound, Bedridden, or Helpless

HOMEBOUND PATIENTS

Within recent years, efforts have been made through research and organized programming, to attend to the oral health needs of the chronically ill and handicapped. Patients of all age groups are confined to hospitals, institutions, nursing homes, skilled nursing facilities, or private homes, and need special adaptations for dental and dental hygiene care. Portable equipment is available and special training for dental personnel is encouraged.

Dental care for the chronically ill must be completed in a variety of surroundings. For the hospitalized, dental clinics frequently are available to provide care for in-patients. Those who are not hospitalized may be confined to their homes or may be able to be transported to the dental office or clinic in a wheelchair, depending on the severity and extent of disability.

Dentists and dental hygienists in private practice have occasion to attend patients confined to their homes. Dental hygiene techniques lend themselves to care for the bedridden since nearly the entire treatment can be completed with manual instruments. Instruction in personal oral preventive procedures has particular significance for the comfort as well as the health of the patient. Suggestions relative to planning and conducting a home visit are included in this chapter.

I. Objectives

A. Aid in preventing dental caries and periodontal diseases which would require extensive treatment.

B. Assist in preventing further complication of the patient's state of health by lessening oral care problems.

C. Contribute to the patient's comfort, mental ease, and general well-being.

D. Encourage adequate personal care procedures, whether performed by the patient or an attendant.

E. Contribute to general rehabilitation or habilitation of the patient.

II. Preparation for the Home Visit

A. Understanding the Patient

1. Consider the characteristics associated with the particular chronic illness or disease.

2. Consider special problems related to age. (For example, for the gerodontic patient see page 624).

3. Review patient's medical history (by telephone, if preliminary visit is not practical) to determine unusual precautions that must be taken. Arrange with physician and dentist when premedication is indicated (pages 99–100).

B. Instruments and Equipment

1. Sterile instruments and other items are transported in the packages in which they were sterilized.

2. Gauze sponges, cotton rolls and pellets, wood points, and dappen dishes are prepared in packages that will be convenient to open and use at the bedside.

3. Substances such as the disclosing agent, postoperative antiseptic, polishing agent, and topical fluoride preparation are carried in small, tightly closed bottles.

4. Coverall: a large plastic drape is of particular importance, since in certain types of illness the patient's coordination during rinsing may be limited. Thoughtfulness in the care of bed linen is appreciated by the patient's attendant.

5. Emesis basin: for patient rinsing. Although a small basin undoubtedly would be available at the home, the kidney-shaped basin facilitates the rinsing process.

6. Lighting: adaptation of available possibilities.

   a. Headlight or reflector: dentist may have as part of the office equipment; with practice, the dental hygienist can learn to use with ease.

   b. Photography spot light: might be available either from the dentist or from the patient's home; need a type with a narrow, concentrated beam.

   c. Gooseneck lamp: might be available in patient's home; need bulb of adequate wattage.

7. Miscellaneous facilities usually available at the home: arrangements must be planned (by telephone) in advance of appointment.

   a. Large towels: for covering pillows.

   b. Types of pillows available which may be firm enough to assist in maintaining patient's head in reasonably stationary position.

   c. Hospital bed: can be adjusted most effectively for patient's position.

C. Appointment Time

Arrange during the patient's usual waking hours at as convenient a time as possible in relation to nursing care and mealtime schedule.

III. Approach to Patient

Since a majority of patients who come to the dental office are active people with good general health, it is sometimes difficult to adjust to the relatively helpless, chronically ill person. There may be a tendency to be oversolicitous, which does not contribute to the development of a cooperative patient.

Usually, a direct approach with gentle firmness is most successful. Establishment of rapport with the patient depends in part on whether the patient has requested and anticipated the appointment or whether those caring for the patient have insisted on and arranged for the visit.

A. Personal Factors

Frequently, the well-adjusted chronically ill person may be more appreciative of the care provided than the patient who comes to the dental office, and may be well aware of the difficulties under which the dental hygienist is working. The cooperation obtained frequently depends on the patient's attitude toward the illness or disability.

A prolonged illness which may have been accompanied by suffering is not conducive to a healthy outlook on life. Monotonous confinement contributes to the development of characteristics such as those listed below.

1. Difficulty in maintaining a cheerful attitude.

2. Bored or dissatisfied with sameness of daily routine.

3. Easily depressed.

4. Discouragement about recovery leads to mental state that retards recovery.

5. Sensitive and easily offended.

6. Demanding; enjoys being waited on if used to having prompt attention to each request.

7. Indifferent to personal appearance and general rules of personal hygiene.

8. Preoccupied with details of medical examinations, tests, treatment, medicaments, and symptoms.

B. Suggestions for General Procedure

1. Request that visitors be asked to remain

out of the room during the appointment to prevent distraction of patient.

2. Introduce each step slowly, to be sure patient knows what is being done.

3. Do not make the patient feel rushed. Listen attentively; socializing is one of the best ways to establish rapport.

4. Regardless of inconvenience of arrangements, two or more appointments should be planned when extensive scaling is required.
   a. Need to avoid tiring the patient.
   b. Need for observing tissue response.
   c. Need to give encouragement in plaque control procedures.

IV. Dental Hygiene Care

A. The Working Situation

Since many patients can be up in a chair or wheelchair at least an hour or two each day, only rarely is it necessary to perform procedures with the patient in bed. For the patient in the chair, a kitchen or large bathroom may be most satisfactory for working. In either situation, ingenuity is needed to arrange patient position, head stabilization, and proper lighting to maintain patient comfort and yet provide access for the operator.

1. *Patient in Bed*
   a. Hospital bed: adjust to lift patient's head to desirable height.
   b. Ordinary bed: use firm pillows to support patient.

2. *Patient in Wheelchair*
   a. Portable headrest may be attached to back of plain chair or wheelchair.
   b. Although it is possible to back the chair against a wall and insert a pillow for the head, it may be better to have patient moved to a davenport or chair where a more stable headrest could be provided.

3. *Small Patient.* Positions for plaque control described on page 704 and shown in figure 50–6 may be applicable for dental hygienist during treatment.

4. *Suggestions for Lighting*
   a. Turn off overhead lighting to reduce shadows in the mouth.
   b. Headlight: usually the most convenient and efficient form of lighting because of concentrated beam.
   c. Head reflector: reflect light from bed lamp attached to bed behind patient's head.
   d. Gooseneck or photographer's light: care must be taken not to direct light into patient's eyes.

5. *Instrument Arrangement.* On towel on table beside bed or chair.

B. Instrumentation

Scaling is complicated by instability of head. A mouth prop may be needed when patient has difficulty in opening.

C. Fluoride Application

Selection of method for fluoride application will vary with the patient and the home situation. The use of self-care techniques will depend on the patient's handicap and the cooperation of the attendant. The most benefit would be obtained from a daily mouthrinse, chewable tablet, or gel application in a mouthguard tray or brush-on (pages 447, 456–458).

V. Patient Instruction

A. Personal Oral Care

Provide specific instruction for attendant of helpless or uncoordinated patient. Demonstrate in patient's mouth. A powered toothbrush may prove valuable for certain patients (pages 353, 702).

B. Dietary Suggestions

1. Need for consultation with physician concerning prescribed diet. When significant relationships of diet to oral health are suspected, they should be reported to the dentist. The patient's problem can then be discussed with the physician and dietary adjustments made.

2. Cariogenic foods should be avoided as snacks. The patient and those who provide the patient's food need specific suggestions for food substitutes that are noncariogenic.

3. Factors influencing suggestions for diet
   a. Patient's appetite may be poor, par-

ticularly if there is discouragement about the state of health.

b. Patient may be finicky in food selection, which may have affected the general nutritional state or have resulted in excessive use of cariogenic foods.

c. Monotony of meals may have lessened the desire to eat.

THE HOSPITALIZED HELPLESS OR UNCONSCIOUS PATIENT

Personal oral care procedures for the hospitalized patient are accomplished by the attendant member of the nursing staff when self-care by the patient is impossible. Planning and conducting an oral health in-service program for the nursing staff and other direct-care people are described on pages 707–710.

Understanding the possible procedures for oral care of hospitalized patients is important to all dental hygienists, whether or not they are employed in a hospital, if they are to appreciate ramifications of dental hygiene care for the many types of patients with special needs.

Skill is required to carry out routine methods of toothbrushing, rinsing, and cleaning of removable dentures for the conscious patient who is able to cooperate. Methods must be adapted when the patient's head cannot be elevated. When the patient's illness or injury involves the oral cavity, the advice and recommendations of the attending oral surgeon are followed.

Maintenance of oral cleanliness for the acutely ill or unconscious patient requires special procedures because of the complete helplessness of the patient. Objectives and methods described below have application for patients with other special needs as, for example, the patient with a fractured jaw (page 661) or severe mental retardation (page 734).

I. Objectives of Care

A. Prevent debris in the mouth from being aspirated and clogging air passages.

B. Minimize the possibility of oral infection.

C. Clean the mouth and provide comfort for the patient.

II. Care of Removable Dentures

A. Remove dentures from the patient's mouth.

It is usual hospital policy to remove dentures when a patient is unconscious.

B. Procedure for removal is described on page 580.

C. Clean the dentures (pages 385–393) and store in water in a covered container by the patient's bedside.

III. General Mouth Cleansing

A. Edentulous and Dentulous

1. Cleanse the mouth at least three times each day to prevent dryness and sordes. Sordes is a crust-like material that collects on the lips, teeth, and gingiva of a patient with a fever or dehydration in a chronic debilitating disease.

2. Apply a lubricant, such as equal parts pure glycerin and lemon juice, to the oral mucosa and the lips. Prepared disposable swabs are available for this purpose.

B. Brushing and Flossing

1. *Patient Who Can Rinse.* When helpless for manipulation of brush or floss but can rinse and expectorate, a patient can be propped upright and an emesis basin used.

2. *Patient Who Cannot Participate:* suction is a necessity. When suction is used, an assistant is needed, except for the suction toothbrush described below (IV).

3. *Brush.* A powered brush may be more efficiently and thoroughly used than a manual brush when an attendant must brush a helpless patient's teeth. A mouth prop can be placed in one side while the other side is retracted.

IV. Toothbrush with Suction Attachment

The toothbrush with attached suction provides an efficient and safe method for patient care.

A. Description of the Brush[1,2]

1. Soft-textured nylon brush with hole drilled between the bristles in the middle of the head of the brush.

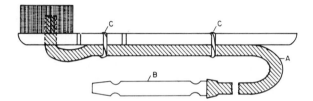

Figure 51–1. Soft toothbrush with suction attachment for care of helpless patient. **A.** Plastic tubing. **B.** Adapter for attachment of tubing to aspirator or suction outlet. **C.** Rubber bands to attach tubing to toothbrush handle. Plastic tube is inserted through a hole in the head of the brush and extended to a level slightly below the brushing plane.

2. Small plastic tubing inserted into hole; end adjusted slightly below level of brushing plane.
3. Other end of tubing passed across back of brush handle and attached to handle by small rubber bands (figure 51–1).
4. Tubing is connected by an adapter to aspirator or suction outlet.

B. Procedure for Use of Brush

The detailed procedure would be outlined for hospital personnel and included in the nursing procedures manual. An abbreviated outline of the basic steps is included here.

1. Preparation of the patient
   a. The patient may be aware of what is going on, although may not respond in a usual manner.
   b. Tell patient that the teeth are going to be brushed.
   c. Turn patient on a side and place a pillow at the back for support.
   d. Place a face towel under patient's chin and over bedding.
2. Attach toothbrush to suction outlet and lay brush on towel near patient's mouth.
3. Place a rubber bite block on one side of the patient's mouth between the teeth. String tied to bite block is fastened to patient's gown with a safety pin.
4. Dip brush in fluoride mouthrinse; turn on suction.
5. Gently retract lip and carefully apply the appropriate toothbrushing procedures; apply suction over each tooth surface with particular care at each interproximal area. Moisten brush frequently.
6. Move bite block to opposite side of mouth and continue brushing procedure.

7. Place brush in cup of clear water to allow water to be sucked through and clear the tubing both during the procedure, if there is clogging, and after brushing to clean the tube.
8. Remove bite block; wipe patient's lips with paper wipe and apply petrolatum.
9. Wash brush and bite block; prepare materials for next use.
10. One toothbrush usually is sufficient for the patient's stay in the hospital.

TECHNICAL HINT

Suction brush (*Aspir-Brush*) available commercially
Ray Graham Association for the Handicapped
Grand Oak Office Center
970 North Oaklawn Avenue (Suite 300)
Elmhurst, Illinois 60126

References

1. Capps, J.S.: New Device for Oral Hygiene, *Am. J. Nursing*, 58, 1532, November, 1958.
2. Tronquet, A.A.: Oral Hygiene for Hospital Patients, *J. Am. Dent. Assoc.*, 63, 215, August, 1961.

Suggested Readings

Anderson, J.L.: Dental Treatment for Homebound and Institutionalized Patients, in Nowak, A.J.: *Dentistry for the Handicapped Patient*. St. Louis, The C.V. Mosby Co., 1976, pp. 211–224.
Bell, C.E., Lasater, T.M., Sawyer, J.F., and Ramirez, A.: Communicating Dental Hygiene Practices to Chronically, Emotionally Ill, Hospitalized Patients, *Am. J. Public Health*, 63, 778, September, 1973.
Duncan, J.L.: Incorporating Oral Hygiene Procedures in Geriatric Nursing Homes, *Dent. Hyg.*, 53, 519, November, 1979.
Ettinger, R.L. and Pinkham, J.R.: Dental Care for the Homebound—Assessment and Hygiene, *Aust. Dent. J.*, 22, 77, April, 1977.
Kamen, S.: A Prototype Service for Nursing Homes, *J. Hosp. Dent. Pract.*, 10, 67, July–September, 1976.
Kerson, J.: Treatment Planning for Patients in Nursing Homes, *J. Am. Dent. Assoc.*, 89, 640, September, 1974.
Lotzkar, S.: Dental Care for the Homebound, in Davidoff, A., Winkler, S., and Lee, M.H.M.: *Dentistry for the*

Special Patient. Philadelphia, W.B. Saunders Co., 1972, pp. 131–155.

Lukens, E.M., Saxton, R.N., and Bolender, C.L.: Development of a Nursing-home Dental Program, *J. Prosthet. Dent.*, *33*, 22, January, 1975.

Maurer, J.: Providing Optimal Oral Health, *Nurs. Clin. North Am.*, *12*, 671, December, 1977.

Niebel, H.H. and Keough, G.: Oral Hygiene Program for Totally Dependent Patients, *Military Medicine*, *137*, 71, February, 1972.

Odom, J.G. and Shipman, B.: The Hospitalized and Homebound Patient, *Dent. Clin. North Am.*, *21*, 647, July, 1977.

Siskind-Houle, B.: The Dental Hygienist's Role in Care of the Elderly, *Dent. Hyg.*, *53*, 507, November, 1979.

Stiefel, D.J., Lubin, J.H., and Truelove, E.L.: A Survey of Perceived Oral Health Needs of Homebound Patients, *J. Public Health Dent.*, *39*, 7, Winter, 1979.

Hospital Patient

Benson, C.M., Maibusch, R., and Zimmer, S.E.: Oral Health of Hospitalized Patients. Part I: An Overview of Oral Hygiene Nursing Care, *Dent. Hyg.*, *54*, 384, August, 1980.

Caveny, M.: The Dental Hygienist in Hospital Practice, *Dent. Hyg.*, *50*, 205, May, 1976.

Emery, C.A.: Hospital Dental Service: A Clinical Evaluation to Determine Its Justification, *J. Am. Dent. Assoc.*, *90*, 1018, May, 1975.

Emery, C.A.: Evaluation of Oral Hygiene in a Hospitalized Population, *Gen. Dent.*, *28*, 54, January–February, 1980.

Gamble, J.W.: The Hospitalized Dental Patient, in Clark, J.W., ed.: *Clinical Dentistry, Volume 1*, Chapter 32. Hagerstown, Maryland, Harper & Row, 1981, pp. 1–29.

Hendler, B.H. and Alling, C.C.: Inpatient Hospital Dentistry, *Dent. Clin. North Am.*, *19*, 595, October, 1975.

Iranpour, B. and Brown, I.S.: Ambulatory Hospital Dentistry, *Dent. Clin. North Am.*, *19*, 587, October, 1975.

Miller, M.: Dental Health Education in the Hospital—A Role for the Dental Hygienist, *Can. Dent. Hyg.*, *13*, 38, Summer, 1979.

Pickard, R.G. and Grigel, M.A.: Provision of Preventive Dentistry in the Hospital Environment, *J. Am. Dent. Assoc.*, *100*, 881, June, 1980.

Salley, J.J., Van Ostenberg, P.R., and Gump, M.L.: Dentistry and Its Future in the Hospital Environment, *J. Am. Dent. Assoc.*, *101*, 236, August, 1980.

Zimmer, S. and Maibusch, R.: Oral Health of Hospitalized Patients: Part II. A Clinical Study, *Dent. Hyg.*, *54*, 423, September, 1980.

52

The Patient with Epilepsy

Epilepsy is not a disease entity, but is rather a term used to describe a symptom or group of symptoms of disordered function of the central nervous system. A person with epilepsy may be susceptible to recurrent involuntary loss of consciousness or awareness with or without convulsive movements or spasms. Some patients may have convulsions without loss of consciousness.

It has been estimated that from .33 to 4.0 percent of the population of the United States have some form of epilepsy. A small percentage are hospitalized.

The patient's medical history should reveal a susceptibility to seizures and the physician must be contacted when additional information other than that provided by the patient is required. The well-controlled patient who is under anticonvulsant therapy usually presents no specific problems. An uncontrolled patient may require special treatment. A knowledge of symptoms is important in all cases, and dental personnel should know and be able to apply emergency measures in or out of the dental office.

Except for effects left by accidents occurring during a seizure, oral manifestations are limited to certain patients being treated with phenytoin (sodium diphenylhydantoin, Dilantin) which may induce a gingival overgrowth. All patients are advised by their physicians to live a moderate life and pay strict attention to general health rules. Care of the oral cavity becomes important both for its relationship to general health and to oral accidents which may occur during a severe convulsion.

DESCRIPTION[1,2,3]

A seizure is a convulsive disorder that results from a transient, uncontrolled alteration in brain function. The effect is an abrupt onset of symptoms which may be of a motor, sensory, or psychic nature, depending on which brain cells are involved.

I. Precipitating Factors That May Occur in Those Not Medicated

A. Arousal of anxiety through some immediate interpersonal conflict or through fantasy of such a conflict.
B. Emotional disturbances from excitement, fear, frustration, or tensions, particularly in teenage patients.
C. Fatigue secondary to sleep deprivation.
D. Sleep or arousal from sleep.
E. Flickering lights, sudden sounds, or other physical or sensory stimuli.

II. Types of Seizures

The two types of seizures are *generalized* and *partial*. Loss of awareness or a change in the level of consciousness is characteristic of generalized seizures. Seizures in which consciousness is not lost are called partial seizures. A patient may have both partial and generalized attacks. The frequency of attacks varies from several a day to one every few years in those who are not completely controlled.

A. Generalized Tonic–Clonic (Grand Mal, Major Epilepsy)

1. *The Aura or Warning*. Lasts from a moment to several seconds and may consist of one of a number of sensations suggested below. Not all patients experience an aura.
   a. Numbness or tingling.
   b. Strange feeling over stomach.
   c. Hallucination of a special sense: flashes of light, noises, peculiar taste or smell.
   d. Twitching or stiffness of certain muscles.
   e. Fear.
2. *The Seizure*
   a. Loss of consciousness: sudden and complete; patient falls. A patient in the dental chair may slide out.
   b. The entire voluntary musculature experiences continuous contraction, which is the *tonic* (tension) phase. The *clonic* movements follow, with intermittent muscular contraction and relaxation.
   c. Muscles of chest and pharynx may contract at same time thus forcing air out which results in a peculiar sound known as the "epileptic cry."
   d. Color: pale at first, then superficial veins become gorged; chest becomes fixed and aeration of blood ceases, leading to cyanosis of face.
   e. Pupils dilate.
   f. Intermittent muscular contractions follow, rapidly at first, then less frequently. If tongue is between the teeth it may be bitten.
   g. The incident lasts from 1 to 3 minutes; the bladder, and rarely the rectum, may be emptied.
   h. Respiration begins to return. Saliva, which previously could not be swallowed, may become mixed with air and appear as foam.
   i. Postconvulsive coma: fixed or sluggish pupils, noisy respiration, profuse perspiration, cyanosed lips, and complete relaxation of body muscles.
   j. Patient emerges in a cloudy state.
3. *Postconvulsive Phase*. Headache, muscle aches, and drowsiness; usually falls into a deep sleep.
4. *Occurrence*. Some patients have seizures only during sleep or an hour or so after waking. Others have a random distribution day and night.

B. Generalized Absence (Petit Mal, Minor Epilepsy)

1. *The Seizure*
   a. Loss of consciousness for 5 to 30 seconds.
   b. Patient usually does not fall; posture becomes fixed; may drop whatever is being held.
   c. May become pale.
   d. May have rhythmic twitching of eyelids, eyebrows, or head.
   e. Attack ends as abruptly as it began; the patient resumes activities: may or may not be aware of attack.
2. *Occurrence*. Most common in children 3 to 15 years of age. Seizures may occur up to as many as 100 times each day. Individual *petit mal* seizures occur more frequently than *grand mal*.

C. Complex Partial (Psychomotor)

1. *The Seizure*
   a. Trance-like state with confusion: usually for few minutes, sometimes for hours.
   b. Consciousness is impaired to varying degrees.
   c. May manifest purposeless movements or actions followed by confusion, incoherent speech, ill humor, bad temper; frequently does not remember what happened during the attack.
2. *Occurrence*. Primarily a disorder of adults and older children.

D. Status Epilepticus

Status epilepticus is a condition in which a series of any type of seizure occurs without the patient regaining total awareness in between. There is danger to life, and emergency medical care is required. To prevent cerebral damage, ventilation and oxygen may be indicated.

III. Etiology[1,2]

Epilepsy is a symptom of a disorder of the central nervous system, the explanation for which is not clear. During infancy, seizures can be related to congenital maldevelopment or a birth injury; while in older children and adolescents, trauma, infections, or idiopathic causes also are possible. In middle age and older, tumors, vascular disease, and the other symptomatic factors listed below are predominant.

A. Idiopathic Epilepsy

1. Genetic predisposition to seizures or to other neurologic abnormalities for which seizure may be a symptom.
2. Includes approximately 75 percent of all epilepsies.
3. Tends to manifest early in life; majority of cases between ages 2 and 14.

B. Symptomatic or Acquired Epilepsy

1. Known cerebral lesion brings about dysfunction leading to seizures.
    a. Brain tumor.
    b. Trauma (head injury).
    c. Infection (meningitis, encephalitis).
    d. Degenerative brain disease.
    e. Alcoholism and drug addiction; seizures are common during drug withdrawal.
2. Occurrence: not related to age, but generally a symptomatic cause is suspected in epilepsy that manifests after age 20.

IV. Personal Factors

There is no characteristic personality of epileptics. A good part of any maladjustment exhibited by the noninstitutionalized patients can be blamed on the attitude of society toward them. They react individually according to their feelings toward themselves and how others look upon their illness.

Occupation may be limited as the person with epilepsy cannot be permitted to participate in activities that provide hazards in the event of a seizure. This is particularly depressing to adults who have acquired epilepsy since reaching the working age and who may be required to change their vocation.

V. Treatment[1,4]

Anticonvulsant drugs are used to control seizures.[5,6] Many drugs are available, and for certain patients a tranquilizer may be prescribed along with the anticonvulsant.

Patients whose etiology is found to be a brain tumor undergo surgery for tumor removal. Anticonvulsant medication is usually necessary following the surgery.

In addition to medication, patients frequently need psychologic or psychiatric support therapy to aid in coping with problems during rehabilitation. Psychologic turmoil may increase the frequency of seizures, which in turn, requires increased amounts of anticonvulsant drugs.

ORAL FINDINGS

Epilepsy in itself produces no oral changes. Specific effects relate to anticonvulsant therapy using phenytoin and to the results of oral accidents during seizures.

I. Gingival Manifestation

Phenytoin-induced gingival overgrowth occurs in 25 to 50 percent of the people using phenytoin for treatment.[7] No other anticonvulsant, in fact, no other drug, produces such an unusual side effect. The condition will be described in detail below.

Phenytoin has been used in the treatment of many conditions other than epilepsy. These include behavior problems, stuttering, headaches, neuromuscular disturbances, and cardiac conditions. When a patient's oral examination shows the presence of gingival enlargement and the drug history shows the use of phenytoin, it cannot be assumed that the patient's problem is epilepsy.

II. Effects of Accidents During Seizures

A. Scars of Lips and Tongue

During generalized tonic–clonic seizures, the oral tissues, particularly tongue, cheek, or lip, may be bitten. Scars may be observed during the extraoral/intraoral examination, and the cause differentiated from other types of healed wounds.

B. Fractured Teeth

During the tonic and clonic movements,

teeth may be clamped and bruxing may be forceful enough to fracture teeth.

PHENYTOIN-INDUCED GINGIVAL ENLARGEMENT (OVERGROWTH)

Gingival enlargement is one of several side effects from treatment with phenytoin. The condition is also called Dilantin hyperplasia, Dilantin-induced hyperplasia, diphenylhydantoin-induced hyperplasia, diphenylhydantoin gingival hyperplasia, Dilantin-induced gingival fibrosis, and phenytoin-induced hyperplasia.

I. Side Effects of Phenytoin

In addition to gingival overgrowth, other side effects may influence dental hygiene appointments. During history preparation and the extraoral/intraoral examination, the effects described below can aid in understanding the patient and planning treatment.

A. General Effects That May Occur[4,5]

Drowsiness, gastric distress, skin rash, ataxia (loss of muscular coordination that may be apparent by an unsteady gait), and restlessness are not uncommon. Increased hair growth may occur in women.

B. Nutritional Influences

Vitamins K, D, and folic acid are affected by anticonvulsant drugs. A megaloblastic anemia can result from a low folic acid blood level, which is described on page 803. Epithelial changes such as glossitis, angular cheilosis, and ulcerations of the lips, tongue, and buccal mucosa, may be observed.[8,9]

C. Fetal Hydantoin Syndrome[10,11]

Children of women receiving anticonvulsant therapy during pregnancy are more susceptible to malformations. They may have craniofacial abnormalities, growth retardation, mental deficiency, congenital heart defects, and cleft lip and/or palate.

II. Occurrence[12]

A. Age

There is a greater incidence in younger patients than in older patients just beginning therapy.

B. Initial Enlargement

The gingiva may start to enlarge within a few weeks or even after a few years following start of drug use.

C. Dosage and Length of Treatment

The size of the dose or the length of treatment are not necessarily factors in the incidence or nature of the gingival enlargement.

D. Sites

The anterior gingiva are usually more affected than the posterior, and the maxillary more than mandibular. Facial and proximal areas are usually larger than lingual and palatal.

E. Edentulous Areas

An overgrowth of tissue may occur in an edentulous area, although this is relatively rare. A source of trauma or irritation from a denture or the presence of retained roots and unerupted teeth has usually been associated.[13]

III. Tissue Characteristics

A. Early Clinical Features

The overgrowth appears as a painless enlargement of interdental papillae with signs of inflammation. Eventually, the tissue becomes fibrotic, pink, and stippled, with a mulberry- or cauliflower-like appearance.

B. Advanced Lesion

With time, the tissue increases in size, extends to include the marginal gingiva, and covers a large portion of the anatomic crown. Often, there are cleft-like grooves between the lobules (figure 52–1).

C. Severe Lesion

Large, bulbous gingiva may cover the enamel, tend to wedge the teeth apart, and interfere with mastication.

D. Microscopic Appearance

During therapy, phenytoin is present in the saliva, blood, gingival sulcus fluid, and dental plaque. The number of fibroblasts and the amount of collagen in the tissue are

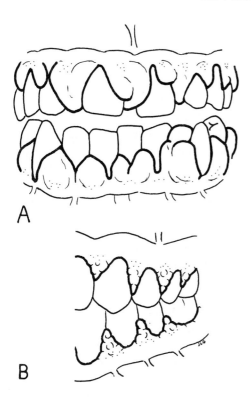

Figure 52–1. Phenytoin-induced gingival enlargement. **A.** Prominent papillary enlargement with cleft-like grooves. Note manner in which the fibrotic tissue has wedged certain teeth apart. **B.** Mulberry-like shape of interdental papillae.

increased. The stratified squamous epithelium is thick, with long rete pegs. Inflammatory cells are in greatest abundance near the base of the pocket.

IV. Complicating Factors

A. Plaque and Gingivitis

Adequate plaque control, particularly starting before the administration of phenytoin, decreases the extent of gingival overgrowth.[14,15] When plaque control efforts are perfected and carried out immediately after surgical removal of the excess gingival tissue, the regrowth can be expected to be minimal or not to occur at all.[16,17]

B. Orthodontic Appliances

The use of phenytoin while wearing appliances can result in marked enlargement of gingival tissue, with the bands and the teeth nearly covered by the overgrowth. There may be gingival bleeding, bad odor from plaque and food retention, and great difficulty in performing plaque control procedures. The united efforts of the dental hygienist, orthodontist, and the periodontist together with a motivated patient are needed if the tissue growth is to be controlled.[18]

C. Other Contributing Factors

Mouthbreathing, overhanging restorations, large carious lesions, calculus, and other plaque-retaining factors encourage gingival overgrowth. Treatment must include removal of overhangs and calculus, and restoration of carious lesions.

V. Treatment of Phenytoin-Induced Gingival Overgrowth

A. Conservative Treatment

Scaling with a concentrated program of plaque control and oral physical therapy may cause early lesions to regress. Gingival curettage may also help during the early stages before the tissue has become fibrotic.

A program of prevention and control should be started prior to, or simultaneously with, initiation of phenytoin administration.

B. Change in Drug Prescription

Phenytoin alone or with phenobarbitol has been a drug of choice for use with patients subject to generalized seizures since the drug was introduced in 1938. Many other drugs are in current use, none of which induces gingival enlargement. If the patient has a severe problem and is faced with embarrassment and social problems because of the appearance of the gingiva, the physician could be approached concerning the possibility of changing the prescription to a different drug. If possible, such a change should be made just prior to gingivectomy or other surgical removal procedure that may be planned.

C. Surgical Removal

Assuming a sufficient band of attached gingiva exists, the usual surgical procedure for tissue removal has been gingivectomy. Prior to surgery, a regulated program of plaque control should be introduced and continued as soon as surgical dressings have been removed.[16,17]

Control is possible, although there may be some slight return of enlarged tissue. A positive pressure device may be used following surgery.

D. Positive Pressure Appliance

The use of a custom fitted rubber mouthpiece designed to exert pressure against the gingival margin has been shown effective for selected patients.[19,20] In one reported study, the wearing of a pressure device was a stimulus to improved personal daily care.[21]

DENTAL HYGIENE CARE

For the patient with epilepsy, general health has special significance, and oral health contributes to general health. For the patient with phenytoin-induced gingival enlargement, emphasis in appointments is on a rigid oral hygiene program if the gingival enlargement is to be kept to a minimum.

I. Patient History

Except in an unusual situation, most patients with epilepsy will have had a thorough medical examination prior to the dental appointment. In preparing the patient history, however, all patients should be asked whether they ever had a seizure or currently do have recurrent or occasional seizures. When there is a positive answer, additional questioning is indicated.

A. History of Seizures

Questioning includes type, frequency, severity, and duration of episodes. The precipitating factors, need for any special premedication, and all information that has application during the dental and dental hygiene appointments must be carefully documented.

B. Medications

The type, dosage, effectiveness in seizure control, and known side effects are recorded. Patients using valproic acid may be subject to blood coagulation defects and should be questioned concerning spontaneous bleeding and ease of bruising.[22] Prior to surgical procedures, deep scaling, and soft tissue curettage, when bleeding can be

expected, blood testing for platelet count and bleeding time provide important information for the prevention of an emergency situation.

II. Patient Approach

A. Provide a calm, reassuring atmosphere.
B. Treat as an ordinary individual with patience and empathy; avoid oversolicitousness.
C. Encourage self-expression particularly if the patient tends to be quiet and withdrawn and has narrowed interests.
D. Do not mistake drowsiness (effect of drugs) for inattentiveness.
E. Recognize possible impairment of memory when reviewing personal oral care procedures.
F. Appeal to patient's lagging interest in personal appearance: develop interest in caring for the mouth; commend all little successes.
G. Drugs used in treatment tend to make patient drowsy; may sleep more than an average person.
   1. Be understanding when patient is late or misses an appointment.
   2. Plan telephone reminder at opportune time if patient is chronically late.

III. Treatment Plan: Instrumentation[23,24]

The treatment needs of a patient with phenytoin-induced gingival enlargement were described above. The dental hygiene treatment, planned within the total treatment plan, depends on whether the patient is just starting phenytoin therapy or, if already receiving phenytoin, the severity of the gingival enlargement.

A. Prior To and At the Start of Phenytoin Therapy

A rigorous plaque control program and complete scaling is introduced in preparation for phenytoin therapy. The patient (and parents) must understand that with controlled oral hygiene and emphasis on all phases of prevention, gingival enlargement can be prevented to a large degree.[14,15,23]

B. Initial Appointment Series for Patient Treated With Phenytoin

Weekly appointments for complete plaque

control instruction, scaling, and curettage are planned with the following objectives:

1. *For Slight or Mild Gingival Overgrowth.* Conservative treatment, including frequent thorough scalings, can be expected to lead to tissue reduction, provided the patient cooperates in daily plaque control. Frequent maintenance appointments can provide function and comfort with a minimum of pocket depths and no signs of inflammation.

2. *For Moderate Gingival Overgrowth.* After the initial series of weekly plaque instruction, scalings, and curettage, reevaluation of the tissue can determine what further procedures may be needed. For a cooperative patient, changing the medication to another anticonvulsant, use of surgical pocket removal, and continuing frequent maintenance appointments can provide an optimum level of oral health.

3. *Severe Fibrotic Overgrowth.* Initial scaling and plaque control are carried out to prepare the mouth for surgical pocket removal. Plans for changing the drug or altering the dose should be discussed with the patient's physician. A pressure device may also be advisable.[17,24]

C. Recall Intervals

Frequent recalls on a 1-, 2- or 3-month plan are indicated, depending on the severity of the gingival enlargement and the ability and cooperation of the patient to maintain the oral health. Most patients need continuing assistance and supervision, and their response depends on the instruction and devotion of the dental personnel.

IV. Treatment Plan: Prevention[12]

Daily plaque removal and fluoride therapy, the use of pit and fissure sealants, and dietary control all have a vital part in the care of the patient with a convulsive disorder. Initiation of preventive measures as soon as possible after the disorder has been diagnosed can contribute to the total health and well-being of the patient.

EMERGENCY CARE

When a seizure occurs, no attempt should be made to stop the convulsion or to restrain the patient. An outline for procedure appears in table 58–1 on page 850. Some additional suggestions regarding patient care during a generalized seizure that are applicable in a dental office are included here.

I. Objectives

A. To prevent body injury.
B. To prevent accidents related to the oral structures, such as:
  1. Tongue bite.
  2. Broken or dislocated teeth.
  3. Dislocated or fractured jaw.
  4. Broken fixed or removable dentures.

II. Preparation for Appointment

When patient's medical history indicates epilepsy, precautions may prevent complications should a seizure occur.
A. Emergency materials should be readied in a convenient place.
B. Have patient remove dentures for duration of appointment.
C. Provide a calm and reassuring atmosphere.

III. First Signs of Seizure

A. Lower the dental chair and tilt back.
B. Check and establish airway.
C. Do not restrain the patient in any way.
D. Clear aside movable dental equipment and sharp, potentially injurious instruments.
E. Turn patient's head gently on side to prevent aspiration of saliva and to prevent the tongue from dropping back. Do not apply force to turn the head while the neck is stiff during the convulsive stage.
F. Check for breathing obstruction.
G. Loosen tight belt, collar, necktie.
H. *Do not* force anything between the teeth. If an instrument becomes clamped between the teeth during a sudden attack, do not attempt to remove it.
I. Observe patient's actions and prepare a report for the patient's dental record as well as for the physician if one is required (page 835 and figure 58–1).

IV. Postconvulsive Phase

A. Allow patient to rest.
B. Talk to the patient in a low, reassuring tone. Ask onlookers to leave the patient in privacy.

C. When there are repeated convulsions, promptly obtain medical help.

D. Check oral cavity for trauma to teeth or tissues. Palliative care can be administered. Should a tooth be broken, it is urgent that the piece be located so that aspiration is prevented.

TECHNICAL HINTS

I. Never use a glass syringe or other breakable instrument when a seizure could occur.

II. When a patient vomits during a seizure, use high-power evacuator with wide tip to remove material from the mouth as a first aid measure against aspiration of vomitus into the airway.

III. Source of Informational Materials
Epilepsy Foundation of America
1828 L Street N.W.
Washington, D.C. 20036

References

1. Glaser, G.H.: The Epilepsies, in Beeson, P.B., McDermott, W., and Wyngaarden, J.B., eds.: *Cecil Textbook of Medicine*, 15th ed. Philadelphia, W.B. Saunders Co., 1979, pp. 851–862.
2. Dreifuss, F.E.: The Nature of Epilepsy, in Wright, G.N., ed.: *Epilepsy Rehabilitation*. Boston, Little, Brown & Co., 1975, pp. 8–27.
3. Malamed, S.F.: *Handbook of Medical Emergencies in the Dental Office*. St. Louis, The C.V. Mosby Co., 1978, pp. 197–207.
4. Rodin, E.A.: Medical Considerations, in Wright, G.N., ed.: *Epilepsy Rehabilitation*. Boston, Little, Brown & Co., 1975, pp. 28–50.
5. Ciancio, S.G. and Bourgault, P.C.: *Clinical Pharmacology for Dental Professionals*. New York, McGraw-Hill, 1980, pp. 147–153.
6. Cowan, F.F.: *Pharmacology for the Dental Hygienist*. Philadelphia, Lea & Febiger, 1978, pp. 344–352.
7. Angelopolous, A.P. and Goaz, P.W.: Incidence of Diphenylhydantoin Gingival Hyperplasia, *Oral Surg.*, *34*, 898, December, 1972.
8. Stein, G.M. and Lewis, H.: Oral Changes in a Folic Acid Deficient Patient Precipitated by Anticonvulsant Drug Therapy, *J. Periodontol.*, *44*, 645, October, 1973.
9. Mallek, H.M. and Nakamoto, T.: Dilantin and Folic Acid Status. Clinical Implications for the Periodontist, *J. Periodontol.*, *52*, 255, May, 1981.
10. Hanson, J.W. and Smith, D.W.: The Fetal Hydantoin Syndrome, *J. Pediatr.*, *87*, 285, August, 1975.
11. Friis, M.L.: Epilepsy Among Parents of Children With Facial Clefts, *Epilepsia*, *20*, 69, February, 1979.
12. Braham, R.L., Casamassimo, P.S., Nowak, A.J., Posnick, W.R., and Steinberg, A.D.: *The Dental Implications of Epilepsy*. United States Department of Health, Education, and Welfare, DHEW Publication Number (HSA) 78-5217, 1977, 18 pp.
13. Dreyer, W.P. and Thomas, C.J.: Diphenylhydantoinate-induced Hyperplasia of the Masticatory Mucosa in an Edentulous Epileptic Patient, *Oral Surg.*, *45*, 701, May, 1978.
14. Hall, W.B.: Dilantin Hyperplasia: A Preventable Lesion, (Abstr.), *J. Periodont. Res.*, p. 36, Supplement 4, 1969.
15. Ciancio, S.G., Yaffe, S.J., and Catz, C.C.: Gingival Hyperplasia and Diphenylhydantoin, *J. Periodontol.*, *43*, 411, July, 1972.
16. King, D.A., Hawes, R.R., and Bibby, B.G.: The Effect of Oral Physiotherapy on Dilantin Gingival Hyperplasia, *J. Oral Path.*, *5*, 1, Number 1, 1976.
17. Donnenfeld, O.W., Stanley, H.R., and Bagdonoff, L.: A Nine Month Clinical and Histological Study of Patients on Diphenylhydantoin Following Gingivectomy, *J. Periodontol.*, *45*, 547, August, 1974.
18. Vandersall, D.C. and Slade, D.: Periodontic/Orthodontic Management of Diphenylhydantoin Gingival Hyperplasia: Case Report, *J. Periodontol.*, *47*, 656, November, 1976.
19. Sheridan, P.J. and Reeve, C.M.: Effective Treatment of Dilantin Gingival Hyperplasia, *Oral Surg.*, *35*, 42, January, 1973.
20. Davis, R.K., Baer, P.N., and Palmer, J.H.: A Preliminary Report on a New Therapy for Dilantin Gingival Hyperplasia, *J. Periodontol.*, *34*, 17, January, 1963.
21. Babcock, J.R.: The Successful use of a New Therapy for Dilantin Gingival Hyperplasia, *Periodontics*, *3*, 196, July–August, 1965.
22. Hassell, T.M., White, G.C., Jewson, L.G., and Peele, L.C.: Valproic Acid: A New Antiepileptic Drug With Potential Side Effects of Dental Concern, *J. Am. Dent. Assoc.*, *99*, 983, December, 1979.
23. Pihlstrom, B.L., Carlson, J.F., Smith, Q.T., Bastien, S.A., and Keenan, K.M.: Prevention of Phenytoin Associated Gingival Enlargement—A 15-month Longitudinal Study, *J. Periodontol.*, *51*, 311, June, 1980.
24. Steinberg, A.D.: Clinical Management of Phenytoin-induced Gingival Overgrowth in Handicapped Children, *Pediatr. Dent.*, *3*, 130, May, 1981.

Suggested Readings

Betts, T.A.: Epilepsy, *Br. Dent. J.*, *143*, 278, October 18, 1977.

Coulter, D.L.: The Unfairness of Life for Children With Handicaps, *J. Am. Med. Assoc.*, *244*, 1207, September 12, 1980.

Goldin, G.J. and Margolin, R.J.: The Psychosocial Aspects of Epilepsy, in Wright, G.N., ed.: *Epilepsy Rehabilitation*. Boston, Little, Brown & Co., 1975, pp. 66–80.

Goldstein, E.P.: Convulsive Disorders, in Nowak, A.J.: *Dentistry for the Handicapped Patient*. St. Louis, The C.V. Mosby Co., 1976, pp. 95–101.

Greiner, A.L. and Rosenthal, A.H.: A Case Report: Prevention of Self-inflicted Trauma During Grand Mal Seizure, *J. Dent. Handicap.*, *3*, 26, Winter/Spring, 1978.

Hauser, W.A. and Kurland, L.T.: The Epidemiology of Epilepsy in Rochester, Minnesota, 1935 Through 1967, *Epilepsia*, *16*, 1, March, 1975.

Phenytoin-induced Gingival Enlargement

Angelopoulos, A.P.: Diphenylhydantoin Gingival Hyperplasia, A Clinicopathological Review. 1. Incidence, Clinical Features and Histopathology, *Can. Dent. Assoc. J.*, *41*, 103, February, 1975.

Angelopoulos, A.P.: A Clinicopathological Review. Diphenylhydantoin Gingival Hyperplasia: 2. Aetiology, Pathogenesis, Differential Diagnosis and Treatment, *Can. Dent. Assoc. J.*, *41*, 275, May, 1975.

Church, H.A. and Dolby, A.E.: The Effect of Dilantin on the Cellular Immune Response to Dento-gingival Plaque Extract, *J. Periodontol., 49*, 373, July, 1978.

Gelb, D.A.: The Management of Dilantin Gingival Fibromatosis, *Periodont. Case Rep., 1*, 16, Number 2, 1979.

Girgis, S.S., Staple, P.H., Miller, W.A., Sedransk, N., and Thompson, T.: Dental Root Abnormalities and Gingival Overgrowth in Epileptic Patients Receiving Anticonvulsant Therapy, *J. Periodontol., 51*, 474, August, 1980.

Harris, M. and Goldhaber, P.: Root Abnormalities in Epileptics and the Inhibition of Parathyroid Hormone Induced Bone Resorption by Diphenylhydantoin in Tissue Culture, *Arch. Oral Biol., 19*, 981, November, 1974.

Hassell, T.M.: Stimulation and Inhibition of Fibroblast Subpopulations by Phenytoin and Phenytoin Metabolites: Pathogenetic Role in Gingival Enlargement, *Pediatr. Dent., 3*, 137, May, 1981.

Hassell, T.M., Dudley, K.H., Hirsch, P.F., Hutchens, L.H., Johnston, M.C., and Moriarty, J.D.: Summary of an International Symposium on Phenytoin-induced Teratology and Gingival Pathology, *J. Am. Dent. Assoc., 99*, 652, October, 1979.

Hassell, T.M., Page, R.C., and Linde, J.: Histologic Evidence for Impaired Growth Control in Diphenylhydantoin Gingival Overgrowth in Man, *Arch. Oral Biol., 23*, 381, May, 1978.

Hassell, T.M., Page, R.C., Narayanon, A.S., and Cooper, C.G.: Diphenylhydantoin (Dilantin) Gingival Hyperplasia: Drug-induced Abnormality of Connective Tissue, *Proc. Nat. Acad. Sci., 73*, 2909, August, 1976.

Israel, H.: Abnormalities of Bone and Orofacial Changes from Anticonvulsant Drugs, *J. Public Health Dent., 34*, 104, Spring, 1974.

Keith, D.A.: Side Effects of Diphenylhydantoin: A Review, *J. Oral Surg., 36*, 206, March, 1978.

Khuen, J.E.: The Use of Dilantin in Association With Oral Healing, *Dent. Hyg., 51*, 61, February, 1977.

Klar, L.A.: Gingival Hyperplasia During Dilantin Therapy: A Survey of 312 Patients, *J. Public Health Dent., 33*, 180, Summer, 1973.

Navarro, R.A. and Correll, P.J.: Plaque Control in Gingival Hyperplasia. Secondary Dilantin Therapy: Report of a Case, *J. Oral Med., 31*, 27, January–March, 1976.

Nuki, K. and Cooper, S.H.: The Role of Inflammation in the Pathogenesis of Gingival Enlargement During the Administration of Diphenylhydantoin Sodium in Cats, *J. Periodont. Res., 7*, 102, Number 2, 1972.

Reynolds, N.C. and Kirkham, D.B.: Therapeutic Alternatives in Phenytoin-induced Gingival Hyperplasia, *J. Periodontol., 51*, 516, September, 1980.

Setterstrom, J.A., Gross, A., D'Alessandro, S.M., and Godat, R.F.: Immunoglobulins in Periodontal Tissues. III. Concentrations of Immunoglobulins in Dilantin-induced and Idiopathic Gingival Hyperplastic Tissues, *J. Periodontol., 51*, 25, January, 1980.

Staple, P.H., Reed, M.J., and Mashimo, P.A: Diphenylhydantoin Gingival Hyperplasia in *Macaca arctoides:* A New Human Model, *J. Periodontol., 48*, 325, June, 1977.

Staple, P.H., Reed, M.J., Mashimo, P.A., Sedransk, N., and Umemoto, T.: Diphenylhydantoin Gingival Hyperplasia in *Macaca arctoides:* Prevention by Inhibition of Dental Plaque Deposition, *J. Periodontol., 49*, 310, June, 1978.

53

The Patient with Mental Retardation

With trends toward deinstitutionalization and emphasis on special training and education in local agencies and schools, more people with mild and moderate mental retardation have appeared as dental and dental hygiene patients in private dental offices and clinics, as well as school and community dental facilities. Dental hygienists in all settings have opportunities to contribute to the health and well-being of this special group.

Approximately 3 percent of the population is affected by mental retardation. Of these, nearly 90 percent are only borderline and mildly retarded, while another 6 percent are moderately retarded. Less than 5 percent are severely or profoundly retarded and, usually, require lifetime custodial care.

I. Definitions

A. Mental Retardation

Mental retardation refers to significantly subaverage general intellectual functioning, existing concurrently with deficits in adaptive behavior and manifested during the developmental period.[1]

In that formal definition, the American Association on Mental Deficiency uses general intelligence tests to clarify *general intellectual functioning*. The levels are explained below, under II.

The term *adaptive behavior* is used to mean the standard of independence and responsibility expected for an individual's age group. *Developmental period* refers to the time from birth to 18 years of age.

B. Mental Deficiency

The term *mental deficiency* may be used interchangeably with mental retardation, although mental deficiency is more frequently used to imply persons of all ages, whether manifested in the developmental period or later.

C. Mental Illness

Mental retardation must not be confused with mental illness. The term mentally ill refers to a person with an emotional disorder. Examples of severe mental illnesses are schizophrenia and psychoses, and examples of less severe mental illnesses are personality disorders and psychoneuroses. The symptoms and methods for treatment of mental illnesses are very different from those of mental retardation.

It is possible for a person with mental retardation to become disturbed or mentally ill. Special treatment would be needed and the attitude and support of professional people can be especially important.

II. Levels of Mental Retardation

The levels of intellectual functioning are designated *mild, moderate, severe,* and *profound.* Standardized intelligence tests are used to determine individual levels. The Intelligence Quotient (IQ) expresses the test results.

From an educational standpoint, the term *educable, trainable, dependent,* and *life support* have been applied. These terms do not strictly coincide with the four categories mild, moderate, severe, and profound, since there are variations in the abilities of individuals and in their backgrounds.

Adaptive behavior is described briefly for each of the categories as they are listed below.[1,2,3,4] An understanding of expected capabilities can help provide necessary background information for teaching basic oral care procedures.

A. Mild Retardation

1. *Educable.* IQ 68 to 52.
2. *Adaptive Behavior*
    a. Child. In special classes for the educable, the child advances to a level of third to sixth grade. Practical skills can be learned.
    b. Adult. At adult level, the individual cares for personal hygiene and other necessities, with reminders. There is good communication, although the attention span and memory are less than average. Activities that do not require involved planning or rapid implementation can be carried out satisfactorily. Most educable individuals can engage in semiskilled or simple skilled work with guidance, and so maintain themselves.

B. Moderate Retardation

1. *Trainable.* IQ 51 to 36.
2. *Adaptive Behavior*
    a. Child. There is a marked developmental lag in the early years, but the child can be trained in personal care and hygiene with help. These children attend classes and learn simple habits and skills, but they do not learn to read and write. They speak in short sentences, and understand best when single-thought, short sentences are used. They participate well in group activities.

    b. Adult. As adults they attend to personal care, with reminders, and have a relatively short attention span and memory. Although they may have problems of coordination, they perform simple tasks and are conscientious about taking responsibility for errands and helpful duties. Although not completely capable of self-maintenance, many do unskilled work with direct supervision.

C. Severe Retardation

1. *Dependent.* IQ 35 to 20.
2. *Adaptive Behavior*
    a. Child. Children at this level can benefit from systematic habit training and may make attempts at personal care and dressing with assistance. They usually walk, use some speech, and respond to directions.
    b. Adult. Adults conform to a daily routine and may help with household and other small tasks, in spite of a limited attention span. Some personal care with supervision is possible.

D. Profound Retardation

1. *Total Dependency.* IQ 19 and below.
2. *Adaptive Behavior*
    a. Child. There are delays in all phases of development, and close supervision and care are necessary.
    b. Adult. Many remain inert and placid throughout the early years and never learn to sit up. A few may learn a few words, but as a group their ability to interact is lacking. Nursing care is needed, and many cannot feed themselves.

ETIOLOGY OF MENTAL RETARDATION

Mental retardation represents a more or less important symptom in well over 200 different conditions. Many of these are rare. A variety of means of classification is found in the literature, and it has been convenient to divide the causes into factors operating before birth, at birth, and after birth before mental development has been completed.

A majority of instances of mental retardation results from prenatal influences; a small number is effected as injuries at birth. It should be appreciated that diagnosis may be complicated and difficult and many cases can only be classified as of unknown origin.

I. Principal Groups of Causes[1]

A. Infections and intoxications.
B. Trauma or physical agent.
C. Disorders of metabolism or nutrition.
D. Gross brain disease (neoplasms).
E. Chromosomal abnormalities.
F. Gestational disorders (prematurity).
G. Environmental.
H. Unknown.

II. Examples During Prenatal Period

A. Infections[5]

Brain damage can result from maternal infection during pregnancy. Serious infections during the first trimester are most likely to cause physical malformations.

1. *Congenital Rubella Syndrome.* German measles virus infection during the first trimester may result in abnormalities, and mental retardation occurs in approximately 50 percent of the infants. The rubella syndrome also may include cataracts, cardiac anomalies, deafness, and microcephaly.

   Immunization with rubella vaccine has reduced the incidence of the disease in the general population. Since more prospective mothers are immune than were in the past, retardation related to the virus infection has been reduced.

2. *Congenital Syphilis.* Transfer of syphilis from the mother leads to numerous symptoms, and when the central nervous system is involved, hydrocephalus, convulsions, and mental retardation can result. Hutchinson's triad, which is associated with the late stage of congenital syphilis, includes deafness, interstitial keratitis, and dental defects. Hutchinsonian incisors, which are notched and tapered, mulberry molars, and microdontia are typical (figure 14–2, page 237).

B. Metabolic Disorders

1. *Phenylketonuria (PKU).*[3] Phenylketon-

uria results from an error of metabolism in which the enzyme necessary for digestion of the amino acid phenylalanine is missing. Severe mental retardation is a consequence. Early recognition of the missing enzyme with early dietary control lessens the severity of retardation. Many states require blood and urine screening tests soon after an infant is born. A diet free from animal and vegetable protein is necessary.

2. *Galactosemia.* Galactosemia is a defect of carbohydrate metabolism in which galactose and lactose cannot be utilized. The condition can be diagnosed by blood test at birth, and with the use of substitutes for foods containing galactose, permanent cerebral damage can be prevented.

3. *Congenital Hypothyroidism.* Cretinism is usually due to partial or complete absence of the thyroid gland at birth. Mental retardation accompanies a variety of physical symptoms related to defective development.

C. Chromosomal Abnormality

Down's syndrome is described in a separate section on page 735.

III. Examples at Birth

A. Mechanical Injury at Birth

Damage leading to mental retardation may have a variety of causes, including difficulties of labor and thrombosis.

B. Anoxia

Asphyxiation from prolonged anoxia may result from labor difficulties.

IV. Examples During Postnatal Period

A. Infections

Cerebral infection may be caused by a wide variety of organisms. Examples of diseases that may have this effect are encephalitis and meningitis.

B. Postnatal Trauma

Accidents of infancy may result in a fractured skull or prolonged unconsciousness.

C. Nutritional Disorder

Dietary imbalances and inadequacies, debilitating diseases, or parasitic diseases, can lead to slow development and retardation.

GENERAL CHARACTERISTICS

I. Physical Features

Since most individuals with mental retardation are in the borderline and mild categories, no unusual physical characteristics should be expected at initial patient evaluation, other than those present in the usual population of normal intelligence.

Within the low moderate, severe, and profound groups certain physical variations appear more frequently. Facial or other characteristics may be pathognomonic for a particular condition or syndrome; that is, there may be an identifying characteristic specific for that condition, which rarely occurs in other syndromes.

Skull anomalies include microcephaly (smaller), hydrocephalus (larger, contains fluid), spherical (occurs in Down's syndrome), conical, or otherwise asymmetrical shapes. Other features such as asymmetries of the face, malformations of the outer ear, anomalies of the eyes, or unusual shape of the nose may be present. Growth and physiologic development are generally delayed.

II. Oral Findings

A higher incidence of oral developmental malformations has been observed, some specifically associated with particular syndromes or conditions. Oral findings that have been observed to occur more frequently in individuals with mental retardation than in people with normal intelligence include the following:

A. Lips

Thickness of the lips is common.

B. Tooth Anomalies

Teeth may be imperfectly formed; eruption patterns may be delayed or irregular.

C. Malocclusion

The incidence of malocclusion is increased. An underdeveloped maxilla may contribute to malocclusion.

D. Periodontal Conditions

Gingivitis and periodontitis are common in individuals with mental retardation. Patients with Down's syndrome have more severe disease than other groups with mental retardation. Surveys have shown that institutionalized patients have more periodontal involvement than noninstitutionalized.[6,7]

E. Habits

There is increased incidence of clenching, bruxing, mouthbreathing, and tongue thrusting.

F. Dental Caries

The same factors are effective in the prevention of dental caries in the special group as in a population of normal intelligence. These include exposure to fluoridation and other forms of fluoride, form and frequency of cariogenic foods in the diet, and the control of dental plaque.

Studies have shown that when all degrees of retardation are grouped together, dental caries incidence is generally higher for noninstitutionalized than for institutionalized patients, particularly among the profoundly retarded group.[8,9,10] Institutionalized individuals have a controlled diet with less food available between meals. They also may have less accessibility to snacks containing refined carbohydrates, except those brought by visitors, which it is to be hoped, may be controllable. The private water supply for many institutions has been fluoridated, which may be equally true of the community water supply where the noninstitutionalized individuals reside.

When the figures for dental caries incidence are separated according to degree of retardation, the severely and profoundly retarded patients have been shown to have significantly more dental caries.[10,11]

Additional references to dental caries surveys are included with the *Suggested Readings* at the end of the chapter.

DENTAL AND DENTAL HYGIENE CARE AND INSTRUCTION

Procedures for patient management and care

of the patient with a disability were described in Chapter 50 with suggestions for various types of adaptations. The patient with mental retardation may have physical and sensory disabilities or systemic disease problems, so that application of information from various chapters can be used during treatment. Patients with any type of mental retardation need basic periodontal therapy consisting of intensive daily plaque control, scaling, curettage, and frequent recall supervision.

In the following pages, the special characteristics and problems of patients with Down's syndrome and the syndrome of autism (Kanner's syndrome) will be described.

DOWN'S SYNDROME

A special and unique group of individuals with mental retardation has a chromosomal abnormality manifested in Down's syndrome or trisomy 21 syndrome. The condition occurs in approximately one in 600 live births.

Formerly, there was an increased incidence of births of babies with Down's syndrome with advancing maternal age. However, in recent years, the average age of mothers of Down's infants has decreased.[12] There is also statistical evidence to show that the father can be the source of the chromosomal abnormality.[13]

Patients with Down's syndrome have a combination of characteristic abnormalities that are relatively constant. They tend to resemble one another.

I. Physical Characteristics[3,14]

A. Stature

Small, with a short neck; awkward, waddling gait; general growth retardation.

B. Head

Microcephaly; flat on facial and occipital sides; short, underdeveloped nose with depressed bridge; scanty hair.

C. Eyes

Oblique slant laterally with narrow opening between eyelids; fold of skin continues from upper eyelid over the inner angle of the eye (epicanthic fold) (figure 53–1). Nearsightedness, eyes crossing inward, and cataracts are common.

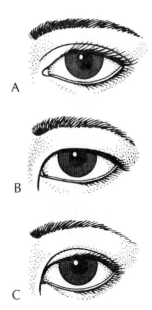

Figure 53–1. Eye characteristic of Down's syndrome. **A.** absence of epicanthic fold, **B.** epicanthic fold in Oriental populations, and **C.** epicanthic fold of person with Down's syndrome. (From Smith, G.F. and Berg, J.M.: Down's Anomaly, 2nd ed. Edinburgh, Churchill Livingstone, 1976.)

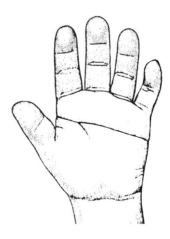

Figure 53–2. Hand of individual with Down's syndrome. Short stubby fingers, little finger curved inward, and a single transverse palmer crease are characteristic. (From Smith, G.F. and Berg, J.M.: Down's Anomaly, 2nd ed. Edinburgh, Churchill Livingstone, 1976.)

D. Hands

Broad, with short stubby fingers. The little fingers are curved inward. A single transverse palmer crease may also be present (figure 53–2).

II. Oral Findings

A. Lips

Habitually, the young person with Down's syndrome holds the mouth open with the tongue protruded. The lips are often thickened, cracked, and dry, which results from excessive bathing in saliva while the mouth is open. Mouthbreathing is common. Since respiratory infections frequently exist, and the tonsils and adenoids are often enlarged, breathing through the nose may not be easy. The incidence of cleft lip, cleft palate, or cleft uvula is greater than in the general population.[15]

B. Tongue

The tongue is generally deeply fissured and appears large. The jaws are narrow and the palate short and narrow, which tends to force the tongue into protrusion and make it appear larger.

C. Teeth

Eruption is delayed and irregular in sequence. There may be microdontia and congenitally missing teeth. Anomalies such as fused teeth and peg lateral incisors occur frequently.

D. Occlusion

Angle's Class III and posterior crossbite are common and relate to the flat face and underdevelopment of the mid-facial region. Frequently, the teeth are spaced apart, partly because certain anomalous teeth are narrow and require less space, and there are missing teeth.

E. Periodontal Disease

Increased susceptibility to plaque and bacterial products is apparent. Periodontal conditions are more severe than can be accounted for by local factors alone. Even at early ages, individuals with Down's syndrome show bone loss and other signs of periodontal disease.[7,16,17]

Necrotizing ulcerative gingivitis (NUG), superimposed over gingivitis or periodontitis, has been found in more patients with Down's syndrome than with other types of mental retardation. Recurrences of NUG contribute to rapid progression of periodontal disease with bone loss.[18]

III. Disease Incidence and Susceptibility

The mortality rate among patients with Down's syndrome is high during their early years because of high susceptibility to respiratory infections, congenital heart lesions, and leukemia. Premature senile dementia is characteristic among older individuals.

A. Susceptibility to Infection

Defects in the body's defense mechanism lead to early infections of a serious nature. The abnormality of immune function continues to be a subject of research.[19,20]

B. Hepatitis

Patients with Down's syndrome have an unusual response to hepatitis B surface antigen (HBsAg). Residents of institutions for mentally retarded individuals have a high incidence of hepatitis B, especially among children with Down's syndrome.[21] The carrier rate is much higher than in the community at large.

As a result of deinstitutionalization and mainstreaming, carriers placed in classrooms with susceptible children and teachers have created a public health problem in certain locations. Serologic surveillance, improvement of classroom personal hygiene, and placing the carrier children in separate classrooms apart from the susceptible children are necessary considerations.[22,23] Teachers who are immune can be assigned to teach in these classrooms. As fewer individuals with mental retardation are placed in institutions, and with the development of a hepatitis B vaccine,[24] problems of the carrier children will be lessened or even eliminated.

Dental office and clinic procedures and precautions for hepatitis control were described on pages 64–65.

C. Leukemia

In children with Down's syndrome and leukemia the death rate is 18 times greater than in the rest of the population. Whereas the peak age for leukemia is 4 years in children of normal intelligence, in Down's syndrome the peak is age 1 year.

D. Congenital Heart Defects

Between 40 and 60 percent of children with Down's syndrome have congenital heart defects. Information from the patient's medical history is used to identify the need for antibiotic premedication for the prevention of infective endocarditis.

IV. Level of Mental Retardation

Generally, the IQ of patients with Down's syndrome is under 50, in the trainable group. Those who have been institutionalized for a long period of time usually will show lower IQ scores.

The rate of mental development becomes progressively slower, and the progress made in training levels off with age. The average IQ for older children and adults ranges from 25 to 50, which may be lower than the score at younger ages for the same individuals. With supervision and help, many children with Down's syndrome learn useful and workable skills in labor and household tasks.

Socially, many of the children are more advanced, and may appear to have more intelligence than actually exists. The characteristics of friendliness and personal interaction are described below. Many people with Down's syndrome are fond of music and have a good sense of rhythm. They enjoy singing, playing an instrument, and listening to music. Background music in the dental office or clinic may be helpful in gaining rapport with these special patients.

V. Personal Characteristics[25]

The newborn baby with Down's syndrome is easily cared for, and is considered a "good" baby by the parents. Later, many of the small children are cheerful, happy, and responsive to learning. Individual differences can be noted, and personality disturbances are not uncommon.

Typical characteristics are listed here which may suggest management approaches for dental and dental hygiene appointments.
A. Like attention; require affection for feeling of security.
B. Cheerful disposition; rarely irritable; easily amused.
C. Sociable; observant; take initiative.
D. Tendency to imitate; mischievous.

E. Periods of stubbornness; obstinate and determined to have their own way. Early parental discipline is necessary. In the dental hygiene appointment, the initial approach can be very important to continued control and cooperation.

SYNDROME OF AUTISM

Autism is a behavioral developmental disability manifested by limited ability to understand and communicate. It appears during the first 36 months of life, but is not the result of the baby's environment as was once thought. Other names commonly used for the condition are Kanner's syndrome, early infantile autism, primary autism, and infantile or childhood autism. Since it is a life-long disability and autistic people live a normal life span, names that refer to infancy or childhood are less accurate.

Although relatively rare, autism occurs in approximately 5 out of every 10,000 births, and is found in males four times more frequently than in females. Children all over the world have been found with autism, and no factor of race, ethnic background, parental intelligence, social class, or parental personality has been shown to be related.

I. Characteristics[26,27]

Autism is a severely incapacitating condition. It is present at birth, but may not be identified specifically for months or years, depending on the age at which the parent brings the child to the physician or other professional person with questions concerning the lack of normal development.

A. Behavioral Features

The symptoms are a result of physical disorders of the brain. The behavioral symptoms include:
1. *Disturbances in Developmental Rates and Sequences.* Physical, social, and language skills appear at abnormal rates.
2. *Disturbances of Responses to Sensory Stimuli.* Any one or a combination of sight, hearing, touch, pain, balance, smell, taste, or posture may be affected.
3. *Disturbances of Speech, Language, and Nonverbal Communication.* Speech and language are absent or delayed, whereas specific thinking capabilities may be

present. When speech develops, it is apt to be atonal, arrhythmic, or stereotyped, with meaningless repetition of words spoken by others. Words are used without attaching the usual meaning to them.

4. *Disturbances in the Ability to Relate to People, Objects, or Events.* Typically, appropriate responses to adults and other children are absent. Objects and toys are not used as normally intended.

Autistic persons have a need for maintenance of sameness, and changes from a specific sequence of events or breakaway from routine may cause discomfort or panic.

B. Intellectual Features

Testing for the IQ has shown that approximately 60 percent have scores below 50, 20 percent fall between 50 and 70, while 20 percent are greater than 70. Typically, an autistic person shows wide variations of scores on different tests at different times.[26]

C. Other Disorders

Autism may occur alone or with other conditions that also have an influence on the central nervous system such as metabolic disturbances, Down's syndrome, or epilepsy. At least 25 percent of children with autism develop seizures between ages 11 and 19.

D. Prognosis

People with autism may live a normal life span, and a few become relatively self-sufficient with regular employment. Symptoms may change with age, and periodic reexamination for reassessment is important.

II. Treatment[28,29]

Since the etiology is not known, treatment has not been specific. A variety of approaches has been tried singly or in combination, depending on the individual's needs. In addition to psychotherapy, behavioral modification, and drugs, special education classes for play therapy and speech therapy may be used.

A. Psychotherapy

Parents of an autistic child are under such stress that emotional disorders of the par-

ents may emerge. Along with supportive counseling, the need for psychotherapy may become evident. The child with autism may also be helped by psychotherapy, although the usefulness would be limited for a severely withdrawn child.

B. Behavior Modification

To provide continuity in behavior modification treatment by a specialist, parents may be trained in the basic procedures and serve as paraprofessionals.[30] The parent has the responsibility for care of an outpatient child for many more hours than the therapist, and learning needs constant reinforcement.

C. Pharmacotherapy[31]

Various psychotropic drugs, hormones, megavitamins, and other pharmaceuticals have been tried. Drug therapy depends on the individual needs, and the main objective is to make the child more receptive to education and other therapies.

Patients may have other drugs in their complete treatment regime, which need consideration during dental and dental hygiene appointments. The patient with seizures may receive phenytoin. Phenytoin-induced gingival overgrowth is described on page 724.

III. Personal Factors and Dental Hygiene Care[29,32]

For many patients with autism, appointments for health care, medical or dental, are frightening, difficult experiences. Because of language disability and lack of communication, anxiety, and limited social contact, dental care may have been neglected.

Although not all autistic patients are difficult to treat, a few are impossible without sedation, general anesthesia, or physical restraints.[33] Hospitalization with general anesthesia is usually considered a last resort since it does nothing to aid in making a cooperative patient for the future.

A. Oral Health Problems

Except when autism is combined with a developmental disability of a different nature, there is no specific oral manifestation.

The general health and factors that must be considered for preappointment planning such as antibiotic premedication are also not manifestations specifically related to autism. A number of factors can contribute to a condition of poor oral health.

1. *Previous Dental Care.* The parent may not have taken the child to obtain care because of fear of the child being hurt, or fear of embarrassment that would result from the behavior of the difficult child. Frustration at home over continuous management of the disabled child could lead a parent to place dental care at a low priority level.

   For the child who had been taken to a dental office or clinic, previous dentists and dental hygienists may not have succeeded in accomplishing treatment of a satisfactory quality.

2. *Dental Caries.* Problems of feeding may have led the parent to lines of least resistance in the serving of foods the child would accept, without regard for nutritive content or dental caries prevention. The child's need for sameness may have been applied to dietary selection. A minimal, limited diet may or may not have had excess carbohydrates. A second factor is the possibility that the rewards used in behavior modification therapy may be carbohydrates. Repetition of cariogenic rewards frequently over long periods could have had a major effect on dental caries development.

3. *Oral Hygiene.* Even a parent or direct-care staff person who is well informed about current plaque control procedures may have had such difficulty in coping with an uncooperative autistic child that daily oral care procedures have never been carried out adequately.

B. Dental Staff Preparation

Advanced review and discussion of the patient's medical, dental, and personal histories, and information from the physician, psychiatrist, teacher, or other persons associated with the patient may be necessary as the dentist and the auxiliaries begin to learn how to work with the patient. Several short orientation appointments may be planned initially.

The same members of the dental team should be involved at each appointment so that the patient will not be disturbed by changes, and time will not be lost in reorientation.[34]

C. Structured Environment

1. Provide the child with predictable and consistent experiences.

2. Create a quiet environment free from sensory stimuli.[35] Avoid use of loud, inconsistent background music, noisy dental apparatus, and irrelevant conversations.

3. Begin with orientation to the setting and to each part of the equipment. The first appointment may not include any instruments, as the patient may not be ready. Patience and firmness are necessary elements. Instruction takes the form of "show–tell–do" repeated many times.

4. Use the parent to help condition the patient. Give the parent a plastic mouth mirror and a few dental films to take home for practice in the mouth each day.

5. Apply behavior modification procedures if the child is trained by that method. Use the parent or therapist-teacher to assist in presenting in a simple step-by-step manner the preventive measures. Reinforcers or rewards are given immediately following each success. By using nonsweet rewards, the parent or teacher can be educated.

TECHNICAL HINTS

I. Informed Consent

Written approval of the treatment plan is obtained from the parent or legal guardian.[4]

II. Source of Materials and Information

American Association on Mental Deficiency
5101 Wisconsin Avenue, N.W.
Washington, D.C. 20016

References

1. Grossman, H.J., ed.: *Manual on Terminology and Clas-*

sification in Mental Retardation, 1977 Revision. Washington, D.C., American Association on Mental Deficiency, 1977, pp. 11–37.

2. Morgan, S.B.: Mental Retardation, in Wessels, K.E., ed.: *Dentistry and the Handicapped Patient*. Littleton, Massachusetts, P.S.G. Publishing Company, 1979, pp. 21–32.

3. Morgan, A.J. and Johnston, M.K.: *Mental Health and Mental Illness*, 2nd ed. Philadelphia, J.B. Lippincott Co., 1976, pp. 145–173.

4. Snow, M.K. and Stiefel, D.J.: *Dental Treatment of the Mentally Retarded*. Disability Dental Instruction, 4919 Northeast 86th Street, Seattle, Washington, 98115, 15 pp.

5. Kamen, S.: Mental Retardation, in Nowak, A.J.: *Dentistry for the Handicapped Patient*. St. Louis, The C.V. Mosby Co., 1976, pp. 39–54.

6. Cutress, T.W.: Periodontal Disease and Oral Hygiene in Trisomy 21, *Arch. Oral Biol.*, *16*, 1345, November, 1971.

7. Tesini, D.A., Cohen, M.M., O'Donnell, J.P., and Clark, E.A.: Comparison of Periodontal Disease in Institutionalized and Noninstitutionalized Mental Retardates, *J. Dent. Res.*, *55*, B-261, Abstract #796, Special Issue B, 1976.

8. Cutress, T.W.: Dental Caries in Trisomy 21, *Arch. Oral Biol.*, *16*, 1329, November, 1971.

9. Sandler, E.S., Roberts, M.W., and Wojcicki, A.M.: Oral Manifestations in a Group of Mentally Retarded Patients, *J. Dent. Child.*, *41*, 207, May–June, 1974.

10. Tesini, D.A.: An Annotated Review of the Literature of Dental Caries and Periodontal Disease in Mentally Retarded Individuals, *Special Care*, *1*, 75, March–April, 1981.

11. Pollack, B.R. and Shapiro, S.: Comparison of Caries Experience in Mentally Retarded and Normal Children, *J. Dent. Res.*, *50*, 1364, September–October, 1971.

12. Holmes, L.B.: Decreasing Age of Mothers of Infants with the Down Syndrome, *N. Engl. J. Med.*, *298*, 1419, June 22, 1978.

13. Magenis, R.E., Overton, K.M., Chamberlin, J., Brady, T., and Lovrien, E.: Parental Origin of the Extra Chromosome in Down's Syndrome, *Hum. Genet.*, *37*, 7, Number 1, 1977.

14. Smith, G.F. and Berg, J.M.: *Down's Anomaly*, 2nd ed. Edinburgh, Churchill Livingstone, 1976, pp. 14–41.

15. Schendel, S.A. and Gorlin, R.J.: Frequency of Cleft Uvula and Submucous Cleft Palate in Patients with Down's Syndrome, *J. Dent. Res.*, *53*, 840, July–August, 1974.

16. Saxén, L., Aula, S., and Westermarck, T.: Periodontal Disease Associated with Down's Syndrome: An Orthopantomographic Evaluation, *J. Periodontol.*, *48*, 337, June, 1977.

17. Brown, R.H.: A Longitudinal Study of Periodontal Disease in Down's Syndrome, *N.Z. Dent. J.*, *74*, 137, July, 1978.

18. Brown, R.H.: Necrotizing Ulcerative Gingivitis in Mongoloid and Non-Mongoloid Retarded Individuals, *J. Periodont. Res.*, *8*, 290, Number 5, 1973.

19. Smith and Berg: op. cit., pp. 141–148.

20. Reiser, K., Whitcomb, C., Robinson, K., and MacKenzie, M.R.: T and B Lymphocytes in Patients with Down's Syndrome, *Am. J. Ment. Def.*, *80*, 613, May, 1976.

21. Blumberg, B.S., Gerstley, B.J.S., Sutnick, A.I., Millman, I., and London, W.T.: Australian Antigen, Hepatitis Virus and Down's Syndrome, *Ann. N.Y. Acad. Sci.*, *171*, 486, September 24, 1970.

22. Bakal, C.W., Marr, J.S., Novick, L.F., Millner, E.S., Goldman, W.D., and Pitkin, O.E.: Deinstitutionalized Mentally Retarded Hepatitis-B Surface Antigen Carriers in Public School Classes: A Descriptive Study, *Am. J. Public Health*, *70*, 709, July, 1980.

23. Bakal, C.W., Novick, L.F., Marr, J.S., Millner, E.S., Goldman, W.D., and Pitkin, O.: Mentally Retarded Hepatitis-B Surface Antigen Carriers in NYC Public School Classes: A Public Health Dilemma, *Am. J. Public Health*, *70*, 712, July, 1980.

24. Gerety, R.J., Tabor, E., Purcell, R.H., and Tyeryar, F.J.: From the National Institute of Allergy and Infectious Diseases, Summary of an International Workshop on Hepatitis B Vaccines, *J. Infect. Dis.*, *140*, 642, October, 1979.

25. Smith and Berg: op. cit., pp. 72–75.

26. National Society for Autistic Children, Board of Directors: A Short Definition of Autism, Adopted, June 27, 1977, New York Society for Autistic Children, 169 Tampa Avenue, Albany, New York 12208.

27. Ritvo, E.R. and Freeman, B.J.: Current Research on the Syndrome of Autism: Introduction. The National Society for Autistic Children's Definition of the Syndrome of Autism, *J. Am. Acad. Child Psychiatry*, *17*, 565, Autumn, 1978.

28. Ornitz, E.M. and Ritvo, E.R.: The Syndrome of Autism: A Critical Review, *Am. J. Psychiatry*, *133*, 609, June, 1976.

29. Robinson, M.D. and Milius, A.C.: Childhood Autism, in Nowak, A.J.: *Dentistry for the Handicapped Patient*. St. Louis, The C.V. Mosby Co., 1976, pp. 102–120.

30. Freeman, B.J. and Ritvo, E.R.: Parents as Paraprofessionals, in Ritvo, E.R., ed.: *Autism. Diagnosis, Current Research and Management*. New York, Spectrum, 1976, pp. 277–285.

31. Fish, B.: Pharmacotherapy for Autistic and Schizophrenic Children, in Ritvo, E.R., ed.: *Autism. Diagnosis, Current Research and Management*. New York, Spectrum, 1976, pp. 107–119.

32. Kopel, H.M.: The Autistic Child in Dental Practice, *J. Dent. Child.*, *44*, 302, July–August, 1977.

33. Braff, M.H. and Nealon, L.: Sedation of the Autistic Patient for Dental Procedures, *J. Dent. Child.*, *46*, 404, September–October, 1979.

34. Gabriel, H.P. and Gluck, R.: Management of an Autistic Child Undergoing Open Heart Surgery, *Pediatrics*, *51*, 251, February, 1973.

35. Swallow, J.H.: The Dental Management of the Autistic Child, *Br. Dent. J.*, *126*, 128, February 4, 1969.

Suggested Readings

Albino, J.E., Schwartz, B.H., Goldberg, H.J.V., and Stern, M.E.: Results of an Oral Hygiene Program for Severely Retarded Children, *J. Dent. Child.*, *46*, 25, January–February, 1979.

Bouter, H.P. and Smeets, P.M.: Teaching Toothbrushing Behaviour in Severely Retarded Adults: Systematic Reduction of Feedback and Duration Training, *Int. J. Rehabil. Res.*, *2*, 61, January, 1979.

Capute, A.J.: Developmental Disabilities, An Overview, *Dent. Clin. North Am.*, *18*, 557, July, 1974.

Cohen, M.M.: Chromosomal Disorders, *Dent. Clin. North Am.*, *19*, 87, January, 1975.

Cudzinowski, L.: von Gierke's Disease: Report of Case, *J. Dent. Child.*, *46*, 53, September–October, 1979.

Ellenor, G.L., Zimmerman, S., and Kriz, J.: An Interdisciplinary Approach to the Dental Care of the Mentally Disabled, *J. Am. Dent. Assoc.*, *97*, 491, September, 1978.

Gellis, S.S., Feingold, M., and Rutman, J.V.: *Atlas of Mental Retardation Syndromes*. United States Department of Health, Education, and Welfare, Division of Mental Retardation, 1968, pp. 2–167.

Gorlin, R.J., Pindborg, J.J., and Cohen, M.M., Jr.: *Syndromes of the Head and Neck*, 2nd ed. New York, McGraw-Hill, 1976, 812 pp.

Goyings, E.D. and Riekse, D.M.: The Periodontal Condition of Institutionalized Children; Improvement Through Oral Hygiene, *J. Public Health Dent.*, 28, 5, Winter, 1968.

Greene, N.M. and Falcetti, J.P.: A Program of General Anesthesia for Dental Care of Mentally Retarded Patients, *Oral Surg.*, 37, 329, March, 1974.

Hamilton, J.: Andy Wants to Be Grown Up: Managing Parental Anxiety, *The Exceptional Parent*, June, 1980 (Reprinted in *J. Am. Dent. Assoc.*, 101, 882, November, 1980).

Heling, B., Shapiro, S., Segal, E., and Hofman, A.: Periodontal and Oral Hygiene Status of Retarded Children in Israel, *Isr. J. Dent. Med.*, 21, 52, April, 1972.

Hunt, N.: *The World of Nigel Hunt; the Diary of a Mongoloid Youth*. New York, Garrett, 1967, 126 pp.

Indresano, A.T. and Rooney, T.P.: Outpatient Management of Mentally Handicapped Patients Undergoing Dental Procedures, *J. Am. Dent. Assoc.*, 102, 328, March, 1981.

King, W.C.: Oral Characteristics of Phenylketonuric Children, *J. Dent. Child.*, 36, 61, January, 1969.

Lindquist, B. and Heijbel, J.: Bruxism in Children with Brain Damage, *Acta Odontol. Scand.*, 32, 313, Number 5, 1974.

Lu, D.P.: Clinical Investigation of Relative Indifference to Pain Among Adolescent Mental Retardates, *J. Dent. Child.*, 48, 285, July–August, 1981.

McCracken, A.: Drool Control and Tongue Thrust Therapy for the Mentally Retarded, *A.J.O.T.*, 32, 79, February, 1978.

Miller, M.: Oral Hygiene Management of the Moderate to Severely Mentally Retarded Child, *Dent. Hyg.*, 53, 265, June, 1979.

Myers, H.M., Dumas, M., and Ballhorn, H.B.: Dental Manifestations of Phenylketonuria, *J. Am. Dent. Assoc.*, 77, 586, September, 1968.

Nowak, A.J.: The Role of Dentistry in the Normalization of the Mentally Retarded Person, *J. Dent. Child.*, 41, 456, November–December, 1974.

Nystrom, E.: A Toothbrushing Program for Trainable Mentally Retarded School Children, *Dent. Hyg.*, 53, 323, July, 1979.

Peterson, D.S., Chiniwalla, N., and Puddhikarant, P.: The Use of Vanity to Improve Oral Hygiene in the Retarded, *Dent. Assist.*, 48, 31, September/October, 1979.

Poole, A.E.: Variation in Protein Structure and Inborn Errors in Metabolism, *Dent. Clin. North Am.*, 19, 47, January, 1975.

Powell, D.: Dental Health Care for the Special Child, *Dent. Hyg.*, 47, 215, July–August, 1973.

Powell, E.A.: A Quantitative Assessment of the Oral Hygiene of Mentally Retarded Residents in a State Institution, *J. Public Health Dent.*, 33, 27, Winter, 1973.

Reynolds, W.E. and Block, R.M.: Evaluating the Effectiveness of Instruction in Oral Hygiene for Mentally Retarded Boys, *J. Public Health Dent.*, 34, 8, Winter, 1974.

Savide, N.L., Blain, S.M., and Jedrychowski, J.R.: The Use of Systematic Desensitization in the Dental Treatment of a Mentally Retarded Adolescent, *J. Dent. Handicap.*, 4, 10, Fall/Winter, 1978.

Schwartz, B.H., Albino, J.E., and Bissell, G.D.: Development and Evaluation of a Dental Health Training Program for Severely Retarded Children, *J. Dent. Handicap.*, 4, 17, Fall/Winter, 1978.

Steinberg, A.D. and Zimmerman, S.: The Lincoln Dental Caries Study: A Three-year Evaluation of Dental Caries in Persons with Various Mental Disorders, *J. Am. Dent. Assoc.*, 97, 981, December, 1978.

Svatum, B. and Gjermo, P.: Oral Hygiene, Periodontal Health and Need for Periodontal Treatment Among Institutionalized Mentally Subnormal Persons in Norway, *Acta Odontol. Scand.*, 36, 89, Number 2, 1978.

Troutman, K.: Behavioral Management of the Mentally Retarded, *Dent. Clin. North Am.*, 21, 621, July, 1977.

Usher, P.J.: Oral Hygiene in Mentally Handicapped Children; a Pilot Study of the Use of Chlorhexidine Gel, *Br. Dent. J.*, 138, 217, March 18, 1975.

Wright, A.D.: Mental Subnormality, *Br. Dent. J.*, 145, 272, November 7, 1978.

Autism

Holroyd, J. and McArthur, D.: Mental Retardation and Stress on the Parents: A Contrast Between Down's Syndrome and Childhood Autism, *Am. J. Ment. Def.*, 80, 431, January, 1976.

Lovaas, O.I., Schreibman, L., and Koegel, R.L.: A Behavior Modification Approach to the Treatment of Autistic Children, *J. Autism Child Schizophr.*, 4, 111, June, 1974.

O'Gorman, G.: Childhood Autism, *Practitioner*, 221, 365, September, 1978.

Down's Syndrome

Claycomb, C.K., Summers, G.W., Hall, W.B., and Hart, R.W.: Gingival Collagen Biosynthesis in Mongolism, *J. Periodont. Res.*, 5, 30, Number 1, 1970.

Gullikson, J.S.: Oral Findings in Children with Down's Syndrome, *J. Dent. Child.*, 40, 293, July–August, 1973.

Khan, A.J., Evans, H.E., Glass, L., Shin, Y.H., and Almonte, D.: Defective Neutrophil Chemotaxis in Patients with Down Syndrome, *J. Pediatrics*, 87, 87, July, 1975.

Kroger, J. and Day, V.: Down's Syndrome: Hygienist's Perspective, *Dent. Hyg.*, 55, 35, March, 1981.

Kroll, R.G., Budnick, J., and Kobren, A.: Incidence of Dental Caries and Periodontal Disease in Down's Syndrome, *N.Y. State Dent. J.*, 36, 151, March, 1970.

Miller, M.F. and Ship, I.I.: Periodontal Disease in the Institutionalized Mongoloid, *J. Oral Med.*, 32, 9, January–March, 1977.

O'Riordan, M.W. and Walker, G.F.: Dimensional and Proportional Characteristics of the Face in Down's Syndrome, *J. Dent. Handicap.*, 4, 6, Fall/Winter, 1978.

Scully, C.: Down's Syndrome: Aspects of Dental Care., *J. Dent.*, 4, 167, July, 1976.

Sznajder, N., Carraro, J.J., Otero, E., and Carranza, F.A.: Clinical Periodontal Findings in Trisomy 21 (Mongolism), *J. Periodont. Res.*, 3, 1, Number 1, 1968.

Tannenbaum, K.A.: The Oral Aspects of Mongolism, *J. Public Health Dent.*, 35, 95, Spring, 1975.

Hepatitis

Blumberg, B.S., Sutnick, A.I., and London, W.T.: Australia Antigen as a Hepatitis Virus, *Am. J. Med.*, 48, 1, January, 1970.

Chaudhary, R.K., Perry, E., and Cleary, T.E.: Prevalence of Hepatitis B Infection Among Residents of an Institution for the Mentally Retarded, *Am. J. Epidemiol.*, 105, 123, February, 1977.

Gust, I.D., Dimitrakakis, M., and Sharma, D.L.B.: The

Prevalence of HBeAg and Anti-HBe in an Institution for the Mentally Retarded, *Aust. N.Z.J. Med.*, 8, 471, October, 1978.

Higgins, G.R., Parker, C.E., Faust, J.A., and Rosenfeld, M.: Hepatitis-Associated (Australia) Antigen and Down's Syndrome, *Am. J. Ment. Def.*, 78, 426, January, 1974.

Madden, D.L., Dietzman, D.E., Matthew, E.B., Sever, J.L., Lander, J.J., and Purcell, R.H.: Epidemiology of Hepatitis B Virus in an Institution for Mentally Retarded Persons, *Am. J. Ment. Def.*, 80, 369, January, 1976.

Madden, D.L., Matthew, E.B., Dietzman, D.E., Purcell, R.H., and Sever, J.L.: Hepatitis and Down's Syndrome, *Am. J. Ment. Def.*, 80, 401, January, 1976.

McMillan, B.C., Hanson, R.P., Golubjatnikov, R., and Sinha, S.K.: Hepatitis-B Surface Antigen and Antibody: Prevalence and Persistence In Institutionalized and Noninstitutionalized Persons, *Public Health Rep.*, 94, 262, June, 1979.

Szmuness, W. and Prince, A.M.: The Epidemiology of Serum Hepatitis (SH) Infections: A Controlled Study in Two Closed Institutions, *Am. J. Epidemiol.*, 94, 585, December, 1971.

Szmuness, W., Prince, A.M., Etling, G.F., and Pick, R.: Development and Distribution of Hemagglutinating Antibody against Hepatitis B Antigen in Institutionalized Populations, *J. Infect. Dis.*, 126, 498, November, 1972.

54

The Patient with a Physical or Sensory Handicap

It is not possible to describe in detail the many diseases of the locomotor system, nervous system, and organs of special senses that have as a symptom or leave as a chronic after effect loss of sensory or motor function in the form of a handicap.

This chapter contains brief descriptions of selected diseases or conditions to illustrate the types of care necessary and the adaptations that must be made by the patient as well as by the professional person during treatment appointments.

General suggestions that may be adapted to a variety of patients with disabilities were described in Chapter 50. From those descriptions, methods and materials can be selected as they apply in the situations created by the different patients included in this chapter and encountered in practice. References and suggested readings are included at the end of the chapter for additional information.

SPINAL CORD DYSFUNCTIONS

Among people disabled by spinal cord dysfunction, paralysis is a common symptom. Paralysis means the loss of power of voluntary movement of a muscle due to interruption of one of the motor pathways from the cerebrum to the muscle fiber.

I. Types of Paralysis

A. Paresis

Paresis means partial paralysis. The term may be used to designate weakness rather than complete paralysis.

B. Quadriplegia (tetraplegia)

Quadriplegia means complete or partial paralysis (paresis) of the trunk and all four extremities.

C. Paraplegia

Paraplegia is complete or partial paralysis of the lower trunk and both lower extremities.

D. Hemiplegia

Hemiplegia means complete or partial paralysis of one side of the body.

E. Triplegia

Triplegia is hemiplegia with the additional paralysis of one limb on the opposite side.

II. Causes of Disruption of Spinal Cord Function

Examples are provided in parenthesis.
A. Trauma (spinal cord injury)

B. Neoplasms (within the cord or extradural)
C. Viral or bacterial infections (poliomyelitis)
D. Progressive degenerative disorders (multiple sclerosis)
E. Vascular accidents (hemorrhage, thrombus, embolus, hematoma)
F. Compression from an arthritic spur (spondylytic osteoarthritis)
G. Congenital anomalies or deformities (myelomeningocele, meningocele, spina bifida)

SPINAL CORD INJURY

Spinal cord injury is the impairment of spinal cord function resulting from the application of an external traumatic force. The effect is partial or complete paralysis to a degree related to the spinal cord level and the extent of the injury.

I. Occurrence

At least one half of the trauma cases result from motor vehicle accidents; other causes are falls, diving accidents, and violence, such as from gunshot or stabbing wounds. Between 80 and 90 percent of the patients are young males between 18 and 25 years of age.

II. The Initial Injury

Total or partial loss of sensory, motor, and autonomic function occurs below the level of injury. The injury may be diagonal and leave one side with better function than the other at that particular level.

A. Types of Injury

Damage to the spinal cord may result from one or more of the following:
1. Fracture, dislocation, or both, of one or more vertebrae.
2. Compression, stretching, bending, or severing of the spinal cord.

B. Emergency Patient Care[1]

At the scene of an accident, severe damage can be done by inexpert care. The patient should be placed in a supine position, but when back injury is suspected, the arms and legs should be straightened with caution. Any twisting motion may produce irreversible injury to the spinal cord by bony fragments cutting into or severing the cord. When transfer is made, the patient must be moved by at least four persons and placed on a board for transport.

C. Spinal Shock

Immediately after the injury, spinal shock causes a complete loss of reflex activity. The result is a flaccid paralysis below the level of injury. The state of spinal shock may last from several hours to 3 months.

III. Characteristics of Spinal Cord Injury

The pattern of signs and symptoms depends on the nature and level of injury to the spinal cord. There are 7 cervical (C), 12 thoracic (T), and 5 lumbar (L) vertebrae, with paired spinal nerves passing out from each.

The areas of the body that are controlled at the different levels are illustrated in figure 54–1. The patient's condition is referred to by the letter C, T, or L, followed by the specific vertebra number where the injury occurred. The most severely handicapped patients have a lesion level above C6, which refers to the sixth cervical vertebral level.

A. Sensorimotor Effects

1. *Complete Lesion.* A complete transection or compression of the spinal cord leaves no sensation or motor function below the level of the lesion.
2. *Incomplete Lesion.* Partial transection or injury of the spinal cord leaves some evidence of sensation or motor function below the level of the lesion. The sensation and motor function usually return within a few hours after injury, and maximum return will occur in 6 months to 1 year.

B. Other Possible Effects

1. Impairment of voluntary bladder and bowel control.
2. Impairment of sexual function.
3. Impairment of vasomotor and body temperature regulatory mechanisms.

IV. Secondary Complications That May Occur[2,3]

Most of the complications described here do not occur in patients with lesions below the T6 level.

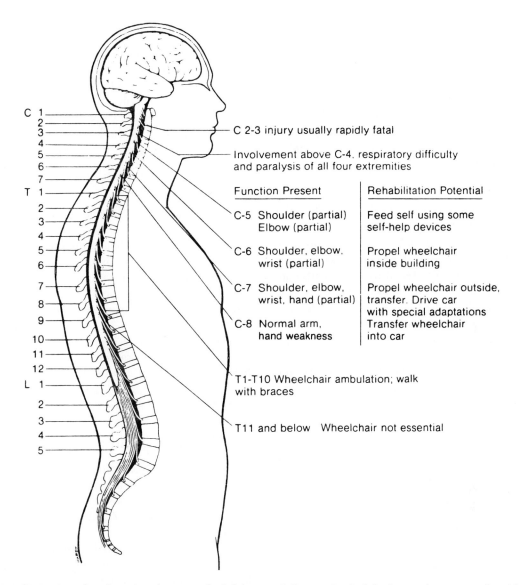

C 2-3 injury usually rapidly fatal

Involvement above C-4, respiratory difficulty
and paralysis of all four extremities

Function Present	Rehabilitation Potential
C-5 Shoulder (partial) Elbow (partial)	Feed self using some self-help devices
C-6 Shoulder, elbow, wrist (partial)	Propel wheelchair inside building
C-7 Shoulder, elbow, wrist, hand (partial)	Propel wheelchair outside, transfer. Drive car with special adaptations
C-8 Normal arm, hand weakness	Transfer wheelchair into car

T1-T10 Wheelchair ambulation; walk
with braces

T11 and below   Wheelchair not essential

Figure 54–1.   Sequelae of spinal cord injury and rehabilitation challenges. On the left, the vertebrae are numbered by C (Cervical), T (Thoracic), and L (Lumbar). Spinal nerves are numbered on the right. The most severely handicapped patients have a lesion level above C6. (From Brunner, L.S. and Suddarth, D.S.: Textbook of Medical-Surgical Nursing, 4th ed. Philadelphia, J.B. Lippincott Co., 1980.)

A. Respiratory Function

Respiratory difficulties may occur. During dental hygiene therapy, attention to patient position and continuous suction to keep passageways clear are vital. Some quadriplegic patients are unable to elicit a functional cough and need assistance. By placing manual pressure over the abdomen, below the diaphragm, after the patient has inhaled, the patient may be assisted while an attempt to cough is made.[3]

B. Tendency for Pressure Sores

A pressure sore or decubitus ulcer is due to pressure exerted on the skin and subcutaneous tissues by bony prominences and the object on which they rest, such as a mattress. The result is tissue anoxia or ischemia. The cutaneous tissue becomes broken or destroyed, which leads to destruction in the subcutaneous tissue. An ulcer forms, which may be very slow to heal, and may become infected by secondary bacterial invasion. Anemia and poor nutrition may also contribute.

Prevention of pressure can be accomplished by the use of padding and by regular turning of the patient. The dental chair can be positioned to prevent pressure. The patient may be asked to bring special padding for the appointment, and also asked to provide instruction for the dental personnel so correct procedures may be followed.

C. Spasticity

As spinal shock subsides, muscle-reflex spasticity develops from a slight to a severe degree. Stimuli such as pressure sores, infections, and sensory irritation may bring on a spasm. Before dental hygiene treatment, the patient should be asked about susceptibility to spasms and to describe the procedure to follow should one occur.

D. Body Temperature

High-level quadriplegic patients are unable to regulate body temperature. A blanket may be needed in colder weather and air cooling during summer. When no air conditioning is available, the patient's temperature should be monitored. In the event of a temperature rise, treatment should be postponed.

E. Vulnerability to Infection

Infections related to elimination, decubitus ulcer, and respiratory problems are the most common.

F. Autonomic Dysreflexia

1. *Definition.* Autonomic dysreflexia, or hyperreflexia, is an *emergency* condition in which the blood pressure increases sharply. It may occur in patients with lesions at T4 or above, but not below that level. A variety of stimuli may precipitate dysreflexia, especially an irritation to the bowel or bladder.

2. *Symptoms*
   a. Increased blood pressure with slowed pulse rate. The blood pressure may rise to 300/160.
   b. Pounding headache.
   c. Flushing, chills, perspiration, stuffy nose.
   d. Restlessness; increased spasticity.

3. *Emergency Care*[3,4]
   a. Position chair upright gradually. Do NOT recline the chair, because increased blood pressure in the brain could result.
   b. Monitor the blood pressure.
   c. Call for medical aid.
   d. Check bladder distension and unclamp catheter.

V. Personal Factors

The typical patient is a young man, possibly a former athlete. Depression and discouragement along with the pain and pressures of treatment and rehabilitation make psychiatric therapy necessary for many patients.

Physical and occupational therapists provide self-care training and preparation for discharge from the rehabilitation hospital. As much responsibility as possible is given the patient for personal care. Daily oral care, which at first may have been carried out by the nursing care staff, gradually should become a part of the daily hygiene routine accomplished by the patient, depending on the cord level of injury.

VI. Dental Hygiene Care

Emergency dental care may be needed during the patient's hospital period of recovery and treatment. Only the most necessary palliative treatment can be provided with portable equipment at the bedside.[5]

By the time the patient is able to be transported to a dental office or clinic, physical and psychologic preparation for daily living will be at a stage where the patient has developed a stable routine.

Most of the information necessary for patient management and instruction is presented in Chapter 50. A few special considerations will be described here.

A. Dental Chair Position

1. Wheelchair transfers (page 691).
2. Chair angle[3]
   a. For the patient with a gravity-drained urinary appliance, the chair may be adjusted to accommodate the drainage, or the patient should be uprighted at intervals to allow drainage to take place. It may be necessary to

empty the bag during the appointment.

b. The chair angle should not be changed abruptly because of the patient's susceptibility to postural hypotension.

c. Change the patient's body position in the chair by lifting and turning at intervals to prevent pressure sores and pain in muscles and joints. The use of padding has already been mentioned earlier in this section.

B. Four-handed Dental Hygiene

An assistant is a necessity. Precautions for the patient with spinal cord injury relate to the problems of respiration, pressure sores, spasms, autonomic dysreflexia, temperature control, and other factors that were described earlier. Assistance is definitely needed in many ways, including the following:

1. Assist in wheelchair transfer and in turning the patient at intervals.

2. Monitor vital signs.

3. Watch the patient for signs of body needs, emergencies.

4. Assist with rubber dam. A rubber dam should always be used for appropriate procedures such as application of topical fluorides, sealants, and polishing of restorations, because of danger of a respiratory complication should materials be inhaled.

5. Suction

   a. Prevent aspiration of foreign materials such as calculus.

   b. Use ultrasonic instruments with great caution, if at all. When unavoidable, care must be taken to prevent aspiration of water, to avoid spraying the throat and stimulating a gag or cough, and to make sure the instrument tip does not overheat.

6. Assist with all procedures to make the total treatment time as brief and efficiently used as possible without sacrificing patient comfort.

C. Disease Control

A complete preventive program with plaque control, fluorides, and nutrition and diet counseling is essential. Frequent recall usually is necessary to motivate, follow up with additional instruction, and assist the patient in carrying out the recommended procedures. Instruction for the direct-care person for the severely injured patient is included.

The technique and procedures described on pages 698–707 can be applied and personalized. Care of removable appliances includes cleaning mouth-held implements.

VII. Mouth-Held Implements

The patient without hands or without the use of hands may utilize the mouth for performing many tasks and the teeth for holding objects. The maintenance of optimum oral health has special significance for these individuals, since many of the same functions could not be accomplished in an edentulous mouth.

Mouth-held appliances have been fabricated that are effective in carrying out a variety of basic procedures and that contribute to increased independence for a person without the use of hands. A device makes possible such activities as pressing light switches, writing, typewriting, dialing a telephone, pushing an elevator button, or turning the pages of a book.

An oral telescoping orthosis has been developed that has advantages over a plain mouthstick.[6] An *orthosis* is a device added to a person's body to restore function, assist weak muscles, correct a deformity, immobilize a part, or substitute for absent motor power. The improved instrument covers the complete dentition, is electrically operated with buttons for control by the tongue, and has a telescoping mechanism to change the operational range.

The formerly used plain mouthsticks, which required gripping the stick with the teeth, damaged the teeth by causing chipping and undue and uneven pressures that led to periodontal trauma. When the appliance was adapted to anterior teeth only, there was tipping and extrusion of the incisors.

A minimum requirement for the preparation of an orthosis is that it cannot damage soft or hard oral tissues. One prerequisite is the use of a sanitary material that can be easily cleaned.[7] Before making impressions for constructing a mouthpiece, periodontal and restorative therapy should be completed and the occlusion adjusted. Plaque control procedures must be effective, and the patient instructed carefully in the importance and methods of oral hygiene and appliance care.

MYELOMENINGOCELE[8]

Spina bifida is a congenital defect or opening in the spinal cord. A portion of the spinal membranes may protrude through the opening with or without spinal cord tissue. When the spinal cord protrudes through the spina bifida, the condition is called *myelomeningocele*.

Embryologically, a neural tube forms during the first month of pregnancy. From the neural tube, the brain, brain stem, and spinal cord arise, and eventually, the vertebrae form and enclose the spinal cord. When a place in the spinal column fails to close, the result is an open defect in the spinal canal which is called a spina bifida. The cause of the failure of the tube to develop and close normally by one month is not known.

I. Types of Deformities

A. Myelomeningocele

A myelomeningocele is a protrusion or outpouching of the spinal cord and its covering (meninges) through an opening in the bony spinal canal. Because there is protrusion of part of the spinal cord and nerve roots, there is flaccid paralysis of the legs and part of the trunk, depending on the level of the protrusion (herniation).

B. Meningocele

A meningocele is a protrusion of the meninges through a defect in the skull or spinal column. Since no neural elements are contained in the protrusion, paralysis is uncommon.

C. Spina Bifida

Spina bifida is a congenital cleft in the bony encasement of the spinal cord. When there is no outpouching of the meninges or spinal cord, it is called *spina bifida occulta*. There are usually no symptoms with spina bifida occulta.

II. Physical Characteristics

Depending on the level of the myelomenin-

gocele, some or all of the signs and physical characteristics listed here may be found.

A. Bony Deformities

Muscle imbalance from paralysis can cause dislocation of the hip, club foot, and spinal curvatures such as humpback (kyphosis), curvature (scoliosis), or swayback (lordosis).

B. Loss of Sensation

Lack of skin sensitivity to pain, temperature, and other sensations can lead to problems of inadvertent burn or trauma unrecognized by the patient or attendant, or pressure sores, described on page 745. Frequent position changes are necessary.

C. Bladder and Bowel Paralysis

Rarely is the herniation low enough so that the nerve supplies to bladder and bowel are not affected. Lack of bowel and bladder control requires continual attention. Kidney infection with loss of kidney function is one cause of shorter life expectancy.

D. Hydrocephalus

Hydrocephalus is a condition in which there is an excessive accumulation of fluid in the brain which dilates the cerebral ventricles, causes compression of brain tissues, and separates the cranial bones as the head enlarges (figure 54–2). Development is slowed, and retardation occurs. Many of these patients have seizures.

A high percentage of children with myelomeningocele have hydrocephalus.

III. Medical Treatment

Surgical, orthopedic, medical, urologic, as well as physical and occupational therapy, may constitute a minimum of specialties involved in the care of a patient with myelomeningocele.

A. Neurosurgery

1. *Closure of the Myelomeningocele.* Surgical closure helps to prevent infections that may otherwise have entered into the spinal cord. Paralysis is not lessened by the surgery.
2. *Treatment of the Hydrocephalus.* Permanent drainage systems may be accomplished in the form of a ventriculoatrial

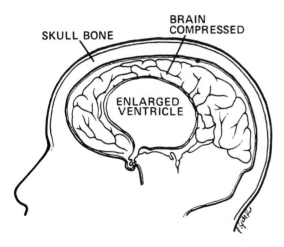

Figure 54-2. Hydrocephalus. The ventricle is enlarged because of the accumulation of fluid. Brain tissues are compressed. (From Bleck, E.E. and Nagel, D.A.: Physically Handicapped Children. A Medical Atlas for Teachers. New York, Grune & Stratton, 1975.)

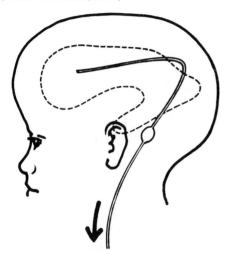

Figure 54-3. Shunt for treatment of hydrocephalus. Fluid is drained by way of a ventriculoatrial or a ventriculoperitoneal shunt. (From Bleck, E.E. and Nagel, D.A.: Physically Handicapped Children. A Medical Atlas for Teachers. New York, Grune & Stratton, 1975.)

shunt between the cerebral ventricle and the atrium of the heart (figure 54-3). Sometimes, drainage by way of the abdomen in the form of a ventriculoperitoneal shunt is used.

B. Orthopedic Surgery

Bracing to support the trunk and lower limbs is used in accord with the extent of the individual's paralysis. Ambulation varies from dependency on a wheelchair, walker, use of crutches or cane, or may be near normal with only foot problems. Orthopedic surgical procedures can assist by reducing or correcting deformities.

IV. Dental Hygiene Care

Management for the physical handicaps of the patient with myelomeningocele can be adapted from the information in Chapter 50. Wheelchair transfers and assistance for patients with crutches were described on pages 691–694. Special adaptations for plaque control techniques will be needed when the cervical or thoracic body level is involved, and the assistance of a parent or aide may be required.

Patients with seizures treated with phenytoin may need gingival treatment for phenytoin-induced gingival overgrowth. The condition is described on page 724.

Patients with shunts will need prophylactic antibiotic premedication prior to all dental and dental hygiene therapy.

CEREBROVASCULAR ACCIDENT (Stroke)

Cerebrovascular accident or stroke is a sudden loss of brain function resulting from interference with the blood supply to a part of the brain. The patient is frequently disabled by changes in motor, communication, and perception functions. Hemiplegia or hemiparesis is common.

I. Etiologic Factors

The stroke may be severe and followed by death within minutes. The less severe attack leaves the patient with symptoms and signs that will be described below. Strokes are usually brought on by one of the following:

A. Thrombosis

A clot within a blood vessel of the brain or neck closes or occludes the vessel and shuts off the oxygen supply to the portion of the brain supplied by that vessel, resulting in cerebral infarction.

B. Cerebral Embolism

A blood vessel is blocked by a clot or other material carried through the circulation from another part of the body.

C. Narrowing of an Artery that Supplies the Brain

The usual cause is atherosclerosis.

D. Cerebral Hemorrhage

A cerebral blood vessel may rupture and bleed into the brain tissues.

E. Predisposing Factors

Patients with certain conditions may be considered "risk" patients, or more susceptible to having strokes. Early diagnosis and treatment for control of the following predisposing factors are necessary in the prevention of stroke and its devastating effects. Risk factors related to atherosclerosis are described on page 784, and hypertension page 781.

1. Atherosclerosis
2. Hypertension, the greatest risk factor that leads to stroke.[9]
3. Aneurysm
4. Heart disease, especially enlarged heart.
5. Diabetes

II. Occurrence

A. Cerebral thrombosis is the most common cause of stroke: it accounts for 50 to 90 percent of strokes in people over 45. Cerebral hemorrhage causes up to 20 percent in the 30 to 60 age group; and aneurysms occur more in younger people between 20 and 30.
B. Stroke is the third leading cause of death in the United States.

III. Signs and Symptoms

The effects of a stroke depend on the location of the damage to the brain as well as the degree or extent of involvement. The side of the face and body affected will be opposite to that of the brain injury.

A. Transient Ischemic Attack

"Little strokes" may last a few minutes to an hour, and may leave no damage. A history of transient attacks is also a possible risk factor or warning.

B. Acute Symptoms of a Stroke

Acute symptoms and emergency procedures are included in table 58–1, page 847.

C. Residual or Chronic Effects

Approximately two thirds of those who survive have some degree of permanent disability. Temporary or permanent loss of thought, memory, speech, sensation, or motion results. The side affected influences the symptoms.

Persons with right hemiplegia have more difficulty with verbal communication and are more apt to be cautious, anxious, and disorganized. Patients with left hemiplegia have difficulty with action requiring physical coordination, and may respond impulsively with overconfidence.[10]

Common signs and symptoms are described briefly here for application during clinical patient care.

1. *Paralysis.* Hemiplegia (one side of the body) or portions such as an arm, leg, or the face.
2. *Articulation.* Difficulty of speech, which may be due to involvement of the tongue, mouth, or throat as well as to brain damage related to the speech centers.
3. *Salivation.* Difficulty in control of saliva complicated by difficulty in swallowing.
4. *Sensory.* Loss in affected parts with superficial anesthesia; or the opposite may occur with increased sensitivity to pain and touch.
5. *Visual Impairment.* Blurred vision, or diminished visual acuity.
6. *Mental Function.* May be unaffected, but slowness, with poor memory and loss of initiative are common. Brain deterioration may occur over a period of time.
7. *Personal Factors.* Personality changes relate to emotional trauma, fear, discouragement, and dependency. Anxiety neuroses and periods of depression, which are not uncommon, may require assistance from a psychiatrist.

IV. Medical Treatment

A. Surgical

Treatment may include surgical correction of aneurysms, clots, or malformations. Newer developments include surgery in the intracranial arteries using an operating microscope to remove very small clots or perform minute grafting to bypass blocked vessels and provide collateral circulation.

B. Physical and Occupational Therapy

Rehabilitation techniques are vital to the patient's functioning.

C. Drugs

Careful recording of the medical history will include the listing of medications. The patient may have a variety of drugs for some or all of the following purposes:
1. Anticoagulant (blood thinner).
2. Antihypertensive (to lower the blood pressure).
3. Thrombolytic (clot dissolving).
4. Vasodilator (to relax the blood vessels of the brain).
5. Steroid (to control brain swelling).
6. Anticonvulsant (for the patient with epilepsy).

V. Dental Hygiene Care

Elective dental treatment is not usually advisable until 6 months or more after a stroke; but if possible, preventive measures and plaque control techniques should be introduced or reinstated early. Regular appointments for preventive care should be initiated as soon as a release can be obtained from the physician.

Patients may be homebound or brought to the clinic or office by wheelchair or walker. Factors described in Chapter 50 apply for the patient who has had a stroke. Every attempt should be made to provide complete care, rather than temporary care which may increase the severity of needs at a later time. For the dental hygienist, this means complete scaling and planing to control the periodontal status.

A. Appointment Procedures

Because of weakness, treatment may best be accomplished in shorter appointments and small increments of instrumentation. The suggestions for appointments (page 688) have already been described. The application of four-handed dental hygiene during instrumentation is necessary for all of the same reasons described for the spinal-cord-injured patient on page 747.

B. Disease Control

Techniques for plaque control may need special adaptations. When the right-handed person is paralyzed on the right side (or the left-handed on the left), development of dexterity for the manipulation of plaque removal implements with the nondominant hand will take time and patience. The patient needs to be as self-sufficient as possible, but should be encouraged to have the paralyzed side deplaqued daily (brush, floss, and supplementary aids) by a family member or other direct-care person for whom instruction is provided.

The paralyzed side of the face tends to sag or droop, and because of inactivity of the tongue on the same side, self-cleansing is ineffective. Lack of sensation hinders the patient from realizing that collection of food debris and tooth deposits may be extensive.

Rinsing is difficult or impossible, so that the preferred method for daily fluoride application may be the use of a gel tray by the direct-care person, or the brushing of the teeth with a fluoride gel. When xerostomia is present, substitute saliva can be recommended (page 680).

Modified handles for toothbrushes and floss holders are shown on page 701. The patient who wears dentures will need a suction cup brush in order to clean the denture with one hand (figure 50–5, page 703).

MUSCULAR DYSTROPHIES[11,12]

The muscular dystrophies are inherited diseases characterized by progressive severe weakness and loss of use of symmetrical groups of muscles. The term *dystrophy* means degeneration and is associated with atrophy and dysfunction.

At least eight syndromes of muscular dystrophy have been separated by clinical and genetic means. The etiology for each type is not known, but the underlying pathologic processes do not differ. Generally, the diseases are limited to skeletal muscles with cardiac muscle only rarely involved.

All of the dystrophies are rare. The two types described below are the more common.

I. Duchenne Muscular Dystrophy (Pseudohypertrophic)

A. Occurrence

The Duchenne type is limited to males and transmitted by female carriers.

B. Age of Onset

The condition becomes apparent during early childhood, usually between 2 and 5 years, always before 10 years.

C. Characteristics

1. Enlargement (pseudohypertrophy) of certain muscles, particularly the calves, is present in early years.
2. Weakness of hips: child falls frequently, has increasing difficulty in standing erect.
3. Lordosis; abdominal protuberance.
4. Gait
   a. Waddling: either walks on toes or flatfoot; a result of muscle contracture.
   b. Balance: precarious; patient arches back in attempt to find center of gravity; gait is slow as balance must be attained with each step.
5. Progressive muscular wasting: eventual involvement of thighs, shoulders, trunk; inactivity is detrimental and increases the individual's helplessness and dependency.
6. Intellectual impairment: average I.Q. in the range of 80 to 90, with some of normal intelligence and others at moderate to severe level of retardation.

D. Prognosis

Disablement severe by puberty; child is confined to a wheelchair. Patients rarely live to reach their third decade.

II. Facioscapulohumeral Muscular Dystrophy

A. Occurrence

Males and females are equally affected.

B. Age of Onset

Between 10 and 18 with an average at 13 years, after puberty. Mild symptoms may appear at later ages.

C. Characteristics

1. Facial muscles involved, particularly the obicularis oris.
2. Scapulae prominent; shoulder muscles weak, difficulty in raising the arms.
3. Eyes: difficulty in closing them completely.

D. Prognosis

Progresses more slowly than the Duchenne type. Most patients live a normal life span, and become incapacitated late in life.

III. Medical Treatment

There is no known specific treatment. Symptoms may be relieved. The patient is encouraged to lead as full a life as possible and keep active. Since inactivity leads to obesity, diet planning is important.

IV. Dental Hygiene Care

Adaptations depend on the patient's disability. Patients may have slight muscular involvement, be ambulatory but have balancing difficulties, be in a wheelchair, or bedridden. Factors described for general consideration of patients with disabilities have application (Chapter 50). Suggestions listed below will be useful for certain patients.

A. Patient Reception and Seating

1. *Assistance for the Walking Patient*
   a. Certain patients do better without assistance, as they have developed their own method of balancing and the merest touch may upset them.
   b. Many gain balance by holding both hands on partially flexed forearm of person walking beside them.
2. *Seating Preparation*
   a. Raise chair: when patient does not have strength to lower himself into chair.
   b. Remove conventional chair arm: allow patient to sit directly.
3. *After Seating Patient:* tilt chair back gently; balance is precarious while sitting as well as standing; patient may fall forward.
4. *Assistance for Patient While Rising from Chair*

a. Stand directly in front of patient: lock arms around lower back and pull forward near hips.

b. Allow patient to sway upper trunk back while rising to standing position.

c. Provide support until balance is obtained for walking.

B. Patient Instruction

1. *Problems of Oral Cleanliness*

   a. Facial muscle weakness may interfere with self-cleansing mechanisms and prevent adequate rinsing by the patient with facioscapulohumeral dystrophy.

   b. Gaping lips: effect on oral tissues similar to that of mouthbreathing.

   c. Weakness of arm and shoulder: difficulty in applying toothbrush. A powered brush or an adapted handle for a regular brush (pages 700–703) may have advantages.

2. *Disease Control*

   a. Instruct parent or other person who cares for patient.

   b. When patient is receiving therapy, solicit assistance and advice from the occupational therapist.

MYASTHENIA GRAVIS

Myasthenia gravis is an immunologic neuromuscular disease characterized by weakness and fatigability of symmetrical voluntary muscles. It is caused by an autoimmune process that results in a defect in nerve impulse transmission at the neuromuscular junctions. In myasthenia gravis, there is a marked reduction in numbers of acetylcholine receptors in each neuromuscular junction when compared to the normal number of receptors.[13] Continuing research will clarify the detailed mechanisms of the immunologic disorder. It is now suggested that more than one disease or syndrome is involved.[14]

The patient with myasthenia gravis has a special significance for dental professionals because the facial and oral parts served by certain cranial nerves are involved early. Muscles of the eyes, facial expression, mastication, and swallowing are affected. In advanced severe forms of the disease, muscle involvement may be extensive and result in total paralysis.

I. Occurrence

Myasthenia gravis may have its onset at any age. The early peak at about age 20 affects females twice as frequently as males. In late adult life more males than females are affected.

II. Signs and Symptoms

A. Early Signs

Weakness of eye movements with double vision (diplopia) and drooping eyelids (ptosis) may be the initial indicators. In certain patients, the disease may progress no farther.

B. Oral and Facial Problems

Involvement of muscles of the face, mastication, and tongue lead to swallowing difficulties (dysphagia) and a lack of facial expression. Disturbed speech and expression, with a weak voice that sounds tired and muffled, are typical. A patient may support the chin with one hand to help during talking.

C. Progressive Involvement

When the muscles that are used during breathing become involved, serious respiratory complications can result. Because of the lack of facial expression, it may be difficult for the patient to convey distress.

Generalized fatigue is usually not so evident in the morning or immediately after rest. Weakness may increase as the day goes by, a factor pertinent to the time selected for dental and dental hygiene appointments.

D. Precipitating Factors

Individual reactions vary, but the more common predisposing, aggravating factors affecting the severity of muscular involvement include emotional excitement, surgical procedures, loss of sleep, alcoholic intake, and especially, infections. Prevention of oral infections and of the need for dental or periodontal surgery contribute to patient stability. Myasthenic crisis is best avoided by elimination and prevention of infection and all precipitating factors.

E. **Types of Crises**

  1. *Myasthenic Crisis*[15]

     a. Cause. A myasthenic crisis may result from increased severity of the disease or it may be precipitated by one of the aggravating factors mentioned above, particularly infection. The relative deficiency of acetylcholine, which leads to the crisis symptoms, can usually be corrected by the physician's administration of anticholinesterase.

     b. Symptoms and signs. There is a sudden inability to swallow, speak, or maintain a patent airway. Marked weakness of respiratory and pharyngeal muscles leads to depression of respiration and obstruction. The patient may also have double vision and drooping eyelids.

     c. Emergency care

        (1) Suction.

        (2) Ventilation: provide a patent airway (pages 838–839).

        (3) Obtain medical assistance; transport to hospital emergency facility.

  2. *Cholinergic Crisis*

     a. Cause. The cholinergic crisis results from excessive doses of anticholinesterase.

     b. Symptoms and signs. There is increased muscle weakness within 30 to 60 minutes of taking the medication, excessive pulmonary secretion, cramps, and diarrhea.

     c. Treatment. No further medication should be taken at that time. Medical assistance is needed promptly. When there are respiratory symptoms, ventilation is urgent.

III. **Medical Treatment**[14]

Medical treatment may have two purposes: (1) to influence the course of the disease, and (2) to induce disease remission. Anticholinesterase agents are used for most patients at intervals during the day. A sustained-release preparation may be used at bedtime, particularly for the patient who awakens with severe weakness.

Current therapy for attempting to induce remission includes surgical removal of the thymus gland, particularly if a tumor of the gland develops, and drug therapy. Steroids and immunosuppressive medications have been shown to benefit selected patients.[14]

IV. **Dental Hygiene Care**

A. **Appointment Factors**[15]

  1. *Time and Length.* Short appointments planned in conjunction with the patient's medication schedule and early in the day, since weakness worsens with activity.

  2. *Recall.* Frequent appointments to aid the patient in obtaining and maintaining freedom from oral infection.

  3. *Preparation for the Appointment.* Office emergency equipment for a possible respiratory emergency must be checked and be in order. Stress reduction procedures should be followed.

     At the outset, the patient should be asked about medication and whether it has been taken on schedule prior to the appointment.

B. **Four-handed Dental Hygiene**

For any patient who is a potential respiratory risk, an assistant is needed to aid in observing the patient and to monitor vital signs. Since the patient with myasthenia gravis may have difficulty in providing a warning of distress, the need for supervision is indicated.

  1. *Suction.* An assistant is needed to maintain the airway, to assure no problem of aspiration, as well as to provide a clean field for efficient instrumentation which will take a minimum length of time. A side effect of the anticholinesterase medication is increased salivation.

  2. *Rubber Dam Application* for appropriate procedures to prevent aspiration of harmful substances.

C. **Patient Instruction for Disease Control**

  1. *Diet Evaluation.* A dietary survey and instruction are recommended. The patient with myasthenia gravis may have difficulty in masticating and swallowing, and adequate food selection for oral health and dental caries prevention may be difficult.

2. *Plaque Control.* Weakness and fatigability may have discouraged the patient's routine daily plaque control efforts. A powered brush or other aids (pages 700–703) might be recommended. Instruction for a family member or other direct-care person may be needed to provide the severely disabled patient with assistance.

MULTIPLE SCLEROSIS

Multiple sclerosis is a degenerative, demyelinating disease characterized by progressive disability. It is also called *disseminated sclerosis.* Sclerosis means hardening, especially by overgrowth of interstitial tissue.

Pathologically, the myelin sheath is destroyed within the white matter of the central nervous system. The sheath degenerates in patches called *MS plaques* and is replaced by sclerotic tissue. There is interference with the transmission of nerve impulses, and frequent involvement of the spinal cord and optic nerves.

The etiology is not known. Research has centered around a possible autoimmune mechanism and an association with viral infections.

I. Occurrence

A. Onset

Usually, the onset is between 20 and 40 years of age, rarely before 15 or after 55 years.

B. Geographic

The disease is more prevalent in cold and temperate climates.

II. Characteristics

A. Initial Symptoms: Vary
1. May be visual impairment, difficulty in coordination, tremor, fatigue, weakness, or numbness of a part of the body.
2. May have a sudden onset of severe illness with paralysis or marked weakness.

B. Course of Disease
1. *Relapses and Remissions.* An attack may last several days or weeks and be followed by a symptom-free period. Physical impairment varies, but the condition worsens with each attack.
2. *Precipitating Factors*
   a. Infection

   Various types of infection, systemic or local, can stimulate a relapse. Oral infections are no exception.
   b. Stress and emotional trauma.
   c. Injury.
   d. Heavy exercise and fatigue.
   e. Pregnancy.

   For certain patients, pregnancy may appear to increase the risk and bring on an attack. Since the effect is more likely to be noticed during the first several months after delivery, fatigue and stress may be the direct precipitating effects.

   Effects of multiple sclerosis on the pregnancy should also be recognized. Possible side effects of medications on the developing fetus should be considered since certain medications used may have to be discontinued if they are teratogenic.
3. *Longevity.* People with multiple sclerosis may live many years. Death is usually the result of an infection, such as of the urinary tract or bronchopneumonia. Fewer than half may eventually become nonambulatory.

C. Physical Symptoms

A wide distribution of areas is affected, which results in a variety of symptoms. Symptoms fluctuate and several years may elapse between attacks. With extended rest, symptoms usually subside.
1. Involuntary motion of eyes (nystagmus); may later become partially or completely blind.
2. Speech disorders: possible loss of speech in advanced stages.
3. Changes in muscular coordination and gait; loss of balance; spasms.
4. Paralysis of one or more extremities; occasionally, facial paralysis.
5. Autonomic derangements such as urinary frequency and urgency; later urinary incontinence.
6. Susceptibility to infection, particularly upper respiratory.
7. Seizures.

D. Personal Factors

1. Optimism and cheerfulness out of proportion to the degree of disability and seriousness of the illness; euphoria or the opposite, leading to depression.
2. Subject to sharp deviations of mood: emotional outbursts with spells of laughing and crying.
3. Poor memory; poor judgment.
4. Passive dependency; lack of responsibility.

III. Medical Treatment

A. No specific treatment since the cause of the disease is unknown.
B. General hygienic care: adequate nutrition, rest, avoidance of strain, prevention of infections.
C. Physical and occupational therapy; exercise, but not strenuous exertion, is very important.
D. Psychotherapy for personality problems and morale building is frequently necessary.
E. Drugs: primarily prescribed for alleviation of symptoms. Immunosuppressants have been tried because of the possibility of an immunologic etiologic factor.
F. Patient should continue in a usual occupation as long as possible; activity should be encouraged.

IV. Dental Hygiene Care

Many factors described in Chapter 50, page 685, have direct application for the patient with a disability associated with multiple sclerosis. For the patient with paraplegia or quadriplegia, items from the section on spinal-cord-injured patients can be used (page 744).

Since relapses may be precipitated by infections, dental hygiene care for the prevention of oral infection assumes particular significance.

A. Appointment Considerations

1. Provide a warm, quiet, comfortable atmosphere. The patient needs to remain relaxed mentally and physically; people around cannot be tense, restless, or noisy.
2. Frequent short appointments contribute to preventing fatigue, emotional stress,

and advanced dental or periodontal conditions.

B. Patient Instruction

1. *Problems of Personal Oral Care*
   a. Involvements of the tongue and facial muscles interfere with the self-cleansing mechanisms.
   b. Paralysis may make grasping and manipulating a toothbrush difficult or impossible. Adaptive aids are described on pages 700–701.
2. *Factors Affecting Teaching*
   a. Slow response of patient; give instruction slowly and simply.
   b. Visual disturbances (pages 764–766).

CEREBRAL PALSY

Palsy means impairment of the ability to control movement, and cerebral palsy means a condition in which injury to parts of the brain has occurred prenatally, natally, or postnatally and resulted in paralysis or disruption of motor parts. Such a condition can occur at any age as a result of brain injury from a variety of causes. It can be caused by anoxia during pregnancy or delivery, maternal infection during pregnancy (for example, rubella), blood type incompatibility, severe nutritional lack during pregnancy, or maternal diabetes endocrine imbalance. Later in infancy, infectious diseases such as meningitis or encephalitis, lead poisoning, direct trauma from accidents, or battering (nonaccidental injury) may be implicated.

Symptoms usually can be observed during the first year after birth, but may not appear for several years. General symptoms that may occur are tense, contracted muscles, uncontrolled movements of limbs, eyes, or head, poor coordination, muscle spasms, problems with hearing and/or seeing, and a lack of manual dexterity.

I. Occurrence

Approximately 3 individuals per 1000 have cerebral palsy in the United States, of which one fifth are seriously disabled.

II. Types and Characteristics[16,17]

Classified by motor activity, six types have been named. In each type, different parts of the brain are damaged, and the symptoms vary respectively. More than 50 percent of those with cerebral palsy are in the spasticity group, 15 to 20 percent are athetoid, and the remainder are divided among the other four types or have mixed types.

A. Spasticity

1. Muscles have increased tone, tension, and activity.
2. Condition characterized by spasms, which are sudden, involuntary contractions of single muscles or groups of muscles.
3. Patient has complete or partial loss of ability to control muscular movement; therefore, movements are awkward and stiff.
4. Activity: lack of control causes patient to fall easily; tends to avoid activity; may gain weight, particularly during teen years; caloric requirement is therefore low.
5. Brain damage to motor area of cerebral cortex (figure 54–4).

B. Athetosis

1. Condition characterized by constant, involuntary unorganized muscular movement.
2. Patient lacks ability to direct muscles in the motions desired; probably the most difficult dental patient.

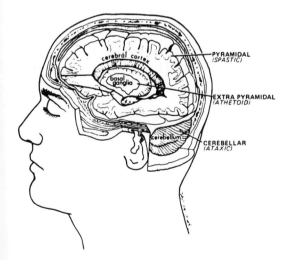

Figure 54–4. Cerebral palsy. Major parts of the brain involved in the three principal types of cerebral palsy. (From Bleck, E.E. and Nagel, D.A.: Physically Handicapped Children, A Medical Atlas for Teachers. New York, Grune & Stratton, 1975.)

3. Grimacing, drooling, and speech defects are common.
4. Factors influencing movements
   a. Effort by patient to control muscle activity results in exaggerated muscle movement.
   b. May be initiated and aggravated by stimuli outside body, such as sudden noises, bright lights, or quick movements by people or things in the area.
   c. Intensity influenced by emotional factors: patient is least in control in an emotionally charged environment such as the dental office.
5. Activity: constantly in motion; burns up energy; usually very thin; caloric requirement of diet is therefore high.
6. Brain damage to basal ganglia (figure 54–4).

C. Ataxia

1. Loss of equilibrium: balance and orientation difficult; walk uncertain; has difficulty in sitting straight.
2. Lack of coordination; needs time to execute changes.
3. Activity: inactive because of balance disturbance; tends to put on weight; caloric requirement in diet is therefore low.
4. Brain damage to cerebellum (figure 54–4).

D. Rigidity

1. Muscles may be rigid and stiff, with resistance to movement and hypertonicity.
2. Tendency to lack of activity.

E. Tremor

Involuntary muscle quivering, which may affect part or all of the body.

F. Flaccidity

1. Hypotonia or atonia of muscles that are flabby and weak.
2. Unable to stand or raise head.
3. Drooling; difficulty in swallowing and chewing; speech problems.

G. Mixed

Various combinations of the six types occur.

III. Conditions Accompanying Motor Activity

In addition to impaired movement, weakness, and lack of coordination, the handicapping conditions listed below may also occur.

A. Mental Retardation

Approximately 50 percent of individuals with cerebral palsy also have mental retardation.

B. Learning Disabilities

Of the 50 percent who are not mentally retarded, many have problems of learning because of sensory defects, especially hearing and seeing, as well as perceptive-cognitive deficiencies. Speech difficulties and inability to move about freely can also contribute to learning problems.

C. Seizures

Between 25 and 30 percent have seizures and undergo related drug therapy.

D. Sensory Disorders

Seeing and hearing problems are not uncommon.

IV. Medical Treatment

Surgical, orthopedic, medical, as well as speech, physical therapy, and occupational therapy may constitute a minimum of specialties involved in the care of a patient with cerebral palsy. Bracing to support the lower limbs, the use of canes, crutches, walkers, or wheelchairs are used to increase function. Surgery may be needed for orthopedic deformities or for correcting eye or ear difficulties.

Patients may use tranquilizers to reduce tension or aid in limiting problems associated with nerve damage. Other medication may include drugs for seizure control. There is no cure for cerebral palsy.

V. Oral Characteristics

A. Disturbances of Musculature

Facial grimacing, abnormal muscle function, facial asymmetry, and problems of mastication and swallowing are common. Opening of the mouth may present problems during dental and dental hygiene therapy as well as during plaque control at home.

B. Malocclusion

There is a high incidence of malocclusion. Oral habits of mouth breathing, tongue thrusting, and faulty swallowing contribute to orthodontic needs.

C. Attrition

Severe, constant, involuntary grinding of teeth wears down tooth structure and restorations. Bruxism is most extensive in the athetoid group.

D. Fractured Teeth

Patients fall frequently; accidents to anterior teeth result.

E. Dental Caries

There may be a slightly higher rate of dental caries, but the same factors are operating for the patient with cerebral palsy as in the physically normal population. Difficulties in maintaining plaque control and problems of mastication, which lead to the use of a soft diet, may predispose to an environment for bacterial plaque formation.

F. Periodontal Disease

Periodontal or gingival diseases are found in a very high percent of patients with cerebral palsy.
1. *Phenytoin-induced Gingival Overgrowth.* When phenytoin is used in the treatment of epilepsy, the patient is susceptible to gingival enlargement. The condition and its prevention are described on page 724.
2. *Predisposing Factors to Periodontal Involvement.* Mechanical difficulties related to plaque control, mouth breathing, and increased food retention because of ineffective self-cleansing all lead to increased periodontal involvement and plaque collection. Many patients with cerebral palsy have heavy calculus deposits.

VI. Dental Hygiene Care

Procedures described in Chapter 50 (page 685) apply in the management of the patient with cerebral palsy. Many special adaptations are needed, and experience contributes to developing the necessary patience and confidence.

Dental hygiene care is complicated by the difficulties the patient has in cooperating and by the oral manifestations listed above. Understanding the physical characteristics is particularly necessary to the success of the appointments. Athetoid movements should not be interpreted as lack of cooperation and a patient's inability to communicate does not mean lack of comprehension.

Dentists occasionally find it necessary to use general anesthesia in a hospital situation for the unmanageable patient.

There are dangers for both the patient and dental personnel which may result from the uncontrolled movement of the patient. The sudden forceful closure of the mouth on the finger of the operator or on a glass mouth mirror, or movement of the patient which diverts a sharp instrument into the patient's tissues, are examples.

Assistance throughout appointments is important. Suggestions for management should be solicited from family or direct-care attendants. Sedation through premedication may be possible, and various restraining procedures may be used (page 694).

Selected patients with cerebral palsy may use a mouth-held instrument as described on page 747. Oral care and preventive measures are vital to this group of patients.

BELL'S PALSY

Bell's palsy is a paralysis of the facial muscles innervated by the facial or seventh cranial nerve. Although the cause is not known, various possible agents have been implicated, including bacterial and viral infections, particularly herpes simplex, trauma from tooth removal, or surgery of the parotid gland area such as the removal of a tumor.

I. Occurrence

Although relatively rare, the incidence increases with each decade of life. Women are more frequently affected than men in younger age groups, but after age 50, it is more common in males.

II. Characteristics[18]

A. Signs and Symptoms

Abrupt paralysis of facial muscles, usually without preceding pain, occurs on one side of the face.
1. *Mouth.* The corner of the mouth droops and there is uncontrollable salivation with drooling.
2. *Eye.* Eyelids cannot be closed. Watering and drooping of the lower lid invite infection.

B. Functional Problems

Speech and mastication are difficult.

C. Prognosis

A majority of patients experience a return to normal within a month, many have a spontaneous recovery. Others may have lasting residual effects or permanent paralysis.

III. Medical Treatment[19]

Without knowledge of the specific etiology, treatment has not been definitive. Temporary palliative measures, such as protecting the eye during sleep and massaging the involved muscles, provide some relief.

A. Drugs

Steroids have been used to improve the prognosis.

B. Surgical[20]

The objectives for surgical procedures have been to improve the appearance, provide facial symmetry with voluntary motion, and provide control of the eye and the mouth. Surgery has included repair of the facial nerve, nerve transplantation and grafting, crossover nerve grafts from the uninvolved side of the face, muscle transfers, and free muscle grafts. Prosthetic rehabilitation has been combined with surgical.

C. Prostheses[21]

Surgery may be contraindicated or unsuccessful, and prosthetic treatment may aid in providing tissue support and assist in speech. Facial symmetry has been improved with the use of removable prostheses.

IV. Dental Hygiene Care

Instruction and frequent appointments to supplement the patient's efforts usually are needed. A removable prosthesis will need daily care since debris and plaque collect readily.

When only the seventh nerve has been affected, sensory responses are still intact. When anesthesia is used on the opposite side, special precautions should be provided for postoperative care until the anesthesia has worn off.

Protective goggles should be worn by the patient. Care is necessary to ensure that calculus, polishing paste, or other foreign material does not enter the eye, since the eyelid lacks its natural ability to close for protection.

PARKINSON'S DISEASE

Parkinson's disease is a progressive disorder of the central nervous system in which there is loss of postural reflexes, slowness of spontaneous movement, tremor, and muscle rigidity. It is also known as *paralysis agitans, Parkinson's syndrome,* and *Parkinsonism.*

Although the cause is not known, the basis for the specific group of symptoms is known. There is degeneration of certain neurons in the substantia nigra of the basal ganglia where posture, support, and voluntary motion are controlled. In addition, there is a severe deficiency of dopamine, one of the substances that participates in nerve transmission.

I. Occurrence

Parkinson's disease affects middle-aged and older persons primarily, with a higher incidence in men than in women. It is fairly common, with an estimated incidence of 1 in every 100 persons over age 60.

II. Characteristics

The signs and symptoms center around tremor, rigidity, and loss or impairment of motor function (akinesia), although all three occur in other conditions which must be differentiated by a physician when a diagnosis is made.

A. General Manifestations

1. Body posture bent, with bent head and general stiffness.
2. Motion and responses slowed; difficulty in keeping balance.
3. A quick shuffling gait.
4. Speech monotonous and slow.
5. Tremor of one or both hands; the fingers may be involved in a pill-rolling motion in which the thumb and index finger are rubbed together in a circular movement. The tremor can be reduced or stopped when the person engages in purposeful action.
6. Intellect is seldom affected except in the very advanced stages.
7. Eventually, after 10 to 20 years, the person may become incapacitated and require complete care.

B. Face and Oral Cavity

1. Expression is fixed and mask-like with diminished eye blinking.
2. Tremor in lips, tongue, neck, and difficulty in swallowing.
3. Excess salivation and drooling.

III. Medical Treatment

A. Drug Therapy

Although there is no known cure for Parkinson's disease, symptomatic control can be accomplished, at least in part, by replenishing the dopamine shortage with Levodopa. Side effects are common, and may indicate an overdose.[22] Orthostatic hypotension and dizziness may be expected and should be considered when adjusting the dental chair.

B. Physical Therapy and Active Exercise[23]

Maintenance of good general health, with plenty of rest and nutritious meals, is encouraged. Professional physical therapy and occupational therapy have particular significance for a patient's well-being.

IV. Dental Hygiene Care

Various adaptations of procedures can be anticipated from knowledge of the physical characteristics noted above. Personal interest, attention, and encouragement contribute to help the patient bear the stresses of the disability.

General suggestions for the gerodontic patient in Chapter 45 may prove useful, as well as suggestions related to physical disabilities in Chapter 50. Special adaptations for plaque control may be needed.

ARTHRITIS

Diseases of the joints, including arthritis, are among the most common causes of chronic illness in the United States. Besides arthritis as a disease entity, arthritic manifestations are produced as part of various other chronic diseases. There may be temporary or permanent, partial or complete disability. A person may suffer from more than one type at a time.

Arthritis means inflammation in a joint. It may occur in an acute or chronic form and may be localized or generalized. When many joints are involved, the term polyarthritis may be applied.

Factors that have been implicated in the etiology of rheumatic and arthritic diseases include infectious agents, traumatic disorders, endocrine abnormalities, tumors, allergy and drug reactions, and inherited or congenital conditions. When the etiology is known, specific medical, physical, and surgical therapies may be available to alleviate pain and disability.

I. Rheumatoid Arthritis[24]

Rheumatoid arthritis is a chronic, immunologic systemic disease in which inflammation of the joints occurs in exacerbations and remissions. The etiology is unknown, and how the inflammation in the joints is initiated remains a question.

A. Occurrence

The onset is between ages 20 and 40, although it may occur at any age. More females than males are affected. It is rare in tropical countries.

B. Signs and Symptoms

1. Joint pain and swelling. Rheumatoid arthritis is a polyarthritis with migratory pain, swelling, tenderness, and warmth in symmetrical joints. Fingers, hands, and knees are usually affected first.
2. Morning stiffness and stiffness after periods of inactivity.
3. Weakness, fatigue, loss of appetite and weight, anemia, low grade fever.
4. Subcutaneous nodules in elbows, wrists, or fingers develop in approximately 20 percent of the patients, and nodules may appear in other body organs.
5. Temporomandibular joint involvement may occur. There may be pain with jaw movements and difficulty in chewing. Ankylosis may develop but is not a common finding.
6. Progressive deformity with limited motion in the more severely involved joints and muscle atrophy adjacent to the joints.

C. Medical Treatment

Without specifically known etiology, therapy is limited to an individualized program involving pain relief, physical and occupational therapy, and overall health maintenance with adequate nutrition. The most widely prescribed drug is aspirin, which is used for its anti-inflammatory effect. Selected patients have been treated by joint replacement surgery.

II. Juvenile Rheumatoid Arthritis

When rheumatoid arthritis occurs in children under 16 years of age, there are differences from the disease in adults. The onset is usually more acute, with prolonged fever and enlargement of spleen and lymph nodes. The inflammation of many joints, particularly knees, wrists, and spine may appear after a few weeks. Figure 54–5 shows the shape of affected fingers. The temporomandibular joint may be involved, with pain and limited oral opening.

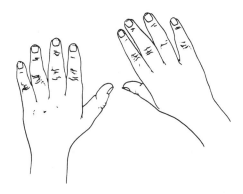

Figure 54–5. Fingers of a child with rheumatoid arthritis. The fingers are tapered from fat central areas. The joint nearest the tip of the finger is the least involved. (From Bleck, E.E. and Nagel, D.A.: Physically Handicapped Children. A Medical Atlas for Teachers. New York, Grune & Stratton, 1975.)

Many patients have complete remissions, some have increasing disability, while others may have mild arthritic symptoms that continue for years. Child patients are encouraged to lead as normal a life as possible. The long-term treatment program includes activity to maintain function and drugs to relieve pain.

III. Degenerative Joint Diseases

Degenerative joint disease (DJD), or osteoarthritis as it is frequently called, affects the weight-bearing joints particularly. Since inflammation is not the basic joint problem, degenerative joint disease is a more accurate term.

No specific etiology is known, but predisposing causes may include repeated trauma, obesity, age changes in the joint tissues, mechanical stresses to the weight-bearing joints, and faulty body posture.[24,25]

A. Occurrence

The onset is between 50 and 70 years of age, with the average onset 20 years later than that of rheumatoid arthritis. As many as 85 percent of people over age 70 have evidence of degenerative joint disease.

B. Symptoms

At first insidious, with slight stiffness of a single joint, the eventual condition leads to much pain, deformity, and limitation of movement.
1. Hips, knees, fingers, vertebrae affected most frequently.
2. Swelling is rare; ankylosis does not occur.
3. Stiffness in the morning on rising and after periods of inactivity; diminishes with exercise.
4. Pain aggravated by temperature changes and bearing body weight.
5. Temporomandibular joint is usually without pain or other clinical symptoms, although crepitation, clicking, or snapping may occur when the joints are exercised.

C. Medical Treatment

Moderate exercise, aspirin or other pain-relieving drug therapy, weight reduction for obese patients, physical therapy, and selected orthopedic surgical procedures compose the general treatments available. Total hip or knee joint replacement has proven satisfactory for many patients, and has been used more widely for DJD than for rheumatoid arthritis.

IV. Personal Factors

With long-range illnesses, patients are frequently discouraged or apprehensive. Certain patients may be worried, pessimistic, or resigned. Some may be impatient and tend to harm themselves by overexercise. A few are irritable, a characteristic related to the pain that has been suffered.

Psychologic causes for temporomandibular joint dysfunction have been demonstrated. In certain instances, treatment of the psychologic factors can result in relief of physical symptoms.[26] Facial abnormalities and occlusal discrepancies have also been implicated in temporomandibular joint problems. Any of these other conditions may occur with arthritis of the joint.

V. Dental Hygiene Care

A high standard of general health contributes to the well-being of the patient with arthritis. Maintenance of oral health contributes to general health.

Adjustments for physical disabilities of the patient with arthritis may be found in Chapter 50. Assistance with ambulation, chair positioning, and other special adaptations will be needed.

A. Patient History

Questions to determine whether the patient has a joint prosthesis should be included in the patient history. Because of the susceptibility to infection at the interface of the bone and the prosthesis, prophylactic antibiotic premedication to prevent bacteremia is essential.[27,28]

B. Instrumentation

For the patient with arthritis of the temporomandibular joint, instrumentation may need adaptations to accommodate a minimal opening of the mouth. Fatigue in the joint may be reduced by rest periods, minimizing the pressure on the mandible, and by overall efficiency to shorten the necessary appointment time. More frequent appointments can contribute to keeping the oral health at a maximum and thus preventing long, difficult scaling sessions.

C. Plaque Control

Because of hand and arm involvement, a patient may have difficulty grasping a toothbrush or lifting the arm for sufficient periods to clean the mouth completely. Adapted brushing procedures may be applied (pages 700–705).

D. Diet and Nutrition

1. No special nutritional factors are known to be associated with the course or treatment of arthritis. Physicians generally recommend a normal, well-balanced diet with a controlled caloric intake for weight control. Encouragement of restriction of sweets and selection of noncariogenic between-meal snacks can help to improve oral health.

2. Dietary analysis: obtaining a food diary for several days to a week can be important for counseling, especially for the gerodontic arthritic patient.

SCLERODERMA
(Progressive Systemic Sclerosis)

Scleroderma is an autoimmune disease of connective tissue in which there is an overproduction of collagen. The most striking physical symptom is the immobility and rigidity of the skin, but inflammation and sclerosis occur throughout the body, which gives the disease the full title of *progressive systemic sclerosis.*

The etiology is not known, but research has been concerned with studying collagen synthesis irregularities, associated immunologic disorders, and microvascular abnormalities. Hereditary factors are not involved.

I. Occurrence

Scleroderma has its onset between ages 30 and 50, but may affect any age, even infants. It may develop over months or years. It is two to five times more common in females.

II. Characteristics

Scleroderma may be localized and involve only the skin, or it may be generalized and involve all body organs. The most notable changes are in the skin, gastrointestinal tract, kidneys, heart, muscles, and lungs. Eventual death is due to renal failure, cardiac failure, pulmonary insufficiency, or intestinal malabsorption. Symptoms vary, and all individuals will not have all the symptoms and signs listed below.

A. General Manifestations

1. *Joints.* Pain, swelling, and stiffness of the fingers and knee joints.
2. *Polyarthritis.* Symmetrical polyarthritis, similar to rheumatoid arthritis.
3. *Skin.* Hard and fixed; ivory-white, yellow, or gray, sometimes with brown pigmentation in the late stages.
4. *Face.* When the face is affected it becomes masklike and expressionless.

B. Oral Characteristics

1. *Lips:* thin, rigid, with oral stricture and difficulty in opening and closing.
2. *Mucosa:* thin, pale, tender, rigid, with poor healing capacity.
3. *Gingiva:* pale, and unusually firm.
4. *Teeth:* mobility is common.
5. *Radiographic Findings:* marked widening of the periodontal ligament spaces. This finding is sometimes considered pathognomonic for scleroderma. It has been observed in as many as 37 percent in a group of patients with systemic sclerosis.[29]
6. *Mastication:* difficult; temporomandibular joint movement is limited.
7. *Tongue:* may be immobile; speech difficult.

III. Medical Treatment

Specific therapy is not known. Medications that retard collagen deposition have not yet been effective for scleroderma. Treatment, therefore, has been directed at specific system complications, physical therapy, and attempts to maintain normal activities.

IV. Dental Hygiene Care

The tightening of the skin and lips limits opening of the mouth and complicates all dental and dental hygiene procedures as well as daily self-care by the patient. Every effort for preservation of the teeth and gingiva in health should be made to prevent the need for extensive treatment.

With oral stricture, the preparation and wearing of dentures would be difficult or impossible as the disease became more severe.[30]

Patients with scleroderma are sensitive to cold and dampness, stress, undue emotional tension, and fatigue. All of these factors can be considered for the dental hygiene appointment.

SENSORY DISORDERS[31,32]

VISUAL IMPAIRMENT

Limitations of sight cover a broad spectrum from the slightly affected to the completely blind with no perception of light. Adaptations during the appointment vary then from a procedure as simple as providing a patient's eyeglasses before demonstrating a toothbrushing procedure to those required for the partially sighted or completely sightless as described in this section.

Loss of sight is a major physical deprivation. In many people, blindness is secondary to a primary condition which may have been the cause of the blindness and in itself may be disabling.

In the United States, "legal blindness" is defined as follows: the central visual acuity is 20/200 or less in the better eye after correction, or visual acuity of more than 20/200 if there is a peripheral field defect in which the widest diameter of the visual field is less than a radius of 10 degrees. Only approximately 3 percent of legally blind people are totally blind. The term legal blindness is a legal, not a medical term, but certification of the degree of severity of blindness is obtained from an ophthalmologist.

I. Causes of Blindness

The five leading causes of blindness are diabetic retinopathy, senile cataracts, senile macular degeneration, glaucoma, and prenatal influences.[33] At least one half of the blindness in children is of prenatal origin. Other causes are injuries, neoplasms, and retrolental fibroplasia. Retrolental fibroplasia was a major cause of blindness in premature infants, but now is rare since it has been shown that it can be prevented by proper control of the oxygen exposure of an infant.

More than 50 percent of new cases of blindness occur in the population over 65 years of age.

II. Personal Factors

Each blind person must be considered in relation to individual aptitudes, interests, abilities, and potentialities, with blindness only one factor involved, and frequently not the most important. No pattern of patient attitudes and personality characteristics can be described. The only thing this group of patients has in common is difficulty in seeing. A few suggestions of factors involved are mentioned below.

A. Child

1. *Learning Ability*
   a. Sensory defects often mask a child's intellectual capacity since responses cannot be the same as in other children.
   b. Blind children may learn to speak later than sighted children and may start school when they are a year or two older.
   c. It takes a blind child longer to cover the same amount of material, therefore there may be a different educational level than for the sighted child of the same chronologic age.
   d. Blind children are deprived of the opportunity to learn by imitation.
2. *Personal Factors.* Environment influences the child's adjustment and parental attitude affects the blind child as it does the sighted child. When the parent is overindulgent and protective, the child may be self-centered, dependent, and emotionally less stable.

B. Adult

The adult who has always been blind or has been so since childhood has made adjustments and may be employed in a limited but useful occupation. The greater number who become blind after adulthood experience an immediate natural reaction of depression and feeling of helplessness.

When loss of vision is incipient, usually shock and upheaval are less, but there may be many years of dread, worry, and anxiety in anticipation. When the patient begins to accept the handicap, efforts for rehabilitation are made easier. Independence and self-confidence should be developed and the pa-

tient must be helped not to become helpless.

III. Dental Hygiene Care

A. Totally Blind

1. *Factors in Patient Care*
   a. A blind person can perceive a new experience readily if told about it in detail.
   b. Because of the visual handicap, the patient must rely more on other senses and cultivate them.
   c. A blind person has to be neat and orderly: if something is put down it must be readily located again.
   d. A blind person does things deliberately and slowly to gain perception and prevent accidents.
   e. Effective conversation with a blind person can best be accomplished by speaking as on a telephone.
   f. A blind person learns to interpret tone of voice and put more reliance on this than people with sight who can watch facial expressions.

2. *Patient Reception and Seating*
   a. Lower dental chair prior to receiving patient; move other dental equipment such as the bracket tray and operating stool from pathway.
   b. Guide to dental chair: patient holds arm and is led without being pushed or pulled (figure 54–6).

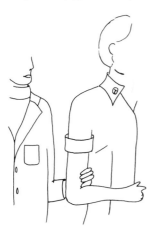

Figure 54–6. Escorting a blind person. The patient holds the arm above the elbow, walks beside and slightly behind. The blind person senses the body motion of the escort for guidance.

   c. Provide forewarnings of potential hazards in the pathway.
   d. Instruct patient of step up to conventional dental chair.
   e. For recall patient: when patient has become familiar with office arrangement from previous appointments, changes should be mentioned to prevent embarrassment.
   f. When leaving operatory during the appointment, explain absence; prevent embarrassment of patient speaking to someone who is not there; speak when reentering the room.

3. *The Dog Guide*
   a. Do not distract a dog guide on duty by speaking to or touching it.
   b. Ask the patient where the best place will be for the dog to stay during the appointment. The dogs are gentle, carefully trained animals, and may lie quietly in a corner of the treatment room as directed by the patient.

4. *Techniques*
   a. Describe each step in detail before proceeding: instruments, materials, and how each will be applied; mention flavors.
   b. Permit patient to handle instruments such as a mouth mirror; this applies particularly to child patient who is not familiar with dental procedures.
   c. Use other instruments of a similar size and shape when describing scalers or explorers since handling sharp instruments would be dangerous for the patient.
   d. Moving rubber cup may be applied to child's finger: when power-driven instruments disturb the patient, a porte polisher may be used when polishing is considered necessary.
   e. Avoid surprise applications of compressed air, water from syringe, or power-driven instruments.
   f. Speak before touching the patient: by maintaining contact of a finger on a tooth or through retraction while changing instruments, repeated orientation is avoided.

g. Rinsing: use evacuator when possible; without evacuation, explain the water syringe or place rinsing cup in the hand each time rather than expect the patient to pick it up from unit; help avoid patient's embarrassment if water is spilled.

5. *Instructions for Patient*
   a. Give instructions clearly and concisely.
   b. Visual aids such as models may be used if described in detail and given to the patient to handle.
   c. Toothbrushing: demonstrate in patient's mouth.
   d. Educational materials have been prepared in braille or on tapes.[34,35]

B. Partially Sighted

People with sight often underestimate the degree of it and fail to realize how useful a little vision can be. Patience in helping a patient make full use of available vision, without oversolicitousness, is important. Although many of the procedures described for the totally blind can be applied to the partially sighted, a few additional hints are suggested below.

Elderly patients with failing sight will rarely admit such a handicap. Sight failure in the aged or lowered vision at any age may be suspected from the patient's unusual squinting, blinking, or lack of continuing attention. Techniques can be adapted without mention of sight to the patient.

1. Avoid glare of operating light in patient's eyes for patient comfort. Sensitivity to light is characteristic of many eye conditions.
2. Do not expect patient to see fine detail as in a radiograph or on a small model.
3. Work patiently and give instruction slowly: patient may have slow visual accommodation.
4. Present the patient's eyeglasses before beginning instruction.

HEARING IMPAIRMENT

When hearing is impaired to the extent that it has no practical value for the purpose of communication, a person is considered deaf. When hearing is defective but functional with or without a hearing aid, the terms "hard of hearing" or "partially deaf" are used.

I. Causes of Hearing Impairment

Inability to hear may be temporary or permanent. A wide variety of factors contribute to deafness. In young children, heredity; prenatal influences, particularly rubella and blood incompatibilities; perinatal conditions, notably birth trauma, and prematurity; and postnatal influences, particularly infectious diseases (meningitis), trauma, and drugs are important causes.

Deafness beginning during school-age years can result from complications of upper respiratory infections. Older people may develop deafness following chronic infection of the middle ear, toxicity from various chemotherapeutic drugs, and trauma. Deterioration of hearing range may occur with aging.

II. Characteristics

A. Major Types

1. *Conductive Hearing Loss*
   a. Part involved: middle ear, external canal, or drum membrane.
   b. Hearing aid: plate behind ear; sound is conducted by bone.
   c. Speech: soft and low; person hears own voice louder than that of others.
2. *Perceptive or Sensorineural Hearing Loss*
   a. Part involved: inner ear; injury to nerves.
   b. Hearing aid: button in ear; sound conducted by air. Hearing aids are more helpful to those with conductive hearing loss.
   c. Speech: loud; person cannot hear own voice.
3. *Combined Conductive and Sensorineural Hearing Loss*
4. *Psychogenic Hearing Loss*
   a. Unrelated to structural changes.
   b. May be a manifestation of an emotional disturbance.

B. Characteristics Suggesting Hearing Impairment

Partial deafness may not have been diagnosed, or certain patients, particularly the elderly, many not admit hearing limitation.

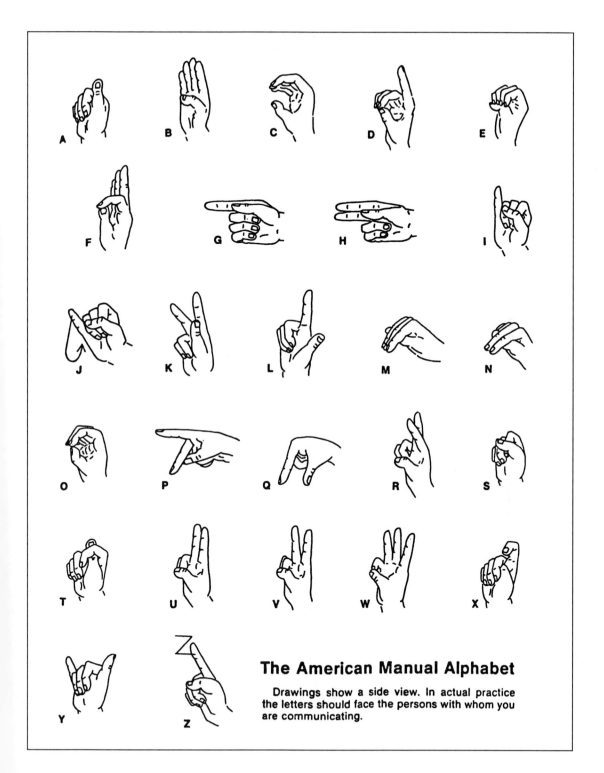

The American Manual Alphabet

Drawings show a side view. In actual practice the letters should face the persons with whom you are communicating.

Figure 54–7. American manual alphabet. Fingerspelling is used in combination with signs and speaking or forming words on the lips. (From Riekehof, L.L.: The Joy of Signing. Springfield, Missouri, Gospel Publishing House, 1978. Reproduced by permission of the publisher.)

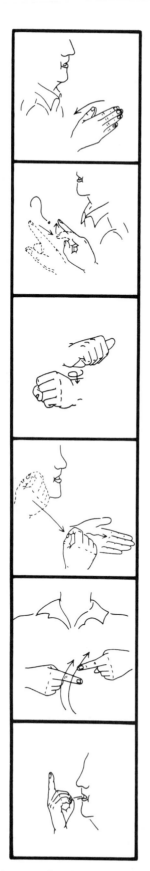

ASK, REQUEST

Place the open hands palm to palm and draw them toward the body.
Origin: Hands held as in prayer.
Usage: *Ask* for help. What is your *request?*

QUESTION

Draw a question mark in the air with the index finger; draw it back and direct it forward as if placing the dot below the question mark.
Usage: That *question* is hard to answer.

ENGAGEMENT, APPOINTMENT, RESERVATION

Make a small circle with the right "A" hand and then place the wrist on the wrist of the left "S" which is facing right.
Origin: Indicating one is bound.
Usage: a dinner *engagement* tonight.
a 4 o'clock *appointment.*
a plane *reservation.*

SECRETARY

Take an imaginary pencil from the ear, write into the left hand and make the "PERSON" ending.
Origin: A person who takes notes.
Usage: Teri is my good *secretary.*

COME

Index fingers rotating once around each other move toward the body. Or, use the open hand in a beckoning motion.
Origin: Using the hands in a natural motion.
Usage: When can you *come* to my home?
Come, I'm waiting for you. (Use second description.)

DENTIST

Place the right "D" at the teeth.
Origin: The initial sign at the teeth.
Usage: Let the *dentist* check your teeth.

Figure 54–8. Examples of signing. (From: Riekehof, L.L.: The Joy of Signing. Springfield, Missouri, Gospel Publishing House, 1978. Reproduced by permission of the publisher.)

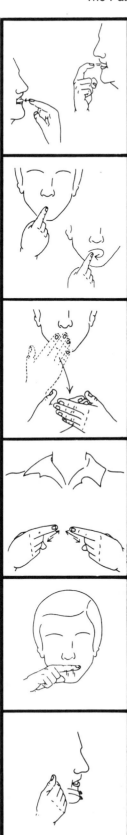

TEETH

Run the tip of the bent index finger across the teeth.
Usage: strong white *teeth*.

TONGUE

Touch the tip of the tongue with the index finger.
Usage: A look at your *tongue* tells the doctor something.

MOUTH

Point to the mouth.
Usage: The dentist looked into my *mouth*.

LIPS

Trace the lips with the index finger.
Usage: Your *lips* are easy to read.

GOOD, WELL

Touch the lips with the fingers of the right hand and then move the right hand forward placing it palm up in the palm of the left hand.
Origin: It has been tasted and smelled and offered as acceptable.
Usage: *good* food; doing *well* at work.

PAIN, ACHE, HURT

The index fingers are jabbed toward each other several times.
Note: This sign is generally made in front of the body but may be placed at the location of the pain, as: headache, toothache, heartache, etc.
Usage: suffered *pain* after the accident; *aching* all over; my knee *hurts*; have an *earache*.

TOOTHBRUSH

Using the index finger as a brush, imitate the motion of brushing the teeth.
Usage: *brushing teeth* twice a day.

DAILY, EVERY DAY

Place the side of the "A" hand on the cheek and rub it toward the chin several times.
Origin: Indicating several tomorrows.
Usage: *daily* bread.
drive to work *every day*.

Clues to the identification of a hearing problem are listed below.

1. Lack of attention; fails to respond to conversational tone.
2. Intentness; strained facial expression; stares at others.
3. Turns head to one side; hearing may be good on one side only.
4. Gives unexpected answer unrelated to question; does one thing when told to do another.
5. Frequently asks others to repeat what was said.
6. Unusual speech tone.
7. Inaccurate pronunciation: characteristic in child who repeats what is heard; with defective hearing, certain sounds are missing in the hearing range.

C. Personal Factors

People with hearing loss tend to have more emotional difficulties than those with sight loss. People with a hearing impairment are inclined to withdraw. They are bothered when they do not know what others are saying. This is mostly true of older people who develop paranoid tendencies and believe that when they cannot hear, other people are talking about them. Children do not have this problem, but live in their own little world and watch others.

III. The Dental Hygiene Appointment

At the initial appointment, the patient may need to be accompanied by a person who can assist with the preparation of the histories and listen while the treatment plan is presented. Lengthy or involved explanations require an interpreter who is familiar with the communication methods of the patient.

A. Patient With Hearing Aid

1. Be careful not to touch a hearing aid when it is operating.
2. Ask patient to turn off or remove a hearing aid when a power-driven dental instrument, particularly an ultrasonic scaler, will be used. The noise can be amplified many times, much to the discomfort of the patient.

B. Patient With Partial Hearing Ability

1. Speak clearly and distinctly; direct speaking to side of "good" ear, if hearing is impaired on one side only.
2. Eliminate interfering noises: from street outside or saliva ejector suction.

C. Lip Reader

1. Be sure patient is looking; do not turn to side; speak directly.
2. Speaker's face must be clearly visible so patient can read lips easily; difficult because dental light is directed to patient's face; operator may have back to window.
3. Speak in normal tone; do not accentuate words; pause more frequently than usual.
4. Do not raise voice; raising voice aggravates the situation; patient may be inclined to withdraw.
5. When patient cannot understand, use alternate words to express the same thought; many letters and combinations of letters look the same on the lips; others are not visible at all.
6. Keep calm; display of irritation or annoyance over difficulties in conversing will discourage or upset the patient.
7. Write proper names or unusual words the patient fails to understand.
8. When wearing a mask is required because of a communicable disease, communication by writing notes will be necessary. If maximum precautions are being observed (page 64), the pencil and paper can be destroyed with the other disposables.

D. Sign Language

Learning basic sign language and finger spelling can provide health personnel with an added communication skill.[31] The American manual alphabet is shown in figure 54–7.[36] A few examples of signs are shown in figure 54–8, and a bibliography of sources is included with the Suggested Readings at the end of this chapter.

E. General Suggestions

1. Written messages. Use a clipboard with a marker-type pen attached, and large paper, at least $8\frac{1}{2} \times 11$ inches. Write large.

2. Do not startle the patient by tapping to gain attention.
3. Watch for patient's motions and facial expressions to determine reaction or discomfort.
4. Teach by demonstration
   a. Open mouth wide each time patient is to open.
   b. Younger child may be taught to rinse by watching and imitating.
   c. Provide reassurance and approval by maintaining eye contact and smiling.
5. Appointment making: Person with a hearing impairment should always have written appointment card to assure complete understanding; appointments made by telephone should be confirmed by mail.
6. Use judgment in prolonging conversation with deaf person: certain patients are under tension and tire easily, whereas others enjoy the opportunity to be the center of attention.

TECHNICAL HINTS

Sources of Materials and Information

National Foundation of Dentistry for the Handicapped
1726 Champa (Suite 422)
Denver, Colorado 80202

Arthritis Foundation
3400 Peachtree Road Northeast (Suite 1101)
Atlanta, Georgia 30326

National Multiple Sclerosis Society
205 East 42nd Street
New York, New York 10017

National Spinal Cord Injury Foundation
369 Elliot Street
Newton Upper Falls, Massachusetts 02164

Spina Bifida Association of America
343 South Dearborn (Suite 319)
Chicago, Illinois 60604

United Cerebral Palsy Associations
66 East 34th Street
New York, New York 10016

American Foundation for the Blind
15 West 16th Street
New York, New York 10011

National Society to Prevent Blindness and Its Affiliates
79 Madison Avenue
New York, New York 10016

National Academy, Gallaudet College
Kendall Green
Washington, D.C. 20002
(Professional Training Program for communication and training in deafness)

References

1. Brunner, L.S. and Suddarth, D.S.: *Textbook of Medical–Surgical Nursing*, 4th ed. Philadelphia, J.B. Lippincott Co., 1980, pp. 1253–1254.
2. Wilson, D.J., McKenzie, M.W., and Barber, L.M.: *Spinal Cord Injury, A Treatment Guide for Occupational Therapists.* Thorofare, New Jersey, Charles B. Slack Inc., 1974, pp. 1–14.
3. Schubert, M.M., Snow, M., and Stiefel, D.J.: *Dental Treatment of the Spinal Cord Injured Patient.* Disability Dental Instruction, 4919 Northeast 86th Street, Seattle, Washington 98115, 34 pp.
4. Trombly, C.A. and Scott, A.D.: *Occupational Therapy for Physical Dysfunction.* Baltimore, The Williams & Wilkins Co., 1977, pp. 305–307.
5. Durnan, J.R. and Thaler, R.: Dental Care for the Patient with a Spinal Cord Injury, *J. Am. Dent. Assoc., 86,* 1318, June, 1973.
6. Cloran, A.J., Lotz, J.W., Campbell, H.D., and Wiechers, D.O.: Oral Telescoping Orthosis: An Aid to Functional Rehabilitation of Quadriplegic Patients, *J. Am. Dent. Assoc., 100,* 876, June, 1980.
7. Blaine, H.H. and Nelson, E.P.: A Mouthstick for Quadriplegic Patients, *J. Prosthet. Dent., 29,* 317, March, 1973.
8. Bleck, E.E.: Myelomeningocele, Meningocele, Spina Bifida, in Bleck, E.E. and Nagel, D.A., eds.: *Physically Handicapped Children—A Medical Atlas for Teachers.* New York, Grune & Stratton, 1975, pp. 181–192.
9. Malamed, S.F.: *Handbook of Medical Emergencies in the Dental Office.* St. Louis, The C.V. Mosby Co., 1978, pp. 184–193.
10. Schubert, M.M., Snow, M.K., Stiefel, D.J., and DeFreece, A.: *Dental Treatment of the Stroke Patient.* Disability Dental Instruction, 4919 Northeast 86th Street, Seattle, Washington 98115, 29 pp.
11. Robbins, S.L. and Cotran, R.S.: *Pathologic Basis of Disease,* 2nd ed. Philadelphia, W.B. Saunders Co., 1979, pp. 1468–1470.
12. Isselbacher, K.J., Adams, R.D., Braunwald, E., Petersdorf, R.G., and Wilson, J.D., eds.: *Harrison's Principles of Internal Medicine,* 9th ed. New York, McGraw-Hill, 1980, pp. 2059–2063.
13. Robbins and Cotran: op. cit., pp. 1471–1472.
14. Drachman, D.B.: Medical Progress: Myasthenia Gravis (First of Two Parts), *N. Engl. J. Med., 298,* 136, January 19, 1978; (Second of Two Parts): *298,* 186, January 26, 1978.
15. Frankel, H.H.: Management of Children with Myasthenia Gravis, *J. Dent. Child., 45,* 151, March–April, 1978.
16. Danforth, H.A., Snow, M., and Stiefel, D.J.: *Dental Management of the Cerebral Palsied Patient.* Disability Dental Instruction, 4919 Northeast 86th Street, Seattle, Washington 98115, 30 pp.

17. Sorenson, H.W.: Physically Handicapped, in Nowak, A.J.: *Dentistry for the Handicapped Patient*. St. Louis, The C.V. Mosby Co., 1976, pp. 23–38.

18. Shafer, W.G., Hine, M.K., and Levy, B.M.: *A Textbook of Oral Pathology*, 3rd ed. Philadelphia, W.B. Saunders Co., 1974, pp. 800–801.

19. Vap, J.G.: Bell's Palsy, *Ear, Nose, Throat J.*, 57, 284, July, 1978.

20. Ewing, J.A. and Endicott, J.N.: Rehabilitation of the Face After Facial-Nerve Paralysis, *Ear, Nose, Throat J.*, 57, 288, July, 1978.

21. Larsen, S.J., Carter, J.F., and Abrahamian, H.A.: Prosthetic Support for Unilateral Facial Paralysis, *J. Prosthet. Dent.*, 35, 192, February, 1976.

22. Ciancio, S.G. and Bourgeault, P.C.: *Clinical Pharmacology for Dental Professionals*. New York, McGraw-Hill, 1980, pp. 152–153.

23. Trombly and Scott: op. cit., pp. 122–123.

24. Robbins and Cotran: op. cit., pp. 1514–1523.

25. Hahn, B.H.: Arthritis, Bursitis, and Bone Disease, in Steinberg, F.U., ed.: *Cowdry's The Care of the Geriatric Patient*, 5th ed. St. Louis, The C.V. Mosby Co., 1976, pp. 11–34.

26. Lupton, D.E.: Psychological Aspects of Temporomandibular Joint Dysfunction, *J. Am. Dent. Assoc.*, 79, 131, July, 1969.

27. Rubin, R., Salvati, E.A., and Lewis, R.: Infected Total Hip Replacement after Dental Procedures, *Oral Surg.*, 41, 18, January, 1976.

28. Mulligan, R.: Late Infections in Patients with Prostheses for Total Replacement of Joints: Implications for the Dental Practitioner, *J. Am. Dent. Assoc.*, 101, 44, July, 1980.

29. White, S.C., Frey, N.W., Blaschke, D.D., Ross, M.D., Clements, P.J., Furst, D.E., and Paulus, H.E.: Oral Radiographic Changes in Patients with Progressive Systemic Sclerosis (Scleroderma), *J. Am. Dent. Assoc.*, 94, 1178, June, 1977.

30. Uthman, A.A., Winkler, S., and Scott, S.J.: The Scleroderma Patient, *J. Oral Med.*, 33, 65, April–June, 1978.

31. Engar, R.C. and Stiefel, D.J.: *Dental Treatment of the Sensory Impaired Patient*. Disability Dental Instruction, 4919 Northeast 86th Street, Seattle, Washington 98115, 65 pp.

32. Kanar, H.L.: The Blind and the Deaf, in Nowak, A.J.: *Dentistry for the Handicapped Patient*. St. Louis, The C.V. Mosby Co., 1976, pp. 121–133.

33. Gish, C.: *Facts about Aging and Blindness*. New York, American Foundation for the Blind, 15 West 16th Street, New York, New York 10011.

34. Braille Volunteers of Huntington, P.O. Box 8097, Huntington, West Virginia 25705

35. State of Iowa Commission for the Blind, 4th and Keosauqua Way, Des Moines, Iowa 50309

36. Riekehof, L.L.: *The Joy of Signing*. Springfield, Missouri, Gospel Publishing House, 1978, p. 15.

Suggested Readings

Been, V.C.: Harborview, *Dent. Hyg.*, 54, 480, October, 1980.

Blacharsh, C.: Dental Aspects of Patients with Cystic Fibrosis: A Preliminary Clinical Study, *J. Am. Dent. Assoc.*, 95, 106, July, 1977.

Corbet, B.: *Options. Spinal Cord Injury and the Future*. Denver, Hirschfeld Press, 1980, 152 pp.

Crinzi, R.A., Palm, N.V., Mostofi, R., and Indresano, A.T.: Management of a Dental Infection in a Patient with Sturge-Weber Disease, *J. Am. Dent. Assoc.*, 101, 798, November, 1980.

Croll, T.P., Greiner, D.G., and Shut, L.: Antibiotic Prophylaxis for the Hydrocephalic Dental Patient with a Shunt, *Pediatric Dent.*, 1, 81, June, 1979.

Garsrud, O.: Therapeutic Dental Aid for Patient with Multiple Sclerosis, *Br. Dent. J.*, 150, 356, June 16, 1981.

Hamada, T., Kobayashi, M., and Yasuyuki, K.: Electromyographic Activity of Masticatory Muscles in Patients with Progressive Muscular Dystrophy (Duchenne type): Relation Between Integrated Electromyographic Activity and Biting Force, *Special Care*, 1, 37, January–February, 1981.

Hartlmaier, K.M.: Mentally and Physically Handicapped Deserve Special Dental Care, *Quintessence Journal*, 1, 27, May, 1979.

Herbold, E.T. and Lindenmuth, J.E.: Communication in Patient Management as Seen in a Patient with Multiple Sclerosis, *J. Am. Dent. Assoc.*, 99, 487, September, 1979.

Jebreil, K.: Palliative Dental Treatment in Primary Amyloidosis, *J. Prosthet. Dent.*, 44, 552, November, 1980.

Koster, S.: Orthodontics for the Handicapped Patient, in Nowak, A.J.: *Dentistry for the Handicapped Patient*. St. Louis, The C.V. Mosby Co., 1976, pp. 331–333.

Larsen, S.J., Carter, J.F., and Abrahamian, H.A.: Prosthetic Support for Unilateral Facial Paralysis, *J. Prosthet. Dent.*, 35, 192, February, 1976.

Libman, R.H., Coke, J.M., and Cohen, L.: Complications Related to the Administration of General Anesthesia in 600 Developmentally Disabled Dental Patients, *J. Am. Dent. Assoc.*, 99, 190, August, 1979.

Marmary Y., Glaiss, R., and Pisanty, S.: Scleroderma: Oral Manifestations, *Oral Surg.*, 52, 32, July, 1981.

Mason, R.M., Helmick, J.W., Unger, J.W., Gattozzi, J.G., and Murphy, M.W.: Speech Screening of Children in the Dental Office, *J. Am. Dent. Assoc.*, 94, 708, April, 1977.

Nezon, E.R. and Liljemark, W.F.: Prevalence of Certain Plaque Organisms in Patients with Cystic Fibrosis: A Clinical Microbiological Investigation, *J. Dent. Res.*, 59, 1993, November, 1980.

Pinkham, J.R.: Practical Considerations for Dental Assessment and Treatment of Mentally and Emotionally Ill Patients, *J. Dent. Handicap.*, 4, 50, Summer, 1979.

Poland, C. and Davis, W.B.: Dental Problems of the Handicapped Child, in McDonald, R.E. and Avery, D.R.: *Dentistry for the Child and Adolescent*, 3rd ed. St. Louis, The C.V. Mosby Co., 1978, pp. 488–503.

Snow, M., Hale, J.M., and Stiefel, D.J.: *Disabled Dental Patients—How Many?* Disability Dental Instruction, 4919 Northeast 86th Street, Seattle, Washington 98115, 11 pp.

Swerdloff, M.: The Problems and Concerns of the Handicapped, *J. Dent. Educ.*, 44, 131, March, 1980.

Wiesjahn, V.: Scoliosis: The Dentist's Role in the Team Approach, *J. Hosp. Dent. Pract.*, 4, 7, January, 1970.

Mouth-held Orthosis

Bartling, D.: Dental Care of Hand-less Persons and the Provision of Mouth-Supported Devices for Their Use, *Quintessence Int.*, 4, 37, August, 1973.

Bartling, D.: Dental Care of Hand-less Persons and the Provision of Mouth-Supported Devices for Their Use (II), *Quintessence Int.*, 4, 47, September, 1973.

Brown, J.P., Chapman, R.P., and Mellor, C.W.: Interchangeable Mouth-held Appliances for the Physically Handicapped Child, *J. Int. Dent. Child.*, 6, 27, December, 1975.

Cloran, A.J.: Telescopic Mouth Instruments for Severely

Handicapped Patients, *J. Prosthet. Dent.*, 32, 435, October, 1974.

Fogg, R.A. and Radell, M.H.: A Removable Oral Prosthetic Appliance for Bell's Palsy: Report of Case, *J. Am. Dent. Assoc.*, 94, 1169, June, 1977.

Grisius, R.J. and Firtell, D.N.: Mouth-controlled Devices to Assist the Handicapped, *J. Hosp. Dent. Pract.*, 13, 107, Third Quarter, 1979.

King, W.C.: Mouthstick Habilitation, *J. Am. Dent. Assoc.*, 87, 839, October, 1973.

Lutwak, E.: A New Mouthstick Prosthesis for Handicapped Patients, *J. Prosthet. Dent.*, 37, 61, January, 1977.

Smokler, J. and Rappaport, S.C.: Mouthstick Prosthesis for a Patient with Arthrogryposis Multiplex Congenita, *J. Prosthet. Dent.*, 42, 316, September, 1979.

Zalkind, M., Mitrani, Z., and Stern, N.: Mouth-operated Devices for Handicapped Persons, *J. Prosthet. Dent.*, 34, 652, December, 1975.

Stroke

Ehrlich, A.: The Stroke Patient, *Dent. Assist.*, 39, 15, October, 1970.

Kleiman, C.S., Zafran, J.N., and Zayon, G.M.: Dental Care for the Stroke Patient, *Dent. Hyg.*, 54, 237, May, 1980.

Selley, W.G.: Dental Help for Stroke Patients, *Br. Dent. J.*, 143, 409, December 20, 1977.

Zafran, J.N. and Zayon, G.M.: Prosthodontics and the Stroke Patient, *J. Am. Dent. Assoc.*, 74, 1250, May, 1967.

Myasthenia Gravis

Bottomley, W.K. and Terezhalmy, G.T.: Management of Patients with Myasthenia Gravis Who Require Maxillary Dentures, *J. Prosthet. Dent.*, 38, 609, December, 1977.

Calcaterra, T.C., Stern, F., Herrmann, C., and Mulder, D.G.: The Otolaryngologist's Role in Myasthenia Gravis, *Trans. Am. Acad. Ophthal. Otol.*, 76, 308, March–April, 1972.

Gallagher, D.M., Erickson, K.L., and Genkins, G.: Current Concepts in the Surgical Treatment of Patients with Myasthenia Gravis, *J. Oral Surg.*, 39, 30, January, 1981.

Grob, D., ed.: Myasthenia Gravis (5th Conference), *Ann. N.Y. Acad. Sci.*, 274, 1–682, May 28, 1976.

Havard, C.W.H.: Progress in Myasthenia Gravis, *Br. Med. J.*, 3, 437, August 25, 1973.

McFarlin, D.E.: Myasthenia Gravis, in Samter, M., ed.: *Immunological Diseases*, 3rd ed. Boston, Little, Brown and Co., 1978, pp. 1383–1399.

Cerebral Palsy

Capute, A.J.: Developmental Disabilities, An Overview, *Dent. Clin. North Am.*, 18, 557, July, 1974.

Hengen, M.: The Role of the Dental Hygienist in the Dental Care of the Cerebral Palsy Patient, *Dent. Hyg.*, 54, 472, October, 1980.

Kanar, H.L.: Cerebral Palsy and Other Gross Motor or Skeletal Problems, in Wessels, K.E., ed.: *Dentistry for the Handicapped Patient*. Littleton, Massachusetts, PSG Publishing, 1979, pp. 33–62.

Kanar, H.L.: Dental Characteristics, in Cruickshank, W.M., ed.: *Cerebral Palsy. A Developmental Disability*, 3rd ed. Syracuse, New York, Syracuse University Press, 1976, pp. 343–368.

Knott, G.P.: Attitudes and Needs of Parents of Cerebral Palsied Children, *Rehabilitation Lit.*, 40, 190, July, 1979.

Koweek, R. and Rosenstein, S.N.: A Comparison of Oral Stereognosis Ability Between Cerebral Palsy Patients with Head and Neck Involvement and Those without This Involvement, *J. Dent. Guid. Counc. Handicap.*, 15, 3, Spring, 1976.

Leary, B.A. and Zucker, S.B.: Teaching Preventive Dentistry to Adolescents with Cerebral Palsy, *Special Care*, 1, 13, January–February, 1981.

Schweyer, K.L.: Intravenous Conscious Sedation: An Alternative Modality in the Management of the Cerebral Palsy Patient, *Gen. Dent.*, 27, 33, May–June, 1979.

Watson, A.O.: Treatment of Cerebral Palsied Patients. A Report on 33 Years of Treatment from 1946 to 1978, *Aust. Dent. J.*, 24, 290, October, 1979.

Parkinson's Disease

Duvoisin, R.: Parkinsonism, *Clinical Symposia*, 28, Number 1, CIBA Pharmaceutical, 1976, 29 pp.

Greer, M.: How to Achieve Maximum Benefit for the Patient with Parkinson's Disease, *Geriatrics*, 31, 89, April, 1976.

Gresh, C.: Helpful Tips You Can Give Your Patients with Parkinson's Disease, *Nursing*, 10, 26, January, 1980.

Walter, D.C. and Barbeau, A.: Parkinson's Disease: The Effect of Levodopa Therapy on the Dentition: Report of a Case, *J. Am. Dent. Assoc.*, 85, 133, July, 1972.

Arthritis

Barriga, B., Lewis, T.M., and Law, D.B.: An Investigation of the Dental Occlusion in Children with Juvenile Rheumatoid Arthritis, *Angle. Orthod.*, 44, 329, October, 1974.

Blackwood, H.J.J.: Pathology of the Temporomandibular Joint, *J. Am. Dent. Assoc.*, 79, 118, July, 1969.

Crum, R.J. and Loiselle, R.J.: Incidence of Temporomandibular Joint Symptoms in Male Patients with Rheumatoid Arthritis, *J. Am. Dent. Assoc.*, 81, 129, July, 1970.

Marbach, J.J.: Arthritis of the Temporomandibular Joints, *Dent. Radiogr. Photogr.*, 42, 51, Number 3, 1969.

Mayne, J.G. and Hatch, G.S.: Arthritis of the Temporomandibular Joint, *J. Am. Dent. Assoc.*, 79, 125, July, 1969.

Seymour, R.L., Crouse, V.L., and Irby, W.B.: Temporomandibular Ankylosis Secondary to Rheumatoid Arthritis, *Oral Surg.*, 40, 584, November, 1975.

Shafer, W.G., Hine, M.K., and Levy, B.M.: *A Textbook of Oral Pathology*, 3rd ed. Philadelphia, W.B. Saunders Co., 1974, pp. 657–661.

Trenwith, J.A. and Beale, G.: Rheumatoid Arthritis in the Temporomandibular Joint, *N.Z. Dent. J.*, 73, 195, October, 1977.

Turpin, D.L. and West, R.A.: Juvenile Rheumatoid Arthritis: A Case Report of Surgical/Orthodontic Treatment, *Am. J. Orthod.*, 73, 312, March, 1978.

Zampelli, M., Salkin, L.M., Vandersall, D.C., and Denbo, J.A.: Rheumatoid Arthritis of the Temporomandibular Joint: Case Report, *J. Periodontol.*, 45, 26, January, 1974.

Visual Impairment

Ball, R.O., Zucker, S.B., and Fretwell, L.D.: Teaching Preventive Dentistry to Patients with Impaired Vision, *J. Dent. Handicap.*, 4, 23, Fall/Winter, 1978.

Greeley, C.B., Goldstein, P.A., and Forrester, D.J.: Oral Manifestations in a Group of Blind Students, *J. Dent. Child.*, 43, 39, January–February, 1976.

Huntley, D.E. and Ralston, B.J.: A Plaque Control Program for Blind Patients, *J. Dent. Handicap.*, 3, 23, Summer, 1977.

Kisby, L.: Understanding the Blind Child, *J. Pedodont.*, 2, 67, Fall, 1977.

Lebowitz, E.J.: An Introduction to Dentistry for the Blind, *Dent. Clin. North Am.*, 18, 651, July, 1974.

Ligh, R.Q.: The Visually Handicapped Patient in Dental Practice, *J. Dent. Handicap.*, 4, 38, Summer, 1979.

Miller, D.D.: The Blind Dentist: Serving the Profession and His Community, *J. Am. Dent. Assoc., 94*, 30, January, 1977.

Morsey, S.L.: Communicating with and Treating the Blind Child., *Dent. Hyg., 54*, 288, June, 1980.

Schnuth, M.L.: Dental Health Education for the Blind, *Dent. Hyg., 51*, 499, November, 1977.

Smith, M.E.: Ophthalmic Aspects, in Steinberg, F.U., ed.: *Cowdry's The Care of the Geriatric Patient,* 5th ed. St. Louis, The C.V. Mosby Co., 1976, pp. 351–363.

Hearing Impairment

Brownstein, M.P.: Dental Care for the Deaf Child, *Dent. Clin. North Am., 18*, 643, July, 1974.

Flynn, P.T. and McGregor, D.K.: Communication Disorders: An Overview and Practices for the Dental Hygienist, *Dent. Hyg., 51*, 455, October, 1977.

Harford, E.R.: Guidelines for Hearing Problems: Substituting Management for Myth, *Geriatrics, 34*, 69, December, 1979.

Mueller, K. and Gantt, D.: Communicating with the Deaf Patient, *J. Dent. Handicap., 3*, 22, Winter/Spring, 1978.

Sign Language

Grossnickle, K., Lehew, D., Odell, D., and Staub, C.: *Take Time to Communicate.* Cumberland, Maryland, Dental Hygiene Program, Allegany Community College, 1981.

Mueller, K.I.: *Clinical Sign Language.* Frankfort, Kentucky, Department for Human Resources, 1977.

O'Rourke, T.J.: *A Basic Vocabulary of American Sign Language for Parents and Children.* Silver Spring, Maryland, National Association of the Deaf, 1977.

Riekehof, L.L.: *The Joy of Signing.* Springfield, Missouri, Gospel Publishing House, 1978.

Roy, H.L.: *Bobby Visits the Dentist.* Washington, D.C., Gallaudet College Press, 1975.

Talley, L.: *Let Your Fingers Do the Talking.* Johnson City, Tennessee, Department of Dental Hygiene, Eastern Tennessee State University, 1981.

55

The Patient with a Cardiovascular Disease

Cardiovascular, as the names implies, includes diseases of the heart and blood vessels. Diseases of the heart are the leading causes of death in the United States, and of these, ischemic heart disease is responsible for at least 90 percent. Death rates from cardiovascular diseases have declined due to improved medical care, development of systems for emergency care, and education in preventive health behavior.[1]

Patients with cardiovascular conditions are encountered frequently in a dental office or clinic and may be from any age group, although the highest incidence is among older people. A heart disease may be present for many years prior to the time symptoms are recognized. The patients seen in the dental office, therefore, range from those with no obvious symptoms to the nearly disabled. In severe cases, the nonambulatory patient may require care in the home.

Classification of the diseases is made either on an anatomic or etiologic basis. In an anatomic system, diseases of the pericardium, myocardium, endocardium, heart valves, and blood vessels are defined. In an etiologic system the diseases are named by the cause. The principal causes of heart diseases are infectious agents, atherosclerosis, hypertension, immunologic mechanisms, and congenital anomalies.

The five major cardiovascular diseases are congenital heart disease, rheumatic heart disease, infective endocarditis, ischemic heart disease, and hypertensive heart disease. Characteristics and symptoms are complex and overlapping. The diseases are described below and their major symptoms and treatment procedures listed.

CONGENITAL HEART DISEASES

Anomalies of the anatomic structure of the heart or major blood vessels result following irregularities of development during the first 9 weeks in utero. The fetal heart is complete by the ninth week.

Early diagnosis is important because between one fourth and one half of the infants born with cardiovascular anomalies require treatment during the first year. Treatment usually involves surgical correction.

I. Incidence

The incidence of congenital heart disease is approximately 8 per 1000 live births. In the school age group, there are 2 to 6 per 1000. More males than females are involved.

II. Types

There are many types of heart defects. The ones that occur most frequently are the ventricular septal defect, patent ductus arteriosus, atrial septal defect, tetralogy of Fallot, and transposition of the great vessels.

A diagram of the normal heart is shown in figure 55–1 to provide a comparison with the anatomic changes that may appear in a defective heart. Congenital anomalies either produce abnormal pathways in the blood flow or interfere with the flow itself. The two most common anomalies will be described.

A. Ventricular Septal Defect

In this type of defect, the left and right ventricles are connected through an opening in their dividing wall (septum). The oxygenated blood from the lung, which is normally pumped by the left ventricle to the aorta and then to the entire body, can pass across to the right ventricle as shown in figure 55–2.

When the opening is very small, only a heart murmur and little disability results. If the opening is large, the heart enlarges to compensate for overwork.

B. Patent Ductus Arteriosus

A patent ductus arteriosus means there is an open passageway (shunt) between the two great arteries that arise from the heart, namely the aorta and the pulmonary artery. Normally, the opening is closed during the first few weeks after birth. When the open-

ing does not close, blood from the aorta can pass back to the lungs, as shown in figure 55–3. The heart compensates in the attempt to provide the body with oxygenated blood and becomes overburdened.

III. Etiology

Causes are genetic, environmental, or a combination.

A. Genetic

In some types of defects heredity is apparent.

B. Environmental

Most congenital anomalies originate between the fifth and eighth week of fetal life when the heart is developing.
1. Rubella (German measles).
2. Drugs
   a. Chronic maternal alcohol abuse. The fetal alcohol syndrome consists of small head, jaws, and eyeballs, fetal growth retardation, developmental delay, and cardiac septal defects.
   b. Thalidomide.
   c. Lysergic acid diethylamide (LSD).
3. Radiation.

IV. Prevention[2]

A. Use of rubella vaccine for childhood immunization. Vaccination confers indefinite immunity. Vaccination for women of childbearing age is highly advised. The vaccine should not be given during pregnancy, and not within 3 months of becoming pregnant, because of potential risks to the fetus.
B. No medications used during pregnancy without prior consultation with the physician.
C. New drug testing to provide physicians with information about drugs that may be teratogenic.
D. Appropriate use of radiologic equipment. A lead apron should be used for oral radiographs.
E. Control of drug and alcohol addictions.
F. Genetic counseling.

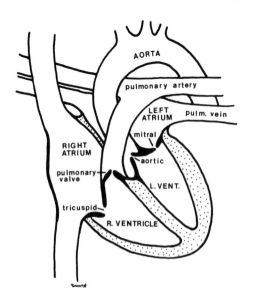

Figure 55–1. Diagram of normal heart to show location of tricuspid, pulmonary, aortic, and mitral heart valves.

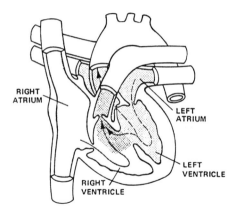

Figure 55–2. Ventricular septal defect. The right and left ventricles are connected by an opening that permits oxygenated blood from the left ventricle to shunt across to the right ventricle and recirculate to the lungs. (From Bleck, E.E. and Nagel, D.A.: Physically Handicapped Children. A Medical Atlas for Teachers. New York, Grune & Stratton, 1975.)

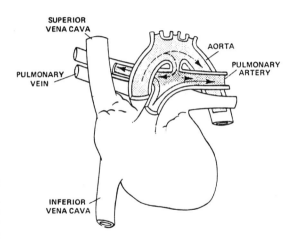

Figure 55–3. Patent ductus arteriosus. An open passageway between the aorta and the pulmonary artery permits oxygenated blood from the aorta to pass back into the lungs. (From Bleck, E.E. and Nagel, D.A.: Physically Handicapped Children. A Medical Atlas for Teachers. New York, Grune & Stratton, 1975.)

V. Clinical Considerations

A. Signs and Symptoms of Congenital Heart Disease

Obvious symptoms are not always apparent in less severe cases. General conditions that may be present and that influence patient management are
1. Easy fatigue.
2. Exertional dyspnea; fainting.
3. Cyanosis of lips and nailbeds.
4. Poor growth and development.
5. Chest deformity.
6. Heart murmurs.

B. Dental Hygiene Concerns

1. *Prevention of Infective Endocarditis* (page 778). Defective heart valves are susceptible to endocarditis from bacteremia produced during oral treatments.
2. *Elimination of Oral Diseases:* maintenance of a high level of oral health.
3. *Preparation for Heart Surgery.* Dental and periodontal infections must be diagnosed and treated prior to surgery. Postoperative infection related to bacteremias of oral origin is a serious risk. After surgery, dental and dental hygiene procedures will require antibiotic protection for all procedures.

RHEUMATIC HEART DISEASE[3,4]

Rheumatic heart disease is a complication following rheumatic fever. A rather high percentage of patients with a history of rheumatic fever have permanent heart valve damage. The damaged heart valve, as in congenital heart disease, is susceptible to infective endocarditis.

I. Rheumatic Fever

A. Incidence

Approximately 90 percent of initial attacks occur between ages 5 and 15. The patient is left susceptible to future attacks, which may cause additional damage to previously damaged heart valves. The tendency to recurrence diminishes with age.

B. Etiology

1. Onset. The onset of acute rheumatic fever usually appears 2 to 3 weeks after a beta-hemolytic Group A streptococci pharyngeal infection.
2. Rheumatic fever and rheumatic heart disease are believed to be immunologic disorders caused by sensitization to antigens of beta-hemolytic Group A streptococci.

C. Prevention

The persistence and severity of the pharyngeal infection are significant in whether or not rheumatic fever follows; therefore, early diagnosis and treatment of streptococcal throat and pharyngeal infections are necessary.[2]

D. Symptoms of Rheumatic Fever

Over a period of several months of low grade fever, the joints, heart muscles, central nervous system, skin, and subcutaneous tissues become involved. All of the symptoms described below disappear with recovery except the cardiac valve damage.

1. *Arthritis.* Migratory polyarthritis is present, which may affect more than one joint at a time. The temporomandibular joint is rarely involved.

2. *Carditis.* In a severe case, death may result from heart failure during the acute stage of rheumatic fever, or valvular damage may be sustained with disability. Severity varies and many do not have heart symptoms at the time of the acute illness, some never, and others may have rheumatic heart disease diagnosed later in life without having had evidence of rheumatic fever.

   The mitral valve is most commonly affected, followed by the aortic valve (figure 55–1). Rheumatic carditis is almost always associated with a significant murmur of insufficiency. The damaged valves are susceptible to infection, leading to infective endocarditis.

3. *Subcutaneous Nodules.* Painless swellings may appear over bony prominences.

4. *Chorea.* Irregular and involuntary actions of muscles, particularly of the extremities and the face, may appear as a late or delayed manifestation.

5. *Erythema Marginatum.* A pink skin rash, which may appear long after the acute stage, tends to be migratory and transient.

II. The Course of Rheumatic Heart Disease

Many factors influence the outlook after rheumatic fever symptoms subside. Usually, no symptoms persist except the effects of the valvular deformity; which is the reason the disease is sometimes called rheumatic valvular disease or chronic valvular heart disease.

A. Symptoms

1. Stenosis or incompetence of valves; most commonly, the aortic and mitral valves.

2. Heart murmur influenced by the amount of scarring of the valves and myocardium.

3. Cardiac arrhythmias.

4. Late symptoms include shortness of breath, elevation of diastolic blood pressure, enlargement of the left ventricle, and increasing signs of cardiac failure.

B. Practice Applications

The significance in dental and dental hygiene practice is the same as for congenital heart disease.

1. Maintenance of a high level of oral health to prevent a need for treatment of advanced disease.

2. Prevention of infective endocarditis by antibiotic premedication.

3. Preparation of the mouth prior to heart surgery to prevent the need for serious therapy after surgery. This applies with greater impact when a heart valve prosthesis is involved.

INFECTIVE ENDOCARDITIS

Infective endocarditis is a microbial infection of the heart valves or endocardium which occurs in proximity to congenital or acquired defects. Subacute infective endocarditis, often called subacute bacterial endocarditis (SBE), is of vital concern in the dental and dental hygiene care of high risk patients with valvular defects.

A bacteremia, or presence of microorganisms in the blood stream, is necessary for the development of infective endocarditis. A transitory bacteremia usually is created during dental hygiene treatment as well as during surgical procedures involving the upper respiratory tract, genitourinary tract, or lower gastrointestinal tract.

Infective endocarditis is a serious disease, the prognosis of which depends on the degree of cardiac damage, valves involved, duration of the infection, and treatment. Patients are prone to develop heart failure leading to death unless the infection is promptly controlled.

Infective endocarditis is characterized by the formation of vegetations composed of masses of bacteria and blood clots on the heart valves. The vegetations may arise on normal valves, but are most likely to occur on previously damaged valves. When a bacteremia occurs, the heart valves may become infected and infective endocarditis can develop.

I. Occurrence

Infective endocarditis is rare in children. The mean age is in the 40 to 50 year range, and more males than females are involved.

A decreased frequency might have been expected over the past years because of the extended use of antimicrobial agents, but this does not appear to have happened.[4] The explanation may be the increased incidence of infective endocarditis related to mainline drug addiction, cardiac surgery, and the increased use of prosthetic valves, all of which invite the implantation of microorganisms in the heart tissues.

II. Etiology

A. Microorganisms[4,5,6]

Almost any species of microorganisms may cause infective endocarditis. Streptococci and staphylococci are responsible in a large majority of cases, with alpha-hemolytic streptococci being the most prevalent. Since yeast, fungi, and viruses have been implicated, the choice of the name "infective" endocarditis is more inclusive than "bacterial" endocarditis.

B. Predisposing Factors

1. *Heart Valve Damage.* Approximately 40 to 60 percent of damaged heart valves result from rheumatic heart disease, and another 10 percent are congenital in origin. Other causes include syphilis, atherosclerosis, and degenerative heart disease.
2. *Heart Surgery.* Infective endocarditis may be a complication of open heart surgery, particularly that associated with valvular prostheses. Intravascular sutures, pacemaker wires, and Teflon-Silastic tubes may also be predisposing factors.
3. *Infection at Portals of Entry.* Infections at sites where microorganisms may enter the blood stream provide a constant source of potential infectious microorganisms. In the oral cavity, organisms enter the stream by way of periodontal and gingival pockets, where multitudes of many species of microorganisms are harbored. An open infection area such as an ulcer caused by an ill-fitting denture may also provide a site of entry.

C. Precipitating Factors

1. *Self-induced Bacteremia.* In the oral cavity, self-induced bacteremias may result from eating, bruxing, chewing gum, or any activity that can force bacteria through the wall of a diseased sulcus or pocket. Bacteremias produced by oral hygiene devices are summarized on page 336.
2. *Trauma to Tissues by Instrumentation.* Bacteremias are created during general or oral surgery, endodontics, periodontal therapy, scaling, curettage, polishing, and particularly, any therapy that causes bleeding. The relationship of bacteremias to scaling and curettage is described on page 508. Bacteremia from use of polishing procedures is included on page 563.

III. Disease Process

A. Bacteremia Initiated

1. Trauma from instrumentation can rupture blood vessels in the gingival sulcus or pocket.
2. Pressure from trauma forces oral microorganisms into the blood stream. Ease of entry of organisms directly relates to the severity of trauma and the severity of the gingivitis or periodontitis.

B. Bacterial Implantation

1. Circulating microorganisms attach to damaged heart valve, prosthetic valve, or other susceptible area.
2. Microorganisms proliferate to form bacterial masses.

C. Subsequent Effects

1. Heart valve becomes inflamed; function is diminished.
2. Clumps of microorganisms (emboli) may break off and spread by way of the general circulation; complications result.

IV. Prevention

Three basic areas for attention in dental and dental hygiene care contribute to the prevention of infective endocarditis. These are identification of risk patients, prophylactic antibiotic coverage for appointment procedures, and working with the patient to improve and maintain a high level of oral health to diminish the frequency and severity of bacteremias.

A. Patient History

1. *Special Content.* It cannot be overemphasized that a careful, complete patient history is needed to detect risk patients. Specific questions should be directed to elicit any history of rheumatic fever and its related symptoms, congenital heart defects, cardiac surgery, presence of prosthetic valves, pacemaker, or previous episode of infective endocarditis.

2. *Consultation with Patient's Physician.* Consultation can be assumed necessary for all patients with a history of rheumatic fever, heart defects, and any other condition suggesting the need for prophylactic antibiotic premedication. Instrumentation, including the use of a probe or explorer during evaluation of the patient, must be withheld until the medical status is cleared.

B. Prophylactic Antibiotic Premedication

1. *Recommended Regimens.* The recommendations of the American Heart Association are outlined on page 100. The American Dental Association Council on Dental Therapeutics has approved the recommendations as they pertain to dentistry.[7,8]

2. *Rationale.* The rationale for giving antibiotics before dental and dental hygiene procedures to risk patients is that these patients are less likely to develop infective endocarditis.

3. *Objectives of the Recommended Regimen*
   a. Prevent bacteremia or reduce the severity and magnitude of it.
   b. Administer antibiotic 30 minutes to 1 hour before, so the blood level at the time of the actual procedure is adequate.

C. Indications for Prophylactic Antibiotics

1. *Heart Disease Risk*
   a. Damaged heart valve (congenital or rheumatic).
   b. Previous episode of infective endocarditis.
   c. Other heart conditions advised by the physician.[6]
   d. Pacemaker. Requirements for a patient with a pacemaker are described on page 790.

2. *Other Conditions.* Patients with a reduced capacity to resist infection, associated with poor healing, immunosuppression, and others listed on pages 99–100 will need antibiotic coverage.

3. *Long-term Penicillin Treatment.* A patient receiving long-term penicillin for rheumatic fever prophylaxis should be given additional coverage because certain microorganisms of the oral cavity become relatively resistant to penicillin.

4. *Prosthetic Heart Valve.* Increased protection over the usual prescription is needed. A combination of penicillin and streptomycin is recommended (page 100).

D. Dental Hygiene Care

Maintenance of a high degree of oral health is very important to each patient susceptible to infective endocarditis. Research has shown that bacteremia following toothbrushing is minimal or absent in clinically healthy tissues.[9]

1. *Instruction.* Instruction in brushing and flossing at initial appointments should be provided while the patient is under antibiotic coverage, particularly if the gingiva show signs of inflammation and bleed readily.

2. *Sequence of Treatment.* Plaque removal instruction should precede instrumentation for scaling and root planing, in order to bring the tissues to as healthy a state as possible. The more severe the disease, the higher incidence of bacteremia during and following instrumentation.

3. *Instrumentation*
   a. Reduce the microbial population

about the teeth and oral mucosa prior to instrumentation by having the patient brush, floss, and rinse thoroughly with a povidone-iodine mouthrinse. By reducing the number of microorganisms, the incidence of bacteremia can be reduced.[10,11]

b. Use particular care in all instrumentation to prevent unnecessary trauma.

HYPERTENSION

Hypertension means an abnormal elevation of blood pressure. It is a symptom, not a disease entity. It is a contributing or risk factor in many vascular diseases, or it may be a result or an effect of underlying pathologic changes.

It has been estimated that one in six Americans has high blood pressure, but that only one-half of those has been diagnosed. Of those whose disease condition has been recognized, many are not being treated or the treatment is inadequate.

Detection of blood pressure for dental and dental hygiene patients has become an essential step in patient evaluation prior to treatment. Early detection, with referral for additional diagnosis and treatment when indicated, can prove to be life saving for certain people. In addition, knowledge of the health problems of patients is needed in order that dental and dental hygiene care can be safe and free from dangers of emergencies which can arise.

I. Etiology

A. Primary or Essential Hypertension

1. *Incidence:* approximately 90 percent of all hypertension is primary or essential.
2. *Cause:* idiopathic; the etiology is unknown.
3. *Predisposing or Risk Factors.*[4,12] Combinations of the factors listed below are more significant than any one alone.
   a. Heredity.
   b. Overweight.
   c. Race: the incidence is higher among black than among white Americans, the illness is more severe, and there is a higher mortality rate at a younger age.[13]
   d. Climate: hypertension is less common in tropical and semitropical countries.
   e. Salt, particularly in excess, in the diet.
   f. Sex: males are more affected before age 45; females slightly more than males in later years.
   g. Age: general increase from birth to age 20; leveling off until 40 years of age, then a slow increase into the older age group.
   h. Cigarette smoking and other risk factors for atherosclerosis are interrelated (page 784).
   i. Oral contraceptives: severe hypertension due to contraceptives is uncommon. Increased hypertension over years of using contraceptives has been shown, particularly when other risk factors are also involved.
   j. Environmental conditions that increase stress factors.

B. Secondary Hypertension

About 10 percent of all hypertension is secondary. A specific cause can be identified, in which the pathologic elevation of blood pressure is secondary to a major underlying disease. Examples are disorders of the kidney, or the adrenal or pituitary glands.

II. Blood Pressure Levels

The blood pressure is the pressure exerted by the blood within the arteries. It is determined by the cardiac output, resistance of the capillary bed, and volume and viscosity of the blood. Diseases can alter each of the parts, and thus alter the blood pressure.

A. Diastolic and Systolic Determinations

The blood pressure is recorded by two determinations, the systolic and the diastolic. During systole, the ventricular contraction forces blood into the arteries.

Systole is followed by diastole, when the ventricles and arteries relax and the ventricles fill with incoming blood in preparation for the next contraction. The normal healthy heart will beat between 60 and 90 times per minute.

B. Determination of Blood Pressure

Procedures for blood pressure determination are described with other vital signs in Chapter 7, pages 107–111.

Blood pressure fluctuates, so that more than one reading is needed. It is recommended that the blood pressure be taken two or three times and the average reading be recorded in the patient's record. When physicians plan treatment for a hypertensive patient, it is customary to study the individual's pattern by making at least three determinations on at least two different days.

C. Standards for Interpretation[14,15]

Systolic and diastolic findings are recorded in the form of a ratio or fraction, for example, 140/90 mm. Hg. The diastolic reading is used as a guide to determine the severity of hypertension as it relates to the need for referral and/or treatment.

Patients with diastolic readings of 115 mm. Hg or over need immediate referral for medical evaluation and treatment. In a dental office or clinic, treatment must be postponed as advised in table 7–1, page 103. Patients with diastolic readings of 90 mm. Hg and over also need referral for additional evaluation and supervision.

Degrees of severity at the different levels are in the following ranges:

200/115 and over	severe high blood pressure
180/105 to 200/114	moderate to severe high blood pressure
140/90 to 180/104	mild high blood pressure
120/80 to 140/89	normal range
90/60 to 120/79	low range

D. Low Blood Pressure

Many healthy people have a normal diastolic pressure under 90 mm. Hg or even under 80 mm. Hg, which may be considered "low blood pressure." Such a level is normal for that person and no clinical problems are evident.

A marked sudden drop in blood pressure is usually associated with an emergency such as severe blood loss, shock, myocardial infarction, or other medical problem. Immediate attention, in the category of a medical emergency, is indicated. Referral to specific procedures can be found in table 58–1, pages 845–852.

E. Postural Hypotension

Postural or orthostatic hypotension is a condition in which fainting, nausea, or feelings of fainting or dizziness occur when a person sits up quickly from a supine position. One predisposing factor for postural hypotension is the medication used for hypertension.[16]

III. Clinical Symptoms of Hypertension

Since hypertension frequently goes unrecognized because of the lack of apparent clinical symptoms, determination of the blood pressure takes on added significance. Knowledge of the possible symptoms can aid dental personnel in watching their patients for early signs, or for identification from the information the patient presents during the preparation of the patient history.

A. High Blood Pressure

Evidence of the following may be present:
1. Headaches.
2. Dizziness, fainting.
3. Shortness of breath, particularly on effort.
4. Disturbances of concentration or memory impairment.

B. Long-standing Severe Elevation of Blood Pressure

Hypertensive crisis is a life-threatening disorder. The brain, eyes, heart, or kidneys may undergo marked changes in function. In the severe state, if any or all of the following are noted, the patient should be referred immediately:
1. Occipital headaches, more severe in the morning.
2. Mental confusion leading to stupor, coma, convulsions.
3. Blurring of vision; possible loss of sight.
4. Severe dyspnea.
5. Chest pains similar to angina pectoris.

C. Major Sequelae

1. Hypertensive heart disease: enlarged heart with eventual cardiac failure.
2. Cerebral vascular accident (stroke, page 749).
3. Hypertensive renal disease.

4. Ischemic heart disease (page 784).

IV. Treatment

A. Goals

1. *Primary Hypertension*
   a. Achieve and maintain diastolic pressure level at 90 or below with minimal adverse effects.
   b. Lower the risk of serious complications and premature death.
2. *Secondary Hypertension.* Surgery or other correction of the cause is needed.

B. Life Style Changes

1. Salt restriction and weight loss may be all that is needed for the control of mild elevations of blood pressure.
2. Correction and elimination of all risk factors related to hypertension and atherosclerosis are needed at all levels of severity of hypertension. Risk factors were listed on page 781.

C. Antihypertensive Drug Therapy[17,18]

1. *Selection of Therapy.* The decision by the physician to prescribe drug therapy at the various levels depends on the severity of the hypertension as well as all factors related to the patient's health.
   a. Diastolic pressure over 105: all patients require drug therapy.[14]
   b. Mild elevations: drugs may be needed when the individual is not willing or able to adhere to the corrective and preventive diet and other risk factor limitations.
2. *Categories of Drugs Used in Therapy*
   a. Diuretics to promote renal excretion of water and sodium ions.
   b. Sympatholytic agents to modify the sympathetic nerve activity.
   c. Vasodilators to act directly on the blood vessels.
3. *Duration.* Management of hypertension must be considered a lifelong endeavor. Periodic monitoring is essential every 3 to 6 months. Dental personnel can encourage their patients to continue treatment even when a normal reading is maintained. Since many antihypertensive drugs have undesirable side effects, the patient may become discouraged and discontinue treatment.
4. *Side Effects.* The effects of the different drugs prescribed vary, but some of the problems confronted by patients may actually influence the behavior at dental and dental hygiene appointments. Cancellation of an appointment could be anticipated. Side effects may include some or all of the following:
   a. Fatigue easily.
   b. Gastrointestinal disturbances including nausea, diarrhea, or cramps.
   c. Xerostomia.
   d. Postural hypotension with dizziness and fainting.
   e. Impotence.
   f. Depression.

V. Hypertension in Children

The blood pressure in normal infants is approximately 70/45 mm. Hg. During childhood and adolescence it rises to reach a level of about 120/80 mm. Hg by age 20.[19]

Children 3 years of age and over need to have blood pressure determinations made at least annually. A variety of cuff sizes are available, and other procedural suggestions are described on pages 107–111.

When a child between ages 3 and 12 has a diastolic pressure greater than 90 mm. Hg, or if over age 12, greater than 100 mm. Hg, further investigation is indicated.[20] Since hypertension has a familial tendency, determining the pressure levels for children of parents known to have hypertension may reveal important information in the health of the child. In one study, 50 percent of the children with elevated blood pressures had parents with hypertension.[21]

HYPERTENSIVE HEART DISEASE[4]

Hypertensive heart disease results from the increased load on the heart because of elevated blood pressure. When the peripheral arterial resistance to the flow of blood pumped from the heart is increased, the blood pressure rises. The heart attempts to maintain its normal output, but to cope with the increased workload resulting from the peripheral resistance, muscle fibers are stretched, and the heart enlarges.

The effect of hypertension on the heart is at

first a thickening of the left ventricle. In later stages, the entire heart is enlarged. This may be discerned by radiographic and medical examination.

Cardiac enlargement has no specific symptoms, but the patient may have symptoms of hypertension such as headaches, weakness, and others listed on page 782. When undiagnosed and untreated, the severity increases and left ventricular congestive failure occurs, resulting from the disturbance of cardiac function.

ISCHEMIC HEART DISEASE

Ischemic heart disease is the cardiac disability, acute and chronic, that arises from reduction or arrest of blood supply to the myocardium in association with disease processes in the coronary arterial system. The heart muscles (myocardium) are supplied through the coronary arteries, which are branches of the descending aorta. Because of the relationship to the coronary arteries, the disease is often referred to as coronary heart disease or coronary artery disease.

Ischemia means oxygen deprivation in a local area from a reduced passage of fluid into the area. Ischemic heart disease is the result of an imbalance of the oxygen supply and demand of the myocardium, which in turn, results from a narrowing or blocking of the lumen of the coronary arteries.

I. Etiology

Other factors may be involved, but the principal cause of the reduction of blood flow to the heart muscle is *atherosclerosis* of the vessel walls, which narrows the lumen, thus preventing the flow of blood.

A. Definition of Atherosclerosis

Atherosclerosis is a disease of medium and large arteries in which atheromas deposit on and thicken the intimal layer of the involved blood vessel. An atheroma is a fibro-fatty deposit or plaque, containing several lipids, especially cholesterol. With time, the plaques continue to thicken and eventually close the vessel. Some plaques calcify, whereas others may develop an overlying thrombus.

B. Predisposing Factors for Atherosclerosis

Each of the risk factors listed here is significant alone. When they occur in combinations, there is increased risk of atherosclerosis, and therefore, of ischemic heart disease. Prevention depends on educational programs along with early identification of persons at risk.[2]

1. Elevated levels of blood lipids; the result of an increased dietary intake of cholesterol, saturated fat, carbohydrate, especially sucrose, alcohol, and calories.
2. Elevated blood pressure.
3. Cigarette smoking.
4. Diabetes.
5. Obesity.
6. Insufficient physical activity.
7. Increased tensions; emotional stress.
8. Family history. Genetic inheritance may not be the factor so much as the perpetuation of familial life-style habits. Diet, smoking habits, tensions, and tendencies toward lack of exercise are typical examples.

II. Manifestations of Ischemic Heart Disease

Ischemic heart disease has three major manifestations. They are angina pectoris, myocardial infarction, and sudden death.

A. Angina Pectoris

Angina pectoris is a symptom complex or syndrome of discomfort in the chest and adjacent areas, which results from transient and reversible myocardial oxygen deficiency. Although other forms of coronary disease may cause similar pain symptoms, approximately 90 percent of angina attacks are related to coronary artery atherosclerosis.

1. *Predisposing Factors.* An attack of angina pectoris may be precipitated by exertion or exercise, emotion, or a heavy meal. In the dental office or clinic, a preventive atmosphere of calmness and quiet can do much to alleviate stress.
2. *Symptoms*
   a. Chest pain. Each person who suffers from angina has a characteristic pattern of pain symptoms. When

changes in the usual pains occur, the physician must be notified.

Commonly, there is thoracic pain, which is substernal and radiates down the left arm and up to the mandible. It may last for seconds or minutes.

The pain is squeezing or crushing, paroxysmal, or pressing, with a feeling of weight on the chest. The patient stops and tends to stiffen.

b. Other symptoms. There may be pallor, faintness, sweating, difficulty in breathing, anxiety, or fear.

3. *Treatment.* A vasodilator, usually nitroglycerin, is administered sublingually.

4. *Procedure During an Attack in the Dental Office*

a. Stop the dental or dental hygiene procedure. Call for assistance and the emergency kit or cart.

b. Seat the patient upright; reassure the patient.

c. Administer nitroglycerin sublingually. Use of the patient's own supply is preferred. Prior to starting procedures of the dental hygiene appointment, the patient's supply should be placed within reach. The patient can be asked when the nitroglycerin was purchased, since the potency is lost after 6 months out of a sealed storage container.

d. Give additional vasodilator. Usually, the first tablet relieves the condition within minutes. When it is suspected that the patient's supply may not be fresh and the first tablet has been ineffective, use of a second tablet from the dental office emergency kit may be advisable.[22]

e. Call for medical assistance. When the response from the second dose of vasodilator is lacking, assume the attack to be a myocardial infarction. Oxygen administration may be indicated.

f. Record vital signs.

g. Recovery. For the patient who recovers without additional medical assistance, allow a rest period before dismissal. Record vital signs again.

5. *Subsequent Dental and Dental Hygiene Appointments.* Make an entry in the patient's permanent record, noting especially any procedures that may have contributed to the attack. Alter procedures to prevent future episodes.

B. Myocardial Infarction

Myocardial infarction is the most extreme manifestation of ischemic heart disease. It is also called *heart attack, coronary occlusion,* or *coronary thrombosis.*

1. *Definition.* Myocardial infarction is a syndrome that results from a sudden reduction or arrest of coronary blood flow. An *infarct* is an area of tissue that undergoes necrosis due to complete interference with blood flow, usually from obstruction of the supplying artery. *Infarction* is the process leading to the development of an infarct.

The most common artery associated with a myocardial infarction is the anterior descending branch of the left coronary artery. That is also the most common site of advanced atherosclerosis.

2. *Etiology.* The immediate cause in many cases is a thrombosis that blocks an artery already narrowed by atherosclerosis. In turn, the blockage creates an area of infarction, which leads to myocardial necrosis of the area. Necrosis of the area can occur within a few hours.

A few patients die immediately or within a few hours. Sudden death may be due to ventricular fibrillation.

3. *Symptoms of Pain*

a. Location. Pain symptoms may start under the sternum, with feelings of indigestion, or in the middle to upper sternum. Pain may last for extended periods, even hours. When the pain is severe, it gives a pressing or crushing heavy sensation and is not relieved by rest or nitroglycerin.

b. Onset. The pain may have a sudden onset, sometimes during sleep or following exercise. The pain may be radial, similar to angina pectoris, which extends to the left arm and mandible.

4. *Other Symptoms.* Cold sweat, weakness and faintness, shortness of breath, nausea, and vomiting may occur. Blood pressure is lowered.

5. *Management During an Attack*
    a. Proceed the same as for angina pectoris: stop dental and dental hygiene treatment, sit the patient up for comfortable breathing, give nitroglycerin, and reassure the patient.
    b. Summon medical assistance as soon as it is known that nitroglycerin does not provide prompt relief. When nitroglycerin does not reduce the angina-like pain within 3 minutes, call both a physician and the ambulance with paramedical personnel.
    c. Record vital signs.
    d. Administer oxygen.
    e. Apply cardiopulmonary resuscitation if indicated while waiting for medical assistance.
    f. Transport to hospital.
6. *Treatment After Acute Symptoms*
    a. Medical supervision. Current medical care for heart attack calls for a shortened rest period with increased activity in keeping with the strength and progress of the patient. Most patients experience extreme fatigue during their convalescence. Medication usually includes an anticoagulant, which complicates dental hygiene treatment.

    Life style changes related to diet, smoking, and stressful activities are essential. Many patients need considerable education, reassurance, and motivation.[23]
    b. Subsequent appointments. Elective dental and dental hygiene appointments are postponed 3 months to 1 year until the patient's physician has given consent. Even when medical clearance has been given, some precautions are needed.

HEART FAILURE

Heart failure is a syndrome in which an abnormality of cardiac function is responsible for the inability or failure of the heart to pump blood at a rate necessary to meet the needs of the body tissues. Because of the collection of fluids in various body organs, the term *congestive heart failure* is used.

I. Etiology

There are many types of causes for heart failure. The causes fall into two categories, namely the underlying and the precipitating causes.

A. Underlying Causes

Examples of cardiovascular disease that result in heart failure are
1. Heart valve damage (rheumatic heart disease, congenital heart disease).
2. Myocardial failure due to an abnormality of heart muscle or secondary to ischemia.

B. Precipitating Causes

Examples that place an additional load on a chronically burdened myocardium are
1. Acute hypertensive crisis (page 782).
2. Massive pulmonary embolism. A thrombus may form in a lower extremity of an inactive person with low cardiac output and circulatory stasis. The thrombus may break loose, and carried by the blood stream, lodge in the pulmonary artery to cause a pulmonary embolism. Severe dyspnea, cyanosis, congestive failure, and shock result.
3. Arrhythmia. An arrhythmia is a heart rhythm irregularity. Ventricular fibrillation is a cardiac arrhythmia in which the muscle fibers contract irregularly. After resuscitation of a person with myocardial infarction, the recurrent arrhythmia, or ventricular fibrillation, is the major risk leading to sudden death.

II. Clinical Manifestations

The clinical manifestations coincide with the parts of the heart involved. Signs and symptoms are different, in general, depending on whether the left or the right side of the heart or both are affected. The general effects are extreme weakness, fatigue, fear, and anxiety.

A. Left Heart Failure

The left side of the heart receives oxygenated blood from the lungs and pumps the blood into the aorta to the rest of the body. A pathologic condition of the left ventricle or the mitral valve would alter output, and there would be respiratory difficulty because of the backup of fluid and blood into the lungs.

Clinical symptoms are more prominent at night. The patient rests better in a sit-up or semi-sit-up position with more than one pillow.

1. *Subjective Symptoms*
   a. Weakness, fatigue.
   b. Dyspnea, particularly evident on exertion. Shortness of breath on lying supine, relieved when sitting up.
   c. Cough and expectoration.
   d. Nocturia.
2. *Objective Symptoms*
   a. Pale, sweating, cold skin.
   b. Breathing obviously difficult.
   c. Diastolic blood pressure increased.
   d. Heart rate rapid.
   e. Anxiety, fear.

B. Right Heart Failure

The right heart receives the venous blood from the vena cava and pumps it to the lungs for oxygenation. Right heart failure shows evidence of systemic venous congestion with peripheral edema. When left heart failure precedes right heart failure, the heart is already congested. Resistance to receiving the venous blood is an additional factor.

1. *Subjective Symptoms*
   a. Weakness, fatigue.
   b. Swelling of feet and/or ankles. The edema progresses to the thighs and abdomen (ascites) in advanced stages of heart failure.
   c. Cold hands and feet.
2. *Objective Symptoms*
   a. Cyanosis of mucous membranes and nailbeds.
   b. Prominent jugular veins.
   c. Congestion with edema in various organs: enlarged spleen and liver; gastrointestinal distress with nausea and vomiting; central nervous system involvement with headache and irritability.
   d. Anxiety, fear.

III. Treatment During Chronic Stages

A patient with an appointment in a dental office or clinic may be receiving a variety of medical treatments. These should be revealed by questioning during preparation of histories. Nearly all patients with heart failure complications will have the following in their medical treatment plan:

A. **Drug Therapy:** usually digitalis and a diuretic.

B. **Dietary Control**
   1. Limited sodium intake to alleviate fluid retention.
   2. Weight reduction.

C. **Limitation of Activity:** depending on severity of the health problem.

IV. Emergency Care for Heart Failure and Acute Pulmonary Edema

A medical emergency that demands urgent attention may occur anywhere. The patient with heart failure or acute pulmonary edema is usually conscious.

A. Position the patient for comfortable breathing: upright.
B. Administer oxygen.
C. Record and monitor vital signs (blood pressure, respiratory rate, and pulse).
D. Reassure the patient.
E. Obtain medical assistance: physician and ambulance.

SUDDEN DEATH

Clinical death that occurs within 24 hours after onset of symptoms is known as sudden death, whereas death within 30 seconds is instantaneous death. Biologic death occurs when permanent cellular damage has been done, primarily from lack of adequate oxygen supply. Biologic death will take place when oxygen delivery to the brain is inadequate for 4 to 6 minutes.

I. Etiology

Nearly all sudden deaths are due to cardiovascular causes, predominantly coronary atherosclerosis. Examples of noncardiac causes are cerebral hemorrhage, drug overdose or toxicity, and pulmonary thromboembolism.

II. Mechanism of Sudden Cardiovascular Death

A. Definition and Description

A majority of sudden deaths are due to

ventricular fibrillation, which is an arrhythmia or absence of heart beat rhythm. Because of many premature beats in which individual muscle bundles fibrillate or contract independently, the ventricle cannot be refilled. Insufficient blood is pumped into the coronary arteries to supply the myocardium. A severe lack of oxygen to the heart muscles causes ventricular standstill, which is one form of cardiac arrest.

B. Clinical Signs of Death

1. Loss of consciousness.
2. No respiration, no pulse, no blood pressure.
3. Dilated pupils.

III. Emergency Care[24,25]

A. Immediate Need: Oxygen

Every second counts, as there are only 4 minutes, or 6 at the most, before enough brain cells die from lack of oxygen to produce "biologic death."

B. Basic Life Support

Details of the procedures are described on pages 837–842.
1. Provide artificial ventilation.
2. Provide artificial circulation.
3. Provide transportation to a hospital.

CARDIAC PACEMAKER[26]

The natural pacemaker, or center where the normal heartbeat is initiated, is the S-A Node (sino-atrial node) located in the right atrium or auricle. From that node, impulses are sent along the muscle walls to stimulate and regulate the contractions of the ventricles, which pump the blood throughout the body. When the natural pacemaker is not functioning or the impulses are interrupted because of heart block, cardiac arrest, various arrhythmias, or other disease conditions, treatment by a cardiologist may include the placement of an artificial pacemaker.

An artificial cardiac pacemaker is a device composed of a pulse generator with a lead (wire) to the myocardium where an electrode is implanted. Impulses are generated to restore and regulate the heartbeat.

I. Description

A. Parts and Power

A permanently implanted pacemaker has electrodes inserted transvenously to the endocardium, usually inside the wall of the right ventricle. Less commonly, the leads may go to the pericardium of the external heart wall.

The electrodes are connected to the power source, a plastic- or metal-encased, hermetically sealed generator, which is implanted under the skin in the thorax or upper abdomen. The area selected depends on the individual condition as determined by the cardiologist (figure 55–4).

Mercury, zinc, or lithium salt batteries are used. Since periodic need for battery replacement has been a major problem, research has been conducted to develop new types, some programmed to permit conservation of energy,[27] and others with rechargeable batteries. Nuclear powered types currently being researched may be expected to last for longer periods of time.

B. Types

1. *Demand.* The demand pacemaker stimulates the heart only when the rate varies from a predetermined norm. By sensing a discrepancy in the electrical signals produced by natural means, the pacemaker sends a signal or stimulus, which regulates the heartbeat.
2. *Fixed Rate.* A preset rate of electrical stimuli is provided independent of the natural heart activity when the natural

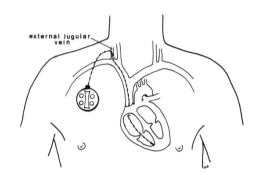

Figure 55–4. Location of cardiac pacemaker. Electrodes are inserted transvenously to the wall of the left ventricle. The power source in the arrangement shown by this diagram is implanted under the skin in the chest.

beat is too slow. Each individual is evaluated for the type best for the condition of the heart. The fixed rate is currently used less frequently than the demand type.

II. Interferences and Their Effects

External electromagnetic interferences can stop or alter the function of a pacemaker. Warning signs in public places are used to identify areas where a person with a pacemaker should not enter, such as where a microwave oven is in operation.

Different models of pacemakers and their sensitivities to interference vary. Newer models are made with a special shielding to protect against interference.

A. General Sources of Interference

Care must be taken relative to microwave ovens, airport screening devices, theft prevention devices, radio transmitters, towers for television and radar, and equipment such as arc welders. Pacemaker wearers are advised to have all equipment checked, kept in good repair, and grounded to prevent electric shock. Devices such as electric shavers and clippers should not be repeatedly turned on and off and should not be operated directly over the implant area.[28]

B. Dental Sources

Ultrasonic scaling units, electrodesensitizing equipment, pulp testers, electric toothbrushes,[29] electrosurgery machines, certain casting equipment, and the Myomonitor,[30] are among the potential sources of interference. Dental devices that apply an electric current directly to the patient are considered those most likely to interfere.

The dental environment has been shown to be a source of moderate electromagnetic interference.[31] All dental equipment should be kept in good repair. Electric devices that contact or can contact the patient should be checked for leakage, since leakage can be a source of interference. Electric appliances need to be earth grounded.

The effect of distance has not been sufficiently researched, hence patients in adjacent dental operatories should be checked before equipment is used.

C. Symptoms of Pacemaker Malfunction

A patient may mention feelings of discomfort. At the same time, the clinician must be aware of possible changes and signs in the event of stopping or altering of a pacemaker.
1. Difficulty in breathing.
2. Dizziness, light headedness, feelings of faintness, or syncope.
3. Changes in pulse rate.
4. Swelling of legs, ankles, arms, wrists.
5. Chest pain.
6. Prolonged hiccoughing.
7. Muscle twitching.

D. Emergency Procedures[32]

In the event a pacemaker should be turned off, immediate action is needed.
1. Turn off all suspected sources of interference.
2. Call for medical assistance; a defibrillator may be needed.
3. Position the patient for cardiopulmonary resuscitation.
4. Open airway, check for breathing, and begin mouth-to-mouth ventilation. The complete procedure is described on page 840.
5. Observation. When the heart is forced to assume its rhythm again as a result of artificial circulation, the pacemaker will be set into action to resume the generation and regulation of the pulse.

III. Appointment Guidelines for a Pacemaker

General procedures for all patients with cardiovascular involvement as described in this chapter apply to the patient wearing a pacemaker. In addition, certain adaptations are recommended.

A. Informed Consent[33]

The signature of the patient or the patient's parent or guardian on a formal statement is a necessary protection against any legal liability in the event of complications or undesirable effects. The patient should receive careful instruction in the anticipated procedures and materials used. Dental and dental hygiene records should be accurate and all-inclusive with a detailed record for each appointment.

B. Patient Histories

The usual health history should be supplemented with information about the type of pacemaker, how long it has been in use, where it is located, the underlying disease condition, and other information pertinent to the patient's safety during dental and dental hygiene appointments. Consultation with the patient's cardiologist is indicated.

C. Prophylactic Antibiotic Premedication

The underlying cardiovascular disease is the basic determinant for use of antibiotic prophylaxis. Infective endocarditis has occurred in patients with pacemakers. The pacemaker wires may serve as a predisposing factor.[5]

Antibiotic prophylaxis may be indicated during the first 6 months following placement of the pacemaker. After implantation, the pulse generator and the electrodes are usually covered by endothelium.[31] Although the patient with a pacemaker appears to be at low risk of endocarditis, the dentist and the cardiologist may choose to use antibiotics to cover dental and dental hygiene procedures.[8]

D. Patient Preparation

1. *Chair Position.* Positioning the patient to support breathing and circulation is important. If the patient experiences difficulty in breathing when in the supine position, the chair back should be elevated to reduce stress.

   There may be some discomfort from wire tension or strain at the implant site if the chair is positioned too far back. That would depend on the location of the pulse generator.

2. *Lead Apron.* Protection of the pulse generator and the lead wires is indicated. A lead apron can serve to interrupt interferences that may be created by electric devices, including handpieces. A lead apron can be heavy and uncomfortable, which may require some consideration.

The importance of grounding and checking all equipment for leakage has been described in II. B., page 789.

E. Radiography

Implantation and monitoring of a pacemaker may have required multiple exposures to radiation. Dental radiation should be limited when possible, and the patient protected by a full-sized lead apron.

F. Instrumentation

The use of manual procedures is advisable. In the absence of specific information, and until the time when all pacemakers are known to be safely shielded, avoidance of power-driven instruments known to cause interference is recommended.

ANTICOAGULANT THERAPY[17,34]

Anticoagulants are used in the treatment of many cardiovascular diseases to prevent embolus and thrombus formation. A prescribed drug may be continued indefinitely in the patient's life as a preventive measure.

Drugs most commonly used are heparin and coumarin derivatives, which act to prevent or delay blood coagulation. Usually, the bleeding time is not altered. Although precautions are needed to prevent hemorrhage, it has been shown that discontinuing the drug can be much more hazardous for the patient than performing the dental and dental hygiene therapy with precautions. When extensive surgical procedures are required, the patient may be hospitalized.

I. Clinical Procedures

A. Consultation

Information about the patient's prothrombin time is obtained from the physician during an initial consultation. The prothrombin time is a test of the coagulation phase of blood clotting used to monitor therapy with anticoagulants. A therapeutic range of $1\frac{1}{2}$ to 2 times the normal level is preferred.

B. Treatment Planning

1. Quadrant scaling and root planing
   a. Treat the most healthy quadrant first. The least bleeding will occur.

b. Teach and emphasize daily plaque control procedures in a series of appointments to prepare the gingival tissue for instrumentation. Healthy, healed tissue does not bleed as readily or as profusely.

2. Determine the prothrombin time within 24 hours before an appointment. The patient can have the test made on the day of a dental appointment by preplanning with the physician and the laboratory.

3. Safe level for dental and dental hygiene procedures is considered to be $1^1/_2$ times the normal, provided precautions are taken during instrumentation and postoperative care.

C. Local Hemostatic Measures

Instrumentation can be performed for most patients without complication, provided precautions are taken to minimize tissue trauma, control bleeding, and not dismiss the patient until bleeding has stopped.

1. *Pressure.* Pressure with sponges or cotton pellets packed interdentally can aid in control.[35]

2. *Suture.* Sutures may be used to close and adapt the tissue interdentally, following deep scaling and gingival curettage.

3. *Periodontal Dressing.* Placement of a dressing is sometimes advisable to provide pressure and protection from trauma, which may initiate postoperative bleeding. Dressing placement is described on pages 546–548.

II. Postoperative Instructions

The practice by oral surgeons of closely observing patients for 6 to 8 hours following a surgical procedure may have application following certain dental and dental hygiene procedures for selected patients. At least, it may be advisable to check with the patient that postoperative instructions are being closely followed.

Postoperatively, the patient is advised to avoid vigorous toothbrushing and rinsing for several hours or until the next day. The use of extraoral icepacks may be helpful. General postoperative instructions may be found on page 599; for the care of an area with a dressing, see page 548.

The use of a soft diet, cool rather than hot foods, and general moderation in activity may be important.

Long-term instruction must emphasize the maintenance of gingival health to prevent future bleeding problems.

HEART SURGERY

Cardiac surgery has become widely used. Patients in dental offices and clinics who have had or will have surgery should be identified and need special procedures. Since the patient with a cardiac prosthesis is at risk for infective endocarditis, all possible dental treatment must be done prior to the date of cardiac surgery and preventive measures must be emphasized.

I. Presurgical

Before elective heart surgery, the patient's mouth should be brought to a state of optimum health, with all sources of infection removed. All restorations and other dental procedures must be completed.

Depending on the type of surgery to be performed, antibiotic prophylaxis will be required. In order that the resistance of the oral flora be decreased prior to the heart surgery, time should elapse between completion of the dental and periodontal therapy, including dental hygiene procedures, before the heart surgery.[36]

Patients requiring heart surgery need information and motivation relative to the importance of oral health in eliminating a potential source of infective endocarditis. Vigilance in a preventive program including plaque control and self-applied fluorides is essential.

II. Postsurgical

A. Recall Appointments

Frequent recall appointments are necessary for supervision and maintenance.

B. Prophylactic Antibiotics

Antibiotic coverage for all procedures for patients with prostheses was described on page 780. Because of the high susceptibility to infective endocarditis, the special regimen for high risk patients includes both penicillin and streptomycin (page 100).[7]

LOCAL ANESTHESIA

Minimization of stress factors is an important

consideration when planning appointments for a patient with a cardiovascular disease. Information from the medical history and from consultation with the patient's physician is needed to understand the patient's risk status.

Apprehension, concern, and long, tiring appointments can stimulate the patient's own discharge of epinephrine, which in turn, increases the heart rate, raises the blood pressure, and puts stress on the entire system. Premedication and anesthesia can reduce such effects.[18]

I. Premedication

A sedative can be prescribed by the dentist or the physician to the advantage of the patient. The premedication selected depends on the individual and the disease condition. Barbiturates, for example, have been used, but possible interaction with other medications taken by the patient must be checked. Although small amounts of barbiturates rarely cause increased blood pressure, pulse rate, or other symptoms, the administration to a patient with untreated, perhaps unrecognized, or drug-controlled hypertension may cause a marked fall in blood pressure or syncope.[37]

A careful medical history, determination of vital signs, with information about currently used medications, previous experiences with drugs, and reference to current drug interaction data are needed.

II. Topical Anesthetic

The use of a topical anesthetic at an injection site for local anesthesia may aid in reducing anxiety. Sufficient time for it to take effect should be allowed. Patient discomfort from injection is minimized.

III. Local Anesthesia

A. Rationale

Anesthesia must be as profound as possible, using as minimum a total dose as possible. When pain is experienced, release of epinephrine by the patient's adrenal glands can occur.

B. Technique

A slow, careful procedure in a calming atmosphere can soothe the patient and alleviate anxiety.

The use of an aspiration technique can prevent direct injection into the venous system. Emergencies that may result are central nervous system stimulation or depression, hypertensive crisis, myocardial ischemia, and cardiac collapse.[17]

C. Use of Vasoconstrictor

1. *Purposes.* The purposes for adding a vasoconstrictor (usually epinephrine) to a local anesthetic solution are to localize the anesthetic at the site and to intensify and prolong the anesthetic effect. Absorption into the systemic circulation is delayed. Despite the importance of these effects, the vasoconstrictor action on the circulatory system can be unfavorable to the patient with cardiovascular problems.

2. *Effect on the Cardiovascular Patient.* The effects are diverse and dependent on the amount and manner of administration. The heart responds with an increased rate, increased blood pressure, and decreased efficiency.[38]

   Sensitivity to the changes is most pronounced in patients using hypertensive drugs, digitalis, and other medications for cardiovascular conditions. Adverse reactions to vasoconstrictors also occur in patients with arrhythmias, atherosclerosis, congestive heart disease, angina pectoris, and recent myocardial infarction.[39]

D. Clinical Application

Whether or not to use an epinephrine-containing local anesthetic has been a subject of controversy and concern. Many physicians do not advise the use of epinephrine for their patients during dental appointments. Differing opinions may be found among dental clinicians and in the literature.[39,40,41,42]

In the past, local anesthetics were not available that did not need epinephrine to enhance the anesthetic effect. Currently, Mepivacaine HCl 3% without vasoconstrictor can provide profound anesthesia for a reasonable operating period. With the advantage of an available anesthetic that is effective without epinephrine, the potential ill effects on the patient's circulation can be avoided. Unless performing in a controlled situation, knowing the patient's condition adequately, and obtaining the approval of the physician as well as the dentist, the use of local anesthesia *without* vasoconstrictor may prove advisable for patients with hypertensive and cardiovascular diseases. If epinephrine is used, the patient's pulse and blood pressure should be monitored.

CONTRAINDICATIONS TO DENTAL AND DENTAL HYGIENE APPOINTMENTS

The opinion and recommendation of the patient's physician provides the final word relative to performing dental and dental hygiene procedures on a particular day. The following four serious conditions are generally considered to be contraindications:[34]

A. Acute or recent myocardial infarction.
B. Unstable or recent onset of angina pectoris.
C. Uncontrolled arrhythmia.
D. Significant uncontrolled hypertension.

TECHNICAL HINTS

I. Record Prescriptions

Record all prescriptions by date, drug, dose, and directions in the patient's permanent record.

II. Determine Status of Prescription

Check that the patient has filled the prescriptions.

III. Prepare for Appointment

Before each appointment for a patient with a cardiovascular disease
A. Determine and record blood pressure.
B. Review patient history and notes relative to previous appointments in order to prepare adequately for the current appointment.
C. Check with the patient to be sure that prescribed medications have been taken and at the proper time.
  1. Antibiotic premedication must be taken one hour before the appointment.
  2. Question the patient concerning drugs that may have been taken on the same day as the appointment, such as a sedative, alcoholic beverage, or other, which

may influence the premedication or the effect of anesthetic to be given.

IV. Source of Materials

Local Heart Association
and
American Heart Association
7320 Greenville Avenue
Dallas, Texas 75231

FACTORS TO TEACH THE PATIENT

I. Hypertension Therapy

Encourage patients who have been diagnosed as hypertensive to continue their prescribed therapy.

II. Stress Reduction Procedures[43]

A. Select an appointment time that is optimum with respect to time of day when the patient is feeling best and may be less fatigued. For most anxious patients, a morning appointment is preferred.
B. Get adequate sleep and rest, and engage in nonfatiguing activities during the 24 hours before the appointment.
C. Use premedication as prescribed for sleeping the night before. A sedative may be prescribed to be taken 60 minutes before an appointment; at the dental office, if possible. When taken at home one hour before, the patient should not drive a car.
D. Allow time to get to the dental office or clinic; bring own reading material, knitting or sewing, or other relaxing activity in the event waiting is unavoidable.
E. Eat breakfast, lunch, or other usual between-meal food and take usual medications on schedule.
F. Do not relay feelings of stress to other members of the family, especially children.

References

1. United States Department of Health, Education and Welfare: *Health—United States.* Washington, D.C., Public Health Service, National Center for Health Statistics, DHEW Publication Number (PHS) 78–1232, 1978, p. 31.
2. Paffenbarger, R.S.: Prevention of Heart Disease, *Postgrad. Med., 51,* 74, January, 1972.
3. Isselbacher, K.J., Adams, R.D., Braunwald, E., Petersdorf, R.G., and Wilson, J.D., eds.: *Harrison's Principles of Internal Medicine,* 9th ed. New York, McGraw-Hill, 1980, pp. 1090–1092.

4. Robbins, S.L. and Cotran, R.S.: *Pathologic Basis of Disease*, 2nd ed. Philadelphia, W.B. Saunders Co., 1979, pp. 663–686.

5. Beeson, P.B., McDermott, W., and Wyngaarden, J.B.: *Textbook of Medicine*, 15th ed. Philadelphia, W.B. Saunders Co., 1979, pp. 386–387.

6. Karchmer, A.W.: Infective Endocarditis, in Conn, H.F., ed.: *Current Therapy*. Philadelphia, W.B. Saunders Co., 1980, pp. 206–212.

7. American Heart Association, Committee on Prevention of Rheumatic Fever and Bacterial Endocarditis: Prevention of Bacterial Endocarditis, *Circulation*, 56, 139A, July, 1977.

8. American Heart Association: Prevention of Bacterial Endocarditis, *J. Am. Dent. Assoc.*, 95, 600, September, 1977.

9. Sconyers, J.R., Albers, D.D., and Kelly, R.: Relationship of Bacteremia to Toothbrushing in Clinically Healthy Patients, *Gen. Dent.*, 27, 51, May–June, 1979.

10. Randall, E. and Brenman, H.S.: Local Degerming with Povidone-iodine. I. Prior to Dental Prophylaxis, *J. Periodontol.*, 45, 866, December, 1974.

11. Brenman, H.S. and Randall, E.: Local Degerming with Povidone-iodine. II. Prior to Gingivectomy, *J. Periodontol.*, 45, 870, December, 1974.

12. Beeson, McDermott, and Wyngaarden: op. cit., pp. 1200–1212.

13. Finnerty, F.A.: Hypertension is Different in Blacks, *J.Am.Med.Assoc.*, 216, 1634, June 7, 1971.

14. United States Department of Health and Human Services: *The 1980 Report of the Joint National Committee on Detection, Evaluation, and Treatment of High Blood Pressure*. United States Department of Health and Human Services, Public Health Service, National Institutes of Health, NIH Publication Number 81-1088, December, 1980.

15. Malamed, S.F.: *Medical Emergencies in the Dental Office*. St. Louis, The C.V. Mosby Co., 1978, p. 22.

16. Ibid., p. 95.

17. Cowan, F.F.: *Pharmacology for the Dental Hygienist*. Philadelphia, Lea & Febiger, 1978, pp., 306–343.

18. American Dental Association, Council on Dental Therapeutics: *Accepted Dental Therapeutics*, 39th ed. Chicago, American Dental Association, 1982, pp. 4–7.

19. Chue, P.W.Y.: Hypertension: Implications for Dentistry, *Dent. Surv.*, 51, 25, May, 1975.

20. National Heart, Lung, and Blood Institute, Task Force on Blood Pressure Control in Children: Recommendations of the Task Force on Blood Pressure Control in Children, *Pediatrics*, 59, 799, Number 5 Supplement, May, 1977.

21. Kowalski, C.I., Randolph, M.F., and Macko, D.J.: A Study of Blood Pressure in Children, *J. Am. Dent. Assoc.*, 97, 966, December, 1978.

22. Malamed: op. cit., p. 295.

23. Horlick, L.: Care and Rehabilitation after Myocardial Infarction, in Conn, H.F., ed.: *Current Therapy*. Philadelphia, W.B. Saunders Co., 1980, pp. 223–227.

24. Dunn, M.J. and Booth, D.F.: *Internal Medicine/Systemic Emergencies*. Baltimore, The Williams & Wilkins Co., 1975, pp. 79–88.

25. Malamed: op. cit., pp. 313–316.

26. Griffiths, P.V.: The Management of the Pacemaker Wearer During Dental Hygiene Treatment, *Dent. Hyg.*, 52, 573, December, 1978.

27. Vera, Z., Janzen, D., and Mason, D.T.: Longevity of Programmable Energy Output Pacemakers. Early Results and Experiences, *Br. Heart J.*, 39, 1364, December, 1977.

28. *Pacing Your Heart*, 1978. Medtronic, Inc., 3055 Old Highway Eight, P.O. Box 1453, Minneapolis, Minnesota, 55440.

29. Escher, D.J., Parker, B., and Furman, S.: Pacemaker Triggering (Inhibition) by Electric Toothbrush, *Am. J. Cardiol.*, 38, 126, July, 1976.

30. Martinis, A.J., Jankelson, B., Radke, J., and Adib, F.: Effects of the Myo-monitor on Cardiac Pacemakers, *J. Am. Dent. Assoc.*, 100, 203, February, 1980.

31. Simon, A.B., Linde, B., Bonnette, G.H., and Schlentz, R.J.: The Individual With a Pacemaker in the Dental Environment, *J. Am. Dent. Assoc.*, 91, 1224, December, 1975.

32. Ore, D.E. and Shriner, W.: When Your Patient Has a Pacemaker, *N.Y. J. Dent.*, 45, 227, August–September, 1975.

33. Dreifus, L.S. and Cohen, D.: Implanted Pacemakers: Medicolegal Implications, *Am. J. Cardiol.*, 36, 266, August, 1975.

34. Glasser, S.P.: The Problems of Patients With Cardiovascular Disease Undergoing Dental Treatment, *J. Am. Dent. Assoc.*, 94, 1158, June, 1977.

35. Carranza, F.A.: *Glickman's Clinical Periodontology*, 5th ed. Philadelphia, W.B. Saunders Co., 1979, pp. 787–788.

36. Santinga, J.T., Fekety, R.F., Bottomley, W.K., Else, B., and Willis, P.W.: Antibiotic Prophylaxis for Endocarditis in Patients With a Prosthetic Heart Valve, *J. Am. Dent. Assoc.*, 93, 1001, November, 1976.

37. Cowan: op. cit., p. 209.

38. Cowan: op. cit., pp. 83–87.

39. American Dental Association, Council on Dental Therapeutics: op. cit., pp. 166–169.

40. Bennett, C.R.: *Monheim's Local Anesthesia and Pain Control in Dental Practice*, 6th ed. St. Louis, The C.V. Mosby Co., 1978, pp. 172–182.

41. Hayden, J. and Jorgensen, N.B.: Complications from Local Analgesia, in McCarthy, F.M.: *Emergencies in Dental Practice*, 3rd ed. Philadelphia, W.B. Saunders Co., 1979, pp. 441–442.

42. Tufts University School of Dental Medicine, Department of Oral and Maxillofacial Surgery: The Use of Vasoconstrictors in Cardiac Patients, *Clinical Handbook*, 1979–1980.

43. Malamed: op. cit., pp. 27–30.

Suggested Readings

Berger, E.N.H.: Attitudes and Preventive Dental Health Behavior in Children with Congenital Cardiac Disease, *Aust. Dent. J.*, 23, 87, February, 1978.

Caccamo, L.P.: The Cardiovascular Patient: A Review of Pathophysiology and Dental Implications, *Special Care*, 1, 88, March–April, 1981.

Chapman, N.L.: Alteration of Nutrition Habits in Ischemic Heart Disease, *Clin. Prev. Dent.*, 2, 9, January–February, 1980.

Dionne, R.A.: The Pharmacological Basis of Pain Control in Dental Practice: Local Anesthetics, *Compend. Cont. Educ. Gen. Dent.*, 1, 229, July–August, 1980.

Dreizen, S., Levy, B., Stern, M., and Bernick, S.: Human Lingual Atherosclerosis, *Arch. Oral Biol.*, 19, 813, September, 1974.

Elliot, R.H.: A Dental Service for Children Suffering from Cardiac Disease, *Br. Dent. J.*, 138, 179, March 4, 1975.

Hollinger, J.O. and Moore, E.M.: Cardiovascular Considerations in General Dentistry, *Dent. Surv.*, 54, 16, October, 1978.

Lynch, M.A., ed.: *Burket's Oral Medicine, Diagnosis and*

Treatment, 7th ed. Philadelphia, J.B. Lippincott Co., 1977, pp. 375–398.

Reuben, B.M.: A Current Practical Review of Local Anesthesia, *Dent. Surv.,* 56, 38, July, 1980.

Roser, S.M. and Rosenbloom, B.: Continued Anticoagulation in Oral Surgery Procedures, *Oral Surg.,* 40, 448, October, 1975.

Scopp, I.W.: An Overview of the Heart Patient in Dental Practice, *N.Y. J. Dent.,* 49, 48, February, 1979.

Sorenson, H.W.: The Pedodontic Patient With Heart Disease, *Dent. Clin. North Am.,* 17, 173, January, 1973.

Sutherland, K.J.: Systemic Problems Affecting Dental Treatment, *Aust. Dent. J.,* 23, 140, April, 1978.

Tocker, J. and Weibert, E.: The Dental Significance of Corticosteroids, Antihypertensive Drugs and Anticoagulants, *Dent. Hyg.,* 49, 11, January, 1975.

Hypertension

Abbey, L.M.: Dealing With the Hypertensive Patient–Dentist–Physician Interaction, *Dent. Surv.,* 54, 26, May, 1978.

Argentieri, R.: Dental Care for the Hypertensive Patient, *N.Y. State Dent. J.,* 44, 55, February, 1978.

Berman, C.L., Giovannoli, R.T., and Modugno, R.J.: Hypertension: The Invisible Epidemic, *J. Prev. Dent.,* 5, 8, September–October, 1978.

Little, J.W. and Jakobsen, J.: Management of the Hypertensive Patient in Dental Practice, *J. Oral Med.,* 29, 13, January–March, 1974.

Newkirk, C.: The Hypertensive Dental Patient: Detection and Treatment, *Dent. Hyg.,* 51, 205, May, 1977.

Simpson, T.H.: The Hypertensive Patient in Dental Practice, *Dent. Assist.,* 44, 16, February, 1975.

Infective Endocarditis

Baumgartner, J.C., Heggers, J.P., and Harrison, J.W.: The Incidence of Bacteremias Related to Endodontic Procedures. I. Nonsurgical Endodontics, *J. Endodont.,* 2, 135, May, 1976.

Curran, J.B., Ogle, R.G., and Waite, D.E.: Infection of Abnormal Heart Valves and Total Joint Prosthesis Following Dental Procedures, *Northwest Dent.,* 55, 192, July–August, 1976.

Elliot, R.H. and Dunbar, J.M.: Antibiotic Sensitivity of Oral Alpha-haemolytic Streptococcus from Children with Congenital or Acquired Cardiac Disease. A Prolonged Survey, *Br. Dent. J.,* 142, 283, May 3, 1977.

Everett, E.D. and Hirschman, J.V.: Transient Bacteremia and Endocarditis Prophylaxis. A Review, *Medicine,* 56, 61, January, 1977.

Hockett, R.N., Loesche, W.J., and Sodeman, T.M.: Bacteraemia in Asymptomatic Human Subjects, *Arch. Oral Biol.,* 22, 91, Number 2, 1977.

Little, J.W.: Management of the Patient With a History of Rheumatic Fever in Dental Practice, *J. Oral Med.,* 33, 47, April–June, 1978.

Macedo-Sobrinho, B.: Infective Endocarditis: Is it Being Neglected Within the Dental Profession? *Clin. Prev. Dent.,* 1, 14, November–December, 1979.

Mostaghim, D. and Millard, H.D.: Bacterial Endocarditis: A Retrospective Study, *Oral Surg.,* 40, 219, August, 1975.

Munroe, C.O. and Lazarus, T.L.: Predisposing Conditions of Infective Endocarditis, *Can. Dent. Assoc. J.,* 42, 483, October, 1976.

Pogrel, M.A. and Welsby, P.D.: The Dentist and Prevention of Infective Endocarditis, *Br. Dent. J.,* 139, 12, July 1, 1975.

Stimmel, H.M., Orchen, J.J., Skaff, D.M., Brown, A.T., and Spedding, R.H.: Penicillin-resistant Alpha-hemolytic Streptococci in Children With Heart Disease Who Take Penicillin Daily, *J. Dent. Child.,* 48, 29, January–February, 1981.

Wright, A.D.: Infective Endocarditis, *Br. Dent. J.,* 144, 351, June 6, 1978.

Pacemaker

American Dental Association Council on Dental Materials and Devices: Possible Electromagnetic Interference With Cardiac Pacemakers from Dental Induction Casting Machines and Electrosurgical Devices, *J. Am. Dent. Assoc.,* 86, 426, February, 1973.

American Heart Association: *Living With Your Pacemaker.* American Heart Association, National Center, 7320 Greenville Avenue, Dallas, Texas 75231.

Hartlmaier, K.M.: The Cardiac Pacemaker and the Dentist, *Quintessence Int.,* 9, 9, June, 1978.

Rezai, F.R.: Dental Treatment of a Patient With a Cardiac Pacemaker, *Oral Surg.,* 44, 662, November, 1977.

Walter, C.: Dental Treatment of Patients With Cardiac Pacemaker Implants, *Quintessence Int.,* 6, 57, August, 1975.

56

The Patient with a Blood Disorder

Oral soft tissue changes, lowered resistance to infection, and bleeding tendencies are major factors to be considered for patients with blood diseases. Oral manifestations of blood disorders are generally exaggerated in the presence of bacterial plaque and local predisposing factors. Dental hygiene care and supervision make an essential contribution to the oral health and comfort of a patient with a blood disease.

I. Oral Findings Suggestive of Blood Disorders

Early signs of systemic conditions frequently appear in the oral soft tissue. The patient's medical history may not reveal the existence of a blood disorder, but the alert dental hygienist may note tissue characteristics suggestive of disease. By calling the findings to the attention of the dentist, an important referral for medical examination may lead to diagnosis and treatment of a serious disease. In addition, the findings of laboratory blood examination may provide essential information for safe and effective dental and dental hygiene therapy.

Listed below are certain oral soft tissue changes that may occur in patients with blood diseases. Many of the findings are not exclusive to systemic blood disorders. The important thing is to recognize change in a previously healthy patient, or what appears to be an exaggerated response in a patient being examined at an initial appointment.

Findings that may indicate a blood disorder including the following:
A. Gingival bleeding, spontaneously or upon gentle probing.
B. History of difficulty in controlling postoperative hemorrhage by usual procedures.
C. History of bruising easily, with large ecchymoses.
D. Numerous petechiae.
E. Marked pallor of the mucous membranes.
F. Atrophy of the papillae of the tongue.
G. Persistent sore or painful tongue (glossodynia).
H. Acute or chronic infections, such as candidiasis, which do not respond to usual treatment.
I. Severe ulcerations associated with a lack of response to treatment.
J. Exaggerated gingival response to local irritants, sometimes with characteristics of necrotizing ulcerative gingivitis (ulceration, necrosis, bleeding, pseudomembrane).

II. The Normal Blood[1]

A. Composition

The blood is composed of 55 percent plasma fluid and 45 percent formed elements. The formed elements are categorized by type into erythrocytes (red blood cells or corpuscles), leukocytes (white blood cells), and thrombocytes (platelets). The red

797

blood cells comprise about 44 percent and the white blood cells 1 percent of the 45 percent total formed elements.

The *hematocrit* is the percentage of packed volume of blood cells, the normal value for which approximates 45 percent, as shown in table 56–1. The test for the hematocrit is commonly used in general health evaluations.

B. Origin

In adults, all blood cells originate in the bone marrow. The erythrocytes and granulocytes pass through a series of transformations from the stem cell (cell of origin), the *hemocytoblast*, and leave the bone marrow as mature cells to enter the circulating blood.

Table 56–1.   Tests Used for Blood Evaluation

Test	*Normal Range**	*Causes of Deviations*

Hemoglobin	Males: 14–18 g./100 ml
	Females: 12–16 g./100 ml
		Increased in
		  Polycythemia
		  Dehydration
		
		Decreased in
		  Anemias
		  Hemorrhage
		  Leukemias

Hematocrit
  (volume of packed
  red cells)
	Males: 40–54%
	Females: 37—47%
		Increased in
		  Polycythemia
		  Dehydration
		
		Decreased in
		  Anemias
		  Hemorrhage
		  Leukemia

Bleeding Time	Duke: 1–3½ minutes
	Ivy: less than 5 minutes
	Modified Ivy: 2½–10 minutes
	  (Mielke template)
		Prolonged in
		  Disorders of platelet function
		  Thrombocytopenia
		  von Willebrand's disease
		  Leukemias
		  Aspirin and certain other drug use

Clotting Time	Glass tube: 4–8 minutes	Prolonged in
		  Vitamin K deficiency
		  Severe hemophilia
		  Anticoagulant therapy
		  Liver diseases

Prothrombin Time
  (P.T.)
	11–15 seconds	Prolonged in
		  Polycythemia vera
		  Prothrombin deficiency
		  Anticoagulant therapy
		  Vitamin K deficiency
		  Liver diseases
		  Aspirin use

Partial Thromboplastin
  Time (P.T.T.)
	68–82 seconds	Prolonged in
		  Hemophilia A and B
		  von Willebrand's disease
		  Anticoagulant therapy

*The normal range varies with the specificity of the technique used. There is also a range variation, depending on the health facility and the laboratory.

The bone marrow also produces the stem cells for the agranulocytes. The lymphocytes and monocytes leave the bone marrow in immature forms and go to the lymphoid tissues for later maturing. In certain blood diseases and cancers, the immature cell forms predominate.

C. Plasma

The constituents of the fluid portion of the blood are similar to those of the connective tissue. There is a two-way exchange at the capillary level. The plasma is comprised 90 percent of water and 10 percent of the following:

1. *Plasma Proteins*
   a. Albumin (functions to maintain tissue fluid pressure).
   b. Gamma globulins (circulating antibodies essential in the immune system).
   c. Beta globulins (transport of hormones, metallic ions, and lipids).
   d. Fibrinogen and prothrombin (blood clotting).
2. *Inorganic Salts:* sodium, potassium, calcium, bicarbonate, chloride.
3. *Gases:* dissolved oxygen, carbon dioxide, and nitrogen.
4. *Substances Being Transported:* hormones, nutrients, waste products, enzymes.

D. Red Blood Corpuscles

1. *Description.* Although usually called red blood cells, these corpuscles have no nuclei. They are biconcave discs which contain hemoglobin. The cells are sensitive and flexible and change shape readily as they pass through small capillaries.

   Table 56–2 contains reference values for blood cells and the names of conditions in which increases or decreases in the normal values occur.
2. *Function.* Hemoglobin carries oxygen to the body cells in the form of oxyhemoglobin. Carbon dioxide is transported from the cells.

   The hemoglobin is measured in grams (g.) per 100 milliliters (ml). Normal values are shown in table 56–1 and range

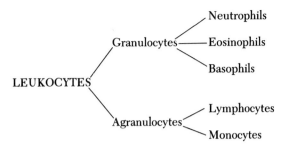

Figure 56–1. Types of leukocytes. Leukocytes are divided into granulocytes and agranulocytes, which are subdivided as shown.

from 12 to 18 g. per 100 ml. The values reflect the anemic state when the hemoglobin is lowered. They also reflect conditions in which the hemoglobin is increased to a level higher than normal.

E. White Blood Cells

1. *Types.* White blood cells are divided into two general groups, the granulocytes and the agranulocytes. Granulocytes have granules in their cytoplasm, whereas the agranulocytes do not. They are further subdivided as shown in figure 56–1.
2. *Functions.* All white cells are amoeboid or motile, which permits them to pass through the walls at the terminal ends of capillaries and into the connective tissue. Their work is done within the connective tissue, where they have phagocytic, immunologic, and other functions related to the inflammatory process.

   The cells respond to an injury or invasion of microorganisms and migrate into the area in large numbers. Neutrophils arrive first and are active in phagocytizing foreign material and microorganisms.

   In reality, the blood is only a transport medium for the white cells as they pass to areas in the connective tissue where their functions are needed. Their numbers and proportions in the blood maintain a constant level in health, as shown in table 56–2. A *differential cell count* of the white blood cells is used in the detection and monitoring of diseased states. Increases and decreases of each cell type

Table 56–2.   Blood Cells Reference Values

Cell Type	Normal Value	Causes of Increase	Causes of Decrease
Red Blood Corpuscles	Male 4.5–6.0 Female 4.3–5.5 million per cu. mm.	Polycythemia Dehydration	Anemias Leukemias Hemorrhage
Total White Blood Cells	5,000–10,000 per cu. mm.	Inflammation Overexertion Polycythemia vera	Aplastic anemia Granulocytopenia Drug poisoning Thrombocytopenia Radiation Severe infections
DIFFERENTIAL **White Cell** **Granulocytes**			
1. Neutrophils (PMNs)	60–70%	Acute infections Myelogenous leukemia Poisoning Erythroblastosis	Aplastic anemia Granulocytopenia
2. Eosinophils	1–3%	Allergic diseases Dermatitis Hodgkin's disease Scarlet fever	Aplastic anemia Typhoid fever
3. Basophils	1%	Certain chronic infections	Aplastic anemia
Agranulocytes **1. Lymphocytes**	20–35%	Lymphocytic leukemia Chronic infections Viral diseases	Aplastic anemia Myelogenous leukemia Radiation
2. Monocytes	2–6%	Monocytic leukemias Tuberculosis Infective endocarditis Hodgkin's disease	Aplastic anemia
Platelets	150,000–400,000 per cu. mm. Wintrobe method: 140,000–440,000 per cu. mm.	Polycythemia vera Chronic myelocytic leukemia Sickle cell anemia Rheumatic fever Hemolytic anemias Bone fractures	Acute severe infections Cirrhosis of the liver Thrombocytopenic purpura Acute leukemias Aplastic anemias Pernicious anemia

can be associated with certain conditions.

F. Agranulocytes

1. *Lymphocytes.* A mature lymphocyte is a small round cell with a round nucleus that nearly fills the cell, leaving only a narrow rim of cytoplasm. Less mature forms are larger, with more cytoplasm.

   In the connective tissue, certain lymphocytes may differentiate into plasma cells which produce and secrete antibody. The *plasma cell* is a relatively large oval cell with an eccentric nucleus. Lymphocytes and plasma cells are common in areas of chronic inflammation.

2. *Monocytes.* A monocyte is a large cell with a bean-shaped or indented nucleus. It is actively phagocytic. In the connective tissue, monocytes differentiate into macrophages which are important in immunologic processes.

G. Granulocytes

1. *Neutrophils.* Neutrophils are the most numerous of all the white blood cells. They are also named polymorphonuclear leukocytes and referred to as "PMNs" or "polys." The nucleus of a neutrophil has three to five lobes connected by thin chromatin threads.

    In circulation, the cells are round, but in the tissues they are more or less amoeboid as they function in phagocytosis. Neutrophils are part of the first line of defense of the body.

2. *Eosinophils.* An eosinophil usually has a two-lobed nucleus and larger, coarser granules than those of a neutrophil. The granules stain a distinct bright pink, so that microscopically, the cells can be readily recognized, even though few in number. The numbers increase markedly during allergic conditions.

3. *Basophils.* In contrast to the eosinophil or neutrophil, the nucleus of a basophil is usually in "U" or "S" form. The functions of the basophil are related to increasing vascular permeability during inflammation, thus permitting phagocytic cells to pass into the area.

H. Platelets

A platelet is a small round or oval formed element without a nucleus. It is approximately one fourth the size of a red blood cell. Platelets are active in the blood clotting mechanism and essential in the maintenance of the integrity of blood capillaries by closing them at a time of injury. After healing, the platelets participate in clot dissolution.

ANEMIAS

Anemia means a reduction of the hemoglobin concentration, the hematocrit, or the number of red blood cells to a level below that which is normal for the individual.[2] As a result of anemia, oxygen-carrying capacity to the cells is diminished.

I. Classification by Etiology

Anemias are usually classified into three groups by general causes. The categories and an example of each are listed below. Later in the chapter, selected specific anemias with their oral implications will be described.

A. Caused by Blood Loss

1. *Acute:* blood loss from trauma or disease.
2. *Chronic.* An internal lesion with constant slow bleeding, usually of gastrointestinal or gynecologic origin can lead to a chronic loss of blood. An *iron deficiency anemia* can result.

B. Caused by Increased Hemolysis

Hemolysis means the destruction of red blood cells. These types of anemias are called "hemolytic anemias" because of the cell destruction.

1. *Hereditary Hemolytic Disorders*
    Example: *Sickle cell anemia,* which belongs to the group of hereditary disorders called the hemoglobinopathies.
2. *Acquired Hemolytic Disorders*
    Examples: drugs, infections, and certain physical and chemical agents that may cause red cell destruction. In the category of antibody-mediated anemia, *erythroblastosis fetalis* occurs when a mother is Rh negative and develops antibodies against a fetus that is Rh positive. It is sometimes called hemolytic disease of the newborn.

C. Caused by Diminished Production of Red Blood Cells

A nutritional deficiency or bone marrow failure may be the reason for diminished production.

1. *Nutritional Deficiency*
    a. Inadequate diet choices or inadequate intake.
    b. Defective absorption from the gastrointestinal tract.
        Example: *pernicious anemia,* which results from a B_{12} vitamin absorption deficiency.
    c. Increased demand for nutrients.
        Example: *iron deficiency anemia,* which may occur during pregnancy or during a growth spurt.
2. *Bone Marrow Failure*
    Example: *aplastic anemia,* which may result from bone marrow failure due to

drug use, irradiation, or chemicals. In aplastic anemia, there is a combination of anemia, neutropenia, and thrombocytopenia, which means a quantitative decrease in all cells formed in the bone marrow.

II. Clinical Characteristics of Anemias

When a patient's medical history shows the presence of anemia, certain general characteristics may be anticipated for which appointment and clinical adaptations may be needed.

The general signs and symptoms are

A. Skin: pale and thin.
B. Weakness, malaise, easy fatigability.
C. Dyspnea on slight exertion, faintness.
D. Headache, vertigo, tinnitus.
E. Dimness of vision, spots before the eyes.
F. Nails become brittle and lose their convexity.
G. Severely ill patient: cardiac failure may result from effects of hypoxia.

IRON DEFICIENCY ANEMIA

Iron deficiency anemia is a hypochromic microcytic anemia, which means there is a hemoglobin deficiency (hypochromic) and the red blood corpuscles are smaller than normal and deficient in hemoglobin (microcytic). In general, it is found more in younger than in older people, and more in females than in males.

I. Causes

A. Malnutrition or malabsorption.
B. Chronic infection.
C. Increased body demand for iron over and above the daily intake. Example: during pregnancy.
D. Chronic blood loss. When iron-deficiency anemia occurs in men or in postmenopausal women, it usually means there is bleeding, and tests are needed to find the internal source.
  1. Causes of internal bleeding
    a. Gastrointestinal diseases such as ulcer, cancer.
    b. Drugs, notably aspirin.
    c. Hemorrhoids.
  2. Excessive menstrual flow.
  3. Frequent blood donations.

II. Signs and Symptoms

A. General

Clinical manifestations of iron deficiency anemia include general weakness, headache, pallor, and fatigue on slight exertion.

B. Oral[3]

1. Pallor of the mucosa and gingiva.
2. Tongue changes
  a. Atrophic glossitis with loss of filiform papillae. In moderate and severe anemia, when the hemoglobin is at 10 or below, the entire tongue is usually involved. In slight anemia (hemoglobin 11 to 12), only the margins and anterior portion of the dorsum may be atrophic.[4]
  b. Glossodynia, more frequent in slight to moderate anemia.
  c. Secondary irritations to the thinned, atrophic mucosa from smoking, mechanical trauma, or hot, spicy foods.

III. Therapy

Iron deficiency anemia is treated with oral ferrous iron tablets. Liquid preparations, which are sometimes used for children, may stain the teeth. Administering the medicine by way of a straw is advised.

MEGALOBLASTIC ANEMIAS

Megaloblastic anemias are characterized by abnormally large (megalo-) red blood corpuscles, many of which are oval shaped. The two principal types of megaloblastic anemias are *pernicious anemia* and *folate deficiency anemia*.

Pernicious anemia is due to a deficiency of vitamin B_{12} and folate deficiency anemia is due to a deficiency of folate, or folic acid. These two vitamins are essential in red blood cell production in the bone marrow. When one or the other is deficient, the basic precursor cell ("-blast") is altered, which leads to a derangement in the formation of red blood cells and abnormal, megaloblastic cells result.[5] A megaloblastic anemia can result from a deficiency of either vitamin B_{12} or folate, or both together.

I. Pernicious Anemia

The implication of "fatality" when the word "pernicious" is used can be misleading, since synthetic vitamin B_{12} is now available for treatment and disease control. The traditional name is still in current use, however.

A. Etiologic Factors

Vitamin B_{12} deficiency can be caused by decreased intake (inadequate diet or impaired absorption) or increased requirement (pregnancy, hyperparathyroidism, disseminated cancer). Pernicious anemia is caused by *impaired absorption* of B_{12} due to failure of production of *intrinsic factor* (IF) by the gastric mucosa.

Pernicious anemia is primarily a disease of people over 40 years of age. Frequently, the reason for lack of production of *intrinsic factor* is either chronic atrophic gastritis or surgical removal or partial removal of the stomach.

In the childhood form of the disease, other causes are in effect, since no gastric abnormality exists. Although more research is needed, there may be either a hereditary inability to produce intrinsic factor, or the intrinsic factor produced may be ineffective.

B. Clinical Findings

1. *General.* Weakness, tingling or numbness of fingers and toes, and weight loss are usually found. Central nervous system involvement may be manifested by difficulty in walking, some lack of coordination, loss of vibratory sense, and mental confusion.

2. *Oral*
   a. Tongue (atrophic glossitis, burning tongue). There may be a painful, inflamed, flabby tongue that is red, smooth, and shiny with loss of filiform papillae. Secondarily, sensitivity to hot or spicy foods and other irritants, and painful swallowing may be expected.
   b. Gingiva and mucosa. Soft tissues may be pale and atrophic, and appear similar to those in a general vitamin B deficiency.

C. Treatment

Vitamin B_{12} is administered by injection twice weekly until the condition is controlled, and then monthly, indefinitely.

II. Folate Deficiency Anemia

Folate deficiency anemia has the same characteristics as pernicious anemia, except clinically, there are no neurologic changes.

A. Etiologic Factors[5]

Folate deficiency can be caused by decreased intake (inadequate diet, impaired absorption), increased requirement (pregnancy, disseminated cancer), or blocked activation (certain drugs impair the utilization of folate).

B. Dietary Factors

Folates are abundant in green vegetables (spinach, lettuce, cabbage, asparagus), yeast, and liver. Only minimal subsistence diets or special diets influenced by factors such as poverty, food fadism, or alcoholism, when the use of alcohol takes precedence over food, are likely to be deficient in folates. Folate deficiency anemia is not uncommon, but may be more frequently related to malabsorption than inadequate intake.

The main sources of vitamin B_{12} are meat and dairy products, that is, all foods containing animal protein. Liver is a rich source and was originally used in therapy before the development of synthetic B_{12}.

SICKLE CELL ANEMIA

Sickle cell anemia is a hereditary form of hemolytic anemia with severe complications involving other body systems. The name is derived from the crescent or "sickle" shape the red blood corpuscles assume when they become deoxygenated.

The disease occurs primarily in the black population and in white populations of Mediterranean origin. The incidence of sickle cell trait (carrier state) is approximately 1 in every 10 American black people. Sickle cell anemia is found in approximately 0.3 to 1.3 percent or one in 400. In certain countries of Africa, the rate may be as high as 30 percent of the population.

Tests are available for screening and diagnosis of those with sickle cell trait. Genetic counseling can play an important role in prevention. Detection of the presence of sickle cell anemia is possible before birth, so that proper observation and supervision of the infant and young child can be provided.

I. Disease Process

Signs and symptoms do not appear until after approximately the sixth month, when hemoglobin has matured. Growth and development may be impaired during the early years. There is a marked susceptibility to communicable diseases, and young children are especially susceptible to· pneumococcal infections.

The disease abnormality is in the type and solubility of hemoglobin. The defective hemoglobin loses oxygen and the red blood corpuscles become distorted into sickled shapes (figure 56–2). Increases in blood fluid viscosity result, and blood stasis occurs, which can lead to thrombosis formation and infarction. The sickled cells may collect in the vital organs and lead to serious involvement and organ enlargement, particularly of the liver and spleen. Chronic changes may occur in any organ system of the body.

II. Clinical Course

A. Severe Hemolytic Anemia

In adults, chronic hemolytic sickle cell disease can be severe. The hematocrit may range between 18 and 30 percent. The life span of red blood corpuscles normally is from 90 to 120 days, whereas in hemolytic anemia such as sickle cell anemia, the red blood corpuscle survival rate is about 10 to 15 days.

B. Sickle Cell Crisis

Periodic recurrences of clinical exacerbations of the disease with periods of remission characterize childhood and adolescence. The acute form of the disease is called the sickle cell crisis.
1. *Precipitating Factors.* Crises may appear at any time with or without stimuli.

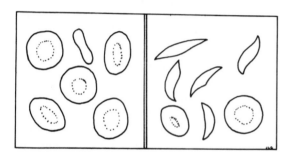

Figure 56–2. Sickle cell anemia. *Left,* diagrammatic drawing of normal red blood cells. *Right,* sickle shapes of red blood cells of a patient with sickle cell anemia.

However, viral or bacterial infections, other systemic diseases, exertion, trauma, temperature changes (dehydration in summer, reflex vasospasm in cold weather) may be specific precipitating factors.
2. *Clinical Signs and Symptoms.* A crisis is characterized by severe pain. Infarctions occur in various tissues and organs. When the central nervous system becomes involved, there may be symptoms of seizure, stroke, or coma.

The effects of a crisis may be reversible to some degree, severe physical conditions can result, or a crisis can be fatal. The high mortality rate in young children may be due to the effects of a crisis or to severe infections.

C. Systemic Changes That May Occur

Chronic changes may occur in any organ system at any age. The kidney is a major organ affected; changes in the cardiopulmonary system can result in enlargement of the heart, heart murmurs, and coronary insufficiency. Ocular disturbances are not uncommon in adults, even leading to blindness. Certain patients may be susceptible to cerebrovascular accidents with hemiplegia.

D. Bone Changes[6]

Bone changes noted in the skeletal bones also may be seen in the mandible.
1. Bone marrow hyperplasia with osteoporosis and loss of trabeculation.
2. Bone abnormalities resulting from thrombosis and infarction.
3. Bone lesions, which result from infection.
4. Generalized bone growth retardation.

E. Treatment[7]

1. *Preventive Procedures*
   a. Folate supplements daily.
   b. Pneumococcal polyvalent vaccine administered to children.
   c. Genetic counseling for those with sickle cell trait.
2. *Treatment for Disease State*
   Supportive and palliative treatments include treatments for specific symp-

toms during crises, such as pain relief and the use of antibiotics for infectious diseases. Oxygen therapy and blood transfusions have limited selective use.

III. Oral Implications

A. Radiographic Findings[6,7]

Although radiographic findings of bone changes cannot be considered exclusive to sickle cell anemia, the high incidence of characteristics listed below provides a relationship that may, in time, contribute to diagnosis. The bone changes can be observed in patients with sickle cell trait as well as sickle cell anemia.

1. Decreased radiodensity; increased osteoporosis.
2. Coarse trabecular pattern with large marrow spaces.
3. Findings in children. Significant bone loss, indicating the presence of periodontitis, was observed in a group of children under 10 years of age.[6]

B. Oral Soft Tissues

The tissues may show the pallor typical of anemias, and because of the specific destruction of tissues in the liver of the patient with sickle cell anemia, the gingiva may have a jaundiced color.

Periodontal evaluation for all ages is likely to reveal pockets, infection, bleeding, and the need for a strict preventive and treatment program.

C. General Suggestions for Appointment Management[7,8]

The objective during therapy is to provide care without precipitating a sickle cell crisis. Particular effort should be made to eliminate infection by such means as wearing gloves and a mask and to minimize exposure of the patient to airborne microorganisms. In general, during a sickle cell crisis, treatment should be limited to emergency relief.

1. Prepare or refer to a comprehensive medical history.
2. Use prophylactic antibiotics. The advice of the patient's physician will be obtained. For a patient so highly susceptible to infection, antibiotics should be considered routine, since any form of tissue manipulation can create a bacteremia.
3. Obtain a hematocrit and a hemoglobin determination immediately prior to each treatment appointment. The patient's physician can provide the interpretation and advise whether the patient is able to have a dental or dental hygiene appointment that day.
4. Use local anesthesia without vasoconstrictor. Creating an area of vasoconstriction may result in localized infarction.[8]
5. Teach and supervise a comprehensive preventive program to minimize oral infection and control etiologic factors. Preventive measures for dental caries may be especially needed since a high incidence of enamel hypomineralization has been noted.[7]

POLYCYTHEMIAS

Polycythemia means an increase in the number and concentration of red blood corpuscles above the normal level. Hemoglobin and hematocrit values are raised. The three general categories are described below.

I. Relative Polycythemia

When there is a loss of plasma without a loss of red blood cells, the concentration of cells increases and a relative polycythemia results. The causes of fluid loss may be conditions such as dehydration, diarrhea, repeated vomiting, sweating, or loss of fluid from burns.

Other contributing factors may be smoking, hypertension, obesity, and stress, particularly in middle-aged males.

II. Polycythemia Vera (Primary polycythemia)[9]

In contrast to "relative" polycythemia, which results from fluid loss, in primary "absolute" or "true" polycythemia, there is an actual increase in the number of circulating red blood corpuscles. In addition to an increased red blood cell count and hemoglobin value, the white cell and platelet counts are also elevated. There is increased viscosity of the blood, which affects the oxygen transport to the tissues.

A. Cause

Polycythemia vera is a neoplastic condition resulting from a bone disorder in which the primitive red cells or stem cells proliferate. It occurs more frequently after age 40 and more in males.

B. Clinical Signs and Symptoms

Clinical manifestations relate to increased blood volume and viscosity and tendencies to thrombosis and hemorrhage.

1. *General.* There is a ruddy cyanosis of the skin with hemorrhagic spots such as petechiae or ecchymoses. The patient suffers from headaches, dizziness, nasal and gastric bleeding, and abdominal pain. Elevated blood pressure and enlarged spleen are found along with high blood test values. A few cases transform into leukemia.
2. *Oral*
   a. Color: deep purplish-red tongue, mucous membranes, and gingiva.
   b. Gingiva: enlarged, with bleeding on slight provocation.

C. Treatment

1. Chemotherapy or radiation.
2. Phlebotomy, in which blood is removed to reduce the total volume, and particularly, the red cell volume of the blood.

D. Dental Hygiene Treatment Consideration

Increased health of the gingival tissues can result from frequent recall for the supervision of personal daily plaque removal procedures. When supplemented by professional treatment, especially calculus removal, bleeding tendencies can be lessened.

III. Secondary Polycythemia[9]

Secondary polycythemia is also called erythrocytosis, which simply means an increase in numbers of red blood cells. The increased red cell production can result from hypoxia, such as occurs in residents of high altitudes.

Another cause for increased numbers of red blood corpuscles is an increase in the body's production of erythropoietin, a hormone essential to stimulate the development of the red blood cells in bone marrow. A variety of diseases and tumors can cause the excess erythropoietin production. Treatment of the underlying condition is necessary to correct the secondary polycythemia.

THE WHITE BLOOD CELLS

Disorders of the white blood cells may occur because of a decrease (leukopenia) or an increase (leukocytosis) in cell numbers. The types of white blood cells were described on page 799 and in table 56-2.

I. Leukopenia

A decrease in the total number of white blood cells results when cell production cannot keep pace with the turnover rate or when an accelerated rate of removal of cells occurs, as in certain disease states.

A. Conditions in which Leukopenia Occurs

1. *Specific Infections.* Typhoid fever, influenza, malaria, measles (rubeola), and German measles (rubella) are examples.
2. *Disease or Intoxification of the Bone Marrow.* Chronic drug poisoning, radiation, and autoimmune or drug-induced immune reactions may be implicated.

B. Agranulocytosis[10]

Agranulocytosis, or malignant neutropenia as it is sometimes called, is a rare, serious disease in which the destruction of bone marrow is so severe that it is irreversible. Drugs or an autoimmune process are the usual causes.

1. *Clinical Course.* With a sharp drop in white blood cells, bacterial invasion may be rapid and acute illness may develop. Malaise, chills, and fever are followed by extreme weakness. With complete depression of the bone marrow, blood cells cannot be produced, and death can occur within a few days.

   Initial therapy involves terminating a toxic drug that may have caused the condition and using antibiotics and other symptom-relieving measures. Bone marrow transplants are the treatment of choice, assuming that a compatible donor is available.

2. *Oral Lesions.* Ulceration in the mouth and pharynx is common in agranulocytosis. Symptoms also include gingival bleeding, increased salivation, and a fetid odor. During the severe illness, only palliative relief is possible, using a soft diet and attempts at cleaning the mouth with a soft toothbrush, possibly a suction brush (pages 718–719).

II. Leukocytosis

An increase in numbers of circulating white blood cells may be caused by inflammatory and infectious states, trauma, exercise, and other conditions listed in table 56–2. The most extreme abnormal cause of leukocytosis is leukemia.

LEUKEMIAS

Leukemias are malignant neoplasias of immature white blood cells. They are characterized by abnormally large numbers of specific types of leukocytes and their precursors located within the circulating blood and bone marrow and infiltrated into other body tissues and organs.

I. Incidence[11]

Cancer of all types is the second leading cause of death in the United States, and leukemias are the seventh leading cause of cancer death in adults. In children under 15 years of age, cancer is second only to accidents as the major cause of death, and leukemia is the leading cause of cancer death for both boys and girls. Between ages 15 and 34, leukemia is still the leading cause of cancer deaths in males, and second only to breast cancer in females.

Certain types of leukemias occur more frequently in specific age groups. For example, 80 percent of leukemias in persons under age 15 are acute lymphocytic leukemias, with a peak of incidence at 4 years of age. In the age group over 60, chronic lymphocytic leukemia predominates.[12]

II. Classification[12]

Leukemias are first named by whether they are acute or chronic, and then subdivided by the maturity and type of white cell predominating, whether myeloid, lymphoid, or monocytic.

In a basic classification, there are the following six types:

1. Acute lymphocytic (lymphoblastic) leukemia (ALL)
2. Chronic lymphocytic leukemia (CLL)
3. Acute myelocytic (myeloblastic) leukemia (AML)
4. Chronic myelocytic leukemia (CML)
5. Acute monocytic (monoblastic) leukemia (A MoL)
6. Chronic monocytic leukemia (C MoL)

III. Etiology

Specific etiology is not known, and extensive research continues. Viral etiology has been demonstrated in laboratory research with animals.

Predisposing factors, or leukemogenic agents, which have been shown to influence the development of certain types, are ionizing radiation, environmental chemical agents, and genetic factors.

IV. Disease Process and Effects

Leukemias are characterized by (1) generalized replacement of bone marrow with proliferating leukemic cells, (2) large numbers of immature white cells in the circulating blood, and (3) widespread infiltrates of white cells throughout the body. The changes that result may be divided into primary and secondary. There are also tertiary effects associated with the treatment given.

A. Primary Changes

The primary changes are those directly related to the increase in numbers of white blood cells.
1. *Bone Marrow.* All of the active red marrow is affected; the marrow is replaced by the neoplastic cells.
2. *Lymph Nodes.* Nodes throughout the body are usually enlarged in all forms of leukemia, due to the accumulation of increased numbers of leukemic cells.
3. *Spleen and Liver.* Both liver and spleen are enlarged, the spleen to the greater degree.
4. *Other Leukemic Infiltrates.* Many organs and tissues become involved, for example the kidneys, adrenals, thyroid, myocardium, and gingiva, which will be described below.

B. Secondary Changes

Secondary changes are the result of complications that arise from the destructive effects of the leukemic infiltrates.

1. *Anemia.* Red cells cannot develop because of the infiltrated bone marrow. Severe anemia can result.
2. *Thrombocytopenia.* Abnormal bleeding tendency is a significant characteristic of all forms of leukemia. The platelet count is very low.
3. *Susceptibility to Bacterial Infection.* Circulating white cells do not have their usual defense capacities.
4. *Osteoporosis.* Expansion of the marrow spaces and changes in the bone by the leukemic infiltrate lead to osteoporosis and radiographic radiolucency. Osseous changes in the maxilla and mandible are not uncommon.

V. Clinical Signs and Symptoms

A. Onset

There are marked differences between the clinical findings of acute and chronic forms of leukemia. The acute diseases appear suddenly and severely, while the chronic types are insidious.

B. General Physical Symptoms

1. Fatigue, pallor, weakness (from anemia).
2. Purpura and ecchymoses of the skin, bleeding from the nose and gingiva (from thrombocytopenia).
3. Fever, indicating an infection (from lowered susceptibility).
4. Headache, nausea, vomiting, and sometimes seizures and coma (from leukemic infiltration of the meninges).

VI. Treatment for Leukemia[13,14]

A. Induction of Remission

The objective at the outset is to return the blood and bone marrow to minimal normal blood test levels.

1. Chemotherapy.
2. Irradiation.

B. Preventive Central Nervous System Therapy

Cranial radiation supplemented by chemotherapy is administered for central nervous system infiltration.

C. Stabilization Therapy

Treatment for anemia, bleeding, infections, and other complications is needed.

D. Continuation Therapy

During remission, therapy must be continued to prevent bone marrow relapse. Cessation of therapy may vary from 2 to 4 years of remission.

Child patients on remission go to school and participate in normal activities. Physically, the only difference is the loss of hair, a side effect of chemotherapy, which is reversible if chemotherapy is completed. Remission periods are used for routine dental and dental hygiene therapy.

E. Bone Marrow Transplant[15]

When indicated, transplants may be performed during remission, while the patient is stronger and the numbers of cancer cells may be fewer. Chemotherapy and total body radiation precede the marrow transplant to eradicate leukemic cells and suppress immunoreactivity.

Marrow from an identical twin or matched sibling to prevent graft-versus-host complications is administered intravenously. Autologous bone marrow has been used, which has been obtained from the patient during a remission period.

VII. Oral Manifestations

A high percentage of patients with leukemia have oral complications. Patients with acute leukemias have more oral problems than those with chronic disease.

The oral lesions may be described as (1) those directly related to the increase in leukemic cells (primary), (2) those related to the complications that result from the leukemic infiltrate (secondary), and (3) those that result from treatment (tertiary).[16]

A. Primary Oral Lesions[12,16]

1. *Leukemic Infiltrate of the Gingiva.* Patients with the monocytic leukemias tend to have more pronounced gingival lesions than with other forms of leukemia.

a. Gingival characteristics. The gingiva is grossly enlarged and bluish red, has blunted papillae and a soft, spongy consistency. The enlargement may be great enough to cover a large portion of the anatomic crown. Since alveolar bone loss is a common finding of all ages,[17] there are deep pockets, both gingival and periodontal. Varying degrees of ulceration and necrosis, sometimes with a pseudomembrane, may be present.

b. Plaque and local irritants. Plaque, materia alba, and calculus aggravate, and therefore increase the severity of, the gingival lesions.

2. *Leukemic Infiltrate of the Pulp.* Pain in the otherwise apparently healthy teeth of patients with acute leukemia has resulted from infiltration of the pulp by leukemic cells. Endodontic treatment can provide prompt relief.[18,19]

B. **Secondary Oral Lesions**

1. *Hemorrhagic Manifestations*
   a. Petechiae and ecchymoses may be observed on the lips, soft palate, floor of the mouth, and buccal and labial mucosa.
   b. Gingival bleeding appears spontaneously or on gentle provocation.

2. *Increased Susceptibility to Infection*
   a. Bacterial, fungal, viral. Many types of organisms may be found in the local areas of infection, which are often associated with severe ulceration. Candidiasis is a common finding with white plaques covering varying degrees of the mucosal surfaces.[16]
   b. Necrotizing ulcerative gingivitis (NUG). NUG superimposed over the gingival condition associated with leukemic infiltration is not uncommon. Characteristics of NUG were described on pages 535–536.

C. **Tertiary Oral Lesions**

Oral complications that result from the use of chemotherapeutic agents include painful ulcerations, spontaneous gingival bleeding, tongue desquamation, xerostomia, and secondary infections. Chemotherapy and its effects were described on pages 676–677. Radiation therapy may also involve the head and neck; and the problems of caries prevention related to xerostomia need attention (pages 675, 680).

VIII. **Dental Hygiene Care**

Selection of procedures centers around the patient's problems of susceptibility to infection and bleeding. During acute exacerbations, the patient is usually very ill, and certain suggestions listed below may apply to hospital care. Consultation with the patient's physician, hematologist, or oncologist is mandatory to explain the oral treatment needed and to obtain information about the hematologic status.

A. **Preparation for Appointments**

1. *Prophylactic Antibiotic Premedication* (page 100). The patient with leukemia is susceptible to infection, and drugs used in therapy are immunosuppressive.

2. *Blood Evaluation.* Complete blood evaluation tests, including a minimum of those listed in table 56–1, are essential shortly before dental and dental hygiene treatment.[16,20] Treatment cannot be performed unless blood levels are within an acceptable range.

3. *Aseptic Techniques.* Patients with leukemia who have had multiple blood transfusions may be carriers of hepatitis. Since the patient is also very susceptible to infection, a two-way emphasis on aseptic technique exists. Procedures as outlined for hepatitis B are recommended (page 64).

B. **Oral Examination**

A careful, thorough examination is needed. This should include probing to evaluate the periodontal status and pulp testing, in addition to percussion and radiographs, to evaluate the teeth. It is not uncommon for dental and periodontal conditions without symptoms to become acute problems during chemotherapy.[18]

C. **Acute Problems During Exacerbation Periods**

1. *Gingival Inflammation.* Palliative treatment for grossly enlarged, bleeding, ul-

cerated gingiva includes frequent warm saline rinses, a nutritious liquid diet with dietary supplements, and plaque removal procedures using a soft toothbrush. A suction toothbrush may be of value in the hospital setting (pages 718–719).

2. *Scaling.* When the platelet and white blood cell counts permit, scaling can be started and may be continued with subgingival scaling and gingival curettage as indicated.[16] NUG therapy as outlined on pages 537–540 can be adapted to the individual's needs.

3. *Post-treatment Instructions.* The objective is to control bleeding. The diet should consist of cold, clear liquids for the first 24 hours, and then cool, soft foods. Since suction can disturb clotting, the use of straws should be avoided. There should be no smoking, and medications that suppress platelet function, such as aspirin, should be avoided. A close follow-up is indicated: the patient should be seen as frequently as possible. A healing time two or three times longer than normal may be expected.

   Treatment of the gingiva by scaling in small segments, supplemented by repeated instruction in brushing and flossing, can allow for gingival lesions to subside.

4. *Candidiasis and Other Oral Infections.* Rinsing with nystatin is usually indicated for Candida infection. Treatment for oral lesions associated with chemotherapy is limited and nonspecific. A mouthrinse containing a topical anesthetic may be necessary to relieve the pain and discomfort from oral mucosal ulcerations while eating.

D. Oral Care During Remission

Complete preventive care with a supervised plaque removal program, daily self-applied fluoride, sealants, dietary control, and any other measure deemed necessary to obtain and maintain optimum oral health for the individual should be instituted during the remission period and followed with regular recall. Complete scaling, planing, and all periodontal therapy must be completed along with dental treatments. Al-

though it may be doubtful that all severe tissue reactions during periods of chemotherapy can be alleviated, much suffering can be prevented if the oral cavity is in a state of health at the outset.

HEMORRHAGIC DISORDERS

Hemorrhagic disorders have in common tendencies to spontaneous bleeding and moderate to excessive bleeding following trauma or a surgical procedure. Spontaneous bleeding occurs as small hemorrhages into the skin or mucous membranes and other tissues, and appears as petechiae or purpura. Moderate to excessive bleeding or prolonged bleeding may follow dental hygiene therapy, including scaling, root planing, or gingival curettage. A history or suspicion of a bleeding problem should be fully evaluated before treatment is started.

I. Detection

A. Patient's Medical and Dental Histories

A carefully prepared medical history can provide specific information about bleeding disorders and the treatment received by the patient. When no specific disease is mentioned, clues to possible hemorrhagic tendencies must be sought out through interview.

A basic health questionnaire (pages 87–89) should include items relative to bleeding, bruising, blood transfusions and for what reasons they were needed, blood disorders, familial blood disorders, and previous abnormal bleeding that may have followed past dental or dental hygiene appointments. Follow-up conversational questioning after "yes-no" answers on a written questionnaire can delve into sufficient detail to determine the need for blood tests before treatment is started.

Additional information is also obtained by consultation with the patient's physician. When blood tests have been made in the past but are not recent, new reports can be requested.

B. Laboratory Blood Tests

Selected basic tests are listed in table 56–1 with their normal values. Additional tests are frequently needed for a thorough evaluation of specific conditions.

Certain tests are needed on the same day as treatment, because blood values may fluctuate. For example, the patient using anticoagulants is required to have a prothrombin time determination within 24 hours of appointment time (page 798). A patient with leukemia also needs immediate preevaluation, as described on page 809.

The types and numbers of tests will vary. For example, the information required prior to subgingival instrumentation and periodontal surgery will depend on the severity of the patient's condition. The opinions of dentists and physicians will differ depending on their previous experiences. For a patient with leukemia, the tests recommended may include a prothrombin time, partial thromboplastin time, thrombin time, fibrinogen level, and platelet count, in addition to routine blood counts and a differential white count.[16]

II. Types of Hemorrhagic Disorders

A. Due to Abnormalities of the Blood Capillaries

In this type of disorder, vascular fragility is increased, which leads to petechial and purpuric hemorrhages in the skin or mucous membranes, including the gingiva. A variety of conditions may cause bleeding as a result of an abnormality of the blood vessel walls, including the following:
1. Severe infections (septicemias, severe measles, typhoid fever).
2. Drug reactions (sulfonamides, phenacetin).
3. Scurvy or vitamin C deficiency (impaired collagen of vessel wall).

B. Due to Platelet Deficiency or Dysfunction

1. *Thrombocytopenia.* A lowered number of platelets may be due to decreased production in the bone marrow. The cause of bone marrow depression may be invasive disease such as leukemia or deficiencies such as folate or vitamin B_{12} deficiency anemias.
2. *Platelet Dysfunction.* A defect in platelet function interferes with the blood clotting mechanism and leads to a prolonged bleeding time. Defects occur as a result of certain hereditary states, uremia, certain drugs, and von Willebrand's disease. An example of drugs that affect platelet function is the salicylates (aspirin).[21-22]

C. Due to Blood Clotting Defects

A possible irregularity or disorder is associated with each of the many clotting factors.
1. *Acquired Disorders*
   a. Vitamin K deficiency. Vitamin K is essential for prothrombin synthesis and factors VII, IX, X.
   b. Liver disease. Nearly all of the clotting factors are produced in the liver. When the liver is not functioning properly, the clotting factors may be altered.
2. *Hereditary Disorders.* There are at least 30 coagulation disorders which are hereditary, each resulting from a deficiency or abnormality of a plasma protein. Clinically, their signs and symptoms are similar. The following three will be described in detail in the next section:
   a. Hemophilia A (factor VIII abnormality).
   b. Hemophilia B (factor IX abnormality).
   c. von Willebrand's disease (von Willebrand factor, which chemically forms a large part of the factor VIII complex. One component affects platelet function).

HEMOPHILIAS

The hemophilias are a group of congenital disorders of the blood clotting mechanism. The partial thromboplastin time is used as a screening test for detecting mild hemophilia (PTT, table 56–1).

The three most common types are classic hemophilia A, hemophilia B or Christmas disease, and von Willebrand's disease. Hemophilias A and B are inherited by males through an x-linked recessive trait carried by females, and von Willebrand's disease is transmitted by an autosomal codominant trait. Rarely is a female affected by hemophilias A or B, but von Willebrand's disease occurs in males and females.

There are approximately 25.8 persons with hemophilia in every 100,000 or 1 in 4,000 males in the United States, of which 80 percent have hemophilia A.[23] Von Willebrand's disease is at least as common as hemophilia A.

I. General Characteristics

A. Level of Clotting Factor

The severity of the disease can be related directly to the level of the clotting factor in the circulating blood. Normal concentrations of the clotting factors are between 50 and 100 percent.

Patients with severe hemophilia have a clotting factor VIII or IX less than 1 percent. They have spontaneous bleeding into muscles, joints, and soft tissues, and severe, prolonged bleeding after minor trauma.

When the hemophilia is less severe, the clotting factor is in the 2 to 5 percent range. Spontaneous bleeding may be only occasional, and gross bleeding after light but definite trauma will occur.

The accepted minimal surgical level of clotting factor is 30 percent. The same percentage would apply for any procedure that caused bleeding, notably subgingival scaling and planing. One hour before treatment, the level may be raised to 100 percent.[24] Consultation with the patient's hematologist is indicated.

B. Symptoms and Effects

1. *Effects of Minor Trauma.* Bleeding and bruising from minor trauma vary, depending on the severity of the disease.
2. *Hemarthroses.* Bleeding into the soft tissue of joints (knees, ankles, elbows) begins in the very young with severe hemophilia. Much swelling, pain, and incapacitation are created. Permanent joint damage can result, and the patient may need splints, braces, or orthopedic surgery. Hemarthroses almost never occur in von Willebrand's disease.[24]
3. *Intramuscular Hemorrhage.* Hemorrhage into the muscles is accompanied by pain and limitation of motion.

4. *Renal Changes.* Abnormalities of renal function and hematuria may occur.
5. *Oral Bleeding.* Bleeding from the gingiva is common and more extensive when periodontal infection is more severe. Because of fear of bleeding, patients may neglect toothbrushing and flossing, which can lead to increased plaque accumulation and inflammation. Small children may injure the oral area when they tumble, and severe bleeding can result.
6. *Neurologic Complications.* Intracranial hemorrhages may occur with or without prior head trauma. Serious functional impairment may result with complications such as epileptic seizures.

II. Treatment[24]

Recent developments in therapy have changed the quality of life and possibly the life span for many people with hemophilia. The use of outpatient clinics and home therapy have nearly eliminated the long and expensive hospitalizations of years past.

A. Factor Replacement Therapy

Clotting factor preparations include *fresh frozen plasma*, which contains all of the clotting factors, *cryoprecipitate*, which contains factor VIII and fibrinogen, and *concentrates* of a variety of products available for reconstitution.

B. Home Infusion Program[25]

Hemophilia care-center teams work with health personnel in the patient's home community to plan and carry out an individual program of instruction for the parents of a young patient and self-care by the patient by age 10, or as soon as the child is capable. The prescribed concentrates of clotting factor can be stored in the home refrigerator and reconstituted as needed for infusion.

The parents and child are taught to recognize the symptoms of the beginning of a bleeding episode or bleeding from injury, and how to administer the treatment. For patients who have bleeding episodes often, such as more than once each week, a prophylactic schedule may be appropriate. Many patients do not require more than one infusion each month, so that routine prophylaxis is not needed.

A sense of security for a patient is provided through contacts with a social worker and local health personnel. Telephone consultations are available on a 24-hour basis with the hemophilia care center, which may be located at a distance. Precautions are taken to arrange for infusion if necessary during school or working hours.

III. Dental Hygiene Care

Although prevention and control of bleeding are the central issues when planning appointments for a patient with hemophilia, other factors also require adaptations and attention. A few of these patients are multihandicapped as a result of internal hemorrhages, which have led to mental and physical problems.

Suggestions for appointments from Chapter 50 may prove useful for the patient who has had hemarthroses and orthopedic treatment. Because early treatment for bleeding episodes has been made possible through home programs and new replacement products, the incidence of physical deformities has been lowered. Older patients would not have had such benefits.

A few patients will have suffered brain damage as a result of cerebral hemorrhage, and may be limited intellectually. Others will have emotional stresses related to the disease and its treatment. New channels for adjustment have opened since the patient has been able to develop the responsibility for self care. This is very much in contrast to previous requirements of long hospitalizations, childhood separation from family and school, and dependency on others.

A. Preparation for Appointments

1. *Preliminary Evaluation.* The patient's medical and dental histories must include the pertinent hemophilic history with information about the type, severity, treatment, medications used for pain and other symptoms, and family history. Additional information from the hematologist contributes to planning safe and effective appointments. Thorough and complete care can contribute in every respect to the health and well-being of the patient.

2. *Premedication*

a. Factor replacement therapy. In preparation for local anesthetic administration, subgingival instrumentation, surgical procedures, or any procedure likely to cause bleeding, replacement therapy is given just prior to the appointment. The patient who is on a home care plan may administer the replacement therapy at home. Reinfusion postoperatively is sometimes indicated.[26,27]

b. Fibrinolytic therapy. Epsilon-aminocaproic acid (EACA) is used to control bleeding after appointments. EACA acts to maintain a fibrin clot after it is formed.[28]

c. Prophylactic antibiotic premedication. Patients with joint prostheses require antibiotic premedication.[29]

3. *Aseptic Techniques.* Many of the blood products used in treatment are prepared from pooled concentrates, which increases the risk of hepatitis. Since patients with hemophilia may be hepatitis carriers, routine precautions for hepatitis should be followed (page 64).

B. Preventive Program

The prevention and control of gingival and dental diseases constitute important aspects of care for patients with hemophilia. Not only are dental and periodontal treatment complicated by necessary special precautions, but spontaneous oral bleeding problems can be at least partially controlled by the elimination of oral diseases.

1. *Parental Instruction.* All possible preventive measures should be started while the child is very young, including fluorides, sealants, plaque control, diet for caries control, and early professional supervision.

2. *Plaque Removal.* Complete instruction is given as for any patient.

a. Flossing. Teach flossing carefully and correctly to prevent cutting the gingiva and inducing proximal bleeding.

b. Aids for handicaps. Patients with limited range of motion may benefit from the special adaptations described on pages 700–702.

C. **Local Anesthesia**

1. *Prevention of Hematomas.* Hematomas may be produced following administration of local anesthesia into loose connective tissue that is highly vascularized. The incidence of hematoma is greatly lessened by the current use of factor replacement therapy. Additional doses of replacement therapy can be used should a hematoma develop.

2. *Inhibitors.* A periodic screening test for circulating inhibitors, antifactor VIII or antifactor IX is necessary for finding the approximately 10 percent of patients with severe hemophilia who have inhibitors. This information is important to have before administering anesthetic or any treatment, since the inhibitor prevents control by replacement therapy. An adjustment in the amount of replacement therapy is needed to prevent hematomas and bleeding following treatment.[30]

3. *Procedure for Local Anesthesia*[27,31]

   a. Elevate the patient's missing factor level to 30 to 50 percent. Higher percentages to 80 or 100 percent may be recommended.[24,28]

   b. Use a continuous aspirating technique as the needle is advanced

      (1) When no blood is aspirated, no additional replacement therapy will be needed.

      (2) When blood is aspirated, observe precautions for possible hematoma and maintain the missing factor level at 30 to 50 percent or higher for 36 to 48 hours following the appointment.

D. **Instrumentation**

All instrumentation is performed carefully but thoroughly to minimize tissue trauma and prevent bleeding. Treatment planning for a series of appointments as described on pages 329–331 is appropriate.

1. *Tissue Conditioning.* When oral care has been neglected and the gingiva are soft, spongy, and plaque and calculus are in abundance, a tissue conditioning program is advised. Patient instruction in plaque control procedures is given, practiced, and repeated as necessary over a series of appointments. All possible motivational devices can be employed (pages 334, 411).

   Supragingival scaling can be completed in small segments. As the tissue begins to shrink, heal, and become more firm, subgingival scaling and root planing can be initiated.

2. *Probing and Periodontal Treatment Planning.* Depending on the bleeding tendencies of the gingival tissues, probing and charting for complete periodontal treatment planning may need to be postponed for a few appointments while tissue conditioning is carried out.

   Many patients can be brought to a state of periodontal health through conservative measures of subgingival scaling, root planing, and gingival curettage. Complete treatment should be accomplished, however; so that if periodontal surgery is indicated, it should not be neglected.[27,32] As with all oral surgery for a patient with hemophilia, coordination with the medical team, and hospitalization when indicated, can provide the patient with safe and effective treatment.

E. **Miscellaneous Treatment Suggestions**[27,32,33]

Techniques and procedures should be analyzed to make sure that all excess trauma to the patient is prevented. The same procedures should be applied to all patients, but with a patient who has a bleeding problem, there is greater significance.

1. *Rubber Dam.* A thin rubber dam may be more gentle to the oral tissues than a heavy one. The use of a Young's frame may eliminate pressure, especially at the corners of the mouth. Rubber dam clamps can be checked for sharp corners, and placed carefully without damage to the gingival tissues.

2. *Film Placement.* Films can cut and press on the mucous membranes. Care in placement must be exercised.

3. *Impressions.* Beading the rims of the trays will protect the mucosa from pres-

sure and damage from a hard, possibly rough, surface (page 171).

4. *Evacuation.* High vacuum suction tips may be sharp. Caution in the use of suction is necessary to prevent pulling the sublingual or other mucosal tissues into the suction tip and causing hematomas.

Selection of a saliva ejector is important. The use of a soft, rubber-padded tip may prevent injury to the sublingual mucosa.

5. *Periodontal Dressing.* After subgingival scaling, planing, and curettage, a periodontal dressing can provide pressure and adapt the tissue against the teeth as an aid for the prevention of postappointment bleeding.

6. *Treatment for Hematoma.* Ice pack application may limit the spread of a hematoma as a temporary measure. Prompt replacement therapy will still be needed.

7. *Aspirin.* Never suggest the use of aspirin for pain relief of a patient with a bleeding disorder. The bleeding tendency is greatly increased by drug-induced platelet dysfunction.

8. *Frequency of Recall.* Frequent recall appointments can aid in keeping the oral tissues in an optimum state of health and help prevent the need for complex dental treatments.

TECHNICAL HINT

Source of Materials
National Hemophilia Foundation
25 West 39th Street
New York, NY 10018

References

1. Borysenko, M., Borysenko, J., Beringer, T., and Gustafson, A.: *Functional Histology.* Boston, Little, Brown & Co., 1979, pp. 35–41.
2. World Health Organization: *Nutritional Anaemias.* WHO Technical Report Series No. 503, Geneva, World Health Organization, 1972, 29 pp.
3. McCarthy, P.L. and Shklar, G.: *Diseases of the Oral Mucosa,* 2nd ed. Philadelphia, Lea & Febiger, 1980, p. 405.
4. Dayal, P.K. and Mani, N.J.: Clinical Aspects of the Tongue in Anemia, *Ann. Dent.,* 38, 21, Spring, 1979.
5. Robbins, S.L. and Cotran, R.S.: *Pathologic Basis of Disease,* 2nd ed. Philadelphia, W.B. Saunders Co., 1979, pp. 733–739.
6. Sanger, R.G. and Bystrom, E.B.: Radiographic Bone Changes in Sickle Cell Anemia, *J. Oral Med.,* 32, 32, April–June, 1977.
7. Sanger, R.G. and McTigue, D.J.: Sickle Cell Anemia—Its Pathology and Management, *J. Dent. Handicap.,* 3, 9, Winter–Spring, 1978.
8. Rouse, L.E. and Hays, G.L.: Dental Considerations in Sickle Cell Anemia, *Gen. Dent.,* 27, 18, November–December, 1979.
9. Robbins and Cotran: op. cit., pp. 742–745.
10. Shafer, W.G., Hine, M.K., and Levy, B.M.: *A Textbook of Oral Pathology,* 3rd ed. Philadelphia, W.B. Saunders Co., 1974, pp. 678–680.
11. Cancer Statistics, 1982. *Ca—A Cancer Journal for Clinicians,* 32, 15, January/February, 1982.
12. Robbins and Cotran: op. cit., pp. 779–789.
13. Smithson, W.A., Gilchrist, G.S., and Burgert, E.O.: Childhood Acute Lymphocytic Leukemia, *Ca—A Cancer Journal for Clinicians,* 30, 158, May/June, 1980.
14. Simone, J.V.: The Treatment of Acute Lymphoblastic Leukaemia, *Br. J. Haematol.,* 45, 1, May, 1980.
15. Fefer, A.: Bone Marrow Transplants in Leukemic Patients in Remission, *Ca—A Cancer Journal for Clinicians,* 30, 45, January/February, 1980.
16. Segelman, A.E. and Doku, H.C.: Treatment of the Oral Complications of Leukemia, *J. Oral Surg.,* 35, 469, June, 1977.
17. Curtis, A.B.: Childhood Leukemias: Osseous Changes in Jaws on Panoramic Dental Radiographs, *J. Am. Dent. Assoc.,* 83, 844, October, 1971.
18. Peterson, D.E. and Overholser, C.D.: Dental Management of Leukemic Patients, *Oral Surg.,* 47, 40, January, 1979.
19. Sela, M.N. and Pisanti, S.: Early Diagnosis and Treatment of Patients with Leukemia, a Dental Problem, *J. Oral Med.,* 32, 46, April–June, 1977.
20. Carey, J.A. and Chilcote, R.R.: Dental Treatment for the Child with Acute Lymphocytic Leukemia 1974, *J. Dent. Child.,* 42, 191, May–June, 1975.
21. American Dental Association, Council on Dental Therapeutics: *Accepted Dental Therapeutics,* 39th ed. Chicago, American Dental Association, 1982, p. 195.
22. Cowan, F.F.: *Pharmacology for the Dental Hygienist.* Philadelphia, Lea & Febiger, 1978, pp. 174–176.
23. Merritt, A.D. and Conneally, P.M.: Hemophilia: Genetics and Counseling, in Hilgartner, M.W., ed.: *Hemophilia in Children.* Littleton, Massachusetts, Publishing Sciences Group, 1976, p. 33.
24. Hilgartner, M.W., ed.: *Hemophilia in Children.* Littleton, Massachusetts, Publishing Sciences Group, 1976, pp. 151–170.
25. van Eys, J.: Home Transfusion for Hemophilia, in Hilgartner, M.W., ed.: *Hemophilia in Children.* Littleton, Massachusetts, Publishing Sciences Group, 1976, pp. 185–200.
26. Currier, G.F., Pribisco, T., and McWilliams, N.B.: Restorative Dentistry in Hemophilic Children, *J. Dent. Handicap.,* 2, 3, Winter, 1976.
27. Evans, B.E. and Aledort, L.M.: Hemophilia and Dental Treatment, *J. Am. Dent. Assoc.,* 96, 827, May, 1978.
28. Needleman, H.L., Kaban, L.B., and Kevy, S.V.: The Use of Epsilon-aminocaproic Acid for the Management of Hemophilia in Dental and Oral Surgery Patients, *J. Am. Dent. Assoc.,* 93, 586, September, 1976.
29. Mulligan, R.: Late Infections in Patients with Prostheses for Total Replacement of Joints: Implications for the Dental Practitioner, *J. Am. Dent. Assoc.,* 101, 44, July, 1980.
30. Abildgaard, C.F.: Management of Inhibitors in Hemophilia, in Hilgartner, M.W., ed.: *Hemophilia in Children.* Littleton, Massachusetts, Publishing Sciences Group, 1976, pp. 171–184.

31. Segelman, A.E.: Protocol for the Management of the Hemophiliac Having Oral Surgery (letter), *J. Oral Surg.*, 36, 423, June, 1978.
32. Chiono, O. and Kasper, C.K.: Hemophilia, in Nowak, A.J.: *Dentistry for the Handicapped Patient.* St. Louis, The C.V. Mosby Co., 1976, pp. 134–150.
33. Evans, B.E., ed.: *Dental Care in Hemophilia.* New York, National Hemophilia Foundation, 1977, 16 pp.

Suggested Readings

Adler, S.S.: Anemia in the Aged: Causes and Considerations, *Geriatrics*, 35, 49, April, 1980.

Carranza, F.A.: *Glickman's Clinical Periodontology*, 5th ed. Philadelphia, W.B. Saunders Co., 1979, pp. 524–537.

Grossman, R.C.: Orthodontics and Dentistry for the Hemophilic Patient, *Am. J. Orthod.*, 68, 391, October, 1975.

Herschfus, L.: Oral Manifestations of Blood Disorders, *J. Oral Med.*, 25, 56, April–June, 1970.

Kerr, D.A. and Ash, M.M.: *Oral Pathology. An Introduction to General and Oral Pathology for Hygienists*, 4th ed. Philadelphia, Lea & Febiger, 1978, pp. 319–334.

Lasser, S.D., Camitta, B.M., and Needleman, H.L.: Dental Management of Patients Undergoing Bone Marrow Transplantation for Aplastic Anemia, *Oral Surg.*, 43, 181, February, 1977.

Little, J.W.: Detection and Management of the Potential Bleeder in Dental Practice, *J. Oral Med.*, 31, 11, January–March, 1976.

Menius, J.W. and Webster, W.P.: Dental Management of Mild Hemophilia with Polycythemia Vera, *Oral Surg.*, 45, 714, May, 1978.

Millard, H.D. and Gobetti, J.P.: Nonspecific Stomatitis—a Presenting Sign in Pernicious Anemia, *Oral Surg.*, 39, 562, April, 1975.

Murphy, N.C. and Bissada, N.F.: Iron Deficiency: An Overlooked Predisposing Factor in Angular Cheilitis, *J. Am. Dent. Assoc.*, 99, 640, October, 1979.

Stamps, J.T.: The Role of Oral Hygiene in a Patient with Idiopathic Aplastic Anemia, *J. Am. Dent. Assoc.*, 88, 1025, May, 1974.

Tyldesley, W.R.: Oral Signs and Symptoms in Anaemias, *Br. Dent. J.*, 139, 232, September 16, 1975.

Vandesteen, G.E., Altman, L.C., and Page, R.C.: Peripheral Blood Leukocyte Abnormalities and Periodontal Disease, *J. Periodontol.*, 52, 174, April, 1981.

Weiss, J.I.: Thrombocytopenic Purpura: The Dentist's Responsibility, *J. Am. Dent. Assoc.*, 87, 165, July, 1973.

Wells, T.J.: A New Concept in the Control of Acute Gingival Hemorrhage, *J. Oral Surg.*, 34, 435, May, 1976.

Hemophilia

Duperon, D.F. and Dobbs, T.M.: Dental Care for Patients with Congenital Haemorrhagic Disorders, *Can. Dent. Assoc. J.*, 42, 269, May, 1976.

Evans, B.E., Irving, S.P., and Aledort, L.M.: Use of Microcrystalline Collagen for Hemostasis after Oral Surgery in a Hemophiliac, *J. Oral Surg.*, 37, 126, February, 1979.

Evian, C.I., Corn, H., Guernsey, L.H., and Rosenberg, E.S.: Complications of Severe Bleeding in a Patient with Undiagnosed Factor XI Deficiency, *Oral Surg.*, 52, 12, July, 1981.

Glogoff, M., Baum, S.M., Sussman, R., Stewart, S., and Stoopack, J.C.: Management of the Hemophilic Oral Surgery Patient, *J. Oral Surg.*, 30, 252, April, 1972.

Kaneda, T., Nagayama, M., Minato, F., Nakahira, H., Nakajima, J., and Shikimori, M.: Problems Involved in Grading the Severity of Hemophilia by Test Results, *J. Oral Surg.*, 36, 956, December, 1978.

Larson, C.E., Chang, J.-L., Bleyaert, A.L., and Bedger, R.: Anesthesia Considerations for the Oral Surgery Patient with Hemophilia, *J. Oral Surg.*, 38, 516, July, 1980.

Leake, D. and Deykin, D.: The Diagnosis and Treatment of Bleeding Tendencies, *Oral Surg.*, 32, 852, December, 1971.

Lorson, E.L., Goldwasser, M.S., Osbon, D.B., and Kirby, R.W.: von Willebrand's Disease: Current Concepts and Report of Case, *J. Oral Surg.*, 34, 655, July, 1976.

Lucas, O.N. and Prescott, G.H.: Hemophilias and Other Hemorrhagic Disorders. Significance of Preventive Dentistry, *Dent. Clin. North Am.*, 19, 63, January, 1975.

Mulkey, T.F.: Outpatient Treatment of Hemophiliacs for Dental Extractions, *J. Oral Surg.*, 34, 428, May, 1976.

Murphy, J.B., Nersasian, R., and Clark, A.: The Management of Drug Induced Gingival Hyperplasia in Mentally Retarded Patients with Hemophilia: A Report of Two Cases, *J. Periodontol.*, 49, 44, January, 1978.

Nakai, T.R., Peterson, J.C., and Law, D.B.: Current Concepts in the Management of the Hemophilic Pedodontic Patient, *J. Dent. Child.*, 41, 361, September–October, 1974.

Nakajima, T., Tomizawa, M., Hasegawa, S., Ohnishi, M., and Tokiwa, N.: Topical Application of Antihemophilic Factor after Dental Extractions in Hemophilic Patients, *J. Oral Surg.*, 36, 873, November, 1978.

Powell, D. and Bartle, J.: The Hemophiliac: Prevention is the Key, *Dent. Hyg.*, 48, 214, July–August, 1974.

Sydney, S.B. and Ross, R.: Periodontal Surgery in a Patient with von Willebrand's Disease, *J. Am. Dent. Assoc.*, 102, 660, May, 1981.

Leukemia

Bodey, G.P.: Oral Complications of the Myeloproliferative Diseases, *Postgrad. Med.*, 49, 115, January, 1971.

Curtis, A.B.: Childhood Leukemias: Initial Oral Manifestations, *J. Am. Dent. Assoc.*, 83, 159, July, 1971.

Deasy, M.J., Vogel, R.I., Annes, I.K., and Simon, B.I.: Periodontal Disease Associated with Preleukemic Syndrome, *J. Periodontol.*, 47, 41, January, 1976.

Ferguson, M.M., Dagg, J.H., and Hunter, I.P.: The Presentation and Management of Oral Lesions in Leukaemia, *Can. Dent. Assoc. J.*, 6, 201, September, 1978.

Goepferd, S.J.: Leukemia and Its Dental Implications, *J. Dent. Handicap.*, 4, 44, Summer, 1979.

Lorson, E.L., Higuchi, K.W., and Osbon, D.B.: Leukemia: The Dentist's Role in Diagnosis, *J. Am. Dent. Assoc.*, 97, 69, July, 1978.

Michaud, M., Baehner, R.L., Bixler, D., and Kafrawy, A.H.: Oral Manifestations of Acute Leukemia in Children, *J. Am. Dent. Assoc.*, 95, 1145, December, 1977.

Pogrel, M.A.: Acute Leukemia. An Atypical Case Presenting with Gingival Manifestations, *Int. J. Oral Surg.*, 7, 119, April, 1978.

Pollack, A.: The Leukaemias, *Br. Dent. J.*, 142, 369, June 7, 1977.

Presant, C.A., Safdar, S.H., and Cherrick, H.: Gingival Leukemic Infiltration in Chronic Lymphocytic Leukemia, *Oral Surg.*, 36, 672, November, 1973.

Reichart, P.A. and Dornow, H.: Gingivo-Periodontal Manifestations in Chronic Benign Neutropenia, *J. Clin. Periodont.*, 5, 74, February, 1978.

Shepherd, J.P.: The Management of the Oral Complications of Leukemia, *Oral Surg.*, 45, 543, April, 1978.

Smith, G.: Initial Oral Signs of Acute Leukemia, *Dent. Hyg.*, 55, 16, April, 1981.

Sonis, A.L. and Sonis, S.T.: The Presence of Lymphoblasts

in the Gingival Crevice of Children with Acute Lymphoblastic Leukemia, *J. Periodontol.*, 52, 276, May, 1981.

Stafford, R., Sonis, S., Lockhart, P., and Sonis, A.: Oral Pathoses as Diagnostic Indicators in Leukemia, *Oral Surg.*, 50, 134, August, 1980.

Takagi, M., Sakota, Y., Ishikawa, G., Kamiyama, R., Nakajima, T., and Nomura, T.: Oral Manifestations of Acute Promyelocytic Leukemia, *J. Oral Surg.*, 36, 589, August, 1978.

Williams, L.T., Peterson, D.E., and Overholser, C.D.: Leukemia and Dental Treatment, *Dent. Hyg.*, 55, 29, April, 1981.

Sickle Cell Anemia

Catena, D.L.: Oral Manifestations of the Hemoglobinopathies, *Dent. Clin. North Am.*, 19, 77, January, 1975.

Daramola, J.O.: Massive Osteomyelitis of the Mandible Complicating Sickle Cell Disease: Report of Case, *J. Oral Surg.*, 39, 144, February, 1981.

Kinsey, R.W., Ballard, J.B., and Matukas, V.J.: Sickle Cell Hemoglobinopathies: A Protocol for Management, *J. Oral Surg.*, 37, 441, June, 1979.

Mourshed, F. and Tuckson, C.R.: A Study of the Radiographic Features of the Jaws in Sickle-cell Anemia, *Oral Surg.*, 37, 812, May, 1974.

Powell, E.A. and Januska, J.R.: Sickle Cell Anemia: Chronology, Natural History, and Implications for Dental Practice, *Quart. Nat. Dent. Assoc.*, 31, 72, July, 1973.

Sanger, R.G., Greer, R.O., and Averbach, R.E.: Differential Diagnosis of Some Simple Osseous Lesions Associated with Sickle-cell Anemia, *Oral Surg.*, 43, 538, April, 1977.

Scopp, I.W.: Sickle Cell Anemia: Dental Implications, *N.Y. J. Dent.*, 48, 87, March, 1978.

Sears, R.S., Nazif, M.M., and Zullo, T.: The Effects of Sickle-cell Disease on Dental and Skeletal Maturation, *J. Dent. Child.*, 48, 275, July–August, 1981.

57

The Patient with Diabetes Mellitus

A preventive dental hygiene program is vital for the patient with diabetes mellitus. The patient with diabetes, particularly one whose condition is unstable or uncontrolled, has a lowered resistance to infection and a delayed healing process. Gingival reactions to bacterial plaque are frequently exaggerated. Periodontal disease tends to develop with increased severity at an earlier age than in the nondiabetic patient.

The presence of infection, including infection in the oral cavity, may intensify the diabetic symptoms and contribute to difficulty in insulin regulation. The dental team, therefore, has a significant responsibility to provide the patient with oral care and instruction for self-care aimed at maintaining health and preventing gingival and periodontal diseases which may be potential sources of infection.

Modifications of dental and dental hygiene procedures for the diabetic patient may be indicated, depending on the severity and control of the diabetes. No treatment involving tissue manipulation, including subgingival probing and scaling, should be attempted until the diabetic state has been confirmed with the patient's physician. Controlled diabetics may be treated as healthy patients. Uncontrolled diabetics need antibiotic premedication.

I. Occurrence[1]

A. Population Involved

Approximately 4.8 million people in the United States have reported diabetes mellitus. In addition, some 5.5 million individuals carry the genetic make-up that can lead eventually to symptomatic diabetes. Together, these figures represent over 5 percent of the population.

B. Age and Other Factors

The prevalence rate increases from 1.3 persons per 1000 under 17 years of age to 78.5 per 1000 aged 65 years and over. The rates are higher in females and in the nonwhite population.

C. Increased Incidence

An increased incidence of diabetes in recent years can be related to various factors including the following:
1. Improved methods of diagnosis.
2. Concentrated professional and community efforts to find undiagnosed cases and bring them to treatment.
3. Increased longevity of life
   a. More people live to the older age groups, when diabetes is more prevalent.
   b. Diabetics live longer because of current modes of treatment; they may marry and have children who inherit a genetic predisposition to the disease.

4. Obesity, with generalized increased food consumption and tendency for less physical exercise.

THE DIABETIC SYNDROME: CLASSIFICATION

Classically, diabetes mellitus is an hereditary disease of metabolism with (1) inadequate production and action of the hormone insulin from the beta cells of the islets of Langerhans in the pancreas; and (2) disorders in the metabolism of carbohydrates, proteins, and fats. The main problem is an inability to utilize glucose, which leads to hyperglycemia, or excess sugar in the blood.

Diabetes is a complex disease that has been shown to be part of a heterogenous group of disorders that have glucose intolerance in common. More than 30 conditions, many of which are rare, have glucose intolerance as a characteristic.

The classification outlined here was prepared by the National Diabetes Data Group in an international workshop.[2] Classification is by clinical symptoms and results of the glucose tolerance test.* Type I and Type II from the classification are described below. Table 57–1 compares the characteristics of the two types.

I. Type I. Insulin-Dependent Diabetes Mellitus (IDDM)

A. Characteristics

1. Insulin deficiency.
2. Dependence on injected insulin to sustain life and prevent ketosis.
3. Abrupt onset of symptoms; usually arises in childhood or puberty, but may occur at any age.

B. Former Names

IDDM has been known as juvenile diabetes, juvenile-onset diabetes, ketosis-prone diabetes, and brittle diabetes.

---

*Oral glucose tolerance test: a generally used test for diagnosis of diabetes. Following the ingestion of a specific amount of glucose in solution, in a nondiabetic the fasting blood glucose rises promptly, then falls to normal within 2 hours. In a diabetic, the blood glucose increase is greater and the return to normal prolonged. (Fasting blood glucose means the glucose determination on a specimen of blood drawn after at least 10 hours of fasting.) Universally accepted test values that define diabetes mellitus have been widely researched and summarized in the literature.[2]

II. Type II. Noninsulin-Dependent Diabetes Mellitus (NIDDM)

A. Characteristics

1. Not dependent on insulin for prevention of ketonuria, and not prone to ketosis.
2. Have minimal or no symptoms and may be asymptomatic for years, with slow disease progression.
3. Onset typical after 35 to 40 years, but may occur in younger individuals.
4. Obese type: represent 80 percent of the diabetic population; condition improves with weight reduction and diet control.
5. Nonobese type: represent 10 percent of the diabetic population.

B. Former Names

NIDDM has been called adult-onset diabetes, maturity-onset diabetes, ketosis-resistant diabetes, maturity-onset-type diabetes of the young.

ACTION OF INSULIN

I. Functions of Insulin

As a powerful hormone, insulin directly or indirectly affects every organ in the body.

A. Facilitates conversion of glucose to fat in adipose tissue.
B. Speeds the conversion of glucose to glycogen in the liver and muscles.
C. Facilitates the transmission of glucose into cells.
D. Speeds the oxidation of glucose within the cells for energy.

II. Effects of Decreased Insulin

In diabetes, insulin is decreased in amount or function.

A. With decreased insulin, less glucose is transmitted through cell walls into the cells.
B. Glucose increases in the circulating blood until a threshold is reached when glucose spills over into the urine.
C. Without glucose in the cells to use for energy, the cells utilize fats.
   1. End products of fat metabolism (ketones) accumulate in the blood.
   2. Ketones are acid. Usually, when they accumulate, they are neutralized in the blood stream. When there is such a large

Table 57–1. Comparison of Characteristics of Insulin-dependent and Noninsulin-dependent Diabetes Mellitus

Characteristic	Insulin-dependent Diabetes Mellitus	Noninsulin-dependent Diabetes Mellitus
Age of Onset	Usually under 25 years; may appear later	Adulthood, particularly over 40 years; may appear at younger ages
Body Weight	Normal or thin	High percent obese at the time of diagnosis
Rate of Onset of Clinical Symptoms	Rapid	Slow
Severity	Severe	Mild
Diabetic Emergency (Ketoacidosis)	Common	Rare
Stability	Unstable	Stable
Insulin Treatment Required	Almost all	Less than 25 percent
Chronic Manifestations	Uncommon before 20 years; prevalent and severe by age 30	Develop slowly with age

quantity, the neutralizing effect is depleted rapidly and an acid condition (acidosis) results.

3. In severe, untreated, or inadequately controlled diabetes, acidosis leads to diabetic coma (ketoacidosis).

III. Insulin Complications

With earlier diagnosis, improved treatment procedures, and better informed patients and their families, there has been a decrease in emergencies. It now becomes increasingly important to recognize the earliest symptoms in order to arrest the development of a crisis stage.

A. Insulin Reaction

Too much insulin (hyperinsulinism), with lower blood glucose.

B. Diabetic Coma (ketoacidosis)

Too little insulin (hypoinsulinism). See table 57–2 for a comparison of the characteristics of insulin reaction and diabetic coma, and the respective treatment procedures.

SIGNS, SYMPTOMS, EFFECTS

I. Signs and Symptoms of Uncontrolled Diabetes

A. The Classic Triad
  1. Increased urine (polyuria).

  2. Excessive thirst (polydipsia).
  3. Increased appetite (polyphagia).
B. Dehydration from fluid loss.
  1. Dry, itchy skin.
  2. Dry mouth; decreased saliva.
  3. Burning tongue.
C. General weakness, drowsiness, fatigue.
D. Weight loss from inability to utilize foods.
E. Elevated blood glucose (hyperglycemia).
F. Glucose in the urine (glycosuria).
G. Slow wound healing; persistent infections such as boils or carbuncles.
H. Pain and/or numbness in the fingers and toes.
I. Changes in vision.

II. Infection and Diabetes

A. Diabetics, particularly the inadequately controlled, are more susceptible to infections.
B. Failure to treat an infection increases the severity of the diabetic state and intensifies the symptoms; can precipitate diabetic coma.
C. With infection present, insulin requirements may increase; with elimination of the infection, it may be possible to decrease the prescribed insulin.
D. Frequently encountered infections involve the urinary tract, skin, lungs (pneumonia or

Table 57–2.   Comparison of Insulin Reaction and Diabetic Coma

	Insulin Reaction *(Hypoglycemia)*	*Diabetic Coma* *(Ketoacidosis)*

History
 	
(Predisposing
Factors)
	Too much insulin
	Too little food: delayed or omitted
	Loss of food by vomiting or diarrhea
	Excessive exercise
		Too little insulin: omission of medication
		   or failure to increase dose when
		   requirements increased
		Too much food
		Infection
		Stress
		Illness of any sort

Cause	Lowered blood glucose with excess
	   insulin in proportion
		Decreased glucose utilization when
		   insufficient insulin leads to prolonged
		   increasing acidosis

Occurrence	In insulin-dependent diabetics
	   particularly the unstable, severe type
		Insulin-dependent person who is poorly
		   controlled, unstable, who omits or
		   reduces insulin for emotional or other
		   reasons

Onset	Sudden Slower when long-acting insulin is used	Gradual, over many hours, even days
Physical Findings	Skin: moist, increased perspiration Hunger Headache Tremor Pallor Dilated pupils Dizziness, staggering gait Weakness	Skin: flushed and dry Nausea, vomiting Lack of appetite Weak, rapid pulse Dry mouth, thirst Soft, sunken eyeballs Increased urination Deep, difficult breathing Abdominal pain
Behavior	Drowsiness Restlessness, anxiety, irritability Incoordination Stupor, confusion Eventual coma, with or without convulsions	Progressive drowsiness Confusion Lethargy Weakness Eventual coma

Treatment	Give sugar to raise the blood glucose
	   level (orange juice, candy, sugar
	   cubes)
	Revival: prompt
	Unconscious or unresponsive: treated by
	   injection of glucagon* or may require
	   intravenous glucose
		Immediate professional care,
		   hospitalization
		Keep patient warm
		Fluids for the conscious patient
		Insulin injection by physician

Prevention	Smooth regulation of diabetes with steady diet, insulin, exercise	Early diagnosis of diabetes Well-indoctrinated, regulated patient

Glucagon is a hormone produced by the alpha cells of the pancreas, which increases blood glucose.

tuberculosis), and the oral cavity, particularly the periodontium.

E. Factors involved: impaired circulation, alterations in carbohydrate and protein metabolisms, altered nutritional state, or abnormal immunologic response.

III. Diabetes in Pregnancy

A. Effects on Mother

Insulin adjustment, carefully supervised prenatal care, and improved obstetric practices have lessened much of the potential danger for the mother.

B. Effects on Offspring

1. Infants are larger; premature births more frequent; incidence of congenital malformations high.
2. High perinatal death rate, less with improved prenatal care.

IV. Long-term Complications

Patients with controlled diabetes may develop complications later than those less well controlled. The principal involvements are in the nervous system (neuropathy), kidney (nephropathy), retina (retinopathy), and blood vessels (arteriosclerosis and atherosclerosis).

Kidney disease is most severe in insulin-dependent diabetes, while atherosclerotic coronary heart disease is common in older persons with diabetes. Retinopathy occurs frequently, and diabetes is a leading cause of blindness in the United States.

V. Personal Factors[3]

A. Impact of Personality on Diabetes

1. Problems during treatment may be related to an imbalance between diet and insulin, but often can be influenced by the patient's conscious or subconscious attempt to resist.
2. Periods of emotional distress bring on alterations in the blood glucose.
3. Changes that lead to acidosis and coma may start during periods of depression, hostility, or anxiety, particularly when such symptoms lead to neglect of diet or insulin.

B. Impact of Diabetes on Personality

1. Reaction to an initial diagnosis may be extremely traumatic with long-range effects, particularly in a child.
   a. Adult patient may suffer fear, frustration, and confusion. Less mature adults show less acceptance, and may reject the diagnosis and try to control their treatment.
   b. Parents of a child with diabetes may be acutely disturbed and experience feelings of guilt and rejection of the "imperfect" child.
2. Adult behavior during the course of treatment can vary from reckless neglect of treatment to the opposite extreme where there can be obsession with details and preoccupation with weighing of foods and extreme attention to personal hygiene.
3. Adolescents may find the restrictions nearly intolerable and their hopes for the future seemingly destroyed. Growing independence and rejection of authority figures (parents and physician) makes diabetes control difficult.
4. Younger children may exhibit feelings of oppression, restriction, or suppressed emotions because of subordination and control by the diabetic regimen.
5. Parents' attitudes influence the diabetic child's adjustment.
   a. Overanxious, overprotective parent may precipitate anxiety states or complete dependence of the child.
   b. Overindulgent parent may indirectly lead the child to exploitation or even complete control.
   c. Indifferent or nonchalant parent may give the child feelings of desertion, neglect, or depression.

TREATMENT FOR DIABETES CONTROL

Objectives in patient care are to correct metabolic disturbances, attain the best possible state of general health, and prevent or postpone complications or chronic effects of diabetes. Treatment methods depend on the severity of the disease, age, activity, vocation, and psychologic needs as well as the nutritional and weight problems of the patient.

I. General Procedures

A. Methods Used

1. Immediate treatment: management of acute symptoms.
2. Elimination of sources of infection, including oral diseases.
3. Patient education: self-care.
4. Diet and exercise.
5. Medication: insulin for the insulin-de-

pendent patient. Oral hypoglycemic agents may be used for selected patients.

6. Personal hygiene: physical and mental.

B. Self-care

There is no known cure for diabetes. The success of treatment depends on the knowledge, understanding, and attitude of the patient, and on how well the condition is managed on a day-to-day basis throughout life.

1. *Instruction.* Continuing instruction must be provided the patient by the health team, including the physician, registered nurse, dietitian, and other specialists. The dentist and dental hygienist participate to instruct and supervise the patient's oral health practices for the prevention and control of oral diseases.

2. *Components of Self-care*

   a. Objectives: to prevent infections and injuries; prevent glycosuria; and maintain the best possible general health.

   b. Specific instruction: the elements of treatment learned and carried out by the individual include diet management, urine testing, technique of insulin injection and sites for it, care of syringe and of insulin, care of the feet to prevent lesions and infections, and what to do in case of acute complications.[4]

   c. Instruction materials: a number of excellent books and other printed materials have been prepared specifically for the patient with diabetes. Review of some of these materials can provide the dental team members with greater insight into the background and knowledge of the patient in preparation for oral health instruction. Addresses for sources of informational materials are included in Technical Hints at the end of this chapter.

II. Diet and Exercise

Diet planning is basic to all diabetic therapy. Exercise is an essential part of the treatment program and contributes to lowering insulin requirements.

A. Fundamentals of the Diabetic Diet

1. *Carbohydrates.* Elimination of concentrated carbohydrates (sugar, frostings, pastries, candy, syrup, and others).

2. *Total Food Intake.* The daily intake may be identical with normal for the patient's age and stature, with appropriate adjustments for growth in the young patient, degree of activity, and occupation. The obese patient should be put on a weight-reduction diet.

3. *Diet Selection*

   a. Individual quantitative need. As the treatment schedule is planned by the physician and dietitian, the individual needs are determined within the framework of the patient's customary diet. The adequate diabetic diet is calculated so that ideal body weight can be obtained and maintained.

   b. Food exchange system. This widely used system groups foods into six categories, namely, bread, meat, vegetable, milk, fruit, and fat. Each patient is instructed in specific selections from each list. Only the specific amounts are to be eaten and other additions cannot be made. Food exchange means that a certain serving from one group can only be exchanged with an equivalent.

   At first, all patients are expected to measure and weigh their food so that the size of proper servings can be learned. Patients with severe diabetes may need to weigh and measure for a longer period or indefinitely.

B. Eating Habits

1. *Distribution of Food.* Daily regimen of eating a prescribed caloric intake is essential to balance insulin and blood glucose.

2. *Meals.* Three spaced, on time, meals and three interval feedings are usually indicated. All food, including that used between meals, is counted into the day's total intake.

3. *Intake of Food.* Patient must eat all the food prescribed at the prescribed times.

Rejected foods or food lost through vomiting must be reported as these may explain changes in glucose balance.

III. Medication

A. Insulin Therapy

1. *Indications.* All patients suffering acute complications (ketoacidosis); most Type I (IDDM) patients; and Type II patients with diabetes too severe for control by diet use insulin. Daily injection is required.
2. *Types of Insulin.* Insulin is classified as short-acting, intermediate-acting, or prolonged-acting.
3. *Dosage.* Depends on the severity of the individual case.
   a. Objective: to attain optimum utilization of glucose throughout each 24 hours.
   b. Factors affecting the need for insulin: food intake, emotional disturbances, variations in exercise, or infections.

B. Oral Hypoglycemic Agents

Oral hypoglycemic agents are used less than in past years because research has revealed significant detrimental side effects.[5] They may still be used when diet control has proved unsuccessful or insulin cannot be used for a reason such as allergy or immune reaction. One group of hypoglycemic agents, the sulfonylureas, act by stimulating insulin release from the beta cells.

ORAL RELATIONSHIPS

The oral mucosa, tongue, and periodontal tissues of a patient with diabetes mellitus may show unusual susceptibility, and tendency toward more marked reactions to injury, infections, and all local irritants than do tissues of nondiabetics. Such a response is related to the general lowered resistance and delayed healing processes.

I. Periodontal Involvement

A. Clinical Findings

Marked periodontal disease may be observed at early ages, particularly in patients with insulin-dependent diabetes. There may be alveolar bone resorption, loss of attachment, pocket formation, and increased tooth mobility, sometimes accompanied by pathologic tooth migration and other signs of trauma from occlusion. Patients with diabetes are more susceptible to periodontal abscess formation.

When the periodontal condition of a patient with well-controlled diabetes is compared with the normal population, the differences are not great. Literature reviews have summarized the various research studies.[6,7,8] It should be recognized that wide differences in disease severity and individual response exist. The lowered resistance and susceptibility to infection truly make the patient with diabetes a "special" patient with respect to periodontal disease prevention and control.

B. Contributing Factors

1. Diabetes acts as a conditioning, modifying, and accelerating factor, with local irritants having an important role in the development of periodontal symptoms.[8]
2. Inadequate plaque control contributes to more severe tissue response because of decreased resistance.

II. Dental Caries

A. Uncontrolled Diabetes

Dental caries rate is generally consistent with the patient's own age group or may be slightly higher related to diminished saliva and dry mouth or to a high carbohydrate diet in the obese.

B. Controlled

With a well-regulated diet, necessarily low in or free of sugar-containing foods, and with a regular eating pattern that excludes permissive and unaccounted-for between-meal snacks, a reduced dental caries experience is frequently observed.

III. Other Oral Findings

In addition to the signs and symptoms of periodontal disease, certain other oral findings may be noted. These occur primarily when diabetes is uncontrolled or poorly controlled. These signs can be important for identifying a previously undiagnosed case of diabetes.

It should be clear that diabetes does not cause oral disease. The conditions listed below relate to or secondarily result from the lowered resistance and susceptibility to infection that is characteristic of the tissues.

A. **Lips:** drying, cracking, angular cheilosis.

B. **Xerostomia:** alteration in microflora, increased plaque formation.

C. **Mucosa:** edematous, red, possibly ulcerated; burning sensations; poor tolerance for removable prostheses.

D. **Dry, Sore Mouth:** may lead to diet alterations incompatible with diabetic diet requirements.

DENTAL HYGIENE CARE

Since infection in the oral cavity can alter the course of diabetes and its treatment, the control of oral diseases has a vital role in the maintenance of the patient's health. Frequent and thorough care, with regular supervision of the patient's self-care, is required. This, in turn, requires gaining the patient's utmost cooperation and confidence.

I. Patient History

To supplement the basic medical history obtained, additional questioning will provide other essential information, such as the type and schedule of medication, dietary requirements, meal schedule, and frequency of medical appointments. History updating at each recall appointment can provide significant new information.

II. Consultation with Physician

Consultation between the dentist and the physician is necessary before any instrumentation involving tissue manipulation is performed.

A. **Information Obtained**

1. Degree of control, stability, and severity of the diabetes; susceptibility of the patient to emergency reactions.
2. Other health problems that may influence oral care.
3. Advice relative to a prescription for antibiotic therapy or sedative in preparation for dental and dental hygiene appointments.
4. Instructions that have been given the patient about diet, personal care, medication adjustment, or other.

B. **Use of Information**

The dental hygienist should study and apply information from the patient history and the physician-dentist consultation in order that dental hygiene phases of care and instruction be conducted in accord with the health requirements of the patient.

III. Appointment Planning

Except for relief of pain or other emergency performed after initial consultation with the physician, treatment, including dental hygiene appointment procedures, should not be started until the diabetes is under control.

Stress, including that created during a dental or dental hygiene appointment, increases glycemia and a tendency toward diabetic acidosis and coma. Appointment planning centers around stress prevention.

In general, the patient with well-controlled diabetes can be treated in the same way as a patient without diabetes. However, a few precautions are indicated.

A. **Time**

1. Choice: morning, $1\frac{1}{2}$ to 3 hours after the patient's normal breakfast and medication, during the descending portion of the blood glucose level curve.
2. Long-acting medication: adjust time accordingly.

B. **Precautions**

1. The patient should not be kept waiting unduly.
2. Do not interfere with the patient's regular meal and between-meal eating schedule.
3. Avoid long periods of stressful procedures: dental and dental hygiene care should be divided into units for short appointments appropriate to the individual's needs.
4. Additional precautions are indicated for the patient with long-term diabetes complications related to atherosclerosis and

other cardiovascular diseases. The needs of the gerodontic patient may be applied. Other chapters of Section VI of this book include information pertinent to the management of the patient with diabetes.

5. Prepare for diabetic emergency when the patient's history reveals diabetic instability or susceptibility to emergencies. Keep sugar cubes or other sweets as part of the office emergency supplies (page 833 and table 58–1, page 848).

C. Maintenance Phase: Recall Frequency

1. Appoint for supervision and examination on a regular 2- to 3-month basis.
2. Probe carefully to detect early gingival bleeding and evidence of pocket formation.
3. Soft tissue examination with attention to areas of irritation related to fixed and removable prosthesis must be carried out at each recall.
4. Calculus and other local irritants cannot be permitted to accumulate; therefore, routine scaling and planing may be required.

IV. Clinical Procedures

A. Instrumentation

1. *Antibiotic Premedication.* Prophylactic antibiotic therapy may be indicated to prevent postoperative infection. The young patient with moderate to severe insulin-dependent diabetes particularly will require guarded attention. Antibiotic protection may be indicated for a patient who has a history of slow healing from previous scaling or any surgical procedure or who has had periodontal abscess formation.
2. *Quadrant or Area Scaling.* When a patient is known to have a healing problem, limiting the number of teeth to be completed at each appointment is recommended. For each area, scaling should be completed insofar as possible. A plaque check and review of personal oral hygiene procedures prior to each scaling will improve the health and con-dition the tissues for succeeding scalings.

With complete scaling and root planing in deep pockets, particularly in areas of furcation involvement, the possibility for periodontal abscess formation may be kept at a minimum.

3. *Aseptic Technique.* Scrupulous procedures for sterile instrument and tray preparation should be the same for all patients. However, it is important to keep in mind the diabetic's susceptibility to infection and take any necessary precautions.
4. *Postoperative Healing.* Undue trauma to tissues must be avoided to encourage postoperative healing without complications.

B. Fluoride Application

When the gingival tissue has been inflamed or scaling has been extensive, it is advisable to postpone a topical fluoride application until the gingival tissue shows improvement following healing and personal oral care by the patient.

V. Patient Instruction

A. Influence of Diabetes Instruction

Many patients with diabetes are already education-oriented since instruction relative to diabetes and self-care procedures by the physician, nurse, and dietitian is an integral part of therapy. Some emphasis on the care of the mouth may have been made. The interrelation of oral tissue infection and the control of diabetes can be reinforced as personal instruction is given.

B. Plaque Control

Self-care measures for plaque control are selected on the basis of individual needs (pages 410–411). Continuing supervision and review of recommended procedures is critical to the patient with diabetes because of increased susceptibility to periodontal tissue involvement.

C. Diet

1. Correlate information about dental caries prevention with the elimination of

concentrated sweets. Since the diabetic diet contains no concentrated sweets, cooperation in caries control measures can be expected.

2. Reinforce principles of a nutritious diet in accord with the instruction provided by the physician, as a contribution to general health. Emphasis on the texture of the diet to avoid soft foods which cling to the teeth and gingiva is important to the periodontal disease-prone patient.

PREVENTION OF DIABETES

When diabetes is detected and treated early, most complications can be minimized, postponed, or possibly prevented. Mass screening has been used for many years to locate those persons who may have diabetes. Both blood and urine tests have been used for screening, but blood tests have been shown to be the most reliable.

In the universal effort of the health professions and community groups to find early diabetes, it is becoming increasingly evident that dental offices and clinics may become important screening centers. The history-taking and oral examination procedures for dental patients can be extremely useful for singling out diabetic suspects. Suspects can then be referred for a blood test, or an initial screening test can be performed in the dental office.

In addition to the objectives related to the health and well-being of individuals and the community health aspects of case finding, the dentist and dental hygienist have a responsibility to seek out diabetic patients in order that safe and successful dental and periodontal treatment, including the phases of care assigned the dental hygienist, may be carried out. Before proceeding with traumatic, stress-creating treatment in an infection-prone patient, every effort should be made to discover the true systemic condition of each patient.

I. Diabetic Suspects Among Dental Patients

A. Patients in a Diabetes-Susceptible Group

From observation and through questions in the patient history, the following may be identified:

1. Individuals with close relatives who have diabetes.
2. Women with abnormal obstetric history; particularly, large babies.
3. Obese persons, particularly in the over-40 age group.
4. Those with eye, kidney, or coronary artery disease.

B. Patients with Symptoms Suggestive of Diabetes

Questions in the patient history can be directed to obtain information such as the following:

1. Weight changes: weight loss with increased appetite.
2. Thirst; frequent urination.
3. Slow healing cuts, bruises, or skin infections such as boils or carbuncles.
4. Pain in extremities: fingers and toes.
5. Fatigue and drowsiness.
6. Most recent blood tests: whether test was made for blood glucose.

C. Repeat of Patient History

With long-standing patients it is not unusual for the history to have been completed at an initial visit without follow-up reviews periodically. Illnesses, hospitalizations, or other involvements, including a diagnosis of diabetes, may have occurred subsequent to the original history record. At each recall appointment, a review history is indicated (page 99).

TECHNICAL HINTS

Sources of Materials and Information

American Diabetes Association
600 5th Avenue
New York, N.Y. 10020

Canadian Diabetic Association
1491 Yonge Street
Toronto, Ontario, M4T 1Z5 Canada

International Diabetes Federation
10, Queen Anne Street
London W1 M OBD, England

References

1. United States Department of Health, Education, and Welfare, Public Health Service: *Diabetes Data Compiled 1977.* Washington, D.C., National Institutes of

Health, DHEW Publication Number (NIH) 78–1468, pp. 8–9.

2. National Diabetes Data Group, Harris, M. and Cahill, G., Chairmen: Classification and Diagnosis of Diabetes Mellitus and Other Categories of Glucose Intolerance, *Diabetes, 28,* 1039, December, 1979.
3. Krall, L.P., ed.: *Joslin Diabetes Manual,* 11th ed. Philadelphia, Lea & Febiger, 1978, pp. 219–222.
4. Ibid., pp. 41–161.
5. Haunz, E.A. and Blaine, M.: Diabetes Mellitus in Adults, in Conn, H.F., ed.: *Current Therapy.* Philadelphia, W.B. Saunders Co., 1981, pp. 437–452.
6. Saadoun, A.P.: Diabetes and Periodontal Disease: A Review and Update, *Periodont. Abstr., 28,* 116, Number 4, 1980.
7. Ranney, R.R.: Pathogenesis of Periodontal Disease, in *International Conference on Research in the Biology of Periodontal Disease.* Chicago, University of Illinois, 1977, pp. 263–265.
8. Stahl, S.S.: The Etiology of Periodontal Disease—Review of Literature, in *World Workshop in Periodontics.* Ann Arbor, Michigan, University of Michigan, 1966, pp. 141–142.

Suggested Readings

Basker, R.M., Sturdee, D.W., and Davenport, J.C.: Patients With Burning Mouths. A Clinical Investigation of Causative Factors, Including the Climacteric and Diabetes, *Br. Dent. J., 145,* 9, July 4, 1978.

Behr, M.T.: Dental Considerations of Most Common Medical Therapy, in Boundy, S.S. and Reynolds, N.J., eds.: *Current Concepts in Dental Hygiene,* Volume 2. St. Louis, The C.V. Mosby Co., 1979, pp. 147–149.

Bussell, S.N., Smales, F.C., Sutton, R.B.O., and Duckworth, R.: Glucose Tolerance in Patients With Lesions of the Oral Mucosa, *Br. Dent. J., 146,* 186, March 20, 1979.

Campbell, M.J.A.: The Effect of Age and the Duration of Diabetes Mellitus on the Width of the Basement Membrane of Small Vessels, *Aust. Dent. J., 19,* 414, December, 1974.

Ciancio, S.G., Golub, L.M., Mosovich, L., Katz, C., and Kleinberg, I.: Urea Levels in the Gingival Crevices of Diabetic and Normal Adolescents, *J. Dent. Res., 56,* 1144, October, 1977.

Ficara, A.J., Levin, M.P., Grower, M.F., and Kramer, G.D.: A Comparison of the Glucose and Protein Content of Gingival Fluid From Diabetics and Nondiabetics, *J. Periodont. Res., 10,* 171, July, 1975.

Friedman, G.J.: Diet in the Treatment of Diabetes Mellitus, in Goodhart, R.S. and Shils, M.E., eds.: *Modern Nutrition in Health and Disease,* 6th ed. Philadelphia, Lea & Febiger, 1980, pp. 977–997.

Goteiner, D.: Glycohemoglobin (GHb): A New Test for the Evaluation of the Diabetic Patient and Its Clinical Importance, *J. Am. Dent. Assoc., 102,* 57, January, 1981.

Grower, M.F., Ficara, A.J., Chandler, D.W., and Kramer, G.D.: Differences in cAMP Levels in the Gingival Fluid of Diabetics and Nondiabetics, *J. Periodontol., 46,* 669, November, 1975.

Keene, J.J.: Arteriosclerotic Changes Within the Diabetic Oral Vasculature, *J. Dent. Res., 54,* 77, January–February, 1975.

Lane, D.S.: Dental Considerations of Diabetes Mellitus, *Dent. Hyg., 53,* 306, July, 1979.

Lynch, M.A., ed.: *Burket's Oral Medicine, Diagnosis and Treatment.* 7th ed. Philadelphia, J.B. Lippincott Co., 1977, pp. 560–567.

Malamed, S.F.: *Handbook of Medical Emergencies in the Dental Office.* St. Louis, The C.V. Mosby Co., 1978, pp. 164–176.

Motegi, K., Nakano, Y., and Ueno, T.: Clinical Studies on Diabetes Mellitus and Diseases of the Oral Region, *Bull. Tokyo Med. Dent. Univ., 22,* 243, September, 1975.

Phagan, P.: Dental Hygiene Therapy for the Diabetic Patient, *Quintessence Journal, 3,* 21, January, 1981.

Pourdeihimi, B., Keene, J.J., Gargiulo, A.W., and Toto, P.D.: Insulin 1¹²⁵ Distribution Within Oral Tissues, *J. Periodontol., 51,* 199, April, 1980.

Smith, M.J.A.: Oral Lichen Planus and Diabetes Mellitus: A Possible Association, *J. Oral Med., 32,* 110, October–December, 1977.

Tasch, E.G., Kennon, S., and Arm, R.N.: Dental Management of the Diabetic Patient, *Q. Natl. Dent. Assoc., 36,* 107, April, 1978.

Wright, A.D.: Diabetes, *Br. Dent. J., 142,* 286, May 3, 1977.

Diabetes in Children

Bay, I., Ainamo, J., and Gad, T.: The Response of Young Diabetics to Periodontal Treatment, *J. Periodontol., 45,* 806, November, 1974.

Bernick, S.M., Cohen, D.W., Baker, L., and Laster, L.: Dental Disease in Children With Diabetes Mellitus, *J. Periodontol., 46,* 241, April, 1975.

Gislen, G., Nilsson, K.O., and Matsson, L.: Gingival Inflammation in Diabetic Children Related to Degree of Metabolic Control, *Acta Odontol. Scand., 38,* 241, Number 4, 1980.

Matsson, L. and Koch, G.: Caries Frequency in Children With Controlled Diabetes, *Scand. J. Dent. Res., 83,* 327, Number 6, 1975.

Ringelberg, M.L., Dixon, D.O., Francis, A.O., and Plummer, R.W.: Comparison of Gingival Health and Gingival Crevicular Fluid Flow in Children With and Without Diabetes, *J. Dent. Res., 56,* 108, February, 1977.

Periodontal Disease

Aleo, J.J.: Diabetes and Periodontal Disease. Possible Role of Vitamin C Deficiency: An Hypothesis, *J. Periodontol., 52,* 251, May, 1981.

Baer, P.N. and Wright, W.E.: Localized Advanced Periodontal Disease in a Juvenile Diabetic: Case Report With a Long-term Follow-up, *Periodontal Case Reports, 2,* 5, Number 1, 1980.

Carranza, F.A., ed.: *Glickman's Clinical Periodontology,* 5th ed. Philadelphia, W.B. Saunders Co., 1979, pp. 509–514, 587, 598, 787.

Cohen, D.W., Friedman, L.A., Shapiro, J., Kyle, G.C., and Franklin, S.: Diabetes Mellitus and Periodontal Disease: Two-year Longitudinal Observations. Part I, *J. Periodontol., 41,* 709, December, 1970.

Frantzis, T.G., Reeve, C.M., and Brown, A.L.: The Ultrastructure of Capillary Basement Membranes in the Attached Gingiva of Diabetic and Nondiabetic Patients with Periodontal Disease, *J. Periodontol., 42,* 416, July, 1971.

Hoge, H.W. and Kirkham, D.B.: Juvenile Diabetes and Periodontitis, *Dent. Surv., 54,* 27, October, 1978.

Hove, K.A. and Stallard, R.E.: Diabetes and the Periodontal Patient, *J. Periodontol., 41,* 713, December, 1970.

Listgarten, M.A., Ricker, F.H., Laster, L., Shapiro, J., and Cohen, D.W.: Vascular Basement Lamina Thickness in the Normal and Inflamed Gingiva of Diabetics and Nondiabetics, *J. Periodontol., 45,* 676, September, 1974.

Manouchehr-Pour, M., Spagnuolo, P.J., Rodman, H.M., and Bissada, N.F.: Impaired Neutrophil Chemotaxis in

Diabetic Patients With Severe Periodontitis, *J. Dent. Res.*, *60*, 729, March, 1981.

McMullen, J.A., Van Dyke, T.E., Horoszewicz, H.U., and Genco, R.J.: Neutrophil Chemotaxis in Individuals With Advanced Periodontal Disease and a Genetic Predisposition to Diabetes Mellitus, *J. Periodontol.*, *52*, 167, April, 1981.

Nichols, C., Laster, L.L., and Bodak-Gyovai, L.Z.: Diabetes Mellitus and Periodontal Disease, *J. Periodontol.*, *49*, 85, February, 1978.

Sánchez-Cordero, S., Hoffman, H., and Stahl, S.S.: Occurrence of Staphylococcus in Periodontal Pockets of Diabetic and Nondiabetic Adults, *J. Periodontol.*, *50*, 109, March, 1979.

Scopp, I.W.: Periodontics and Diabetes, *N.Y. J. Dent.*, *47*, 9, January, 1977.

Sznajder, N., Carraro, J.J., Rugna, S., and Sereday, M.: Periodontal Findings in Diabetic and Nondiabetic Patients, *J. Periodontol.*, *49*, 445, September, 1978.

58

Emergency Care

It is relatively easy to be skillful in techniques that are repeated frequently. Emergency care is performed only occasionally, and in instances that involve lifesaving measures, may be performed once in many years. To be prepared for that rare moment is difficult, but the public expects an individual trained in a health profession to be able to act in an emergency. Periodic review of procedures is necessary if application is to be effective.

Emergencies may occur within or in the vicinity of a dental office or clinic. Readiness involves not only having knowledge of proper procedures, but equipment kept in a convenient place. A quick, handy reference of emergency measures is important, which may be in the form of a posted chart with characteristic symptoms and related treatment.

The information included in this chapter is basic, and presented without an attempt to mention all types of emergencies that may arise, particularly those of involved traumatic injuries. The principal objectives are to list the symptoms and treatment of the more common emergencies that can occur and to provide a list of the equipment that should be readily available. It is assumed that other references will be kept in the dental office and that all dental personnel will familiarize themselves with such sources of information.

As an auxiliary to the dentist, the dental hygienist should be familiar with all procedures required in emergencies. Resuscitation involving techniques such as drug injection or tracheotomy would be carried out by the dentist. Knowledge of procedures and required equipment or materials is necessary in order that the dentist may have immediate and efficient assistance.

PREVENTION OF EMERGENCIES

The permanent record of any patient with a possible risk factor can be identified by printing in large letters in a conspicuous place on the outside of the folder the name of the special condition. Prior to each appointment, the record should be reviewed so that preparatory steps can be taken.

Prevention of emergencies requires preparedness, alertness, and anticipation. Some of the procedures that contribute to meeting the requirements are described here.

I. The Patient History

The carefully prepared and regularly updated medical and personal history, with adequate follow-up consultation with the patient's physician for integration of dental and medical care, can prevent many emergencies by alerting dental personnel to the individual patient's needs and idiosyncrasies. Factors that should be included in the patient's history have been listed on pages 90–91 and include:

A. Knowledge of specific physical conditions that may lead to an emergency.

B. Knowledge of diseases for which the patient is or has been under the care of a physician and the type of treatment, including medications.

C. Information concerning allergies or drug reactions.

II. Rapport and Stress Minimization

Stress and anxiety are the basis for many of the common emergencies that occur in a dental office or clinic. The office atmosphere and the warmth and sincerity of the personnel can help a patient feel wanted and secure.

Reduction of stress includes the following:[1]

A. Appointment Scheduling

1. Time of appointment planned in accord with personal health requirements.
2. Waiting time minimized.
3. Check usual meal time and previous meal for prevention of hunger anxiety or hypoglycemia.
4. Limit length of appointment to the patient's durability.

B. Medication

1. Premedication when indicated and recommended by the physician and dentist.
2. Pain control during treatment.
3. Patient's own prescriptions. Patients who are subject to emergencies should be instructed to bring their own prescribed medicines, for example, the patient with asthma or one who is subject to attacks of angina pectoris.
4. Postoperative instructions for prevention and/or relief of discomfort.

III. Observation and Vital Signs

A. Extraoral Examination

The general appearance of the patient on the day of the appointment may reveal indicators that encourage preparation for emergencies.

B. Vital Signs Monitored and Recorded in the Patient's Record (pages 103–111)

IV. Prevention of Accidents to Face and Eyes[2,3]

Protective eyeglasses are recommended for every patient and for the operator and assistants at all appointments (page 52). Face and eye accidents that occur during dental and dental hygiene procedures can result in serious disability, loss of working time, and an injured patient may justifiably take legal action. The effects of the preventive measures listed here apply to either a patient or a member of the dental staff.

A. Protective full coverage glasses should be worn by all dental personnel and patients at each appointment (figure 4–2, page 52).

B. Instruments, medications, and materials being transferred must be carried around the periphery, never over a patient's face.

C. Attention and care must be paid during the use of handpieces, ultrasonic scalers, and other power-driven instruments or implements that create aerosols, splatter, and ejected debris. Handpieces and ultrasonic scalers should be turned on and off only inside the oral cavity. Power-driven instruments should not be in operation while they are being inserted or removed from the patient's mouth. Aerosol production was described on pages 16–17.

D. Appropriate working distance from the operating field to the faces of dental and dental hygiene operators should be maintained. A distance of 14 to 16 inches from the patient's mouth to the operator's eyes is recommended (page 71). The faces and eyes of operator and assistant should not be positioned within the danger zone close to the patient's mouth.

E. Rubber dam should be used for all appropriate procedures to protect the patient's tissues, prevent aspiration, and provide the operator with improved access and visibility.

EMERGENCY MATERIALS AND PREPARATION

Organization is a key concept in being prepared for an emergency. Group planning and individual acceptance of responsibility can provide the team with efficiency, composure, and freedom from fear at the time of crisis.

I. Communication: Telephone Numbers for Medical Aid

Telephone numbers should be posted near

each extension from which outside calls can be made.
A. Rescue squads with paramedics (fire, police, flying squad, or 911 in many cities in the United States).
B. Ambulance service.
C. Nearest hospital emergency room.
D. Poison information center.
E. Physicians
  1. Patient's physician should be listed in the permanent record in a standard, convenient place.
  2. Physicians available for emergency calls.

II. Equipment for Use in an Emergency

Every dental office or clinic should have an emergency kit or cart,[4] and everyone in the office must be familiar with its contents. The kit should be in order, its contents replenished and old materials replaced as needed.

The emergency equipment should be portable and kept in a place readily accessible to all treatment rooms. Materials are kept separate from other office supplies and plainly marked. Materials included are selected to accomplish emergency treatment by current methods.

The items listed below imply proper training in their use. A team should work out additions to the list in keeping with their training and abilities.

A. Basic Equipment

  1. Portable positive pressure oxygen delivery system with clear face masks (child and adult sizes).
  2. AMBU resuscitation bag with mask.
  3. Plastic oral airways (adult and child sizes) for a team trained in their correct use.
  4. Blood pressure cuff and stethoscope.
  5. Cricothyrotomy needle.
  6. Suction tips with large diameter, such as tonsil and adenoid tips. Tips must have rounded edges so they may be placed into the pharynx without danger of cutting the mucous membrane.
  7. Disposable sterile syringes: 2, 5, and 10 ml. capacities with disposable needles for intravenous, intramuscular, and subcutaneous injections.
  8. Packaged alcohol wipes or swabs.
  9. Thermometer.
  10. Tourniquets: made of rubber or latex tubing. The blood pressure cuff also may be used as a tourniquet.
  11. Penlight or flashlight.
  12. Scissors.
  13. Commercial cold pack (nonrefrigerated quick-forming cold bag.)
  14. Brown paper bags.
  15. Blanket.
  16. Board: 12 by 24 inches to place under patient in a soft dental chair for cardiopulmonary resuscitation.
  17. Blank forms: *Record of Emergency* (figure 58–1) with pen.

B. Bandages and Dressings

Dressings are purchased in individual packages and maintained in the sealed sterile state.
  1. Adhesive bandages.
  2. Sterile dressings in sealed envelopes: 2 × 2 inches, and 4 × 4 inches.
  3. Rolled bandage: 1-inch (5 yards); 2-inch (5 yards).
  4. Adhesive tape.
  5. Gauze sponges (4 × 4 inches).
  6. Inflatable splints (assorted sizes).

C. Noninjectable Treatment Items

  1. Respiratory stimulant: aromatic ammonia in vaporoles (gray color wrapper). Since this may be a frequently used item, additional vaporoles kept in each treatment room in a universally selected place can facilitate action for a patient with syncope.
  2. Antihypoglycemic: sugar cubes or packages, hard candies.
  3. Vasodilator: nitroglycerin tablets (0.3 mg.) or amyl nitrite vaporoles (yellow wrapper).
  4. Bronchodilator: epinephrine mistometer (inhaler).
  5. Sterile eye irrigating solution.
  6. Bicarbonate of soda.

D. Drugs

All dental personnel must be familiar with the emergency drugs maintained in the particular office or clinic. The purpose and method of administration for each should be clearly identified with the container. A com-

RECORD OF EMERGENCY

NAME _____   DATE _____   TIME _____

ADDRESS _____

Onset of Emergency _____
CPR Started _____
Ambulance Called _____
Ambulance Arrived _____

Pertinent Medical History _____

Hospital Called _____
Physician Called _____
Patient Left Office _____

Description of Emergency _____

Attended by: Self _____
                    Relative _____
                    Other _____

Time							
Blood Pressure							
Pulse							
Respiration							
Pupils							
Skin—color —temperature							
Level of Consciousness							
Medication (specify)							
Other Treatment (specify)							

Comments and Summary   Personnel Attending

Figure 58–1. Record of emergency. Prepared in duplicate, one copy can accompany patient to emergency center and the second copy can remain in the patient's dental record file.

partmentalized clear plastic cabinet or box can be particularly useful for this purpose, since the labels and instructions can be seen from the outside and efficient selection can be made.

The replacement date must appear clearly on each item with a limited shelf life. When narcotics are included in the list of drugs available for emergencies, storage in a less accessible place than an emergency kit and purchase in small amounts are indicated to prevent them from being stolen easily.

Drug categories and examples of each that may be kept in a dental office or clinic for use by the dentist are listed below.[5]

1. *For Acute Allergic Reaction:* epinephrine 1:1000.
2. *Anticonvulsant:* Diazepam or a barbiturate such as pentobarbital.
3. *Antihistamine:* Chlorpheniramine or diphenhydramine HCl (Benadryl).
4. *Analgesic:* Morphine sulfate or Meperidine (Demerol).
5. *Vasopressor:* Methoxamine.
6. *Corticosteroid:* Hydrocortisone sodium succinate (Solu-Cortef).
7. *Antihypoglycemic:* 50% dextrose solution (for unconscious patient).

III. Record of Emergency

Figure 58–1 shows an example of a form that can be used to record the essential information during an emergency. Such a form can be printed into pads for the convenience of having a carbon copy to place in the patient's permanent record when the original accompanies the patient to a hospital or other medical facility.

A. Purposes

1. Organize data collected during the emergency.
2. Serve as a time reference during the monitoring of vital signs.
3. Prepare a record from which the medical personnel can interpret the patient's condition at the time of transfer from the dental facility.

B. Uses

1. Evaluation for planning dental and dental hygiene appointments so that future

emergencies for the patient can be avoided.
2. Provide a reference in the event legal questions arise. A well-kept record can be vital, and each emergency, however insignificant the incident may seem, should be recorded.[6,7]

IV. Practice and Drill

A. Staff Instruction

Each member of the clinic or office staff must be thoroughly familiar with the location, purpose, effect, and application of each item of equipment and its source.

B. Assignments

Specific responsibilities are assigned to each staff member. Each must know the order of procedures in an emergency. Moments count, and there is no time for fumbling or discussion.

C. Flow Chart

Figure 58–2 is an example of possible distribution of duties when four people are available to attend the patient, and figure 58–3 when there are three people. Although the chart can be posted for study, it must be memorized by the persons concerned. There would not be time in a real emergency to consult a flow chart.

1. *Advantages*
   a. Organization for efficient use of personnel.
   b. Sharing responsibility relieves pressure.
   c. Duties can be carried out quietly, without excess discussion.
   d. Necessary work gets done without duplication and without omissions.
2. *Preparation.* The preparation of a flow chart and the assignment of all duties related to emergencies should be a result of the planning of the whole team together.
3. *Substitutions.* Because a staff member may be absent from the scene at the time of an emergency, each person should know the duties for all positions so that substitutions can be made and doubling of duties accomplished.

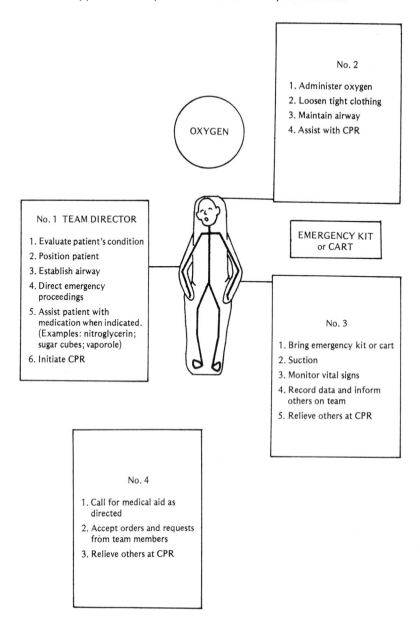

No. 2
1. Administer oxygen
2. Loosen tight clothing
3. Maintain airway
4. Assist with CPR

OXYGEN

No. 1 TEAM DIRECTOR
1. Evaluate patient's condition
2. Position patient
3. Establish airway
4. Direct emergency proceedings
5. Assist patient with medication when indicated. (Examples: nitroglycerin; sugar cubes; vaporole)
6. Initiate CPR

EMERGENCY KIT or CART

No. 3
1. Bring emergency kit or cart
2. Suction
3. Monitor vital signs
4. Record data and inform others on team
5. Relieve others at CPR

No. 4
1. Call for medical aid as directed
2. Accept orders and requests from team members
3. Relieve others at CPR

Figure 58–2. Emergency team flow chart: four people. Suggested distribution of responsibilities to be memorized and practiced. Note position of oxygen and emergency kit or cart. Compare with figure 58–3, flow chart for three people.

D. Drills

1. Regular reviews and rehearsals for each type of emergency should be made. These should be conducted on a "surprise" basis at least once a month. The dentist can use a specific code call when there is an intercom or other message system.

2. Practice in the use of all procedures, including oxygen administration, resuscitation, and airway maneuvers, as well as specific positioning of a patient for all emergencies, is indicated.

3. Equipment and materials can be checked at the time of the drill to assure their availability and that each is in working order. Outdated supplies can be replaced. One staff member should be in charge of the emergency supplies.

E. New Staff Member

1. Assignment of duties and practice for the

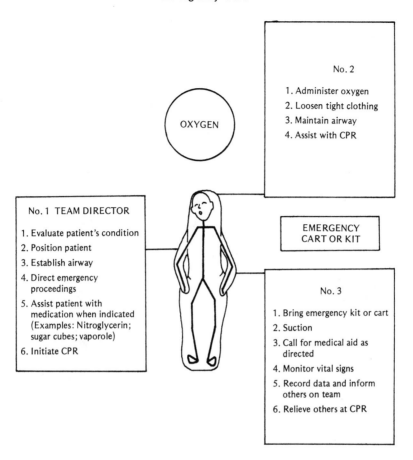

No. 2

1. Administer oxygen
2. Loosen tight clothing
3. Maintain airway
4. Assist with CPR

OXYGEN

No. 1 TEAM DIRECTOR

1. Evaluate patient's condition
2. Position patient
3. Establish airway
4. Direct emergency proceedings
5. Assist patient with medication when indicated (Examples: Nitroglycerin; sugar cubes; vaporole)
6. Initiate CPR

EMERGENCY CART OR KIT

No. 3

1. Bring emergency kit or cart
2. Suction
3. Call for medical aid as directed
4. Monitor vital signs
5. Record data and inform others on team
6. Relieve others at CPR

Figure 58–3. Emergency team flow chart: three people. Compare duties of person in position no. 3 with duties of people in positions no. 3 and no. 4 in figure 58–2.

new member should be a part of the first working day's orientation.

2. New members must be expected to renew certificates by taking necessary refresher courses within a specified time. Such a procedure would not be necessary in a state where a renewal certificate is required for annual licensure.

F. Procedures Manual

A loose-leaf manual, reviewed and updated three or four times each year, can provide a valuable study and work reference. It is particularly useful during the orientation of a new member.

The notebook can contain work assignments and check lists for equipment and resources. Direct reference information concerning specific emergencies with their symptoms and initial treatment, may be placed in alphabetic order in a specially color-coded section. Members of the team can keep the manual current by bringing references and notes from readings and courses.

BASIC LIFE SUPPORT[8,9]

Sudden cessation of effective respiration and circulation must be treated immediately. Without breathing and heart action, oxygen cannot be carried to the cells and a deficiency occurs immediately. The lack of oxygenated blood affects the pupils within a minute, therefore the response of the eyes to light is an important sign. *Irreversible brain tissue damage results in 4 to 6 minutes in the absence of oxygenated blood.*

Basic patient care in an emergency is defined by the letters A-B-C-D, which are the objectives for the treatment:

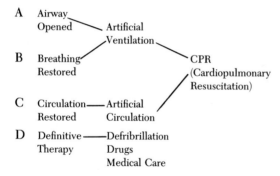

A Airway
   Opened ———— Artificial
                  Ventilation
B Breathing
   Restored   CPR
                            (Cardiopulmonary
                             Resuscitation)
C Circulation—— Artificial
   Restored   Circulation
D Definitive ——Defibrillation
   Therapy   Drugs
                 Medical Care

It is necessary to keep calm and act promptly, but not hastily. The incorrect procedure may be more harmful than none at all. It is assumed that each dental auxiliary will have participated in courses in emergency procedures and resuscitation techniques while in school and periodically since graduation for refresher, renewal, and updating. This section is intended to provide an outline for reference and review. The steps described are carried out in rapid succession.

I. Determine State of Consciousness

A. Unconscious Patient

1. *Shake the Shoulder and Shout.* If fractures are suspected, the shake must be gentle. The unconscious patient will not respond.
2. *Apply Sensory Stimulation.* The patient will not respond to sensory application such as pinching.

B. Call Loudly for Help

When available, use an alert (buzzer) system of an office or clinic.

C. Proceed to Treat

1. *Unconscious Patient:* position for resuscitation.
2. *Conscious Patient:* determine specific conditions (table 58–1).

II. Position Unconscious Patient

Figure 58–4 shows the four basic positions. The correct position in each emergency situation must be learned.

A. Supine: head on level with heart, feet slightly raised (figure 58–4C).

The supine position is most frequently used. The exceptions for particular types of emergencies are included in table 58–1.

B. Exceptions for Special Consideration

1. *Pregnancy.* During the third trimester, place patient on her side to prevent pressure on the vena cava.
2. *Severe Facial Injury.* Turn on side to lessen danger of blood, debris, and displaced parts from falling into the throat and to permit drainage of fluids.

AIRWAY

I. Open Airway

A. Remove Dental Chair Head Support

A round or wedge-shaped accessory head or shoulder support should be removed to

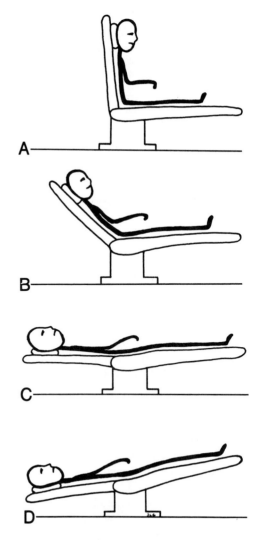

Figure 58–4. Basic patient positions. **A.** Upright. **B.** Semi-upright. **C.** Supine or horizontal with the brain on the same level as the heart. **D.** Trendelenburg, with the brain lower than the heart and the feet slightly elevated.

permit the head to lie flat and the chin to be raised without resistance.

B. Tilt Head Back

1. Head tilt: place palm of hand on patient's forehead to apply backward pressure.
2. Head tilt with chin lift: palm of hand on forehead to apply backward pressure; fingertips (not thumb) of other hand under chin with light pressure on mandible to bring chin up.
3. Head tilt with neck lift: palm of hand on forehead to apply backward pressure; other hand beneath neck near back of skull to lift and support (figure 58–5). Apply pressure gently: danger of causing cervical spine injury.

II. Check Breathing

A. Place ear over patient's mouth and nose while looking at chest.
B. LOOK for chest movement.
C. LISTEN for and FEEL air from nose and mouth.
   1. Unconscious with no breathing: continue airway procedures.
   2. Unconscious and breathing: monitor vital signs, determine other specific conditions.

III. Jaw Thrust

A. Indications

1. First procedure when there is a sus-pected neck injury. It can be done without extending the neck.
2. Second procedure when breathing does not start after airway is opened by usual procedures.

B. Procedure

1. From the top of the patient's head, grasp angles of the mandible, lift and displace it forward; tilt head back.
2. Open lips to allow mouth breathing.
3. Pain from this maneuver may bring response from the patient.

IV. Recheck Breathing (Repeat Step II.)

A. Listen for Possible Obstruction

1. Partial obstruction: noisy air flow.
2. Complete obstruction
   a. Cannot hear or feel airflow.
   b. No inflation during ventilation.

B. Second Operator

1. Loosen tight collar and belt.
2. Monitor and record vital signs.

C. Airway Open

Proceed with artificial ventilation.

BREATHING

I. Clear the Mouth

Turn the patient's head to the side to clear the mouth of mucus, vomitus, and other foreign

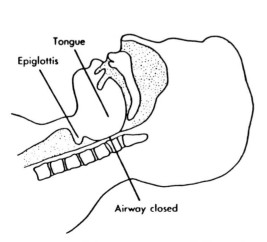
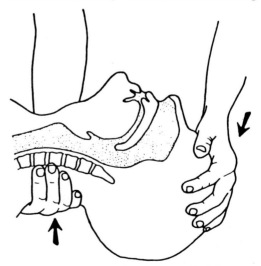

Figure 58–5. Head tilt to open airway. *Left,* Unconscious person with tongue falling against posterior wall of pharynx and obstructing the air passage. *Right,* Head tilted by placing one hand under the neck and the other hand on the forehead to open the airway. Note tongue lifted from pharyngeal wall. (From: Malamed, S.F.: Handbook of Medical Emergencies in the Dental Office. St. Louis, The C.V. Mosby Co., 1978.)

material. Use suction, gauze, and finger. Dentures should be left in place to provide support for mouth-to-mouth ventilation.

II. Position

A. Mouth-to-Mouth

Pinch the nose closed with thumb and index finger of hand on patient's forehead. Continue to maintain backward pressure.

B. Mouth-to-Nose

When necessary because of oral condition or impossibility of opening the mouth, or when a tight seal cannot be made, the mouth is held closed and the nose is used.

III. Rescue Breathing

A. Take a breath and apply a wide open mouth over the patient's mouth to make a tight seal. Watch chest for movement.
B. Deliver *four* quick breaths within 5 seconds without waiting for deflation. The purpose is to provide a positive pressure in the lungs.
C. Remove mouth and take in fresh air between each ventilation. The operator must take care not to become hyperventilated by taking too many deep breaths.

IV. Check Pulse

Check carotid pulse (for operator working alone). Determine whether artificial circulation is needed.

V. Repeat the Ventilations

A. Adult: repeat every 5 seconds (12 per minute).
B. Child: 18 to 20 times per minute, using more shallow breaths, depending on the size of the child.
C. Effective artificial ventilation is noted when the patient's chest rises with each ventilation.

CARDIAC COMPRESSION
(Artificial Circulation)

The principle is that rhythmic pressure applied over the lower half of the sternum compresses the heart to produce artificial circulation. The procedure is also called *external cardiac compression*.

I. Check Pulse

A. Lone Operator

1. Check carotid pulse on side of neck near operator's position quickly, between ventilations.
2. Patient with pulse: continue artificial ventilation as long as necessary, until recovery or help arrives.
3. *Patient without pulse: begin artificial circulation immediately.*

B. Team (figures 58–2 and 58–3)

1. Blood pressure and pulse are monitored while other person checks airway and begins ventilation.
2. Proceed with team approach for cardiopulmonary resuscitation.

II. Position

A. Patient is in Supine Position

When working in a dental chair, lower the chair to its lowest position and place a board or other firm flat object under the patient's back to provide a solid surface for compression.[10]

B. Locate Point for Pressure

1. Run middle finger of hand I along the lower edge of the rib cage to the notch in the midline. Hand I is the nondominant hand.
2. With middle finger in the notch and index finger beside it, place the heel of hand II next to the index finger on the midline of the sternum.
3. Place heel of hand I on top of hand II with the fingers in the same direction. Link and close the fingers.
4. Turn the fingers up so that only the heel of hand II is on the patient (figure 58–6).

III. Compression

A. Lean forward over the positioned hands, arms straight, until shoulders are directly over the sternum.

B. Use a firm, steady, vertical pressure (not a blow). The sternum moves down $1\frac{1}{2}$ to 2 inches (figure 58–6).

C. Hold the pressure at the bottom of each stroke very briefly to allow the heart to empty; release pressure but maintain contact and position of the hands.

D. Repeat at a rate of 60 times per minute when there are two operators.

E. Make compressions smooth and uninterrupted, with compression and relaxation of equal duration.

F. Use natural weight of upper body to prevent pushing from the shoulders or depending on arm strength.

G. As the heart is compressed between the sternum and the spine (figure 58–6), blood is forced out of the heart into the circulation.

H. Release of pressure allows blood to flow into the heart.

I. An interruption in compression results in a return of blood flow to zero.

IV. Length of Treatment

A. Signs of recovery: pupils constrict when exposed to light, normal skin color returns, patient may gasp or show other sign of breathing, and the body may move or wiggle.

B. Do not stop heart compressions while patient is being transported to the hospital.

C. When circulation and breathing appear to have returned, do not leave patient: watch for need to continue resuscitation in case of relapse.

V. Coordinated Activity

A. Lone Operator

1. Provide ventilation and compressions.
2. Use rate of 15 to 2: 15 compressions followed by 2 quick lung inflations.
3. Compress at the rate of 80 per minute to make up the time utilized for inflations.
4. Check carotid pulse and pupil response every few minutes.

B. Two Operators

1. First person begins airway, breathing, and circulation as described above.
2. Second person calls for medical assistance and ambulance, then promptly takes over either ventilation or circulation.
3. Use coordinated rhythm of 1 to 5: one lung inflation after 5 compressions. The rhythm of the compressions must not be interrupted for ventilation, or for exchange of places.

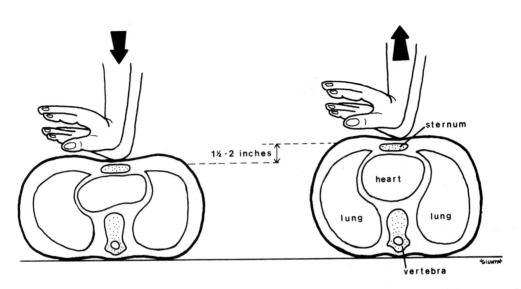

Figure 58–6. External cardiac compression. *Right,* Hands in position on midline of the sternum with fingers turned up. *Left,* Application of firm vertical pressure compresses the heart. Pressure is released while hands are held in position for the next compression. Compressions are repeated at a rate of 60 per minute for an adult.

C. Three Operators

1. Third person seeks medical aid, as the other two proceed with rescue efforts (figure 58–3).
2. Monitor vital signs, observe eye response periodically.
3. Take over ventilation or compressions at intervals.

VI. Child Patient (Infants under 1 year; child to 8 years)

A. Airway

For a neck lift, place fingers under neck and shoulders; lift gently. A chin lift is preferred.

B. Pulse

For an infant use the brachial pulse (upper arm on inside, midway between elbow and armpit).

C. Ventilation

1. Cover nose and mouth to make seal.
2. Use 4 quick gentle breaths: watch chest rise.
3. Ventilate an infant 20 times per minute; a child, 15 times.

D. Chest Compressions

Note small size of chest, higher position of heart, and faster heart rate. Compressions must be accompanied by rescue breathing.
1. Apply pressure near middle of the sternum, higher than for an adult.
2. Infant: use 2 to 3 fingers to compress ½ to 1 inch; 100 per minute.
3. Child: larger child may require the heel of one hand to compress 1 to 1½ inches; 80 per minute.

VII. Sequelae

Cardiopulmonary resuscitation must be continued until medical assistance arrives or the patient begins to recover. When the patient is transported to a hospital, resuscitation must continue.

When recovery occurs in the dental office, the patient can be moved to a couch for rest, but must be watched carefully. The cause of the emergency must be determined and additional treatment provided when indicated.

The *Record of Emergency* with monitored vital signs should accompany the patient to the medical care facility for reference by the persons assuming responsibility. The carbon copy for the patient's dental files is marked clearly with recommendations for prevention of future emergencies.

OXYGEN ADMINISTRATION

Oxygen is an important agent, useful in most emergencies when respiratory difficulty is apparent. *Oxygen is not indicated when there is hyperventilation*, since the patient has increased air, and is in need of carbon dioxide.

I. Equipment

A. Parts

Oxygen resuscitation equipment consists of an oxygen tank, a reducing valve, a flow meter, tubing, mask, and a positive pressure bag. The *E* cylinder, which can provide oxygen for 30 minutes, is the minimum size recommended. Smaller tanks provide too little oxygen for a real emergency, and larger tanks are less portable.

B. Directions

Clear, readable directions should be permanently attached to the tank. Practice is a definite part of team drills.

II. Procedure

A. Position patient in supine.
B. Clear debris from the oral cavity and establish an airway.
C. Apply mask. Use full-face clear mask when available.
D. Adjust oxygen flow so that the positive pressure bag remains filled.
E. To force oxygen into the lungs, manually compress the bag intermittently at 3- to 5-second intervals to provide 15 to 20 respirations per minute. Watch chest rise and fall. When the chest does not rise and fall, recheck airway for obstruction.
F. Observe skin color and respirations for return to normal.
G. Adaptation: when patient is breathing but respirations are shallow or otherwise deficient, compress bag in harmony with each inspiration of the patient to increase the depth and volume of breaths.

AIRWAY OBSTRUCTION[11,12]

I. Prevention

With thought and planning, care can be exercised to prevent aspiration of objects by a patient during a dental or dental hygiene appointment. A few of the procedures that contribute to this are as follows:

A. Position the patient in supine during examination and treatment. The throat is closed (figure 58–5).

B. Use rubber dam for all appropriate procedures.

C. Use a length of floss to tie to small objects such as a rubber dam clamp or a bite block. Floss hangs out from angle of lips.

D. Use low-speed handpiece to prevent splashing or spinning masses of agents into the throat.

E. Have assistant use aspirator for various procedures that involve large pieces of calculus, copious blood clots, excess saliva, excess water for ultrasonic scaling, restorative materials, and other potentially inhalable items.

F. Attention to mobile permanent or exfoliating primary teeth that could be inadvertently displaced.

II. Recognition of Airway Obstruction

Immediate recognition is essential. Differentiation from other emergencies such as fainting, heart attack, or stroke, in which a sudden respiratory failure may also occur, may be necessary when no object or material was involved that could have been inhaled.

When there is no doubt that an object has been inhaled, medical aid must be obtained. A radiograph may be needed to confirm the location of a radiopaque object.

A. Signs and Symptoms of Partial Obstruction

1. Poor air exchange with gasping and noisy respirations.

2. Patient clutches throat; has expression of panic and distress.

3. Patient's face may become red or the patient may show evidence of cyanosis.

4. Increased breathing difficulty.

B. Complete Obstruction

1. Patient attempts to breathe but is unable to obtain air exchange, cough, or speak.

2. No noise in larynx or pharynx.

3. Substernal retraction of the diaphragm.

4. Dilated pupils.

5. Cyanosis.

6. Unconsciousness.

III. Outline of Treatment

An airway must be established within 3 to 5 minutes to prevent permanent brain damage from oxygen deficiency. With total obstruction, the patient may become unconscious within a few seconds.

Treatment begins with the A, B, C of basic life support, unless inhalation of a specific item was observed. When the inspiration is known, the operator may proceed directly to attempt to dislodge the obstruction.

A. Let patient cough when possible.

B. Open airway, which distinguishes degree of obstruction, partial or complete.

C. Use manual maneuvers
   1. Back blows.
   2. Abdominal thrusts.

D. Check mouth and throat for foreign bodies (finger sweep). Repeat back blows and thrusts.

E. Unconscious patient
   1. Check breathing.
   2. Artificial ventilation. May need slow, full, forceful ventilation for a partially obstructed airway.
   3. Cardiopulmonary resuscitation as indicated.

F. Obtain medical assistance; transport to hospital emergency.

IV. Back Blows

A. Patient Standing or Sitting

1. Position
   a. Patient in a dental chair will sit up and turn sidewards; a very tall person should sit down for a short operator.
   b. Operator is at the side and slightly behind; patient bends forward.

2. Deliver four sharp blows with the heel of the hand to the patient's spine between the shoulder blades.

3. Place hand on chest for support of the patient during the blows.

B. Patient in Supine Position

1. Position
   a. Supine with feet slightly elevated.
   b. Roll the patient so the chest leans against the operator's leg for support.
2. Operator reaches over to deliver four blows to center upper back.

C. Child

A small child can be held face down over the operator's forearm with the head supported in the hand. Four back blows are delivered with the heel of the hand between the shoulder blades, using much less force than for an adult. With continued head and neck support, the child is turned over for chest thrusts.

V. Manual Abdominal Thrust

Four manual thrusts are made to the upper abdomen, or in selected cases, the chest. The abdominal thrust should not be used for a woman during pregnancy or for a very obese person.

The thrusts are given to provide pressure against the diaphragm which will compress the lungs. In turn, the pressure in the lungs is increased, which forces air through the trachea and may force out the obstructing object.

A. Patient Standing or Sitting

1. From behind, operator wraps arms around the waist of the patient. Make a fist with the nondominant hand.
2. Hold thumb side of the fist on the patient's upper abdomen above the navel and below the xiphoid. Grab the fist with the other hand.
3. Press the fist four times into the abdomen with quick upward thrusts.

B. Patient in Supine Position

1. Open the airway and turn the head to the side.
2. Stand beside and facing the head of the chair when the patient is in the dental chair. On the floor, a more direct thrust can be applied from astride the patient.
3. Hold the heel of one hand over the upper abdomen, with the other hand on top.
4. Apply four quick thrusts.

C. Child

The body is positioned with the head slightly lower than the trunk. Two or three fingertips on the middle of the sternum are pressed into the chest with four quick thrusts. Finger sweeps are avoided except when the object is actually seen.

VI. Chest Thrust

As mentioned before, the chest thrust is not used routinely, but is only recommended when it is not possible to use the abdominal thrust, such as during pregnancy and for very obese individuals.

A. Patient Standing or Sitting with Operator Behind

1. From behind, wrap arms around chest of the patient at level of armpits.
2. Make a fist with the nondominant hand. Position the thumb side of the fist on the sternum. The thrust should definitely not be made on the ribs or on the xiphoid because fracture is possible.
3. Grasp the fist with the other hand and apply four quick backward thrusts.

B. Patient in Supine Position

1. Open the airway and turn the head to the side.
2. Position hands on the lower sternum in the same position as for external cardiac compression (page 840 and figure 58–6).
3. Apply four quick downward thrusts.

VII. Finger Sweep

After each series of back blows and abdominal thrusts, an attempt should be made to remove the offending object by examination of the mouth and throat and by using the fingers, gauze, or suction appropriately. Care must be taken not to force the object deeper.

A. Position the Head

Turn the patient's head to one side, open the mouth, and lift the tongue and lower jaw with the thumb and index finger of the nondominant hand.

B. Index Finger Sweep

1. Slide the index finger along the buccal mucosa and deep into the throat to the base of the tongue.

2. Anticipate contact with an object, move slowly, with care not to push the object farther into the throat.
3. Hook the end of the finger under and around to remove the object.

C. Repeat

Repeat back blows, abdominal thrusts, and finger sweep several times.

SPECIFIC EMERGENCIES

Certain systemic disease conditions and physical injuries require specific treatment during an emergency. In table 58–1, the *Emergency Reference Chart,* a variety of conditions are listed with their symptoms and treatment procedures. Some of the same conditions have been described in detail in Section VI of this book.

Table 58–1. Emergency Reference Chart

Emergency	Signs/Symptoms	Procedure

All Cases		1. Determine consciousness (shake and shout)
		 2. Place in supine position
		 3. Identify major problem
		   A. Airway
		   B. Breathing
		   C. Circulation
		 4. Act in accord with findings
		 5. Summon assistance

Respiratory Failure	Labored or weak respirations or cessation of breathing Cyanosis or ashen-white with blood loss Pupils dilated Loss of consciousness	Position: supine, head turned to side Check for and remove foreign material from mouth Establish airway Mouth-to-mouth breathing Monitor vital signs: blood pressure, pulse, respirations Administer oxygen
Airway Obstruction	Good air exchange, coughing, wheezing	Sit patient up Loosen tight collar, belt No treatment: let patient cough
Partial	Poor air exchange, noisy breathing, weak, ineffective cough, difficult respirations, gasping Patient is panicky	Reassure patient Treat for complete obstruction (page 843)
Complete	Gasping with great effort; no noises Patient clutches throat Unable to speak, breathe, cough Cyanosis Dilated pupils	*Conscious patient* 4 back blows (page 843) 4 manual thrusts (page 844) Finger sweep for foreign body Repeat as needed
	Unconscious in 10 seconds after complete obstruction occurs	*Unconscious patient* Position: supine Open airway; maintain tilted head Check breathing Attempt to ventilate Roll patient with chest against operator's leg or knees to administer 4 back blows Turn patient on back for 4 manual thrusts Finger sweep Attempt to ventilate Repeat blows, thrusts, sweep Call for medical assistance

Table 58–1. *continued*

Emergency	Signs/Symptoms	Procedure
Hyperventilation Syndrome	Lightheadedness, giddiness Anxiety, confusion Dizziness Overbreathing (25 to 30 respirations per minute) Feelings of suffocation Deep respirations Palpitations (heart pounds) Tingling or numbness in the extremities	Terminate oral procedure Remove rubber dam and objects from mouth Position upright or best for comfortable breathing Loosen tight collar Reassure patient Ask patient to breathe deeply (7 to 10 per minute) into a paper or plastic bag adapted closely over nose and mouth. (Carbon dioxide is indicated, NOT oxygen.)

Hemorrhage	Prolonged bleeding
	  a. Spurting blood: artery
	  b. Oozing blood: vein
		Compression over bleeding area
		  a. Apply gauze pack with pressure
		  b. Bandage pack into place firmly where possible
		Severe bleeding: digital pressure on pressure point of supplying vessel
		Watch for shock symptoms

	Bleeding from tooth socket	Pack with folded gauze; do not dab Have patient bite down firmly Do not rinse
	Bleeding of an extremity	Elevate the part: support with pillows or substitute Apply tourniquet only when limb is amputated, mangled, or crushed
	Nosebleed	Tell patient to breathe through mouth Apply cold application to nose Press nostril on bleeding side for a few minutes Plug nostril with gauze (not cotton); leave end hanging out Advise patient not to blow the nose for an hour or more
Syncope (fainting)	Pale, gray face, anxiety Dilated pupils Weakness, giddiness, dizziness, faintness, nausea Profuse cold perspiration Rapid pulse at first, followed by slow pulse Shallow breathing Drop in blood pressure Loss of consciousness	Position: Trendelenburg Loosen tight collar, belt Place cold, damp towel on forehead Crush ammonia vaporole under patient's nose Keep warm (blanket) Monitor vital signs: blood pressure, pulse, respirations Keep airway open May require oxygen Keep in supine position 10 minutes after recovery to prevent nausea and dizziness Reassure patient, especially during recovery

Table 58–1. *continued*

Emergency	Signs/Symptoms	Procedure
Shock	Skin: pale, moist, clammy Rapid, shallow breathing Low blood pressure Weak, may be restless Nausea, vomiting Thirsty, if shock is from bleeding Eventual unconsciousness if untreated	Position: Trendelenburg Keep quiet and warm Monitor vital signs: blood pressure, respirations, pulse Keep airway open Administer oxygen Summon medical assistance

Stroke
(cerebrovascular
  accident)
	Premonitory
	  Dizziness, vertigo
	  Transient paresthesia or weakness
	    one side
	  Transient speech defects
	Serious
	  Headache (with cerebral
	    hemorrhage)
	  Breathing labored, deep, slow
	  Chills
	  Paralysis one side of body
	  Nausea, vomiting
	  Convulsions
	  Loss of consciousness
	    (slow or sudden onset)
		Conscious patient
		  Turn patient toward affected side; semi-
		    upright
		  Loosen clothing about the throat
		  Reassure patient; keep calm, quiet
		  Monitor vital signs: blood pressure,
		    pulse, respirations
		  Administer oxygen when there is a
		    respiratory difficulty
		  Do not give stimulant, sedative, or
		    narcotic
		  Clear airway; suction vomitus because
		    the throat muscles may be paralyzed
		  Seek medical assistance promptly
		
		Unconscious patient
		  Position: supine
		  Basic life support
		  Cardiopulmonary resuscitation if
		    indicated

**Cardiovascular
  Diseases**
	Symptoms vary depending on cause	*For all patients*
		  Be calm and reassure patient
		  Keep patient warm and quiet; restrict
		    effort
		  Call for medical assistance

Angina Pectoris
(page 784)
	Sudden crushing, paroxysmal pain in
	  substernal area
	Pain may radiate to shoulder, neck,
	  arms
	Pallor, faintness
	Shallow breathing
	Anxiety, fear
		Position: upright, as patient requests, for
		  comfortable breathing
		Place nitroglycerin sublingually
		Administer oxygen if needed
		Reassure patient
		
		Without prompt relief after a second
		  nitroglycerin, treat as a heart attack.

**Myocardial
  Infarction**
(heart attack)
(page 785)
	Sudden pain similar to angina pectoris,
	  which also may radiate, but of longer
	  duration
	Pallor; cold, clammy skin
	Cyanosis
	Nausea
	Difficulty in breathing
	Marked weakness
	Anxiety, fear
	May lose consciousness
		Position: with head up for comfortable
		  breathing
		Symptoms are not relieved with
		  nitroglycerin
		Monitor vital signs: blood pressure, pulse,
		  respirations
		Administer oxygen if needed
		Alleviate anxiety; reassure
		Call for medical assistance for transfer to
		  hospital

Table 58–1. *continued*

Emergency	Signs/Symptoms	Procedure
Heart Failure (page 786)	Difficult or labored breathing Pulmonary congestion with cough. May cough up blood Rapid, weak pulse Dilated pupils May have chest pain	Urgent medical assistance needed Place patient in upright position Make patient comfortable: cover with blanket Administer oxygen Reassure patient
Cardiac Arrest	Skin: ashen gray, cold, clammy No pulse No heart sounds No respirations Eyes fixed, with dilated pupils; no constriction with light Unconscious	Position: supine Basic life support Check oral cavity for debris or vomitus; leave dentures in place for a seal Begin cardiopulmonary resuscitation: minutes count (page 840)

Adrenal Crisis (cortisol deficiency)	Anxious, stressed
	Mental confusion
	Pain in abdomen, back, legs
	Muscle weakness
	Extreme fatigue
	Nausea, vomiting
	Lowered blood pressure
	Elevated pulse
	
	Loss of consciousness
	Coma
		Conscious patient
		    Terminate oral procedure
		    Call for help and emergency kit
		    Position patient in supine with legs slightly raised
		    Request telephone call for medical assistance
		    Administer oxygen
		    Monitor blood pressure and pulse
		    Administration of glucocorticosteroid as determined by dentist
		
		Unconscious patient
		    Position patient in supine with legs slightly raised
		    Basic life support
		    Try ammonia vaporole when cause is undecided
		    Administer oxygen
		    Summon medical assistance
		    Administration of glucocorticosteroid as determined by dentist
		    Transport to hospital

Insulin Reaction (hyperinsulinism) (hypoglycemia)	Sudden onset
	Skin: moist, cold, pale
	Confused, nervous, anxious
	Bounding pulse
	Salivation
	Normal to shallow respirations
	Convulsions (late)
		Conscious patient
		    Administer oral sugar (cubes, orange juice, candy)
		    Observe patient for one hour before dismissal
		    Determine time since previous meal, and arrange next appointment following food intake
		
		Unconscious patient
		    Basic life support
		        Position: supine
		        Airway maintenance
		        Administer oxygen
		        Monitor vital signs
		    Summon medical assistance
		    Administer intravenous glucose

Table 58–1. *continued*

Emergency	Signs/Symptoms	Procedure

Diabetic Coma (ketoacidosis) (hyperglycemia)	Slow onset
	Skin: flushed and dry
	Breath: fruity odor
	Dry mouth, thirst
	Low blood pressure
	Weak, rapid pulse
	Exaggerated respirations
	Coma
		Conscious patient
		   Terminate oral procedure
		   Obtain medical care: hospitalization indicated
		   Keep patient warm
		
		Unconscious patient
		   Basic life support
		   Urgent medical assistance needed

Allergic Reaction
1. Delayed[14]
	Skin
	   Erythema (rash)
	   Urticaria (wheals, itching)
	   Angioedema (localized swelling of mucous membranes, lips, larynx, pharynx)
	
	Respiration
	   Distress, dyspnea
	   Wheezing
	   Extension of angioedema to larynx: may have obstruction due to swelling of vocal apparatus
		Skin:
		   Administer antihistamine
		Respiration:
		   Position: upright
		   Administer oxygen
		   Epinephrine
		
		Airway obstruction
		   Position: supine
		   Airway maintenance
		   Epinephrine
		Summon medical assistance

2. Immediate
 	
   Anaphylaxis (anaphylactic shock)
	Skin
	   Urticaria (wheals, itching)
	   Flushing
	Nausea, abdominal cramps, vomiting, diarrhea
	Angioedema
	   Swelling of lips, membranes, eyelids
	   Laryngeal edema with difficult swallowing
	Respiration distress
	   Cough, wheezing
	   Dyspnea
	   Airway obstruction
	   Cyanosis
	Cardiovascular collapse
	   Profound drop in blood pressure
	   Rapid, weak pulse
	   Palpitations
	   Dilation of pupils
	
	Loss of consciousness (sudden)
	   Cardiac arrest
		Rapid treatment needed
		Position: supine (except when dyspnea predominates)
		Administer oxygen
		Basic life support
		Monitor vital signs
		Epinephrine
		Cardiopulmonary resuscitation
		
		Summon medical assistance; transfer to hospital

Table 58–1.   *continued*

Emergency	Signs/Symptoms	Procedure
Local Anesthesia Reactions 1. Psychogenic	Reaction to injection, not the anesthetic Syncope Hyperventilation syndrome	See above in this table Page 846 (syncope) Page 846 (hyperventilation)
2. Allergic (very rare)	Anaphylactic shock Allergic skin and mucous membrane reactions Allergic bronchial asthma attack	See above in this table Page 849
3. Toxic Overdose	Effects of intravascular injection rather than increased quantity of drug are more common	

	a. Stimulation phase
	   Anxious, restless, apprehensive, confused
	   Rapid pulse and respirations
	   Elevated blood pressure
	   Tremors
	   Convulsions
		Mild reaction
		   Stop injection
		   Position: supine
		   Loosen tight clothing
		   Reassure patient
		   Monitor blood pressure, heart rate, respirations
		   Administer oxygen
		   Summon medical assistance

	b. Depressive phase
	   Follows stimulation phase
	   Drowsiness, lethargy
	   Shock-like symptoms: pallor, sweating
	   Rapid, weak pulse and respirations
	   Drop in blood pressure
	   Respiratory depression or respiratory arrest
	   Unconsciousness
		Severe reaction
		   Basic life support: maintain airway
		   Continue to monitor vital signs
		   Cardiopulmonary resuscitation
		   Administration of anticonvulsant

Epileptic Seizure 1. Generalized tonic–clonic (*Grand mal* page 722)	Anxiety or depression Pale, may become cyanotic Muscular contractions Loss of consciousness	Position: supine. Do not attempt to move from dental chair Make safe by placing movable equipment out of reach Do not force anything between the teeth. A soft towel or large sponges may be placed while mouth is open Open airway; monitor vital signs Allow patient to sleep during postconvulsive stage Do not dismiss the patient if unaccompanied
2. Generalized absence (*Petit mal* page 722)	Brief loss of consciousness Fixed posture Rhythmic twitching of eyelids, eyebrows, or head May be pale	Take objects from patient's hands to prevent dropping

Table 58–1. *continued*

Emergency	Signs/Symptoms	Procedure
Burns[15]		*First and Second Degree Burns*
1. First degree	Skin reddened Swelling Pain	Do not give food or liquids. Anticipate nausea Be alert for signs of shock Do not apply ointment, grease, or bicarbonate of soda
2. Second degree (partial thickness)	Skin reddened, blisters Swelling Wet surface Pain (more than third degree) Heightened sensitivity to touch	Immerse in cool water to relieve pain Do not apply ice Gently clean with a mild antiseptic (pHisoHex) Dress lightly with bandage Elevate burned part Obtain medical assistance
3. Third degree (full thickness)	Leathery look Insensitive to touch	Request medical assistance and transport system Treat for shock Basic life support: maintain airway Check for other injuries Wrap in clean sheet; transport
4. Chemical burn	Reddened, discolored	Immediate, copious irrigation with water for one-half hour Check directions on container from which the chemical came, for antidote or other advice Burn caused by an acid may be rinsed with bicarbonate of soda; burn caused by alkali may be rinsed in weak acid such as acetic (vinegar) Medical assistance advised or obtained
Internal Poisoning[16]	Signs of corrosive burn around or in oral cavity Evidence of empty container or information from patient Nausea, vomiting, cramps	Be calm and supportive Basic life support: airway maintenance Artificial ventilation (inhaled poison) Record vital signs Induce vomiting if patient is conscious by giving plain water and gagging with a finger Do not induce vomiting if caustic, corrosive, or petroleum products have been ingested Avoid nonspecific and questionably effective antidotes, stimulants, sedatives, or other agents, which may do more harm Obtain medical assistance

Table 58–1.   *continued*

Emergency	Signs/Symptoms	Procedure
Foreign Body in Eye	Tears Blinking	Wash hands Ask patient to look down Bring upper lid down over lower lid for a moment; move it upward Turn down lower lid and examine: if particle is visible remove with moistened cotton applicator Use eye cup: wash out eye with mild boric acid solution or plain water When unsuccessful, seek medical attention: prevent patient from rubbing eye by placing gauze pack over eye and stabilizing with adhesive tape
Chemical Solution in Eye	Tears Stinging	Irrigate promptly with copious amounts of water. Continue for 15 to 20 minutes
Dislocated Jaw	Mouth is open: patient is unable to close	Stand in front of seated patient Wrap thumbs in towels and place on occlusal surfaces of mandibular posterior teeth Curve fingers and place under body of the mandible Press down and back with thumbs and at same time pull up and forward with fingers (figure 58–7) As joint slips into place, quickly move thumbs outward Place bandage around head to support jaw
Facial Fracture	Pain, swelling Ecchymosis Deformity, limitation of movement Crepitation on manipulation Zygoma fracture: depression of cheek Mandibular fracture: abnormal occlusion	Place patient on side Basic life support Support with bandage around face, under chin, and tied on the top of the head (Barton) Seek prompt transport to emergency care facility
Tooth Forcibly Displaced (avulsed tooth)	Swelling, bruises, or other signs of trauma, depending on the type of accident	Instruct patient or parent to rinse tooth gently in cool water and place in water or wrap in wet cloth Bring to the dental office or clinic *immediately* The longer the time lapse between avulsion and replantation, the poorer the prognosis

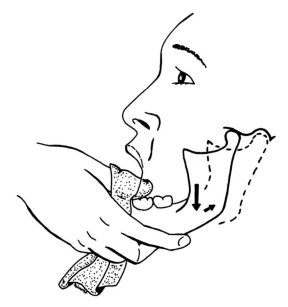

Figure 58–7.   Treatment of a dislocated jaw. With thumbs wrapped in towels and placed on the occlusal surfaces of the mandibular teeth, the fingers are curved under the body of the mandible. The jaw is pressed down and back with the thumbs while pulling up and forward with the fingers to permit the condyle to pass over the articular eminence into its normal position in the glenoid fossa. As the jaw slips into place, the thumbs should be moved quickly outward.

TECHNICAL HINTS

I. Precautions During Mouth-to-Mouth Ventilation

Infection may be transmitted or acquired.[13] Dental personnel need to gain proficiency in the use of mechanical CPR equipment to prevent unnecessary contact with ill, debilitated patients or those known or suspected to be carriers of a disease. Periodic personal tests for syphilis, hepatitis, and tuberculosis are advisable.

II. Care of Drugs

A. Label each with information about shelf-life and due-date for replacement. Nitroglycerin, for example, must be changed at 6 months.

B. Check weekly to maintain emergency kit in workable order.

C. Test oxygen equipment regularly to guard against leaks in tubing and to insure a supply of oxygen.

D. Dispose of an out-of-date narcotic drug in the presence of a witness to prevent question that the drug may have been stolen.

III. Eye Safety

In addition to eye protection during working hours, professional people should wear protective glasses for activities outside the practice area, such as for sports, hobbies, and other potentially harmful activities.

IV. Medic Alert Identification

Identification for patients with medical problem: a metal emblem worn as a bracelet or a pendant is available to provide specific information pertinent to an emergency that may arise. Information about the emblems is available by writing the Medic Alert Foundation International, Turlock, California, 95380. In addition to noting patients who are wearing the identification and recording the fact along with other information in the patient history, other patients can be given information about the service.

V. Sources of Materials and Information:

American Heart Association
7320 Greenville Avenue
Dallas, Texas 75231

American National Red Cross
17th and D Streets
Washington, D.C. 20006

References

1. Malamed, S.F.: *Handbook of Medical Emergencies in the Dental Office*. St. Louis, The C.V. Mosby Co., 1978, pp. 27–30.
2. Cooley, R.L., Cottingham, A.J., Abrams, H., and Barkmeier, W.W.: Ocular Injuries Sustained in the Dental Office: Methods of Detection, Treatment, and Prevention, *J. Am. Dent. Assoc.*, 97, 985, December, 1978.
3. Hartley, J.L.: Eye and Facial Injuries Resulting from Dental Procedures, *Dent. Clin. North Am.*, 22, 505, July, 1978.
4. Booth, D.F. and Dunn, M.J.: Systemic Emergencies, in Dunn, M.J., ed.: *Dental Auxiliary Practice*, Module 4. Baltimore, The Williams & Wilkins Co., 1975, pp. 71–72.
5. Malamed: op. cit., pp. 32–48.
6. American Dental Association, Council on Dental Therapeutics: *Accepted Dental Therapeutics*, 39th ed. Chicago, American Dental Association, 1982, pp. xxv–xxvii.
7. Sheppard, G.A.: Legal Aspects of Emergencies, in McCarthy, F.M.: *Emergencies in Dental Practice*, 3rd ed. Philadelphia, W.B. Saunders Co., 1979, pp. 698–738.
8. American Heart Association, 1979 National Conference on Cardiopulmonary Resuscitation and Emergency Cardiac Care: *Standards and Guidelines for Cardiopulmonary Resuscitation (CPR) and Emergency Cardiac Care (ECC)*, *J.Am.Med.Assoc.*, 244, 453, August 1, 1980.

9. American National Red Cross: *Cardiopulmonary Resuscitation.* Washington, D.C., American National Red Cross, 1981, 57 pp.

10. Quinn, T.W.: Cardiopulmonary Arrest, in McCarthy, F.M.: *Emergencies in Dental Practice*, 3rd ed. Philadelphia, W.B. Saunders Co., 1979, pp. 421–433.

11. American Red Cross: *First Aid for Foreign Body Obstruction of the Airway.* The American National Red Cross, 1978, 30 pp.

12. American Heart Association: *A Manual for Instructors of Basic Cardiac Life Support.* Dallas, Texas, American Heart Association, 1981, pp. 61–68.

13. Hendricks, A.A. and Shapiro, E.P.: Primary Herpes Simplex Infection Following Mouth-to-Mouth Resuscitation, *J.Am.Med.Assoc.*, 243, 257, January 18, 1980.

14. Malamed: op. cit., pp. 251–274.

15. Munster, A.M.: Physical and Chemical Injuries, in Conn, H.F., ed.: *Current Therapy.* Philadelphia, W.B. Saunders Co., 1980, pp. 903–910.

16. Arena, J.M.: Acute Miscellaneous Poisoning, in Conn, H.F., ed.: *Current Therapy*, Philadelphia, W.B. Saunders Co., 1980, p. 921.

Suggested Readings

American Dental Association, Council on Dental Therapeutics: *Accepted Dental Therapeutics*, 39th ed. Chicago, American Dental Association, 1982, pp. 59–79.

Barkmeier, W.W., Cooley, R.L., and Abrams, H.: Prevention of Swallowing or Aspiration of Foreign Objects, *J. Am. Dent. Assoc.*, 97, 473, September, 1978.

Brand, M.K.: CPR for Oral Health Professionals: A Dental Team Training Course, *Dent. Hyg.*, 54, 475, October, 1980.

Capello, J. and Wheatley, F.: Medical Emergencies: the Dental Team Approach, *Dent. Surv.*, 53, 24, August, 1977.

Chue, P.W.Y.: The Hyperventilation Syndrome: Diagnosis and Management, *Dent. Surv.*, 51, 31, December, 1975.

Chue, P.W.Y.: Transient Loss of Consciousness: Common Faint or Serious Symptom? *Dent. Surv.*, 51, 40, November, 1975.

Chue, P.W.Y.: Emergency Management of Cardiac Arrest, *Dent. Surv.*, 51, 36, April, 1975.

Croll, T.P., Brooks, E.B., Schut, L., and Laurent, J.P.: Rapid Neurologic Assessment and Initial Management for the Patient with Traumatic Dental Injuries, *J. Am. Dent. Assoc.*, 100, 530, April, 1980.

Department of Health, Education, and Welfare, Project ACORDE: *Management of Dental Office Emergencies.* Quercus Corporation, 2768 Pineridge Road, Castro Valley, California, 94546, July, 1976, 51 pp.

D'Eramo, E.M.: Emergency Drills for the Anesthetic Team, *Anesth. Prog.*, 23, 13, January–February, 1976.

Dietz, E.R.: Dental Office Emergencies, *Dent. Assist.*, 47, 30, November/December, 1978.

Eisenberg, M.S., Copass, M.K., Hallstrom, A., Cobb, L.A., and Bergner, L.: Management of Out-of-Hospital Cardiac Arrest, *J.Am.Med.Assoc.*, 243, 1049, March 14, 1980.

Freeman, N.S., King, R.A., Plezia, R.A., and Shearer, H.T.: Office Emergencies: An Outline of Causes, Symptoms, and Treatment, *J. Am. Dent. Assoc.*, 94, 91, January, 1977.

Goldman, H.S.: Hazards in the Dental Workplace, *Clin. Prev. Dent.*, 2, 18, September–October, 1980.

Greenfield, W.: Medical Emergencies in the Dental Office, in Boundy, S.S. and Reynolds, N.J., eds.: *Current Concepts in Dental Hygiene, Volume 2.* St. Louis, The C.V. Mosby Co., 1979, pp. 69–81.

Hendler, B.H. and Rose, L.F.: Common Medical Emergencies: A Dilemma in Dental Education, *J. Am. Dent. Assoc.*, 91, 575, September, 1975.

Leonard, M.S.: Office Emergencies, in Waite, D.E., ed.: *Textbook of Practical Oral Surgery*, 2nd ed. Philadelphia, Lea & Febiger, 1978, pp. 82–94.

Lewis, J.E.S.: A Simple Technique for Reduction of Longstanding Dislocation of the Mandible, *Br. J. Oral Surg.*, 18, 52, March, 1981.

March, N.F. and Matthews, R.C.: New Techniques in External Cardiac Compressions. Aquatic Cardiopulmonary Resuscitation, *J.Am.Med.Assoc.*, 244, 1229, September 12, 1980.

Matukas, V.J. and McCallum, C.A.: Medical Emergencies in the Dental Office, in Clark, J.W., ed.: *Clinical Dentistry, Volume 1*, Chapter 30. Hagerstown, Maryland, Harper & Row, 1981, pp. 1–17.

Mosby, E.L.: Managing Emergencies in the Dental Office, *U.S. Navy Med.*, 68, 22, June, 1977.

Neal, S.C.: Medical Emergencies in the Dental Office, in Castano, F.A. and Alden, B.,A., eds.: *Handbook of Clinical Dental Auxiliary Practice*, 2nd ed. Philadelphia, J.B. Lippincott Co., 1980, pp. 261–281.

Needleman, H.L. and Berkowitz, R.J.: Electric Trauma to the Oral Tissues of Children, *J. Dent. Child.*, 41, 19, January–February, 1974.

Needleman, M.S., McLaughlin, D.K., Orner, G., and Mumma, R.D.: Eye Hazards Among a Dental School Population, *J. Dent. Educ.*, 41, 573, September, 1977.

Perks, E.R.: The Diagnosis and Management of Sudden Collapse in Dental Practice, Part 1. The Incidence of Emergencies, *Br. Dent. J.*, 143, 196, September 20, 1977.

Schultz, R.C. and Oldham, R.J.: An Overview of Facial Injuries, *Surg. Clin. North Am.*, 57, 987, October, 1977.

Stamps, J.T. and Muth, E.R.: Reducing Accidents and Injuries in the Dental Environment, *Dent. Clin. North Am.*, 22, 389, July, 1978.

Vincent, J.W.: Reduction of Luxation of the Temporomandibular Joint—An Extraoral Approach, *J. Prosthet. Dent.*, 44, 445, October, 1980.

Woodworth, J.V. and Woodworth, C.E.: Emergency! The Dentist's Role in Prevention and Treatment, Part Two, *Gen. Dent.*, 26, 46, July–August, 1978.

Anaphylaxis

Chue, P.W.Y.: Emergency Management of Anaphylactic Reactions, *Dent. Surv.*, 51, 32, July, 1975.

Gill, C. and Michaelides, P.L.: Dental Drugs and Anaphylactic Reactions, *Oral Surg.*, 50, 30, July, 1980.

Glauda, N.M., Henefer, E.P., and Super, S.: Nonfatal Anaphylaxis Caused by Oral Penicillin: Report of Case, *J. Am. Dent. Assoc.*, 90, 159, January, 1975.

Seskin, L.: Anaphylaxis Due to Local Anesthesia Hypersensitivity: Report of Case, *J. Am. Dent. Assoc.*, 96, 841, May, 1978.

Thurm, P.S.: Anaphylaxis, *Dent. Hyg.*, 53, 21, January, 1979.

Emergency Kit or Cart

American Dental Association, Council on Dental Therapeutics: Emergency Kits, *J. Am. Dent. Assoc.*, 87, 909, October, 1973.

American Dental Association, Council on Dental Therapeutics: Office Emergencies and Emergency Kits, *J. Am. Dent. Assoc.*, 101, 305, August, 1980.

Lee, P.W.: A Practical Emergency Kit for the Dental Office, *Can. Dent. Assoc. J.*, 41, 225, April, 1975.

McGivern, B.E.: The Office Emergency Cart, *J. Oral Surg.*, *37*, 436, June, 1979.

Schijatschky, M.: Basic Emergency Kit, *Quintessence Int.*, *6*, 71, March, 1975.

Local Anesthesia Complications

Alling, C.C.: Local Anesthesia, in Clark, J.W., ed.: *Clinical Dentistry, Volume 1,* Chapter 24. Hagerstown, Maryland, Harper & Row, 1981, pp. 1–10.

Bennett, C.R.: *Monheim's Local Anesthesia and Pain Control in Dental Practice,* 5th ed. St. Louis, The C.V. Mosby Co., 1974, pp. 154–196.

Booth, D.F. and Dunn, M.J.: Local Anesthesia, in Dunn, M.J. ed.: *Dental Auxiliary Practice,* Module 5. Baltimore, The Williams & Wilkins Co., 1975, pp. 45–50.

Covino, B.G. and Giddon, D.B.: Pharmacology of Local Anesthetic Agents, *J. Dent. Res., 60,* 1454, August, 1981.

Giovannitti, J.A.: Evaluation of Local Anesthetic Hypersensitivity Reactions, *Clin. Prev. Dent., 3,* 20, January–February, 1981.

Giovannitti, J.A. and Bennett, C.R.: Assessment of Allergy to Local Anesthetics, *J. Am. Dent. Assoc., 98,* 701, May, 1979.

Hayden, J. and Jorgensen, N.B.: Complications from Local Analgesia, in McCarthy, F.M.: *Emergencies in Dental Practice,* 3rd ed. Philadelphia, W.B. Saunders Co., 1979, pp. 434–448.

Hayes, S.M.: Allergic Reaction to Local Anesthetic: Report of a Case, *Gen. Dent., 28,* 30, January–February, 1980.

Kramer, H.S. and Mitton, V.A.: Complications of Local Anesthesia, *Dent. Clin. North Am., 17,* 443, July, 1973.

Perks, E.R.: The Diagnosis and Management of Sudden Collapse in Dental Practice, Part III. Collapse in the Dental Chair Under Local Anesthesia, *Br. Dent. J., 143,* 307, November, 1977.

Reuben, B.M.: A Current Practical Review of Local Anesthesia, *Dent. Surv., 56,* 38, July, 1980.

Stone, J. and Kaban, L.B.: Trismus after Injection of Local Anesthetic, *Oral Surg., 48,* 29, July, 1979.

Prefixes, Suffixes, and Combining Forms

a-, an- absence, lack, without, e.g. *a*morphous
ab- from, away, e.g. *ab*normal
ad- (change d to c,f,g,p,s, or t before words beginning with those consonants) to, toward, e.g., *ad*hesion, *ac*cretion
adeno- gland, e.g. *adeno*fibroma
-algia pain, e.g., neur*algia*
ambi- on both sides, e.g. *ambi*dexterity
ana- up, excessive, again, e.g. *ana*bolism
angio- vessel, e.g. *angio*ma
anti- against, e.g. *anti*dote
aqu-, aqua- water, e.g. *aqu*eous
arthro-, arth- joints, e.g. *arth*ritis
-ase denotes an enzyme, e.g. dextrin*ase*
-asthenia weakness, e.g. my*asthenia* gravis
auto-, aut- self, e.g. *auto*transplant

bi- two, twice, double, e.g. *bi*furcation
bio-, bi- life, living, e.g. *bio*psy
-blast formative cell, e.g. osteo*blast*
-brachy- short, e.g. *brachy*dactylic
brady- slow, e.g. *brady*cardia
bucc- cheek, e.g. *bucc*inator

calc- stone, calcium, lime, e.g. *calc*ification
cardio-, cardi- heart, e.g. *cardio*vascular
cata- down, against, e.g. *cata*bolism
-cele swelling, protrusion, hernia, e.g. meningo*cele*
cephalo-, cephal- head, e.g. *cephalo*metry
cerebro-, cerebr- brain, e.g. *cerebr*al palsy
cheilo-, cheil- lip, e.g. *cheil*itis
chloro-, chlor- pale green, e.g. *chloro*phyll
chromo-, chromat- color, pigmentation, e.g. *chromo*genic
-cidal killing, e.g. bacteri*cidal*
-clast break up, divide into parts, e.g. osteo*clast*

-clus- shut, e.g. oc*clus*ion
co-, com-, con-, cor- with, together, e.g. *con*genital
coll- glue, e.g. *coll*oid
contra- opposite, e.g. *contra*lateral
cryo-, cry- cold, freezing, e.g. *cryo*therapy
cuti- skin, e.g. *cuti*cle
cyan- blue, e.g. *cyan*otic
-cyto-, -cyt- cell, e.g. leuko*cyte*

-dactyl, dactylo- fingers, e.g. *dactyl*edema
de- down, away from, separation, e.g. *de*calcification
denti-, dent- tooth, e.g. *dent*ition
-derm-, -derma- skin, e.g. hypo*derm*ic
di- twice, two, e.g. *di*plopia
dia- (drop *a* before words beginning with a vowel) through, apart, e.g. *dia*phragm
dis- separation, opposite, taking part, e.g. *dis*infect
disto-, dist- posterior, distant from center, e.g. *dis*tobuccal
-drome course, e.g. syn*drome*
dur- hard, e.g. in*dur*ation
dys- bad, ill, difficult, e.g. *dys*trophy

ecto-, ect- without, outer side, e.g. *ecto*derm
-ectomy surgical removal, e.g. gingiv*ectomy*
-emia (-aemia) blood condition, e.g. bacter*emia*
en- in, on, into, e.g. *en*demic
endo- inside, e.g. *endo*dontics
entero-, enter- intestine, e.g. *entero*toxin
epi- upon, after, in addition, e.g. *epi*dermis
erythro-, eryth- red, e.g. *eryth*ema
ex- beyond, from, out of, e.g. *ex*udate
extra- outside of, beyond the scope of, e.g. *extra*cellular

faci-   face, e.g. *faci*al
-ferent   carry, bear, e.g. af*ferent*
fibro-, fibr-   fibers, fibrous tissue, e.g. *fibro*blast
fract-   break, e.g. *fract*ional

galacto-, galact-   milk, e.g. *galact*ose
gastro-, gastr-   stomach, e.g. *gastr*itis
-gen-   produced, e.g. glyco*gen*
genio-   chin, lower jaw, e.g. *genio*plasty
germ-   bud, early growth, e.g. *germ*inal
gero-   old age, e.g. *gero*dontics
glosso-, gloss-   tongue, e.g. *gloss*itis
gluco-, gluc-   glucose, e.g. *gluc*oneogenesis
glyco-, glyc-   sweet, e.g. *glyc*erin
gnatho-, gnath-   jaw, e.g. *gnatho*dynamometer
-gnosis   knowledge, e.g. prog*nosis*
-gram, -graph   write, draw, e.g. radio*graph*ic
gran-   grain, particle, e.g. *gran*uloma
gyn-, gyne-, gynec-   woman, e.g. *gynec*ology

hemi-   half, e.g., *hemi*section
hemo-, (haemo-)   blood, e.g. *hemo*rrhage
hepato-, hepat-   liver, e.g. *hepat*itis
hetero-, heter-   other, different, e.g. *hetero*genous
histo-, hist-   tissue, e.g. *histo*logy
homo-, homeo-   like, similar, e.g. *homeo*stasis
hydro-, hydr-   water, e.g. *hydro*cephalic
hyper-   abnormal, excessive, e.g. *hyper*trophy
hypno-, hypn-   sleep, e.g. *hypn*otic
hypo-, hyp-   deficiency, lack, below, e.g. *hypo*tonic
hystero-, hyster-   uterus or hysteria, e.g. *hyster*ectomy

-ia   state or condition, e.g. glycosur*ia*
-ic   of, pertaining to, e.g. gastr*ic*
idio-   one's own, separate, distinct, e.g. *idio*pathic
in-   not, without, e.g. *in*activate
infra-   beneath, below, e.g. *infra*orbital
inter-   between, among, e.g. *inter*cellular
intra-   within, into, e.g. *intra*oral
ischo-, isch-   suppression, stoppage, e.g. *isch*emia
iso-   equality, similarity, e.g. *iso*tonic
-ist   one who practices, holds certain principles, e.g. hygien*ist*
-itis   inflammation, e.g. dermat*itis*

-ject-   throw, e.g. in*ject*ion
juxta-   next to, near, e.g. *juxta*position

karyo-, kary-   nucleus of a cell, e.g. *karyo*lysis
kerato-, kerat-   horny, keratinized tissue, e.g. *kerat*inization
kin-   move, e.g. *kin*etic

labio-   lip, e.g. *labio*version
lacto-, lact-   milk, e.g. *lact*ation
laryngo-, laryn-   larynx, e.g. *laryn*gitis
later-   side, e.g. *later*oversion
leuko-, leuk-   white, e.g. *leuk*oplakia
linguo-, lingu-   tongue, e.g. *lingu*al
lipo-, lip-   fat, fatty, e.g. *lip*oma
-logy   doctrine, science, e.g. periodonto*logy*

lympho-, lymph-   lymph, e.g. *lymph*angioma
-lysin, -lysis, -lytic   dissolving, destructive, e.g. hemo*lysis*

macro-, macr-   enlargement, elongated part, e.g. *macro*dontia
mal-   bad, ill, e.g. *mal*nutrition
-megalo-, -megal-   large, great, e.g. *megalo*blast
melano-   dark-colored, relating to melanin, e.g. *me-lano*genesis
meningo-, mening-   meninges, e.g. *mening*itis
meno-   month, e.g. *meno*pause
mes-, medi, mesio-   middle, intermediate, e.g. *meso*derm
meta-, met-   over, beyond, transformation, e.g. *me-ta*bolism
metro-, metra-   uterus, e.g. *metro*fibroma
-metry   measure, e.g. cephalo*metry*
micro-, micr-   small, e.g. *micro*organism
mono-   one, single, e.g. *mono*saccharide
morpho-, morph-   form, shape, e.g. *morph*ology
muco-, muc-   relating to mucous membrane, e.g. *muco*gingival
myo-, my-   muscle, e.g. *myo*cardium

naso-   nose, e.g. *naso*palatine
necr-   death, e.g. *necr*otic
neo-, ne-   new, recent, e.g. *neo*plasm
nephro-, nephr-   kidneys, e.g. *nephr*itis
neuro-, neuri-, neur-   pertaining to nerves, e.g. *neur*asthenia
nucleo-, nucle-   pertaining to nucleus, e.g. *nucleo-*protein

ob-   (change b to c before words beginning with c) against, toward, e.g. *oc*clusion
odonto-, odont-   tooth, e.g. *odont*algia
-oid   like, resembling, e.g. ameb*oid*
-oma   swelling, tumor, e.g. lip*oma*
-opia, -opy   sight, eye defect, e.g. my*opia*
oro-   mouth, oral, e.g. *oro*nasal
ortho-, orth-   straight, normal, e.g. *ortho*dontics
-osis   condition, state, e.g. cyan*osis*
osteo-, oste-   bone, e.g. *osteo*porosis
oto-, ot-   ear, e.g. *oto*plasty
-ous   full of, having, e.g. aque*ous*
ovi-, ovo-, ovu-   egg, e.g. *ovu*lation

pan-   all, every, general, e.g. *pan*acea
para-   beyond, beside, near, e.g. *para*site
patho-, path-   disease, e.g. *patho*gnomonic
pedia-, pedo- (paedo-)   child, e.g. *pedo*dontics
per-   throughout, completely, e.g. *per*cussion
peri-   around, near, e.g. *peri*apical
phago-   to eat, e.g. *phago*cytic
-phile, -phil   loving, e.g. hemo*phil*ia
phlebo-, phleb-   vein, e.g. *phleb*itis
-phobe, -phobia   fear, dread, e.g. photo*phobia*
-plas-   mold, shape, e.g. gingivo*plas*ty
plasmo-, -plasm   form, e.g. cyto*plasm*
-plegia, -plexy   paralysis, stroke, e.g. hemi*plegia*
-pnea, (-pnoea)   breathing, e.g. dys*pnea*

pneumo- air, lung, e.g. *pneumo*thorax
-poiesis, -poietic production, e.g. erythro*poietic*
poly- many, much, e.g. *poly*saccharide
pont- bridge, e.g. *pont*ic
post- behind, after, e.g. *post*natal
pre- before, in front of, e.g. *pre*maxilla
pro- before, in front of, e.g. *pro*gnathic
proprio- one's own, e.g. *proprio*ceptive
proto- first, e.g. *proto*plasm
pseudo- false, deceptive, e.g. *pseudo*membrane
psycho-, psych- mind, mental processes, e.g. *psycho*somatic
pulmo- lung, e.g. *pulmo*nary
pur-, pyo- pus, e.g. *pur*ulent, *pyo*rrhea
pyro- fever, heat, e.g. *pyro*genic

re- back, again, e.g. *re*gurgitate
-renal kidney, e.g. ad*renal*
retro- back, backward, behind, e.g. *retro*molar
-rhage breaking, bursting forth, profuse flow, e.g. hemor*rhage*
-rhea, (-rhoea) flow, discharge, e.g. pyor*rhea*
rhino-, rhin- nose, e.g. *rhin*itis
rube- red, e.g. *rube*lla

sarco- flesh, muscle, e.g. *sarco*ma
-sclero- hard, e.g. *sclero*derma

-scopy examination, inspection, e.g. micro*scopy*
semi- half, partly, e.g. *semi*permeable
sial-, sialo- saliva, e.g. *sialo*graphy
somat-, somato-, -some body, e.g. chromo*some*
-squam- scale, e.g. de*squam*ative
stomat- mouth, e.g. *stomat*itis
sub- beneath, under, deficient, e.g. *sub*acute
super- above, upon, excessive, e.g. *super*numerary tooth
syn- with, together, e.g. *syn*drome

tachy- swift, e.g. *tachy*cardia
tact- touch, e.g. *tact*ile
thermo- heat, e.g. *thermo*phile
thrombo-, thromb- clot, coagulation, e.g. *thromb*in
trans- beyond, through, across, e.g. *trans*plantation
tropho-, trophic nutrition, nourishment, e.g. hyper*trophic*
-tropic turning toward, changing, e.g. hydro*tropic*

-ule diminutive, small, e.g. tub*ule*
-uria urine, e.g. glucos*uria*

vaso- blood vessels, e.g. *vaso*dilation
vita- life, e.g. *vita*min

xero- dry, e.g. *xero*stomia

Glossary

This brief glossary includes primarily the words that have been used but not defined in the text. Those defined in the text may be located through the Index. The meaning of words from the basic medical and dental sciences frequently can be determined from the list of word prefixes, suffixes, and combining forms on the previous pages. A medical dictionary should be an important adjunct to guide professional reading.

A

Abscess: a localized, circumscribed collection of pus.

Absorption: taking up of fluids or other substances by the skin or mucous surfaces; passage of substances to the blood, lymph, and cells from the alimentary canal after digestion.

Abutment: a tooth used for the support or retention of a fixed or removable prosthesis.

Accessory: subordinate, attached, or added for convenience.

Acid: a chemical substance which in aqueous solution undergoes dissociation with the formation of hydrogen ions; pH less than 7.0.

Acidogenic: acid-forming or producing.

Acne vulgaris: a chronic inflammatory disease of the sebaceous glands which appears on the face, back, and chest in the form of eruptions.

Acquired characteristics: those obtained after birth, as a result of environment.

Acuity: sharpness or clearness, especially of the special senses.

Acute: having rapid onset, short, severe course, and pronounced symptoms; opposite of chronic.

Adenopathy: swelling or enlargement of lymph nodes.

Adsorption: a process believed to be physical in nature in which molecules of a gas or liquid condense or adhere on the surface of another substance.

Aerobe: a microorganism that requires free oxygen to exist.

Agar: gelatin extracted from seaweed, used as a nutrient solidifying agent in bacteriologic culture media; constituent of a reversible hydrocolloid impression material.

Agglutination: state of being united; adhesion of parts; clumping, as bacteria or other cells.

Alkali: a strong water-soluble base; see **Base.**

Allergen: an antigenic substance that produces hypersensitivity, which may be inhaled, ingested, or injected, or may produce a reaction upon contact with the skin.

Allergy: a hypersensitive state gained from exposure to a specific substance or allergen, re-exposure to which causes a heightened capacity to react.

Alloy: a substance composed of a mixture of two or more metals.

Alopecia: loss of hair.

Amalgam: an alloy of two or more metals, one of which is mercury.

  Dental amalgam: an alloy of silver, tin, copper, zinc, and mercury, used for dental restorations.

Ameloblast: epithelial cell of the enamel organ which functions in the formation of enamel.

Amorphous: lacking specific form or shape; unorganized.

Ampere: unit of quantity of electric current.

Amylase: an enzyme that converts starch into sugar.

Anaerobe: a microorganism that requires complete or almost complete absence of free oxygen to exist.

  Facultative anaerobe: microorganism that can exist under either aerobic or anaerobic conditions.

  Obligative anaerobe: microorganism that can exist only in the complete absence of free oxygen because oxygen is toxic to it.

Analgesia: absence of sensibility to pain; loss of sensibility to pain without loss of consciousness; first stage of general anesthesia.

Anaphylaxis: an acute, severe, allergic reaction characterized by sudden collapse, shock, or respiratory and circulatory failure following the injection of an allergen; increased susceptibility to an allergen resulting from previous exposure to it.

Anemia, nutritional: deficiency anemia; caused by some deficiency or fault in the diet or in nutrition.

Anesthesia: loss of feeling or sensation.

General anesthesia: an irregular, reversible depression of the cells of higher centers of the central nervous system that makes the patient unconscious and insensible to pain.

Local anesthesia: loss of sensibility to pain in a specific area, not accompanied by loss of consciousness.

Topical anesthesia: a form of local anesthesia, whereby free nerve endings in accessible structures are rendered incapable of stimulation by application of an anesthetic drug directly to the surface of the area.

Aneurysm: dilation of an artery.

Anhydrous: containing no water.

Ankylosis: union or consolidation of two similar or dissimilar hard tissues previously adjacent but not attached, as a tooth and its surrounding bone.

Anodontia: congenital absence of teeth; failure of teeth to form; may be partial or complete.

Anodyne: any agent that neutralizes or relieves pain.

Anomaly: deviation from the normal.

Anorexia: diminished appetite; aversion to food.

Anoxia: oxygen deficiency; a condition in which the cells of the body do not have or cannot utilize sufficient oxygen to perform normal function.

Antibiotic: a chemical substance derived from fungi or microorganisms which, in dilute solutions, can destroy or inhibit the growth of bacteria and other microorganisms; used in the treatment of infectious diseases of man, animals, and plants.

Antidote: a medicine or other remedy for counteracting the effects of a poison.

Apatite: inorganic compound with a complex formula containing calcium and phosphate; makes up the inorganic portion of bones and teeth.

Fluorapatite: containing fluoride radical.

Hydroxyapatite: containing hydroxyl radical.

Aphasia: loss of the power of expression by speech, writing, or signs or of comprehension of spoken or written language, due to injury or disease of the brain centers.

Aphtha: a little ulcer.

Aphthous ulcer: aphthous stomatitis; canker sore, vesicle that ruptures after one or two days and forms a depressed, spherical, painful ulcer with elevated rim.

Aqueous: watery; prepared with water.

Armamentarium: the equipment, such as books, materials, and instruments essential to professional practice.

Dental hygiene armamentarium: all the instruments and equipment used during a dental hygiene procedure.

Dental hygiene instrumentarium: set of instruments used for a particular operation by the dental hygienist.

Articulation: the place where two or more bones of the skeleton join or unite; bony joint which may or may not be movable.

Artifact: in radiography, a substance or structure not naturally present in living tissues, but of which an authentic image appears in a radiograph; a blemish or an unintended radiographic image that may result from the faulty manufacture, manipulation, exposure, or processing of an x-ray film.

Asepsis: condition in which septic, infective, putrefactive material is absent; exclusion of microorganisms.

Asphyxia: suffocation or a temporary state of lifelessness as a result of cessation of breathing.

Aspirator: an apparatus employing suction.

Astringent: a substance that causes contraction or shrinkage and arrests discharges.

Atom: the small particle of an element that is composed of protons, neutrons, and electrons.

Atrophy: a degenerative process characterized by diminution in size and wasting away of cells or of an organ, generally associated with an interference in nutrition.

Attenuation: reducing, thinning, or weakening; reduction of the virulence of a virus or pathogenic microorganism, as by successive culture or repeated inoculation; in radiography, the process by which a beam of radiation is reduced in energy when passing through some material.

Attrition: gradual wearing away of tooth structure resulting from mastication.

Audiologist: a specialist in evaluation and rehabilitation of those whose communication disorders center in whole or in part in the hearing function.

Autoclave: an apparatus for effecting sterilization by high temperature obtained from steam under pressure.

Autograft: an autologous graft in which the tissue is obtained from the same individual.

Autonomic (involuntary) nervous system: a division of the nervous system that supplies the sensory innervation for the smooth muscles, heart, and glands. It is divided into the parasympathetic (craniosacral) and the sympathetic (thoracolumbar) systems.

Auxiliary: giving support; helping; aiding; assisting.

B

Backscatter: radiation deflected by scattering processes at angles greater than 90 degrees to the original direction of the beam of radiation.

Bacteremia: presence of bacteria in the blood

stream. It may be transient, intermittent, or continuous.

Bacterial spore: a resistant form of bacteria encapsulated by a thick cell wall which enables the cell to survive in environments unfavorable to immediate growth and division; not a reproductive mechanism.

Bactericidal: capable of destroying bacteria.

Bacteriostatic: capable of inhibiting the growth and multiplication of bacteria.

Barodontalgia (Aerodontalgia): the sudden acute pain response in a tooth under reduced barometric pressure, notably during space flight.

Base: a chemical substance that in solution yields hydroxyl ions and reacts with an acid to form a salt and water. A base turns red litmus paper blue and has a pH higher than 7.0.

Bevel: the inclination one line or surface makes with another when they are not at right angles.

Bifid: cleft into two parts or branches.

Biopsy: the removal and examination, usually microscopic, of a section of tissue or other material from the living body for the purpose of diagnosis.

Bite-wing radiographic survey: dental radiographs that show the coronal portions of maxillary and mandibular teeth, used for detecting deviations in the structure or form of the proximal surfaces of teeth and the crest of the interdental bone.

Body mechanics: proper balance of the skeleton by muscular alignment which favors function with the least amount of expended energy; refers to a dynamic position as opposed to **posture,** which is alignment in a rigid position.

Bruxism: a neurogenically related habit of grinding, clenching, or clamping the teeth. Damage to the teeth and attachment apparatus can result.

Buffer: any substance in a fluid that tends to lessen the change in hydrogen ion concentration (reaction), which otherwise would be produced by adding acids or alkalis.

Burnish: to make smooth and bright; to polish by friction.

C

Calcification: the process by which organic tissue becomes hardened by a deposit of calcium and other inorganic salts within its substance.

Cancer: malignant and invasive neoplasm.

Canker sore: see **Aphthous ulcer.**

Carbohydrate: organic compound of carbon, hydrogen, and oxygen: includes starches, sugars, cellulose; formed by plants and used for growth and source of energy.

Carcinoma: a malignant neoplasm of epithelial origin.

Caries: see **Dental caries.**

Cariogenic: caries producing; conducive to caries.

Carious: affected with caries or decay; in dentistry, a carious lesion is a cavity in a tooth which is the result of dental caries.

Carrier: an infected person who harbors a specific infectious agent in the absence of discernible clinical disease and serves as a potential source of infection.

Cartilage: firm, elastic, flexible connective tissue which is attached to articular bone surfaces and which forms certain parts of the skeleton.

Cassette: light-tight container in which x-ray films are placed for exposure to x-radiation; usually backed with lead to eliminate the effect of backscatter radiation.

Cataract: a clouding or opacity of the lens of the eye which leads to blurring of vision and eventual loss of sight.

Caustic: an agent that burns or corrodes; destroys living tissue; having a burning taste.

Cauterize: to burn, corrode, or destroy living tissue by means of a caustic substance, heated metal, or an electric current.

Central ray: a hypothetical x-ray whose direction of travel corresponds to the geometric center of a useful beam of x-radiation.

Cephalometer: an orienting device for positioning the head for radiographic examination and measurement.

Cephalometrics: scientific study of the measurements of the head.

Cephalometry: measurement of the bony structure of the head using reproducible lateral and anteroposterior radiographs.

Cheilosis: a condition marked by fissuring and dry scaling of the surface of the lips and angles of the mouth; characteristic of riboflavin deficiency.

Chorea: a nervous disorder characterized by irregular and involuntary action of the muscles of the extremities and the face.

Chronic: characterized by a long, slow course, as compared with acute.

Clean: freedom from or removal of all matter in which microorganisms may find favorable conditions for continued life and growth.

Clinic: an establishment where patients are admitted for study and treatment by a group of practitioners.

Clinical: pertaining to a clinic or to the actual observation and treatment of patients, as distinguished from theoretic or experimental.

Coagulation: changing of a soluble into an insoluble protein; process of changing into a clot.

Coaptation: proper adaptation or union of parts to each other, such as the ends of a fractured bone or the edges of a wound without overlap.

Col: concavity of the interdental gingiva; ridge-shaped depression between two peaks formed by the facial and lingual papillae.

Commissure: angle or corner of eye or lips.

Communicable: capable of being transmitted from one person to another.

Compatible: capable of existing together in harmony; with medications, suitable for simultaneous administration.

Conduction: the transfer of sound waves, heat, nerve influences, or electricity.

Cone: an accessory device on a dental x-ray machine designed to indicate the direction of the central axis of its x-ray beam and to serve as a guide in establishing a desired source-to-film distance. Such "cones" may be conical or cylindrical in form; provision for beam collimation and/or added filtration may be incorporated in the construction of the "cone."

Congenital: existing at or before birth.

Contagious: communicable; transmissible by contact with an infected or sick person.

Contaminate: to render impure by contact or mixture; in sterile technique, to introduce microorganisms.

Contracture: shortening or distortion; permanent, as from shrinkage of muscles, or temporary, from sudden stimulus.

Convalescence: the gradual recovery of health and strength after illness.

Corrode: to eat away or wear away, as by rust, causing deterioration of a substance.

Crepitation: a crackling sound; noise made by rubbing together the ends of a broken bone.

Cryosurgery: surgery performed with the use of decreased temperature.

Cryotherapy: therapeutic application of cold.

Cryptogenic: of obscure, doubtful, or undeterminable origin.

Current: the number of electrons per second passing a given point on a conductor. Electrons are negatively charged and move toward the positive.

Cuticle, primary: a delicate membrane covering the crown of a newly erupted tooth; produced by the ameloblasts after they produce the enamel rods. Also called Nasmyth's membrane.

Cyanosis: blueness of the skin due to insufficient oxygenation of the blood.

Cyst: a sac, normal or pathologic, containing fluid or other material.
  Dentigerous cyst: formed by a dental follicle, containing one or more well-formed teeth.
  Radicular cyst: an epithelial-lined sac, formed at the apex of a pulpless tooth, containing cystic fluid.

D

Debridement: removal of debris, foreign material, or devitalized tissue.

Decalcification: process by which calcium salts and other inorganic substances are removed.

Defibrillator: an agent or measure, for example an electric shock, that arrests fibrillation of the ventricular muscle and restores the normal beat.
  Fibrillation: exceedingly rapid contractions that replace normal contractions.

Deglutition: the act of swallowing.

Dehiscence: isolated area in which a root is denuded of bone when the denuded area extends to the margin of the bone. Compare with **Fenestration.**

Dehydration: removal of water; the condition that results from undue loss of water.

Dental caries: a disease of the calcified structures of the teeth, characterized by decalcification of the mineral components and dissolution of the organic matrix.

Dental prosthetic laboratory procedures: the steps in the fabrication of a dental prosthesis that do not require the presence of a patient for their accomplishment.

Dental public health: see under **Public health.**

Denticle: a pulp stone; relatively large body of calcified substance in the pulp chamber of a tooth.

Dentition: the kind, size, and arrangement of the teeth.
  Mixed dentition: combination of both primary and permanent teeth present in the oral cavity; state occurs when the first permanent molars erupt and extends until the last primary tooth is exfoliated.
  Permanent dentition: the natural teeth which must function throughout adult life.
  Primary (deciduous) dentition: the first teeth; normally will be shed and replaced by permanent teeth.
  Succedaneous dentition: permanent teeth that erupt in positions of exfoliated primary teeth.

Denture: an artificial substitute for missing natural teeth and adjacent tissues.
  Complete denture: a dental prosthesis that replaces the entire dentition and associated structures of the maxilla and/or mandible.
  Partial denture: a dental prosthesis that restores one or more but not all of the natural teeth and/or associated parts and that is supported by the teeth and/or mucosa. It may be removable or fixed.

Denudation: laying bare; surgical or pathologic removal of epithelial covering.

Desensitization: process of removing reactivity or sensitivity.

Desquamation: shedding or casting off, as of the superficial epithelium of mucous membrane or skin; a normal physiologic process.

Detergent: agent that cleanses.

Detritus: debris that adheres to tooth, gingival, and mucosal surfaces.

Devitalize: to deprive of vitality or of life; in dentistry, to destroy the vitality of the dental pulp.

Diagnosis: a scientific evaluation of existing conditions; the process of determining by examination the nature and circumstances of a diseased condition; the decision reached as to the nature of a disease.
  Differential diagnosis: the art of distinguishing one disease from another.

Diastema: a space or cleft; in dentistry, a space between teeth.

Diet: the customary allowance of food and drink taken by a person from day to day.
  Bland diet: meal plan in which all food that can cause chemical, mechanical, or thermal irritation is avoided.

Dietary: a regular or systematic scheme of diet.

Digital: of, pertaining to, or performed with a finger.

Dilate: to make wider or larger; cause to expand.

Dislocation: see **Luxation.**

Distilled water: water that has been subjected to a process of vaporization and subsequent condensation for purification.

Distortion: (radiographic) deviation of a radiographic image from the true outline or shape of an object or structure.

Donor site: area from which tissue is obtained during surgical procedures such as for a graft.

Dorsum: The back surface or a part similar to the back in position.

Duct: a passage with well-defined walls; especially a tube for the passage of excretions or secretions.

Dysarthria: disturbance of articulation due to emotional stress or to paralysis, incoordination, or spasticity of the muscles used for speaking.

Dyslexia: impairment in the ability to read.

Dysplasia: abnormal development or growth; an alteration in adult cells characterized by variations in their size, shape, and organization.

Dyspnea: difficult or labored breathing.

E

Ecchymosis: black and blue discoloration of the skin caused by the escape of blood from the vessels into the tissues; bleeding into the subcutaneous tissues.

Ecology: the science that deals with the study of the environment and the life history of organisms.

Ectopic: out of place. An **ectopic pregnancy** is one that occurs elsewhere than in the cavity of the uterus.

Edema: collection of abnormally large amounts of fluid in the intercellular spaces, causing swelling.

Pitting edema: pressure on edematous area causes pits, which remain for prolonged period after pressure is released.

Edentulous: without teeth.

Emaciation: condition of excessive leanness or wasted body tissues.

Embolism: sudden blocking of an artery or vein by a clot or obstruction which has been brought to its place by the blood current.

Embryo: the fetus in its earlier stages of development, especially before the end of the second month.

Emesis basin: a basin, usually kidney shaped, used for receiving material expectorated or vomited.

Emollient: softening or soothing; an agent used to soften the skin or other body surface.

Endemic: present in a community or among a group of people; the continuing prevalence of a disease as distinguished from an epidemic.

Endocardium: the endothelial lining membrane of the heart.

Endodontics: that branch of dentistry concerned with the etiology, diagnosis, and treatment of diseases of the dental pulp and their sequelae.

Endometrium: the mucous membrane lining the uterus.

Enzyme: an organic compound, frequently protein in nature, which can accelerate or produce by catalytic action some change in a specific substance.

Ephebodontics: dentistry for the individual undergoing the transition from childhood to adulthood, that is, the period of life known as adolescence.

Epidemic: the occurrence in a community or region of a group of illnesses of similar nature, clearly in excess of normal expectancy and derived from a common source.

Epithelialization: growth of epithelium over a denuded surface.

Epithelize, epithelialize: to cover or become covered with epithelium.

Erosion: progressive loss of tooth structure by a chemical process without the aid of bacteria; area is smooth, hard, and shiny.

Eruption: the act of breaking out, appearing or becoming visible; a visible pathologic lesion of the skin, marked by redness, swelling, or both.

Tooth eruption: the combination of movements of a tooth both before and after the emergence of its crown into the oral cavity, which serves to bring it and maintain it in occlusion with the tooth or teeth of the opposing arch.

Erythema: abnormal redness of the skin due to local congestion; may result from inflammation or excess exposure to x-ray.

Erythrocyte: red blood corpuscle; specialized cell for the transportation of oxygen.

Escharotic: corrosive; capable of producing sloughing.

Ethics: the science of right conduct; a system of rules or principles governing the conduct of a professional group planned by them for the common good of man; the principles of morality.

Etiology: the science or study of the cause of disease; that which is known about the causes of a disease.

Euphoria: well-being; absence of pain or distress; an abnormal or exaggerated sense of well-being.

Exfoliate: to fall off in scales or layers; in dentistry, to shed primary teeth.

Exodontics: that branch of dentistry concerned with the removal of teeth.

Exostosis: a bony outgrowth from the surface of bone.

Extirpation: complete removal or eradication of a part; in dentistry, the removal of the dental pulp from the pulp chamber and root canal.

Exudate: the material composed of serum, fibrin, and white blood cells in variable amounts, formed as a reaction to injury of tissue and blood vessels.

F

Febrile: pertaining to fever; feverish.

Fenestration: isolated area in which a root is denuded of bone when the marginal bone is intact. Compare with **Dehiscence.**

Fermentable: term applied to a substance that is capable of undergoing chemical change as a result of the influence of an enzyme; usually applied to substances that break down to an acid or an alcohol; applied to carbohydrate breakdown to form acid in the dental plaque.

Fetus: the unborn offspring in the uterus, after the second month.

Film badge: a pack containing a radiographic film or films to be used for the detection and measurement of radiation exposure in personnel monitoring.

Fistula: a narrow passage or duct leading from one cavity to another, as from a periapical abscess to the oral cavity.

Flora: the entire plant life of a geographic area; used to indicate the microorganisms that live together in a specific location.

Oral flora: the microorganisms that inhabit the oral cavity of an individual, usually saprophytic, and that live together in a symbiotic relationship.

Fluoridization: application of fluoride solution to the teeth; compare with fluoridation, in which the fluoride content of the community water supply is adjusted.

Fog: darkening of the whole or part of a developed radiograph from sources other than the radiation of the primary beam to which the film was exposed.

Chemical fog: darkening due to imbalance or deterioration of processing solutions.

Light fog: darkening due to unintentional exposure to light to which the emulsion is sensitive, either before or during the processing.

Radiation fog: darkening due to radiation from sources other than intentional exposure to the primary beam; for example, scatter radiation, or film storage not protected from radiation.

Follicle (dental): the sac that encloses the developing tooth before its eruption.

Forceps: a two-bladed instrument with handles for pulling, compressing, or grasping.

Frenectomy: complete removal of a frenum.

Frenotomy: partial removal of a frenum.

Frenum: a narrow fold of mucous membrane passing from a more fixed to a movable part, as from the gingiva to the lip, cheek, or undersurface of the tongue, serving in a measure to check undue movement of the part.

Friable: easily broken or crumbled.

Furcation: area or region lying between and at the base of two or more anatomically divided roots.

G

Germicide: anything that destroys bacteria; applied especially to chemical agents that kill disease germs, but not necessarily bacterial spores: applied to both living tissue and inanimate objects.

Gerodontics: that branch of dentistry which treats all problems peculiar to the oral cavity in old age and the aging, including clinical problems of senescence and senility.

Gestation: pregnancy.

Gingivectomy: the surgical removal of diseased gingiva to eliminate periodontal pockets.

Gingivoplasty: the surgical contouring of the gingival tissue to produce the physiologic architectural form necessary for the maintenance of tissue health and integrity.

Glaucoma: a disease of the eye marked by intense intraocular pressure, which can result in hardness of the eye, atrophy of the retina, cupping of the optic disk, and blindness.

Glossitis: inflammation of the tongue.

Gnathodynamometer: an instrument for measuring the force exerted in closing the jaws.

Graft: tissues transferred from one site to replace damaged structures in another site.

Free graft: tissue for grafting is completely removed from its donor site.

Pedicle graft: the graft remains attached to its donor site. See also **Autograft; Heterograft; Homograft.**

Grit: the size of abrasive particles determined by the number of particles which, end to end, equal one inch; fine, stony, hard particles used for grinding.

H

Habilitation: application of measures that will assist a person in obtaining a state of health, efficiency, and independent action; make over in an improved form.

Halitosis: offensive or bad breath, may be related to systemic disease or uncleanliness of the oral cavity.

Health: state of complete physical, mental, and social well-being, not merely the absence of disease.

Hemangioma: a benign tumor composed of newly formed blood capillaries filled with blood.

Hematoma: a blood clot formed from blood that has been released by trauma or pathology and that accumulates within a tissue.

Hemoglobin: the protein coloring matter of the red blood cells; conveys oxygen to the tissues; occurs as oxyhemoglobin in arterial blood and reduced hemoglobin in venous blood.

Hemorrhage: bleeding; an escape of blood from the blood vessels.

Hemostat: an instrument or other agent used to arrest the escape or flow of blood.

Hepatitis: inflammation of the liver.

Heredity: the inheritance of resemblance, physical qualities, or diseases from a familial predecessor; the passage of characteristics from one generation to its progeny by genetic linkage.

Heterograft: a heterologous graft in which the tissue is obtained from another species.

Homeostasis: the state of equilibrium in the living body with respect to various functions and to the chemical compositions of the fluids and tissues.

Homograft: a homologous graft in which the tissue is obtained from a different individual of the same species.

Hone: a fine grit stone used for sharpening a cutting instrument (noun); to sharpen (verb).

Hydrogen peroxide: clear, colorless liquid which is a strong oxidizing and bleaching agent.

Hygiene: the science that deals with the preservation of health.

Hygroscopic: capable of readily absorbing and retaining moisture.

Hyperkeratosis: abnormal increase in the thickness of the keratin layer (stratum corneum) of the epithelium. **Benign hyperkeratosis** is one of the most common white lesions of the oral mucous membrane.

Hyperplasia: increase in size of a tissue or organ caused by the increase in number of cells in normal arrangement.

Hypertension: Pathologic elevation of the blood pressure.

Hypertonic: having excessive tone, tonicity, or activity.

  Hypertonic solution: one that has a higher molecular concentration than another with which it is compared; of greater concentration than isotonic.

Hypertrophy: increase in size of a tissue or organ caused by the increase in size of its cells.

Hypnotic: inducing sleep.

Hypocalcification: deficiency in the mineral content of a calcified tissue, for example in the enamel, results from disturbance in the maturation phase during development; may be due to systemic, local, or hereditary factors.

Hypoplasia: defective or incomplete development; enamel hypoplasia results when the enamel matrix formation is disturbed.

Hypotonic: having diminished tone, tonicity, or activity.

  Hypotonic solution: one that has a lesser molecular concentration than another to which it is compared; of less concentration than isotonic.

Hypoxia: insufficient oxygen in the air, blood, or tissue.

I

Iatrogenic: caused by inadvertent or erroneous diagnosis and/or treatment by a professional.

Idiopathic: self-originated; of unknown cause.

Idiosyncrasy: any tendency, characteristic, or the like, peculiar to an individual.

Immunity: an inherited, congenital, or naturally or artificially acquired ability to resist the occurrence and effects of a specific disease.

  Acquired immunity: that possessed as a result of having and recovering from a disease or from building up resistance against vaccines, toxins, or toxoids.

  Natural immunity: that inherited by the child from the mother or from the race.

  Passive immunity: that possessed as a result of injection of antibodies or antitoxins of serum from an immune individual or lower animal.

Implant: a material or body part that is grafted or inserted within body tissues.

Implantation: the placement within body tissues of a foreign substance, for example metal or plastic, for restoration by mechanical means. In dentistry, a foreign material placed into or onto the jawbone to support a crown, partial or complete denture.

Incipient: beginning to exist; coming into existence.

Incubation: the keeping of a microbial or tissue culture in an incubator to facilitate development.

Incubation period: used to denote the time between exposure to a communicable disease and the appearance of clinical symptoms.

Inert: without intrinsic active properties; no inherent power of action, motion, or resistance.

Infarct: a circumscribed portion of tissue that has suddenly been deprived of its blood supply by embolism or thrombosis and that results in necrosis of the tissue.

Infection: invasion of the body by pathogenic microorganisms and the body's response to the microorganisms and their toxic products; transfer of disease from one part to another or one person to another.

Inflammation: reaction of living tissue to injury; a defense reaction of the body characterized by heat, redness, swelling, pain, and loss of function.

Inhibitor: a substance that arrests or restrains physiologic, chemical, or enzymatic action or the growth of microorganisms.

Inoculation: introduction of microorganisms or some substance into living tissues or culture media; introduction of a disease agent into a healthy individual to induce immunity.

Inorganic: not characterized by organization of living bodies or vital processes; also, pertaining to compounds not containing carbon, except cyanides and carbonates.

Insidious: coming on gradually or almost imperceptibly; as in a disease, the onset of which is gradual, with a more serious effect than is apparent.

Intensifying screen: a card or plastic sheet coated with fluorescent material, positioned in a cassette to contact the film in radiography, so that the visible light from its fluorescent image, when exposed to radiation, will add to the latent image being produced directly by radiation, on a film sensitive to both visible light and x-rays.

Intermaxillary: between the maxilla and the mandible.

In vitro: outside the living body: in a test tube or other artificial environment.

In vivo: in the living body of a plant or animal.

Ion: an electrically charged atom or group of atoms.

  Anion: negatively charged ion, which passes to the positive pole in electrolysis.

  Cation: positively charged ion, which passes to the negative pole in electrolysis.

I.Q.: Intelligence Quotient; the relationship between intelligence and chronologic age.

Irrigation: the flushing or washing out of anything with water or other liquid for the purpose of making it moist, diluting another substance present, or cleaning the area.

Ischemia: local decrease in the blood supply to tissues due to obstruction of inflow of arterial blood.

Isotonic: having a uniform tonicity or tension.

Isotonic solution: one which has the same molecular concentration as another with which it is compared.

J

Jaundice: condition in which there are bile pigments in the blood and deposition of bile pigments in the skin and mucous membranes with resulting yellowish appearance.

Jurisprudence: the science of law, its interpretation and application.

K

Kaolin: a fine white clay; used in pharmacy in ointments and for coating pills.

Keratin: a protein material formed as a transformation product of the cellular proteins of the flat cells on the surface of the epithelium; form of protective adaptation to function.

Keratinization: process of formation of a horny protective layer on the surface of stratified squamous epithelium of certain body surfaces including the epidermis and masticatory oral mucosa.

Kilovoltage: in x-ray machines, the potential difference between the anode and cathode of an x-ray tube.

L

Laceration: a wound produced by tearing or irregular cutting.

Latent: concealed, not apparent, potential.

Lesion: an alteration of structure or of functional capacity due to injury or disease.

Lethargy: condition of drowsiness or sleepiness.

Leukocyte: white blood corpuscle; a formed element of the blood consisting of a colorless mass of protoplasm, having ameboid movements and involved in the destruction of disease-producing microorganisms.

Leukoplakia: white plaque formed upon the oral mucous membrane from surface epithelial cells; potentially a premalignant surface lesion, characterized by hyperkeratosis of the stratified squamous epithelium.

Local: restricted to one spot or area; not generalized.

Luxation: a dislocation. For example, dislocation of the temporomandibular joint occurs when the head of the condyle moves anteriorly over the articular eminence and cannot be returned voluntarily.

Lymphadenopathy: disease process affecting a lymph node or lymph nodes.

M

Macroglossia: enlargement of the tongue.

Malaise: any vague feeling of illness, uneasiness, or discomfort.

Malignant: as applied to tumors: grow rapidly, infiltrate into normal structures, metastasize, and if untreated, invariably lead to death.

Malnutrition: a condition of the body resulting from an inadequate supply or impaired utilization of one or more food constituents.

Mandrel: a spindle, axle, or shaft designed to fit a dental handpiece for the purpose of supporting a revolving instrument.

Manifestation: that which is made evident, especially to the sight and understanding.

Oral manifestation: a symptom or sign of a disease in the oral cavity.

Manikin: model of the human body or a part; used for teaching purposes.

Massage: manipulation of tissues for remedial or hygienic purposes with the hand or other instrument; the systematic application of frictional rubbing and stroking to the gingival tissues for cleansing purposes, for increasing the circulation of blood through the tissues, and for increasing the keratinization of the surface epithelium.

Mastication: a series of highly coordinated functions that involve the teeth, tongue, muscles of mastication, lips, cheeks, and saliva, in the preparation of food for swallowing and digestion.

Matrix: the form or substance within which something originates, takes form, or develops; intercellular substance of a tissue.

Amalgam matrix: a thin metal form, usually stainless steel, adapted to a prepared cavity to supply the missing wall so the amalgam will be confined when condensed into the cavity preparation.

Maxillofacial: pertaining to the jaws and the face.

Maxillofacial prosthetics: the art and science of anatomic, functional, and cosmetic reconstruction, utilizing nonliving substitutes, of those regions in the maxilla, mandible, and face that are missing or defective.

Medication: use of medicine or medicaments for treatment of a disease.

Metabolism: the sum total of the chemical changes occurring in the body; chemical process of transforming foods into complex tissue elements and of transforming complex body substances into simple ones, along with the production of heat and energy.

Anabolism: the building up of tissue; maintenance and repair of the body.

Catabolism: the breaking down of tissue into simpler constituents for energy production and excretion.

Micron: unit of linear measurement; one-thousandth of a millimeter.

Milliliter: one-thousandth part of a liter, usually abbreviated **ml.** It is approximately equal to one cubic centimeter.

Miscible: capable of being mixed.

Monitoring: the overall surveillance of a patient by methods employing the senses of touch, sight, hearing, or smell or by means of devices that operate chemically, physically, or electronically to measure the adequacy of the various physiologic functions.

Morphology: the science that deals with form and structure without regard to function.

Mucin: secretion of the mucous or goblet cell; a polysaccharide protein which, combined with water, forms a lubricating solution called mucus; contained in saliva.

Myocardium: heart muscle; muscular substance of the heart.

N

Nasmyth's membrane: see **Cuticle, primary.**

Necrosis: cell or tissue death within the living body.

Neoplasm: a new growth comprised of an abnormal collection of cells, the growth of which exceeds and is uncoordinated with that of the normal tissues. See **Cancer** and **Malignant.**

Nidus: the point of origin or focus of a process.

Nosocomial: denotes a disorder associated with being treated in a hospital, which is unrelated to the primary reason for being in the hospital.

Nostrum: a quack, patent, or secret remedy.

Nutrition: sum of processes by which an animal or plant absorbs or takes in and utilizes food substances; ingestion, digestion, absorption (of products of digestion) of food materials through mucous membranes of the alimentary tract, transportation by blood and lymph to body cells where they are used or stored.

O

Obese: excessively fat.

Obstetrician: a physician who specializes in the management of pregnancy, labor, and the period of confinement after delivery.

Obtundent: having the power to dull sensibility or soothe pain; a soothing or partially anesthetic medicine.

Odontalgia: toothache; pain in a tooth.

Odontoblast: connective tissue cell that functions in the formation of dentin.

Olfactory: pertaining to the sense of smell.

Oncology: study or science of neoplastic growth.

Ophthalmologist: physician with specialized training and experience who specializes in the diagnosis and treatment of eye diseases; one versed in **ophthalmology,** the sum of knowledge concerning the eye and its diseases. (Obsolete term: oculist.)

Optician: technician who grinds and fits lenses; a maker of optical instruments or glasses.

Optometrist: one who practices **optometry,** the measurement of visual acuity and the fitting of glasses to correct visual defects; a term adopted by opticians who prescribe and fit glasses.

Oral surgery: that part of dental practice which deals with the diagnosis and surgical and adjunctive treatment of the diseases, injuries, and defects of the human jaws and associated structures.

Orthodontics: that area of dentistry concerned with the supervision and guidance of the growing dentition and correction of the mature dentofacial structures, and includes those conditions that require movement of teeth and/or correction of malrelationships of jaws and teeth and malformations of their related structures.

Orthopnea: difficulty in breathing in a horizontal position.

Orthosis: a device added to a person's body to substitute for absent motor power, restore function, assist weak muscles, position or immobilize a part, or correct deformities.

Osmosis: the passage of a solvent through a semipermeable membrane into a solution of higher molecular concentration, thus equalizing the concentrations on either side of the membrane.

Osteoblast: cell whose activity initiates the formation of new bone.

Osteoclast: large multinucleated cell that brings about the resorption of bone; found only during the process of active bone or root resorption.

Osteoectomy, ostectomy: removal of tooth-supporting bone for correction of pockets and nonphysiologic bony contours.

Osteomyelitis: acute or chronic inflammation of the bone marrow or of the bone and marrow.

Osteoplasty: reshaping of bone; **alveoloplasty,** plastic contouring of the alveolar process to achieve physiologic contours in the bone and gingival tissues.

Osteoporosis: abnormal decrease in density of bone by the enlargement of its canals or the formation of abnormal spaces.

Otolaryngologist: medical specialist who treats the ears, throat, pharynx, larynx, nasopharynx, and tracheobronchial tree.

P

Palliative: affording relief but not cure.

Pallor: paleness.

Palpitation: rapid beating of the heart.

Parasympathetic nervous system: craniosacral division of the autonomic nervous system.

Parenteral: route of administration other than by the alimentary canal, that is, by intravenous, intramuscular, or subcutaneous means.

Pathogenesis: the course of development of disease, including the sequence of processes or events from inception to the characteristic lesion or disease.

Pathogenic: causing disease: disease-producing.

Pathognomonic: a sign or symptom significantly unique to a disease as to distinguish the disease from other diseases.

Pedodontics: that branch of dentistry concerned with the etiology, diagnosis, and treatment of oral diseases of children.

Periapical: around the apex of a tooth.

Periapical tissues: the tissues surrounding the apex of a tooth, including the periodontal ligament and the alveolar bone.

Pericardium: the membranous sac that contains the heart.

Pericoronitis: inflammation of the soft tissues surrounding the crown of an erupting tooth; frequently seen in association with erupting mandibular third molars and usually accompanied by infection.

Periodontal care: for the patient with periodontal disease: consists of effective treatment for the elimination of disease and the creation of conditions conducive to the maintenance of periodontal health.

Periodontal care, maintenance phase: after or between phases of active therapy: requires close supervision to prevent recurrence of periodontal disease; includes control of calculus formation, diet, plaque control, and oral physical therapy supervision, follow-up radiographs, and complete operative care.

Periodontics: that branch of dental practice comprising the prevention, diagnosis, and treatment of diseases of the surrounding and supporting structures of the teeth.

Periodontium: the tissues that surround, support, and are attached to the teeth; includes gingiva, cementum, periodontal ligament, and alveolar bone.

Periodontology: the clinical science that deals with the periodontium in health and disease; that branch of dentistry concerned with the etiology, diagnosis, and treatment of diseases of the supporting structures of the teeth.

Petechia: minute hemorrhagic spot, of pinhead to pinpoint size, in the skin.

Petri plate: a small, shallow dish of thin glass with a loosely fitting, overlapping cover, used for plate cultures in microbiology.

pH: symbol commonly used to express hydrogen ion concentration, the measure of alkalinity and acidity. Normal (neutral) pH is 7.0. Above 7.0 the solution is alkaline; below, acid.

Phosphorescence: emission of radiation by a substance as a result of previous absorption of radiation of shorter wave length; contrasts with fluorescence in that the emission may continue for a time after cessation of the ionizing radiation.

Physiologic saline solution: a 0.9% sodium chloride solution, which exerts an osmotic pressure equal to that exerted by the blood, and thus is compatible with blood.

Pipette: a slender, graduated tube for measuring and transferring liquids from one vessel to another.

Placebo: an indifferent substance in the form of a medicine, given for the suggestive effect; an inert compound, identical in appearance with material being tested in experimental research, in which the participants or researchers may or may not know the identity.

Plasma: fluid portion of the blood (serum and fibrinogen) without formed elements; fluid portion of the lymph without its corpuscles or cells.

Pontic: the suspended member of a fixed partial denture; it replaces the lost natural tooth, restores its functions, and usually occupies the space previously filled by the natural crown.

Precipitate: to cause a substance in solution to separate out in solid particles (verb); that which is separated out is called the precipitate (noun).

Predisposition: a concealed but present susceptibility to disease which may be activated under certain conditions.

Predisposing factor: a factor that renders a person susceptible to a disease or condition.

Premaxilla: the intermaxillary bone situated in front of the maxilla proper; carries the incisor teeth.

Premedication: preliminary treatment, usually with a drug, to prevent untoward results which may be effected by the operation to be performed.

Prescribe: to designate or recommend a remedy for administration; to direct in writing the dosage, preparation, and dispensing of a remedy or drug.

Primate space: diastema or gap in tooth row occasionally observed in primary dentition. Characteristic of almost all species of primate except man. Maxillary primate spaces accommodate mandibular canines and mandibular primate spaces accommodate maxillary canines when teeth are in occlusion. Reduced length of canines accompanied man's evolution, so canines no longer protruded beyond occlusal level and diastema was no longer functional.

Prognosis: a forecasting of the probable course and termination of a disease and the response to treatment; the prospect of recovery from a disease as indicated by the nature and symptoms of the case.

Proliferation: reproduction or multiplication of similar forms.

Prone: flat, prostrate; **prone position,** lying flat.

Prosthesis: artificial replacement for a missing part.

Prosthodontics: prosthetic dentistry; that branch of dental art and science pertaining to the restoration and maintenance of oral function by the replacement of missing teeth and adjacent structures by artificial devices. See also **Maxillofacial prosthetics.**

Protective barrier: a barrier of radiation-absorbing material such as lead, concrete, or plaster which serves to reduce radiation hazards.

Protein: any one of a group of complex organic nitrogenous compounds widely distributed in plants and animals which form the principal constituents of cell protoplasm. They are essentially combinations of alpha amino acids and their derivatives.

Proteolytic: effecting the digestion of proteins.

Protoplasm: the only known form of matter in which life is apparent; it composes the essential material of all plant and animal cells.

Protrusion: condition of being thrust forward, as the protrusion of the anterior teeth.

Psychiatry: that branch of medicine which deals with the diagnosis and treatment of mental diseases.

Psychosomatic: pertaining to the mind-body relationship; having body symptoms of a psychic, emotional, or mental origin.

Ptyalin: an enzyme occurring in the saliva which converts starch into maltose and dextrose.

Public health: the science and art of preventing disease, prolonging life, and promoting physical health and efficiency through organized community efforts.

    Dental public health: art of preventing and controlling dental diseases and promoting oral health through organized community efforts.

Pulp stone: see **Denticle.**

Pulpectomy: removal of the pulp chamber and root canals of a tooth.

Pulpotomy: the removal of a portion of the pulp of a tooth, usually meaning the coronal portion.

Purpura: escape of blood into the skin and mucous membranes, forming petechiae and ecchymoses.

Purulent: containing, consisting of, or forming pus.

Pus: a fluid product of inflammation, which consists of a liquid containing leukocytes and the debris of dead cells and tissue elements liquified by the proteolytic and histolytic enzymes that are elaborated by polymorphonuclear leukocytes.

Pyorrhea: a purulent discharge; discharge of pus. Formerly a name for advanced, severe periodontal disease.

Q

Quadrant: any one of the four parts or quarters of the dentition, with the dividing line of the maxillary or mandibular teeth at the midline between the central incisors.

R

Radiation, ionizing: any electromagnetic or particulate radiation capable of producing ions, directly or indirectly, in its passage through matter.

Radiolucent: a substance, which because of its lack of density, permits the passage of x-rays with only very little resistance; radiolucent objects appear dark on radiographs.

Radiopaque: a substance, which because of its density, resists the passage of x-rays; radiopaque objects appear light on radiographs.

Radioresistant: relatively resistant to injury by ionizing radiation.

Radiosensitive: relatively susceptible to injury by ionizing radiation.

Raphe: a ridge, furrow, or seam-like union between two parts or halves of an organ or structure.

Rarefaction: being or becoming less dense.

Recession: gradual drawing away of a tissue or part from its normal position, as the progressive exposure of the root surface by an apical shift of the gingiva.

Rectification: conversion of alternating current to direct current.

Recurrent: returning after intermissions.

Rehabilitation: restoration to former state of health, efficiency, and independent action; regeneration.

Remission: a decrease or arrest of the symptoms of a disease; also the period during which such decrease occurs.

Replantation: replacement of a traumatically or otherwise removed tooth back into its own alveolar socket.

Resection: operation in which a part of a tissue or an organ is removed.

    Root resection: removal of a root from a multi-rooted tooth.

    Hemisection: removal of half of a tooth.

Resorption: removal of bone or tooth structure by pressure; gradual destruction of dentin and cementum of the root, as the primary teeth prior to shedding; in orthodontic tooth movement, bone formation on one side compensates for resorption of bone on the other side.

Resuscitation: restoration of life or consciousness; restoration of heartbeat and respiration.

Rh factor: agglutinogens of red blood cells responsible for isoimmune reactions such as occur in erythroblastosis fetalis and incompatible blood transfusions; erythroblastosis fetalis results when a mother is Rh negative and develops antibodies against the fetus which is Rh positive.

Rheostat: an appliance for regulating the resistance and thus controlling the amount of current entering an electric circuit; the dental unit control is located in a device operated by the foot.

Rheumatic: pertaining to or affected with **rheumatism,** which is a general term pertaining to conditions characterized by inflammation or pain in muscles or joints.

Roentgen (R): an international unit of quantity of radiation based on the ability of x-rays to ionize air.

Rubefacient: reddening of the skin; an agent that reddens the skin by producing active or passive hyperemia.

Ruga: ridge, wrinkle, fold.

    Palatal rugae: the irregular ridges in the mucous membrane covering the anterior part of the hard palate.

S

Sarcoma: malignant neoplasm of connective tissue elements.

Sclerosis: abnormal hardening or thickening of tissue, especially as a result of inflammation or disease of the interstitial substance.

Sedative: a drug that allays activity, excitement, apprehension.

Senescence: process or condition of growing old; physiologic aging not necessarily related to chronologic age.

Senile: of or pertaining to old age; characteristic of old age.

Senility: old age; feebleness of body and mind occurring with old age.

Septum: a dividing wall, partition, or membrane.

Sequestrum: a piece of necrosed bone that has become separated from the surrounding bone; usually the necrosed bone is being expelled from the body.

Serrated: having a sawlike edge.

Serum: the clear, liquid part of blood separated from its more solid elements after clotting; the blood plasma from which fibrinogen has been removed in the process of clotting.

Shelf-life: the length of time a substance or preparation can be kept without changing its chemical structure or other properties.

Slough: a mass of dead tissue in, or cast out of, living tissue.

Space maintainer: a fixed or removable appliance used to replace missing primary teeth to prevent drifting of surrounding teeth until eruption of permanent teeth.

Splint: any apparatus, appliance, or device used to prevent motion or displacement of fractured or movable parts.

Dental splint: appliance designed to immobilize and stabilize mobile teeth.

Spore: see **Bacterial spore.**

Stabile: not moving, stationary, resistant; opposite of labile.

Heat stabile (thermostabile): resistant to moderate degrees of heat.

Stannous: containing tin.

Stenosis: a narrowing of a channel or an aperture, especially a narrowing of one of the cardiac valves.

Sterile: aseptic, free from microorganisms.

Stomatitis: inflammation of the oral mucosa, due to local or systemic factors.

Subclinical: without clinical manifestations; said of early stages of a disease.

Subluxation: partial or incomplete dislocation. See **Luxation.**

Submerged tooth: one which is below the line of occlusion and may be ankylosed; intrusion; infraocclusion.

Supernumerary tooth: extra tooth; one which is in excess of the normal number.

Suppuration: formation of pus.

Sympathetic nervous system: that part of the autonomic (involuntary) nervous system which arises in the thoracic and the first three lumbar segments of the spinal cord.

Syndrome: a group of symptoms and signs which, when considered together, characterize a disease or lesion.

Systemic: pertaining to or affecting the whole body.

T

Tactile: pertaining to the touch; perceptible to the touch.

Tarnish: surface discoloration on a metal, usually the result of oxidation.

Technician, dental laboratory: a technician who performs any type of dental laboratory procedure not requiring the presence of a patient. See also **Dental prosthetic laboratory procedures.**

Teratogenic: causing abnormal development.

Teratoma: a neoplasm composed of multiple tissues, including tissues not normally found in the organ in which it arises.

Therapeutic: pertaining to the treating or curing of disease; curative.

Therapy: the treatment of disease.

Threshold: that amount of stimulus which just produces a perceptible sensation.

Pain threshold: that amount of stimulus which just produces a sensation of pain.

Threshold exposure: the minimum exposure that will produce a detectable degree of any given effect.

Thrombosis: the formation, development, or presence of a thrombus.

Thrombus: a plug or clot in blood vessel or in one of the cavities of the heart formed by coagulation of the blood and remaining at the point of its formation.

Tic: an involuntary purposeless movement of muscle which usually occurs under emotional stress; a twitching, especially of facial muscles.

Tincture: an alcoholic solution of a drug or other chemical substance.

Tone: the normal degree of vigor and tension; a healthy state of a part.

Tonguetie: abnormal shortness of the frenum of the tongue resulting in limitation of the motion of that organ.

Tonus: the slight, continuous contraction of muscle, which in skeletal muscle aids in the maintenance of posture and the return of blood to the heart. See **Tone.**

Topical: on the surface; pertaining to a particular spot; local.

Topography: the detailed description and analysis of the features of an anatomic region or of a special part.

Toxin: any poisonous substance of microbial, vegetable, or animal origin that causes symptoms after a period of incubation; can induce the elaboration of specific antitoxins in suitable animals.

Tracheotomy: surgical operation to provide an artificial opening into the trachea.

Transformer: an electrical device that increases or reduces the voltage of an alternating current by mutual induction between primary and secondary coils or windings.

Transplant: tissue removed from any portion of the body and placed at a different site.

Transplantation: implanting a tissue or organ which has been taken from another part of the same body or from another person.

Autotransplant: transfer of a tooth from one alveolus to another in the same mouth.

Trauma: an injury; damage; impairment; external violence, producing body injury or degeneration.

Trauma from occlusion (traumatic occlusion): the

injury to periodontal tissues caused by occlusal forces.

Treatment: the management and care of a patient for the purpose of curing a disease or disorder.

Tremor: involuntary trembling or quivering.

Trendelenburg position: supine, inclined at an angle of 45 degrees so that the head is slightly lower than the heart.

Trismus: motor disturbance of the trigeminal nerve, especially spasm of the masticatory muscles, which causes difficulty in opening the mouth.

U

Urticaria: hives; nettle rash; an eruption of itching wheals usually of systemic origin. It may be due to a state of hypersensitivity to foods or drugs, foci of infection, physical agents (heat, cold, light, friction), or psychic stimuli.

V

Vehicle: a substance possessing little or no medicinal action, used as a medium to confer a suitable consistency or form to a drug.

Vincent's disease: trench mouth; necrotizing ulcerative gingivitis.

Virulent: capable of causing infection or disease.

Viscosity: stickiness; ability of a fluid to resist change in shape or arrangement during flow.

Volatile: tending to evaporate readily.

Volt: unit of electromotive force sufficient to cause a current of one ampere to flow through a resistance of one ohm.

Voltage: the potential or electromotive force of an electric charge, expressed in volts.

Vulcanite: a hard rubber prepared by vulcanizing India rubber with sulfur; formerly used for making removable dentures.

W

Wheal: an acute circumscribed transitory area of edema of the skin; an urticarial lesion. See **Urticaria.**

Whitlow: a purulent infection or abscess involving the end of a finger; also called a felon.

X

Xerostomia: dryness of the mouth due to functional or organic disturbances of the salivary glands.

Appendix

Table A–1. Tooth Development and Eruption: Primary Teeth

		Hard Tissue Formation Begins (weeks in utero)	Enamel Completed (months after birth)	Eruption (months)	Root Completed (year)
Maxillary	Central Incisor	14	$1\frac{1}{2}$	10 (8–12)	$1\frac{1}{2}$
	Lateral Incisor	16	$2\frac{1}{2}$	11 (9–13)	2
	Canine	17	9	19 (16–22)	$3\frac{1}{4}$
	First Molar	$15\frac{1}{2}$	6	16 (13–19 boys) (14–18 girls)	$2\frac{1}{2}$
	Second Molar	19	11	29 (25–33)	3
Mandibular	Central Incisor	14	$2\frac{1}{2}$	8 (6–10)	$1\frac{1}{2}$
	Lateral Incisor	16	3	13 (10–16)	$1\frac{1}{2}$
	Canine	17	9	20 (17–23)	$3\frac{1}{4}$
	First Molar	$15\frac{1}{2}$	$5\frac{1}{2}$	16 (14–18)	$2\frac{1}{4}$
	Second Molar	18	10	27 (23–31 boys) (24–30 girls)	3

From Lunt, R.C. and Law, D.B.: A Review of the Chronology of Eruption of Deciduous Teeth, *J. Am. Dent. Assoc.*, 89, 872, October, 1974.

Table A–2. Tooth Development and Eruption: Permanent Teeth

		Hard Tissue Formation Begins	*Enamel Completed (years)*	*Eruption (years)*	*Root Completed (years)*
Maxillary	Central Incisor	3–4 mos.	4–5	7–8	10
	Lateral Incisor	10 mos.	4–5	8–9	11
	Canine	4–5 mos.	6–7	11–12	13–15
	First Premolar	$1\frac{1}{2}$–$1\frac{3}{4}$ yrs.	5–6	10–11	12–13
	Second Premolar	2–$2\frac{1}{4}$ yrs.	6–7	10–12	12–14
	First Molar	at birth	$2\frac{1}{2}$–3	6–7	9–10
	Second Molar	$2\frac{1}{2}$–3 yrs.	7–8	12–13	14–16
	Third Molar	7–9 yrs.	12–16	17–21	18–25
Mandibular	Central Incisor	3–4 mos.	4–5	6–7	9
	Lateral Incisor	3–4 mos.	4–5	7–8	10
	Canine	4–5 mos.	6–7	9–10	12–14
	First Premolar	$1\frac{3}{4}$–2 yrs.	5–6	10–12	12–13
	Second Premolar	$2\frac{1}{4}$–$2\frac{1}{2}$ yrs.	6–7	11–12	13–14
	First Molar	at birth	$2\frac{1}{2}$–3	6–7	9–10
	Second Molar	$2\frac{1}{2}$–3 yrs.	7–8	11–13	14–15
	Third Molar	8–10 yrs.	12–16	17–21	18–25

From Wheeler, R. C.: *Dental Anatomy, Physiology and Occlusion*, 5th ed. Philadelphia, W.B. Saunders Co., 1974.

Table A–3. Average Measurements of the Primary Teeth
(in millimeters)

		Overall Length	Length of Crown	Length of Root	Width of Crown (mesial-distal at widest point)
Maxillary	Central Incisor	16.0	6.0	10.0	6.5
	Lateral Incisor	15.8	5.6	11.4	5.1
	Canine	19.0	6.5	13.5	7.0
	First Molar	15.2	5.1	10.0	7.3
	Second Molar	17.5	5.7	11.7	8.2
Mandibular	Central Incisor	14.0	5.0	9.0	4.2
	Lateral Incisor	15.0	5.2	10.0	4.1
	Canine	17.5	6.0	11.5	5.0
	First Molar	15.8	6.0	9.8	7.7
	Second Molar	18.8	5.5	11.3	9.9

From Black, G. V.: *Descriptive Anatomy of the Human Teeth*, ed. 4, Philadelphia, Pa., The S. S. White Dental Manufacturing Company, according to Zeisz, R. C. and Nuchols, J.: *Dental Anatomy*. St. Louis, The C.V. Mosby Co., 1969, p. 458.

Table A–4. Average Measurements of the Permanent Teeth
(in millimeters)

		Overall Length	Length of Crown	Length of Root	Width of Crown (mesial-distal at widest point)
Maxillary	Central Incisor	23.5	10.5	13.0	8.5
	Lateral Incisor	22.0	9.0	13.0	6.5
	Canine	27.0	10.0	17.0	7.5
	First Premolar	22.5	8.5	14.0	7.0
	Second Premolar	22.5	8.5	14.0	7.0
	First Molar	B* 19.5 L 20.5	7.5	B 12 L 13	10.0
	Second Molar	B 17.0 L 19.0	7.0	B 11 L 12	9.0
	Third Molar	17.5	6.5	11.0	8.5
Mandibular	Central Incisor	21.5	9.0	12.5	5.0
	Lateral Incisor	23.5	9.5	14.0	5.5
	Canine	27.0	11.0	16.0	7.0
	First Premolar	22.5	8.5	14.0	7.0
	Second Premolar	22.5	8.0	14.5	7.0
	First Molar	21.5	7.5	14.0	11.0
	Second Molar	20.0	7.0	13.0	10.5
	Third Molar	18.0	7.0	11.0	10.0

From Wheeler, R. C.: *Dental Anatomy, Physiology and Occlusion,* 5th edition. Philadelphia, W.B. Saunders Co., 1974, p. 20.

*B = Buccal measurement; L = Lingual measurement

Index